D0857933

The Pelvic Floor
Its function and disorders

Commissioning Editor: Sue Hodgson
Project Development Manager: Paul Fam
Project Manager: Rory MacDonald
Designer: Andy Chapman
Illustration Manager: Mick Ruddy
Illustrator: Marion Tasker
Cover Illustration: Richard Tibbitts

The Pelvic Floor

Its function and disorders

Edited by

John Pemberton MD
Professor of Surgery
Consultant, Colon and Rectal Surgery
Mayo Graduate School of Medicine
Mayo Clinic and Mayo Foundation
Rochester, MN, USA

Michael Swash MD FRCP MRCPath
Professor of Neurology
Queen Mary's School of Medicine and Dentistry
University of London
Consultant Neurologist, Royal London Hospital
London, UK

Michael M Henry MB FRCS
Consultant Surgeon
Department of Surgery
Chelsea and Westminster Hospital
London, UK

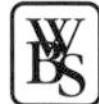
W.B. SAUNDERS

LONDON EDINBURGH NEW YORK PHILADELPHIA ST LOUIS SYDNEY TORONTO 2002

WB SAUNDERS
An imprint of Harcourt Publishers Limited

First published 2002

ISBN 0 7020 2307 8

British Library Cataloguing in Publication Data
A catalogue record for this book is available from the British Library

Library of Congress Cataloging in Publication Data
A catalog record for this book is available from the Library of Congress

Note
Medical knowledge is constantly changing. As new information becomes available, changes in treatment, procedures, equipment and the use of drugs become necessary. The editors and the publishers have taken care to ensure that the information given in this text is accurate and up to date. However, readers are strongly advised to confirm that the information, especially with regard to drug usage, complies with the latest legislation and standards of practice.

Existing UK nomenclature is changing to the system of Recommended International Nonproprietary Names (rINNs). Until the UK names are no longer in use, these more familiar names are used in this book in preference to rINNs, details of which may be obtained from the British National Formulary.

The publisher's policy is to use **paper manufactured from sustainable forests**

Printed in China by RDC Group Limited

Contents

Contributors

Paul Abrams MD FRCS
Professor of Urology
Bristol Urological Institute
Southmead Hospital
Bristol, UK

Edwin P Arnold PhD(Lon) MBChB(NZ) FRCS(Eng) FRACS
Associate Professor of Urology
Christchurch School of Medicine and Health Sciences
Christchuch, New Zealand

David C C Bartolo MS FRCS
Consultant Colorectal Surgeon
Department of Surgery
Royal Infirmary of Edinburgh
Edinburgh, UK

Clive I Bartram FRCS FRCP FRCR
Professor of Gastrointestinal Radiology
St Mark's Hospital
Harrow, UK

Barbara K Bruce PhD
Consultant, Assistant Professor
Department of Psychiatry and Psychology
Mayo Clinic
Rochester, MN, USA

Michael Camilleri MD MPhil(Lon) FRCP(Lon) FRCP(Edin) FACP FACG
Professor of Medicine and Physiology
Consultant in Gastroenterology
Division of Gastroenterology and Hepatology
Mayo Clinic
Rochester, MN, USA

Linda Cardozo MD FRCOG
Professor of Urogynaecology
Department of Obstetrics and Gynaecology
King's College Hospital
London, UK

J Quentin Clemens MD
Assistant Professor of Urology
Co-director, Section of Voiding Dysfunction and Female Urology
Northwestern University Medical School
Chicago, IL, USA

Tim A Cook DM FRCS(Gen)
Consultant Colorectal Surgeon
Gloucestershire Royal Hospital
Gloucester, UK

John O L DeLancey MD
Norman F Miller Professor of Gynecology
Department of Obstetrics and Gynecology
University of Michigan Health System
Ann Arbor, MI, USA

A James Eccersley MA FRCS(Eng)
Specialist Registrar
The Royal London Hospital
London, UK

Paul Enck PhD
Director of Research
University Hospital of General Surgery
Tuebingen, Germany

James W Fleshman MD
Attending Physician
Barnes Jewish Hospital
Washington University Medical Center
St Louis, MO, USA

Clare J Fowler MBBS MSc FRCP
Consultant in Uro-Neurology
Department of Uro-Neurology
National Hospital for Neurology and Neurosurgery
London, UK

Michelle Fynes MD MRCOG
Consultant Gynaecologist and Subspeciality Fellow in Urogynaecology
The Royal Women's Hospital
Carlton
Victoria, Australia

R W Hagger MD
Department of Surgery
St George's Hospital
London, UK

Steve Halligan MB BS MD MRCP FRCR
Consultant Radiologist
Intestinal Imaging Centre
St Mark's Hospital
Harrow, UK

Michael M Henry MB FRCS
Consultant Surgeon
Department of Surgery
Chelsea and Westminster Hospital
London, UK

Patrick Hogston BSc(Hons) FRCS FRCOG
Consultant Gynaecologist
Department of Obstetrics and Gynaecology
St Mary's Hospital
Portsmouth, UK

Gert Holstege MD PhD
Professor of Anatomy
Department of Anatomy and Embryology
University Hospital Groningen
Groningen, Netherlands

Lennox Hoyte MD MSEE
Assistant Professor of OB/Gyn and Radiology
Brigham and Women's Hospital
Boston, MA, USA

Michael L Kennedy BSc(Hons)
Clinical Fellow
Anorectal Physiology Unit
St George Hospital
Sydney, Australia

Davinder Kumar MD FRCS
Colorectal and General Surgeon
St George's Hospital
London, UK

Leo P Lawler MB DABR FRCR
Radiologist
Mallinckrodt Institute of Radiology
St. Louis, MO, USA

Deborah J Lightner MD
Assistant Professor of Urology
Mayo Graduate School of Medicine
Mayo Clinic
Rochester, MN, USA

David Z Lubowski FRACS
Associate Professor
Department of Colorectal Surgery
St. George Hospital
Sydney, Australia

A D H Macdonald
Former Senior House Officer
Department of Surgery
Royal Infirmary of Edinburgh
Edinburgh, UK

Edward J McGuire BSMD
Professor of Surgery
University of Michigan
Ann Arbor, MI, USA

Alan P Meagher FRACS
Consultant Colorectal Surgeon
St Vincent's Hospital
Sydney, Australia

Neil Mortensen MD FRCS
Professor and Consultant Surgeon in Colorectal Surgery
Department of Colorectal Surgery
John Radcliffe Hospital
Oxford, UK

Frauke Musial PhD
Assistant Professor of Psychology
Heinrich-Heine University
Duesseldorf, Germany

Christine Norton MA(Cantab) RGN
Nurse Specialist (Continence)
St Mark's Hospital
Harrow, UK

P Ronan O'Connell MD FRCSI
Consultant Surgeon
Mater Misericordiae Hospital
Dublin, Ireland

Colm O'Herlihy MD FRCPI FRCOG FRANZCOG
Professor of Obstetrics and Gynaecology
University College
Dublin, Ireland

John H Pemberton MD
Professor of Surgery
Consultant, Colon and Rectal Surgery
Mayo Graduate School of Medicine
Mayo Clinic and Mayo Foundation
Rochester, MN, USA

Peter E P Petros MBBS(Syd) D Med Sc(Uppsala) DS(UWA) FRCOG FRANZCOG CU
Department of Gynaecology
Royal Perth Hospital
Perth, Australia

Simon Podnar MD MSc
Assistant Professor of Neurology
Division of Neurology
University Medical Centre
Ljubljana, Slovenia

Eamonn M M Quigley MD FRCP FACP FACG FRCPI
Professor of Medicine and Human Physiology
National University of Ireland
Cork, Ireland

John M Reynard DM MA FRCS(Urol)
Consultant Urologist
Churchill Hospital
Oxford, UK

Peter Sagar MD
Consultant Surgeon
The General Infirmary at Leeds
Great George Street, Leeds, UK

Judith A M L Sie MD
Department of Anatomy and Embryology
University Hospital Groningen
Groningen, Netherlands

Christopher D Sletten PhD
Assistant Professor of Psychology
Mayo Comprehensive Pain Rehabilitation Center
Mayo Clinic
Rochester, MN, USA

Jonathan Sullivan MBBS FRCS
Specialist Registrar in Urology
Royal Devon and Exeter Hospital
Exeter, UK

Michael Swash MD FRCP MRCPath
Professor of Neurology
Queen Mary's School of Medicine and Dentistry
University of London
Consultant Neurologist, Royal London Hospital
London, UK

Michael J Swinn MD BS BSc MSc FRCS
Registrar, Department of Uroneurology
National Hospital for Neurology and Neurosurgery
London, UK

Lawrence A Szarka MD
Senior Associate Consultant
Division of Gastroenterology and Hepatology
Mayo Clinic
Rochester, MN, USA

W Grant Thompson MD FRCPC
Emeritus Professor of Medicine
University of Ottawa
Ontario, Canada

Philip Toozs-Hobson MBBS MRCOG
Consultant Urogynaecologist and Obstetrician
Birmingham Women's Hospital
Birmingham, UK

Eboo Versi MA Dphil(Oxon) MB Bc(Cantab) MRCOG
Medical Director, Urology and Women's Health
Pharmacia Corporation
Peapack, NJ, USA

David B Vodušek MD DSc
Professor of Neurology
Division of Neurology
University Medical Centre
Ljubljana, Slovenia

Steven D Wexner MD
Chief of Staff, Chairman and Residency Director
Department of Colorectal Surgery
Cleveland Clinic Florida
Weston, FL, USA

Norman S Williams MS FRCS
Professor and Director of Surgery
Academic Department of Surgery
Royal London Hospital
London, UK

Rong H Zhao MD PhD
Research Fellow
Department of Colorectal Surgery
Cleveland Clinic Florida
Weston, FL, USA

Preface

The term 'pelvic floor disorders' was used by us in a broad sense, some 20 years ago, in defining the functional relationships of a number of different clinical problems, including urinary and fecal incontinence, constipation, other disorders of micturition, prolapse of pelvic organs and certain pelvic pain syndromes. This term included dysfunction, therefore, of both smooth and striated muscle, as well as in the connective tissues. The interaction of injury to these structures, and to the nerve supply of the pelvic floor musculature, in childbirth, and from other causes, was recognised. In the years that have elapsed since these concepts were reviewed in our earlier book *Coloproctology and the Pelvic Floor* there has been much new work in understanding the pathogenesis of this group of conditions, and especially in their medical and surgical management. In addition, the mechanism involved in maintaining normal structure and function, and the changes that lead to the progressive onset of disorders such as prolapse and incontinence are now becoming better understood. New methods of imaging and new ideas regarding surgical management have especially contributed to this new knowledge.

In order to provide an up to date account of the several pelvic floor disorders and their treatments we believed a fresh approach was needed. This entirely new book *The Pelvic Floor* sets out to address the syndromes of pelvic floor dysfunction from the perspective of the different specialty interests involved in the care of patients afflicted with pelvic floor disorders. In taking this approach we encouraged our authors to take individual paths, and have not attempted to confine or censor their contributions, once the direction of their individual chapters had been defined. This freedom allowed controversy to be clearly expressed, as in the differing views held by some of our contributors concerning some aspects of pathogenesis and treatment. The contribution of imaging to understanding pelvic floor disorders, and its increasing role in clinical investigation and management, is perhaps one of the more obvious examples of this. We believe that expressions of differing views is important and we welcome them. The book contains a number of algorithms concerning pathogenesis, investigation and management of the main pelvic floor disorders. These are intended to act as reference points around which the chapter content can be considered. We hope they prove useful.

Our contributors range through the relevant specialties, including physiology, anatomy, diagnostic imaging, surgery, nursing, gynecology and obstetrics, urology, coloproctology and neurology. It is a distinguished group indeed. They come from academic centers in several continents. It is itself remarkable that so many different specialties maintain an interest in this group of disorders. This is perhaps a tacit acknowledgement of the complexity of the anatomical and functional correlates of pelvic floor function in health and disease. Pelvic floor disorders lead to much misery and discomfort and their prevention and management is important in all societies. We have labored over this book in the belief that it will contribute to the effort to find the best way of addressing these issues. The reader will find there are many areas of incomplete understanding, and we hope these will stimulate some to further investigation and research. Only by careful investigative work will advances be made.

We have enjoyed the task of preparing this volume for publication. We have learned much from our contributors, and thank them for their careful work in preparing their chapters, and especially for so enthusiastically taking on this task. The views of our readers will be received with interest.

John H Pemberton
Michael Swash
Michael M Henry

August 2001

Acknowledgements

Firstly we thank our contributors for their attention to detail, and for so generously giving their time to the preparation of their contributions to this book. They are all acknowledged experts in their field and we are honored they have contributed to this book. The tireless efforts of our friends at Harcourt in the persons of Sue Hodgson, Paul Fam and Rory MacDonald have in no small way contributed to this book. In this day of mega publishers, confusing hierarchies and short cuts to expertise, Sue and her staff have been truly the exception and we remain grateful for their persistence and friendship. The book design has been carefully considered in house, and the publisher's artists have been most helpful and accommodating in developing the algorithms and various other aspects of the book's design. We have relied enormously on email communication in organising the book's contents, but there is no substitute for editorial and publishers' meetings when planning content and finalising detail, and we have enjoyed these occasions.

We would like at this time to pay tribute to our teachers and mentors in England and in the USA, without whom we would not have developed our interest in the pelvic floor and its disorders. The cross-specialty fertilisation of ideas that we have experienced in our research, in conferences, and in clinical practice has been of fundamental importance. The late Sir Alan Parks was especially influential in using the old St Mark's Hospital to our interest in working across the specialty divide. Our Research Fellows, from many different countries, have been important in shaping our ideas in many different ways – a number of them are contributors to this volume. These efforts were among the catalysts that sparked efforts in the United States. Sid Phillips played a key role in the USA with his thoughtful, challenging and rigorous approach to motility research in general and anorectal motility in particular. His kind and selfless efforts formed the basis for the work at Mayo, the interest of a dedicated group of fellows, and sparked others to pursue similar goals at several centers in the United States with an interest in anorectal motility, pelvic floor physiology and dysfunction.

JHP
MS
MMH

SECTION 1

Algorithms

Chapter 1

Algorithms

John H Pemberton, Michael Swash, Michael M Henry, Deborah J Lightner

The algorithms illustrated here are intended to be general guidelines which physicians and surgeons might use to diagnose and potentially manage sometimes quite difficult patients with disordered colonic and pelvic floor function. By no means is every last detail included, much less discussed and physicians seeing many incontinent and constipated patients will always encounter individuals who 'fall off ' the algorithmic tree. But by and large, most patients although challenging, can be diagnosed, which in turn facilitates categorizing them into more homogeneous groups which then can be managed appropriately with medication, biofeedback, surgery, and more likely than not, a combination of all three.

ALGORITHM 1 Investigation and management of fecal incontinence

Algorithm 1 takes the fecally incontinent patient and attempts to determine if there is a neurologic, traumatic, or a combined abnormality present. Category specific treatment is then indicated.

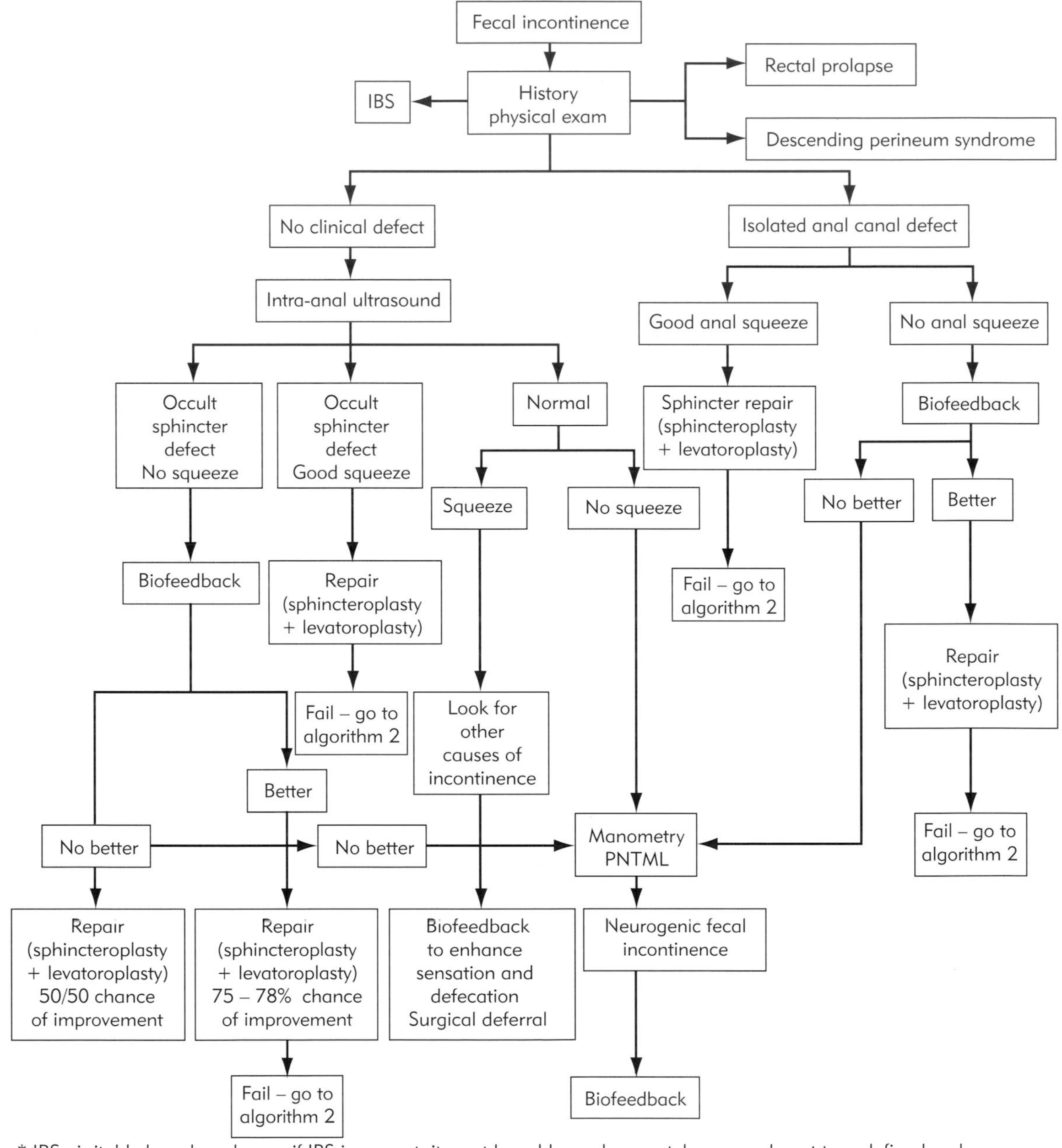

* IBS=irritable bowel syndrome; if IBS is present, it must be addressed separately, preponderant type defined and managed aggressively; diarrhoea predominant IBS with explosive defecation of stool and gas renders operations on the anal sphincter futile.

ALGORITHM 2 Options after failed primary management of fecal incontinence

More aggressive management techniques are illustrated in Algorithm 2. Patients failing more straightforward treatment (Algorithm 1) may then be offered these more 'cutting edge' interventions. Primary sources of Algorithms 1 and 2 are Chapters 6, 13, 16, 17, 24, 26, 27, and 28.

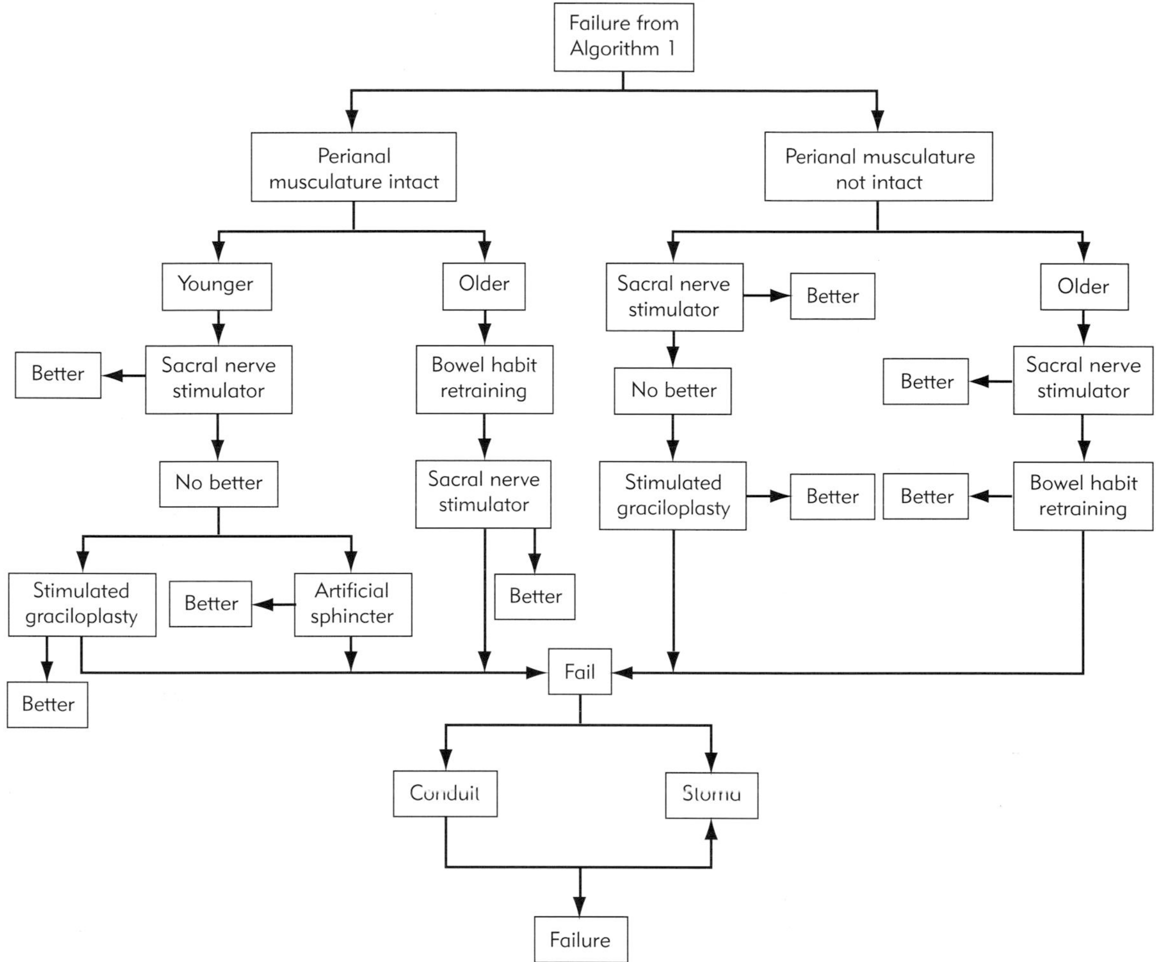

ALGORITHM 3 Evaluation of constipation

Algorithm 3 takes a patient who complains of constipation through a diagnostic evaluation, the aim of which is to categorize patients into homogeneous groups.

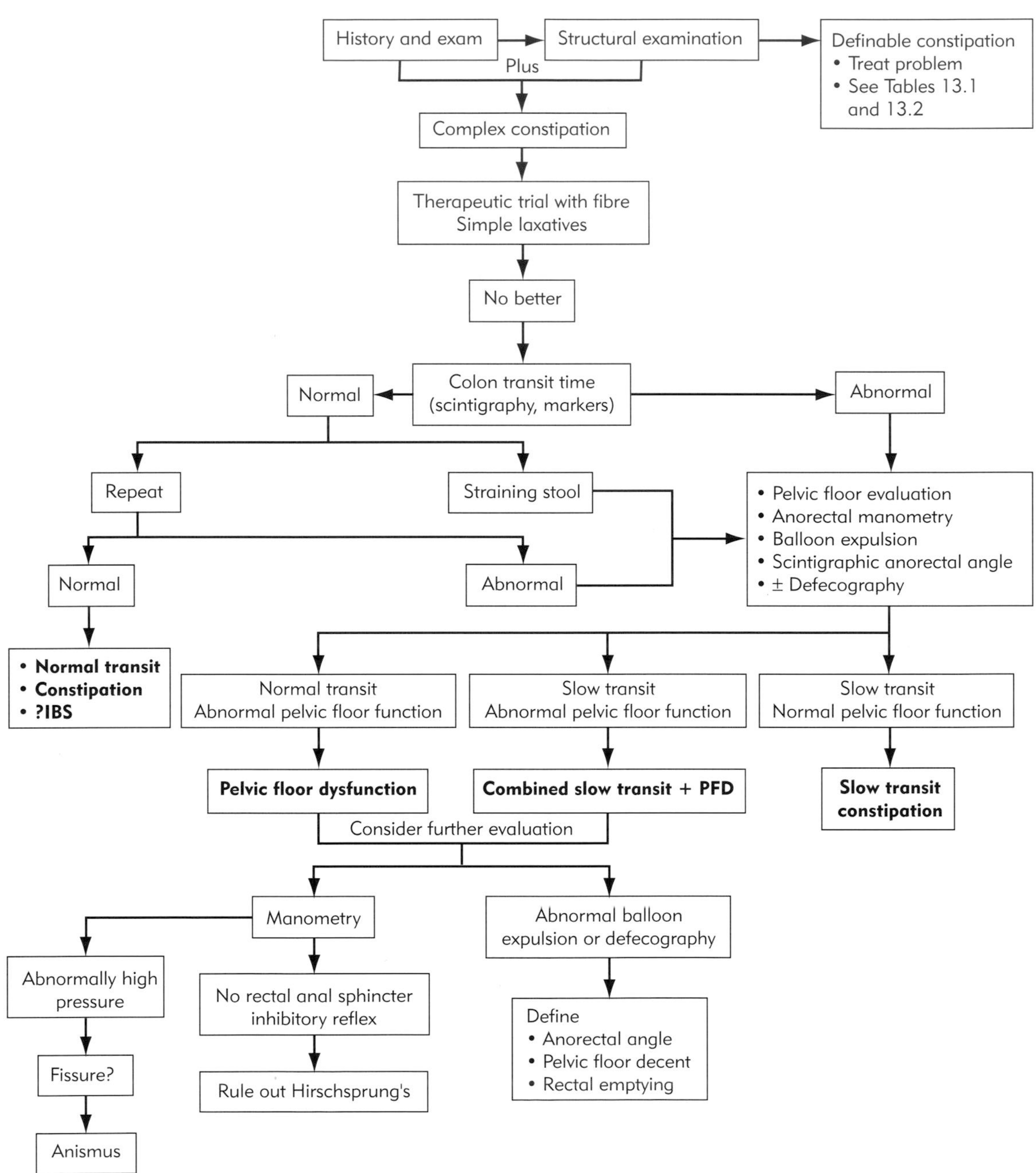

ALGORITHM 4 Management of slow transit contipation

Algorithm 4 illustrates the treatment of slow transit constipation.

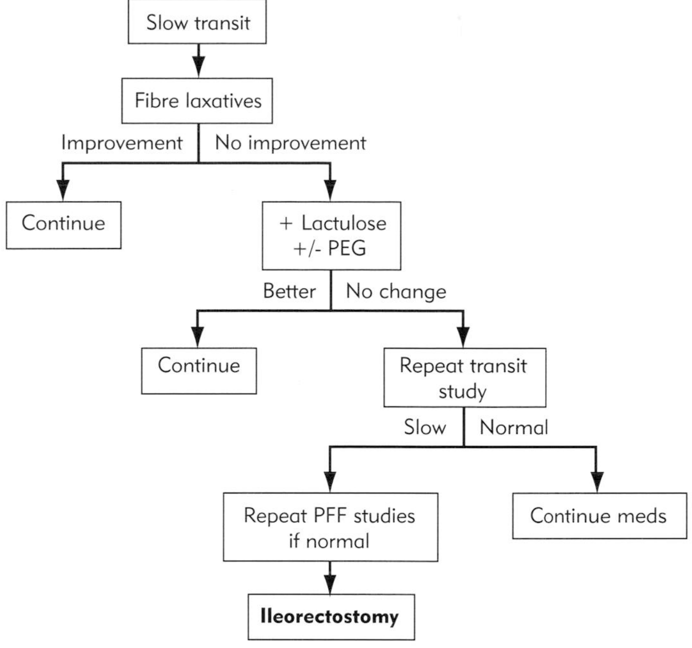

ALGORITHM 5 Posterior pelvic floor dysfunction

Algorithm 5 depicts the treatment of posterior pelvic floor disorders.

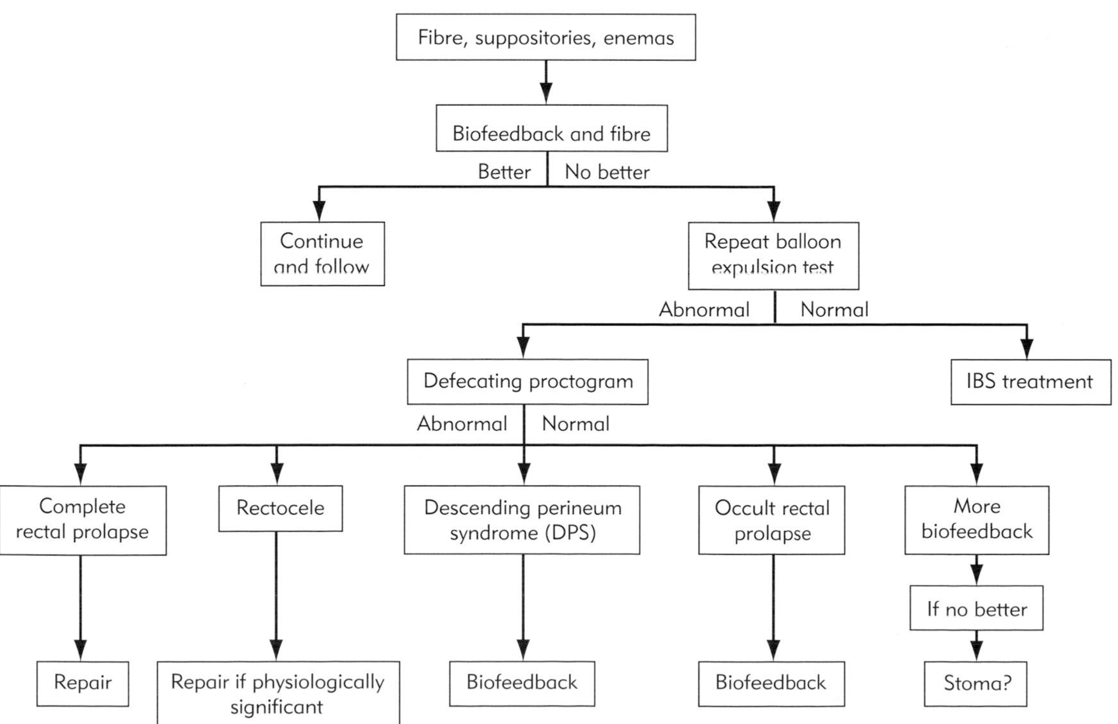

ALGORITHM 6 Complex posterior pelvic floor disorders

Algorithm 6 illustrates the treatment of a combined disorder slow transit plus pelvic.

The primary sources for Algorithms 3, 4, 5, and 6 are Chapters 5, 6, 7, 8, 9, 14, 16, 17, 22, 24, 27 and 28.

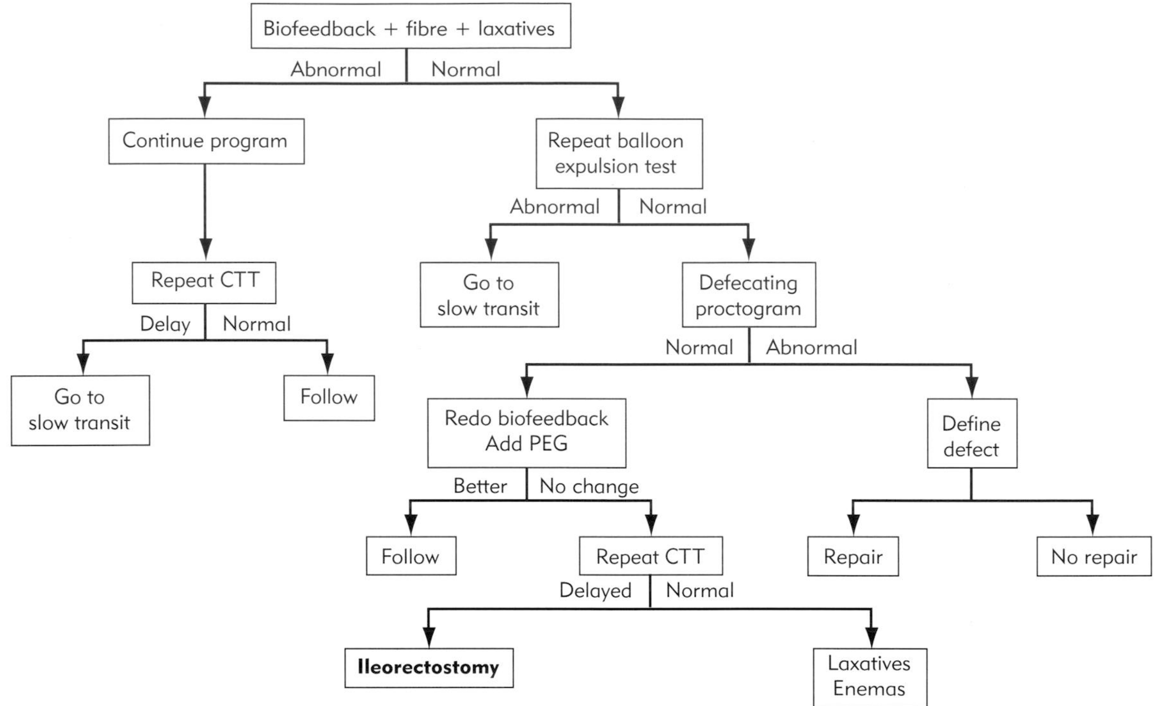

ALGORITHM 7 Urinary stress or urge incontinence

Algorithm 7 illustrates diagnosis pathways for stress and urge incontinence.

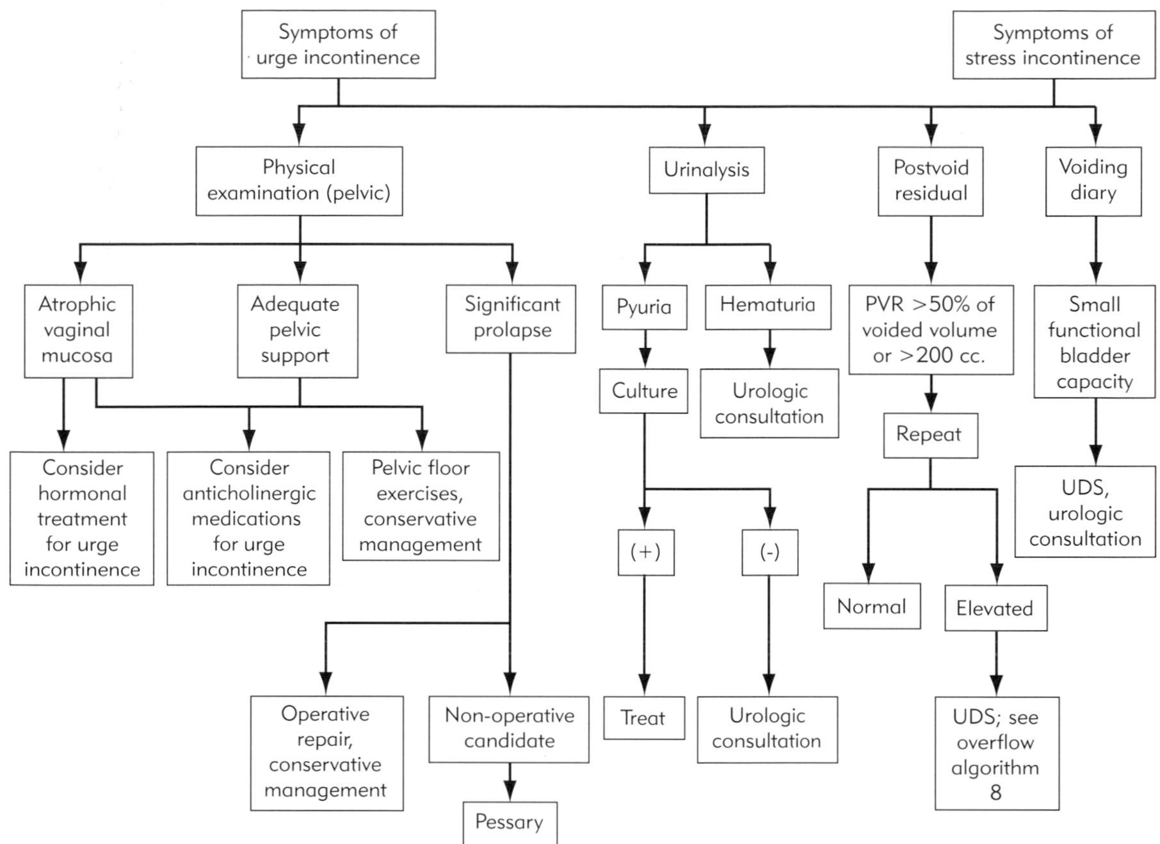

* In males with outlet symptoms: consider prostate cancer and obtain a serum PSA

ALGORITHM 8 Urinary overflow symptoms

Algorithm 8 outlines the diagnosis and treatment of overflow incontinence.

- Symptoms of overflow incontinence*
  - Physical examination (pelvic)
    - Significant prolapse
      - Operative repair
      - Pessary
  - Palpable bladder, and/or high postvoid residual
  - Urodynamics, urologic consultation
    - ↑ Pressure, ↓ flow
      - Outlet obstruction
        - Adrenergic antagonist medications
        - Surgical treatment of distorted anatomy (TURP, prolapse repair)
    - ↑ Pressure, ↓ flow
      - Atonic bladder
        - Precipitating factor
          - Stop or reduce medications
          - Treat constipation
          - Recent surgery
            - Temporary intermittent catheterization
            - Stop or reduce narcotics
          - Spinal cord injured patient
            - Neuro urologic consult
        - No precipitating factor
          - Intermittent catheterization (ambulatory patient)
            - Long term catheterization is a treatment of last resort
          - Timed voiding
          - Neuromodulation

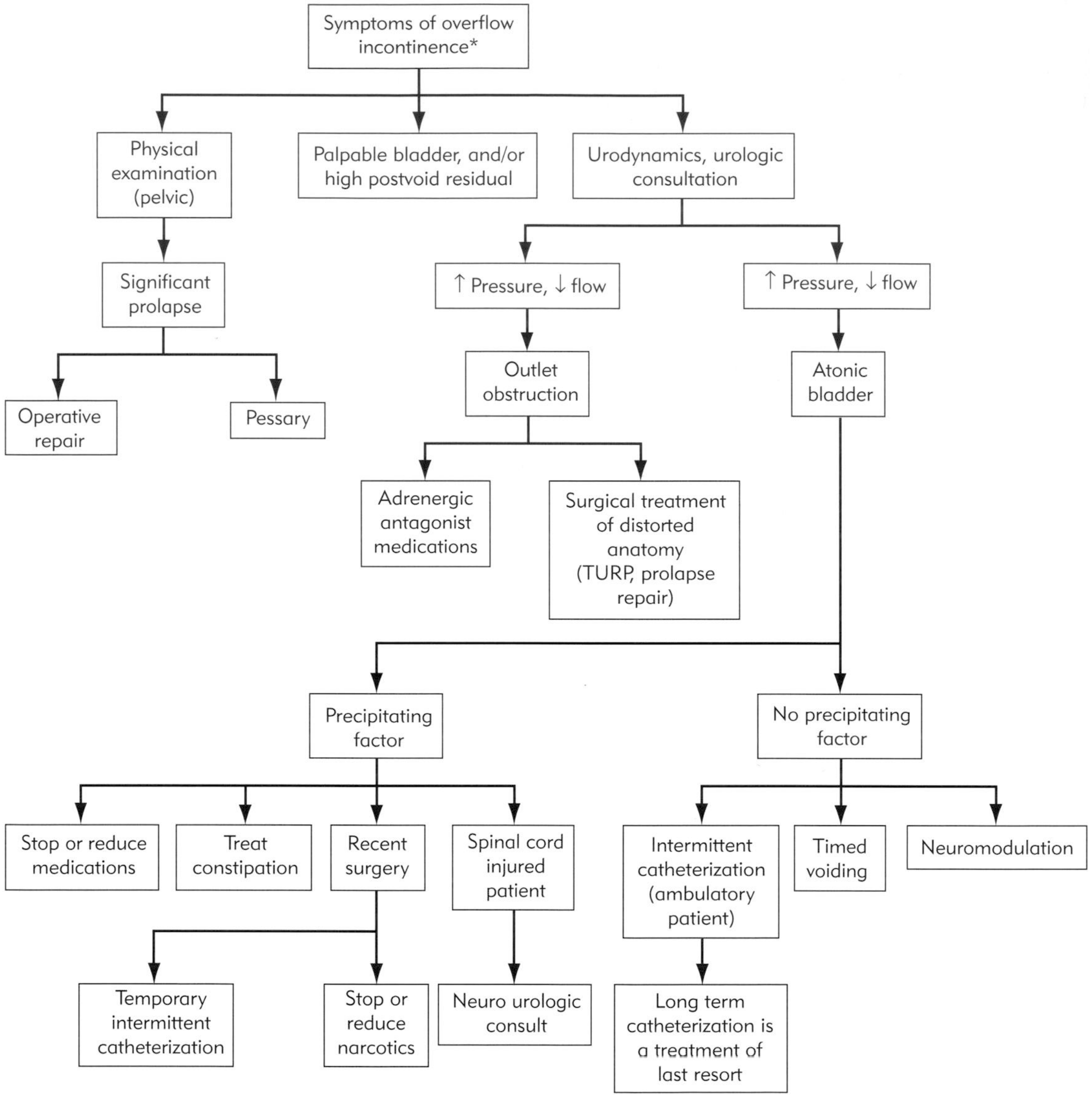

ALGORITHM 9 Acute urinary symptoms

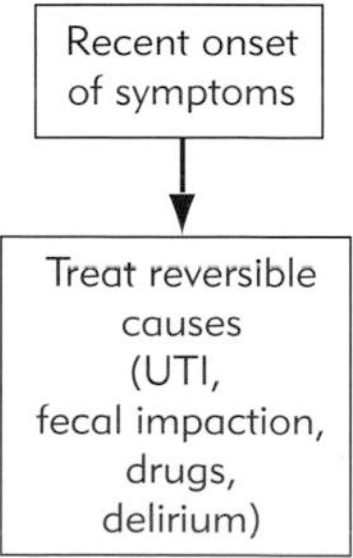

SECTION 2

The normal pelvic floor

Chapter 2

Anterior pelvic floor in the female

John O L DeLancey

INTRODUCTION

Pelvic organ prolapse and urinary incontinence are debilitating problems that prevent women from enjoying a full and active life. These problems arise due to injuries and deterioration of the muscles, nerves and connective tissue that support and control normal pelvic organ function. Although it is clear that incontinence and prolapse increase with age,[1] there is no hour during a woman's life when these structures are more vulnerable than during the time a woman delivers a child. This chapter will address the normal structure and function of the genitourinary system in women and consider the effects of vaginal delivery on the structural integrity of the pelvic floor support system. The anal sphincter and intestinal tract will be discussed in a subsequent section of this book. This section will focus specifically on how the pelvic organs are held in their normal positions and how the neural integration of pelvic muscle and pelvic visceral function affect urinary continence and prolapse of the vagina and uterus.

FEMALE GENITOURINARY SYSTEM

GENITAL TRACT AND PELVIC FLOOR

The pelvic organs, when removed from the body, exist only as a limp and formless mass. Their shape and position in living women is determined by their attachments to the pubic bones through the muscles and connective tissue of the pelvis. The actions of their muscular walls and sphincters require connection to the peripheral and central nervous systems. The structure of these supports and connections are important to our understanding of pelvic floor dysfunction. In discussing these issues I have chosen the broad use of the term pelvic floor to include all the structures supporting the abdominal and pelvic cavity rather than the restricted use of this term to refer to the levator ani group of muscles.

The pelvic floor consists of several components lying between the pelvic peritoneum and the vulvar skin. These are (from above downward) the peritoneum, viscera and endopelvic fascia, levator ani muscles, perineal membrane and external genital muscles. The eventual support for all of these structures comes from their connection to the bony pelvis, and its attached muscles. The viscera are often thought of as being supported by the pelvic floor, but are actually a part of it. Through connections to the pelvis by such structures as the cardinal and uterosacral ligaments, and the pubocervical fascia, the viscera play an important role in forming the pelvic floor.

The female pelvis can naturally be divided into anterior and posterior compartments (Fig. 2.1). The genital tract, through its lateral connections to the pelvic walls, forms the division between these two regions while the

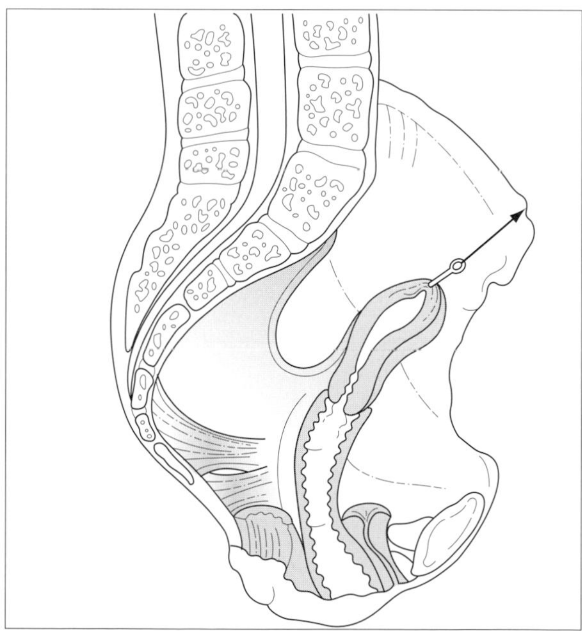

Figure 2.1 Compartments of the pelvis. The vagina, connected laterally to the pelvic walls, divides the pelvis into an anterior and posterior compartment. Copyright DeLancey 1998, based on Sears PS. The fascia surrounding the vagina, its origin and arrangement. *Am J Obstet Gynecol* 1933;**25**:484–92.

levator ani muscles form the bottom of the pelvis. The organs are attached to the levator ani muscles when they pass through the urogenital hiatus and are supported by these connections.

Endopelvic fascia

The top layer of the pelvic floor is provided by the endopelvic fascia that attaches the pelvic organs to the pelvic walls.[2,3,4] Because this layer is a combination of the pelvic viscera and the endopelvic fascia, it will be referred to as the *viscero-fascial* layer. It is common to speak of the fasciae and ligaments alone, separate from the pelvic organs as if they had a discrete identity, yet unless these fibrous structures have something to attach to (the pelvic organs), they can have no mechanical effect.

On each side of the pelvis the endopelvic fascia attaches the cervix and vagina to the pelvic wall (Fig. 2.2). This fascia forms a continuous sheet-like mesentery – extending from the uterine artery at its cephalic margin to the point at which the vagina fuses with the levator ani muscles below. The part that attaches to the uterus is called the *parametrium* and that which attaches to the vagina, the *paracolpium.*

The parametria are made up of what we clinically refer to as the cardinal and uterosacral ligaments.[5,6] These are two different parts of a single mass of tissue. The uterosacral ligaments are the visible and palpable medial margin of the cardinal–uterosacral ligament complex.

Although we name these tissues 'ligaments' and 'fasciae' they are *not* the same type of tissue seen in the

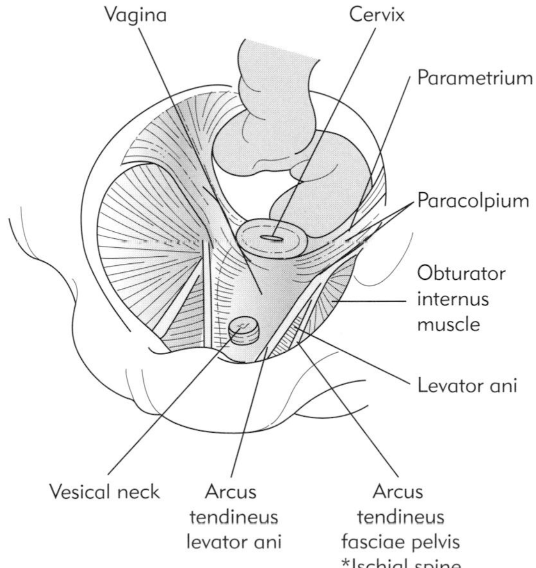

Figure 2.2 Supportive tissues of the cervix and upper vagina. The bladder has been removed above the vesical neck. Copyright DeLancey 1998.

'fascia' of the rectus abdominus muscle or the ligaments of the knee; both of which are made of dense regular connective tissue. These supportive tissues consist of blood vessels, nerves and fibrous connective tissue and can be thought of as mesenteries that supply the genital tract bilaterally. Their composition reflects their combined function as neurovascular conduits as well as supportive structures.

The structural effect of this arrangement is most evident when the uterine cervix is pulled downward with a tenaculum as is done during a D & C or pushed downward during a laparoscopy. After a certain amount of descent within the elastic range of the fascia, the parametria become tight and arrest the further cervical descent. Similarly, downward descent of the vaginal apex after hysterectomy, is resisted by the paracolpia. The fact that these ligaments do not limit the downward movement of the uterus in normal healthy women is attested to by the observation that the cervix may be drawn down to the level of the hymen with little difficulty.[7]

Although it is traditional to focus attention on the ligaments that suspend the uterus, the attachments of the vagina to the pelvic walls are equally important and are responsible for normal support of the vagina, bladder, and rectum even after hysterectomy. The location where these supports are damaged determines whether a woman has a cystocele, rectocele, or vaginal vault prolapse and understanding the different characters of this support helps understand the different types of prolapse that can occur.

The upper two thirds of the vagina is suspended and attached to the pelvic walls by the paracolpium after hysterectomy.[4] This paracolpium has two portions (Fig. 2.3). The upper portion (level I) consists of a relatively long sheet of tissue that suspends the vagina by attaching it to the pelvic wall (Fig. 2.4). In the mid-portion of the vagina, the paracolpium attaches the vagina laterally and more directly to the pelvic walls (level II). This attachment stretches the vagina transversely between the bladder and rectum and has functional significance. The structural layer that supports the bladder ('pubocervical fascia') is composed of the anterior vaginal wall and its attachment through the endopelvic fascia to the pelvic wall. It is not a separate layer from the vagina as sometimes inferred, but is a combination of the anterior vaginal wall and its attachments to the pelvic wall. Similarly, the posterior vaginal wall and endopelvic fascia (rectovaginal fascia) form the restraining layer that prevents the rectum from protruding forward, blocking formation of a rectocele. In the distal vagina (level III) the vaginal wall is directly attached to surrounding structures without any intervening paracolpium. Anteriorly it fuses with the urethra, posteriorly with the perineal body, and laterally with the levator ani muscles.

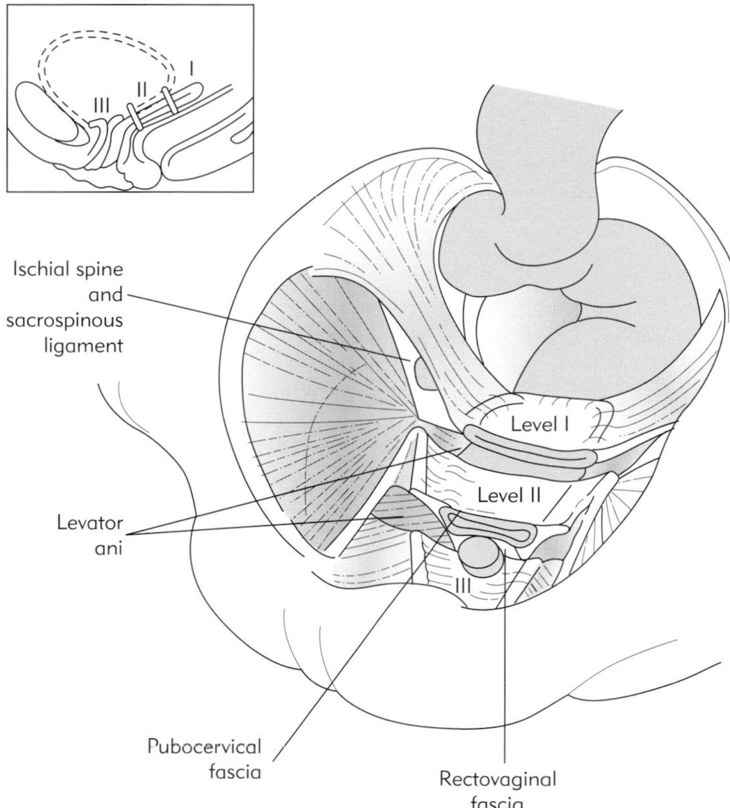

Figure 2.3 Levels of vaginal support after hysterectomy. Level I (suspension) and level II (attachment). In level I the paracolpium suspends the vagina from the lateral pelvic walls. Fibers of level I extend both vertically and also posteriorly towards sacrum. In level II vagina is attached to arcus tendineus fasciae pelvis and superior fascia of levator ani. From DeLancey JOL. Anatomic aspects of vaginal eversion after hysterectomy. *Am J Obstet Gynecol* 1992;166:1717–28, with permission.

Damage to the upper suspensory fibers of the paracolpium causes a different type of prolapse from damage to the mid-level supports of the vagina. Defects in the support provided by the mid-level vaginal supports (pubocervical and rectovaginal fasciae) result in cystocele and rectocele while loss of the upper suspensory fibers of the paracolpium and parametrium is responsible for development of vaginal and uterine prolapse. These defects occur in varying combinations and this variation is responsible for the diversity of clinical problems encountered within the overall spectrum of pelvic organ prolapse

Levator ani muscles

Any connective tissue within the body may be stretched by subjecting it to constant force. Skin expanders used in plastic surgery stretch the dense and resistant dermis to extraordinary degrees and flexibility exercises practiced by dancers and athletes elongate leg ligaments with as little as 10 minutes of stretching a day. Both of these observations underscore the malleable nature of connective tissue when subjected to force over time. If the ligaments and fasciae within the pelvis were subjected to the continuous stress imposed on the pelvic floor by the great weight of abdominal pressure, they would stretch. This stretching does not occur, because the pelvic floor muscles close the pelvic floor and carry the weight of the abdominal and pelvic organs, preventing constant strain on the ligaments.

Below the viscero-fascial layer is the levator ani group of muscles. (Fig. 2.5)[8] They have a connective tissue covering on both superior and inferior surfaces called the superior and inferior fasciae of the levator ani. When these muscles and their fasciae are considered together, the combined structure is called the pelvic diaphragm.

The levator ani muscle consists of two portions, the pubovisceral muscle and the iliococcygeus muscle.[9,10] The pubovisceral muscle is a thick, U-shaped muscle whose ends arise from the pubic bones on either side of

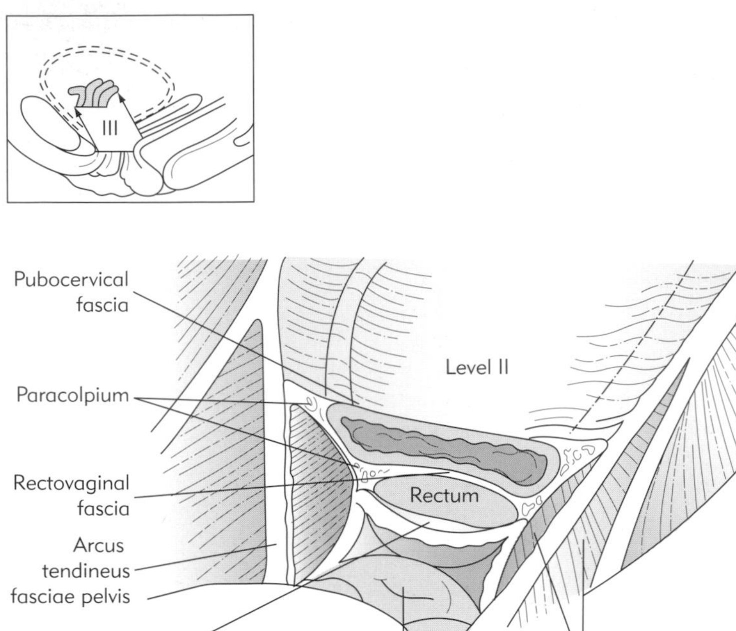

Figure 2.4 Close up of the lower margin of level II after a wedge of vagina has been removed (inset). Note how the anterior vaginal wall, through its connections to the arcus tendineus fascia pelvis, forms a supportive layer clinically referred to as the pubocervical fascia. From DeLancey JOL. Anatomic aspects of vaginal eversion after hysterectomy. *Am J Obstet Gynecol* 1992;**166**:1717–28.

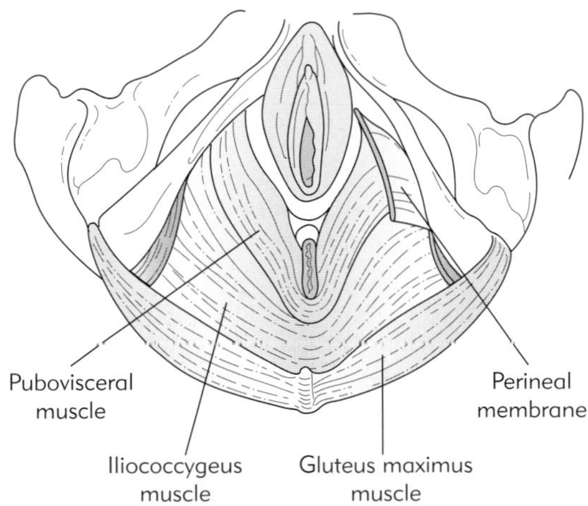

Figure 2.5 Levator ani muscles seen from below. The cut edge of the perineal membrane ('urogenital diaphragm') can be seen on the left of the specimen. Copyright DeLancey, 1994.

the midline and pass behind the rectum forming a sling-like arrangement. This portion includes both the pubococcygeus and puborectalis portions of the levator ani. Laterally, the iliococcygeus arises from a fibrous band on the pelvic wall (arcus tendineus levator ani) and forms a relatively horizontal sheet that spans the opening within the pelvis and forms a shelf on which the organs may rest.

The pubovisceral muscle has several components. The pubococcygeus muscle is the most cephalic portion of the levator and passes from the pubic bones to insert on the inner surface of the coccyx. It comprises only a small portion of the overall levator complex. Clinicians have often referred to the entire pubovisceral muscle under the term pubococcygeus. The pubococcygeus portion of the levator ani muscles actually connects two relatively immovable structures (pubis and coccyx) and, therefore, could not be expected to contribute substantially to supporting the pelvic organs. The puborectalis portion of the pubovisceral muscle passes beside the vagina, the lateral vaginal walls are attached to it. The muscle then continues dorsally where some fibers insert into the rectum between the internal and external sphincter while others pass behind the ano-rectal junction. The vagina attaches to the medial portion of the pubovisceral muscle and the fibers between the vagina and pubic bone are referred to as the pubovaginalis muscle. These muscle fibers are responsible for elevating the urethra during pelvic muscle contraction, but muscle fibers of the levator have no direct connection to the urethra itself.

The opening within the levator ani muscle through which the urethra and vagina pass (and through which prolapse occurs), is called the *urogenital hiatus* of the levator ani. The rectum also passes through this opening, but because the levator ani muscles attach directly to the anus it is not included in the name of the hiatus. The hiatus, therefore, is bounded ventrally (anteriorly) by the pubic bones, laterally by the levator ani muscles and dorsally (posteriorly) by the perineal body and external anal sphincter. The normal baseline activity of the levator ani muscle keeps the urogenital hiatus closed. It squeezes the vagina, urethra and rectum closed by compressing them against the pubic bone and lifts the floor and organs in a cephalic direction.

The levator ani muscles have constant activity[11] similar to other postural muscles. This continuous contraction is similar to the continuous activity of the external anal sphincter muscle and closes the lumen of the vagina in a similar way that the anal sphincter closes the anus. This constant action eliminates any opening within the pelvic floor through which prolapse could occur and forms a relatively horizontal shelf on which the pelvic organs are supported.[12,13]

The interaction between the pelvic floor muscles and the supportive ligaments is critical to pelvic organ support. As long as the levator ani muscles function properly the pelvic floor is closed and the ligaments and fasciae are under no tension. The fasciae simply act to stabilize the organs in their position above the levator ani muscles. When the pelvic floor muscles relax or are damaged, the pelvic floor opens and the vagina lies between the high abdominal pressure and low atmospheric pressure. In this situation it must be held in place by the ligaments. Although the ligaments can sustain these loads for short periods of time, if the pelvic floor muscles do not close the pelvic floor then the connective tissue must carry this load for long periods of time and will eventually fail to hold the vagina in place.

This support of the uterus has been likened to a ship in its berth floating on the water attached by ropes on either side to a dock.[14] The ship is analogous to the uterus, the ropes to the ligaments, and the water to the supportive layer formed by the pelvic floor muscles. The ropes function to hold the ship (uterus) in the center of its berth as it rests on the water (pelvic floor muscles). If, however, the water level were to fall far enough that the ropes would be required to hold the ship without the supporting water, the ropes would all break. The analogous situation in the pelvic floor involves the pelvic floor muscles supporting the uterus and vagina that are stabilized in position by the ligaments and fascias. Once the pelvic floor musculature becomes damaged and no longer holds the organs in place, the connective tissue fails.

Perineal membrane and external genital muscles

In the anterior pelvis, below the pelvic diaphragm, is a dense triangularly shaped membrane called the perineal membrane (urogenital diaphragm). It lies at the level of the hymenal ring, and attaches the urethra, vagina, and perineal body to the ischiopubic rami (Figs 2.6 and 2.7). Just above the perineal membrane are the compressor

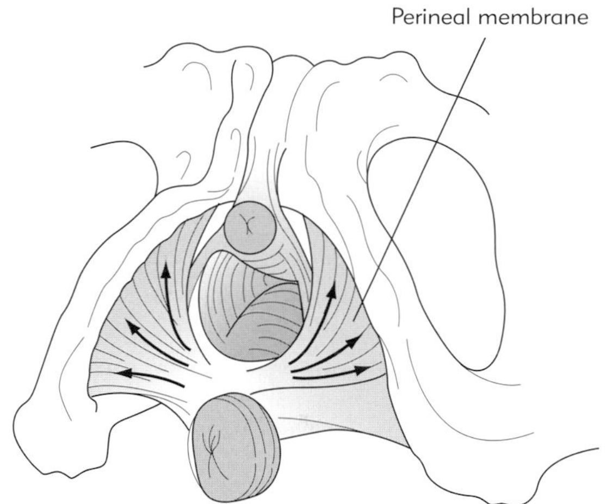

Figure 2.6 The perineal membrane spans the arch between the ischiopubic rami with each side attached to the other through their connection in the perineal body. From DeLancey JOL. Structural anatomy of the posterior compartment as it relates to rectocele. *Am J Obstet Gynecol* 1999;**180**:815–23.

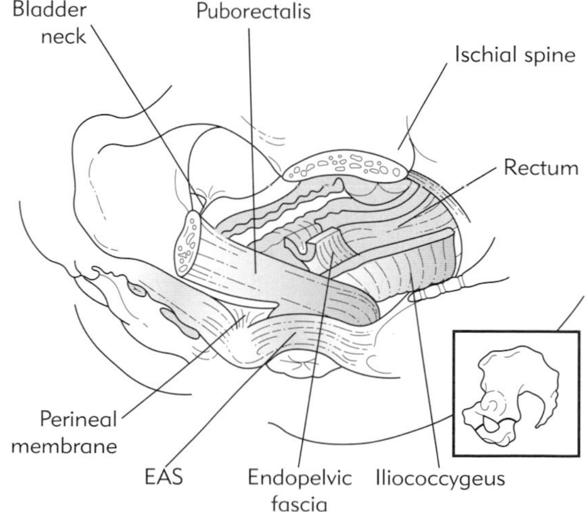

Figure 2.7 Lateral view of the pelvis showing the relationships of the puborectalis, iliococcygeus and pelvic floor structures. From DeLancey JOL. Structural anatomy of the posterior compartment as it relates to rectocele. *Am J Obstet Gynecol* 1999;**180**:815–23.

urethrae and urethrovaginal sphincter muscles, previously discussed as part of the striated urogenital sphincter muscle.

The term perineal membrane replaces the old term urogenital diaphragm, reflecting more accurate recent anatomical information.[15] Previous concepts of the urogenital diaphragm show two fascial layers, with a transversely oriented muscle in between (the deep transverse perineal muscle). Observations based on serial histology and gross dissection, however, reveal a single connective tissue membrane, with muscle lying immediately above. The correct anatomy explains the observation that pressures during a cough are greatest in the distal urethra,[16,17] where the compressor urethra and urethrovaginal sphincter can compress the lumen closed in anticipation of a cough.[18]

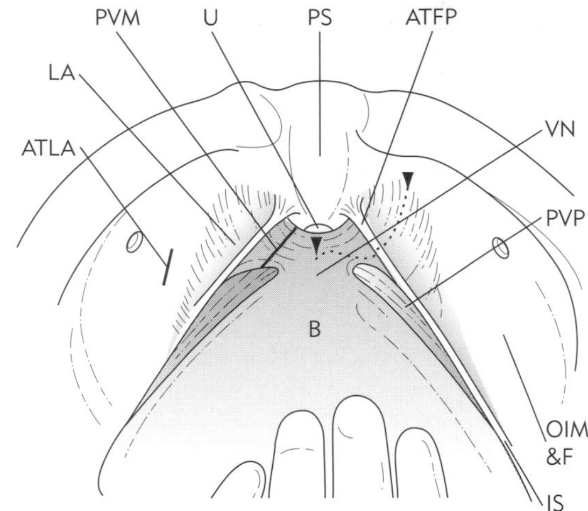

Figure 2.8 Space of Retzius (drawn from cadaver dissection). Pubovesical muscle (PVM) can be seen going from vesical neck (VN) to arcus tendineus fasciae pelvis (ATFP) and running over the paraurethral vascular plexus (PVP). ATLA, arcus tendineus levator ani; B, bladder; IS, ischial spine; LA, levator ani muscles; OIM&F, obturator internus muscle and fascia; PS, pubic symphysis; U, urethra. Dotted lines indicated plane of section of Figure 2.16. Reprinted with permission Alan R. Liss Co. from *Neurol Urodynam* 1989;**8**:53.

Position and mobility of the urethra

The position and mobility of the bladder and urethra are important to urinary continence.[19] Because these two organs are formless when removed from the body, they must depend on their attachments to the pelvic floor for their shape and position. Fluoroscopic examination has shown that the upper urethra and vesical neck are normally mobile structures while the distal urethra remains fixed in position.[20,21] Both the pelvic floor muscles and the pelvic fasciae therefore, determine the support and fixation of the urethra.

Urethral position is determined both by attachments to bone and also to the levator ani muscles. The role of the connection between the urethral supports and to the levator ani is probably more important than previously thought for the following reasons. The resting position of the proximal urethra is high within the pelvis, some three centimeters above the inferior aspect of the pubic bones.[22] Maintenance of this position would best be explained by the constant muscular activity of the levator ani. In addition, the upper two thirds of the urethra is mobile[20,21,23] and under voluntary control. At the onset of micturition, relaxation of the levator ani muscles allows the urethra to descend, and obliterates the posterior urethrovesical angle. Resumption of the normal tonic contraction of the muscle at the end of micturition returns the vesical neck to its normal position.

The anterior vaginal wall and urethra arise from the urogenital sinus, and are intimately connected. The support of the urethra depends, not on attachments of the urethra itself to adjacent structures, but upon the connection of the vagina and periurethral tissues to the muscles and fascia of the pelvic wall. Surgeons are most familiar with seeing this anatomy through the space of Retzius and this view is also helpful in understanding urethral support (Fig. 2.8). On either side of the pelvis, the arcus tendineus fascia pelvis is found as a band of connective tissue attached at one end to the lower sixth of the pubic bone, 1 cm from the midline, and at the other end to the ischial spine. The anterior portion of this band lies on the inner surface of the levator ani muscle that arises some 3 cm above the arcus tendineus fasciae pelvis. Posteriorly, the levator ani arises from a second arcus, the arcus tendineus fasciae levatoris ani, which fuses with the arcus tendineus fasciae pelvis near the ischial spine.

The layer of tissue that provides urethral support has two lateral attachments, a fascial attachment and a muscular attachment[24] (Fig. 2.9). The fascial attachment of the urethral supports connects the periurethral tissues and anterior vaginal wall to the arcus tendineus fasciae pelvis and has been called the paravaginal fascial attachments by Richardson.[25] The muscular attachment connects these same periurethral tissues to the medial border of the levator ani muscle. These attachments allow the levator ani muscle's normal resting tone to maintain the position of the vesical neck, supported by the fascial attachments. When the muscle relaxes at the onset of micturition, it allows the vesical neck to rotate downward to the limit of the elasticity of the fascial attachments, and then contraction at the end of micturition allows it to resume its normal position.

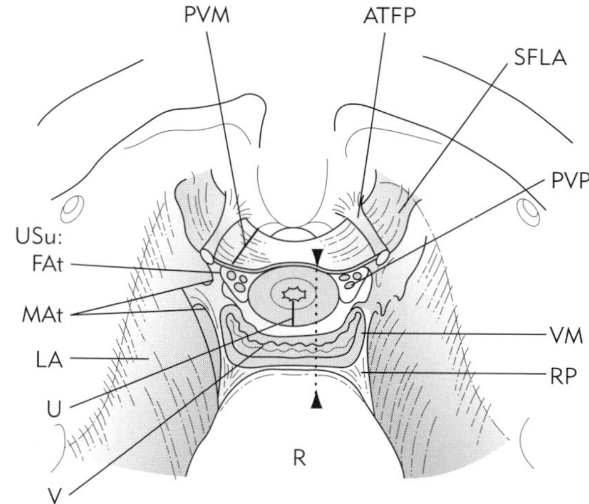

Figure 2.9 Relationship of the supportive tissues of the urethra (USu) to the pubovesical muscles (PVM). Cross section of the urethra (U), vagina (V), arcus tendineus fasciae pelvic (ATFP), and superior fascia of levator ani (SFLA) just below the vesical neck (drawn from cadaver dissection). Pubovesical muscles (PVM) lie anterior to urethra and anterior and superior to paraurethral vascular plexus (PVP). The urethral supports (USu) ('the pubo-urethral ligaments') attach the vagina and vaginal surface of the urethra to the levator ani muscles (MAt, muscular attachment) and to the superior fascia of the levator ani (FAt, fascial attachment). Additional abbreviations: LA, levator ani muscles; R, rectum; RP, rectal pillar; VM, vaginal wall muscularis. Reprinted with permission Alan R. Liss Co. from *Neurol Urodynam* 1989;**8**:53.

Also within this region are the pubovesical muscles. These are extensions of the detrusor muscle.[26–28] They lie within connective tissue, and when both muscular and fibrous elements are considered together, they are called the pubovesical ligaments in much the same way that the smooth muscle of the ligamentum teres is referred to as the round ligament (Fig. 2.9). Although sometimes the terms pubovesical ligament and pubourethral ligament have been considered to be synonymous, the pubovesical ligaments are different structures from the urethral supportive tissues. Fibers of the detrusor muscle are able to undergo great elongation and these weak tissues are therefore not suited to maintain urethral position under stress. In addition, they run in front of the vesical neck rather than underneath it, where one would expect supportive tissues to be found. It is not surprising, therefore that these detrusor fibers are no different in stress incontinent patients, than those without this condition.[29] The tissues that support the urethra are separated from the pubovesical ligament by a prominent vascular plexus, and are easily separated from them. Rather than supporting the urethra, the pubovesical muscles may be responsible for assisting in vesical neck opening at the onset of micturition by contracting to pull the vesical neck forward as some have suggested.[30]

This mechanism influences incontinence, not by determining how high or how low the urethra is, but how it is supported. In examining anatomic specimens, simulated increases in abdominal pressure reveal that the urethra lies in a position where it can be compressed against the supporting hammock by rises in abdominal pressure (Figs 2.10 and 2.11). In this model, it is more the stability of this supporting layer under the urethra than the height of the urethra that determines stress continence. In an individual with a firm supportive layer the urethra would be compressed between abdominal pressure and pelvic fascia in much the same way that you can stop the flow of water through a garden hose by stepping on it and compressing it against an underlying sidewalk. If, however, the layer under the urethra becomes unstable and does not provide a firm backstop for abdominal pressure to compress the urethra against, the opposing force that causes closure is lost and the occlusive action diminished. This latter situation is similar to trying to stop the flow of water through a garden hose by stepping on it while it lies on soft soil.

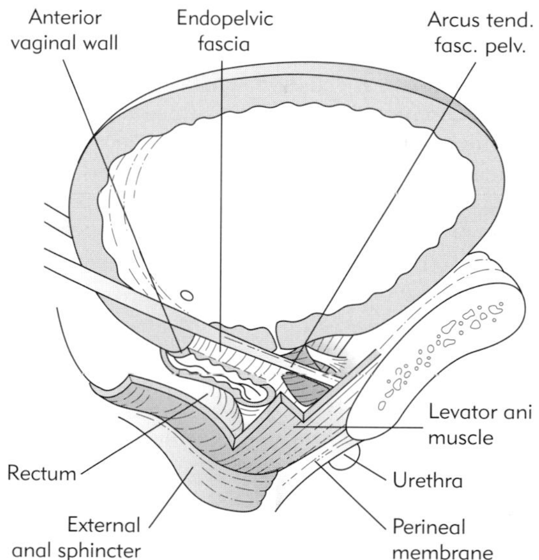

Figure 2.10 Lateral view of the pelvic floor structures related to urethral support seen from the side in the standing position, cut just lateral to the midline. Note that windows have been cut in the levator ani muscles, vagina, and endopelvic fascia so that the urethra and anterior vaginal walls can be seen. From DeLancey JOL. Structural support of the urethra as it relates to stress urinary incontinence: the hammock hypothesis. *Am J Obstet Gynecol* 1994;**170**:1713–20.

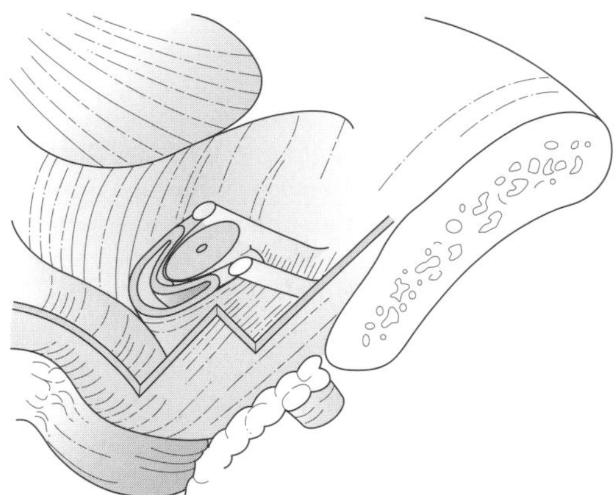

Figure 2.11 Lateral view of pelvic floor with the urethra, vagina and fascial tissues transected at the level of the vesical neck drawn indicating compression of the urethra by downward force (arrow) against the supportive tissues indicating the influence of abdominal pressure on the urethra (arrow). From DeLancey JOL. Structural support of the urethra as it relates to stress urinary incontinence: the hammock hypothesis. *Am J Obstet Gynecol* 1994;**170**:1713–20.

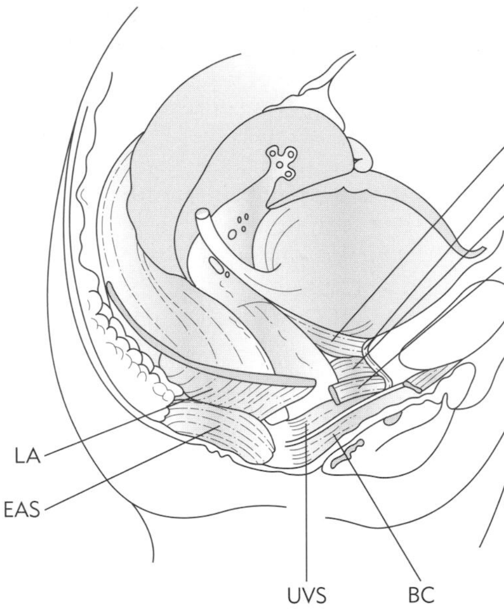

Figure 2.12 Lateral view of the pelvis showing the bladder neck, urethra and levator ani muscles. Portions of the levator ani muscles have been removed. BC, bulbocavernosus muscle; CU, compressor urethrae; DL detrusor loop; EAS, external anal sphincter muscle; LA, levator ani muscle; PVM, pubovesical muscle; US, urethral sphincter; UVS, urethrovaginal sphincter muscle. Copyright DeLancey 1996.

FUNCTIONAL ANATOMY OF THE LOWER URINARY TRACT

The inseparable link between structure and function found in living organisms is one of the common themes found in biology. The anatomy and clinical behavior of the lower urinary tract exemplify this immutable link. The following descriptions are intended to offer a brief overview of some clinically relevant aspects of lower urinary tract structure that help us understand the normal and abnormal behavior of this system (Fig. 2.12).

The lower urinary tract can be divided into the bladder and urethra. At the junction of these two continuous, yet discrete structures, lies the vesical neck. This hybrid structure represents that part of the lower urinary tract where the urethral lumen traverses the bladder wall before becoming surrounded by the urethral wall. It contains portions of the bladder muscle, and also elements that continue into the urethra.

The vesical neck is considered separately because of its functional differentiation from the bladder, and the urethra.

Bladder

The bladder consists of the detrusor muscle, covered by an adventitia and serosa over its dome, and lined by a submucosa and transitional cell epithelium. The muscular layers of the detrusor are not discrete, but in general, the outer and inner layers of the detrusor musculature tend to be longitudinal, with an intervening circular-oblique layer.

Two prominent bands on the dorsal aspect of the bladder form one of the landmarks of the detrusor musculature.[26] They are derived from the outer longitudinal layer and pass beside the urethra to form a loop on its anterior aspect, called the detrusor loop. On the anterior aspect of this loop, some detrusor fibers leave the region of the vesical neck and attach to the pubic bones and pelvic walls. These are called the pubovesical muscles that have been described above (Fig. 2.8).

Trigone

Within the bladder there is a visible triangular area known as the vesical trigone. Its apices are formed by the two ureteral orifices and the internal urinary meatus. The base of the triangle, the interureteric ridge, forms a useful landmark in cystoscopic identification the ureteric orifices. This triangular elevation is caused by the presence of a specialized group of smooth muscle fibers that lie within the detrusor, and arise from a separate embryological primordium. They are continuous above with the ureteral smooth muscle,[31] and below, continue down the urethra. In addition to their visible triangular elevation, these muscle fibers form a ring inside the detrusor loop at the level of the internal urinary meatus.[32] Some fibers continue down the dorsal surface of the urethra and lie between the ends of the U-shaped striated sphincter muscles of the urethra. These smooth muscle fibers of the trigone are clearly separable from those of the detrusor by the smaller size of their fascicles and greater density of surrounding connective tissue. The mucosa over the trigone frequently undergoes squamous metaplasia and therefore differs from that in the rest of the bladder. The circumferential distribution of the trigonal ring fibers at the vesical neck might contribute to closure of the vesical neck's lumen at this area, but its role has yet to be fully elucidated.

Urethra

The urethra holds urine in the bladder and is therefore an important structure that helps determine urinary continence. It is a complex tubular viscus extending below the bladder. In its upper third it is clearly separable from the adjacent vagina, but its lower portion is fused with the wall of the latter structure. Embedded within its substance are a number of elements that are important to lower urinary tract dysfunction. Their locations are summarized in Table 2.1.[33]

Striated urogenital sphincter

The outer layer of the urethra is formed by the muscle of the striated urogenital sphincter (Fig. 2.12) which is found from about 20–80% of total urethral length (measured as a percentage of the distance from the internal meatus to the external meatus). In its upper two thirds, the sphincter fibers lie in a primarily circular orientation, while distally, they leave the confines of the urethra and either encircle the vaginal wall as the urethrovaginal sphincter, or extend along the inferior pubic ramus above the perineal membrane (urogenital diaphragm) as the compressor urethrae. This muscle is composed largely of slow twitch muscle fibers[34] which are well suited to maintaining the constant tone exhibited by this muscle. In addition, voluntary muscle activation increases in urethral constriction during times when increased closure pressure is needed. In the distal urethra, this striated muscle compresses the urethra from above, and proximally, it constricts the lumen. Studies of skeletal muscle blockade suggest that this muscle is

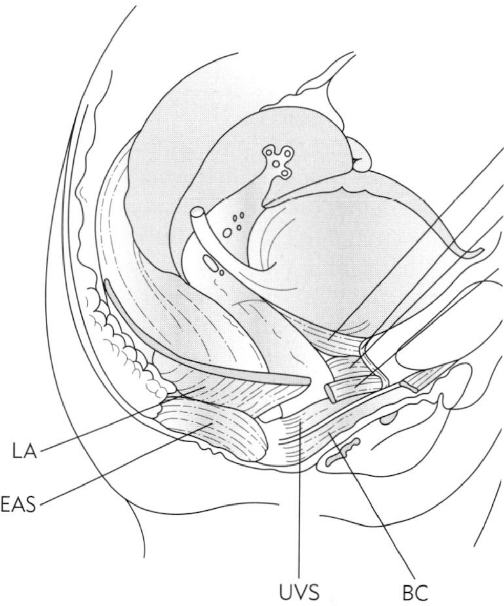

Figure 2.12 Lateral view of the pelvis showing the bladder neck, urethra and levator ani muscles. Portions of the levator ani muscles have been removed. BC, bulbocavernosus muscle; CU, compressor urethrae; DL, detrusor loop; EAS, external anal sphincter muscle; LA, levator ani muscle; PVM, pubovesical muscle; US, urethral sphincter; UVS, urethrovaginal sphincter muscle. Copyright DeLancey 1996.

Table 2.1 Topography of urethral and paraurethral structures[a,c]

Approximate location[b]	Region of the urethra	Paraurethral structures
0–20	Intramural urethra	Urethral lumen traverses the bladder wall
20–60	Mid-urethra	Sphincter urethrae muscle Pubovesical muscle Vaginolevator attachment
60–80	Perineal membrane	Compressor urethrae muscle Urethrovaginal sphincter muscle
80–100	Distal urethra	Bulbocavernosus muscle

[a]Smooth muscle of the urethra was not considered.
[b]Expressed as a percent of total urethral length.
[c]Reprinted with permission from the American College of Obstetricians and Gynecologists. *Obstet Gynecol* 1986;68:91.

responsible for approximately one third of resting urethral closure pressure.[35]

Urethral smooth muscle

The smooth muscle of the urethra is contiguous with that of the trigone and detrusor, but can be separated from these other muscles on embryological, topographical and morphological grounds.[32,36] It is an inner longitudinal layer, and a thin outer circular layer, with the former being by far the more prominent of the two (Figs 2.13 and 2.14). They lie inside the striated urogenital sphincter muscle, and are present throughout the upper four fifths of the urethra. The configuration of the circular muscle suggests a role in constricting the lumen, and the longitudinal muscle may help shorten and funnel the urethra during voiding.

Submucosal vasculature

Lying within the urethra is a surprisingly well developed vascular plexus that is more prominent than one would expect for the ordinary demands of so small an organ[37]. (Fig. 2.13). These vessels have been studied in serial reconstruction by Huisman[32] who has demonstrated the presence of several specialized types of arteriovenous anastomoses. They are formed in such a way that the flow of blood into large venules can be controlled to inflate or deflate them. This would assist in forming a watertight closure of the mucosal surfaces, and offer the possibility of rapid increases in their filling from the pressure on the abdominal vessels which supply them. Occlusion of the arterial inflow to these venous reservoirs has been shown to influence urethral closure pressure.[35] In addition, these appear to be hormonally sensitive,[32] and may help to explain some individuals' response to oestrogen supplementation.

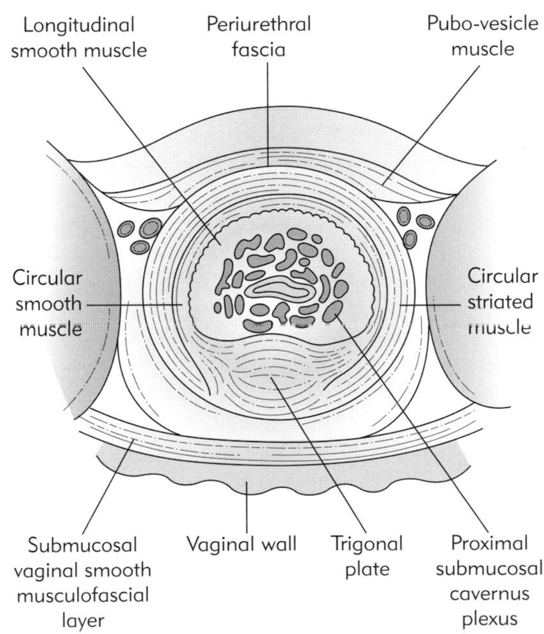

Figure 2.13 Cross section of the mid-urethra modified from Huisman (1983). From Strohbehn K, DeLancey JOL. The anatomy of stress incontinence. *Oper Tech Gynecol Surg* 1997;**2**:5–16, WB Saunders.

Mucosa

The mucosal lining of the urethra is continuous above with the transitional epithelium of the bladder, and with the non-keratinizing squamous epithelium of the vestibule below. This mucosa shares a common derivation from the urogenital sinus with the lower vagina and vestibule. Like these other areas, its mucosa is hormonally sensitive, and undergoes significant change depending on its state of stimulation.

Connective tissue

In addition to the contractile and vascular tissue of the urethra, there is a considerable quantity of connective tissue interspersed within the muscle, and the submucosa. This tissue has both collagenous and elastin fibers. Studies which have sought to abolish the active aspects of urethral closure have suggested that the non-contractile elements contribute to urethral closure.[32] It is difficult, however to study these tissues' function specifically, because there is no specific way to pharmacologically or surgically block their action.

Glands

A series of glands are found in the submucosa primarily along the dorsal (vaginal) surface of the urethra[38] (Fig. 2.15). They are most concentrated in the lower and middle thirds, and vary in number. The location of urethral diverticula, which are derived from cystic dilation of these glands, follows this distribution being most common distally, and usually originating along the dorsal surface of the urethra. In addition, their origin within the submucosa indicates that the fascia of the urethra must be stretched and attenuated over their surface, and indicates the need for its approximation after diverticular excision.

Vesical neck

The term 'vesical neck' is both a regional and functional one as previously discussed. It does not refer to a single anatomical entity. It denotes that area, at the base of the bladder, where the urethral lumen passes through the thickened musculature of the bladder base. Therefore, it is sometimes considered as part of the bladder muscula-

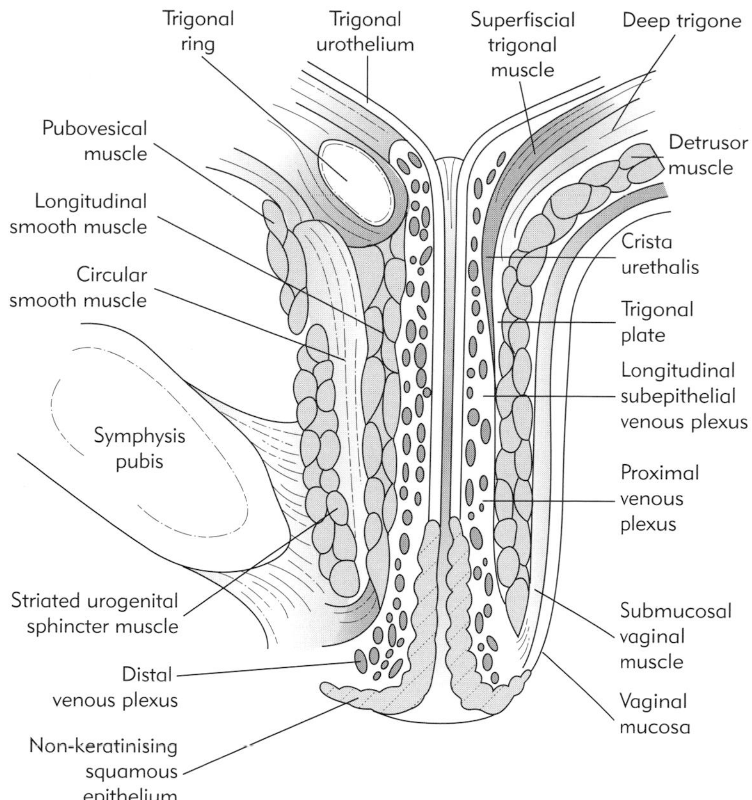

Figure 2.14 Sagittal section of the mid-urethra modified from Huisman (1983). From Strohbehn K, DeLancey JOL. The anatomy of stress incontinence. *Oper Tech Gynecol Surg* 1997;2:5–16, WB Saunders.

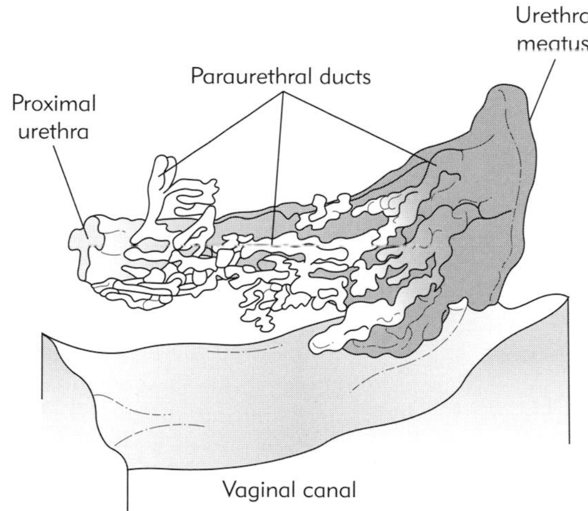

Figure 2.15 The detailed anatomy of the paraurethral glands from wax plate reconstruction showing the predominance of ducts on the vaginal side of the urethra and the larger ducts near the external urinary meatus. From: Huffman J. Detailed anatomy of the paraurethral ducts in the adult human female. *Am J Obstet Gynecol* 1948;55:86–101.

ture, but also contains the urethral lumen studied during urethral pressure profilometry. It is a region where the detrusor musculature, including the detrusor loop, surrounds the trigonal ring and the urethral meatus.

The vesical neck has come to be considered separately from the bladder and urethra because it has unique functional characteristics. Specifically, sympathetic denervation or damage of this area results in its remaining open at rest,[39] and when this happens in association with stress incontinence, simple urethral suspension is often ineffective in curing this problem.[40]

Functional terms

There are a number of terms which have arisen to describe functional units within the vesicourethral unit based upon radiographic observations of the activities of these viscera. The term extrinsic continence mechanism, or external sphincteric mechanism, usually refers to that group of structures which respond when an individual is instructed to stop their urine stream. The two phenomena observed during this effort are a constriction of the urethral lumen by the striated urogenital sphincter, and an elevation of the vesical neck caused by contraction of the levator ani muscles as will be described below. The intrinsic continence mechanism, then consists of the structures which lie within the vesical neck, and which are not specifically activated by contraction of the voluntary muscles. It is this system which fails in patients whose vesical neck can be seen to be open at rest.

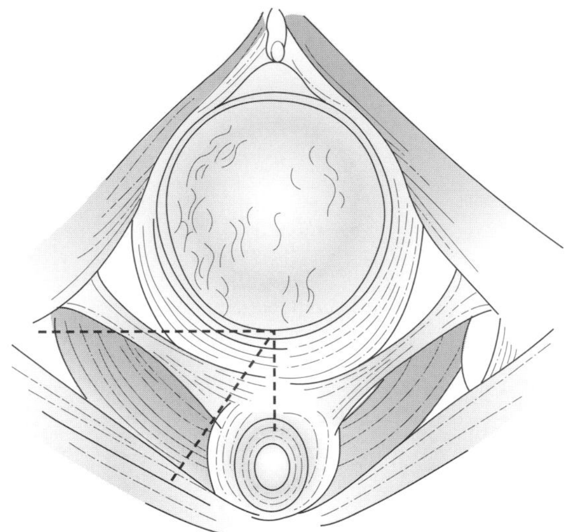

Figure 2.16 Perineal view of the perineal membrane and introitus as the fetal head attempts to dilate the introitus. This results in downward descent of the pelvic floor.

CHILDBIRTH

Despite the miraculous nature of vaginal delivery in the human, relatively few scientific data are available about the changes that occur in the structures of the pelvic floor as the fetal head is delivered. Although scientific study of this phenomenon is in its infancy, extensive experience with observation at birth can provide a reasonable picture of this event. The basic phenomenon involves the passage of an approximately 10-cm diameter fetal head through the ligaments and muscles of the pelvic floor outlined in the previous section.

There is clear evidence that vaginal delivery increases the likelihood of both urinary incontinence and pelvic organ prolapse. Foldspang's epidemiological study[41] shows that urinary incontinence is approximately 2 to 3-fold more likely after vaginal delivery and Timonen's study[42] shows that there is a higher prevalence of pelvic organ prolapse in parous patients with prolapse than there are in the general population.

WHAT HAPPENS DURING NORMAL DELIVERY?

The expulsive forces of the uterus and bearing down efforts increase in abdominal pressure to force the fetus toward the vaginal orifice. The fetal head dilates the vaginal canal and pushes the structures of the pelvic floor downward. The head must pass through the relatively narrow opening in the levator ani muscles (urogenital hiatus) and the perineal membrane (Fig. 2.16). This process of pushing the head through this small opening drives the pelvic floor down (Fig. 2.17). Early in the second stage of labor, the resting tone of the levator ani muscles hold the pelvic floor in place, but with increasing pelvic floor descent and muscular relaxation this situation changes.

Eventually, the muscles lengthen to the point that the elastic limit of their fascial coverings (the superior fascia and the inferior fascia of the levator ani muscles) is reached and further descent is stopped. In addition, the elastic limit of the perineal membrane is reached. Since its two sides unite through the connective tissue of the perineal body,[43] the downward descent of the perineal body is limited by these attachments to the pubic bones. The head must then stretch this opening by causing elongation of the connective tissue sufficient to reach a diameter of 10 cm or circumference of approximately 31 cm.

As the head pushes downward through the outlet, substantial stresses are placed on the perineal membrane and the connection of its two sides through the perineal body. The degree of stress depends upon the resistance of the tissues and the amounts of force that must be applied in order dilate the introital structures. If the tissues are stretchy and yielding then relatively little stress is placed on the perineal membrane and perineal body, while if they are stiff and rigid, then it requires more force in order to achieve dilatation.

BLADDER POSITION DURING DELIVERY

Although there is no specific data set on the pelvic floor in general, observations have been made about the bladder and bladder neck relative to the fetal head during parturition.[44] At the onset of labor, the bladder base and urethrovesical junction are found anteriorly in the pelvis. They are at the level of a line from the lower border of the pubic symphysis to the sacral tip. These relationships do not change significantly during dilatation of the cervix and thinning of the lower uterine segment.

Late in labor, as the fetal head descends into the pelvis, the bladder base is rolled upwards in front of the presenting part. The bladder base comes to be in a line with the urethra as they move towards the upper border of the pubic symphysis. In normal instances there does not seem to be significant upward motion of the bladder neck or lengthening of the urethra. However, there are substantial variations from one patient and one birth to another. Specifically when the pelvis is relatively small

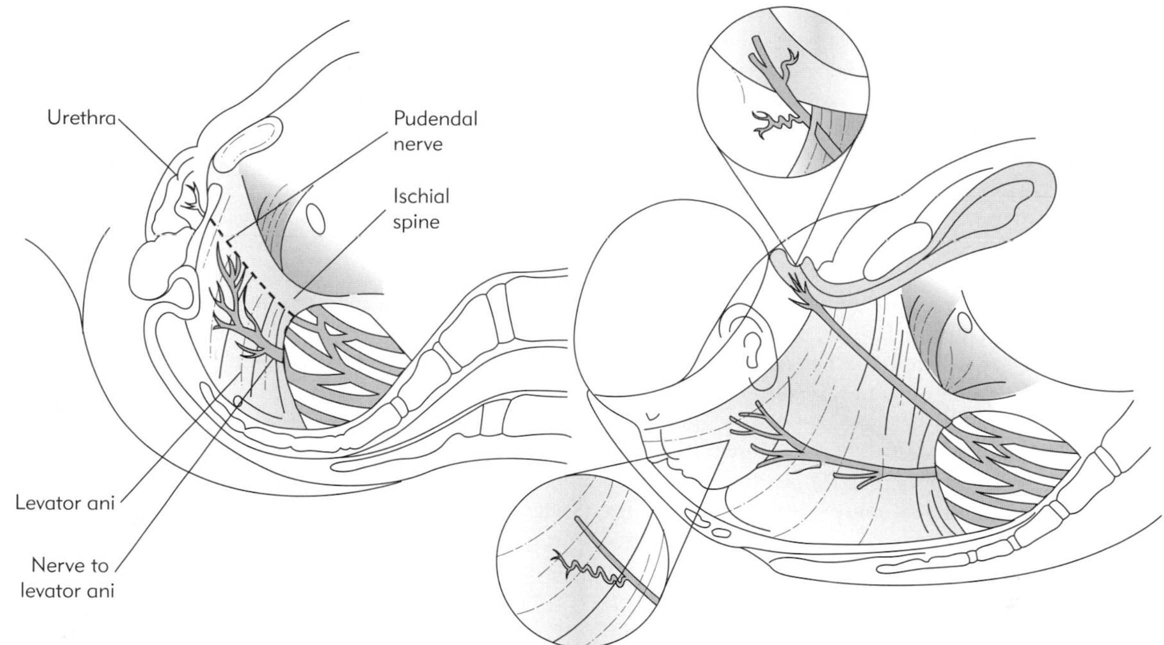

Figure 2.17 Perineal structures, nerves, and vaginal birth. The left panel shows the anatomy of the nerve to the levator ani muscle and pudendal nerve relative to the levator ani muscles as they are prior to vaginal delivery. The right side reveals the situation at the time of vaginal delivery. Note the significant downward descent of the pelvic floor muscles that may stretch or potentially disrupt fibers of these muscles' nerve supply. Copyright DeLancey 1999.

and there is mid-pelvic arrest of the presenting part, the bladder may lift very high to the upper level of the pubic symphysis and the urethra may be lengthened. The specific point at which injury to the urethra or to its supports occurs, however, could not be clarified by these studies.

MECHANISM OF INJURY

How is the pelvic floor damaged as the fetal head passes through it? The commonly held idea that vaginal wall stretching is one of the primary sources of damage is illogical. The uterine cervix starts labor at 1 cm of dilatation (3.1 cm circumference) and stretches to 10 cm of dilatation (31 cm circumference) at the time of delivery; a 10-fold increase in connective tissue length. The cervix, as early as 6 weeks after delivery, has reformed its normal size and consistency. The vagina undergoes much less stretching than the uterine cervix because it begins at 5 cm of dilatation (15.5 cm circumference) and must only go to 10 cm (31 cm); a 2-fold increase in connective tissue length. This is five times less stretching than the cervix undergoes. If the vagina stretches, it should be expected to return to normal.

It has often been assumed that the cardinal and uterosacral ligaments are ruptured because of presumed downward traction on these structures during labor. On closer examination, however, this idea is implausible. The cervix starts at the level of the ischial spines at the beginning of labor and stays at that level throughout labor and delivery. During the process of cervical dilatation, the cervix comes ever closer to the pelvic sidewalls. Because the cardinal and uterosacral ligaments attach the cervix to the pelvic sidewall, the narrowing distance between the cervix and the pelvic side wall must relieve the strain on these structures during labor rather than putting increased stress on them.

What are the normal changes that occur in the pelvic floor as the fetal head passes through the vagina and what injuries might occur during this process? There is little to suggest that damage to the pelvic floor would occur until the head actually engages the pelvic floor. Compression on the pelvic sidewall can cause nerve injury in this area known as maternal obstetrical paralysis, but this is extremely rare. It did occur in the past with very long labors, but is virtually never seen in contemporary obstetrical practice. The structures of the pelvic floor are subjected to force once the head descends below +1 station and encounters the actual structures of the pelvic floor. At this point the fetal head pushes the pelvic floor downwards as it tries to dilate the relatively narrow opening in the vagina. During this process the structures surrounding the vagina are pushed downwards. This would be expected to increase the length of both the nerves to the levator ani muscle as well as the pudendal nerve (Fig. 2.17). The more narrow and rigid the vaginal orifice, the more downward force is needed in order to accomplish dilatation. This, therefore, would lead to greater degrees of descent and potentially more nerve injury. Furthermore, the pressures within the pelvis that occur between the fetal head and the pelvic sidewall could possibly cause compression injury to the pudendal nerve. At the present time, whether nerve disruption or nerve compression is the mechanism of well studied pudendal nerve dysfunction is not known.

How could episiotomy prevent damage? Incising the narrow introital structures opens the diameter of the pelvic outlet by twice the length of the incision. Once this is done, the relaxed opening requires less force to accomplish delivery so that less force is applied to the muscles and fascial tissues. Surgical repair of the incised tissues can then be carried out to restore their continuity. Midline episiotomy as practiced in the United States, however, carries a significant increased likelihood of causing a 3rd or 4th degree laceration, and so the use of this intervention must be balanced against the risk of increased sphincter damage. Mediolateral episiotomy, although avoiding the increase in 3rd and 4th degree laceration rate, does carry significant morbidity for the mother in terms of pain and potential infection. At the present time, long-term information about the use of episiotomy is not available. Current studies that have claimed to disprove utility of episiotomy have only followed patients for a few months and clearly this is not long enough to assess the effectiveness in preventing a condition that usually becomes most clinically manifest 20–30 years after delivery. In addition, an episiotomy may be performed too late after damage has already happened and therefore assessment not only of the use of episiotomy but also of the timing of episiotomy would be appropriate. At the present time, data from randomized trials do not, however, suggest any substantial protection against stress incontinence with commonly used episiotomy practice. Older studies[45–47] have shown that use of episiotomy as a part of a more global attempt to prevent pelvic floor damage have proven effective in lessening pelvic floor damage.

STUDIES OF PELVIC FLOOR DAMAGE

Several studies have been carried out which reveal changes to the pelvic floor after vaginal delivery. Women after vaginal delivery have a lower perineum than nulliparous women or women delivered by cesarean section and also have longer pudendal nerve terminal motor latencies.[48] In addition, changes in the motor units of women studied before and after birth reveal evidence of damage.[49] Furthermore, the strength of the levator ani muscle is less following vaginal delivery,[50] but does show significant recovery in the late puerperium. At the present time most of the studies carried out in this area have emphasized evaluations at 2 months afterwards, but it must be recognized that this has not allowed the full recovery of pelvic floor to finalize before it has been investigated. The importance of prolonged follow-up was demonstrated by Sampselle's study where full pelvic floor function was not restored until approximately 6 months to a year after delivery. This time course would be consistent with the rate of nerve re-growth given the length of the pudendal nerve and nerve to the levator ani muscle. After this recovery, there can be further deterioration of the pelvic floor[51] and the eventual outcome may not be known for several years.

Actual muscle disruption also occurs at the time of vaginal birth. DeLee[52] discussed this in his textbook on obstetrics. Levator muscle injuries have been seen using magnetic MRI scans in symptomatic multiparous women.[53] Histological changes of muscle damage have also been shown in this area[54,55] and are related to failed surgery.[56] This area needs more research, as it is likely to reveal direct information about the injuries associated with urinary incontinence and pelvic organ prolapse.

There is further information concerning vaginal birth in the posterior compartment that will be covered in sections of this book related to that area.

REFERENCES

1. Olsen AL, Smith VJ, Bergstrom JO, Colling JC, Clark AL. Epidemiology of surgically managed pelvic organ prolapse and urinary incontinence. *Obstet Gynecol* 1997;**89**:501–6.
2. Ricci JV, Thom CH. The myth of a surgically useful fascia in vaginal plastic reconstructions. *Quart R Surg Obstet Gynecol* 1954;2:261–3.
3. Uhlenhuth E, Nolley GW. Vaginal fascia a myth? *Obstet Gynecol* 1957;**10**:349–58.
4. DeLancey JOL. Anatomic aspects of vaginal eversion after hysterectomy. *Am J Obstet Gynecol* 1992;**166**:1717–28.
5. Range RL, Woodburne RT. The gross and microscopic anatomy of the transverse cervical ligaments. *Am J Obstet Gynecol* 1964;**90**:460–67.
6. Campbell RM. The anatomy and histology of the sacrouterine ligaments. *Am J Obstet Gynecol* 1950;**59**:1–12.
7. Bartscht KD, DeLancey JOL. A technique to study cervical descent. *Obstet Gynecol* 1988;**72**:940–43.
8. Dickinson, RL. Studies of the levator ani muscle. *Am J Dis Women* 1889;**22**:897–917.
9. Lawson JON. Pelvic anatomy. I. Pelvic floor muscles sphincters. *Ann Roy Coll Surg* 1974;**54**:244–52.
10. Lawson JON. Pelvic anatomy. II. Anal canal and associated sphincters. *Ann Roy Coll Surg* 1974;**54**:288–300.
11. Parks AG, Porter NH, Melzak J. Experimental study of the reflex mechanism controlling muscles of the pelvic floor. *Dis Colon Rect* 1962;5:407–414.

12. Berglas B, Rubin IC. Study of the supportive structures of the uterus by levator myography. *Surg Gynecol Obstet* 1953;**97**:677–92.
13. Nichols DH, Milley PS, Randall CI. Significance of restoration of normal vaginal depth and axis. *Obstet Gynecol* 1970;**36**:251–6.
14. Paramore RH. The uterus as a floating organ. In: *The statics of the female pelvic viscera*, London: HK Lewis, 1918: Chapter 2, 12–15.
15. Oelrich TM. The striated urogenital sphincter muscle in the female. *Anat Rec* 1983;**205**:223–32.
16. Hilton P, Stanton SL. Urethral pressure measurement by microtransducer: The results in symptom-free women and in those with genuine stress incontinence. *Br J Obstet Gynaecol* 1983;**90**:919–33.
17. Constantinou CE. Resting and stress urethral pressures as a clinical guide to the mechanism of continence in the female patient. *Urol Clin North Am* 1985;**12**:247–58.
18. DeLancey JOL. Structural aspects of the extrinsic continence mechanism. *Obstet Gynecol* 1988;**72**:296–301.
19. Hodgkinson CP. Relationships of the female urethra in urinary incontinence. *Am J Obstet Gynecol* 1953;**65**:560–73.
20. Muellner SR. Physiology of micturition. *J Urol* 1951;**65**:805–810.
21. Westby M, Asmussen M, Ulmsten U. Location of maximum intraurethral pressure related to urogenital diaphragm in the female subject as studied by simultaneous urethrocystometry and voiding urethrocystography. *Am J Obstet Gynecol* 1982;**144**:408–412.
22. Noll LE, Hutch JA. The SCIPP line – an aid in interpreting the voiding lateral cystourethrogram. *Obstet Gynecol* 1969;**33**:680–89.
23. Jeffcoate TNA, Roberts H. Observations on stress incontinence of urine. *Am J Obstet Gynecol* 1952;**64**:721–38.
24. DeLancey JOL. Structural support of the urethra as it relates to stress urinary incontinence: the hammock hypothesis. *Am J Obstet Gynecol* 1994;**170**:1713–20.
25. Richardson AC, Edmonds PB, Williams NL. Treatment of stress urinary incontinence due to paravaginal fascial defect. *Obstet Gynecol* 1981;**57**:357–62.
26. Gil Vernet S. *Morphology and function of the vesico-prostato-urethral musculature*. Italy: Edizioni Canova Treviso, 1968.
27. Woodburne RT. Anatomy of the bladder and bladder outlet. *J Urol* 1968;**100**:474–87.
28. DeLancey JOL. Pubovesical ligament: A separate structure from the urethral supports (pubo-urethral ligaments). *Neurourol Urodynam* 1989;**8**:53–62.
29. Wilson PD, Dixon JS, Brown ADG, Gosling JA. Posterior pubo-urethral ligaments in normal and genuine stress incontinent women. *J Urol* 1983;**130**:802–805.
30. Power RMH. An anatomical contribution to the problem of continence and incontinence in the female. *Am J Obstet Gynecol* 1954;**67**:302–314.
31. Woodburne RT. The ureter ureterovesical junction and vesical trigone. *Anat Rec* 1965;**151**:243–9.
32. Huisman AB. Aspects on the anatomy of the female urethra with special relation to urinary continence. *Contrib Gynecol Obstet* 1983;**10**:1–31.
33. DeLancey JOL. Correlative study of paraurethral anatomy. *Obstet Gynecol* 1986;**68**:91–7.
34. Gosling JA, Dixon JS, Critchley HOD, Thompson SA. A comparative study of the human external sphincter and periurethral levator ani muscles. *Br J Urol* 1981;**53**:35–41.
35. Rud T, Anderson KE, Asmussen M, Hunting A, Ulmsten U. Factors maintaining the intraurethral pressure in women. *Invest Urol* 1980;**17**:343–7.
36. Droes, JThPM. Observations on the musculature of the urinary bladder and urethra in the human foetus. *Br J Urol* 1974;**46**:179–85.
37. Berkow SG. The corpus spongiosum of the urethra: its possible role in urinary control and stress incontinence in women. *Am J Obstet Gynecol* 1953;**65**:346–51.
38. Huffman J. Detailed anatomy of the paraurethral ducts in the adult human female. *Am J Obstet Gynecol* 1948;**55**:86–101.
39. McGuire EJ. The innervation and function of the lower urinary tract. *J Neurosurg* 1986;**65**:278–85.
40. McGuire EJ. Urodynamic findings in patients after failure of stress incontinence operations. *Prog Clin Bio Res* 1981;**78**:351–60.
41. Foldspang A, Mommsen S, Lam GW, Elving L. Parity as a correlate of adult female urinary incontinence prevalence. *J Epidemiol Commun Health* 1992;**46**:595–600.
42. Timonen S, Nuoranne E, Meyer B. Genital prolapse: etiological factors. *Ann Chir Gynecol Fenn* 1968;**57**:363–70.
43. DeLancey JOL. Structural anatomy of the posterior compartment as it relates to rectocele. *Am J Obstet Gynecol* 1999;**180**:815–23.
44. Malpas P, Jeffcoate TNA, Lister UM. The displacement of the bladder and urethra during labor. *J Obstet Gynaecol Br Empire* 1949;**56**:949–59.
45. Gainey HL. Postpartum observation of pelvic tissue damage. *Am J Obstet Gynecol* 1943;**45**:457–66.
46. Gainey HL. Postpartum observation of pelvic tissue damage: further studies. *Am J Obstet Gynecol* 1955;**70**:800–7.
47. Ranney B. Decreasing numbers of patients for vaginal hysterectomy and plasty. *S D J Med* 1990;**43**:7–12.
48. Snooks SJ, Swash M, Setchell M, Henry MM. Injury to innervation of pelvic floor sphincter musculature in childbirth. *Lancet* 1984;ii:546–50.
49. Allen RE, Hosker GL, Smith ARB, Warrell DW. Pelvic floor damage and childbirth: a neurophysiological study. *Br J Obstet Gynaecol* 1990;**97**:770–9.
50. Sampselle CM, Miller JM, Mims BL, DeLancey JO, Ashton-Miller JA, Antonakos CL. Effect of pelvic muscle exercise on transient incontinence during pregnancy and after birth. *Obstet Gynecol* 1998;**91**:406–12.
51. Snooks SJ, Swash M, Mathers SE, Henry MM. Effect of vaginal delivery on the pelvic floor: a 5-year follow-up. *Br J Surg* 1990;**77**:1358–60.
52. DeLee JB. The principles and practice of obstetrics. In: *The accidents of labor: injuries to he parturient canal*, 7th edn. Philadelphia: WB Saunders, 1938: Chapter 57, 818–64.
53. Kirschner-Hermanns R, Wein B, Niehaus S, Schaefer W, Jakse G. The contribution of magnetic resonance imaging of the pelvic floor to the understanding of urinary incontinence. *Br J Urol* 1993;**72**:715–8.

54. Koelbl H, Strassegger H, Riss PA, Gruber H. Morphologic and functional aspects of pelvic floor muscles in patients with pelvic relaxation and genuine stress incontinence. *Obstet Gynecol* 1989;**74**:789–95.
55. Dimpfl T, Jaegar C, Mueller-Felber, *et al.* Myogenic changes of the levator ani muscle in premenopausal women: The impact of vaginal delivery and age. *Neurourol Urodynam* 1998;**17**:197–206.
56. Hanzal E, Berger E, Koelbl H. Levator ani muscle morphology and recurrent genuine stress incontinence. *Obstet Gynecol* 1993;**81**:426–9.

Chapter 3

Urinary storage and voiding

Edwin P Arnold

INTRODUCTION

The lower urinary tract functions to store the urine continuously presented to it via the ureters from the kidneys, and at an appropriate time and place, to empty itself completely via the urethra. This chapter will discuss the storage and voiding function of the bladder, and the symptoms and clinical associations of dysfunctions which can occur. The International Continence Society has produced recommendations concerning standardization of terminology and tests used in assessing lower urinary tract function.[1]

ANATOMICAL CONSIDERATIONS

BLADDER

The bladder is a hollow viscus sited in the pelvis and supported by the pelvic floor and associated endo-pelvic fascia and pubo-urethral ligaments, and indirectly by ligaments supporting the uterus, or the prostate. The role of these ligaments has been questioned by Gosling (1996).[2] The bladder is lined by a specialized transitional cell epithelium. The dome has a smooth muscle coat with no distinct layering and this forms a meshwork over the surface of the bladder. The muscle cells apparently slide over each other with passive or active changes in bladder volume. It has a dome, and a bladder base or trigone, and a bladder neck with a structure differing in males and females.

TRIGONE AND URETEROVESICAL SPHINCTER

At its junction with the bladder, the outer longitudinal coat of the ureter splits to allow for the ureteric meatus in the bladder. The medial fibers decussate with those of the opposite side to produce the superficial trigonal muscle and proximally produce the inter-ureteric ridge. The fibers fan out over the trigone and continue on down the urethra. Contraction of this trigonal muscle flattens the ureteric meatus after each wave of ureteric peristalsis passes and prevents reflux of urine into the ureters. The oblique passage of the ureter through the muscle wall of the bladder produces a shutter effect, also helping to prevent vesico-ureteric reflux, when the bladder pressure rises during voiding.

BLADDER NECK

In the male there is a physiological sphincter of circular smooth muscle at the bladder neck under sympathetic adrenergic control. It functions as a genital sphincter at the time of ejaculation, and closes to prevent retrograde ejaculation of semen into the bladder, and to direct distally the seminal fluid emitted into the posterior urethra. It also serves as a urinary sphincter mechanism during storage and remains shut throughout. During a prostatectomy the bladder neck is rendered incompetent and postoperatively there is a risk of retrograde ejaculation or reduced volume of semen about which the patient must be warned preoperatively.[3] A simple bladder neck incision or transurethral incision of the prostate has a lower incidence of retrograde ejaculation than a prostatectomy. If the distal urethral sphincter is compromised as after a fractured pelvis and urethral disruption, continence can be maintained by the bladder neck sphincter. If a patient with a history of previous ruptured urethra and damage to the external sphincter subsequently develops bladder outlet obstruction and requires a prostatectomy, caution is required at the time of surgery to avoid stress incontinence.

In the female there is no anatomical ring of muscle at the bladder neck, and urethral pressure profiles show no significant rise in pressures at the bladder neck level. The bladder neck is closed in around 75% of continent young nulliparous women.[4] The remaining 25% of young women with an open bladder neck were not incontinent, so that by assumption continence in them would depend solely on the efficiency of the distal urethral sphincter mechanism. The bladder neck is open in 50% of perimenopausal continent women.[5]

Division of the hypogastric plexus and the sympathetic supply to the seminal vesicles and bladder neck in the male is sometimes unavoidable during a retroperitoneal lymph node dissection as is carried out for the management of metastatic testis tumors, and this results in paralysed ejaculation and an incompetent bladder neck. Incontinence of urine does not occur, because the distal mechanism remains intact.

Prior to the development of the contraceptive pill, women with severe dysmenorrhoea were sometimes treated by presacral neurectomy to destroy afferent pain pathways. While paralysing the sympathetic supply to the urethra, this apparently did not result in urinary incontinence. Neurohistochemical staining shows sparse adrenergic endings in the female bladder neck and urethra.

URETHRA

Smooth muscle

Most of the urethral smooth muscle is longitudinally disposed[6] and contraction of it should cause urethral shortening and hence widening. It would seem therefore to have a role during voiding rather than contributing to continence. There is a thin, unimpressive layer of circular smooth muscle outside the longitudinal layer, which may contribute to urethral closure.

Striated external urethral sphincter and pelvic floor

As the bladder fills, tension in its wall rises, and this is signaled to the cord via A delta afferents. The result is progressive increase in electromyographic (EMG) activity in the external urethral sphincter during filling, so that urethral closure pressure progressively increases. When the desire to void becomes urgent, voluntary contractions of the external sphincter assist the maintenance of continence by increasing urethral closure pressure, and by lowering detrusor pressure by reflex inhibition of the detrusor via the pontine micturition center.

Female

The female external urethral sphincter is a signet ring-shaped striated muscle incorporated into the wall of the urethra outside the smooth muscle layer. The bulk of it is anterior and it is relatively thin posteriorly where it is adjacent to the anterior vaginal wall. It is a postural muscle with predominantly small diameter slow twitch fibers capable of maintaining a sustained contraction and contributing to the urethral closure pressure. It is supplied by the pudendal nerve. Voluntary interruption of the voiding stream can be achieved by contraction of the striated external urethral sphincter and pelvic floor.

The urethra, vagina and rectum all pass between the medial edges of the levator ani pelvic floor diaphragm. The medial fibers of puborectalis have a dominance of slow twitch fibers also, whereas the remainder of the levator ani has mainly fast twitch fibers, as do most voluntary muscles in the body. The pelvic floor and its ligamentous supports have been described in Chapter 2.

According to Gosling (1996),[2] the medial fibers of levator ani attach to the lateral wall of the vagina and so contraction moves the lateral vaginal walls anteriorly and with them the anterior vaginal wall and the urethra, so that the urethra becomes compressed against the posterior wall of the pubis. These features are becoming clearer through magnetic resonance imaging.[7,8]

Male

In the male the external striated urethral sphincter is pear-shaped, its apex reaching the apex of the prostate while its base extends inferiorly to the membranous urethra. As in the female, it can be used to voluntarily interrupt the voiding stream. After prostatectomy it is the only sphincter mechanism remaining, as the bladder neck will have been ablated. It may be damaged at the time of a TUR of the prostate or at open prostatectomy, and it may then cause stress incontinence. It is at greater risk of surgical compromise during a radical prostatectomy for prostate cancer, but can also be damaged by radical radiotherapy. The external urethra and its sphincter can be disrupted with a fractured pelvis.

Inner urethral wall softness

Within the muscular tube of the urethra there is a mucosa with epithelium, blood vessels and connective tissue, all of which are under the influence of estrogens in women. In low estrogen states after the menopause, the epithelium becomes thinned and the mucosa less vascular, and the softness and bulk of these tissues are reduced. These features reduce urethral resistance and contribute to the rising incidence of sphincter incompetence and leakage with aging. Administering estrogens as hormone replacement therapy in postmenopausal women can increase vascularity and reduce the symptoms of burning, discomfort and urgency, but is not of value in the treatment of urinary incontinence.

Previous vaginal wall or pelvic surgery or radiotherapy can result in scarring and predispose to stress incontinence.

INNERVATION

The predominant neurotransmitter in the bladder is acetylcholine. Stimulation studies *in vitro* and histochemical staining shows that there are also a number of non-adrenergic non-cholinergic (NANC) neurotransmitters present. These include vaso-active intestinal peptide (VIP), calcitonin gene-related peptide (CGRP), Substance P (SP) and adenosine tri-phosphate (ATP). Colocalization is common and has been elegantly demonstrated by Smet *et al.* (1997).[9] They noted that some patients with detrusor instability demonstrate increases in a specific class of nerve fiber containing CGRP and SP. VIP nerves are probably efferent, whereas CGRP and CGRP/SP and neurokinin A (NKA) nerves are probably sensory.

Peripheral innervation

The peripheral nerve supply derives from three sources:

Parasympathetic nerve supply

Cell bodies of efferent fibers lie in the intermedio-lateral horn of the S2, S3 and S4 segments of the spinal cord but predominantly S3. Preganglionic fibers reach the pelvic plexus in front of the piriformis muscle and are joined there by postganglionic sympathetic fibers. Parasympathetic ganglion cells are situated on the bladder wall or intramurally. Postganglionic axons provide cholinergic excitatory inputs to the bladder smooth muscle. The intramural ganglion cells also receive input from sympathetic postganglionic fibres which allows for modulation of excitability. Sensation of bladder filling is mediated by afferents which travel via the pelvic nerve to the sacral dorsal root ganglia of the same segments.

Somatic sacral nerves

Efferents from S3 and some from S2 and S4 supply motor input to the urethral and anal sphincters and to the pelvic floor. Cell bodies for the urethral sphincter lie in the anterior horn (Onuf 's nucleus). The fibres travel in the pudendal nerves and also directly to the superior surface of the levator ani and supply that muscle.

Afferents mediating sensation from the urethra and pelvic floor travel via the pudendal nerve; their cell bodies lie in the dorsal root ganglia and central connections reach the dorsal horn of the spinal cord at the level of S2, S3 and S4.

Sympathetic supply

Cell bodies for the efferents lie in the T11–L2 segments of the cord. Preganglionic fibers synapse in prevertebral ganglia. The postganglionic adrenergic efferents travel via the superior to the inferior hypogastric plexus, and thence reach the bladder to modulate the excitatory status by inhibiting intramural ganglion cells. Other fibers provide excitatory input to smooth muscle at the bladder neck and urethra and to the seminal vesicle and prostatic glands.

Central connections

The dominant center for control of the bladder and pelvic floor lies in the rostral pons. It receives inputs from the pelvic floor and bladder. Descending fibers travel via bulbo-spinal tracts to the vesical efferent neurons and also to Onuf 's nucleus. The neural mechanisms are considered in detail in Chapter 8.

Pelvic reflexes

The structures of the pelvic floor share similar innervation and it is not surprising that bladder, genital and anorectal dysfunctions often coexist; dysfunction in one may influence another. Excitatory and inhibitory reflexes are observed frequently. For example:

- Bladder filling can cause increased rhythmic activity in a rectal pressure line at standard urodynamics.
- The manual evacuation of bowel contents in a spinal cord injury patient may initiate a bladder contraction.
- During a bladder contraction, squeeze of the glans penis, or voluntary contraction of the pelvic floor, can inhibit the detrusor.
- Reflex activity in the bladder can be suppressed by electrical stimulation of pelvic afferents using vaginal/anal electrodes, or by magnetic stimulation applied transcutaneously over the sacrum.[10]

STORAGE

FUNCTIONAL ASPECTS

The significance of the findings of urodynamic studies must always take into account the patient's presenting symptoms. Routine application of urodynamics to evaluate clinical problems with storage and voiding became established in the early 1970s. In addition to the exigencies imposed by the circumstances of a urodynamic study and the presence of catheters, there is also considerable intra-individual variation in both symptoms and measurements. The findings should be regarded as qualitative rather than quantitative.

During normal bladder filling the urine is stored at a low pressure, while the urethra is maintained in the closed position at rest and during any rises in intra-abdominal pressure due to movement, coughing or straining.

As the bladder is an intra-abdominal organ, a pressure sensor inside its lumen records the sum of abdominal pressure and the pressure produced by any detrusor contraction. By accepting the approximation that rectal pressure records reflect intra-abdominal pressure, subtraction of the rectal pressure (abdominal pressure) from total bladder pressure (intravesical pressure) gives an estimate of the pressure produced by the detrusor (intrinsic detrusor pressure).

Compliance

During filling the detrusor pressure may stay flat or in some patients it rises gradually to 10–15 cm of water pressure at maximal functional capacity (350–500 ml). The process is termed receptive relaxation or creep and is expressed as the volume during filling per unit pressure rise (mL/cm pressure rise). Compliance is influenced by the presence of non-contractile elements of elastin and collagen, and inter-cellular substances and cytoskeleton, as well as by myohypertrophy.

The reduced compliance seen in obstruction is mainly due to structural changes in the bladder wall with increased deposition of elastin and collagen secondary to the obstruction. In an experimental model of bladder outlet obstruction in guinea pigs, perfusion in calcium-free solution to abolish muscle contraction did not change the compliance.[11] The dose-response curve to atropine of muscle strips from patients with benign prostatic hyperplasia did not differ according to whether the compliance was normal or reduced.[12]

The significance of a cystometric finding of low compliance is not entirely clear. During filling studies it is often the first indication of the presence of detrusor instability on subsequent provocative testing, e.g. further filling or passive posture change. The increased bladder wall tension will increase afferent input to the spinal cord and increase the excitability of the reflex. Women with detrusor instability and no neurological disorder had a significantly lower compliance than those with stable bladders.[13]

Compliance is reduced in defunctioned states, e.g. after an indwelling catheter or urinary diversion, or if there is fibrosis in the wall as might occur postsurgery to the bladder, or after radiotherapy. It is also reduced if pelvic masses press on the bladder, e.g. in the case of pregnancy, ovarian tumors etc.

Because of the stiffness of the bladder wall, bladder wall tension will rise progressively resulting in increased frequency in amplitude of afferent responses signaled to the central nervous system, and this may be sufficient to fire off an involuntary contraction or to lower the threshold so that posture changes and rapid filling might then precipitate an involuntary contraction.

In an analysis of 170 men with lower urinary tract symptoms of moderate to severe grade according to the IPPS, and a flow rate of less than 15 ml per second, compliance decreased significantly with increasing age and reducing flow rate, with increasing voiding pressure, and with the presence of detrusor instability.[14]

An increased compliance and a large bladder capacity can be seen in some diabetic patients with autonomic neuropathy, and in cauda equina lesions where the voiding efficiency is lost in addition to the filling changes. Anticholinergic drugs like the tricyclic antidepressants can act in a similar fashion.

Filling sensations

During filling people with normal bladder function can often distinguish three types of sensation: a first sensation of filling, a first desire to void (FDV), and a strong desire to void (SDV).[15] Wyndaele noted that the first sensation of filling occurred at around 40% of SDV and the first desire to void at 60% of SDV. There was a small but significant increase in detrusor pressures observed from the volume at first sensation of filling, to that at first sensation to void and to the strong desire to void in that study.

Usually patients can distinguish between sensory and motor types of urgency. Sensory urgency refers to the SDV which if neglected is quite uncomfortable or even painful. At the extremes of life in young children and in the elderly or those with reduced mobility, urinary infections can give rise to sensory urge incontinence simply because it is too painful to hold on. Motor urgency refers to an SDV which if unheeded might risk urge incontinence. It is deemed 'motor' because at cystometry, the sensation of urgency usually is correlated with unstable detrusor contractions. In normal people motor urgency can occur occasionally without risking leakage, but it is an altogether different and more compelling sensation than is simply the strong desire to void. Long-term ambulatory monitoring in asymptomatic individuals has demonstrated detrusor instability in 38%.[16]

Mechanoreceptors on A delta fibres result in electrical activity in afferent fibers travelling via the pelvic nerve and this activity increases in amplitude and frequency with bladder filling. The sensation can be suppressed voluntarily until the bladder becomes uncomfortably full.

Bladder filling sensations are mediated mainly via pelvic nerve afferents while the sensation of SDV may be mediated via the pudendal nerve. There are A delta mechanoreceptors in parallel with detrusor muscle and these are activated by both active and passive stretch. Pain is mediated via unmyelinated C fibers. Bladder inflammation can result in local liberation of nerve growth factor (NGF) and substance P (SP) from macrophages and epithelial cells.[17] Retrograde axonal transport of NGF to dorsal horn neurons can result in 'windup' and central sensitivity as a cause for the chronic pelvic pain syndrome.

The sensation of urgency to void is poorly understood. The tension receptors are in parallel with the circumference of the bladder and are fired by passive stretch and active muscle contraction. Some have argued that the presence of urine in the posterior urethra when the bladder neck is open can cause urgency, but this concept was not confirmed by Sutherst and Brown (1978).[18] Prolapse of the bladder base is often associated with urgency which resolves after surgical correction of the prolapse.[19] In some patients urgency arises after surgery behind the bladder neck as in a pubovaginal sling.[20]

Urgency might arise whenever local changes in tension in the bladder wall occur as it would with any deformity of the bladder outline, or with rhythmic contractions or with the 'fibrillation' type contraction described as micromotion by Coolsaet *et al.* (1993).[21] Such micromotions would not necessarily raise the bladder pressure, but could alter local wall tension and potentially cause urgency.

Detrusor overactivity

The overactive bladder (OAB) is a term used to describe the symptoms of frequency, urgency and urge incontinence. It is not a urodynamic diagnosis. The International Continence Society (ICS) has defined the overactive bladder as one which exhibits the cystometric occurrence of involuntary contractions during filling or provoked by coughing or posture change and which the patient is unable to inhibit. Where a neurological cause has been demonstrated, this is termed *detrusor hyperreflexia*. In the absence of any known or detectable neurological disorder, it is termed *detrusor instability*.

During filling the bladder may be *normal* or *stable*, or *overactive*:

- Normal
- Overactive
  - Detrusor hyperreflexia (if known neuropathy)
  - Detrusor instability (if no neuropathy)
  - Associated with:
    Bladder outlet obstruction
    Urinary tract infections in the very young, and the frail and elderly
    Idiopathic as in many women with urinary incontinence.

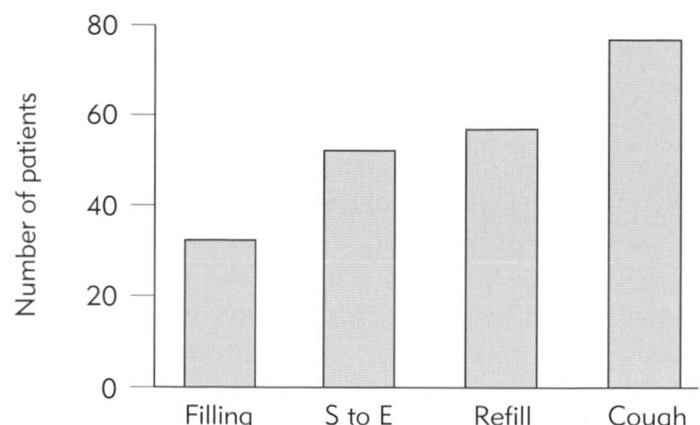

Figure 3.1 Detection of detrusor instability in 77 wet women during a series of provocative tests: rapid filling, passive posture change from supine (S) to erect (E), coughing, and refilling in the erect posture. (Arnold 1974.)

Provocation of detrusor overactivity

FILLING RATE

The bladder fills physiologically at a rate of 1–2 ml per minute and up to 5–10 ml per minute depending on fluid intake and other factors. To fill the bladder at any higher rate is unphysiological, but undertaking long-term ambulatory monitoring tests (LTAM) is beyond the logistic capabilities of most cystometry units, except for research purposes.

In non-neurological patients some cystometry units use ultra-rapid filling (150 ml per minute or more), and the incidence of instability is in fact lower than on LTAM where physiological rates apply, rather than the reverse. On the other hand, in neurological patients especially those with spinal cord injury, the bladder is sensitive to rapid fill and most cystometry units keep the filling rate to 10–20 ml per minute in order to more closely approximate the normal circumstances.

TEMPERATURE OF INFUSED FLUID

The iced water test stimulates capsaicin-sensitive C fiber afferents and can trigger a micturition reflex. Cystometry using iced water has been used to provoke a flaccid neurological bladder to determine if spinal reflex activity has returned after a period of spinal shock. It is usually negative in neurologically normal controls, but it is positive in only 56% of patients with suprasacral spinal cord lesions.[22] It has been shown positive in 12 of 17 (71%) of non-neurogenic males with bladder outlet obstruction, compared with three of 44 non-obstructed individuals. These authors suggest this is due to plasticity of bladder afferents in outlet obstruction and a role for nerve growth factor as a mediator has been suggested.[23]

POSTURE AND VESICOVASCULAR REFLEXES

The normal stable bladder is not provoked to contract by changing posture. However, it can be seen (Fig. 3.1) that the incidence of detrusor instability can be expanded by incorporating various provocative tests.[24] In many women with urinary incontinence, the urgency and urge incontinence is precipitated by the act of standing from a seated or lying position.

The reason for this common effect of posture change is conjectural, but might imply a mass discharge of sympathetic activity in the cord, needed to counter the effects of gravity on lowering the blood pressure. This activity could spread and render hypersensitive the micturition center, in the reverse fashion to that occurring in spinal cord injury patients with autonomic dysreflexia (Fig. 3.4).

The increased incidence of detrusor instability on LTAM might be explained by postural influences during normal daytime activities, or detrusor reflex excitability.

Pathogenesis of detrusor instability

There is discussion about the cause of these waves of unstable bladder contraction. It may lie in increased sensitivity of the micturition reflex induced by rhythmic contractions, or micromotion of muscle cells in the bladder wall and firing of their associated afferents,[21] or it may arise within the central or peripheral nervous system. Perhaps the cause is both myogenic and neurogenic.[25,26,27]

Rhythmic contractions occur in isolated muscle strips and are of increased frequency and amplitude in obstructed bladders, in those from patients with neurological lesions, and in animal studies of obstruction.[28] There was also post-junctional sensitivity to agonists (acetylcholine) in both groups and an increase in atropine resistance on electrical stimulation. Electron microscopy studies show partial denervation and some axonal degeneration.[29] The cause of the denervation seen in obstruction has been debated. One theory is that higher bladder pressures result in mucosal and muscle ischemia, and this causes axonal denervation over time. The ischemia might also be responsible for causing the overactive bladder with aging.

For rhythmic contractions to produce a pressure rise, this would have to involve an afferent nerve-mediated reflex response acting at pelvic plexus or cord level and increased reflex excitability, and a coordinated detrusor contraction. An alternative explanation is to invoke a rapid spread of excitation throughout the bladder from muscle cell to muscle cell. This could be mediated by spread of depolarization currents from cell to cell across points of close contact. Some support for the latter comes from experimental studies in the pig with post-obstructed instability, in which tetrodotoxin administered to paralyse nerve conduction did not abolish rhythmic contractions; nor did division of all the sacral nerve roots.[30,25]

The neurogenic theory of the cause of detrusor instability invokes the central nervous system in initiating and/or coordinating the uninhibited detrusor contraction. Bates (1974)[31] showed that anesthetic instillations into the bladder of patients with detrusor instability could abolish contractions, as could also a caudal anesthetic. The main central control area of the brain for continence and voiding is in the rostral pons where a lateral center controls continence, and voiding is controlled by a medial center. Experimental work has been confirmed in the human by PET scanning,[32] indicating the 'on–off' switch of the micturition reflex sited in the pons. The reflex is modulated and inhibited by higher center control. Uninhibited detrusor contractions can arise in lesions involving higher centers where inhibition is lost, and in these cases there is coordination of bladder contraction with urethral relaxation. In lesions of the spinal cord, however, when the bladder contracts there is often intermittent spasm of the striated muscle of the urethra (detrusor-sphincter dyssynergia).

Many have considered that the presence of detrusor instability is a qualitative observation, the height of the contraction having no direct bearing on the severity of the symptoms. Others have attempted to quantify it by defining a detrusor activity index.[33] More work needs to be done to evaluate these findings.

The incidence of detrusor instability is quite variable on conventional cystometry. Long-term ambulatory monitoring of detrusor activity is a more sensitive method of diagnosing detrusor instability.[34]

There is a rising incidence of detrusor instability with aging in both men and women.[35] Dyssynergic bladder neck obstruction occurs at a younger age than prostatic obstruction but there is a wide span of ages affected, and a rising incidence of detrusor instability with increasing age (Fig. 3.2).[36]

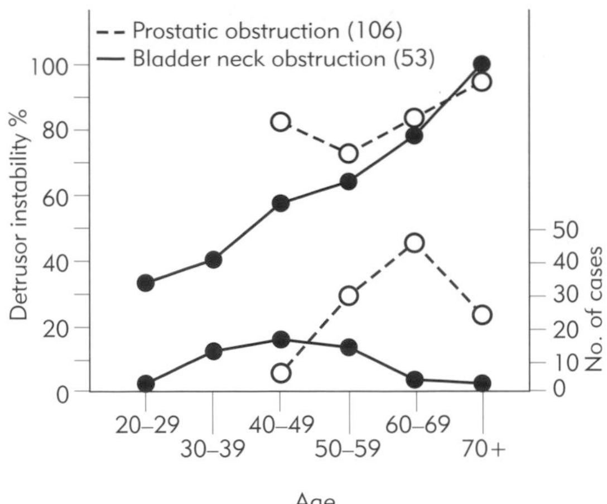

Figure 3.2 Rising incidence of detrusor instability in men with bladder outlet obstruction at bladder neck, or due to prostatic enlargement. (Arnold 1980.)

There is an increased incidence of detrusor instability (78%) in the face of increased bladder pressures during voiding in men with bladder outlet obstruction.[36] This resolves in about a third of cases after relief of obstruction, but persists in the remainder either as phasic detrusor contractions, or as a reduced compliance. Obstruction is a variable independent of age causing detrusor instability. Experimental work shows that rats with obstruction develop detrusor instability as a response.[25] Relief of obstruction after prostatectomy returns cystometry to stable in approximately a third of cases.[36] Detrusor instability which persists might be due to the aging process.

Mucosal permeability

It has been a generally held view that the transitional cell lining of the urinary tract is relatively urine-proof and impermeable. The relative impermeability has been ascribed to the presence of an intact glycosaminoglycan (GAG) layer on the surface of the epithelium. When this is lost as in patients with interstitial cystitis and chronic inflammation and tumors, the mucosa can become more permeable to ions and substances in the urine, including potassium. The urinary concentration of potassium is approximately 10 times that of serum, and if the GAG layer is lost, potassium can diffuse across the mucosa and depolarize smooth muscle cells leading to urgency and/or detrusor contractions.[37,38]

Ultrastructural changes in human bladder epithelium in patients with urinary tract infections, bladder tumors and interstitial cystitis were studied by Eldrup *et al.* (1983)[39] and they showed solute transport through the urothelium, ascribing this to leaky type junctions on electron microscopy studies.

It has been accepted that small molecules up to a certain size (probably less than 20 000 Daltons) may pass through the epithelium. This has been the basis of treating superficial bladder tumors with intravesical instillation of various anti-cancer drugs like doxorubicin hydrochloride and mitomycin C. Molecules like oxybutynin can also be absorbed across the bladder mucosa.

Iontophoresis, or electromotive induction has been used to encourage the transport of drugs from the bladder lumen across the epithelium. For success, such a drug must be water-soluble, electrically stable and ionized. The technique has been used to facilitate local anesthesia of the bladder and to enhance delivery of medication or chemotherapy for bladder tumors. The subject has been reviewed by Kohn and Kaplan (1998).[40]

Urethra and pelvic floor during bladder filling

The striated external urethral sphincter is capable of maintenance of urethral closure as it is composed largely of postural type muscle with slow twitch characteristics. As the bladder fills urethral closure pressure increases secondary to the increased firing of efferents down the pudendal nerve. This effect is triggered by increased afferent discharge from the bladder leading to stimulation of Onuf 's nucleus in the sacral cord, and reflex activation of the urethral sphincter.

Coughing and straining result in transiently increased intra-abdominal pressure, and because the bladder and proximal urethra are both intra-abdominal, there is transmission of the cough induced abdominal pressure to the urethra. Because the rise in urethral pressure precedes by about 250 milliseconds the increase in abdominal pressure, and may exceed it,[41] the pressure 'transmission' is at least in part, active.

In men in whom a spinal cord injury has occurred above T10, the bladder neck is shut until the bladder contracts reflexly. Where the lesion is between T10 and T12 and hence above the sacral center, but involving the sympathetic outflow to the bladder, it is sometimes open, presumably due to reduced sympathetic stimulation in the absence of a detrusor contraction (personal observation). Non-neurological patients who have had a sympathectomy during a retroperitoneal lymph node dissection for testis tumor management, provide a good model of the effect of sympathetic denervation on the urinary competence of the bladder neck sphincter mechanism. The genital sphincter function is paralysed, and there is failure of emission and ejaculation in such patients.

Men with cauda equina lesions may also have bladder neck incompetence for reasons which are not entirely clear, even when cystography is done early after the injury, before any effects of the paralysis of the striated muscles of the pelvic floor could result in descent and bulging of the perineum and opening of the bladder neck.

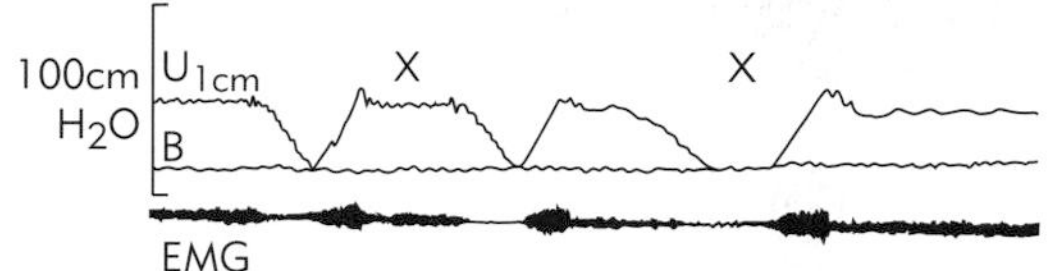

Figure 3.3 Urethral instability: spontaneous relaxation of urethral sphincter. Urethral pressures (U) drop together with silent EMG, in the presence of a normal stable bladder (B). (McGuire 1978, reproduced with permission.)

Urethral instability refers to spontaneous relaxations in urethral closure pressure in the absence of any associated detrusor contractions. It can result in wide opening of the proximal urethra and sudden leakage.[42] This phenomenon and its significance are poorly understood.

The urethral pressure falls:

- just prior to a detrusor contraction associated with voluntary voiding;
- just prior to an unstable bladder contraction;
- spontaneously in the absence of a detrusor contraction (urethral instability) .

STORAGE SYMPTOMS

Daytime frequency and nocturia

The time between voids varies both between and within individuals depending on a host of factors, including fluid intake. It seems reasonable to suggest that, for purposes of empirical definition, a person who can last up to 3 hours or more between voids, does *not* have significant frequency.

The bladder diary in which the patient records the time and volume voided and any leakage episode during a 3–5 day period, is an invaluable if underused demonstration of that person's bladder function, and can corroborate or otherwise the patient's history.

The causes of increased frequency of voiding are listed below:

Causes of frequency

1. *Increased urine production*
   (a) Excessive intake
   (b) Drugs
      - Caffeine
      - Alcohol
      - Diuretics
   (c) Osmotic diuresis – diabetes
   (d) Renal tubular failure
      - Postobstructive diuresis
   (e) Diabetes insipidus

2. *Bladder irritability*
   (a) Sensory
   - Urinary infection
   - Bladder tumors
   - Stones
   - Radiotherapy

   (b) Motor
   - Overactive detrusor dysfunction
     - Neuropathy, e.g. tethered cord
     - Detrusor instability
       Idiopathic
       Associated with bladder outlet obstruction
       Enuresis with diurnal urinary incontinence
3. *Anxiety, thyrotoxicosis*
4. *Cold weather.*

The ambient temperature has a significant influence on voiding frequency as is observed by most people.[43,44]

Causes of nocturia

This is defined as the number of times the desire to void wakens the patient during sleep. Nocturia is a more troublesome symptom than daytime frequency because it interferes with sleep. Apart from the causes of daytime frequency which also can produce nocturia, there are additional causes for nocturia, tabulated below:

1. Increased fluid reabsorption from limbs when recumbent
   - Congestive heart failure – overt or subclinical
   - Postural hypotension
     (seen frequently in spinal cord injury)
2. Poor sleep
3. Reduced tubular reabsorption of water
   - Osmotic effects, e.g. diabetes
   - Antidiuretic hormone (ADH): loss of diurnal rhythm.

Suprapubic pain and burning

Visceral pain from the bladder is often poorly localized in the suprapubic area. The dome of the bladder is sensitive to stretch, and/or spasm. An intravesical pressure of around 38 cm of water was found painful by most subjects[45] and this would be lower in those with urinary infections. Bladder spasms such as those which occur in some patients with indwelling catheters, are a most unpleasant symptom due to involuntary bladder contractions where the bladder is in effect trying to expel the residual urine and the catheter balloon.

Cautery of bladder tumors in the vault is not painful to all subjects but is to some, perhaps if the overlying peritoneum is also involved with the noxious stimulus.

Primary hyperalgesia can be felt suprapubically, or may be referred to the urethra/vagina/perineum in women, or to the testes, inguinal canal and perineum in men.[45] Painful stimuli arising in the pelvis, particularly repetitive ones like those recurring in endometriosis, can lead to 'windup' and central sensitization. Secondary hypersensitivity and allodynia can follow. Inflammation may lead to C fiber afferent stimulation which leads to progressive build-up in amplitude and duration, and up-regulation or dorsal horn neurons. Responses vary according to previous inputs, but increases for both visceral and somatic afferents.[45]

Nerve growth factor (NGF) may be a mediator in the 'windup' process. It is increased in the bladder epithelium in patients with sensory urgency, chronic inflammation and interstitial cystitis, but not in controls with genuine stress incontinence without urgency.[17] NGF is also present in muscle cells of the detrusor when obstructed.[46] Instillation of NGF into the bladder can upregulate dorsal horn neurons by retrograde axonal transport.

In addition to peripheral inflammation sensitizing the spinal cord, there is some evidence that pathology in the cord can cause peripheral inflammation. Pseudo-rabies virus (PRV) injected into the tail muscle of the rat causes inflammation in dorsal horn neurons from which PRV can be demonstrated, but also produces a flaccid bladder and hemorrhagic cystitis in which no PRV can be detected.[47]

Urinary incontinence

Enuresis

Patients with monosymptomatic persistent primary enuresis have a low incidence of detrusor instability (2 out of 11) on conventional cystometry, although clearly for the bladder to empty at night requires an involuntary contraction. Of those who had both nocturnal and diurnal enuresis, 36 of 37 had detrusor instability on conventional cystometry.[48] Those patients presenting in later life for assessment of incontinence, who had a past history of enuresis beyond the age of 7 but who had subsequently become dry, had a high incidence of detrusor instability (14 out of 16 men) or 87%, and 17 out of 26 women, or 65%. This suggests that those individuals who overcome the enuresis later than usual, might have a hyperexcitable micturition reflex, overt in early childhood and which can be inhibited in young adult life, but which can become unmasked later.[49]

Some children with monosymptomatic persistent primary enuresis have an abnormal rhythm of antidiuretic hormone (ADH) production, with loss of the normal reduced urine output at night. Such children can be helped by a prescription of ADH analogs such as DDAVP.

Secondary enuresis refers to bedwetting after an interval of greater than 6 months being dry. In children one needs to consider urinary tract infections, tethered cord syndrome and psycho-social factors in the etiology. In adults one should consider the possibility of chronic retention of urine with overflow, as can occur with bladder outlet obstruction, or the flaccid bladder of a cauda equina lesion.

Urinary incontinence later in life

This is a common problem, and increases in both sexes with increasing age. Continence depends on factors tending to cause leakage being outweighed by those factors producing and maintaining urethral closure.

GENUINE STRESS INCONTINENCE (GSI)

Stress incontinence is a symptom but also a sign and a diagnosis. The symptom refers to leakage of urine if associated with any increase in intra-abdominal pressure. This may be a sudden increase as in a cough, laugh or sneeze, or more prolonged as in lifting and bending. Leakage is linked directly with the abdominal pressure rises and ceases when this pressure ceases to operate, so it is often of a small volume at the time of the rise in pressure.

Some women complain of being 'always wet'. If a person wears protective underwear, it may be difficult to be certain always of the circumstances resulting in leakage, however in most cases women can differentiate between stress and urge incontinence.

For patients who are always wet both in bed and when up and about, one must suspect either gross sphincter incompetence, or a fistula bypassing the sphincter mechanisms, e.g. vesicovaginal, ureterovaginal, or urethrovaginal fistula – in which the bladder neck is already incompetent. If the bladder neck is competent, a urethrovaginal fistula would leak only during voiding and may not be suspected by the patient. An ectopic ureter opening into the urethra below the sphincter, or into the vagina, should be suspected in a child who has been wet continuously day and night.

Genuine stress incontinence refers to incompetence of the urethra causing demonstrable leakage due to rises in abdominal pressure, e.g. on coughing or straining, but in the absence of any detrusor instability detectable on cystometry. Despite the absence of any identifiable bladder neck sphincter muscle in women, the bladder neck is usually cough and strain competent, but cannot always be relied on even in nulliparous under 25-year-old women, many of whom do occasionally leak urine on significant cough, laugh, sneeze or trampolining etc.[50]

Following childbirth there is an increased incidence of urinary incontinence due to incompetence of the distal urethral sphincter. There is evidence that this is due, in part, to stretch damage to the nerve supply of the urethral (and anal) sphincters during vaginal delivery. See also Chapter 4.

Prolapse and GSI often coexist, and have as a common cause, weakness of the sphincter and pelvic floor as a result of nerve damage. The prolapse does not cause incontinence and indeed may mask it. When the pelvic diaphragm is stretched or denervated, the pelvic organs can prolapse into the vagina resulting in any of the following alone or in combinations. Anteriorly, there may be a urethrocele, or cystocele. From above uterine descent or vault prolapse after hysterectomy can occur, while posteriorly an enterocele containing small bowel can prolapse through the pouch of Douglas, or below this a rectocele can occur. The same factors causing weakness of the levators can cause weakness of the urethral and/or anal sphincters, and subsequent urinary or flatus/fecal incontinence.

If a cystocele is present, during coughing and straining this can obstruct the urethra so that leakage does not happen, but it may be masking an underlying sphincter weakness. This can be revealed if a surgical approach to repair the cystocele is undertaken without surgical focus on the incontinent urethra. In one study of 22 continent women with severe prolapse, an occult incontinence as above was found on urodynamic testing in 13 (60%).[51] Frequency, nocturia and urgency symptoms occurred in nine of 22 of these patients (41%). Repair of the prolapse in a selected group of patients was noted to improve frequency and urgency symptoms in 107 of 140 women (76.4%).[19]

When prolapse results in a rotational descent so that the urethra is below the pelvic diaphragm, it may be outside the influence of the pressure zone that enables closure to occur when abdominal pressure rises during coughing and straining.

URGE INCONTINENCE

Women with symptoms of urgency and urge incontinence, frequency and nocturia (OAB), but no stress incontinence, will most often be shown to have detrusor instability on standard cystometry. Those with mixed stress and urge incontinence and frequency and nocturia will show instability in about 30% of cases, while in those with symptoms of stress incontinence alone the incidence of instability is well under 10%.

The incidence of instability is higher when long-term ambulatory studies are conducted. In asymptomatic women 38% were shown to have detrusor instability.[16] In a group of incontinent women with genuine stress incontinence defined by standard cystometry, 43% had detrusor instability on long-term ambulatory monitoring.[52]

In many patients with mixed stress and urge incontinence, after operation the stress incontinence is cured but the urge incontinence persists. In several reports, the outcome of surgery for female urinary incontinence has been negatively prejudiced by the presence of detrusor instability detected preoperatively.[53] The same deleterious effect was noted in a recent study from Bristol comparing outcomes on the basis of detrusor instability detected at standard cystometry and that detected after long-term ambulatory monitoring (LTAM),[52] indicating that detrusor instability is a negative factor whichever way it is detected.

Detrusor instability may arise *de novo* postoperatively; however, some of those thought to have a stable bladder on standard cystometry preoperatively, might well have been shown to have detrusor instability if they had undergone LTAM preoperatively.

Dissection behind the bladder neck as occurs during a pubovaginal sling might damage the neural plexuses there, and be the reason for *de novo* detrusor instability which appears to have a higher incidence postoperatively than that which would occur after a Burch colposuspension.[53,20]

DETRUSOR HYPERREFLEXIA

Many neurological disorders can result in detrusor overactivity. In children spinal dysraphism is becoming less common, but tethered cord syndrome should be considered when a child develops secondary enuresis with or without lower limb symptoms, particularly in the 6 to 10-year-old age group as the spine elongates. In adult life the commonest causes are multiple sclerosis, Parkinson's disease, cerebrovascular accidents, and spinal cord injury.

Symptoms of urgency and urge incontinence, frequency and nocturia and a poor stream, and voiding only small amounts frequently, are often indistinguishable from those symptoms associated with prostatic obstruction. Full urodynamic investigation is needed in patients with neurological disorders to determine if outlet obstruction might be present, before considering any operative intervention. If obstruction is proven and uninhibited bladder contractions are demonstrated at preoperative cystometry, it remains reasonable to offer a prostatectomy but it is important to ensure the patient is aware that the urge incontinence might not improve. Detrusor hyperreflexia increases in incidence with age as does nocturia in both sexes (Figure 3.2). It is often associated with a bladder of impaired contractility (DHIC).[54]

Electron microscopic studies have shown the anatomical basis on which these factors of functional problems might occur. In neurological bladders there are often bizarre forms of hypertrophy of individual cells, axonal degeneration and increase in intercellular substances.[55]

Autonomic dysreflexia

This syndrome affects people with spinal cord injury, predominantly of the upper thoracic cord. Clinically, any

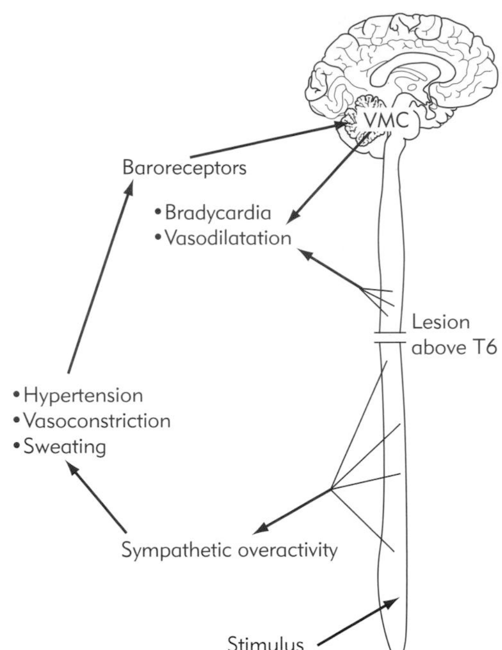

Figure 3.4 Pathogenesis of autonomic dysreflexia.

significant afferent input to the cord below the lesion, can result in a mass sympathetic efferent discharge. This vasoconstricts vessels in the skin and viscera and causes hypertension and headaches, which may be both alarming and dangerous. The hypertension is sensed by afferents in the aortic arch and carotid sinus which relay via the Vagus nerve to the vasomotor center. In turn this causes vasodilatation and sweating of skin above the lesion in the head and neck and slowing of the pulse. This can occur during cystometry, when the bladder is contracting spontaneously. The symptoms can be treated by sublingual nifedipine, or long-term by administering oral terazosine.[56]

VOIDING

At an appropriate time and place and when a person desires to pass urine, the first event is voluntary relaxation of the urethral sphincter and the pelvic floor. This is followed by the detrusor contraction, with opening of the bladder neck and urethra which also shortens. Voiding commences when the detrusor pressure exceeds the urethral closure pressure. Both detrusor contraction and urethral relaxation continue until the bladder is completely empty.

Anxiety and a failure of relaxation affects a proportion of males who find it difficult to void normally in a public urinal. This is common enough to fall within the spectrum of normal, and contributes to the delay in starting. The main delay arises while the activation of the micturition reflex is occurring and while the detrusor pressure is increasing, to reach urethral opening pressure.

Reflex inhibition of the urethral smooth muscle and striated muscle maintain urethral relaxation during voiding. The relative role of smooth and striated components is not fully understood. The urethral smooth muscle is predominantly longitudinal, so the contraction will lead to shortening and widening of the urethra, rather than assisting in its closure.

DETERMINANTS OF PRESSURE AND FLOW

Flow will occur when the detrusor pressure exceeds the opening pressure of the urethra. The flow rate is determined by the degree of excitation of the micturition reflex, bladder muscle contractility factors, and factors influencing the urethral resistance.

Neural mechanisms

Voiding is initiated voluntarily by relaxation of the external urethral sphincter and pelvic floor. Afferents fired by the relaxation of the pelvic floor feed back to the pontine micturition center and are a powerful drive to switch on the detrusor contraction by long-routed spino-bulbo-spinal reflexes. This reflex is enhanced by afferents in the urethra sensing urine flow, and the urethra remains relaxed and coordinated at the pontine level until emptying is complete.[57]

Voluntary interruption of the voiding stream can be achieved by voluntary contraction of the external urethral sphincter and pelvic floor. This causes an isometric detrusor pressure rise (clinical 'stop test'). It is followed by reflex inhibition of the detrusor, involving pelvic floor afferents.

Neurological causes for a slow flow and increased postvoid residual urine (PVR) include the autonomic neuropathy associated with diabetes, and cauda equina lesions, and drugs with anticholinergic properties, e.g. tricyclic antidepressants.

Patients with chronic retention may have an increased sensory threshold when tested by electrical stimulation of the dorsal nerve of the penis/clitoris, or of the bladder neck using a catheter-mounted electrode.[58]

Bladder muscle contractility factors

The bladder contraction is mediated by parasympathetic efferents which are predominantly cholinergic. A small proportion of the force developed is mediated by neither adrenergic nor cholinergic (NANC) neurotransmission. The proportion of NANC transmission increases in the presence of bladder outlet obstruction.

The force of bladder contraction is unchanged or less in patients with bladder outlet obstruction, while the velocity of contraction is slower.[59] The ultrastructural basis for this was found to be myohypertrophy, increase in intercellular substances, including elastin and collagen, and axonal degeneration. These changes can result in detrusor hyperreflexia and impaired contractility (DHIC) also noted in the aging process.[54]

Some drugs impair detrusor contractility, especially anticholinergics like oxybutynin, and tricyclic antidepressants.

Contractility will be reduced when voiding with only a small volume in the bladder because the rate of shortening of an arc on the circumference of the spherical bladder increases exponentially as the bladder volume falls.

Many studies have documented the observation patients have made that when voiding small amounts the flow is slower than if volumes of 150 ml or more are voided. In addition, voiding flow rates tend to be slower if volumes greater than 600 ml are voided. Attempts to normalize flows where less than 150 ml are voided have studied the rate of rise of the flow rate against time.[60]

Poor contractility has been invoked as the cause of low pressure non-obstruction (LPNOB) with a reduced flow rate but a non-elevated detrusor pressure. Some of these cases may be due to a less than complete excitation of the micturition reflex. Variability in reflex excitation leads to variable pressures and some difficulty in defining equivocal from obstructed cases.[61]

With aging some patients develop a combination of detrusor hyperreflexia and impaired contractility (DHIC) associated with urge incontinence together with voiding dysfunction, a slow flow rate and a postvoid residual.[54] The ultrastructural basis for this appears to be smooth muscle hyperplasia, and some areas of atrophy, axonal degeneration and increased deposition of elastin and collagen between muscle bundles.[55]

Changes in urethral resistance

The urethral response to a forced passive dilatation is a steep pressure increase followed by decay until a new equilibrium is reached. This pattern is dependent on the velocity and degree of dilatation due to the visco elastic properties of the periluminal tissues, including striated muscle and collagen.[62]

The intra-individual variability of flow rate is in part due to variations in urethral resistance. These may be due to varying tonus in the smooth muscle at the bladder neck and within the prostate in men, or to varying degrees of relaxation of the rhabdo-sphincter and pelvic floor in both sexes. The volume of non-contractile elements may also vary, for example the vascularity, congestion and glandular activity of the prostate, or varying estrogen status affecting the female urethra.

Mechanical increases in urethral resistance occur with urethral strictures. These may cause a fine high pressure/high velocity flow maintaining the cast distance while the flow rate may be reduced. The urethral stricture has to be quite narrow before it will interfere with the flow rate (<14 Ch).

In women, outlet obstruction can be due to distal urethral stenosis, meatus stenosis, or a urethral diverticulum which fills during voiding and progressively increases the degree of obstruction. Sometimes obstruction can be caused by urethral 'kinking' due to rotational descent where a prolapse is present.

Sphincter-active voiding refers to an intermittent stream caused by abnormal sphincter activity during voiding (Fig. 3.5). The sphincter should remain relaxed throughout voiding, but incoordination can occur as a result of urinary tract infections and reflex urethral spasm because of burning and then sphincter-active voiding patterns remain after clearance of the infection. The sphincter spasm can inhibit the detrusor contraction and lead to increased postvoid residual.[63]

Sphincter-active voiding can result in high pressures within the bladder and risk damage to the upper urinary tracts. Reflux nephropathy can occur in previously normal kidneys in those who had a supranuclear spinal cord injury.[64]

Detrusor-external urethral sphincter dyssynergia can occur also in patients with spinal cord injury. Coordination appears to require function of an intact pons with its integrated long-routed reflexes.[65,57]

After a urinary infection in children, especially boys under 2 years of age, urodynamic studies show quite high voiding pressures, often over 150 cm of water, presumably due to detrusor-sphincter dyssynergia. These children outgrow the abnormal pattern of voiding and pressures return to normal later in childhood.[66]

Neural plasticity in adults as a result of windup can alter neuronal circuits and lead to spread of dysfunction to segments above and below the initiating level, and to impaired bowel and bladder emptying as well as sexual function.

Intra-individual variations of flow/pressure

Urodynamic definitions use intrinsic detrusor pressure at peak flow to define the presence or absence of obstruction. Some have argued that when a steady state exists and the urethra is open with a continuous column of urine to the meatus, that the drive for voiding would be the total intravesical pressure which includes abdominal pressure as well as the intrinsic detrusor component.

Using abdominal straining in order to void is a feature of some areflexic bladders. The flow pattern is characteristically intermittent and stops occur when the patient needs to take another breath. It gives a characteristic flow appearance.

Home uroflowmetry studies emphasize again the variability of flow observed by patients. Flow rate during the night is often slower than by day as observed by Golomb *et al.* (1992)[67] and Boci *et al.* (1999).[68] This may be partly due to variations in the degree of excitation of the micturition reflex, and partly to variable relaxation of the external urethral sphincter.

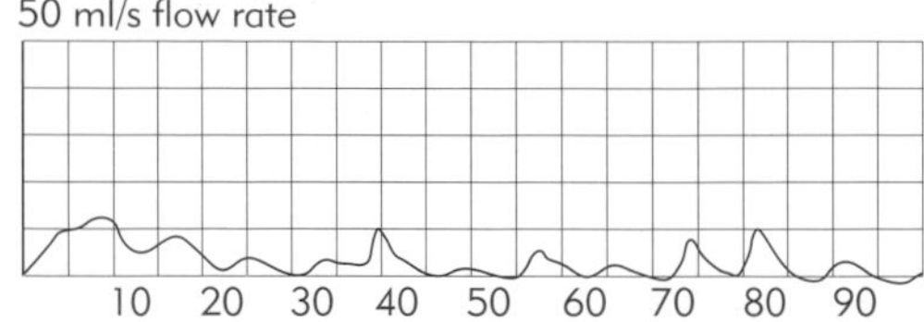

Figure 3.5 Intermittent flow pattern. This could be caused by abdominal straining to void, or by sphincter-active voiding.

Flow rate protocols have been established in some prostate clinics so that adequate volumes can be voided and the flow repeated, but also to compare the rate and pattern in three separate flow voids.[69]

Long-term ambulatory studies of voiding using suprapubic catheters show that voiding occurs at higher pressures and better flows when compared with conventional cystometry studies.[16] This suggests more optimal firing of the micturition reflex under more normal circumstances.

It has been assumed in some urodynamic circles, that the micturition reflex fires off maximally each time. However, this is not so. Many women and some men void more slowly at the time of video urodynamics because of the embarrassment. If they then void in privacy but with the pressure flow lines in position, the flow rate improves. This can be either because the urethra relaxes better and the voiding pressure is lower than before, or because voiding pressures are higher for the better flow indicating a greater degree of activation of the neural reflex (Fig. 3.6).

This variation in detrusor pressure brings into question the accuracy of diagnosing obstruction based on only one study. Some variation in diagnosis of obstruction was shown by Tammela *et al.* (1999)[61] when three separate voids were analysed. They found that of 187 men with lower urinary tract symptoms (LUTS), 125 (67%) were obstructed by Abrams–Griffiths nomogram at the first void, but this dropped to 111 (59%) obstructed at the time of the third pressure flow study done at the same investigation.

EFFICIENCY OF BLADDER EMPTYING AND POSTVOID RESIDUAL URINE

The normal bladder empties to completion during volitional micturition. The detrusor contracts and continues to do so while the urethra remains relaxed, until emptying is complete.

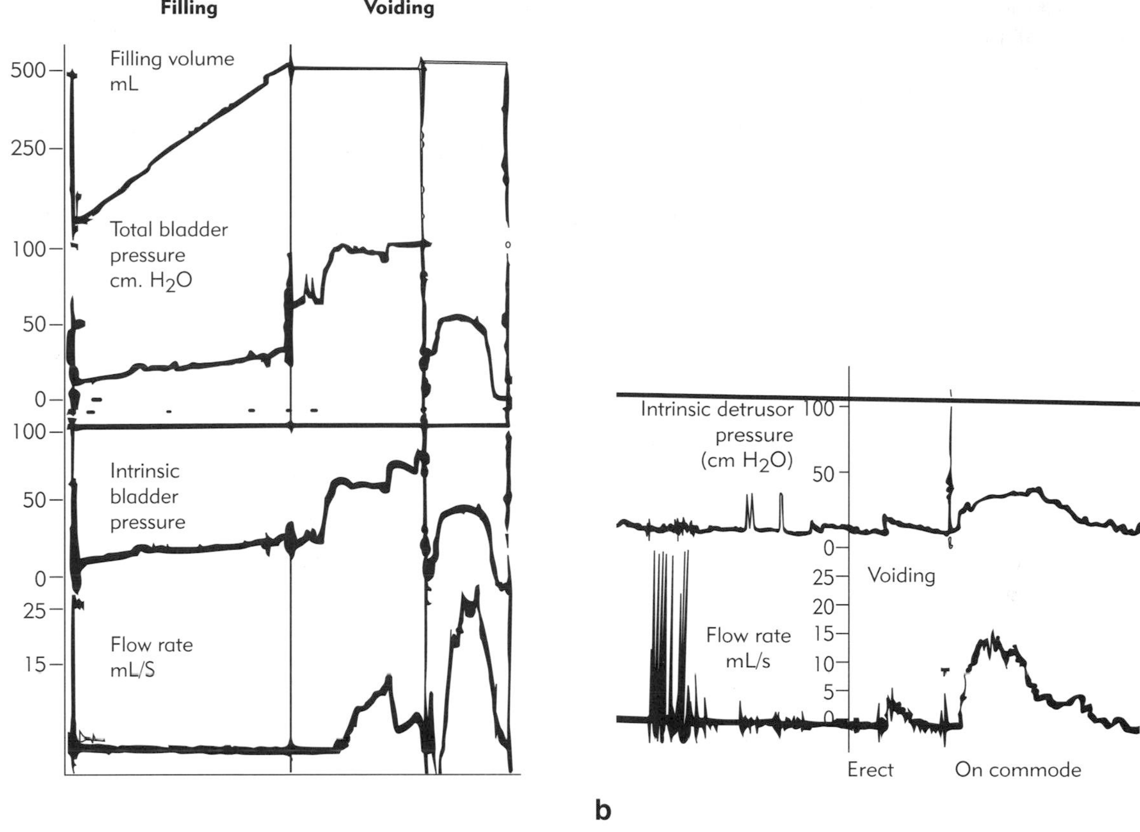

Figure 3.6 Flow rate improvement when voiding in privacy compared to voiding for a video urodynamic study: (a) Improved flow rate and lower voiding pressure due to urethral relaxation; and (b) Improved flow rate due to higher detrusor pressure.

The sensation of incomplete emptying is not uncommon in both men and women. No correlation was found between this sensation and the presence of postvoid residual in studies by Bruskewitz *et al.* (1982)[70] and Reynard *et al.* (1998).[71] Men with chronic retention may be quite unaware that they do not completely empty their bladders.

Some women when voiding in a public toilet often perch or hover above the toilet seat and because of this only a proportion of the bladder volume is emptied, due to inhibition by their surroundings.[72]

Women in the elderly age group if confined to bed, often do not empty their bladders efficiently when perched on a bedpan, or if it is painful to move as after a fractured femur etc. Chronic retention and overflow can lead to urinary tract infections and need a catheter. After a period of continuous drainage, voiding usually resumes in a normal fashion when the patient is mobilized.

The efficiency of emptying is variable within any individual and single measurements are probably unhelpful in reaching a diagnosis.[73] The presence of a postvoid residual does not indicate obstruction nor does its absence rule it out.[74] Postvoid residual does not correlate with symptoms, prostatic size or urethral resistance.[75]

The efficiency of emptying may fall with aging, sphincter-active voiding, or as a result of bladder outlet obstruction.

Compensation and decompensation

The detrusor pressure rises in obstruction 'compensating' for the slow flow rate and follows the hyperbolic curve of the Hill equation relating force and velocity.

'Decompensation' after a period of compensation has been invoked to explain postvoid residual in a similar fashion to left ventricular failure occurring as an end result of long-standing hypertension.

In obstructed voiding the detrusor pressure falls off and may leave a residual urine. It has been argued that the reason for this is that the work that the bladder is able to do in any one voiding cycle is limited.[76,77] Progression to acute urinary retention occurs infrequently. However, the contraction strength of the bladder *in situ* or of muscle strips *in vivo* is unchanged or even slightly reduced in obstruction.[59,78]

Inhibition of micturition reflex

Contraction of the striated urethral sphincter reflexly inhibits the detrusor. This can be observed at urodynamic evaluation during the clinical 'stop test' where the patient is asked to voluntarily interrupt the voiding flow part-way through emptying. It is also seen in patients with sphincter-active voiding. The reflex might be inhibited during obstructed micturition by high intraurethral pressures.

Chronic retention of urine

This has been arbitrarily defined as a PVR greater than 300 ml.

In males this can arise from a high pressure bladder outlet obstruction. The upper tracts are at risk of back pressure effects with ureteric dilatation and hydronephrosis. These patients do well after prostatectomy. There is a group of low pressure–low flow patients in chronic retention who do not risk damage to their upper tracts, but who do poorly following prostatectomy.[79]

TERMINAL DRIBBLING, AND AFTER-DISCHARGE OF URINE

Towards the end of the stream there is often a terminal dribbling until the voiding flow ceases. This can occur in both men and women. The rate of shortening of the circumference of the bladder increases exponentially with bladder emptying, so where little volume remains the efficiency of the contraction will reduce and the flow will slow (see Figure 3.5).

In men some leakage of urine following adjusting clothing after voiding is quite common. Mostly it is due to urine 'pooling' in the urethra because of:

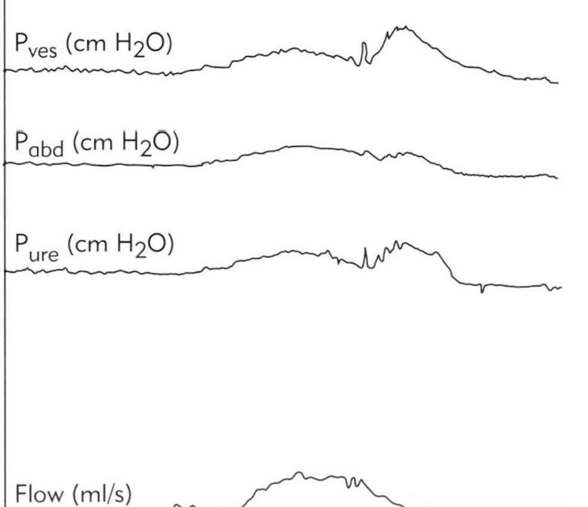

Figure 3.7 'After-contraction' is a detrusor contraction after voiding is complete. (Hoebeke *et al.* 1996, reproduced with permission.)

- inefficient emptying by bulbo-spongiosus contractions;
- not allowing enough time to empty the urethra;
- constriction of the penile urethra by tight underwear or the elastic waistband under the penis, or a trouser zip not opening far enough back in order to avoid urethral compression.

The annoying wetness of underwear and trousers can be avoided by digital stripping of the urethra, and avoiding any restrictive clothing.

In some women because of local vulval anatomy, during voiding some urine may reflux into the vagina. This will leak out on resuming the standing position.

An 'after-contraction', refers to an involuntary detrusor contraction after voiding is completed. It is an uncommon finding in both sexes and also in children, but is consistent with detrusor instability. (Fig. 3.7)[80]

LOWER URINARY TRACT SYMPTOMS (LUTS) AND THEIR SIGNIFICANCE

LUTS

Terms such as 'prostatism', or 'obstructive' or 'irritative' symptoms should no longer be used, as groups of symptoms do not correlate with any specific diagnosis. If symptoms are to be grouped, it is preferable to speak of *storage symptoms* and *voiding symptoms*. Indeed the International Prostate Symptom Score (IPPS) would be better termed International Urinary Symptom Score (IUSS) as the same symptoms occur in women.[81,82]

Several studies have failed to find any correlation between IPPS scores and obstruction as defined by pressure flow studies and the Abrams–Griffiths nomogram[83] even when two to three studies have been performed on the same individual.[61]

BURNING AND PAIN ON MICTURITION

The area of the trigone and posterior urethra appear to have mechanoreceptors and pain (nociceptive) endings. Inflammation and an acid pH result in discomfort referred to the urethral meatus, and may cause associated burning during voiding.

In patients with cystitis, burning is felt in the urethra and at its meatus during voiding. The symptom is rapidly improved by alkalinizing the urine well in advance of the inflammation resolving with concomitant administration of antibiotics. Patients with suprapubic catheters in whom solutions of varying pH were instilled and who were then asked to void, could not distinguish between acid or alkaline pH. Some sensation of temperature of the solution was appreciated by some. Burning requires both inflammation and an acid pH (personal observation).

The symptom can be observed also in patients with a stone in the lower end of the ureter where increased sensitivity of the urethral meatus is felt. This area and the lower end of the ureter share the nerve supply of S_2 and S_3, and voiding can result in a hypersensitive state as urine passes over the external meatus.

Patients with reflux rarely feel pain in the affected loin, although some do. Some patients with a double J ureteric stent between bladder and renal pelvis which allows reflux, do notice loin pain on voiding.

REFERENCES

1. Abrams P, Blaivas JG, Stanton SL, *et al.* The standardisation of lower urinary tract function recommended by the International Continence Society. *Int Urogynecol J* 1990;**1**:45–58.
2. Gosling JA. The structure of the bladder neck, urethra and pelvic floor in relation to female urinary incontinence. Editorial *Int Urogynecol J* 1996;**7**:177–8.
3. McConnell JD, *et al.* Direct outcomes – sexual dysfunction. In: McConnell JD (ed). *Benign prostatic hyperplasia: diagnosis and treatment.* Clinical Practice Guidelines. US Department of Health and Human Services, AHCPR (94-0582), 1994:99–103.
4. Chapple CR, Helm CW, Blease S, *et al.* Asymptomatic bladder neck incompetence in nulliparous females. *Br J Urol* 1989;**64**:357–79.
5. Versi E, Cardozo LD, Studd J. Distal urethral compensatory mechanisms in women with an incompetent bladder neck who remain continent and the effect of the menopause. *Neurourol Urodyn* 1990;**9**:579–90.
6. Gosling JA, Dixon JS, Humpherson JR. *Functional anatomy of the lower urinary tract.* Churchill Livingstone, Edinburgh, 1983.
7. Klutke C, Golomb J, Barbaric Z, *et al.* The anatomy of stress incontinence: magnetic resonance imaging of the female bladder neck and urethra. *J Urol* 1990;**143**:563–6.
8. Christensen LL, Djurhuus JC, Constantinou CE. Imaging of pelvic floor contractions using magnetic resonance imaging. *Neurourol Urodyn* 1995;**14**:209–216.
9. Smet PJ, Moore KH, Jonavicius J. Distribution and colocalisation of calcitonin gene related peptide, tackykinins and VIP in normal and idiopathic unstable human urinary bladder. *Lab Invest* 1997;**77**:37–49.
10. Sheriff MKM, Shah PJR, Fowler C, *et al.* Neuromodulation of detrusor hyperreflexia by functional magnetic stimulation of the sacral roots. *Br J Urol* 1996;**80**(78):39–46.
11. Macneil HF, Brading AF, Williams JH. Cause of low compliance in a guinea pig model of instability and low compliance. *Neurourol Urodyn* 1992;**11**:47–52.
12. Yokoyama O, Mita E, Ishiura Y, *et al.* Bladder compliance in patients with benign prostatic hyperplasia. *Neurourol Urodyn* 1997;**16**:19–27.
13. Harris RL, Cundiff GW, Theofrastous JP, *et al.* Bladder compliance in neurologically intact women. *Neurourol Urodyn* 1996;**15**:483–8.
14. Madersbacher S, Pycha A, Klinger CH, *et al.* Interrelationships of bladder compliance with age, detrusor instability and obstruction in elderly men with urinary tract symptoms. *Neurourol Urodyn* 1999;**18**:3–15.
15. Wyndaele JJ. The normal pattern of perception of bladder filling during cystometry studied in 38 young healthy volunteers. *J Urol* 1998;**160**:479–81.
16. Robertson AS, Griffiths CJ, Ramsden PD. Bladder function in healthy volunteers: ambulatory monitoring and conventional urodynamics. *Br J Urol* 1994;**73**:242–9.
17. Lowe EM, Anand P, Terenghi G, *et al.* Increased nerve growth factor levels in the urinary bladder of women with idiopathic sensory urgency and interstitial cystitis. *Br J Urol* 1997;**79**:572–7.
18. Sutherst JR, Brown M. The effect on the bladder pressure of sudden entry of fluid into the posterior urethra. *Br J Urol* 1978;**50**:406–409.
19. Hastwell GB. Psychogenic pelvic pain, or occult prolapse syndrome? *Med J Austral* 1986;**144**:405–406.
20. Tanagho EA. Urinary stress incontinence: surgical treatment. *Int Urogynecol J* 1998;**9**:1–2.
21. Coolsaet B, van Duyl WA, van Os-Bossagh P, *et al.* New concepts in relation to urge and detrusor instability. *Neurourol Urodyn* 1993;**12**:463–71.
22. Hellström PA, Tammela TLJ, Kontturi MJ, *et al.* The bladder cooling test for urodynamic assessment: analysis of 400 examinations. *Br J Urol* 1991;**67**:275–9.
23. Chai TC, Gray ML, Steers WD. The incidence of a positive iced water test in bladder outlet obstructed patients: evidence of bladder neuronal plasticity. *J Urol* 1998; **160**:34–8.
24. Arnold EP. Cystometry: postural effects in incontinent women. *Urol Internat* 1974;**29**:185–6.
25. Brading AF, Turner WH. The unstable bladder: towards a common mechanism. *Br J Urol* 1994;**73**:3–8.
26. Brading AF. A myogenic basis for the overactive bladder. *Urology* 1997;**50**:(6A Suppl.):57–67.
27. de Groat WC. A neurological basis for the overactive bladder. *Urology* 1997;**50**:(6A Suppl.):36–52.
28. Sibley GNA. Development in our understanding of detrusor instability. *Br J Urol* 1997;**80**:Suppl.1:54–61.
29. Elbadawi A, Yalla SV, Resnick NM. Structural basis of geriatric voiding dysfunction. IV. Bladder outlet obstruction. *J Urol* 1993;**150**:1681–95.
30. Sethia KK. The pathophysiology of detrusor instability. D.M. Thesis, Oxford 1988.
31. Bates CP. Continence and incontinence: a clinical study of the dynamics of voiding and of the sphincter mechanism. *Ann Roy Coll Surg Eng* 1974;**49**:18–35.
32. Blok BFM, Holstege G. The central control of micturition and continence: implications for urology. *Br J Urol* 1999;Suppl.**2**:1–6.
33. van Waalwijk van Doorn ESC, Ambergen AW, Janknegt RA. Detrusor activity index: quantification of detrusor activity by ambulatory monitoring. *J Urol* 1997;**157**:596–9.
34. Webb RJ, Griffiths CJ, Ramsden PD, *et al.* Measurement of voiding pressures on ambulatory monitoring: comparisons with conventional cystometry. *Br J Urol* 1990;**65**:152–4.
35. Finkbeiner AE. The aging bladder. *Int Urogynecol J* 1993;**4**:168–74.
36. Arnold EP. *Bladder responses to outlet obstruction.* PhD Thesis 1980, University of London.

37. Parsons CL, Stein PC, Bidair M, *et al.* Abnormal sensitivity to intravesical potassium in interstitial cystitis and radiation cystitis. *Neurourol Urodyn* 1994;**13**:515–20.
38. Hohlbrugger G. Leaky urothelium and/or vesical ischaemia enable urinary potassium to cause idiopathic urgency/frequency syndrome and urge incontinence. *Int Urogynecol J* 1996;**7**:242–55.
39. Eldrup J, Thorup J, Nielsen SL, *et al.* Permeability and ultrastructure of human bladder epithelium. *Br J Urol* 1983;**55**:488–92.
40. Kohn IJ, Kaplan SA. Where we stand with iontophoresis in urology. *Contemp Urol* 1998;**10**:37–50.
41. Constantinou CE, Govan DE. Spatial distribution and timing of transmitted and reflexly generated urethral pressures in healthy women. *J Urol* 1982;**127**:964–9.
42. McGuire EJ. Reflex urethral instability. *Br J Urol* 1978;**50**:200–204.
43. Geirsson G, Sommar S, Lindstrom S, *et al.* Temperature sensitivity of the bladder cooling reflex in man. *Neurourol Urodyn* 1990;**9**:354–5.
44. Burton G. Urine temperature changes as the bladder fills and in a cold environment. *Neurourol Urodyn* 1992;**11**:297–8.
45. McMahon SB, Dmitrieva N, Koltzenburg M. Visceral pain. *Br J Anaesthes* 1995;**75**:132–44.
46. Steers WD, Kolbeck S, Creedon D, *et al.* Nerve growth factor in the urinary bladder of the adult, regulates neuronal form and function. *J Clin Invest* 1991;**88**:1709–1715.
47. Doggweiler R, Jasmin L, Schmidt RA. Neurogenically mediated cystitis in rats: an animal model. *J Urol* 1998;**160**:1551–6.
48. Whiteside CG, Arnold EP. Persistent primary enuresis: a urodynamic assessment. *Br Med J* 1975;**1**:364–7.
49. Moore KH, Richmond DH, Parys BT. Sex distribution of adult idiopathic detrusor instability in relation to childhood bedwetting. *Br J Urol* 1991;**68**:479–82.
50. Wolin LH. Stress incontinence in young healthy nulliparous female subjects. *J Urol* 1969;**101**:545–9.
51. Rosenzweig BA, Pushkin S, Blumenfeld D, *et al.* Prevalence of abnormal urodynamic test results in continent women with severe genito-urinary prolapse. *Obstet Gynecol* 1992;**79**:539–42.
52. Eckford SD, Bailey RA, Jackson SR, *et al.* Occult post-operative detrusor instability – an adverse prognostic feature in genuine stress incontinence surgery. *Neurourol Urodyn* 1995;**14**:487–8.
53. Vierhout ME, Mulder AFP. Persistent detrusor instability after surgery for concomitant stress incontinence and detrusor instability: a review. *Int Urogynecol* 1993;**4**:237–9.
54. Resnick NM, Yalla SV. Detrusor hyperactivity with impaired contractile function. An unrecognised but common cause of incontinence in elderly patients. *JAMA* 1987; **257**:3076–81.
55. Elbadawi A, Yalla SV, Resnick NM. Structural basis of geriatric voiding dysfunction. II. Ageing detrusor: normal versus impaired contractility. *J Urol* 1993;**150**:1657–67.
56. Vaidyanatha S, Soni BM, Sett P, *et al.* Pathophysiology of autonomic dysreflexia: longterm treatment with terazosine in adult and paediatric spinal cord injury patients manifesting recurrent dysreflexic episodes. *Spinal Cord* 1998;**36**:761–70.
57. de Groat WC. Anatomy and physiology of the lower urinary tract. *Urol Clin North Am* 1993;**20**:383–401.
58. Parys BT, Machen DG, Woolfenden KA, *et al.* Chronic urinary retention – a sensory problem? *Br J Urol* 1988;**62**:546–9.
59. Griffiths DJ. The mechanics of the urethra and of micturition. *Br J Urol* 1973; **45**:497–507.
60. Marshall VR, Ryall RL, Austin ML, *et al.* The use of urinary flow rates obtained from voided volumes less than 150 mls in assessment of voiding ability. *Br J Urol* 1983; **55**:28–33.
61. Tammela TLJ, Schafer W, Barrett DM, *et al.* and the Finasteride Urodynamic Study Group. Repeated pressure-flow studies in the evaluation of bladder outlet obstruction due to benign prostatic enlargement. *Neurourol Urodyn* 1999;**18**:17–24.
62. Baji P, Thind P, Nordsten M. Passive urethral resistance to dilatation in healthy women: an experimental simulation of urine ingression in the resting urethra. *Neurourol, Urodyn* 1995;**14**:115–23.
63. van Gool JD. Dysfunctional voiding: a complex of bladder/sphincter dysfunction, urinary tract infection and vesico-ureteric reflux. *Acta Urol Belg* 1975;**63**:27–33.
64. Arnold EP, Fukui J, Anthony A, *et al.* Bladder function following spinal cord injury: a urodynamic analysis of the outcome. *Br J Urol* 1984;**56**:172–7.
65. Mahony DT, Laferte RO, Blais DJ. Integral storage and voiding reflexes: Neurophysiologic concepts of continence and micturition. *Urology* 1977;**9**:95–106.
66. Sillen U, Bachelard M, Hansson S, *et al.* *Video cystographic recordings in infants after acute pyelonephritis.* International Children's Continence Society Monograph. Tunbridge Wells: Wells Medical, 1996:129–32.
67. Golomb J, Lindner A, Siegel Y, *et al.* Variability and circadian changes in home uroflowmetry in patients with BPH compared to normal controls. *J Urol* 1992; **147**:1044–7.
68. Boci R, Fall M, Walden M, Knutson T, *et al.* Home uroflowmetry: improved accuracy in outflow assessment. *Neurourol Urodyn* 1999;**18**:25–32.
69. Abrams PH. The urine flow clinics. In: Fitzpatrick JN (ed). *Conservative treatment of BPH.* Edinburgh: Churchill Livingston, 1991:33–43.
70. Bruskewitz RC, Iversen P, Madsen PO. Value of post-void residual urine determinations in evaluation of prostatism. *Urology* 1982;**20**:602–604.
71. Reynard JM, Yang Q, Donovan JL, *et al.* The ICS–'BPH' Study: Uroflowmetry, lower urinary tract symptoms and bladder outlet obstruction. *Br J Urol* 1998;**82**:619–23.
72. Moore KH, Richmond DH, Sutherst JR, *et al.* Crouching over the toilet seat: prevalence among British gynaecological outpatients and its effect upon micturition. *Br J Obstet Gynaecol* 1991;**98**:569–72.
73. Birch NC, Hirst G, Doyle PT. Serial residual urine volumes in men with prostatic hypertrophy. *Br J Urol* 1988;**62**:571–5.
74. Dorflinger T, Bruskewitz RC, Jensen KME, *et al.* Predictive value of low maximum flow rate in benign prostatic hyperplasia. *Urology* 1986;**27**:569–73.
75. Cetinel B, Turan T, Talat Z, *et al.* Update evaluation of benign prostatic hyperplasia: When should we offer prostatectomy? *Br J Urol* 1994;**74**:566–71.

76. Schafer W. Urethral resistance? Urodynamic concepts of physiological and pathological bladder outlet function during voiding. *Neurourol Urodyn* 1985; **4**:161–201.
77. Schafer W. Analysis of active detrusor function during voiding with the bladder working function. *Neurourol Urodyn* 1991;**10**:19–35.
78. Gilling PJ, Arnold EP. Contractility of detrusor muscle from patients undergoing elective transurethral resection of the prostate. *Br J Urol* 1991;Proceedings, p. 400.
79. George NJR, Feneley RCL, Roberts JG. Identification of the poor risk patient with prostatism and detrusor failure. *Br J Urol* 1986;**58**:290–95.
80. Hoebeke PB, van Gool JD, van Laeke E, *et al.* The after-contraction in paediatric urodynamics. *Br J Urol* 1996;**78**:780–82.
81. Lepor H, Machi G. Comparison of AUA symptom index for unselected males and females between fifty-five and seventy-nine years of age. *Urology* 1993;**42**:36–40.
82. Chai TC, Belville WD, McGuire EJ, *et al.* Specificity of AUA voiding symptom index: comparison of unselected and selected samples of both sexes. *J Urol* 1993; **150**:1710–13.
83. Chapple CR. Correlation of symptomatology, urodynamics, morphology and size of the prostate in benign prostatic hyperplasia. *Curr Opin Urol* 1993;**3**:5–9.

Chapter 4

Childbirth and pelvic floor injury

Michelle Fynes, Colm O'Herlihy, P Ronan O'Connell

INTRODUCTION

Obstetric trauma is the most important etiological factor in the pathogenesis of fecal incontinence in women. The emotional, psychological and social problems which this causes can be both embarrassing and debilitating. Symptoms of pelvic floor dysfunction and altered fecal or urinary continence are common but frequently unrecognized sequelae of vaginal delivery. Postpartum pelvic floor morbidity represents a large and currently unaddressed health need. Incontinence symptoms are often transient following first vaginal delivery, but successive vaginal deliveries may be associated with recrudescence or deterioration in symptoms. This may have a significant impact on maternal health and well-being. This chapter focuses on the mechanisms of obstetric injury to the pelvic floor. We review the incidence and risk factors for dysfunctional pelvic floor symptoms and incontinence and the influence of obstetric risk factors and mode of delivery on these problems.

PARTURITION AND THE PELVIC FLOOR

Substantial evidence exists for a direct effect of the sex hormones on gastrointestinal function.[1] Estrogen and progesterone receptors have been identified in intestinal smooth muscle[2] and in the striated muscles of the pelvic floor.[3] The serum levels of these two sex steroid hormones are consistently elevated during pregnancy and fall to non-pregnant levels within 72 hours of delivery.[4] Progesterone relaxes gastrointestinal muscle *in vitro* and the administration of estradiol and progesterone *in vitro* reduces intestinal transit.[5] *In vivo* evidence, however, has provided inconsistent data on the influence of these two hormones on gut motility and function. Some studies demonstrate a lowered resting pressure in the esophageal sphincter in pregnancy and others have shown no change.[6] Similarly, contradictory evidence exists on changes in gut motility induced by variation in sex steroid hormone levels during the menstrual cycle.[7] Alteration in the levels of sex steroids are far greater in magnitude in pregnancy than during the menstrual cycle and a direct effect on gut motility in pregnancy can, therefore, not be excluded. Constipation and defecatory difficulty are common symptoms in pregnancy and while they may be due in part to the mechanical effects of the gravid and enlarging uterus, the early onset of symptoms in pregnancy in some women suggests other predisposing factors, which may be endocrine.[8]

Pregnancy itself has not been demonstrated to influence anal sphincter morphology or function in studies combining anal endosonography and anal manometry.[9] Electrodiagnostic studies to evaluate the effect of pregnancy on pudendal nerve function have not been undertaken. The lack of any significant effect of pregnancy on pudendal nerve function may be inferred from studies following elective cesarean section which have not found any increase in abnormal pudendal nerve function following delivery.[10]

Estrogen and progesterone receptors are also present in the lower urinary tract and vagina. Symptomatic cytological and urodynamic changes in the lower urinary tract have been demonstrated during the menstrual cycle, in pregnancy and following the menopause.[11,12] The effects of pregnancy on the lower urinary tract have been extensively studied and have shown how physiologically high progesterone levels affect the ureters, bladder and urethra. During pregnancy, a physiological dilatation of the ureters, which is more common on the right side, is attributable to the smooth muscle relaxant effects of progesterone and the obstructive effects of the gravid uterus. This dilatation increases the risk of urinary stasis, voiding difficulty and lower urinary tract infection, which can, in turn, lead to ascending pyelonephritis, which is a significant risk factor for preterm delivery.

Cystometry during pregnancy demonstrates an increase in bladder capacity and compliance and comparable changes have been demonstrated in the luteal phase of the menstrual cycle when progesterone levels are also elevated.[13] Pregnant women commonly complain of stress incontinence and this has also been attributed to elevated progesterone levels. Urethral pressure profile studies during pregnancy demonstrate no change in closure pressures despite high circulating progesterone levels.[11]

Relaxin is an ovarian polypeptide which peaks during late pregnancy and labor and leads to connective tissue remodeling in the cervix and pelvic floor muscles. Softening and physiological separation of the pelvic ligaments and pubic symphysis facilitates descent and delivery of the fetal head. Although connective tissue changes occur to a variable extent throughout the pelvis, only cervical remodeling has been extensively evaluated and has been shown to follow an alteration of the water/collagen ratio from 20% to 80%.[14] This change primarily occurs through the breakdown of intercellular fibrous bridges and an increase in intracellular and extracellular water content. Modifications in collagen structure are also recognized[15] which increase tissue elasticity to facilitate tissue stretching rather than tearing during labor and delivery. Failure of this connective tissue remodeling process may be associated with an increased risk of tissue injury, a hypothesis which is currently being evaluated.

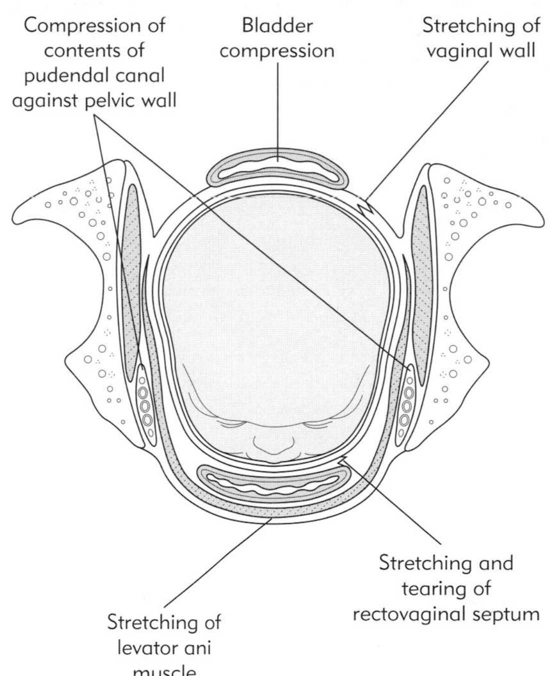

Figure 4.1 Diagrammatic representation of the mechanism of pelvic floor injury during vaginal delivery.

MECHANISM OF OBSTETRIC INJURY

MECHANICAL INJURY

Injury to the anal sphincter mechanism during childbirth may arise secondary to direct disruption of the anal sphincter muscles and or through traction neuropathy of the pudendal nerves.[16,17] The pudendal nerves are fixed at the ischial spines before entering Alcock's canal which predisposes them to traction injury during the late first and second stages of labor as the fetal head reaches the pelvic floor (Fig. 4.1).[16] Pudendal nerve injury may occur at any point along the nerve pathway, from the ventral roots of S2,3,4 to the terminal branches supplying the external anal sphincter.[18,19] Injury to the pudendal nerves is usually secondary to traction, although neural disruption may arise with instrumental delivery.[16] The most important risk factor for mechanical injury to the anal sphincter muscles is first vaginal delivery.[17,20] In contrast, pudendal nerve injury is more common with successive vaginal deliveries, which may have a cumulative effect resulting in symptoms of altered continence many years following childbirth.[19,21]

Disruption of the anal sphincter muscles is best assessed by anal ultrasound examination (Fig. 4.2). This is usually performed using a high frequency (10 MHz) endoanal probe.[16] Sultan *et al.* (1993) performed endoanal ultrasound 6 weeks postpartum on 79 primiparous women and identified anal sphincter defects in 28 (35%).[17] Sphincter defects were not identified in those women delivered by cesarean section. Rieger *et al.* (1998) performed sonography upon 53 primiparous women at a median interval of five weeks following delivery and identified anal sphincter defects in 15 (41%) of the 37 women who delivered vaginally.[22] Again, there were no sphincter defects identified in the remaining 13 women delivered by cesarean section.[22] Most women with postpartum fecal incontinence symptoms have an identifiable anal sphincter defect at endosonography.[16,17,21] Deen *et al.* (1993) studied 46 patients with altered fecal continence and found that 40 (87%) had a recognizable anal sphincter defect on ultrasound.[23] Similarly, Sultan *et al.* (1993) found sphincter defects in nine of 10 primiparous women with fecal incontinence in their study population.[17]

Several authors have documented the incidence of symptoms in women who have undergone primary repair of recognized anal sphincter injury ('third degree tear') at the time of delivery.[24,25,26] In a series of 84 patients interviewed by Wood *et al.* (1998), fecal incontinence symptoms were reported by 21 (25%) who had sustained a previous third degree tear.[27] Crawford *et al.* (1993) performed a telephone survey of 70 women 9–12 months following vaginal delivery, 35 of whom had undergone primary repair of a recognized third degree tear and 35 matched controls.[25] Incontinence of flatus was significantly more prevalent after primary repair of a recognized third degree tear compared with the control group.[25] Haadem *et al.* (1997) surveyed 41 women by postal questionnaire on average 20 years following

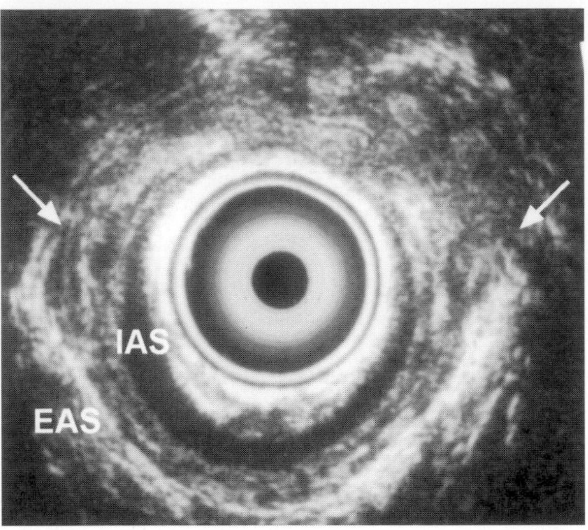

a

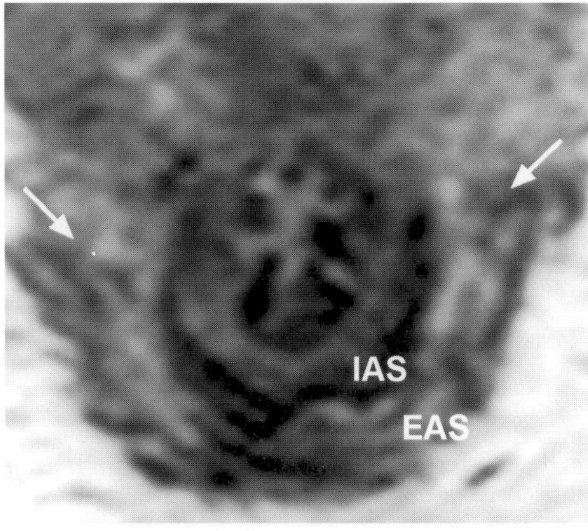

b

Figure 4.2 (a) Trans-anal ultrasound and corresponding MRI image (b) demonstrating persistent full thickness disruption of the external anal sphincter muscle following primary repair of a recognized third degree tear.

primary repair of a recognized anal sphincter tear and 38 matched controls;[26] altered fecal continence was reported by 18 (43%) of those with a history of anal sphincter disruption, compared with only seven (18%) of the matched controls. Similarly, Tetzchner *et al.* (1996) questioned 72 women with documented anal sphincter injury at delivery and found that 42% had persistent symptoms of fecal incontinence at review up to two to four years later.[28]

It is noteworthy, however, that only a small minority of anal sphincter defects found at postpartum endosonography are associated with symptoms.[16,17] In Sultan's study (1993), 28 women had recognizable anal sphincter defects, of whom nine (32%) reported altered fecal continence postpartum.[17] It is suggested that such occult sphincter injuries may progress to be symptomatic in later life.[17,18,19] The number of these injuries, however, is far greater than the documented prevalence of incontinence in the community, and hence many must remain asymptomatic. Their true clinical significance remains uncertain.

PUDENDAL NERVE INJURY

Pudendal nerve function following vaginal delivery may be assessed using the St Mark's endo-anal technique to determine pudendal nerve terminal motor latency (PNTML) on the right and left sides or by using needle electromyography. The latter technique yields more information regarding the type and severity of nerve injury present as well as the prognosis for recovery.[18,19,21]

The hypothesis that childbirth might be a major factor in initiating denervation of the continence mechanism was first investigated by Snooks *et al.* (1984), who found evidence of neuropathic injury in 42% of women following vaginal delivery, but no evidence of pudendal nerve injury in women delivered by cesarean section.[18,19] None of the subjects had sustained a direct injury to the external anal sphincter during delivery. Recovery of pudendal nerve function was observed in 60% subjects 2 months postpartum with persistent evidence of nerve injury in the remainder.[18,19]

OBSTETRIC RISK FACTORS

VAGINAL DELIVERY

Two large prospective investigations have evaluated the mechanism of anal sphincter injury during childbirth and the incidence of altered fecal continence symptoms postpartum.[17,20] In the largest of these comprising a cohort of 184 primiparous women, Donnelly *et al.* (1998) reported altered fecal continence in 25% of women six weeks following first vaginal delivery.[20] Similarly, Sultan *et al.* (1993) identified altered fecal continence in 13% of primiparous and 23% of multiparous women at 6 weeks following vaginal delivery.[17] The most common mechanism of injury in both studies was mechanical disruption of the anal sphincter muscles or combined nerve and muscle injury.

INSTRUMENTAL VAGINAL DELIVERY

Forceps delivery has been shown to be associated with a significantly increased risk of mechanical anal sphincter injury and altered fecal continence.[16,17,20,21,29,30] In a prospective evaluation of primiparas using postpartum endoanal ultrasound to assess sphincter integrity, Donnelly *et al.* (1998) showed that instrumental delivery, predominantly using forceps, was associated with an eight-fold increase in risk of anal sphincter injury.[20] The evidence for an association between vacuum extraction vaginal delivery and anal sphincter injury is less conclusive.[29]

Sultan *et al.* (1998) reviewed 44 women, 5 years following randomization to forceps or vacuum delivery.[29] They identified significantly lower rates of anal sphincter injury among the women delivered by vacuum extraction, compared with forceps delivery, although there was no significant difference in symptoms of altered fecal continence between the two groups. In a large study comprising 349 women, 97% underwent instrumental delivery using vacuum extraction; this instrument correlated significantly with symptoms of altered fecal continence at 5 months postpartum but not at nine months.[31]

In MacArthur's (1997) questionnaire study of 906 women, vacuum extraction and forceps delivery both emerged as significant risk factors for symptomatic fecal incontinence.[32] Preliminary results from a prospective randomized comparison of forceps versus vacuum delivery suggests that both instruments increase the risk of anal sphincter trauma with no statistically significant differences in the rate of postpartum fecal incontinence for these two modes of instrumental delivery.[33] The most significant risk factor for anal sphincter injury and postpartum fecal incontinence however, arises where an attempted vacuum delivery ends with a forceps delivery.[33]

CESAREAN SECTION

Elective pre-labor cesarean section is not associated with the development of postpartum anal incontinence.[10,20] On the other hand, MacArthur *et al.* (1997), reported six cases where new bowel symptoms developed following delivery by emergency cesarean section.[32] An assessment of 34 women who had undergone cesarean section without attempted vaginal delivery, showed that anorectal physiology was unchanged in women delivered by elective cesarean section or by cesarean early in labor.[10] In contrast, emergency cesarean section later in labor may sometimes be associated with altered fecal continence through neuropathic injury.[10] Fynes *et al.* (1998) found prolongation of the pudendal nerve terminal latency and reduction in anal squeeze pressures when intrapartum cesarean delivery occurred after a cervical dilatation greater than 8 cm.[10] Cesarean delivery in labor may not be sufficient to prevent recurrence or new symptoms of fecal incontinence in women with previously symptomatic or occult anal sphincter injury.[21,10]

EPIDURAL ANALGESIA

Over the past 20 years epidural anesthesia has emerged as a major form of pain relief for labor and delivery. The rate of epidural use varies between centers with reported incidences of between 25–70%. The increase in popularity of epidural use has been attributed to the effectiveness of epidural when compared with other forms of pain relief and its ability to restore self-control to the parturient mother.[34,35]

Several studies have examined the impact of epidural analgesia upon pelvic floor function. It has been widely recognized that epidural analgesia leads to an increase in duration of the first and second stages of labor.[13,36] Further investigation by Donnelly *et al.* found that, by prolonging the second stage of labor, epidural analgesia can lead to a significant risk of injury to the anal sphincter mechanism. They reported an increased risk of pudendal nerve injury and of symptoms of altered fecal continence.[13,36] Epidural analgesia correlates with a significant increase in the risk of anal sphincter injury, with one study reporting a two-fold relative risk compared with a control group who did not receive an epidural block.[36] A recent study by Robinson *et al.* suggests that this association is a consequence of the more frequent use of forceps delivery and episiotomy in women in the epidural group.[37]

An increase in pudendal neuropathy is a significant finding associated with epidural analgesia. One study found an increase in pudendal nerve terminal motor latency in the left pudendal nerve when compared to the right, which may be due to the propensity of midwives to nurse patients with epidural analgesia in the left lateral position.[10] Childbirth carries many risks to the perineum and while epidural blockade is an effective and reliable source of pain relief, it can lead to a sequence of events which impact adversely upon the continence mechanism.

PERINEAL LACERATION

Perineal lacerations are classified as first degree (vaginal mucosa/perineal skin), second degree (extending into the perineal muscles), third degree (involving the external anal sphincter) and fourth degree, extending into the rectal mucosa. Perineal laceration is an important cause of postpartum maternal morbidity, the rate of which is significantly increased with second and third degree injuries. Spontaneous perineal laceration is more common with first vaginal delivery and instrumental delivery. Rotational or high forceps procedures may be particularly associated with extensive tissue trauma. Perineal laceration increases the risk of hematoma, infection or granulation tissue formation. Hematoma secondary to extension into the ischiorectal fossa may result in significant postpartum anemia. Long-term sequelae include persistent perineal pain and dyspareunia.

THIRD DEGREE PERINEAL INJURY

Third degree perineal tears have until recently been considered uncommon complications of childbirth, recognized following 0.6% of vaginal deliveries.[38] Postpartum anal endosonography, however, has identified occult anal sphincter injury in up to one third of women following first vaginal delivery.[26,38] Some reports have also noted an apparent increase in the rate of recognized third degree perineal injury (0.6–2.0%) with increased vigilance in regard to examination of the perineum following delivery.[33]

The most significant risk factor for third degree perineal injury is first vaginal delivery. This may reflect the relative inelasticity of the perineum in primiparous women.[26,33,38] More than 50% of all third degree tears occur with instrumental delivery, although this complication is recognized in fewer than 5% of all instrumental deliveries.[38] Forceps appears to be associated with a higher rate of third degree perineal injury compared to ventouse delivery.[39] Significant perineal injury is more likely to occur when instrumental delivery is performed for failure to advance in the second stage of labor.[33] In contrast, in women who have had a previous vaginal delivery, the most significant risk factor is fetal macrosomia.[26,33,38] Previous third degree tear also predisposes to further anal sphincter injury and incontinence with subsequent delivery.[21]

Almost half of all third degree tears at spontaneous vaginal delivery occur despite an episiotomy.[38] The type of episiotomy influences the risk of anal sphincter injury, with midline incisions associated with a much higher rate of third degree injury compared with medio-lateral episiotomy.[41] The timing and size of the episiotomy may also be significant factors which require further evaluation. There is certainly no evidence to suggest that elective episiotomy in women with a previous third degree tear protects against further anal sphincter injury.

Poor technique of repair and lack of operator expertise have been implicated as the primary factors responsible for persistent sphincter disruption and incontinence following primary obstetric anal sphincter repair. Conventional primary repair of third degree perineal injury by obstetricians involves an end-to-end approximation of the torn muscle fragments using 'figure-of-eight' sutures.[38] Prospective evaluations using anal endosonography to assess anatomical integrity of the anal sphincter muscles following primary obstetric repair using this repair technique had identified persistent anal sphincter defects in up to 85% of patients.[26,33,38] Colorectal surgeons generally favour an overlapping repair technique, with long-term success rates in excess of 80%. Sultan *et al.* evaluated primary overlapping obstetric anal sphincter repair in 32 women and demonstrated persistent endosonographic anal sphincter defects in only 15% postpartum.[41] On the other hand, in a prospective observational study by Fitzpatrick *et al.* (1999) comparing overlapping to approximation repair of obstetric anal sphincter disruption, there were no significant differences in the rates of postpartum anal sphincter defects between the two groups. Although it has been suggested that colorectal surgeons should perform all primary sphincter repairs, there are no reported series to date to indicate that the outcome is any different to that in experienced obstetric hands. Other factors which may contribute to persistent postpartum anal sphincter disruption include infection, constipation and defecatory straining which may result in breakdown or pull-through of the repaired anal sphincter ends.

EPISIOTOMY

Episiotomy is the most common surgical procedure performed in obstetrics. Advocates of routine use suggest that it reduces the duration of the second stage of labor, the incidence of perineal laceration, urinary incontinence, third degree perineal injury, intracranial fetal hemorrhage and asphyxia.[42] Meta-analysis does not substantiate these claims and the only consistent advantage of routine episiotomy is a reduction in the incidence of anterior perineal lacerations.[43] Anterior lacerations however, are associated with minimal perineal morbidity and not related to the development of postpartum urinary incontinence.[44]

The impact of episiotomy on the risk of anal sphincter damage is controversial. Poen *et al.* (1997) in a study of 120 women found that medio-lateral episiotomy was associated with fewer third degree tears.[36] Elective episiotomy, however, in women with previous third degree perineal injury has not been shown to reduce the risk of further anal sphincter injury or incontinence. In contrast to previous reports, Sultan *et al.* (1994) found episiotomy to be associated with an increased risk of internal and external anal sphincter injury.[38] Signorello *et al.* (2000) reviewed 626 women 6 months following delivery and found a three-fold increase in fecal incontinence in women following midline episiotomy compared to those who had a spontaneous perineal laceration.[41] Right mediolateral episiotomy is associated with a lower rate of extension into the external anal sphincter muscles than midline procedures, which should probably be abandoned, on current evidence.[37] An ideal episiotomy rate has not been determined but probably lies in the region of 20–30%; lower rates may be associated with increased morbidity.[42]

OBSTETRIC GENITAL FISTULA

Obstetric genital fistulas are common in the developing world where 50–100 000 new cases are diagnosed each year.[45] In West Africa the problem has reached epidemic proportions. Only 15% of women in these areas have access to antenatal care. Maternal mortality is 6–10/1000 compared with 11 per 100 000 in Europe and genitourinary fistula complicates 3–4 per 1000 deliveries.[46] The most common risk factors include first vaginal delivery, obstructed labor, early age at marriage and subsequent first pregnancy with an immature pelvis[47] (Figs 4.3 and 4.4).

A number of specialized fistula hospitals have been established to address this issue, at which the anatomical closure rates for fistula surgery exceed 90%.[48] Typically this combines a layered vaginal closure technique with a Martius labial fat graft. Persistent urinary and fecal incontinence remains a common postoperative problem. Murray *et al.* reported postoperative urinary incontinence following successful fistula closure in 58% of women and fecal incontinence in 39%; the site or size of the fistula did not influence the risk of postoperative urinary or fecal incontinence and 19% of these women also reported severe defecatory difficulty requiring digital evacuation.[49]

Urodynamic assessment performed upon women following successful fistula repair identified genuine stress incontinence in 50%, detrusor instability in 6% and mixed urinary incontinence in 44%. Duc to poor bladdcr compliance and bladder hypersensitivity only a small percentage of women are suitable for adjuvant urinary continence surgery and the lack of access to anticholinergic medication and physiotherapy makes management of the latter group difficult.[49]

To date, the mechanism of fecal incontinence in these women remains unclear. One in four were found to have significant foot drop secondary to perineal nerve palsy and sciatic plexus injury, which occurs as a consequence of high obstruction at the pelvic inlet and traumatic forceps delivery.[45] These associated neuropathies would suggest an anal sphincter injury which is predominantly neurological rather than mechanical.

In contrast, obstetric genital fistulas are uncommon complications of childbirth in more affluent countries. Approximately 1–2 per 100 000 deliveries are complicated by vesico-vaginal fistula which usually follows cesarean delivery or cesarean hysterectomy. Recto-vaginal fistula is a recognized association with 3% of third and fourth degree vaginal tears.[50] The relationship with episiotomy is lower, occurring in <0.1% primigravid deliveries,[51] although coexistent anal sphincter defects are common.[52] Recto-vaginal fistulas usually present with recurring perineal sepsis, persistent foul smelling discharge or passage of flatus per vaginam. Surgical repair with the trans-anal endorectal advancement flap technique offers good results in > 90% of obstetric cases[51] and the majority of fistulas do not recur. If they do, repeated endorectal flap techniques are usually successful in establishing a cure.

INCONTINENCE AND DYSFUNCTIONAL PELVIC FLOOR SYMPTOMS

URINARY INCONTINENCE

Urinary incontinence is identified in 4% of nulliparous women under 35 years.[54] Not just the process of delivery but pregnancy itself is strongly associated with the development of urinary incontinence symptoms. In primiparous pregnancy at 16 weeks, 9% women report symptoms of stress urinary incontinence and beyond 34

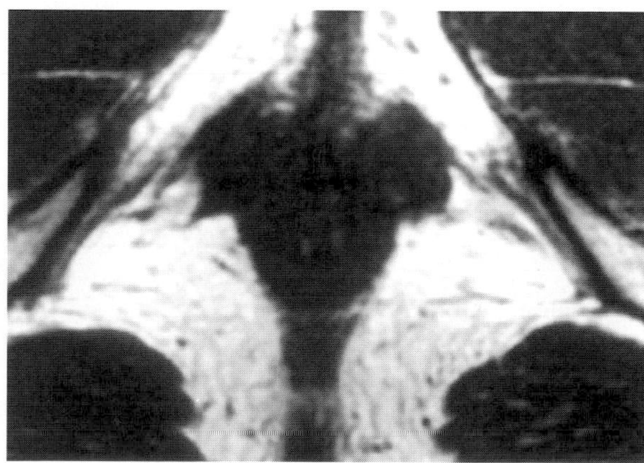

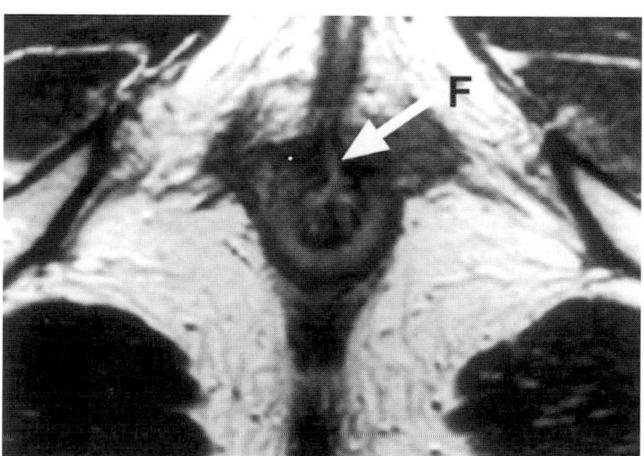

Figure 4.3 MRI images (a) pre- and (b) post-gadolinium contrast demonstrating an unrecognized obstetric rectovaginal fistula.

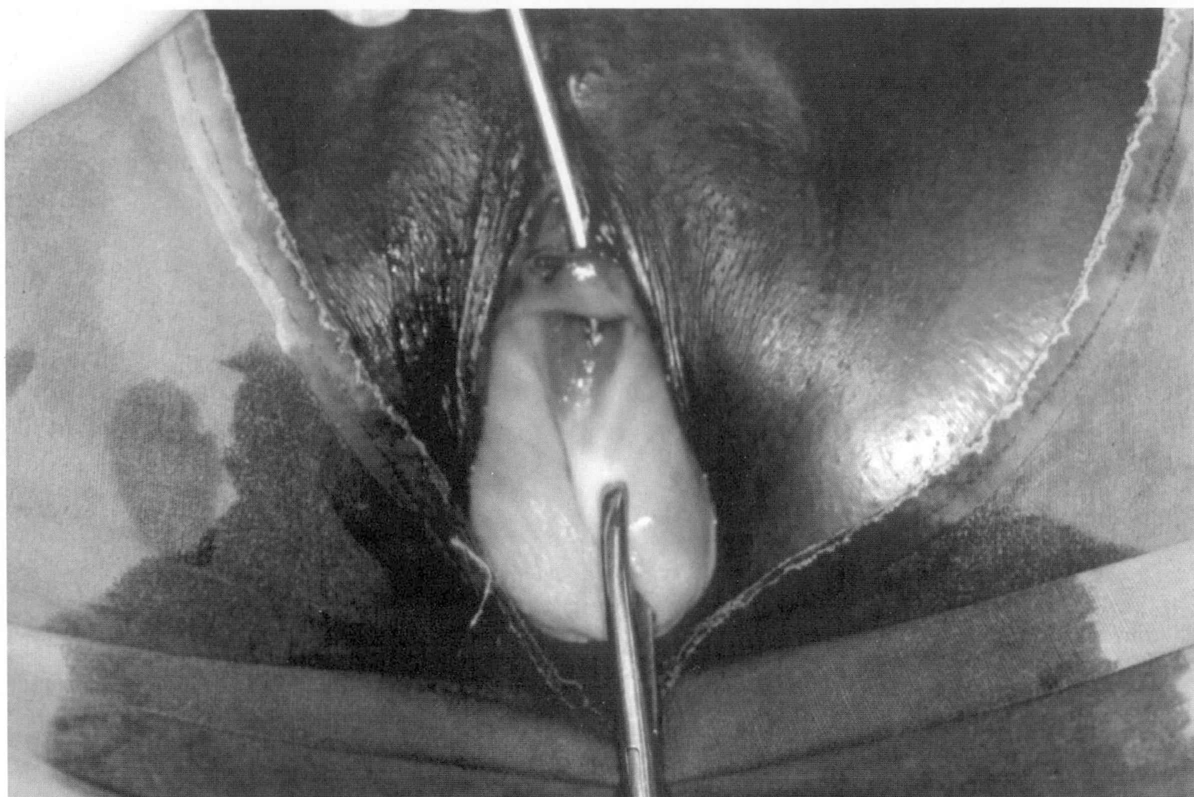

Figure 4.4 Circumferential obstetric urethrovaginal fistula. The bladder neck is completely detached from the bladder base.

weeks gestation > 40% report significant stress urinary leakage at least once a week[53,54] (Fig. 4.5). The incidence of ongoing urinary incontinence at 6–8 weeks postpartum is comparable to that in the third trimester.[53] Over 50% of women recover in the early puerperium, with only 15% reporting persistent urinary incontinence at 3 months.[53,54] Voiding dysfunction occurs to some degree in 10–15% postpartum patients.[56] The incidence of self-reported urinary incontinence is low following delivery with only 8% women presenting for postpartum assessment and treatment.[56]

The most important obstetric risk factors for postpartum urinary incontinence are first vaginal delivery, prolonged second stage, forceps delivery, episiotomy, third degree perineal injury and fetal weight over 4 kg.[1,2,5] Age over 30 years at first delivery, increased BMI exceeding 30 and cigarette smoking are also significant independent risk factors. Epidural analgesia increases the likelihood of postpartum voiding difficulty.[55,57,58] First cesarean delivery reduces the risk of genuine stress incontinence, but cumulative cesarean delivery leads to an increased incidence of urge urinary incontinence.[28,57] In contrast, the incidence of urinary incontinence is not increased with cumulative vaginal deliveries.[59,60]

One of the most significant and often unrecognized problems following third degree perineal injury is stress urinary incontinence,[59] a problem which is identified in 50% women with fecal incontinence following primary repair of recognized obstetric anal sphincter injury and 32% women have persistent urinary incontinence 2–4 years postpartum. The risk of urinary incontinence is related to the extent of anal sphincter injury and is significantly increased with full thickness disruption.[59]

In contrast to anal incontinence, the association between urinary incontinence and childbirth has been less well studied, although a similar neuromuscular mechanism has been implicated. In part, this is due to the fact that trauma to the urethra and bladder is less obvious during labor and delivery. In addition, the neuromuscular function of the intrinsic and extrinsic urethral musculature is more difficult to evaluate and there are no current published studies describing urodynamic evaluation in pregnancy or the early postpartum period.[58]

The mechanism of urinary incontinence in pregnancy remains unclear, but may be due to a combination of endocrine and mechanical factors. While changes in circulating progesterone levels may result in reduced

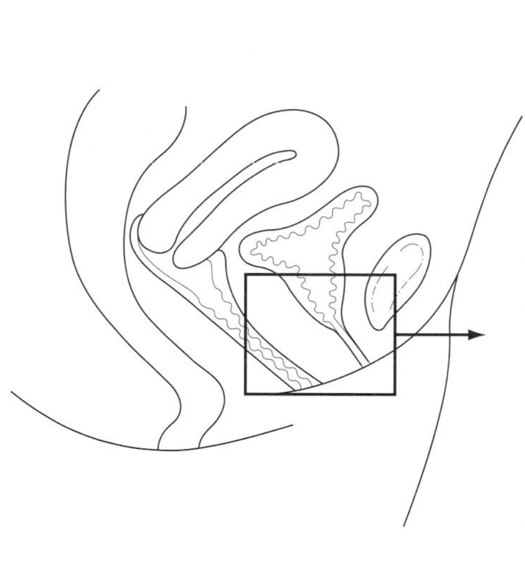

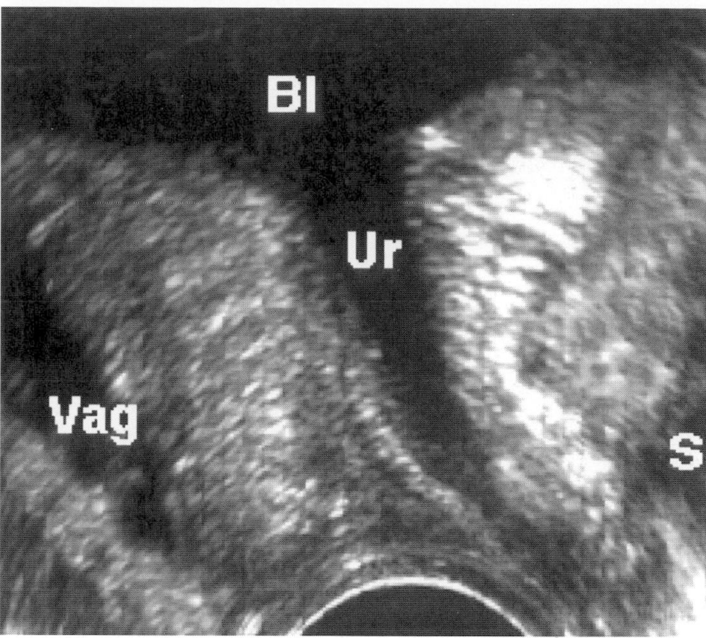

Figure 4.5 Translabial ultrasound demonstrating loss of angulation of the bladder neck secondary to disruption of the pubourethral ligament and bladder neck patency in association with genuine stress incontinence following vaginal delivery.

ureteric peristalsis predisposing to stasis, increased circulating relaxin levels and subsequent pelvic floor remodelling may increase the risk of stress urinary incontinence symptoms. In addition, mechanical factors may increase the risk of stress urinary incontinence in the second trimester but predispose to voiding difficulty and detrusor instability as the base of the bladder is drawn up into the abdominal cavity with advancing gestation. Further prospective studies are required to evaluate the mechanisms of urinary incontinence in pregnancy and postpartum.

All women should be questioned regarding altered urinary incontinence symptoms at their postnatal visit. Pelvic floor exercise therapy and sensory biofeedback therapy using vaginal cones are associated with significant improvement or resolution of symptoms in over 70% of urinary incontinent patients in the first 6 months postpartum.[60] For those with loss of proprioceptive awareness and an inability to target and contract the pelvic floor muscles, electrical stimulation and biofeedback therapy may be appropriate at this stage. Urodynamic assessment should be offered to women with significant urinary incontinence persisting for 6 months after delivery. Surgical intervention can be offered when persistent significant stress urinary incontinence is supported by urodynamic evaluation and where conservative treatment has failed.

While over 100 procedures have been described for the management of stress urinary incontinence, the Burch colposuspension remains the procedure of choice (Fig. 4.6). This operation is associated with an 85% continence rate at 10 years and will also correct coexistent anterior vaginal wall prolapse, it may be performed through an open or laparoscopic incision. While several new continence procedures have been described recently, including the tension-free vaginal tape (TVT) involving placement of a trans-vaginal polypropylene mesh, these interventions require further long-term evaluation before they are routinely adopted. Women who have undergone successful surgical correction of incontinence should subsequently be delivered by elective cesarean section because further vaginal delivery increases the risk of recurrence.

FECAL INCONTINENCE

Several investigations have evaluated the prevalence of fecal incontinence following childbirth.[31,32,63] MacArthur *et al.* (1997) surveyed 1667 postpartum women by postal questionnaire, of whom 906 responded and agreed to be interviewed. In this cohort, 4% reported new symptoms of altered fecal continence after delivery, of whom only 14% had spontaneously consulted a doctor about these symptoms.[32] Similarly, Ryhammer *et al.* (1995) interviewed a cohort of 242 women postpartum and found that 5% had developed frank fecal incontinence.[62] Neither of these postnatal surveys included specific questions regarding loss of flatal control. Symptoms of passive incontinence, however, are more common post-

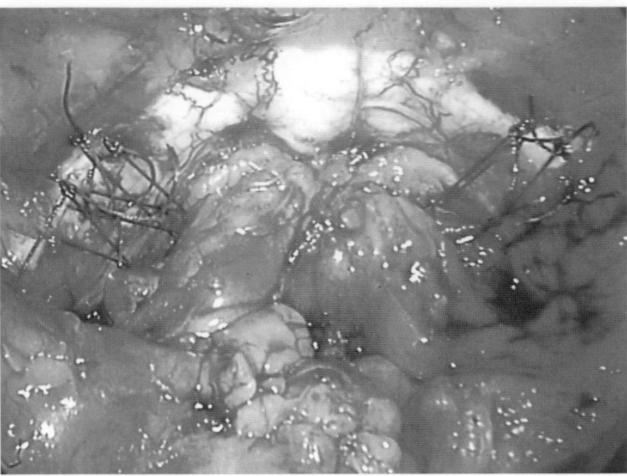

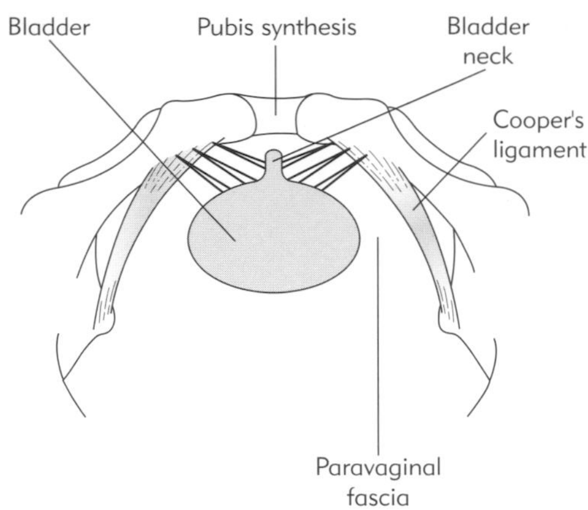

Figure 4.6 Laparoscopic Burch colposuspension demonstrating re-attachment of the paravaginal fascial to the iliopectineal ligament on both sides for the correction of genuine stress incontinence and cystocele. PS: public symphysis; BN: bladder neck; B: bladder; CL: Cooper's iliopectineal ligament; PVF: paravaginal fascia.

partum and relate to the loss of control of liquid stool and flatus. While passive fecal incontinence symptoms have been described as 'minor incontinence', they may prove socially very embarrassing and cause profound psychosexual difficulties. Zetterstrom *et al.* (1999) surveyed 349 primiparous women by postpartum questionnaire and reported episodic frank fecal incontinence in 1% and reduced flatal control in 26% at 9 months following delivery.[30] As stated above, two large prospective investigations have evaluated both the mechanism of anal sphincter injury during childbirth and the incidence of altered fecal continence symptoms postpartum.[17,20] In a cohort of 184 primiparous women, Donnelly *et al.* (1998) reported altered fecal continence in 25% women 6 weeks following first vaginal delivery,[20] while Sultan *et al.* (1993) identified altered fecal continence in 13% of primiparous and 23% multiparous women 6 weeks following vaginal delivery;[17] both concluded that mechanical disruption of the anal sphincter muscles or combined nerve and muscle injury was the predominant mode of injury.

PERINEAL DESCENT SYNDROME AND UTEROVAGINAL PROLAPSE

Perineal descent and vaginal laxity are common findings in women following vaginal delivery and may persist for several months. These changes may be asymptomatic or associated with dragging perineal discomfort. Defecatory difficulty and constipation are commonly associated symptoms, together with an inability to target or localize the pelvic floor muscles and a reduction in vaginal sensation.[62,63] This syndrome is rarely identified in nulliparous women or following elective cesarean section.

It is estimated that 50% of women have some degree of genital prolapse, of whom 10–20% are symptomatic and this increases with age.[64] Uterovaginal prolapse is one of the most common benign gynecological conditions requiring surgical correction and accounts for more than 60% of all gynecological surgical procedures in elderly women.[65] The incidence of hospital admission for uterovaginal prolapse is 2 per 1000 person years of risk.[66] The condition demonstrates a 30% familial concordance and other risk factors include parity, obesity, chronic cough, constipation and defecatory difficulty. In contrast to incontinence, forceps delivery, episiotomy and birthweight are not independent risk factors.[66,67]

The pathogenesis of prolapse is related to disruption of the fascial supports of the uterus and vagina during childbirth, mechanical or neurological injury to the pelvic floor muscles and disruption or denervation of vaginal smooth muscle.[62,68] Fascial defects commonly occur in mid-anterior or posterior vaginal walls, resulting in cystocele or rectocele formation. Multiple fascial defects are common, however, and lateral detachment of the vaginal wall from the arcus tendineus is often associated with significant vaginal prolapse. Defecatory difficulty and straining in the presence of pudendal nerve injury or rectocele may result in further traction on the pudendal nerves and cumulative neurological injury.[62]

In addition, vaginal dissection during prolapse surgery has been demonstrated to be associated with postoperative electromyographic changes (EMG). Recurrence following prolapse surgery is high.[70] Aging leads to further denervation and loss of mechanical pelvic floor support. It is not clear why some parous women are predisposed to symptomatic prolapse and incontinence, but differences in connective tissue metabolism may be a contributory factor. A reduction in cellularity and increase in collagen fibers has been identified in 70% of women with uterovaginal prolapse, compared with 20% of controls.[70,71] Further research is required to evaluate the role of connective tissue changes on the development of pelvic floor prolapse and the influence of pudendal nerve injury on outcome following prolapse surgery and risk of recurrence.

DEFECATORY DIFFICULTY AND CONSTIPATION

Constipation and defecatory difficulty are common problems reported during pregnancy. The pathogenesis in pregnancy may be related to changes in colonic motility due to the effect of increased circulating progesterone levels. In advanced pregnancy the mechanical effects of an enlarged uterus and pelvic floor remodeling may also contribute to defecatory straining.[72] Constipation in pregnancy is more common in multiparous compared with nulliparous women. Marshall *et al.* (1999) reported constipation in 26% of primiparous women compared with 42% of multiparous subjects.[8] The common use of postpartum codeine-based analgesia may also exacerbate this problem and this may be a particular problem in the management of women following primary repair of obstetric anal sphincter injury.

PERINEAL PAIN AND DYSPAREUNIA

Sleep *et al.* (1987) reported significant perineal pain in 8% women at 3 months following normal vaginal delivery[44] and other investigators have reported comparable rates of perineal pain in postpartum women.[32,56] Sleep *et al.* noted an overall rate of dyspareunia in 15% of women at 3 years postpartum.[44] Routine use of episiotomy is one of the most common factors associated with postpartum perineal morbidity.[16] Choice of suture material may be an important factor and polyglycolic acid sutures are effective in reducing postpartum pain and dyspareunia. Wound edema is common within the first 24 hours after delivery and the use of a subcuticular suture can reduce discomfort. Careful postnatal assessment should be carried out to exclude infection, hematoma and granulation tissue formation, which may be overlooked with the practice of early postnatal discharge.

Protracted breastfeeding may lead to significant atrophy of the genital tract and cause dyspareunia. It is effectively treated using topical estrogen therapy. Significant perineal pain in the early puerperium in the absence of infection may be successfully treated with local pulsed laser therapy or ultrasound. Persistent postnatal perineal pain associated with defined scar tissue may benefit from local injection combining a corticosteroid with hyaluronidase and local anesthesia. Rarely, perineal reconstruction and vaginoplasty are required for patients with severe scarring and/or vaginal stenosis following childbirth. When extensive, these procedures may be performed using a levator flap advancement technique or donor fascial allograft. Vaginal dilators may be required for a short term postoperatively. The importance of early recognition and treatment of significant perineal pain and dyspareunia cannot be overemphasized. Left untreated, these problems may lead to significant postnatal depressive symptoms and long-term psychosexual difficulties.

NEUROMODULATION AND BIOFEEDBACK THERAPY

The management of obstetric-related incontinence has been problematic, with an expectant approach often adopted. For patients with frank incontinence and demonstrable external anal sphincter defects, early surgical repair is indicated. Dietary manipulation using a low-residue diet to reduce the amount of fluid in the stool and anti-diarrheal agents, also plays an important role.

Conservative management has traditionally been recommended for postpartum fecal and urinary incontinence. Kegel first described the effects of pelvic floor exercises on stress urinary incontinence postpartum.[74] While Kegel exercises are frequently requested for postpartum urinary and fecal incontinence, the response to therapy has been demonstrably poor.[75,76]

Biofeedback therapy is a behavioral technique using external equipment to demonstrate and alter physiological events using auditory or visual feedback. Conventional postpartum sensory biofeedback therapy for the treatment of fecal incontinence combines standard Kegel exercises with a sensory feedback signal, employing either a perineometer or vaginal cones.[60] Biofeedback improves urinary and fecal incontinence symptoms subjectively[60,66] but no changes have been demonstrable in anal canal pressures as detected by manometry. The differential response in subjective versus objective outcome measures highlights the subjectivity of continence scores and illustrates the complexity of the continence mechanism, in which psychological factors play an important role in determining symptom severity.

The ability to target damaged muscle and initiate a minimal voluntary contraction is a prerequisite for effective biofeedback training.[60] Women with postpartum incontinence frequently have difficulty in initiating and coordinating voluntary contraction of the pelvic floor muscles. This difficulty may be secondary to a loss of cortical awareness following vaginal delivery, in addition to neuromuscular injury.[75,76]

Electrical stimulation has been shown to be associated with significant improvement in urinary continence scores following treatment.[60] Combined biofeedback and electrical stimulation using an endo-anal probe leads to both subjective symptom improvement and objective improvement in anal canal pressures over a 3-month treatment period.[60] Combined therapy may be of particular benefit in women with obstetric neuromuscular injury. Electrical stimulation may inhibit further muscle atrophy and biofeedback may enhance neuromuscular re-education, thus helping to preserve and augment anal sphincter function and fecal continence.

While surgical repair remains the primary treatment for those women with extensive anatomical injury, augmented biofeedback training may be used as an adjunct to surgery. In less severe injuries, augmented biofeedback may improve fecal continence and co-ordination of pelvic floor muscle activity.

CUMULATIVE VAGINAL DELIVERY

Two large prospective investigations have assessed risk factors for fecal incontinence after a second vaginal delivery. Fynes *et al.* (1999) reported that women with transient fecal incontinence or 'occult' anal sphincter defects after first vaginal delivery were at significant risk of developing sustained fecal incontinence following second vaginal delivery.[21] In this study, the greatest risk factor for mechanical anal sphincter injury was first vaginal delivery. In contrast, second vaginal delivery was associated with an increase in pudendal nerve injury, as evidenced by prolongation of PNTML values. These data support Snooks *et al.* hypothesis (1984 and 1990) that successive vaginal delivery is associated with an increased incidence of pudendal nerve injury.[18,19]

Fynes *et al.* also identified full thickness anal sphincter disruption following first vaginal delivery as the most significant risk factor for altered fecal continence. Women with full thickness occult anal sphincter disruption had higher risk of developing new symptoms of altered fecal continence with second vaginal delivery.[21] In addition, all women with persistent symptoms of fecal incontinence following first vaginal delivery deteriorated with subsequent vaginal delivery and 42% of those with transient symptoms following first delivery recurred with second vaginal delivery.[21] Bek *et al.* (1992) found that transient incontinence after a recognized anal sphincter tear during first delivery led to a 7% risk of persistent fecal incontinence following second vaginal delivery.[24] Haadem *et al.* also reported that symptoms of fecal incontinence may persist up to 20 years following obstetric anal sphincter rupture.[26]

THE MENOPAUSE

Although the menopause is considered a risk factor for urinary incontinence, the prevalence of incontinence symptoms is not increased in the perimenopausal period. Oral estrogen therapy confers no short-term continence benefit and is associated with a consistent increase in stress urinary incontinence in women aged over 60 years.[59] This apparent lack of benefit may be related to the progestagen component of current HRT regimens. Further research is required to evaluate the dose-related effect, if any, of estrogen therapy alone and the relative influence of progestagens on the urinary continence mechanism. Estrogen therapy has been demonstrated to have a beneficial effect with regard to a reduction in recurrent urinary tract infection and sensory urgency symptoms associated with genital tract atrophy.[78]

Similarly, the onset of the menopause is recognized as a significant predisposing factor to the development of altered fecal continence in women, an effect related to estrogen withdrawal.[79] Estrogen receptors have been identified in significantly greater numbers in the external anal sphincter muscle compared with the rectus sheath of premenopausal women, compared to male controls.[80] One small prospective observational study has demonstrated significant subjective improvement in fecal incontinence symptoms and an objective increase in anal canal pressures in postmenopausal women following 6 months estrogen therapy.[80,81] Further research is required to evaluate the role of estrogen therapy in postmenopausal fecal incontinence as part of a prospective randomized controlled trial.

PELVIC FLOOR DYSFUNCTION AND AGING

The elderly comprise the most rapidly enlarging sector of the population in western societies, with an 18% increase in those aged over 75 years expected in the next two decades. Twelve percent of women greater than 65 years complain of urinary incontinence compared with 9% of those less than 65 years of age. The female to male prevalence ratio is 8:1.[82,83] Although almost half complain of a significant impact on their daily activities, less than 40% present for evaluation and treatment.[83] Similarly, the prevalence of fecal incontinence is between 9 and 17% in women aged over 75 years. The onset of fecal or urinary incontinence is also frequently cited as the reason why families seek permanent residential placement of an elderly relative and is believed to affect almost 35% of women in permanent psychogeriatric care.[82,84] The female to male predominance in the prevalence data is attributed to the cumulative effects of aging estrogen deficiency and pre-existing obstetric anal sphincter injury and pelvic floor dysfunction.

PREVENTION OF OBSTETRIC PELVIC FLOOR INJURY AND INCONTINENCE

Fecal incontinence predominantly affects parous women. Physicians should be aware that their patients will often not volunteer these symptoms unless specifically asked. The most significant risk for mechanical injury to the anal sphincter mechanism is first vaginal delivery and the risk of mechanical anal sphincter injury is increased in the presence of recognized third degree perineal injury and instrumental delivery. Multiparous vaginal delivery may be associated with cumulative injury to the pudendal nerve while other specific risk factors for pudendal nerve injury include prolonged second stage of labor and instrumental delivery.

Every effort should be made to ensure a normal vaginal delivery through the active management of labor by experienced midwives and obstetricians. Skill is needed to avoid prolonged second stage of labor without increasing the instrumental delivery rate. When instrumental delivery is indicated, expertise in the use of both the forceps and vacuum extraction is necessary to minimize the risk of sphincter injury. Consideration of emergency cesarean section may be necessary if the delivery is likely to be particularly difficult.

Appropriate use of episiotomy is important and the ideal episiotomy rate appears to lie between 20% and 30%. Higher rates do not appear to confer any advantage and lower rates have been demonstrated to increase perineal morbidity. A right mediolateral incision is preferable to a midline episiotomy, which is associated with a higher rate of extension into the anal sphincter muscles and should be avoided. Adequate training of obstetric personnel is needed in the recognition of anal sphincter disruption when it occurs because currently many cases are missed. Perineal repair should be performed using an appropriate technique and suture material. Third degree perineal tears should be repaired by experienced senior obstetric personnel only. Direct opposition of the sphincter may be equally as good as an overlapping technique, although further evaluation is required to assess the functional outcome. The perineum should be inspected carefully in the postnatal period and early treatment instituted for patients with poor healing or anatomical distortion.

All women should be specifically questioned with regard to dysfunctional pelvic floor symptoms and altered fecal and urinary continence at their postnatal visit. Those who have undergone primary repair of a recognized third degree tear should be reviewed in a dedicated clinic in which detailed clinical and physiological assessment is available for women with altered urinary or fecal continence in the early postpartum period. Dietary manipulation and anti-diarrheal agents play an important role. Care should be taken to avoid protracted postpartum straining at defecation, because this may exacerbate pudendal nerve injury and predispose to other pelvic floor problems.

Electrical stimulation and biofeedback therapy are appropriate for patients who have loss of proprioceptive awareness of the pelvic floor muscles. Success with conservative treatment is excellent, with over 70% women demonstrating symptomatic improvement during the first 6 months postpartum. Persistent fecal incontinence symptoms in the presence of a significant anal sphincter defect require a delayed overlapping anal sphincter repair which offers an improved functional outcome in excess of 80% cases. The presence of pudendal nerve injury appears to constitute a poor prognostic factor for outcome. Adequate counseling should be provided regarding the risks of subsequent vaginal delivery and an informed choice made with regard to mode of further delivery in women with identifiable continence difficulties.

Women with persistent symptoms of fecal incontinence or who have undergone surgery for fecal or urinary incontinence should undergo elective cesarean delivery in subsequent pregnancy. There is no justification for a policy of cesarean section for every woman with a history of sphincter injury, as repeated cesarean delivery merely increases other forms of maternal morbidity. Aging and the menopause may effect deterioration in pre-existing continence symptoms or result in the onset of new symptoms superimposed on pre-existing occult childbirth injury. Estrogen replacement can offer significant improvement in postmenopausal with fecal incontinence symptoms.

REFERENCES

1. Kamm MA. Reproductive hormones and motility. *Motility* 1991;**14**:12–14.
2. Singh S, Poulson P, Hanby A, Wright NA, Sheppard MC, Langman MJS. Expression of oestrogen receptors and an oestrogen induced protein in large bowel mucosa and cancers. *Gut* 1992;33:34.
3. Knudsen UB, Laurberg S, Danielson CC. Influence of bilateral oopherectomy and estrogen substitution on the striated anal sphincter in adult female rats. *Scand J Gastroenterol* 1991;**26**:731–36.
4. Donaldson A, Nicolini U, Symes EK, Rodeck CH, Tannirandorn Y. Changes in concentration of cortisol, dehydroepiandrosterone sulphate and progesterone in fetal and maternal serum during pregnancy. *Clin Endocrinol* 1991;**35(5)**447–51.
5. Ganiban G, Besselman D, Harcelrode J, Murthy SNS. Effect of sex steroids on total gastrointestinal transit in male rats. *Gastroenterology* 1985;**88**:1713.
6. Hey VMF, Cowley DJ, Ganguli PC, Skinner LD, Ostick DJ, Sharp DS. Gastro-oesophageal reflux in late pregnancy. *Anesthesia* 1977;**32**:372–7.
7. Kamm MA, Farthing MJG, Lennard-Jones JE. Bowel function and transit rates during the menstrual cycle. *Gut* 1989;**30**:605–608.
8. Marshall K, Thompson KA, Walsh DM, Baxter GD. Incidence of urinary incontinence and constipation during pregnancy and postpartum: survey of current findings at

the Rotunda Lying-in Hospital. *Br J Obstet Gynaecol* 1998;**105**:400–402.

9. Sultan AH, Kamm MA, Hudson CN, Bartram CL. Effect of pregnancy on anal sphincter morphology and function. *Int J Colorect Dis* 1993;**8**:206–209.
10. Fynes M, Donnelly V, O'Connell PR, O'Herlihy C. Caesarean delivery and anal sphincter injury. *Obstet Gynaecol* 1998;**92**:496–500.
11. Van Geelen JM, Doesberg WH, Thomas CMG, Martin CB. Urodynamic studies in the normal menstrual cycle. The relationship between hormonal changes in the menstrual cycle and urethral pressure profiles. *Am J Obstet Gynecol* 1981;**141**:384–92.
12. Tapp AJS, Cardozo LD. The postmenopausal bladder. Br J Hosp Med. 1986;**35**:20–2.
13. Youseff AF. Cystometric studies in gynecology and obstetrics. *Obstet Gynecol* 1956;**3**:181–8.
14. Lepert PC. Anatomy and physiology of cervical ripening. *Clin Obstet Gynecol* 1995;**38**:267–79.
15. Kelly RD. Pregnancy maintenance and parturition: the role of prostaglandin in manipulating the immune and inflammatory response. *Endocr Rev* 1994;**15**:684–706.
16. Kamm MA. Obstetric damage and faecal incontinence. *Lancet* 1994;**344**:730–733.
17. Sultan A, Kamm M, Hudson C, Thomas J, Bartram C. Anal sphincter disruption during vaginal delivery. *N Eng J Med* 1993;**329**:1905–11.
18. Snooks SJ, Swash M, Setchell M, Henry MM. Injury to innervation of pelvic floor sphincter musculature in childbirth. *Lancet* 1984;**ii**:546–50.
19. Snooks SJ, Swash M, Mathers SE, Henry MM. Effect of vaginal delivery on the pelvic floor: a five year follow-up. *Br J Surg* 1990;**77**:1358–60.
20. Donnelly V, Fynes M, Campbell D, Johnson H, O'Connell PR, O'Herlihy C. Obstetric events leading to anal sphincter damage. *Obstet Gynaecol* 1998;**92**:955–961.
21. Fynes M, Donnelly V, O'Connell PR, O'Herlihy C. The effect of second vaginal delivery on anal sphincter function and faecal continence: a prospective study. *Lancet* 1999;**354**:983–6.
22. Rieger N, Schloithe A, Saccone G, Wattchow D. A prospective study of anal sphincter injury due to childbirth. *Scand J Gastroenterol* 1998;**33**:950–55.
23. Deen KI, Kumar D, Williams JG, Olliff J, Keighley MRB. The prevalence of anal sphincter defects in faecal incontinence: A prospective endosonic study. *Gut* 1993;**34**:685–8.
24. Bek KM, Laurberg S. Risks of anal incontinence from subsequent vaginal delivery after a complete obstetric anal sphincter tear. *Br J Obstet Gynaecol* 1992;**99**:724–6.
25. Crawford L, Quint E, Pearl M, De Lancey J, Incontinence following rupture of the anal sphincter during delivery. *Obstet Gynecol* 1993;**82**:527–31.
26. Haadem K, Gudmundsson S. Can women with intrapartum rupture of anal sphincter still suffer after-effects two decades later? *Acta Obstet Gynecol Scand* 1997;**76**:601–603.
27. Wood J, Amos L, Rieger N. Third degree anal sphincter tears: risk factors and outcome. *Aus NZ J Obstet Gynaecol* 1998;**38**:414–17.
28. Tetzschner T, Sorensen M, Lose G, Christiansen J, Anal and urinary incontinence in women with obstetric anal sphincter rupture. *Br J Obstet Gynaecol* 1996;**103**:1034–40.
29. Sultan AH, Johannson RB, Carter JE. Occult anal sphincter trauma following randomized forceps and vacuum delivery. *Int J Gynecol Obstet* 1998;**61**:113–19.
30. Sultan AH, Kamm MA, Bartram CI, Hudson CN. Anal sphincter trauma during instrumental delivery. *Int J Gynecol Obstet* 1993;**43**:263–70.
31. Zetterstrom J, Lopez A, Anzen B, Dolk A, Norman M, Mellgren A. Anal incontinence after vaginal delivery: a prospective study in primiparous women. *Br J Obstet Gynaecol* 1999;**106**:324–30.
32. MacArthur C, Bick DE, Keighley MRB. Faecal incontinence after childbirth. *Br J Obstet Gynaecol* 1997;**104**:46–50.
33. Fitzpatrick M, Fynes M, Cassidy M, Behan M, O'Connell PR, O'Herlihy C. Prospective study of the influence of parity and operative technique on the outcome of primary anal sphincter repair following obstetric injury. *Eur J Obstet Gynecol Reprod Biol* 2000;**89**:159–63.
34. Enkin M, Keirse MJNC, Chalmers I. *A guide to effective care in pregnancy and childbirth.* Oxford: Oxford University Press, 1994:221 pp.
35. Alexander JM, Lucas MJ, Ramin SM, McIntire DD, Leveno KJ. The course of labor with and without epidural analgesia. *Am J Obstet Gynecol* 1998;**178**:516–20.
36. Poen AC, Felt-Bersma RJF, Dekker GA, Deville W, Cuesta MA, Meuwissen SGM. Third degree obstetric perineal tears: risk factors and the preventive role of mediolateral episiotomy. *Br J Obstet Gynaecol* 1997;**104**:563–6.
37. Robinson JN, Norwitz ER, Cohen AP, McElrath TF, Lieberman ES. Epidural analgesia and third or fourth degree lacerations in nulliparas. *Obstet Gynecol* 1999; **94**:259–62.
38. Sultan AH, Kamm MA, Hudson CN, Bartram CI. Third degree obstetric anal sphincter tears: risk factors and outcome of primary repair. *BMJ* 1994;**38**:887–91.
39. Johanson RB, Rice C, Doyle M, *et al.* A randomized prospective study comparing the new vacuum extractor policy with forceps delivery. *Br J Obstet Gynaecol* 1993;**100**:524–30.
40. Signorello LB, Harlow BL, Chekos AK, Repke JT. Midline episiotomy and anal incontinence: retrospective cohort study. *B M J* 2000,**320**:8:86–90.
41. Sultan AH, Monga AK, Kumar D, Stanton SL. Primary repair of obstetric anal sphincter rupture using the overlap technique. *Br J Obstet Gynaecol* 1999;**106**:318–23.
42. Thacker SB, Banta DH. Benefits and risks of episiotomy: an interpretive review of the English language literature 1860–1980. *Obstet Gynecol Surv* 1983;**38**:322–38.
43. Wooley RJ. Benefits and risks of episiotomy: a review of the English language literature since 1980. *Obstet Gynecol Surv* 1991;**50**:806–35.
44. Sleep J, Grant A. West Berkshire perineal management trial: three year follow-up. *B M J* 1987;749–51.
45. Elkins TE. Fistula surgery: past, present and future directions. *Int Urogynecol J* 1997; **8**:30–35.
46. Hilton P, Ward A. Epidemiological and surgical aspects of urogenital fistulae: a review of 25 years' experience in southeast Nigeria. *Int Urogynecol J* 1998;**9**:189–94.

47. Danso KO, Martey JO, Wall LL, Elkins TE. The epidemiology of genitourinary fistulae in Kumasi, Ghana, 1997-1992. *Int Urogynecol J* 1996;**7**:117–20.
48. Goh JT. Genital tract fistula repair on 116 women. *Aust NZ J Obstet Gynaecol* 1998; **38**:158–61.
49. Murray C, Fynes M, Goh J, Carey M. A prospective observational study of the outcome following delayed primary repair of obstetric genital fistula at a fistula hospital. *Br J Obstet Gynaecol* (in press).
50. Ventkatesh KS, Ramanujau PS, Larson DM. Anorectal complications of delivery. *Dis Colon Rectum* 1989;**32**:1039–41.
51. Beynon CL. Midline episiotomy as a routine procedure. *J Obstet Gynecol Commonwealth* 1974;**81**:126–30.
52. Laurberg S, Swash M, Henry MM. Delayed external sphincter repair for obstetric tear. *Br J Surg* 1988;**75**:786–8.
53. Chaliha C, Kahia V, Stanton SL, Monga A, Sultan AH. Antenatal prediction of postpartum urinary and fecal incontinence. *Obstet Gynecol* 1999;**84**:689–94.
54. Morkved S, Bo K. Prevalence of urinary incontinence during pregnancy and postpartum. *Int Urogynecol J* 1999;**10**:394–8.
55. Sand PK, Bowen IW, Ostergard DR. Urinary tract in pregnancy. Gynecological urology and urodynamics: theory and practice 1985; p. 283.
56. Glazener CMA, Abdalla M, Stroud P, Naji S, Templeton *et al.* Postnatal maternal morbidity: extent, causes, prevention and treatment. *Br J Obstet Gynaecol* 1995;**103**:282–7.
57. Viktrup L, Lose G, Rolff M, Varfoed K. The symptom of stress incontinence caused by pregnancy or delivery in primiparas. *Obstet Gynecol* 1992;**79**:945–9.
58. Handa VL, Harris TA, Ostergard DR. Protecting the pelvic floor: obstetric management to prevent incontinence and pelvic organ prolapse. *Obstet Gynecol* 1996;**88**:470–78.
59. Thom DH, Brown JS. Reproductive and hormonal risk factors for urinary incontinence in later life: a review of the clinical and epidemiological literature. *J Am Geriat Soc* 1998;**46**:1411–17.
60. Fynes M, Marshall K, Cassidy M, Behan M, O'Connell PR, O'Herlihy C. A randomised controlled trial of the effect of biofeedback therapy on anorectal physiology and faecal continence. *Dis Colon Rectum* 1999;**42**:753–8.
61. Ryhammer AM, Bek KM, Laurberg S. Multiple vaginal deliveries increase the risk of permanent incontinence of flatus and urine in normal premenopausal women. *Dis Colon Rectum* 1995;**38**:1206–1209.
62. Snooks SJ, Barnes PRH, Swash M. Damage to the innervation of the voluntary anal and periurethral sphincter musculature in incontinence: an electrophysiological study. *J Neurol Neurosurg Psychiat* 1984;**47**:1269–73.
63. Snooks SJ, Swash M, Henry M. Electrophysiologic and manometric assessment of failed postnatal repair for anorectal incontinence. *Dis Colon Rectum* 1984;**27**:733–6.
64. Bek RP, Nordstrom L. A twenty-five year experience with 519 anterior colporrhaphy procedures. *Obstet Gynecol* 1991;**78**:1011–18.
65. Symmonds RE, Williams TJ, Lee RA, Webb MJ. Posthysterectomy enterocele and vaginal vault prolapse. *Am J Obstet Gynecol* 1981;**140**:852–9.
66. Mant J, Painter R, Vessey M. Epidemiology of genital prolapse: observations from the Oxford Family Planning Association study. *Br J Obstet Gynaecol* 1997;**104**: 579–85.
67. Chiaffarino F, Chateroud L, Dundelle M, *et al.* Reproductive factors, family history, occupation and risk of genital prolapse. *Eur J Obstet Gynecol Reprod Biol* 1999;**82**: 63–67.
68. Allen RE, Hosker GL, Smith ARB. Warrel DW. Pelvic floor damage and childbirth: a neurophysiological study. *Br J Obstet Gynaecol* 1990;**97**:770–79.
69. Benson JT. Neurophysiology of the female pelvic floor. *Curr Opin Obstet Gynecol* 1994;**6**:320–323.
70. Makinen J, Kahari VM, Soderstrom KO, *et al.* Collagen synthesis in the vaginal connective tissue of patients with and without uterine prolapse. *Eur J Obstet Gynecol Reprod Biol* 1987;**42**:319–25.
71. Makinen J, Soderstrom KO, Kiilholma P, Hirvonen T. Histological changes in the vaginal connective tissue of patients with and without uterine prolapse. *Arch Gynecol* 1986;**239**:17–20.
72. Brubaker L. Rectocele. *Curr Opin Obstet Gynecol* 1996;**8**:376–9.
73. Olah KS. Episiotomy repair-suture material and short-term morbidity. *J Obstet Gynecol* 1990;**10**:503–505.
74. Kegel AH. Physiological therapy for urinary stress incontinence. *JAMA* 1951;**146**: 915.
75. Bump RC, Glenn Hurt W, Fantl JL, Wymann JF. Assessment of Kegel pelvic muscle exercise performance after brief verbal instruction. *Am J Obstet Gynecol* 1991;**165**: 322–9.
76. Enck P. Biofeedback training in disordered defecation: a critical review. *Dig Dis Sci* 1993;**38**:1953–60.
77. Eriksen PS, Rasmussen H. Low dose 17B oestrodiol vaginal tablets in the treatment of atrophic vaginitis: a double-blinded placebo controlled study. *Euro J Obstet Gynecol Reprod Biol* 1992;**44**:137–44.
78. Parks AG. Anorectal incontinence. *Proc R Soc Med* 1975;**68**:681–90.
79. Haadem K, Ling L, Ferno M, Graffner H. Estrogen receptors in the external anal sphincter. *Am J Obstet Gynecol* 1991;**164**:609–610.
80. Donnelly V, O'Connell PR, O'Herlihy C. The influence of oestrogen replacement on faecal incontinence in postmenopausal women. *Br J Obstet Gynaecol* 1997; **104**:311–15.
81. Khullar V, Cardozo L. Incontinence in the elderly. *Curr Opin Obstet Gynecol* 1998; **10**:391–4.
82. Brocklehurst JC. Urinary incontinence in the community – analysis of a MORI poll. *B M J* 1993;**306**:832–4.
83. Kemp FM, Acheson RM. Care in the community; elderly people living alone at home. *Commun Med* 1989;**11**:21–26.
84. Kok AL, Voorhorst FJ, Burger CW, VanHouten P, Kenemans P, Janssens J. Urinary and fecal incontinence in community residing elderly women. *Age Aging* 1992; **21**:211–215.

Chapter 5

Colon, rectum, anus, anal sphincters and the pelvic floor

Tim A Cook, Neil Mortensen

Understanding normal continence mechanisms and the process of defecation together with changes that occur in disorders of these processes requires a basic knowledge of the anatomy, physiology and pharmacology of the organs involved. This chapter has a broad remit but sets out to discuss the anatomy and embryology of the colon, rectum and anus. Their blood supply and innervation will be covered and a description of the arrangement of enteric neural plexuses will be given. Finally the pharmacology of the internal anal sphincter (IAS) and the sensory innervation of the anal canal and rectum will be described.

ANATOMY OF THE COLON, RECTUM AND ANUS

The large intestine extends from the terminal ileum to the anus. It comprises the cecum, colon, rectum and anus. The colon is approximately 150 cm long although there is considerable variation between individuals. Its largest caliber is about 7.5 cm at the cecum from where it gradually diminishes as it passes distally to the junction of the sigmoid colon and rectum. The caliber of the rectum is much greater just above the anal canal.

In line with the rest of the gastrointestinal tract, the large bowel wall is made up of mucosa, submucosa, muscularis propria and, above the peritoneal reflection in the pelvis, of serosa. The smooth muscle coat (muscularis propria) is arranged in two layers; an inner circular layer and an outer longitudinal layer. In the cecum and colon, this longitudinal layer is concentrated in three bands which are equidistant from each other and are termed the taenia coli. The bowel wall between the taenia coli is thin and this may account for the great capacity of the colon and cecum to undergo distension. The taenia coli are shorter than the overall length of the colon and cause the circular muscle coat to be puckered with the production of typical haustral sacculations. The taenia extend from the base of the appendix at the cecum (the former has a complete longitudinal muscle coat) to the junction of the sigmoid colon and rectum at which point the three bands coalesce to form a complete longitudinal muscle coat in the rectum. With the exception of the appendix, cecum and rectum, the large intestine is peppered with peritoneum covered fatty projections called appendices epiploicae. These are most numerous along the taenia and are relatively flat in the right-sided colon but elongated and pedunculated in the sigmoid.

CECUM

There is considerable variation in the disposition of the colon between individuals, particularly in those portions with a mesocolon. The cecum lies in the right iliac fossa and is usually covered with peritoneum but in a small percentage of individuals this peritoneal covering is deficient and the cecum lies in direct contact with iliacus. The appendix projects from the lowest part of the cecum. The ileum opens into the large intestine through the ileocecal valve which is positioned medially and posteriorly. The valve consists of an upper and lower segment or lip which is semilunar in shape and projects into the cecum. The valve prevents reflux from the cecum into the ileum, but also acts as a sphincter to prevent rapid transit of ileal contents into the cecum. Barium enema studies frequently demonstrate an incompetent ileocecal valve in the absence of pathology.

ASCENDING COLON

The ascending colon is approximately 15 cm long and runs upward from the cecum to the hepatic flexure. It is invested with peritoneum on its anterior, medial and lateral sides, but posteriorly is devoid of peritoneal covering and as a consequence maintains a relatively fixed position. It usually lies in direct contact with iliacus, quadratus lumborum and the origin of the transversus abdominus below and the inferior pole of the right kidney above. Anteriorly it is related to the small intestine and the right edge of the greater omentum. Just below the right lobe of the liver, the colon turns sharply downwards and forwards to form the *hepatic flexure* and the transverse colon passes from this point across the abdomen to the left upper quadrant where it again curves acutely on itself to form the *splenic flexure*.

TRANSVERSE COLON

The transverse colon forms a loop that hangs down immediately below the stomach and is approximately 45 cm long. Proximally, it is related to the right kidney, second part of the duodenum and head of the pancreas on its posterior margin. The remainder of the transverse colon is completely invested in peritoneum and is connected to the inferior border of the pancreas and the lower pole of the left kidney by the transverse mesocolon which divides the abdominal cavity into supracolic and infracolic compartments. Loops of small bowel lie behind the transverse colon including the duodenojejunal flexure. Immediately above this part of the colon lies the stomach and, at its distal portion, the spleen. The greater omentum hangs down from the greater curve of the stomach in front of the transverse colon and is loosely attached to the colon and mesocolon. The splenic flexure is situated higher than the hepatic flexure. It is covered with peritoneum anteriorly but is in direct contact with the left kidney posteriorly. It is also connected to the diaphragm by a band of peritoneum termed the phrenicocolic ligament.

DESCENDING COLON

From the splenic flexure the large intestine becomes the descending colon and runs downwards between psoas and quadratus lumborum as far as the iliac crest, a distance of about 25 cm. On its anterior, medial and lateral aspects it is covered by peritoneum but posteriorly it lies in direct contact with the left kidney, quadratus lumborum, transversus abdominis, iliacus and psoas. The descending colon lies posteriorly in the abdominal cavity and like the ascending colon is relatively fixed in its position. At the iliac crest the colon turns medially and anteriorly in front of iliacus and psoas to become the sigmoid colon.

SIGMOID COLON

The sigmoid colon extends from the lower end of the descending colon to the upper end of the rectum. It forms a loop that varies greatly in its length but averages approximately 40 cm. It is completely surrounded by peritoneum which forms the mesocolon. The mesocolon diminishes in length from its centre to the ends of the loop such that the sigmoid colon is fixed at its junctions with the descending colon and rectum. The mesocolon has an inverted V-shaped attachment to the pelvic walls. The upper limb runs from the medial margin of the left psoas to the midline crossing the left ureter and iliac vessels. The lower limb extends vertically downwards in front of the sacrum. The central portion of the sigmoid colon enjoys a considerable range of movement and as a consequence its relationship with other structures is variable.

RECTUM

The junction of the sigmoid colon and rectum is usually at the level of the sacral promontory. The junction is distinguished by the loss of complete peritoneal covering, absence of a true mesocolon, absence of appendices epiploicae and divergence of the three taenia coli to form a continuous longitudinal muscle layer. The rectum is approximately 15–20 cm long and ends at the top of the anal canal. The upper third of the rectum is covered by peritoneum anteriorly and laterally. The middle third of the rectum is covered only anteriorly and the lower third has no covering as the peritoneum is reflected forward at the base on to the back of the seminal vesicles and bladder, or the vagina and uterus in the female, to form the rectovesical and recto-uterine pouch (of Douglas) respectively. The anterior peritoneal reflection lies approximately 8 cm from the perineal skin in men and 5–8 cm women. Full thickness rectal prolapse is associated with an abnormally deep rectovaginal pouch.

The rectum sits in the hollow anterior to the lower sacrum. The rectum thus passes downwards and posteriorly, then downwards and finally downwards and anteriorly before passing backwards and inferiorly to become the anal canal at the pelvic floor. The anorectal junction is situated 2–3 cm in front of and below the tip of the coccyx. The rectum also has lateral curves which vary in prominence. The upper and lower curves are convex to the right and the middle one concave to the left. The angulations of the rectum on the concave side of each of these curves is accentuated by three transverse mucosal folds (valves of Houston) which partially encircle the rectum.

Fascial relations of the extraperitoneal rectum

Behind the rectum lies the mesorectum containing blood vessels and lymphatics. This is loosely bound down to the front of the sacrum and coccyx by connective tissue. The mesorectum and rectum can be separated from the sacrum by sharp dissection and this is known as the *mesorectal plane*. Once mobilized, the mesorectum remains invested in a thin layer of fascia, the so-called fascia propria. The sacrum and coccyx are also covered in a thicker fascia which extends downwards and forwards on the upper aspect of the anococcygeal ligament and is known as the *fascia of Waldeyer*. As one extends laterally many texts describe fibrous condensations passing from the pelvic fascia on the side wall of the pelvis to the rectum. These lateral ligaments of the rectum contained the middle rectal arteries and were thought to provide support for the rectum. Their division was believed to be essential in the mobilization of the rectum from the pelvis. However, in recent years, many colorectal surgeons have questioned the existence of such clearly defined ligaments. In a recent study of 28 cadavers no connective tissue crossed from the side wall of the pelvis in ten cases. The remaining 18 pelves had only insubstantial connective tissue strands and only 17 middle rectal arteries were identified, always unilaterally. Fourteen of these vessels crossed from the pelvic side wall independent of any other structure.[1] Anteriorly, the rectum is covered with a layer of visceral pelvic fascia which extends from the anterior peritoneal reflection to the urogenital diaphragm. This condensation is called the *fascia of Denonvilliers* and lies between the rectum posteriorly and prostate and seminal vesicle or vagina anteriorly. Recent work has suggested that this is a poorly defined layer but nerves thought to be important in the control of bladder and erectile function and ejaculation have been identified in this fascia.[2]

ANAL CANAL

Historically descriptions of the anal canal have varied. Two definitions of the anal canal exist; a longer 'surgical' anal canal (approximately 4 cm) and a shorter (approximately 2 cm) 'embryological' one. The short anal canal is said to extend from the anal valves to the anal margin. This description is based on the belief that the anal valves and the pectinate or dentate line represent the site of breakdown of the cloacal membrane during development.

The longer anal canal extends from the level of the levator ani where the rectum passes backwards and inferiorly through the pelvic floor. This corresponds to the distal end of the dilated rectum and is also nearest the center of the region of highest intraluminal pressure. Active contraction of the puborectalis maintains the angle between the rectum and anal canal. In combination, these factors suggest that the long anal canal is at least useful as a physiological concept

Epithelial lining

The lining of the anal canal varies along its length due to its embryological derivation. The skin of the buttock is continuous with the anal margin and this continues to the level of the lower border of the internal anal sphincter. Histologically, the lining is stratified squamous keratinising epithelium containing hair follicles, sweat glands and sebaceous glands. Beyond this and extending up to the level of the anal glands, is a stratified squamous epithelium, which is non-keratinising and lacks hair follicles, sebaceous glands and sweat glands. Above this is the anal transition zone, which is an area of variable epithelial structure, with columnar and stratified squamous epithelium often being mixed. Fenger introduced a definition of the anal transition zone as 'the zone interposed between uninterrupted crypt bearing colorectal-type mucosa and uninterrupted squamous epithelium below'. In a study of 113 anal canals using alcian blue Fenger showed that the ATZ was generally located above the dentate line extending for an average of 9 mm.[3] In a few cases the ATZ extended below the dentate line. Using computer mapping, more recent data have suggested that the length of the anal transition zone may in fact be considerably shorter than first thought.[4] The top of the anal canal is lined with rectal mucosa-type columnar epithelium. The short ATZ has implications for the length of columnar epithelial cuff left following restorative proctocolectomy.

Vertical mucosal folds called anal columns are found in the upper anal canal. Each column contains a terminal radical of the superior rectal artery. The columns are joined together at their inferior margin by crescentic folds called the anal valves. The anal valves lie halfway along the anal canal and above each valve lies a pit or sinus. These are of surgical importance in the development of anal fistulae following infection in an anal sinus.

ANAL SPHINCTERS

Internal anal sphincter

The internal anal sphincter is continuous with the circular muscle coat of the rectum superiorly and ends with a well-defined rounded edge 6–8 mm above the anal margin. Muscle fibers have been shown to be grouped into discrete elliptical bundles that lie obliquely in the upper part of the sphincter with their transverse axis running internally and downwards giving them an imbricated arrangement. In the lower part of the sphincter the arrangement becomes more horizontal or even inclines slightly upwards.

Conjoint longitudinal muscle

The longitudinal muscle layer of the lower rectum becomes concentrated into anterior and posterior bands at the level of the pelvic floor. A few fibers connect these bands to the perineal body and coccyx. At the anorectal junction the longitudinal muscle blends with fibers of the pubococcygeus to form the conjoint longitudinal muscle layer. The main layer of longitudinal fibres lies between the internal and external sphincters. Traced downwards it breaks up opposite the lower border of the internal anal sphincter and fibrous septae fan out passing through the external anal sphincter ultimately attaching to the skin of the lower anal canal and perianal region.[5] An additional fine layer of longitudinal fibers has been identified in the submucosal layer. Fine and Lawes suggested that it was concentrated beneath the anal valves and called it the muscularis mucosae ani.[6] Parks[7] gave an alternative description suggesting that by means of a longitudinal band of fibers, which he termed the mucosal suspensory ligament, the lining of the anal canal was firmly attached to the underlying tissue. Goligher[8] however found no evidence of this suspensory ligament in his studies on the sphincters.

External anal sphincter

The external anal sphincter complex of muscles is derived from the posterior part of the cloacal sphincter. In the past the muscle has been divided into three parts; the subcutaneous part was regarded as a multifascicular ring of striated muscle with no anterior or posterior attachment. The superficial part was regarded as an elliptical muscle attached to the coccyx posteriorly and the deep part was thought to be intimately associated with the puborectalis.[5] The lower border of the external sphincter extends beyond the inferior margin of the internal sphincter to become subcutaneous. Its fibers are traversed by the fibrous extensions of the conjoint longitudinal layer. Oh and Kark[9] have emphasized differences between the male and female sphincters and have also pointed out that there are differences in arrangement of fibers in the anterior, posterior and lateral positions. Recent data using endoanal ultrasound have suggested a deficiency in the external sphincter at the upper end of the anal canal.[10]

Bogduk[11] has recently reviewed the anatomy of the external sphincter and emphasized the work of Shafik who suggested that the external sphincter is made up of a series of three loops.[12] The upper loop is made up if the external sphincter and puborectalis and its limbs are attached to the pubis. The middle loop is made up of the mid-portion of the sphincter and attached posteriorly to the coccyx. Other workers have suggested that, anteriorly, fibers decussate in the perineal body and can be traced into the bulbospongiosus and the deep transverse perinei.[11] The basal loop was thought to attach to the skin anterior to the anus but it was acknowledged that it contained some circumferential fibers. It is also penetrated by the tendinous fibers of the conjoint longitudinal layer. Figure 5.1 shows the arrangement of the external sphincter proposed by Bogduk[11] based on the observations from previous studies.

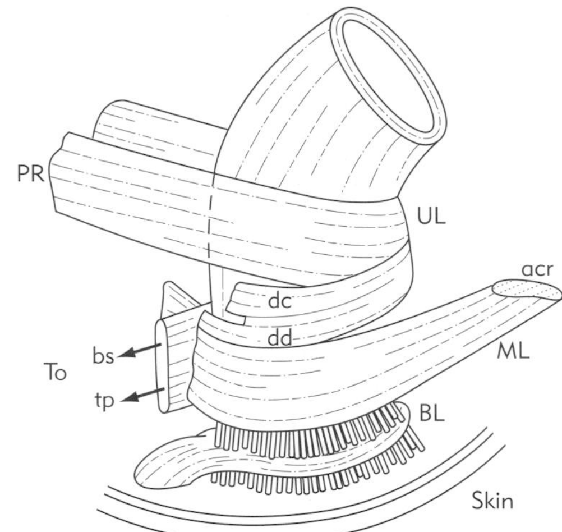

Figure 5.1 Arrangement of the fibers of the external anal sphincter (from Bogduk[11]). PR, puborectalis; UL, upper loop; dc, decussating fibers of puborectalis that blend with the longitudinal muscle of the rectum; dd, decussating fibers that join the perineal body; ML, middle loop; acr, anococcygeal raphe; bs, bulbospongiosus; tp, deep transverse perinei; BL, basal loop, perforated by fibers of the conjoint longitudinal layer.

PELVIC FLOOR

The pelvic floor is principally made up of a pair of compound muscular sheets, composed of predominantly striated muscle and usually referred to as the levator ani. The pelvic floor is defective in the midline where viscera pass through it. In front of the rectoanal flexure lies the *perineal body*. This is a complex fibromuscular wedge between the anal canal and urogenital viscera. Posterior to the rectoanal junction lies the anococcygeal body (also called the anococcygeal plate) which extends from the anal canal to the caudal part of the vertebral column. This body is made up of the presacral fascia, the anococcygeal ligament (the tendinous insertion of the pubococcygeus) which blends with the anococcygeal ligament, the midline attachment of iliococcygeus and most superficially, fibers of the puborectalis intermingling with the external sphincter which attaches to the coccyx.

Thompson[13] originally described three parts to the levator ani muscle based on their origin from a component of the pubic bone and referred to as pubo-, ilio- and ischiococcygeus. The peripheral attachment of the levator ani is a linear one extending from the body of the pubis to the ischial spine.

It is now more conventional to divide the muscle into four parts (Figure 5.2),[14] although ichiococcygeus is a rudimentary muscle in man and represents little more than the sacrospinous ligament. Puborectalis arises from the lower part of the back of the symphysis pubis and forms a loop around the recto-anal flexure. As previously noted, its fibers are closely associated with the deep part of the external sphincter and indeed on histological sectioning it is difficult to distinguish between the two. However, a more recent histological and clinical study has highlighted an anatomical plane of separation between the external sphincter and puborectalis.[15] It was proposed that this plane was important in the spread of suppurative anal lesions. Puborectalis has no posterior attachment to the vertebral column and the loop acts to pull the recto-anal flexure forward accentuating the angle. Fibers of pubococcygeus arise from the pubis and the anterior part of the obturator fascia in continuity with those of puborectalis.

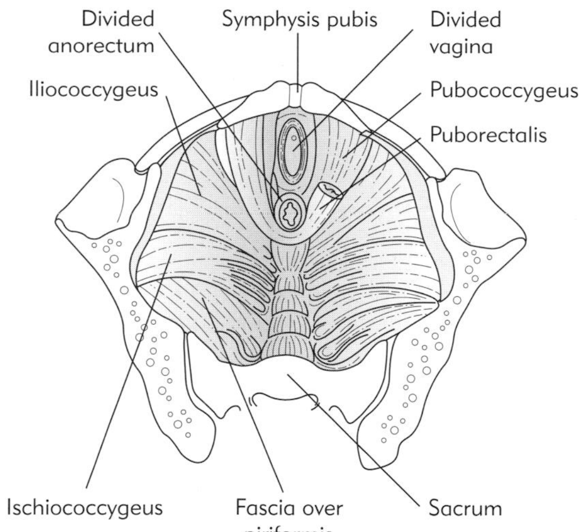

Figure 5.2 Pelvic view of the levator ani to show the four main components: ischiococcygeus, iliococcygeus, pubococcygeus and puborectalis (from Keighley[14]).

Its fibers are directed almost horizontally backwards as a flat band which lies superior to the innermost fibres of iliococcygeus. The main body of the fibers attach to a flattened tendon which inserts behind the rectum on the ventral surface of the coccyx and lies on the anococcygeal raphe formed by the iliococcygeus.

The third part of the levator ani is the iliococcygeus. This is a thin muscle which takes its origin from the medial surface of the ischial spine and posterior part of the fascia covering obturator internus. It partially overlaps the pubococcygeus to insert below it on the lateral surfaces of the terminal portion of the coccyx, the tip of the coccyx and the anococcygeal raphe. The fourth part of the levator ani muscle is the ischiococcygeus, sometimes known as coccygeus. The muscle arises from the tip and posterior surface of the ischial spine and inserts into the lateral surface of the lower part of the sacrum and upper coccyx. In man it is a small muscle with just a few fibers lying on the surface of the sacrospinous ligament.

DEVELOPMENT OF THE COLON, RECTUM AND ANUS

The colon develops from the midgut and hindgut. In addition to the small bowel, midgut derivatives include the cecum and appendix, ascending colon and proximal two thirds of the transverse colon. The hindgut gives rise to the remaining colon, rectum and upper part of the anal canal. Initially the midgut is suspended from the dorsal abdominal wall by a short mesentery but this rapidly increases in length to form a U-shaped loop by the sixth week of embryonic development, herniated into the umbilical cord. Early in the sixth week a small diverticulum appears on the caudal limb of the U-loop and this later develops into the cecum and appendix. Thereafter it is possible to distinguish between the large and small intestine. Until the fifth month the diverticulum has a conical appearance, but after this time there is an expansion of the proximal portion to form the cecum whilst the distal part remains rudimentary becoming the appendix. The cranial portion of the U-loop grows rapidly to form the small intestine which becomes coiled. The caudal portion extends less rapidly.

Within the umbilical cord the midgut undergoes rotation of 90 degrees counterclockwise around the axis of the superior mesenteric artery. By the third month the abdominal cavity has grown sufficiently to accommodate the viscera and the hernia undergoes rapid reduction. The small bowel re-enters first and further rotation of 180 degrees occurring at this stage resulting in the descending colon taking its position on the left side where it loses its mesentery and effectively becomes a retroperitoneal structure. This further rotation also results in the relationship of the superior mesenteric artery with the third part of the duodenum. The cecum is the last part of the intestine to re-enter the abdominal cavity and initially lies on the front of the small bowel but subsequent growth carries it dorsally and to the right where it lies in contact with the liver, ventral to the duodenum. During the terminal months of pregnancy the cecum descends into the right iliac fossa and the ascending colon so formed loses its mesentery as it becomes flattened against the posterior abdominal wall.

Hindgut derivatives are supplied by the inferior mesenteric artery. The terminal portion of the hindgut is called the cloaca. This is an endoderm-lined cavity that is in contact with the surface of the ectoderm. The cloacal membrane is comprised of the cloacal endoderm and the ectoderm of the proctodeum or anal pit. Partitioning of the cloacal membrane takes place during the fifth to seventh week of development when the *urorectal septum* grows down between the hindgut and allantois to fuse with the cloacal membrane. The area of fusion becomes the perineal body and separates the dorsal anal membrane from the larger ventral urogenital membrane. The anal membrane breaks down by the eighth week of gestation establishing the anal canal and bringing the caudal part of the gut into communication with the amniotic cavity.

The urorectal septum also divides the cloacal musculature into anterior and posterior parts. The posterior portion develops into the external anal sphincter whilst the anterior part becomes the superficial transverse perinei, the bulbospongiosus, the ischiocavernosus and the urogenital diaphragm. This explains why one nerve, the pudendal nerve, supplies all the musculature into which the cloacal sphincter divides.

Much has been written about the embryological origin of different parts of the anal canal. It is easy to appreciate that there is a contribution from both the endoderm and ectoderm, but the junction between the two is less well defined. It was originally believed that the anal valves represented the site of breakdown of the anal membrane. However, more recent evidence suggests that membrane disappears before the development of the anal valves. Nobles[16] studied the fate of the anal membrane in a series of human embryos. The anatomical relationship between the early stages of development and the adult form are only approximate because the sphincters migrate through this region during development; the internal sphincter moving distally and the external sphincter growing upwards. Nobles identified a mixture of epithelial types which gradually expands to occupy 15 mm of the canal lining. It was suggested that the attachment of the anal membrane underwent differentially rapid growth to be represented by the whole of this anal transition zone. The more recent findings that the anal transition zone is usually a much narrower segment[4] perhaps fits better with the concept of a thin membrane breaking down.

There are few data on the development of the external anal sphincter and the levator ani. The external anal sphincter is found in human embryos after 8 weeks gestation.[16] The sphincter and the levator ani are thought to develop from hypaxial myotomes. Although closely associated, embryo studies suggest that the external sphincter and levator ani arise from two distinct primordia.[17] Comparative anatomical studies have established the presence of two distinct muscle groups.[18] They are the 'sphincter' group and a lateral 'compressor' group. The latter connects the rudimentary pelvis to the caudal end of the vertebral column and are termed the 'pelvicaudal' muscles. Comparative data have been extensively reviewed by Wendell-Smith[18] who believes that the puborectalis is a ventrally tethered part of the sphincter cloacae complex. Its close relationship with the medial pelvicaudal muscles and its secondary attachment to the pubis has led to confusion in the past. However, this suggestion is further supported by Lawson[19] who showed that the puborectalis was separate from and outside the plane of what he referred to as the puboanalis/iliococcygeus muscle layer. More recent work on 18 human embryos has suggested that puborectalis is a portion of the levator ani, its primordium being common with the ilio- and pubococcygeus muscles.[20] Puborectalis was clearly distinct form the external sphincter by the end of the second month of gestation.

BLOOD SUPPLY

The colon receives its arterial supply from two main branches of the aorta reflecting its embryological development. The superior mesenteric artery supplies the midgut derivatives, the cecum, ascending colon and most of the transverse colon in addition to the small intestine and part of the duodenum. The inferior mesenteric artery supplies the hindgut derivatives; distal transverse colon, descending and sigmoid colon, rectum and upper part of the anal canal.

The superior mesenteric artery arises at the level of the L1 vertebra. It passes behind the splenic vein and neck of the pancreas to pass in front of the uncinate process of the pancreas and third part of the duodenum. Passing along the root of the mesentery it gives off the ileocolic artery to supply the terminal ileum, cecum and appendix. The right colic artery originates from the root of the superior mesenteric artery often in common with the ileocolic or middle colic artery. It runs on the posterior abdominal wall to the medial border of the ascending colon. Descending branches anastomose with the colic branches of the ileocolic artery and ascending branches with a branch of the middle colic artery.

The middle colic artery is the most proximal branch of the superior mesenteric artery. It travels to the right of the midline in the transverse mesocolon and divides into right and left branches to supply most of the transverse colon. The right branch anastomoses with the ascending branch of the right colic artery and the left with a branch of the left colic artery from the inferior mesenteric arterial supply.

The inferior mesenteric artery arise from the aorta at the level of the L3 vertebra. It runs beneath the peritoneal floor to the pelvic brim. On crossing the pelvic brim it becomes the superior rectal artery. The left colic artery arises from the inferior mesenteric artery and divides into an ascending and descending branch which supply the splenic flexure and descending colon. The sigmoid arteries are three or four branches of the inferior mesenteric artery which arise from a common origin and supply the sigmoid colon.

Running around the concave border of the colon is a single arterial trunk called the *marginal artery*. Branches of the superior and inferior mesenteric arteries contribute to it and a potential watershed area is the splenic flexure or the junction between these two vessels.

The major blood supply to the rectum and anal canal is from the superior and inferior rectal arteries. The middle rectal artery also supplies this region of the bowel but its significance has been debated. The superior rectal artery is a direct continuation of the inferior mesenteric artery. It gives off branches to the recto sigmoid and upper rectum before dividing at the level of S3 into right and left branches. These descend on either side of the lower rectum. Each vessel further divides into a series of smaller arteries which extend down beyond the level of the ano-rectal ring. There is a paucity of vessels in the midline in the lower rectum suggesting that there is little in the way of anastomoses between the two collaterals. This has also been put forward as a potential cause of leakage following low anterior resection.

The middle rectal arteries are branches of the anterior division of the internal iliac artery. When present they pass medially and forwards below the peritoneal reflection to reach the rectal wall. They were previously thought to run in the so-called lateral ligaments, but there has been a move away from this term amongst surgeons operating on the rectum. The existence of the middle rectal artery in cadaveric specimens has been debated with a vessel found in 12–70% of cases.[1,21,22]

The inferior rectal arteries are branches of the internal pudendal artery which cross the ischiorectal fossa and divide to send their branches through the external anal sphincter to reach the distal part of the anal canal. These branches run proximally in the submucosa and there seems to be a paucity in the posterior midline, similar to that described for the superior rectal artery. It has been suggested that anal fissures are ischemic in origin arising as a result of this deficiency in the blood supply to the anal canal posteriorly.[23,24] The extent of intramural anastomoses between the arteries supplying the lower rectum and anal canal has been debated and is likely to vary considerably between individuals. Other vessels such as the median sacral artery and inferior vesical arteries also supply the rectum but their contributions are small and variable. However, following division of the superior and middle rectal arteries at the time of anterior resection it is quite clear that the distal rectum and anal canal are able to survive.

The venous drainage of the colon, rectum and anal canal runs in the main with the arterial supply. The inferior mesenteric vein runs up to join the splenic vein. The superior mesenteric vein also joins the splenic vein to form the portal vein.

INNERVATION

The colon, rectum and anal canal are innervated by both the sympathetic (from the eleventh and twelfth thoracic and the lumbar segments) and parasympathetic (from the vagus and first, second and third sacral segments) components of the autonomic nervous system. Sympathetic nerves have an inhibitory effect on colon electal peristalsis in secretions, whereas parasympathetic stimulation increases them. The nerves pass to the colon with its blood supply. The sympathetic supply to the colon is two-fold, by the lumbar part of the sympathetic trunk and via the celiac plexus. Branches arise from all the lumbar ganglia to join the celiac, aortic and superior hypogastric plexuses. Fibers from the third and fourth ganglia join with fibers from the aortic plexus to form the superior hypogastric plexus. The plexus divides into the right and left hypogastric nerves which run down into the pelvis to join the inferior hypogastric plexuses lying posterolaterally on the pelvic side wall.

Fibers from the vagi pass to the celiac plexus. They pass with the blood vessels to the colon in the midgut distribution. Parasympathetic supply of the left colon, rectum and anus comes from the second, third and fourth sacral nerves, the pelvic splanchnic nerves or nervi erigentes. These fibers pass to the two inferior hypogastric plexuses. Parasympathetic fibers to the sigmoid and descending colon pass upward to the superior hypogastric plexus and then to the inferior mesenteric artery by which they are distributed to the colon. The branches of the inferior hypogastric plexuses are wholly visceral and run in leashes of nerves bound up in condensed fibrous tissue. They are accompanied by the visceral branches of the internal iliac arteries. While it is well established that sympathetic vasoconstrictor fibers accompany all arteries to the pelvic viscera, there remains much ignorance as to the course of the motor and sensory fibers to these organs.

The cell bodies of the neurons controlling the striated muscle of the external anal sphincter lie in the ventral horn of the spinal cord at S2 and are sometimes known as Onuf's nucleus.[25] There is evidence of cross-over of fibers so that unilateral cord transection does not abolish tonic discharge.[26] Motor fibers to the external anal sphincter pass in the pudendal nerve (S2 and S3) and, if present, the perineal branch of S4.

Cadaveric studies have suggested that the nerve supply of puborectalis is via the pudendal nerve on its perineal surface. In contrast the remainder of the levator ani receives its supply from the sacral plexus on its pelvic surface. However *in vivo* studies have shown differential contractions of the external anal sphincter and puborectalis during spinal stimulation at L1. Whilst this calls into question the results of post-mortem studies the findings may still be compatible if the supply to puborectalis were via the perineal branch of S4. The *in vivo* findings are, however, consistent with puborectalis and the external sphincter having different embyological origins.[20]

THE MYENTERIC PLEXUS

Although gastrointestinal function is modified by the sympathetic and parasympathetic inputs described above, in the early part of this century, it was recognized that peristalsis could be recorded in whole lengths of isolated animal intestine. This gives rise to the concept of an intramural intrinsic nervous system termed the enteric nervous system (ENS) which primarily controls gastrointestinal motility.[27] The ENS consists of two major plexuses of interconnecting ganglia, the myenteric (Auerbach's) plexus and the submucosal (Meissner's) plexus. The myenteric plexus is innervated by postganglionic sympathetic fibers from the thoracolumbar outflow described above. The parasympathetic innervation consists of the craniosacral outflow via the vagus and splanchnic nerves to postganglionic cell bodies with the bowel wall. The number of neurons in the ENS approximates to that of the central nervous system. It contains entire reflex pathways which permit peristaltic contractions independent of extrinsic innervation. The following types of enteric neuron therefore exist; sensory neurons which monitor the factors such as tension in the bowel wall or the chemical nature of luminal contents; interneurons forming links between enteric neurons; and motor neurons which alter the mechanical activity of the intestine.

STRUCTURE AND ORGANIZATION

The myenteric plexus is situated between the circular and longitudinal layers of the muscularis propria. It consists of a network of nerve strands and small ganglia. There is variation in size between different regions of the gut, but the ganglia of the myenteric plexus are usually larger than those of the submucosal plexus. The myenteric plexus has been subdivided into the primary, secondary and tertiary plexuses. The primary plexus comprises the ganglia and internal strands while the interconnecting nerve strands constitute the secondary plexus. The finer nerve bundles that intertwine between these two plexuses form the tertiary plexus (see Furness and Costa[28]).

The general organization of the myenteric plexus is different in the distal part of the colon compared with the rest of the gastrointestinal tract. Bundles containing myelinated nerve fibers called shunt fascicles lie upon the plexus of the ganglia. These have been shown to convey fibers from the dorsocranial part of the inferior hypogastric plexuses (pelvic plexus) and contain both myelinated and unmyelinated fibers. The myelinated fibers are thought to be parasympathetic afferents and sympathetic efferents, while the unmyelinated fibers arise from the intrinsic nerves of the plexus.[29]

Electron microscopic studies of the ganglia of the myenteric plexus reveal tightly packed cell bodies, enteric glia and cell processes similar to those found in the brain.[30] Although not fully established, this arrangement may be important to the glial functions of uptake and release of transmitter substances and buffering of extracellular potassium concentration. The myenteric plexus is also similar to the central nervous system in its diversity of the types of neurons and axon terminals found in the plexus.

Classification of myenteric neurons

Dogiel classified enteric neurons into three types:

- Type I cells were described as being flattened and had several irregular dendrites and one long thin process which could be traced to the internodal strands. The axonal processes passed through up to four ganglia before entering the circular muscle coat and were said by Dogiel to be motor neurons.
- Type II cells were star- or spindle-shaped with 3–10 dendrites that extended to other ganglia and beyond. These were believed to be sensory neurons.
- Type III cells had processes of intermediate length which branched around the ganglia cells of the same or adjacent ganglia.

More recent work has attempted to further classify enteric neurons based on neuronal size, location of neurons, relationship to satellite cells and ultrastructural appearance. The relationship between the ultrastructure and function is not fully established.

Projections of myenteric neurons

The majority of studies on projections of enteric neurons have relied upon immunohistochemical techniques although electrophysiological studies have earlier revealed some general features of the circuitry in relation to intrinsic reflex pathways in the gut. Much of the work has been performed in guinea pig small intestine where it has been shown that motor neurons for the circular muscle layer are located in the myenteric plexus whereas those for the mucosa are found in the submucosal plexus. Furthermore, both cranial and caudal projections have been identified as well as communicating fibers between the myenteric and submucosal plexuses.[28]

Nerve fibers from the wall of the intestine synapse with cells in the prevertebral ganglia.[31] As many as 30% of nerve fibers found in the mesentery of the small intestine arise from nerve cells within the gut wall. It has been suggested that many of these axons are afferent processes involved in the peripheral intestino-intestinal inhibitory reflex.

NEUROCHEMISTRY OF THE MYENTERIC PLEXUS

Using atropine and a selection of adrenergic antagonists it became evident in the early 1960s that inhibitory transmission in the gastrointestinal tract was mediated by transmitters that had non-adrenergic, non-cholinergic (NANC) properties.[32,33] Since then a large population of NANC nerves have been identified which have both an inhibitory or excitatory effect on intestinal smooth muscle. The nature of the putative NANC neurotransmitters and/or neuromodulators localized in the enteric plexus has been the subject of much investigation but are thought to include purine nucleotides such as adenosine 5′-triphosphate and 5-hydroxytryptamine, amino acids and peptides.[34]

Over the past 30 years a large number of short-chained peptides have been identified in the mammalian ENS. Much of the early evidence for the presence of these peptides in the myenteric nerves rests on immunohistochemical studies. More recently specific antagonists of these peptides have permitted pharmacological and electrophysiological assessment of them. However, much of the data relate to animal studies and there are fewer results of studies performed in human tissue. The list of putative transmitters in the ENS is ever expanding but the peptides include substance P,[35] vasoactive intestinal peptide (VIP),[36] neuropeptide Y,[37] calcitonin gene related peptide,[38] enkephalins,[39] galanin,[40] somatostatin[41] and pituitary adenylate cyclase-activating peptide (PACAP).[42] This list is not meant to be exhaustive, but nevertheless gives an indication of the wide variety of substances that have been proposed to influence gastrointestinal motility. The exact role of many of these compounds remains obscure.

Immunohistochemical studies have also demonstrated the coexistence of these transmitters.[43] Although the significance of this phenomenon also remains unclear it is possible that the coexistence of multiple messengers may provide a mechanism for relaying differential responses and increasing the amount of information transmitted at synapses. There is growing evidence that one agent may act to modify the release of another transmitter at a given nerve terminal.

Over the past 10 years the molecule that has received greatest attention as a putative enteric neurotransmitter is nitric oxide (NO). It had been recognized since the early 1980s that acetylcholine cause vascular smooth muscle to relax only in the presence of the endothelium.[44] An agent called endothelium-derived relaxing factor (EDRF) was shown to be responsible for this effect and Palmer *et al.*[45] later showed that EDRF and NO were equivalent. Nitric oxide was originally implicated as a neuronal messenger in the central nervous system in the late 1970s.[46] Neuronal production of NO was confirmed in studies on rat synaptosomal cytosol[47] and bovine brain cytosol[48] in which addition of L-arginine resulted in the formation of NO and L-citrulline which was accompanied by stimulation of soluble guanylate cyclase. Bredt and colleagues subsequently isolated neuronal nitric oxide synthase (NOS, the enzyme responsible for the generation of NO) from rat cerebellar homogenates and determined its distribution in the central nervous system immunocytochemically.[49,50] NOS activity was associated exclusively with a discrete population of nerves. The realization that NO was a likely neurotransmitter in the central nervous system prompted further investigation of NANC neurotransmission in the gastrointestinal tract.

NITRIC OXIDE AND THE GASTROINTESTINAL TRACT

The rat anococcygeus muscle, although not strictly speaking a gastrointestinal muscle, receives an excitatory adrenergic and inhibitory NANC innervation and has been used extensively to study NANC neurotransmission. N^G-monomethyl-L-arginine (L-NMMA, a methyl derivative of L-arginine) was shown to reduce NANC nerve-mediated relaxation, an effect reversed in the presence of L-arginine.[51,52] L-NMMA also increased basal tone suggesting that there may be tonic release of NO. Following these reports, results of studies of NANC neurotransmission elsewhere in the gastrointestinal tract began to appear.

Ileocolic sphincter

The canine ileocolic sphincter has been one of the most extensively investigated preparations. Bult *et al.*[53] reported crucial experiments showing that stimulation of NANC nerves released a factor whose biological actions were similar to NO and which was inactivated by O_2^- and hemoglobin, inhibited by Nω-nitro-L-arginine (L-NOArg) and potentiated by L-arginine. Responses in biological assay tissue to adenosine triphosphate (ATP) or VIP were different from those elicited by the nerve-produced factor. In addition, responses to both the factor and exogenous NO were enhanced in the presence of superoxide dismutase, whereas those to ATP and VIP were unaffected.[54,55] These data support a role for NO over ATP or VIP as the major inhibitory transmitter.

Colon

Better availability of tissue has permitted more extensive study of human colon. NO has been implicated in the NANC responses for both colonic circular muscle[56,57] and longitudinal muscle from the taenia coli.[58] The anatomical distribution of NOS neurons in the colon has been studied in animals[59] and humans[60] and supports a role for NO as an important neurotransmitter. Middleton *et al.*[61] suggested that the distal colonic circular muscle was under tonic neural inhibition mediated by NO.

Rectum and internal anal sphincter

NO has been implicated in NANC relaxations in porcine rectal circular muscle and human rectal circular and longitudinal muscle.[62–64] Differential staining for NOS between the layers correlates well with responses to electrical stimulation.[65] NANC nerve-mediated relaxations are also thought to be mediated by NO in opossum[66] and human IAS.[67] O'Kelly showed that electrical field stimulation of IAS tissue caused relaxation in the presence of guanethidine and atropine. This effect was blocked by L-NOArg and reversed by L-arginine but not D-arginine (Fig. 5.3).

ANAL TONE AND THE INTERNAL ANAL SPHINCTER

The maintenance of continence is a complex process of inter-relating factors and is covered in detail in the following chapter. However, the anal sphincters contribute

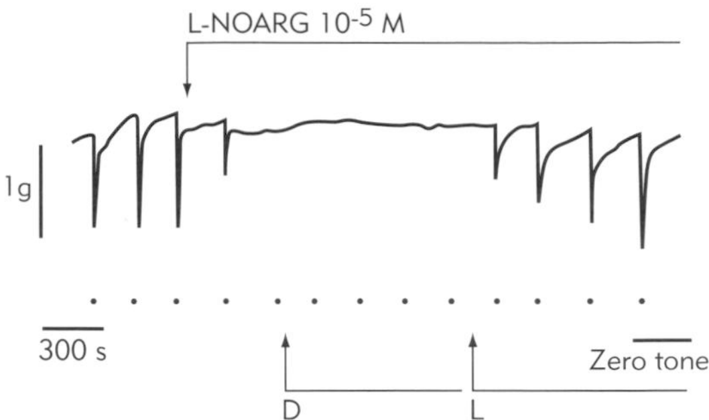

Figure 5.3 *In vitro* **effect of Nω-nitro-L-arginine (L-NOARG) on nerve-mediated relaxation (• = 10 V, 0.5 ms duration, 8 Hz, 1 s train) of internal anal sphincter smooth muscle strips. Its action was antagonized by L-arginine (L) but not D-arginine (D) (from O'Kelly** ***et al.***[67]**).**

to a region of high intraluminal pressure in the anal canal which deserve highlighting. The high pressure zone results principally from the activity of the internal and external anal sphincters. IAS function has been investigated in various ways including *in vivo* studies on patients and healthy volunteers and by *in vitro* techniques using isolated smooth muscle strips. These *in vitro* experiments provide useful information about the types of receptors and intrinsic nerves involved in the motility of the sphincter *in vivo*.

Ganglion cells are sparsely distributed in the region of the anal canal. However, there is an abundance of nerve fibers innervating the smooth muscle cells of the IAS and the concentration of noradrenaline (norepinephrine), the sympathetic neurotransmitter is twice that found in the colon.

Gaskell[68] proposed that gastrointestinal sphincter muscle had an excitatory sympathetic input and inhibitory parasympathetic innervation. This contrasts with the remainder of the gastrointestinal tract. Although when Gaskell first proposed his theory the evidence for it was sparse, over the ensuing years *in vitro* and *in vivo* experiments have shown that sympathetic nerve stimulation or application of the neurotransmitter, noradrenaline can contract the IAS.

The IAS generates a high degree of tone in the resting state and is responsible for 50–85% of overall resting anal tone.[69,70] This is due to both intrinsic myogenic activity[71] and extrinsic adrenergic innervation.[70] Direct local anesthetic blockade of the pudendal nerve, which paralysed the external anal sphincter[69] was used to assess the contribution of the two sphincters to overall anal tone during various degrees of rectal distension. The external sphincter exerted a greater effect during periods of substantial rectal distension.

In vivo experiments have demonstrated that anal tone falls by around 50% following sympathetic blockade by high (T6–T12) spinal anesthesia[72] an effect that was not seen when the sphincter is relaxed after rectal distension. A similar fall in anal pressure was observed following infusion of the α-adrenoceptor antagonist phentolamine.[73] These data suggest that there is a tonic excitatory sympathetic discharge to the IAS. Stimulation of sympathetic fibers running in the presacral nerves during operations has been shown to both increase[74] and decrease IAS tone.[75] The reason for this discrepancy is unclear, but may reflect differences in the stimulation parameters or the influence of background sympathetic activity.

Frenckner and Ihre[72] also assessed the effect of low spinal anesthesia (L5–S1) on anal pressure and suggested that parasympathetic nerves have very little effect on sphincter tone *in vivo*. Although Gutierrez and Shah[73] established that infusion of bethanecol, a muscarinic agonist, in healthy volunteers caused a relaxation of the IAS and fall in anal pressure, their data do not provide evidence for release of cholinergic agents from parasympathetic nerves, but rather that muscarinic receptors on or near IAS smooth muscle cause relaxation.

The IAS has a higher resting pressure than the non-sphincteric rectal smooth muscle above and gives a rapid relaxation in response to the appropriate proximal stimulus. Relaxation does not however depend upon the arrival of a wave of peristalsis from above. The tone is measured as intraluminal pressure within the anal canal and maximum resting tone shows great individual variation ranging from 30–120 cmH_2O compared with a mean resting tone of about 5 cmH_2O in the rectum.

RECTOANAL INHIBITORY REFLEX

This reflex refers to relaxation of the IAS that occurs almost immediately when the rectum or rectosigmoid is distended and is followed by spontaneous recovery. By causing a reduction in anal pressure, rectal contents can come into contact with the specialized sensory epithelium of the anal canal, a process known as ano-rectal sampling. It is dependent upon mechanoreceptors in the rectum and it is generally agreed that the reflex is independent of higher neural centers. Indeed, a normal reflex is observed following division of the hypogastric nerves suggesting that it is entirely located within the bowel wall. However, it seems likely that the reflex can be modulated by extrinsic nerves and this is supported by the observation that presacral nerve stimulation caused IAS relaxation similar to that produced by rectal distension.

Patients with Hirschsprung's disease have no ganglion cells in variable lengths of rectum and colon and IAS relaxation is not elicited following rectal distension in these patients. O'Kelly *et al.* suggested that NO might be important in mediating the recto-anal inhibitory reflex. NOS- containing neurons were identified in the lower rectum of patients undergoing resection for cancer where the recto-anal inhibitory reflex was present[76] but NOS activity was not identified in the myenteric plexus of patients with Hirschsprung's disease.[77]

Further support for this theory was provided in an elegant study by Stebbing *et al.*[78] using a neuronal tracing technique. In the guinea pig, wheatgerm agglutinin conjugated to horseradish peroxidase was injected into the IAS. Transported tracer was demonstrated in neurons of the myenteric ganglia of the distal rectum and all labeled neurons showed co-localization with nitric oxide synthase. Furthermore the guinea pig was demonstrated to exhibit a recto-anal inhibitory reflex; *in vivo* and *in vitro* studies demonstrated that NANC relaxations of guinea pig IAS muscle strips were mediated by NO.

PHARMACOLOGY OF THE INTERNAL ANAL SPHINCTER

The high pressure region of the anal canal is in part due to the intrinsic myogenic properties of the IAS smooth muscle. Much of the information regarding this tissue comes from *in vitro* experiments. Such studies have shown that strips of IAS develop tone that is resistant to tetrodotoxin, a neurotoxin.[79] This is in contrast to rectal smooth muscle strips which after a period of equilibration relax completely, i.e. develop no tone. Tone in the IAS was also associated with slow sinusoidal activity in smooth muscle cells.[80]

The effects of adrenergic agonists are well documented. IAS strips contract to noradrenaline, have a variable response to adrenaline and relax to isoprenaline. Analysis of these responses using appropriate adrenoceptor antagonists have shown that contractions are mediated via α-receptors and relaxations via β-receptors. Contractions to noradrenaline and adrenaline (epinephrine) can be converted to relaxations by the addition of an α-receptor antagonist. Dopamine contracts the IAS.

Burleigh *et al.*[79] have shown that acetylcholine has a predominantly inhibitory effect on IAS smooth muscle acting through muscarinic receptors. This relaxation was thought in part to be due to intrinsic nerve stimulation. O'Kelly *et al.*[81] suggested that muscarinic receptors were present on NO-releasing nerves since inhibitors of nitric oxide synthase attenuated the response to carbachol (a cholinergic analog). In contrast to the findings of Burleigh *et al.*[79] tetrodotoxin had no effect and it was suggested that the muscarinic receptors were present in the nitrergic nerve terminals. Contractions to muscarinic agonists have been observed and may reflect either damage to the intrinsic nerves during retrieval and preparation or by the presence of a small population of excitatory muscarinic receptors similar to those found in the adjacent smooth muscle of the circular muscle of the rectum.

Nicotine and dimethylphenylpiperazinium (DMPP) cause relaxation of IAS strips.[82] This was thought to be due either to release of an isoprenaline-like substance, or due to release of noradrenaline in close proximity to β-receptors.[83] The observation that when sphincter muscle strips preincubated with [^{3}H]noradrenaline relax to noradrenaline there is simultaneous increase in tritiated material supports the latter theory.

Morphine is thought to exert its antidiarrheal effect both by an increase in non-propulsive intestinal activity and contraction of the sphincters. Neither morphine nor loperamide have an effect on the tone of isolated sphincter strips and it has been suggested that they act via intrinsic nerves rather than directly on the smooth muscle or the central nervous system.[84]

In vitro experiments on IAS strips have shown that electrical field stimulation (EFS) resulted in relaxation of the smooth muscle.[79] These relaxations are abolished by tetrodotoxin indicating that they are nerve mediated. Addition of guanethidine and atropine to block adrenergic and cholinergic effects had no effect on the response to EFS indicating that relaxation was mediated by NANC nerves. Nitric oxide has been proposed as the principal NANC transmitter in human IAS although in other animals it appears to interact with peptides such as PACAP and VIP.[42] Carbon monoxide is another gas which has been shown to have an inhibitory effect on opossum IAS.[85]

It is beyond the scope of this chapter to list and discuss all the putative transmitters in the IAS. However a summary of the principal transmitters and their effects is shown in Fig. 5.4. A basic knowledge of the pharmacology of the IAS has a clinical application. The realization that NO may play a role in IAS relaxation led on to the use of nitric oxide donors (e.g. glyceryl trinitrate (GTN)) in the management of anal fissure. Fissures are associated with a raised resting anal pressure secondary to increased IAS tone. Treatment had traditionally been surgical with the aim of reducing sphincter tone by dividing the lower portion of the IAS. However, concerns over subsequent long-term incontinence stimulated interest in pharmacological manipulation of sphincter pressure. Topical application of GTN has been shown to reduce resting anal pressure and heal anal fissures.[86] Other agents that reduce anal pressure include bethanechol[73] and indoramin (α-adrenoceptor antagonist).[87] The effect of bethanechol on anal pressure confirms the *in vitro* observations of cholinergic analogs on IAS strips although the site of action has not been determined. Enthusiasm for pharmacological manipulation of the IAS led on to attempts at increasing anal tone. Topical phenylephrine, an α-adrenoceptor agonist, has recently been shown to increase anal pressure without a concomitant rise in blood pressure.[88] It was suggested that this may be useful in the treatment of incontinence.

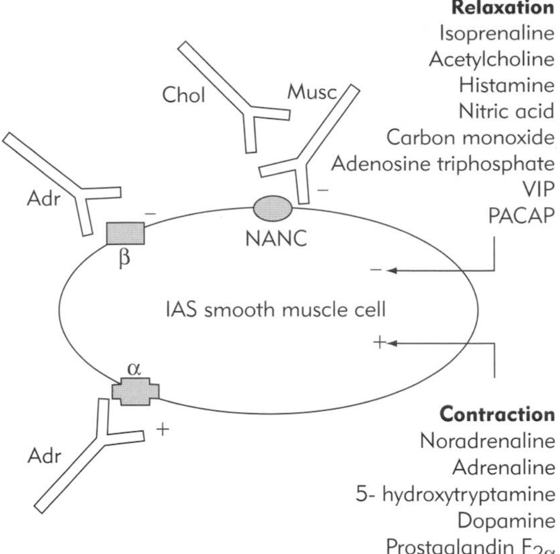

Figure 5.4 Diagram to show which nerves and drugs act on isolated internal anal sphincter smooth muscle. Adr, adrenergic; Chol, cholinergic; Musc, muscarinic receptor.

Work by the same group has shown that in a group of 12 patients with nocturnal incontinence and an ileoanal pouch, although a measured rise in maximum resting pressive was seen in all patients, improvement in symptoms was noted in only half of them.[88a] Nevertheless, pharmacological treatment of sphincter dysfunction represents a great advance in the management of these anal disorders as it avoids surgery in a significant proportion of patients.

ANORECTAL SENSATION

RECTAL SENSATION

Modalities of rectal sensation

Unlike anal sensation the modalities of rectal sensation are indistinct. Like the rest of the colon it is insensitive to stimuli such as pain or touch but is sensitive to distension. Goligher and Hughes[89] described two types of sensation. Using balloon distension of the rectum and colon they showed distension of the rectum up to 15 cm from the anal verge gave a sensation of rectal fullness producing a desire to defecate – *rectal-type sensation*. The sensitivity of the rectum to this form of distension was greatest in the ampulla immediately above the anal sphincters. Distension of the sigmoid colon produced purely abdominal or flatulent sensation referred to the suprapubic or left iliac fossa region – *colonic-type sensation*. The pressure required to elicit rectal-type sensation was less than that required to elicit colonic-type sensation suggesting that the rectum is more sensitive to this type of stimulation. The difference in sensitivity of the rectum and colon is seen under normal conditions. During peristalsis the colon generates intraluminal pressures of up to 50 cmH_2O but this usually produces no sensation other than occasional slight discomfort. Pain is only experienced when peristalsis becomes greatly exaggerated. In contrast, the rectum is able to detect small quantities of flatus and reliably distinguish them from feces.

No recognizable sensory nerve endings have been identified in the bowel wall and it is not yet known where the nerve endings are situated which transmit sensation from the colon and rectum. The absence of specific receptors in the rectal mucosa may account for the poor discriminatory quality of rectal sensation. It has also been suggested that sensation may be due to stimulation of nerve endings in adjacent pelvic structures such as the pelvic floor. This is supported by the finding that patients undergoing low anterior resection with coloanal anastomosis sometimes experience rectal-type sensation, something that does not occur following abdominoperineal excision of the rectum.[90]

Nerve pathways

The nerve supply to the rectum and sigmoid colon is from sympathetic fibers originating in the T7–L2 segments and parasympathetic fibers from S2–4 segments. Goligher and Hughes[89] showed that rectal sensation was unaffected by bilateral and total sympathectomy or by bilateral hemorrhoidal nerve block, but that it was abolished parasympathetic blockade using low spinal anesthesia affecting the first sacral segment. Colonic sensation was unaffected by this spinal anesthesia. This suggests that sensation of rectal distension is mediated through parasympathetic fibers to S2–4 whereas sensation of colonic distension occurs via the sympathetic system.

ANAL SENSATION

Modalities of anal sensation

The modalities of anal sensation can be more precisely defined and have been studied in detail by Duthie and Gairns[91] on healthy volunteers.

The anal canal is extremely sensitive to *touch* from the anal verge to a level between 0.25 and 0.75 cm above the anal valves. The level of stimulus can be distinguished although localization cannot be made. *Pain* in the form of pin-prick sensation is felt more distinctly in the anal canal than the perianal skin. The highest level of sensation is between 0.5 and 1.5 cm above the anal glands and is usually higher than the level for touch. *Cold and heat* are also felt more distinctly in the anal canal than perianal skin with the upper limit of sensation above the anal valves. Longitudinal and rotatory *movement* of an object with the anal canal can be precisely defined. The perianal skin has a similar degree of sensitivity to these stimuli as dorsum of the finger.

Receptors for anal sensation

Duthie and Gairns[91] also carefully assessed the distribution of specific sensory receptors in post-mortem specimens of perianal skin and rectum (Fig. 5.5). The innervation of the perianal skin is similar to other areas of hairy skin elsewhere in the body. Hair follicles are densely innervated by myelinated nerves and whilst there are free intra-epithelial nerve endings there are no organized nerve endings.

Within the anal canal there is regional variation of innervation. The anal margin contains only a few hair follicles. Innervation is similar to the perianal skin although organized nerve endings similar to Krause end-bulbs, which are in close anatomical relationship with hair follicles, help to distinguish this region.

The anal canal is more richly innervated than the anal margin. Large diameter free nerve endings are also found in close relationships with the epithelium and are of a loosely coiled type. More complex forms are found around the anal transition zone. In addition to free nerve endings there are other specific nerve endings which are summarized in Table 5.1.

Nerve pathways

Sensation for the anal canal is by the inferior hemorrhoidal branches of the pudendal nerve to the S2–4 sacral roots. Of these S3 appears to be most important for normal discriminatory functions and continence.

Sampling reflex

Duthie and Bennett[92] suggested that following rectal distension there was a transient relaxation of the upper anal canal permitting rectal contents to come into contact with the lining of the upper anal canal. It was thought

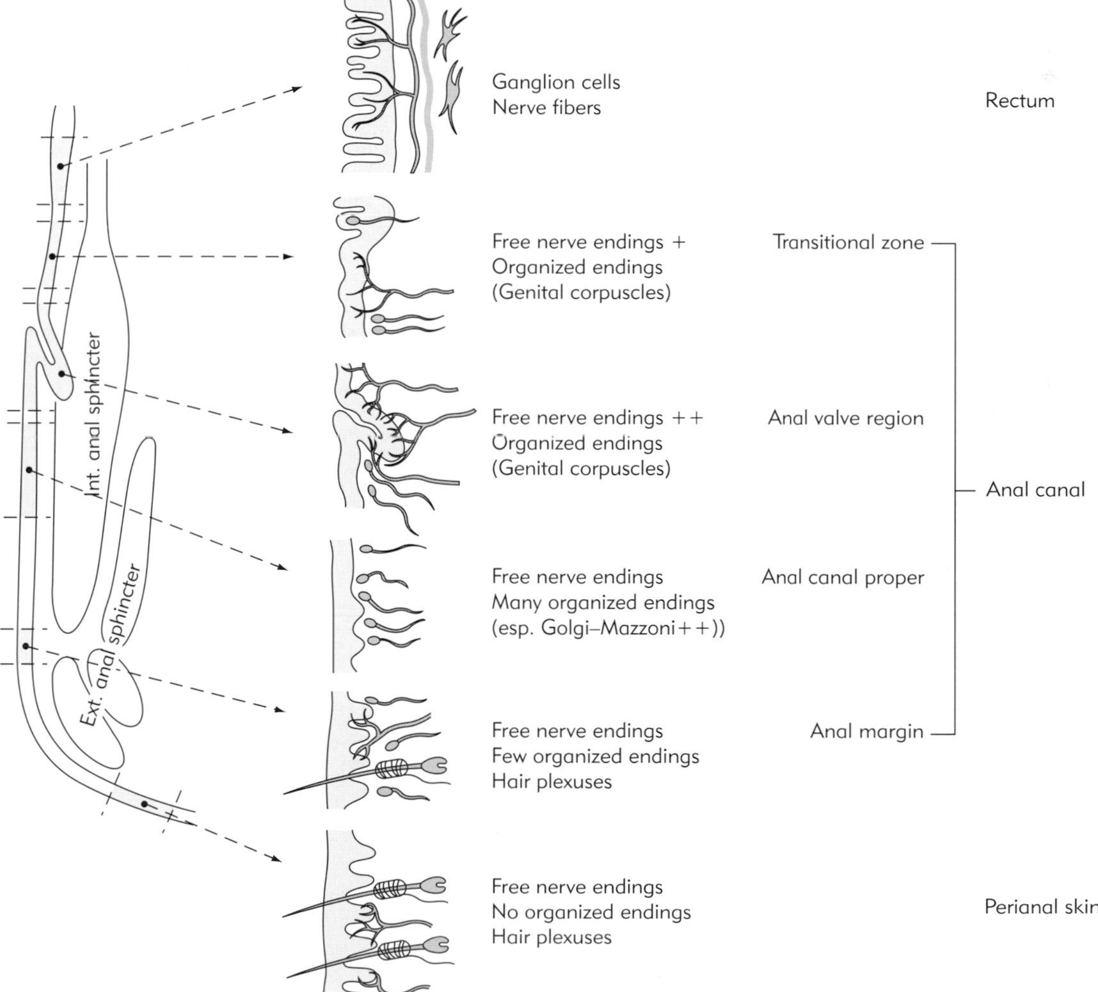

Figure 5.5 Diagramatic representation of sensory nerve endings in the anal canal and perianal skin (from Duthie and Gairns[91]).

Table 5.1 Summary of specific sensory receptors in the anal canal

Receptor	Occurrence	Location	Sensory modality
Meissner's corpuscles	Infrequent	Dermal papillae	Touch
Krause end-bulbs	Numerous	Deep dermis	Acute sensitivity to cold
Genital corpuscles	Numerous	Dermal papillae	Friction
Golgi–Mazzoni bodies	Numerous	Deep	Tension and pressure
Pacinian corpuscles	Infrequent	Deep, close to IAS	Tension and pressure

that the nature of the rectal contents could be discriminated and that this sensory information was believed to be important in the maintenance of continence. This brief relaxation of the upper anal sphincter is termed the sampling reflex. Ambulatory manometry has confirmed that this occurs in a healthy population but is observed less frequently in patients with incontinence.[93]

Application of local anesthetic to the anal canal was not associated with incontinence in healthy individuals but an increase in IAS pressure was observed.[94] Anal canal sensation is diminished following mucosectomy during restorative proctocolectomy but this is not associated with functional impairment.[95] These data suggest that sensory impairment in the anal canal leads to functional disturbance only in the presence of ano-rectal motor dysfunction. Miller *et al.*[96] suggested that sensitivity to temperature change may also be important in discrimination between flatus, liquid and solids. All regions of the anal canal were sensitive to changes in temperature and a significantly reduced sensitivity to temperature was observed in patients with idiopathic incontinence. It has since been suggested that the temperature gradients between the rectum and anal canal are much smaller than the threshold necessary to produce a conscious appreciation of temperature change in the anal canal of healthy individuals.[97] It therefore seems less likely that there is conscious appreciation of the temperature of rectal contents coming into contact with the anal canal during the normal sampling reflex. Maintenance of continence is in fact multifactorial and involves not only ano-rectal sensation, but also sphincters, the pelvic floor and proximal colonic motility and abnormalities of any of these can lead to disorders of evacuation or incontinence.

REFERENCES

1. Jones OM, Smeulders N, Wiseman O, *et al.* Lateral ligaments of the rectum: an anatomical study. *Br J Surg* 1999;**86**:487–9.
2. Kourambas J, Angus DG, Hosking P, *et al.* A histological study of Denonvilliers' fascia and its relationship to the neurovascular bundle. *Br J Urol* 1998;**82**:408–10.
3. Fenger C. The anal transitional zone. Location and extent. *Acta Pathol Microbiol Scand A* 1979;**87a**:379–86.
4. Thompson-Fawcett MW, Warren BF, Mortensen NJM. A new look at the anal transition zone with reference to restorative proctocolectomy and the columnar cuff. *Br J Surg* 1998;**85**:1517–21.
5. Milligan ET, Morgan CN. Surgical anatomy of the anal canal. *Lancet* 1934;**ii**:1150–6.
6. Fine J, Lawes CHW. On the muscle fibres of the anal submucosa with special reference to the pecten band. *Br J Surg* 1940;**27**:723–7.
7. Parks AG. The surgical treatment of haemorrhoids. *Br J Surg* 1956;**43**:337–51.
8. Goligher JC. Surgical anatomy of the anus, rectum and colon. In: Goligher JC (ed). *Surgery of the anus, rectum and colon.* London: Ballière Tindall, 1984:1–47.
9. Oh C, Kark AE. Anatomy of the external anal sphincter. *Br J Surg* 1972;**59**:717–23.
10. Bollard RC, Phillips K, Luidow S, *et al.* Defective versus normal female anal sphincter anatomy. *Br J Surg* 1998;**85**:1566–7 (Abstract).
11. Bogduk N. Issues in anatomy: the external anal sphincter revisited. *Aust NZ J Surg* 1996; **66**:626–9.
12. Shafik A. A new concept of the anatomy of the anal sphincter mechanism and the physiology of defecation. The external anal sphincter: a triple-loop system. *Invest Urol* 1975; **12**:412–9.
13. Thompson P. *The myology of the pelvic floor: a contribution to human and comparative anatomy.* London: McCorquodale, 1899.
14. Keighley MRB. Anatomy and physiology. In: Keighley MRB, Williams NS (eds). *Surgery of the anus, rectum and colon.* London: WB Saunders, 1993.
15. Fucini C, Elbetti C, Messerini L. Anatomic plane of separation between external anal sphincter and puborectalis muscle. *Dis Colon Rectum* 1999;**42**:374–9.
16. Nobles VP. The development of the human anal canal. *J Anat* 1984;**138**:575.
17. Tichy M. The development and organization of the sphincter ani externus and the adjacent part of the levator ani muscle in man. *Folia Morphol Praha* 1984;**32**:113–20.
18. Wendell-Smith CP. *Studies on the morphology of the pelvic floor.* PhD thesis: University of London, UK, 1967.
19. Lawson JO. Pelvic anatomy. I. Pelvic floor muscles. *Ann R Coll Surg Engl* 1974;**54**:244–52.
20. Levi AC, Borghi F, Garavoglia M. Development of the anal canal muscles. *Dis Colon Rectum* 1991;**34**:262–6.
21. Thomson WH. The nature of haemorrhoids. *Br J Surg* 1975;**62**:542–52.
22. Ayoub SF. Arterial supply to the human rectum. *Acta Anat Basel* 1978;**100**:317–27.

23. Klosterhalfen B, Vogel P, Rixen H, *et al.* Topography of the inferior rectal artery: a possible cause of chronic, primary anal fissure. *Dis Colon Rectum* 1989;**32**:43–52.
24. Lund JN, Binch C, McGrath J, *et al.* Topographical distribution of blood supply to the anal canal. *Br J Surg* 1999;**86**:496–8.
25. Schroder HD. Onuf's nucleus X: a morphological study of a human spinal nucleus. *Anat Embryol Berl* 1981;**162**:443–53.
26. Wunderlich M, Swash M. The overlapping innervation of the two sides of the external anal sphincter by the pudendal nerves. *J Neurol Sci* 1983;**59**:97–109.
27. Langley JN. *The autonomic nervous system.* Cambridge: Heffer, 1921.
28. Furness JB, Costa M. *The enteric nervous system.* London: Churchill Livingstone, 1987.
29. Christensen J, Stiles MJ, Rick GA, *et al.* Comparative anatomy of the myenteric plexus of the distal colon in eight mammals. *Gastroenterology* 1984;**86**:706–13.
30. Llewellyn-Smith IJ, Furness JB, Wilson AJ, *et al.* Organization and the fine structure of enteric ganglia. In: Elvin EG (ed). *Autonomic ganglia.* New York: Wiley, 1983:145–82.
31. Macrae IM, Furness JB, Costa M. Distribution of subgroups of noradrenaline neurons in the celiac ganglion of the guinea-pig. *Cell Tiss Res* 1986;**244**:173–80.
32. Burnstock G, Campbell G, Rand MJ. The inhibitory innervation of the taenia of the guinea-pig caecum. *J Physiol Lond* 1966;**182**:504–26.
33. Furness JB, Costa M. The nervous release and the action of substances which affect intestinal muscle through neither adrenoreceptors nor cholinoreceptors. *Philos Trans R Soc Lond B Biol Sci* 1973;**265**:123–33.
34. Hoyle CHV, Burnstock G. Neuromuscular transmission in the gastrointestinal tract. In: Wood JD (ed). *Handbook of physiology – the gastrointestinal system I.* Bethesda MD: American Physiological Society, 1989:435–64.
35. Crowe R, Kamm MA, Burnstock G, *et al.* Peptide-containing neurons in different regions of the submucous plexus of human sigmoid colon. *Gastroenterology* 1992;**102**:461–7.
36. Lynn RB, Sankey SL, Chakder S, *et al.* Colocalization of NADPH-diaphorase staining and VIP immunoreactivity in neurons in opossum internal and sphincter. *Dig Dis Sci* 1995;**40**:781–91.
37. Hellstrom PM, Lundberg JM, Hokfelt T, *et al.* Neuropeptide Y, peptide YY, and sympathetic control of rectal tone and anal canal pressure in the cat. *Scand J Gastroenterol* 1989;**24**:231–43.
38. Domoto T, Yang H, Bishop AE, *et al.* Distribution and origin of extrinsic nerve fibers containing calcitonin gene-related peptide, substance P and galanin in the rat upper rectum. *Neurosci Res* 1992;**15**:64–73.
39. Costa M, Brookes SJ, Steele PA, *et al.* Neurochemical classification of myenteric neurons in the guinea-pig ileum. *Neuroscience* 1996;**75**:949–67.
40. Rattan S, Tamura W. Role of galanin in the gastrointestinal sphincters. *Ann NY Acad Sci* 1998;**863**:143–55.
41. Keast JR, Furness JB, Costa M. Somatostatin in human enteric nerves. Distribution and characterization. *Cell Tissue Res* 1984;**237**:299–308.
42. Chakder S, Rattan S. Involvement of pituitary adenylate cyclase-activating peptide in opossum internal anal sphincter relaxation. *Am J Physiol* 1998;**275**:G769–77.
43. Wang YF, Mao YK, Fox Threlkeld JE, *et al.* Colocalization of inhibitory mediators, NO, VIP and galanin, in canine enteric nerves. *Peptides* 1998;**19**:99–112.
44. Furchgott RF, Zawadzki JV. The obligatory role of endothelial cells in the relaxation of arterial smooth muscle by acetylcholine. *Nature* 1980;**288**:373–6.
45. Palmer RM, Ferrige AG, Moncada S. Nitric oxide release accounts for the biological activity of endothelium-derived relaxing factor. *Nature* 1987;**327**:524–6.
46. Deguchi T. Endogenous activating factor for guanylate cyclase in synaptosomal-soluble fraction of rat brain. *J Biol Chem* 1977;**252**:7617–9.
47. Knowles RG, Palacios M, Palmer RM, *et al.* Formation of nitric oxide from L-arginine in the central nervous system: a transduction mechanism for stimulation of the soluble guanylate cyclase. *Proc Natl Acad Sci USA* 1989;**86**:5159–62.
48. Schmidt HH, Wilke P, Evers B, *et al.* Enzymatic formation of nitrogen oxides from L-arginine in bovine brain cytosol. *Biochem Biophys Res Commun* 1989;**165**:284–91.
49. Bredt DS, Hwang PM, Snyder SH. Localization of nitric oxide synthase indicating a neural role for nitric oxide. *Nature* 1990;**347**:768–70.
50. Bredt DS, Snyder SH. Isolation of nitric oxide synthetase, a calmodulin-requiring enzyme. *Proc Natl Acad Sci USA* 1990;**87**:682–5.
51. Gillespie JS, Liu XR, Martin W. The effects of L-arginine and NG-monomethyl L-arginine on the response of the rat anococcygeus muscle to NANC nerve stimulation. *Br J Pharmacol* 1989;**98**:1080–2.
52. Li CG, Rand MJ. Evidence for a role of nitric oxide in the neurotransmitter system mediating relaxation of the rat anococcygeus muscle. *Clin Exp Pharmacol Physiol* 1989;**16**: 933–8.
53. Bult H, Boeckxstaens GE, Pelckmans PA, *et al.* Nitric oxide as an inhibitory non-adrenergic non-cholinergic neurotransmitter. *Nature* 1990;**345**:346–7.
54. Boeckxstaens GE, Pelckmans PA, Bult H, *et al.* Evidence for nitric oxide as mediator of non-adrenergic non-cholinergic relaxations induced by ATP and GABA in the canine gut. *Br J Pharmacol* 1991;**102**:434–8.
55. Boeckxstaens GE, Pelckmans PA, Ruytjens IF, *et al.* Bioassay of nitric oxide released upon stimulation of non-adrenergic non-cholinergic nerves in the canine ileo-colonic junction. *Br J Pharmacol* 1991;**103**:1085–91.
56. Boeckxstaens GE, Pelcksmans PA, Herman AG, *et al.* Involvement of nitric oxide in the inhibitory innervation of the human isolated colon. *Gastroenterology* 1993;**104**:690–7.
57. Burleigh DE. Ng-nitro-L-arginine reduces nonadrenergic, noncholinergic relaxations of human gut. *Gastroenterology* 1992;**102**:679–83.
58. Tam FS, Hillier K. The role of nitric oxide in mediating non-adrenergic non-cholinergic relaxation in longitudinal muscle of human taenia coli. *Life Sci* 1992;**51**:1277–84.
59. Nichols K, Staines W, Krantis A. Nitric oxide synthase distribution in the rat intestine: a histochemical analysis. *Gastroenterology* 1993;**105**:1651–61.

60. Nichols K, Staines W, Krantis A. Neural sites of the human colon colocalize nitric oxide synthase-related NADPH diaphorase activity and neuropeptide Y. *Gastroenterology* 1994; **107**:968–75.
61. Middleton SJ, Cuthbert AW, Shorthouse M, *et al.* Nitric oxide affects mammalian distal colonic smooth muscle by tonic neural inhibition. *Br J Pharmacol* 1993;**108**:974–9.
62. Stebbing JF, Brading AF, Mortensen NJ. Nitrergic inhibitory innervation of porcine rectal circular smooth muscle. *Br J Surg* 1995;**82**:1183–7.
63. Stebbing JF, Brading AF, Mortensen NJ. Nitrergic innervation and relaxant response of rectal circular smooth muscle. *Dis Colon Rectum* 1996;**39**:294–9.
64. Stebbing JF, Brading AF, Mortensen NJ. Role of nitric oxide in relaxation of the longitudinal layer of rectal smooth muscle. *Dis Colon Rectum* 1997;**40**:706–10.
65. Stebbing JF, Brading AF, Mortensen NJ. Distribution of neuronal nitric oxide synthase immunoreactivity in the muscularis propria of the human rectum. *Dis Colon Rectum* 1996;**39**: A43 (Abstract).
66. Rattan S, Sarkar A, Chakder S. Nitric oxide pathway in rectoanal inhibitory reflex of opossum internal anal sphincter. *Gastroenterology* 1992;**103**:43–50.
67. O'Kelly T, Brading A, Mortensen N. Nerve mediated relaxation of the human internal anal sphincter: the role of nitric oxide. *Gut* 1993;**34**:689–93.
68. Gaskell WH. *The involuntary nervous system.* New York: Longman, 1920.
69. Frenckner B, Euler CV. Influence of pudendal block on the function of the anal sphincters. *Gut* 1975;**16**:482–9.
70. Lestar B, Penninckx F, Kerremans R. The composition of anal basal pressure. An *in vivo* and *in vitro* study in man. *Int J Colorectal Dis* 1989;**4**:118–22.
71. Dickinson VA. Maintenance of anal continence: a review of pelvic floor physiology. *Gut* 1978;**19**:1163–74.
72. Frenckner B, Ihre T. Influence of autonomic nerves on the internal and sphincter in man. *Gut* 1976;**17**:306–12.
73. Gutierrez JG, Shah AN. Autonomic control of the internal anal sphincter in man. In: von Trappen G (ed). *Vth International symposium on gastrointestinal motility.* Leuven: Typoff Press, 1975:363–73.
74. Carlstedt A, Nordgren S, Fasth S, *et al.* Sympathetic nervous influence on the internal anal sphincter and rectum in man. *Int J Colorectal Dis* 1988;**3**:90–5.
75. Lubowski DZ, Nicholls RJ, Swash M, *et al.* Neural control of internal anal sphincter function. *Br J Surg* 1987;**74**:668–70.
76. O'Kelly TJ, Davies JR, Brading AF, *et al.* Distribution of nitric oxide synthase containing neurons in the rectal myenteric plexus and anal canal. Morphologic evidence that nitric oxide mediates the rectoanal inhibitory reflex. *Dis Colon Rectum* 1994;**37**:350–7.
77. O'Kelly TJ, Davies JR, Tam PK, *et al.* Abnormalities of nitric-oxide-producing neurons in Hirschsprung's disease: morphology and implications. *J Pediat Surg* 1994;**29**:294–300.
78. Stebbing JF, Brading AF, Mortensen NJ. Nitric oxide and the rectoanal inhibitory reflex: retrograde neuronal tracing reveals a descending nitrergic rectoanal pathway in a guinea-pig model. *Br J Surg* 1996;**83**:493–8.
79. Burleigh DE, D'Mello A, Parks AG. Responses of isolated human internal anal sphincter to drugs and electrical field stimulation. *Gastroenterology* 1979;**77**:484–90.
80. Bouvier M, Gonella J. Electrical activity from smooth muscle of the anal sphincteric area of the cat. *J Physiol Lond* 1981;**310**:445–56.
81. O'Kelly TJ, Brading AF, Mortensen NJ. Nitric oxide mediates cholinergic relaxation of human internal anal sphincter muscle *in vitro. Gut* 1992;**33**: A48 (Abstract).
82. Parks AG, Fishlock DJ, Cameron JD, *et al.* Preliminary investigation of the pharmacology of the human internal anal sphincter. *Gut* 1969;**10**:674–7.
83. Friedmann CA. The action of nicotine and catecholamines on the human internal anal sphincter. *Am J Dig Dis* 1968;**13**:428–31.
84. Read M, Read NW, Duthie HL. Effects of loperamide on anal sphincter function in patients complaining of chronic diarrhoea with faecal incontinence and urgency. *Dig Dis Sci* 1982;**27**: 807–14.
85. Rattan S, Chakder S. Inhibitory effect of CO on internal anal sphincter: heme oxygenase inhibitor inhibits NANC relaxation. *Am J Physiol* 1993;**265**:G799–804.
86. Lund JN, Scholefield JH. A prospective, randomised, double blind, placebo-controlled trial of glyceryl trinitrate in anal fissure. *Lancet* 1997;**349**:11–14.
87. Pitt J, Boulos PB, Henry MM, *et al.* The effect of α-adrenoceptor blockade on the anal canal profile in patients with anal fissures. *J Physiol* 1997;**499**:78–9P (Abstract).
88. Carapeti EA, Kamm MA, Evans BK, *et al.* Topical phenylephrine increases anal sphincter pressure. *Br J Surg* 1999;**86**:267–70.
88a. Carupeti EA, Kamm MA, Nicholls RJ, Philips RK. Randomized, controlled trial of topical phenylephrine for fecal incontinence in patients after ileoanal pouch construction *Dis Colon Rectum* 2000;**43**:1059–63
89. Goligher JC, Hughes ES. Sensibility of the rectum and colon. Its role in the mechanism of anal incontinence. *Lancet* 1951;**i**:543–7.
90. Lane RH, Parks AG. Function of the anal sphincters following colo-anal anastomosis. *Br J Surg* 1977;**64**:596–9.
91. Duthie HL, Gairns FW. Sensory nerve endings and sensation in the anal region in man. *Br J Surg* 1960;**47**:585–95.
92. Duthie HL, Bennett RC. The relation of sensation in the anal canal to the functional sphincter length: a possible factor in anal incontinence. *Gut* 1963;**4**:179–82.
93. Miller R, Bartolo DC, Cervero F, *et al.* Anorectal sampling: a comparison of normal and incontinent patients. *Br J Surg* 1988;**75**:44–7.
94. Read MG, Read NW. Role of anorectal sensation in preserving continence. *Gut* 1982;**23**: 245–7.
95. Miller R, Bartolo DC, Orrom WJ, *et al.* Improvement of anal sensation with preservation of the anal transition zone after ileoanal anastomosis for ulcerative colitis. *Dis Colon Rectum* 1990;**33**:414–8.
96. Miller R, Bartolo DC, Cervero F, *et al.* Anorectal temperature sensation: a comparison of normal and incontinent patients. *Br J Surg* 1987;**74**:511–5.
97. Rogers J. Anorectal temperature sensation: a comparison of normal and incontinent patients. *Br J Surg* 1987;**74**:1189 (Letter).

Chapter 6

Fecal continence and defecation

David C C Bartolo, A D H Macdonald

INTRODUCTION

The social dysfunction reported by patients presenting with the failure of either continence or defecation shows how important these mechanisms are to normal life. The complexity of the mechanisms involved explains the difficulty in managing these patients when control is lost.

Research approaches to fecal continence have been broad and varied and have shown that normal function depends on a number of important factors including a high-pressure zone formed by functioning anal sphincters, anorectal sensation, the anal sampling reflex, rectal compliance and stool consistency. This chapter seeks to integrate these various facets into a comprehensive picture of current understanding of fecal incontinence before ending with a discussion of defecation.

MECHANISMS OF CONTINENCE

Normal anal continence is a complex process involving integration of somatic and visceral muscle function with sensory information under local, spinal and central nervous system control. Continence is dependent on stool consistency, rectal distensibility and sphincter function. It also depends on the sensory input from the anal canal and rectum. Assessment therefore cannot concentrate on any one modality, but should be global and encompass all aspects of function, which contribute to normal control. The physiological function of the pelvic floor is to create a sphincter and to resist the forces of raised intra-abdominal pressure, which would in turn tend to cause herniation of the pelvic floor.

A number of theories have been proposed to try to explain continence. In 1965 Phillips and Edwards[1] put forward the flutter valve theory that suggested a mechanism analogous to the physiological gastroesophageal sphincter. They argued that intra-abdominal forces were transmitted to the lower rectum forming a high-pressure zone, which prevented descent of stool into the anal canal. However, Duthie (1975)[2] demonstrated that the high-pressure zone was in fact below the level of the pelvic floor/levator mechanism in the anal canal and that a flutter valve mechanism such as the above was not anatomically possible.

Parks (1975)[3] developed the concept of the flap valve theory. This worked on the premise that an acute ano-rectal angle allowed the transmission of intra-abdominal forces to the anterior rectal wall and thereby prevented the passage of feces into the anal canal. It was suggested that the anterior rectal wall was forced down onto the upper anal canal by raised intra-abdominal pressure, thus denying feces access to the anal canal. The rationale for this hypothesis was most probably based on the observation that the anterior rectal wall was visualized occluding the passage of a proctoscope during this investigation. Indeed, this led to Parks' ideas on the role of the normal ano-rectal angle of approximately 90 degrees in maintaining continence. Furthermore, he described loss of continence in patients with perineal descent and rectal prolapse in his papers on the descending perineum syndrome.[4] He went on to develop the operation of postanal repair to restore the ano-rectal angle in the hope of improving continence.

Both of these theories provided an explanation of how a non-sphincteric mechanism could function and would allow the pressure of the rectum to exceed that of the anal canal with maintenance of continence. In fact several reports subsequently showed that many patients with incontinence had normal ano-rectal angles, and moreover, restoration of continence following successful sphincter repair was not correlated with a more acute angle. Indeed, success was observed in some reports of patients with a more obtuse angle.[5–7] As a result of some of these observations, Bartolo and co-workers combined physiological studies with radiographic imaging of the rectum.[8] Solid-state microtransducers recorded rectal pressures and fine wire electrodes measured the muscle activity of the muscles of the pelvic floor. Valsalva maneuvers were performed after the rectum had been filled with liquid thus stressing the anal sphincters. Radiographic imaging of the rectum showed that the anterior rectal wall was separated from the top of the anal canal when the rectum was full of liquid contrast material. Even during Valsalva maneuvers, the anterior rectal wall was not driven into the anal canal. In fact, continence was observed to be dependent on sphincteric action, since rectal pressures rose during the maneuvers, and the sphincters in turn compensated by raising anal pressures as recorded by the microtransducers, and reflected by the rise in electromyographic activity recorded from the external anal sphincter and puborectalis muscles. Thus, it was concluded that continence was sphincteric and dependent on the external anal sphincter and the puborectalis muscles.

These observations are supported by the findings of Ferrara *et al.* who found that prolonged rises in rectal pressures generated by rectal motor complexes are invariably accompanied by a rise in mean anal canal pressure and contractile activity.[9] This in turn maintains a greater pressure in the anal canal relative to the rectal pressure, a gradient that helps to preserve sphincter continence. Of some interest, is the further observation that this relationship is retained after ileal pouch-anal anastomosis; rising intra-pouch pressures are accompanied by rises in anal canal pressure and contractile activity.[10]

Patients who had undergone successful sphincter repair for incontinence showed no change in the ano-rectal angle but increased resting and squeeze pressures in the anal canal. Similar results where found in patients who had undergone postanal repair or anterior sphincteroplasty and levatorplasty. It appeared that the altered ano-rectal angle observed in incontinence represented weakness in the puborectalis muscle.

Bannister *et al.*[11] confirmed the above findings in Valsalva maneuvers and Womack *et al.*[7] demonstrated that restoration of the ano-rectal angle was not required for successful outcome following a postanal repair.

ANO-RECTAL SENSATION

Continence is dependent on an awareness of rectal filling and perception of the quality of rectal contents, be they solid or liquid or gas. This allows appropriate decisions to be made as to whether to pass gas, defer evacuation, or to proceed urgently to the nearest toilet facility. The rate of rectal filling and the state of the rectal wall will have independent influences on the ability to retain feces and distinguish between feces and flatus.[12]

Duthie and Gairns[13] were the first workers to study the nerve fibers found in the rectum and anus. They found no intra-epithelial nerve endings in the rectum. However, the anal canal contained a high density of free nerve endings and organized sensory cells such as Meissner's corpuscles, Golgi–Mazzoni bodies, Krause end bulbs and genital corpuscles which responded to touch, pressure, temperature and friction respectively. These were particularly concentrated in the transitional zone. They correlated their histological findings with sensory studies showing that the anal canal had similar discriminatory properties to the tip of the index finger to light touch, pain and temperature. The rectum was insensitive to these variables.

Rectal distension with balloon catheters produces the sensation of rectal fullness.[14] In the absence of sensory nerve endings in the rectal mucosa it is thought that stretch receptors in the pelvic floor musculature respond to rectal distension.[15] The fact that following coloanal anastamosis[15] and after restorative proctocolectomy[16] patients still maintain the ability to detect rectal filling supports this theory. Alternative hypotheses are that there are receptors in the pelvic sidewalls, which respond to rectal fullness. The most plausible theory is that the anal canal and sphincter respond to sampling of rectal contents, and in particular to the frequency with which it relaxes in response to rectal pressure waves which in turn will induce anal relaxation. Voluntary contraction of the sphincter during urgent calls to stool is almost certainly the result of profound recto-anal internal sphincter inhibition leaving continence dependent on external sphincter and puborectalis activity.

THE ANAL SAMPLING REFLEX

The ability to distinguish between flatus and feces is essential for continence. Duthie and Bennet[17] suggested that the contents of the rectum, which could only register distension, could be identified if they came into contact with the sensitive lining of the anal canal. Pressure measurements in the anal canal have shown rectal distension causes reflex relaxation of the internal anal sphincter.[18] Internal anal sphincter relaxation can also be induced by electrical stimulation of the rectum producing an identical reflex response.[19] This is known as the recto-anal inhibitory reflex. The relaxation of the internal anal sphincter with simultaneous contraction of the external anal sphincter allows the contents of the rectum to come into contact with the sensitive transitional zone of the anal canal, whilst preserving continence. This physiological process has led some to refer to the process as the anal sampling reflex.

Miller *et al.*[5,6] carried out *in vivo* studies during which they made pressure recordings from the rectum and anal canal and observed that sampling of rectal contents occurs up to seven times per hour in normal individuals. These recording techniques demonstrated relaxation of the internal anal sphincter, which in turn allowed access of rectal contents to the proximal anal canal. Simultaneous contraction of the external anal sphincter prevented incontinence.

Impaired anal sensation has been demonstrated in patients with a wide range of ano-rectal disorders including hemorrhoids, incontinence, prolapse, obstructed defecation and slow transit constipation, but not in subjects with anal fissures,[20] where heightened anal sensation was observed. Anal sensitivity has also been shown to decrease with age in women, particularly after the menopause, increasing the risks of fecal incontinence.

Finding that the loss of the anal sampling reflex is associated with poor function following anterior resection is supportive of the reflex maintaining continence. However, it has also been shown that patients who have undergone restorative proctocolectomy for ulcerative colitis with excision of the anal transition zone, which resulted in decreased anal sensation, had no functional impairment.[16] Furthermore, it would be expected that the effectiveness of the anal sampling reflex might be diminished by the application of lignocaine gel to the anal canal. In fact a study by Read and Read[21] showed that continence to 1.5 liters of normal saline infused into the rectum was not altered following presumed local anesthesia of the anal canal lining. However, this study was carried out in healthy volunteers, with perfect continence, who may therefore have been able to compensate for loss of sensation. In addition, the absorption of the gel into the anal canal lining may not have been complete.

Surgical procedures, which relocate the anal transitional zone, from the preoperative prolapsed state back to its more correct anatomic position such as sphincter repair and rectopexy for prolapse, are associated with a lowering of the threshold for mucosal electro-sensitivity, suggesting improved anal sensation.[23,24]

THE HIGH-PRESSURE ZONE

A high-pressure zone is found in the anal canal during the resting state.[24,25] Peak pressures are found 2 cm from the anal verge.[26] The pressure zone is formed by the actions of both the internal and external anal sphincters, but predominantly by the former. Their relative contributions to this zone have been established by studying the effects of general anesthesia with the use of muscle relaxants[25] and by pudendal nerve blockade.[27] These two studies showed that the internal anal sphincter contributed to 70% and 85% of resting tone respectively. Residual EMG activity remained in the external anal sphincter in the subjects under general anesthetic and would explain the difference between these two groups.

Resting anal pressures are similar in both sexes, but men have longer anal sphincters and can achieve higher squeeze pressures for longer periods when compared with women.

The anal cushions are considered to have a role in maintaining fecal continence. They have an arterial blood supply, and behave rather like erectile tissue, in that the spaces may fill with blood and empty depending on the tonic state of contraction of the internal anal sphincter. Thus when the sphincter is relaxed, they become engorged, and blood leaves them when it is contracted. The three cushions form a seal, which occludes the anal canal and makes it watertight. A circular tube would be much more difficult to close effectively. This may explain why some patients experience a deterioration of continence after hemorrhoidectomy. The cushions are thought to contribute up to 15% of the anal canal resting pressure and may have a role to play in the high anal pressures seen in patients with hemorrhoids.[28–32]

THE INTERNAL ANAL SPHINCTER

The internal anal sphincter (IAS) is continuous with the circular muscle of the rectum, although its physiological behavior is different to the circular muscle of the colon.[33] The IAS exhibits a continuous state of tonic contraction *in vivo* and *in vitro*.[34] When stimulated, a stronger state of contraction is elicited than when the same stimulus is applied to the circular muscle of the colon.[35]

Electrophysiological studies have demonstrated slow sinusoidal waves with a frequency of 16 cycles a minute that are propagated through the sphincter. Although pressure waves occur at the same frequency, they are not necessarily in phase with one another.[36] Neither general anesthesia nor the paralysis of the external anal sphincter is associated with any effect on the slow wave frequency.[37] Ultraslow waves, which are superimposed on the slow waves can be found in some subjects and occur with a frequency of 0.5–1 per minute.[37]

Ambulatory recordings of the electromyographic activity of the IAS were made using fine wire electrodes, which once in place were not felt. Solid-state transducers were used to measure pressures in the rectum and also positioned to measure upper and lower anal canal pressures. A computerized technique was used to allow analysis of ano-rectal motility during normal activity away for the laboratory setting. This enabled us to correlate the electrical slow wave frequency with pressure changes. During rises in anal sphincter pressure, the frequency of the slow wave electrical activity increased. Moreover, during the recto-anal inhibitory elicited either by balloon distention or by the sensation of the passage of flatus, the anal pressures fell and this was associated with the abolition of slow wave internal EMG activity. On the other hand, no such correlation was found for the amplitude of EMG activity.[38]

Studies in patients with a deficiency or failure of the IAS have confirmed its important role in fecal incontinence. Complete division of the IAS is associated with fecal soiling and incontinence to flatus in up to 40% of patients. Partial internal sphincterotomy is associated with such incontinence in up to 15% of subjects. Patients with idiopathic fecal soiling are often found to have thinning of the IAS when endoanal ultrasonography is performed. Ultrasonography has enhanced our understanding of disorders of the internal sphincter. Thus, degeneration may occur spontaneously or in prolapse, defects are identifiable after fistula surgery and after inappropriate hemorrhoidectomy. They are frequently seen following obstetric trauma. Recent years have witnessed interest in applying drugs to modify internal sphincter function with the use of nitric oxide donors such as glyceryl trinitrate and isosorbide mononitrate to lower internal sphincter pressure in the treatment of fissures. Calcium channel blockers like diltiazem relax the IAS for the duration of their chemical activities while toxins like botulinum produce a more sustained inhibition of function lasting several weeks.

IAS sphincter relaxation after the initiation of the recto-anal inhibitory reflex was found to be prolonged and more pronounced in incontinent subjects, and this abnormality has been used to stimulate the trial of agents like phenylephrine to augment sphincter function by increasing α-adrenergic activity within the internal sphincter. These measures to augment IAS function have been less successful to date as a consequence of degeneration or myoelectrical desensitization of the smooth muscle, but have been of benefit in the treatment of some patients with ileal pouches who experience nocturnal leakage.

THE EXTERNAL ANAL SPHINCTER AND THE PUBORECTALIS MUSCLE

The external anal sphincter (EAS) forms a ring of muscle around the anal canal and is continuous above with the puborectalis muscle. Recordings from both muscles show that they are both activated together during voluntary contractions of the pelvic floor and during coughing and straining.[27,39–47] This suggests these muscles function together. Although the EAS consists of striated muscle under voluntary control, it is continuously active, which is unusual for such muscles. Measurements from the EAS during sleep show that electromyographic activity is decreased and this is associated with a fall in anal canal pressure but rectal pressure also decreases, allowing continence to be preserved. Floyd and Walls[39] made these observations in 1953, and Walls later demonstrated muscle spindles in the EAS and puborectalis, which was consistent with their reflex mechanisms, and explained their role in preventing herniation of the pelvic contents together with sphincteric activity.

During activity, the EMG responses from the external sphincter increase not only during voluntary contractions, but also during coughing or straining, during exertion such as lifting or during the performance of a Valsalva maneuver. This is all consistent with reflex increased activity mediated via the spinal cord, and reflected by the finding of muscle spindles as outlined above.

EFFECTS OF VARIOUS INFLUENCES ON THE EXTERNAL ANAL SPHINCTER

Tabes dorsalis

In tabes dorsalis, Lissauer's tract or the dorsal nerve root is destroyed so that proprioceptive afferent pathways are damaged. A voluntary contraction can be maintained but is ataxic and driven by supra-segmental input. In tabetic patients, the resting EMG is silent, and activity only occurs following voluntary recruitment or contraction of the sphincter.[42,48,49]

Transection of the spinal cord above the third lumbar segment

Resting EMG activity is normal in such patients, but there can be no voluntary increment. During coughing or raised intra-abdominal pressure, the EMG activity increases in the EAS indicating a reflex pathway via the spinal cord below the level of transection.

Cutaneous stimulation

Stimulation of the perianal skin excites a reflex contraction of the external anal sphincter.[50] It is a polysynaptic response, which is absent in patients with lesions or injuries affecting the nerve supply to anal sphincter, but is preserved in patients following transection of the spinal cord above the third lumbar segment, indicating it is a spinal reflex. It was formerly considered that the reflex latency could be used as a measure of nerve damage in patients with neurogenic incontinence, but this was not borne out by subsequent work because of the polysynaptic pathway. Moreover, it was not possible accurately to discriminate between direct stimulation and reflex responses unless the stimulus was applied to one side or the other.[51]

Rectal distention

Distention of the rectum results in an initial burst of EMG activity following distention with 50 mL of air. This response precedes the reflex inhibition of the IAS described above.[31,52,53] Pudendal nerve blockade abolishes it, and suggests it is a reflex response from the external sphincter.[47,54]

After the initial burst of EMG activity, there is a sustained increase in EAS EMG activity, which persists throughout the period of rectal distention. This EMG activity is also present in patients with transection of the spinal cord above the lumbar segments indicating that cortical control is not involved. Volumes between

150–200 mL will produce constant relaxation or complete inhibition of the EMG recorded from the EAS.

Straining

Kerremans[46] distinguished four patterns of EMG activity on straining as in defecation: (i) a sudden abolition of all electrical activity; (ii) a larger number of patients produced an initial burst of activity lasting for one to two seconds followed by reduced activity for the duration of the straining effort; (iii) some patients showed greatly increased activity for the duration of straining; a few patients had bursts of polyphasic potentials. In all, 80% of his study group showed either temporary or sustained increased activity. Parks and co-workers described an initial burst followed by sustained inhibition. This was also seen in paraplegic patients suggesting the reflex response was inhibition, and that voluntary contraction required some cortical input. These observations should be considered when making a diagnosis of anismus. This finding has been ascribed to explain many different constipative and defecatory disorders, and indeed a whole biofeedback industry has been generated to try and abolish what is clearly a physiological finding, or at best an artefact that is induced by the circumstances of the laboratory. The presence of EMG needles in the anal sphincter is far from physiological. Ihre[47] carried out balloon expulsion tests with simultaneous EMG and manometry and found that 11 of 16 patients expelled a rectal balloon. In eight, the EMG was inhibited, while in three expulsion occurred despite continued EMG activity.

Anal canal distention

Pulling on the anal canal increases EMG activity, and this increase is maintained for the duration of the contraction. It is further increased following cessation of traction, and this has been termed the closing reflex. In paraplegic subjects, the increased EMG response was not seen. This suggests that the normal defecatory response is inhibition, and was overshadowed by a cortical response in subjects with intact nervous systems. It is unlikely that the sustained increase in activity seen during anal distention is part of normal defecation. Indeed in our ambulatory studies, normal defecation was associated with sphincter inhibition. What is important is the reflex closure of the anal canal at the end of defecation.

RECTAL FILLING AND COMPLIANCE

The ability of the rectum to distend and store feces is an important component of continence. Filling of the rectum is first detected at a volume of between 11 and 68 ml. The maximal tolerated volume is usually in the region of 300 ml, but can range from 220 to 510 ml.[55] Rectal distention initiates regular contractions in the rectal wall[56,57] which ultimately prompt the desire to defecate once tolerance is exceeded.[47] As the rectum fills it distends, allowing the pressure to remain relatively unchanged as filling occurs. When measured, the compliance of the rectum has a wide range from 4 to 14 ml/cm H_2O in normal subjects. The compliance of the rectum is greatest during the early stages of filling and decreases as the rectum fills.

A reduction of rectal compliance is associated with an increase in urgency to defecate and also in frank fecal incontinence, even when the sphincter is otherwise normal. Conditions in which this may arise include pelvic radiation,[55] inflammatory bowel disease,[38] and the presence of a rectal neoplasm. The replacement of a non-compliant rectum with the formation of a neorectum allows continence to be restored.[15,16] Loss of rectal sensation is associated with incontinence when rectal filling occurs and rectal pressures may rise and exceed a weakened sphincter before the subject is aware of the need to defecate. In others, rectal pressure increases are pathologically elevated due to smooth muscle hypertrophy which is a response to denervation, These high pressures may overcome a normal sphincter and lead to incontinence, but the subject will experience urgency if the sensory innervation is intact. Orrom et al[58] reported that in incontinent patients with complete rectal prolapse a much smaller volume of rectal distention produced sustained internal sphincter inhibition than in normal subjects. This could be due to sustained internal sphincter inhibition or damage to the internal anal sphincter.

STOOL CONSISTENCY AND VOLUME

The ideal stool is soft and well formed. Volunteers have been shown to pass large deformable stools with greater ease than small hard pellets. Semisolid stool is more efficiently evacuated from the rectum than either solid or liquid stool.[59] Residual stool in the rectum is more likely to cause soiling than if the rectum is efficiently emptied.

High volume and liquid stool can cause incontinence in normal subjects. A severe episode of diarrhea can produce such a situation. In addition, the discrimination between flatus and feces is less exact, which can lead to accidental incontinence. Small hard pellets of stool can accumulate in the rectum and cause marked distention without the urge to defecate and may be associated with incontinence.

DEFECATION

Despite extensive research, the defecation mechanism is still poorly understood. Stool entering the rectum from the sigmoid colon is detected by stretch receptors in the pelvic floor or rectal wall, which produce the urge to defecate as previously discussed. This starts as an intermittent sensation that becomes more constant and ends with pelvic discomfort. The recto-anal inhibitory response is initiated and the anal sampling reflex is used to distinguish stool from flatus, while continence is preserved by contraction of the external anal sphincter. If defecation is not convenient, contraction of the pelvic floor muscles, and the puborectalis, propels feces proximally back into the sigmoid colon. The internal sphincter then regains its tone and returns to the contracted state, thus allowing defecation to be postponed.

The squatting position increases the ano-rectal angle and straightens out the axis of the rectum and anal canal to allow more efficient transmission of force through the bowel lumen. In addition, inhibition of the muscles of the pelvic floor allows the perineum to descend by approximately 2 cm.

For defecation to take place, the pressure in the rectum must exceed the pressure in the anal canal. In combination with internal and external sphincter relaxation the intra-abdominal pressure rises by the performance of a Valsalva maneuver and the bolus of feces is propelled out of the body.

Debate surrounds whether or not contractile waves spread through the rectal wall and aid the expulsion of feces. Rectal complexes have been described, but most authorities feel their contribution to defecation is minimal when compared to abdominal straining. However, recent work has shown that distention of the rectosigmoid junction with balloons causes contraction of the rectum. This has been termed the rectosigmoid-rectal reflex and may be important for defecation.

Completion of defecation is achieved by a closing reflex that contracts the external anal sphincter. This was demonstrated by Porter[41] who applied traction to the anal canal with a finger. EMG activity was seen to increase during this procedure. When the traction was released, a sudden burst of EMG activity followed corresponding to contraction of the EAS and was termed the closing reflex. Similarly, deflation of rectal balloons mimicking rectal emptying is associated with EAS contraction. Simultaneous contraction of the IAS propels any residual feces back into the rectum leaving the anal canal clear.

The appreciation of rectal filling probably depends on many factors including sampling within the anal canal, rectal receptors mediating filling, pelvic floor receptors, and perhaps other unrecognized factors. The awareness of filling persists after replacement of the rectum by either colon or ileum. It is however modified. This awareness persists despite the absence of the recto-anal inhibitory reflex. The absence of the latter does not necessarily exclude the role of anal sensation in appreciating rectal or neo-rectal contents. This is often in spite of mucosectomy to the dentate line, with resultant impairment of anal canal sensation.[60]

REFERENCES

1. Phillips SF, Edwards DAW. some aspects of anal continence and defaecation. *Gut* 1965;**6**:396–405.
2. Duthie HL. Dynamics of the rectum and anus. *Clin Gastroenterol* 1975;**4**(3):467–77.
3. Parks AG. Anorectal incontinence. *Proc Roy Soc Med* 1975;**68**:681–90.
4. Parks AD, Porter NH, Hardcastle JD. The syndrome of the descending perineum. *Proc Roy Soc Med* 1966;**59**:477–82.
5. Miller R, Bartolo DCC, Locke-Edmunds JC, Mortenson NJMcC. A prospective study of conservative and operative treatment for faecal incontinence. *Br J Surg* 1988;**75**:101–105.
6. Miller R, Orrom WJ, Cornes H, *et al.* Anterior sphincter plication and levatorplasty in the treatment of faecal incontinence. *Br J Surg* 1989;**76**:1058–60.
7. Womack NR, Morrison JFB, Williams NS. Prospective study of the effects of post anal repair in neurogenic faecal incontinence. *Br J Surg* 1988;**75**:48–52.
8. Bartolo DCC, Roe AM, Locke-Edmunds JC, *et al.* Flap valve theory of anorectal incontinence. *B J Surg* 1986;**73**:1012–14.
9. Ferrara A, Pemberton JH, Hansen RB. Relationship between anal canal tone and rectal motor activity. *Dis Colon Rectum* 1993;**34**:4.
10. Ferrara A, Pemberton JH, Hansen RB. Preservation of continence after ileoanal anastomosis by the coordination of ileal pouch and anal canal motor activity. *Am J Surg* 1992; **163**:83–9.
11. Bannister JJ, Gibbons C, Read NW. Preservation of faecal continence during rises in intra-abdominal pressure: is there a role for the flap valve? *Gut* 1987;**28**:1242–5.
12. Goligher JC, Hughes ESR Sensibility of the rectum and colon. Its role in the mechanism of anal continence. *Lancet* 1951;**i**:543–8.
13. Duthie HL, Gairns FW. Sensory nerve endings and sensation in the anal region of man. *Br J Surg* 1960;**47**:585–95.
14. Winkler G. Remarques sur la morphologie et l'innervation du muscle releur de l'anus. *Arch Anat Histol Embryol* 1958;**41**:77–95.
15. Lane RHS, Parks AG. Function of the anal sphincter following colo-anal anastomosis. *Br J Surg* 1977;**64**:596–9.
16. Keighley MRB, Yoshioka K, Kmiott W, Heyer F. Physiological parameters influencing functions in restorative proctocolectomy and ileo-pouch-anal anastomosis. *Br J Surg* 1988;**75**:997–1002.
17. Duthie HL, Bennett RC. The relation of sensation in the anal canal to the functional anal sphincter: a possible factor in anal continence. *Gut* 1963;**4**:179–82.
18. Miller R, Lewis GT, Bartolo DCC, *et al.* Sensory discrimination and dynamic activity in the anorectum: evidence using a new ambulatory technique. *Br J Surg* 1988;**75**:1003–1007.
19. Kamm MA, Lennard-Jones JE, Nicholls RJ. Evaluation of the intrinsic innervation of the internal anal sphincter using electric stimulation. *Gut* 1989;**30**:935–8.

20. Roe AM, Bartolo DCC, Mortenson NJ, McC. New methods for assessment of anal sensation in various anorectal disorders. *Br J Surg* 1986;**73**:310–312.
21. Read MG, Read NW. Role of anorectal sensation in preserving continence. *Gut* 1982;**23**:345–7.
22. Duthie GS, Bartolo DCC. A comparison between marlex and resection rectopexy. *Neth J Surg* 1989;**41**:136–9.
23. Duthie GS, Bartolo DCC. Is improvement of continence after rectopexy for rectal prolapse dependent on improved sphincter function or post operative constipation? *Gut* 1989;**30**:A1466.
24. Bennett LRC, Duthie HL. The functional importance of the internal sphincter. *Br J Surg* 1964;**51**:355–7.
25. Duthie HL, Watts J. Contribution of the external anal sphincter to the pressure zone in the anal canal. *Gut* 1965;**6**:64–8.
26. Duthie HL. Anal continence. *Gut* 1971;**12**:844–52.
27. Freckner B, von Euler C. Influence of pudendal block on the function of the anal sphincters. *Gut* 1975; **16**:482–9.
28. Arabi Y, Alexander-Williams J, Keighley MRB. Anal pressure in haemorrhoids and fissure. *Am J Surg* 1977;**1**:608–610.
29. Bennett LRC, Friedman MHW, Goligher JC. Late results of haemorrhoidectomy by ligature and excision. *Br Med J* 1963;**ii**: 216–219.
30. Gibbons CP, Trowbridge EA, Bannister JJ, Read NW. Role of anal cushions in maintaining continence. *Lancet* 1986;**i**:886–88.
31. Hancock BD. Internal sphincter and the nature of haemorrhoids. *Gut* 1977;**18**:651–6.
32. Schuster MM, Hendrix TR, Mendeloff AI. The internal anal sphincter response: manometric studies on its normal physiology, neural pathways and alteration in bowel disorders. *J Clin Invest* 1963;**42**:196–207.
33. Hancock BD, Smith K. The internal anal sphincter and the Lord's procedure for haemorrhoids. *Br J Surg* 1975;**62**:833–6.
34. Kerremans R. Electrical activity and mobility of the internal anal sphincter. An *'in vivo'* electrophysiological study in man. *Acta Gastroenterol Belg* 1968;**31**: 465–82.
35. Burleigh DE, D'Mello A, Parks AG. Responses of isolated human internal anal sphincter to drugs and electrical field stimulation. *Gastroenterology* 1979;**77**: 484–90.
36. Weinbeck M, Altaparmacov I. Is the internal anal sphincter controlled by a myoelectric mechanism? In: Christensen J (ed.) *Gastrointestinal mobility*. New York: Raven Press, 1980:487–93.
37. Wankling W, Brown B, Collins C, Duthie H. Basal electrical activity in the anal canal in man. *Gut* 1968; **9**:457–60.
38. Duthie GS, Miller R, Bartolo DCC. Internal anal sphincter electromyographic frequency is related to anal canal resting pressure. Both are reduced in idiopathic faecal incontinence. *Gut* 1990;**31**:A619.
39. Floyd W, Walls E. Electomyography of the sphincter ani externus in man. *J Physiol* 1953;**122**:599–600.
40. Taverner D, Smiddy FG. An electromyographic study of the natural function of the external anal sphincter and pelvic diaphragm. *Dis Colon Rectum* 1959;2: 153–60.
41. Porter NH. Physiological study of the pelvic floor in rectal prolapse. *Ann Roy Soc Med* 1962;**286**:379–404.
42. Parks AG, Porter NH, Melzak J. Experimental study of the reflex mechanism controlling the muscles of the pelvic floor. *Dis Colon Rectum* 1962;**5**:407–414.
43. Melzak J, Porter NH. Studies on the reflex activity of the external sphincter ani in spinal man. *Paraplegia* 1984;**1**:277–96.
44. Chantraine A. Electromyographic des sphincters stries uretral et anal humains. Etude descriptive et analytique. *Rev Neurol* 1966;**115**:396–403.
45. Chantraine A, Balthazar D. Electromyographie des sphincters stries uretral et anal chez l'enfant normal – étude descriptive et analytique. *Electromyography* 1968;**8**:312–17.
46. Kerremans R. *Morphological and physiological aspect of continence and defaecation*. Arsica, Brussels: Editions.
47. Ihre T. Studies in anal function in continent and incontinent patients. *Scand J Gastroenterol* 1974;**9 (Suppl)**:25.
48. Walton JN. Disorders of the spinal cord and cauda equina. In: *Brain's diseases of the nervous system*, 8th edn. Oxford University Press, Oxford: 1977;751.
49. Struppler A, Burg D, Erbel F. The unloading reflex under normal and pathological conditions in man. In: Desmedt JE (ed.) *New developments in electromyography and clinical neurophysiology*, vol. 3. Basel: Karger, 1973;603–617.
50. Rossolimo G. Der Anal Reflex: Physiologie und Pathologie. *Neurol Cent Blatt Leipzig* 1891; **9**:257–9.
51. Bartolo DCC, Jarratt JA, Read MG, *et al.* Why are geriatric patients incontinent of faeces? *Clin Sci* 1983;**75** (Suppl) 1–10.
52. Gaston EA. The physiology of fecal continence. *Surgery, Gynaecol Obstet* 1948;**87**:280–90.
53. Ustach TJ, Tobon F, Hambrecht T, *et al.* Electrophysiological aspects of human sphincters in function. *J Clin Invest* 1970;**49**:41–4.
54. Varma KK, Stephens D. Neuromuscular reflexes of anal continence. *Aust N Z J Surg* 1972;**41**:263–72.
55. Varma JS, Smith AN, Busuttil A. Correlation of clinical and manometric abnormalities of rectal function following chronic radiation injury. *Br J Surg* 1985;**72**:872–5.
56. Connell AM. The mobility of the pelvic colon, *Gut* 1961;**2**:175–86. Denny-Brown D, Robertson EG. An investigation of the nervous control of defaecation. *Brain* 1935;**58**:256–310.
57. Scharli AF, Kieswetter WB. Defaecation and continence: some new concepts. *Dis Colon Rectum* 1970;**13**:81–107.
58. Orrom WJ, Duthie GS, Bartolo DCC, *et al.* A physiological study of rectal prolapse and rectal intussusception: a comparison of continent and incontinent patients. (Personal communication).
59. Ambroze WL, *et al.* The effect of stool consistency on rectal and neorectal emptying. *Dis Colon Rectum* 1993;**34**:1.
60. Öresland T, Fasth S, Akervall S, *et al.* Manovolumetric and sensory characteristics of the ileoanal J Pouch as compared to healthy rectum with particular reference to function. *Br J Surg* 1990;**77**:803–806.

Chapter 7

Colonic motility and colonic function

Eamonn M M Quigley

Colonic motility should, in theory, sub-serve colonic homeostatic functions.[1–3] These include important roles in absorption, storage and defecation. Thus, the colon performs an important role in fluid and electrolyte absorption, especially in those circumstances where these functions are compromised in the small intestine. More recently, the concept of colonic salvage has been extended beyond water and electrolytes with the recognition of the role of the colon in carbohydrate and bile salt absorption. The colon is also home to a vast and varied bacterial flora whose role continues to be elucidated. It is becoming increasingly clear that this flora has important beneficial functions and that its composition may be influenced in turn by colonic and intestinal motor activity. Sarna[1] stressed three important differences between the colon and the small intestine which might well contribute to its unique motor properties. These included; firstly, the colon is never empty and is thus in a constant digestive state, secondly, its contents are more viscous than elsewhere in the gastrointestinal tract and, finally, its role in defecation implies a significant role for voluntary control and feedback to the rest of the gut.

While studies in a variety of animal models, as well as *in vitro* recordings, have contributed significantly to our understanding of the generation and regulation of colonic motor patterns, this review will confine itself to colonic motor activity and function in man. In contrast to other areas of the gastrointestinal tract, colonic motor activity has received relatively little attention due, in large part, to its relative inaccessibility and to several technical factors which continue to complicate recordings of colonic motor activity, *in vivo*, in man. Thus, recordings of colonic motility have been, variably, performed following introduction of the recording assembly in either an antegrade or retrograde direction, in the prepared and unprepared colon, with or without prior colonoscopy to place the catheter assembly, on a restricted or unrestricted diet, for short or prolonged periods and with a variety of manometric assemblies. Several other factors including stress, exercise, sleep and the menstrual cycle may also significantly influence colonic motor activity. It has been assumed that differences between protocols, based on variations in one or more of these parameters, may explain, in large part, the considerable differences in motor patterns recorded in a variety of studies.

COLONIC MOTOR ACTIVITY

PHASIC MOTOR ACTIVITY

Recordings of motor and myoelectrical activity, in a number of animal species, have identified three phasic contractile (or myoelectrical spiking) events: short-duration (i.e. <15 s duration) contractions (or spikes), long-duration (i.e. 40–60 s) contractions and giant migrating (GMC), or high-amplitude propagating (HAPC), contractions. These may, in turn, occur as isolated events or in bursts and may or may not propagate.[1] Recordings of colonic motor activity in normal man have, in contrast, yielded highly variable results.[1–11] Thus, while, in general, human colonic motility features periods of alternating quiescence and activity, some have failed to reveal any further level of organization in 24-hour recordings.[5] Others, in contrast, have described several discrete motor events, including individual phasic contractions, propagating contractions (both ante-grade and retro-grade), propagating bursts of contractions and, most recognizable of all, high amplitude propagating contractions (HAPCs) (Fig. 7.1).[7,9–11] The electrical equivalents of HAPCs have also been described in man in intra-luminal myo-electrical recordings.[12,13]

Several factors which might explain these variable findings have already been mentioned. Lemann and colleagues, for example, compared motor activity recorded without prior preparation with that recorded following colonic cleansing with a polyethylene glycol (PEG)-based solution.[10] While preparation did increase the frequency of HAPCs there were no other significant differences between the prepped and unprepped colon. In keeping with a number of other prolonged recordings, they found that colonic motility was, for the most part, apparently unorganized and featured periods of quies-

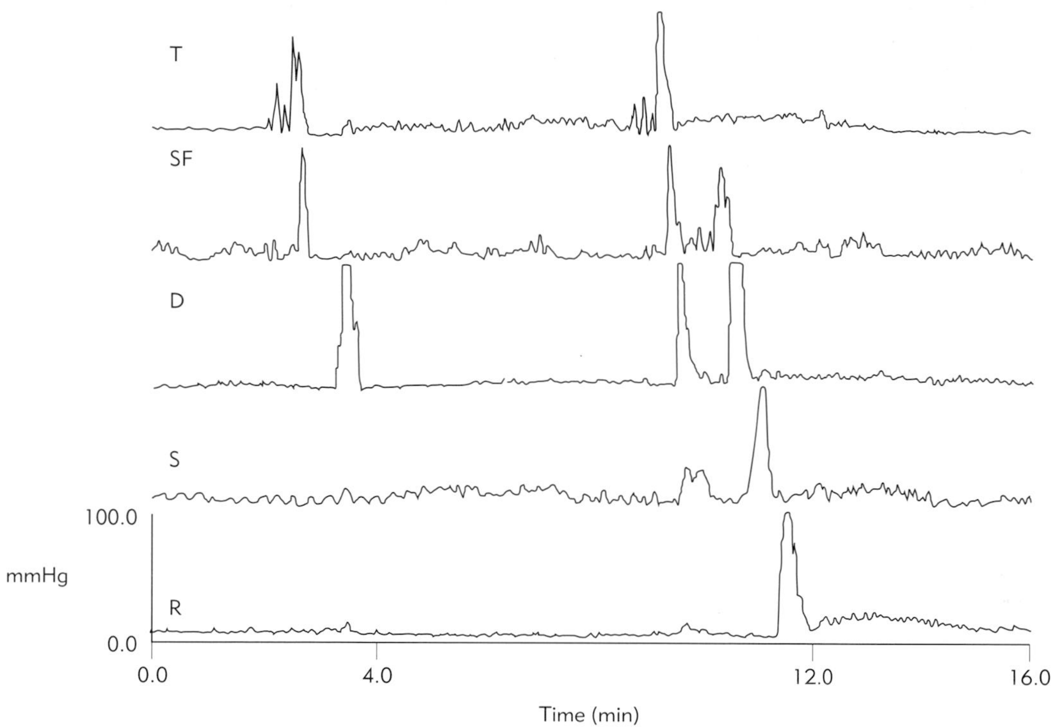

Figure 7.1 Three high amplitude propagated contractions (HAPCs) recorded postprandially in a child. Note propagation from transverse (T) through splenic flexure (SF), descending (D) and sigmoid (S) to rectum (R). (From Di Lorenzo *et al.*[15] with permission.)

cence alternating with periods of irregular activity. Most contractions occurred in bursts which lasted from 1 to 30 minutes and occurred at a frequency of 3 to 6 cycles per minute. HAPCs were, however, clearly identified and, in their study, occurred at a frequency of 5.4 events per 9-hour recording period. Particular importance has been attached to the HAPC given the recognition of its highly propulsive nature, its association with, either the conscious sensation of an urge to defecate,[10,14] or the passage of flatus,[10] and the suggestion that their absence may serve as a marker of colonic motor dysfunction.[15,16] The frequency of this motor event appears, however, to be highly variable, varying anywhere from less than two to as many as 6.9 per 24 hours, in different studies.[5,10,14,17–19] These events typically originate in the cecum or ascending colon and propagate into the sigmoid colon at a velocity of about 1 cm per minute. HAPCs vary with age and are significantly more common in young children.[20] They are stimulated, not only by PEG solutions,[10] and distention[21] but also by laxatives, such as bisacodyl and cascara,[22–24] a further potential explanation for between-study variations in HAPC frequency. Recordings of rectal motor activity have identified intermittent bursts of phasic motor activity – termed the rectal motor complex[25,26] (Fig. 7.2). This complex is unrelated to the migrating complex[27,28] and its physiological significance remains unclear.[28]

The gastro-colonic reflux

Discrepancies between studies are further illustrated by observations on the colonic response to a meal, the so called *gastro-colonic reflex*. While its appellation is, indeed, a misnomer, as the response may be elicited in gastrectomized subjects, the gastro-colonic response has received considerable attention due, in large part, to the frequency of meal-related symptoms among those with presumed disorders of colonic motor function. Initially, most studies of this phenomenon were confined to the recto-sigmoid region:[4,29–33] explorations of the motor response to a meal in other regions of the colon have provided conflicting data and have suggested that several factors may influence the nature and the intensity of this response.[5–7,34–40] These include the anatomical location of the recording site within the colon, the size, composition and consistency of the meal[36] and the rate of delivery of intestinal contents to the colon.[41]

In the recto-sigmoid region, three phases of this response were identified: immediate (up to 11 min) (Fig.

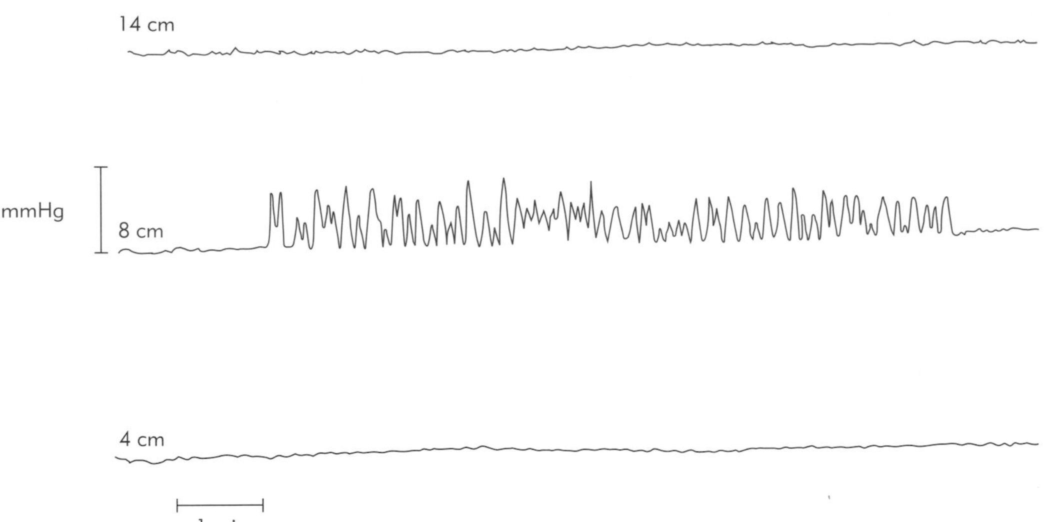

Figure 7.2 The rectal motor complex – a burst of phasic contractions, typically recorded from a single recording site in the rectum. Note catheter location based on distance from anal verge. (From Prior *et al.*[28], with permission.)

7.3), early (up to 60 min) and late (assumed to represent the arrival of chyme into the colon).[1,2] Components of this response have been variably described in the rest of the colon. Steadman and colleagues identified the immediate and early components of this phasic response.[42] Jouet and colleagues noted a postprandial increase in motility index within 30 minutes of meal ingestion in the left colon; they did not record a late component[9] (Fig. 7.3). Ford and colleagues recorded an immediate response in the transverse colon alone; in the sigmoid the response was delayed for 20–30 minutes.[40] Moreno-Osset and colleagues recorded an immediate

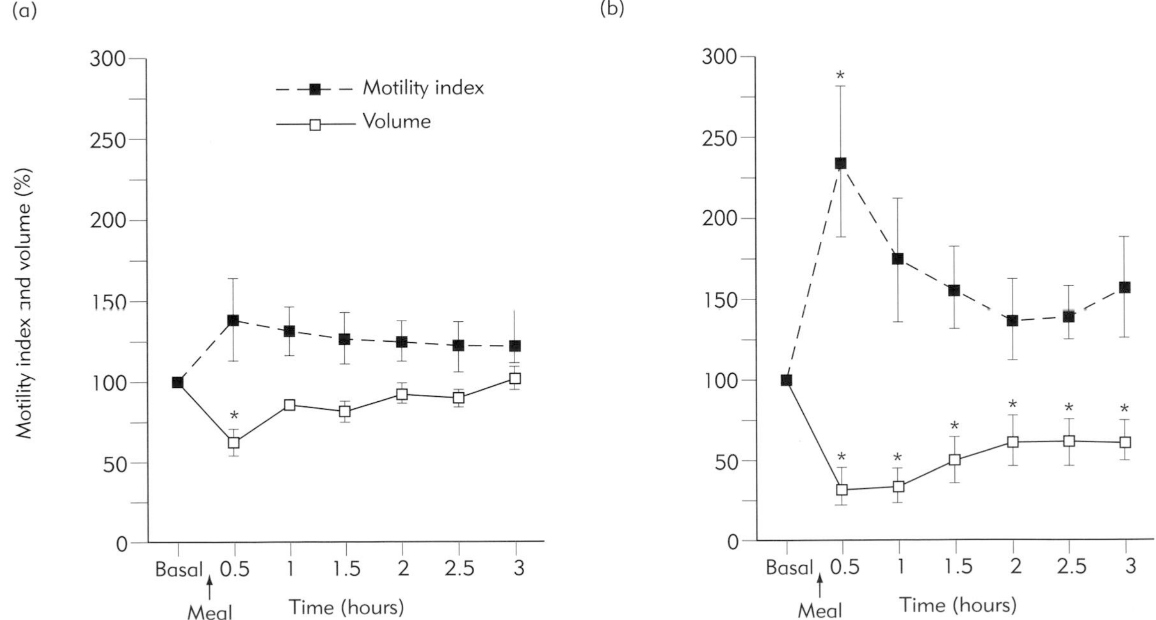

Figure 7.3 Phasic motor and tonic responses to meal ingestion in the proximal (a) and distal (b) colon. Tone recorded by changes in barostat bag volume. *Note*: (i) significant, early increase in motility index in distal colon alone. (ii) Significant increase in tone (decrease in bag volume) in both proximal and distal colon but response greater and more prolonged in distal colon. (From Jouet *et al.*[9] with permission.)

increase in non-propagating contractile activity in the descending, sigmoid and transverse colon and noted that transit of contents followed pressure gradients generated by phasic activity in the various parts of the colon.[34]

The relative intensity of this postprandial response within various parts of the colon has also proven highly variable. Thus, while Lemann and colleagues recorded an increase in motility index throughout the colon, with the exception of the sigmoid, following meal ingestion,[10] Ford and colleagues[40] and Jouet and colleagues,[9] in direct contrast, found that the postprandial increase in motility index was greatest in the sigmoid colon (Fig. 7.3); in yet another study the response was most intense in the descending colon.[37]

Retrograde movement of colon contents

The issue of *retrograde movement*, especially in the right colon, has also been proven contentious. Cannon was perhaps the first to describe prominent retrograde activity in the ascending colon and emphasized its importance in promoting mixing and absorption.[43] While retrograde contractile activity has not been identified with any degree of consistency within any part of the colon in man, studies of transit have identified retrograde (orad) movement of content. Movement of content, in a retrograde direction, from the descending colon or splenic flexure has been identified in response to meal ingestion in some[34,44] but not in other[45] studies.

Diurnal variations

Others have examined *diurnal variations* in colonic motor activity: some have failed to reveal any significant temporal fluctuations in motor activity[5] while others reported motor quiescence during sleep, followed by a clearly recognizable increase in motility either on waking spontaneously in the morning, or on rousing the subject from sleep.[46]

Effect of exercise

Perhaps reflecting the intrinsic variations in colonic motor activity, studies of the *effects of exercise* have also proved variable.[47–50] Rao and colleagues reported a suppression of colonic motility during exercise with a significant post-exercise increase in propagated activity.[47] Others, in contrast, either reported no effect,[50] or the limitation of an exercise-related effect on motility to the ascending colon alone,[48] or to the ascending and descending colon.[49]

Effect of stress

Rao and colleagues also examined the *response of the colon to stress*.[51] Physical stress was associated with the onset of simultaneous contractions whereas psychological stress was more likely to induce propagated activity. Interestingly, the return to baseline motor activity was slower following psychological than physical stress.

Fluctuations in blood sugar do not appear to exert a significant effect on colonic tone or contractility, nor does hyperglycemia suppress the gastro-colonic response.[52] Using a 6-lumen catheter assembly with individual recording sites at 3–4 cm: intervals, Daly and colleagues studied the postprandial response in the recto-sigmoid region, in some detail, and provided some insights into the challenges that colonic manometry faces.[31] During fasting, motor activity in this part of the colon was characterized, primarily, by the presence of contractions isolated to a single recording site. Meal ingestion led to a general increase in motility index (Fig. 7.4) but the most striking change was an increase in the frequency of contractions which occurred simultaneously in at least three channels. This observation emphasizes yet another factor which may significantly influence the outcome of colonic motility recordings; namely, the positioning and spacing of recording sites. Clearly, the ability to recognize contractile activity and, in particular, to define both the occurrence and the extent of propagation will be directly related to the number and proximity of recording sites. Colonic diameter may also influence the fidelity of recordings of phasic contractile events; Van der Ohe and colleagues suggested that the accuracy of such recordings was reduced when the diameter of the colonic lumen exceeded 5–6 cm.[53]

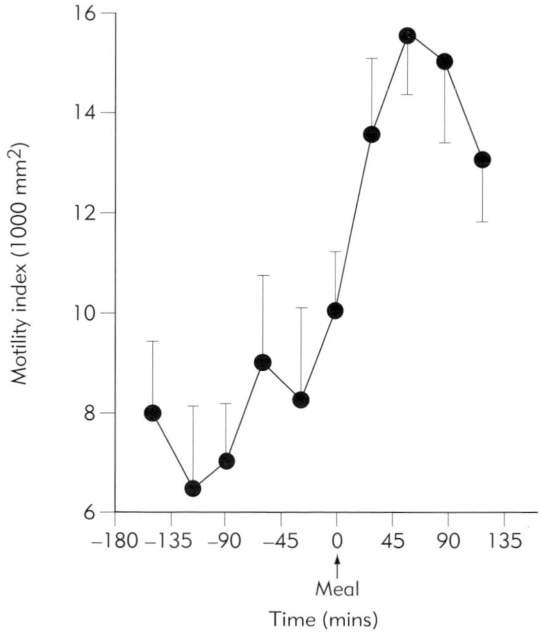

Figure 7.4 Postprandial motor response – recto-sigmoid colon. Note prompt increase in motility index following meal ingestion. (From Daly *et al.*[31] with permission.)

TONE

The advent of innovative methodologies, such as the barostat, now permits prolonged recordings of tone and compliance from various parts of the colon. These systems have also been employed to study the sensory response to colonic distention. It is clear that tone is an important function of this organ and may, indeed, explain some of the difficulties, described above, in attempting to relate motor patterns, derived by conventional methods to colonic function.

Steadman and colleagues provided the first detailed insights into colonic tone in normal individuals.[42] In recordings of tone from the ascending, transverse and descending colon they identified a clear disassociation between changes in tone and intra-luminal pressure wave activity. Tone was at its lowest level during sleep and rose on waking (Fig. 7.5). At rest, tone appeared similar in the sigmoid and transverse colon but was lower in the ascending colon. Ford and colleagues also recorded a similar level of resting tone in the sigmoid and transverse colon, though compliance was greater in the latter.[40]

A variable regional response to meal ingestion has been reported. Steadman and colleagues recorded an immediate, though slowly progressive, postprandial increase in tone.[42] Jouet and colleagues found that the postprandial increase in tone was greater in the distal than the proximal colon[9] (Fig. 7.3), whereas Ford and colleagues recorded exactly the reverse[40] and Steadman and colleagues failed to identify any regional differences.[42] Ford and colleagues noted that the initial change in tone in the ascending colon was related to ileal emptying, from 30 to 105 minutes after meal ingestion the increase in tone was associated with the transfer of contents to the ascending colon.[40]

Jouet and colleagues studied the response in the ascending colon and failed to identify a postprandial relaxation of the right colon, analagous to that identified in the terminal ileum[9] (Fig. 7.3). Instead, they found that tone increased throughout the colon in response to a meal but noted the occurrence of retrograde movement of content which followed pressure gradients, in turn, generated by regional differences in the magnitude of this tonic response. Accordingly, a greater increase in tone in the left colon favored a distal-to-proximal movement of content. Thus, pressure gradients generated by tonic and/or phasic contractile events rather than discrete propulsive waves may be responsible for a significant component of transit of content from one part of the colon into another.

Of interest, given the increasing attention focused on the important role of short chain fatty acids (SCFAs), in

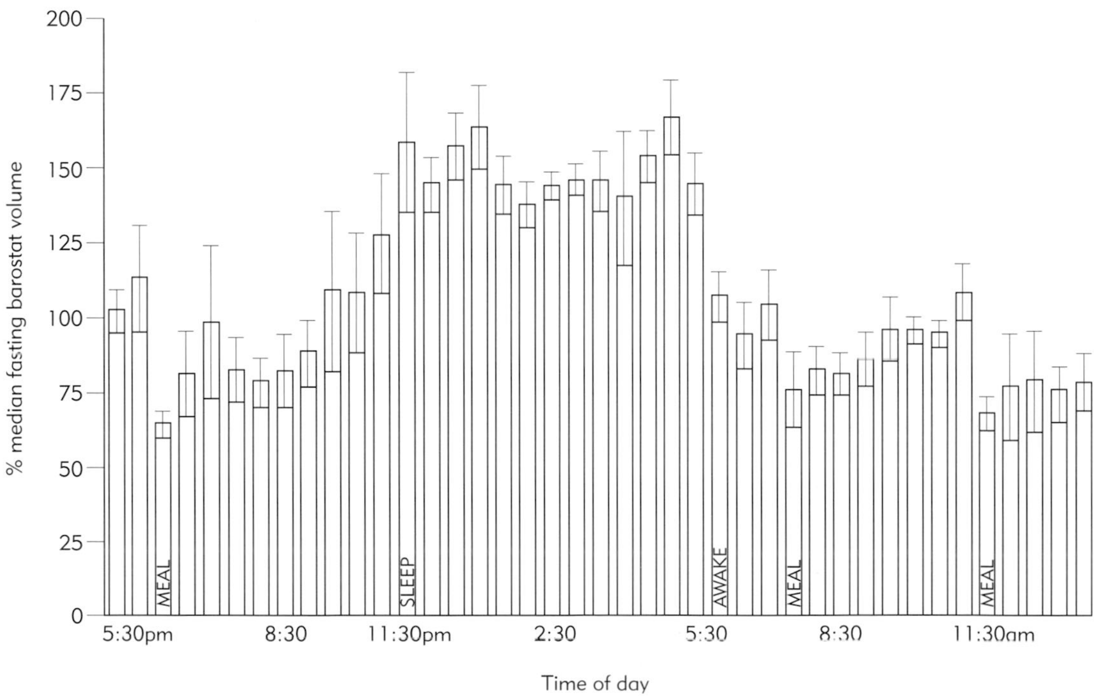

Figure 7.5 Prolonged recording of colonic tone. Note tone is lowest at night, rises on waking and following meal ingestion. Tone measured by changes in barostat balloon volume (i.e. decrease in volume = increase in tone) (From Steadman *et al.*[42], with permission.)

colonic physiology,[54,55] tone may also be augmented by the intraluminal instillation of the SCFA, oleic acid.[56] Colonic distensibility can be augmented by the administration of anti-diarrheal drugs; an observation which may explain, in part, their mode of action.[57] Finally Lagier and colleagues failed to identify any significant age-related change in rectal tone or compliance.[58]

COLONIC TRANSIT

Transit is a more direct measure of true 'function' and, as such, may provide more relevant insights into how the colon participates in storage, transport and defecation.[44,45,59–65] In normal individuals, total transit time through the colon is approximately 35 hours[62] with approximately equal residence times in the right, left and recto-sigmoid portions of the colon.[64] Transit is more rapid in males than in females[62,66,67] but does not, however, appear to be particularly affected by the menstrual cycle.[68] There appears to be a reasonable correlation between colon transit time and stool consistency.[41,69,70] Transit of colonic contents could, in theory, be influenced by a number of factors including the nature of the intra-luminal contents, the degree of loading of the colon and rate and pattern (i.e. continuous infusion versus bolus administration) of loading. Preparation is also important; for example, studies of transit in the unprepared colon have failed to identify retrograde movement,[45] whereas similar studies performed in the prepared colon have recognized bi-directional movement of a marker instilled at the level of the splenic flexture.[34] Studies of differential, or regional, transit times within the colon have provided insights into the function of the various parts of the colon. These suggest an important role for the ascending and transverse colon in storage, with solids being stored preferentially in the ascending colon[45,64] and liquids in the transverse colon. In contrast, the descending colon is viewed primarily as a passive conduit.

In their scintigraphic studies, Proano and colleagues noted that ascending colon emptying was characterized by an initial lag period followed by a phase of linear emptying.[64] They also delineated the ascending and transverse colon as the primary storage areas, with the descending colon functioning as a conduit.

Following food ingestion, the cecum and ascending colon empty and the distal large bowel begins to fill. Ingested tablets also demonstrate stasis in the right colon.[71] Transit is rapid through the descending colon; luminal contents are then stored in the recto-sigmoid colon for many hours.[64]

Given the important role of the colon in fluid conservation,[72,73] Hammer and Phillips[41] and Kamath and colleagues[74] examined the colonic response to fluid loading in great detail. On loading, the ascending colon will accommodate approximately 200 ml; when this volume is exceeded fluid begins to spill into the transverse colon. The head of the solid component moves with liquid whereas the remaining solids move more slowly. The rate of transit of ascending colon contents into, and their residence time in, the transverse colon are governed by the rate of instillation of material into the ascending colon. Following slow infusion, for example, the transverse colon can accommodate stool for in excess of 9 hours, confirming a major storage function for this part of the colon. Thereafter, contents move quickly through the descending colon, only to be further retained in the recto-sigmoid region. Interestingly, and in contrast to other regions, the duration of retention in the recto-sigmoid appeared independent of the rate of movement through the rest of the colon. This observation suggests the potential for the recto-sigmoid to play a key compensatory role to prevent diarrhea when transit through the other segments is accelerated. In these same studies, infusion of up to 500 ml into the right colon did not alter stool frequency or weight.[41] Variations in stool consistency and water content correlated with total colon transit times.

For methological reasons, studies of colonic transit have usually been performed in isolation from studies of colonic motility or tone and direct correlations between these parameters are, therefore, few and far between. Lemann and colleagues examined motility-transit correlations in detail.[10] During fasting they recorded very little organized motor activity: little movement of contents occurred. Following meal ingestion, there was an increase in non-propagating activity which was associated with a gradual movement of contents from the descending colon, in both a retrograde direction into the transverse colon and ante-grade into the sigmoid. Approximately, 50% of subjects developed propagating activity postprandially and this was associated with the rapid movement of contents. Some stool was transported from the splenic flexure to the sigmoid; in others there was retrograde transit from the cecum and ascending colon into the terminal ileum. Attempts to correlate these functions with motor patterns have proven problematic; mainly related to highly variable results from colonic manometry. While some have described prolonged bursts of contractions propagating over short distances as being characteristic of the ascending colon, in keeping with its storage and absorptive functions, others have failed to identify any level of organization in phasic motor activity in any part of the colon.

The difficulties inherent in establishing motility-transit relationships in this organ were exemplified by one study which revealed that a low fat meal was more likely to increase the colonic motility index than a high fat meal; yet neither resulted in any increase in propulsive activity.[75]

MOTILITY AND DEFECATION

Studies which have examined the relationships between motility, transit and defecation have emphasized the participation, not just of the rectum, but of the right and left colon in this process. Thus, in one study, defecation was associated with the distal movement of 13% of the contents of the right colon and, in another, by evacuation of 20% of the contents of the right colon.[76] Lemann and colleagues noted that HAPCs and especially HAPCs which occurred in bursts, were associated with discomfort, an urge to defecate and by the passage of flatus[10] but Herbst and colleagues noted that only 45% of all episodes of defecation were preceded by propagated wave activity.[77] Bassotti looked at correlations between motility and the passage of flatus.[78] Passage of flatus in response to the installation of gas into the rectum was accompanied by an increase in rectal pressure, relaxation of the anal sphincter and propagated colonic contractions (Fig. 7.6). The spontaneous passage of flatus was also associated with propagated contractions but these were of lesser amplitude.[78] Kumar and colleagues noted that the majority of spontaneous expulsions were associated with anal sphincter contraction; not relaxation.[79]

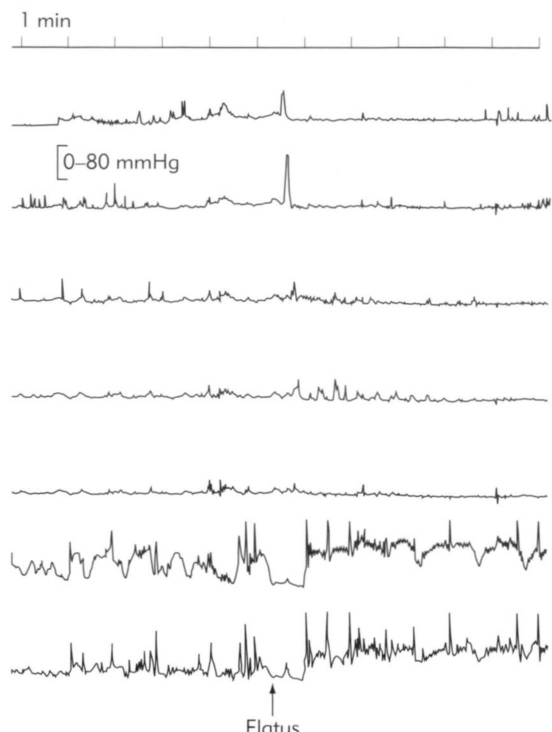

Figure 7.6 Colonic and anorectal motor response to passage of flatus induced by intracolonic instillation of air. Note propagating contraction originating at most proximal recording site (splenic flexure) and migrating through mid-descending, sigmoid (third and fourth sensors into rectum (fifth sensor) associated with relaxation of the anal sphincter (sixth and seventh sensors). (From Bassotti *et al.*[78], with permission.)

THE ILEO-COLONIC JUNCTION

In humans, true tone is inconsistent at the ileo-cecal sphincter. While earlier studies had suggested the presence of sustained tone and tonic responses typical of a gastrointestinal sphincter at the ileo-colonic junction (ICJ),[80] subsequent, prolonged, recordings in intact man failed to confirm these findings and suggested that the motor function of this region may rely, instead, upon coordination of phasic motor activity between the ileum, ileo-colonic junction and proximal colon.[81–83] Accordingly, it was proposed that the ileo-colonic junctional region, including the terminal ileum, the ileocecal valve and the very proximal colon, demonstrated regional motor specialization and behaved as a specialized motor unit. Within this region, unique motor patterns which included discrete clustered contractions and a distinctive motor event variously termed as a prolonged propagating contraction (PPC) or a high amplitude rapidly propagating pressure wave (very similar to the colonic HAPC) promoted aboral movement of chyme and minimized colo-ileal bacterial reflux.[81] Interestingly, in man, and in contrast to other species, migrating motor complex activity, the dominant motor pattern in the fasting small intestine, is not prominent in this region and only a minority of phase 3 complexes reach the terminal ileum.[81] Dinning and colleagues, in studies performed in subjects with temporary defunctioning ileostomies, again proposed the presence of a true sphincter at the ileo-colonic junction.[84] At rest, the ICJ generated a pressure gradient of 9.1 mmHg in their studies; tone was augmented on meal ingestion and on distention of the cecum. The issue of sphincteric function remains, therefore, unresolved.

In a manner analagous to the gastroesophageal junction, it is also evident that ileo-cecal junctional competency is also, in part, related to the integrity of a variety of other factors, including ligamentous attachments and the ileo-colonic angulation.[85,86] In support of a primary role for propulsive events, rather than fluctuations in sphincter tone, in generating colonic filling from the human ileum, studies of transit have failed to identify significant delay at the ICJ, but have revealed that colonic filling occurs largely in discrete boluses; most of these events occur within one hour of a meal.[63] As is the case in the ascending colon, the ileo-colonic junction does not discriminate in emptying rate or pattern between liquids and solids, whereas the distal ileum does.[87] Spiller and colleagues examined the ileal response to food ingestion and confirmed a postprandial increase in ileal emptying, but suggested that this was consequent upon a meal-related increase in ileal flow which led, in turn, to the accumulation of chyme in the terminal ileum and appeared unrelated to the occurrence of either the migrating motor complex or distinctive ileal motor patterns.[88] Ileal motility and emptying are stimulated by installation of short chain fatty acids supporting the hypothesis that specialized ileal motor patterns function to minimize colo-ileal reflux.[89] Indeed, studies of the terminal ileal motor response to a meal revealed findings more in keeping with a reservoir, than a propulsive function[63,90]; on meal ingestion there was a brief tonic and phasic response in the terminal ileum followed by a period of relaxation which lasted for over 2 hours.[91]

CONCLUSIONS

Our understanding of colonic motor function remains incomplete. Manometric studies have proven especially problematic in this organ and appear limited in their ability to reflect the motor function of the colon. Studies of transit suggest, indeed, that discrete contractile events may be but one of several mechanisms that can generate the movement of colonic contents. Alterations in tone and the generation of pressure gradients between adjacent colonic segments may be at least as important in determining the progress of luminal material through the colon.

REFERENCES

1. Sarna SK. Physiology and pathophysiology of colonic motor activity. Part one of two. *Dig Dis Sci* 1991;**36**:827–62.
2. Sarna SK. Physiology and pathophysiology of colonic motor activity. Part two of two. *Dig Dis Sci* 1991;**36**:998–1018.
3. O'Brien MD, Phillips SF. Colonic motility in health and disease. *Gastro Clin North Am* 1996;**25**:147–62.
4. Dinoso VP Jr, Murthy SNS, Goldstein J, Rosner B. Basal motor activity of the distal colon: a reappraisal. *Gastroenterology* 1983;**85**:637–42.
5. Soffer EE, Scalabrini P, Wingate DL. Prolonged ambulant monitoring of human colonic motility. *Am J Physiol* 1989 (*Gastrointest Liver Physiol* **20**); **257**:G601–G606.
6. Kock NG, Hulten L, Leandoer L. A study of the motility in different parts of the human colon. Resting activity, response to feeding and prostigmine. *Scand J Gastroenterol* 1968;**3**:163–9.
7. Bassotti G, Crowell MD, Whitehead WE. Contractile activity of the human colon: lessons from 24 hour studies. *Gut* 1993;**34**:129–33.
8. Reddy SN, Bazzochi G, Chan S. Colonic motility and transit in health and ulcerative colitis. *Gastroenterology* 1991;**101**:1289–97.
9. Jouet P, Coffin B, Lemann M, Gorbatchef C, Franchisseur C, Jian R, Rambaud J-C, Flourie B. Tonic and phasic motor activity in the proximal and distal colon of healthy humans. *Am J Physiol* 1998;**274** (*Gastrointest Liver Physiol* **37**) G459–G464.
10. Lemann M, Flourie B, Picon L, Coffin B, Jian R, Rambaud JC. Motor activity recorded in the unprepared colon of healthy humans. *Gut* 1995;**37**:649–53.
11. Narducci F, Bassotti G, Gaburri M, Morelli A. Twenty-four hour manometric recording of colonic motor activity in healthy man. *Gut* 1987;**28**:17–25.
12. Bueno L, Fioramonti J, Frexinos J. Colonic myoelectrical activity in diarrhoea and constipation. *Gastroenterology* 1980;**27**:381–89.
13. Dapoigny M, Trolese J-F, Bommelaer G. Myoelectric spiking activity of right colon, left colon and rectosigmoid of healthy humans. *Dig Dis Sci* 1988;**33**:1007–1012.
14. Hardcastle JD, Mann CV. Physical factors in the stimulation of colonic peristalsis. *Gut* 1970;**11**:41–6.
15. Di Lorenzo C, Flores AF, Reddy SN, Snape WJ Jnr, Bazzocchi G, Hyman PE. Colonic manometry in children with chronic intestinal pseudo-obstruction. *Gut* 1993;**34**:803–807.
16. Bassotti G, Betti G, Erbella GS, Cavalletti ML, Pelli MA, Morelli A. Prolonged manometric investigation of the colon in research on chronic constipation. *Ital J Gastroenterol* 1991;**23**:13–15.
17. Ford MJ, Camilleri M, Wiste JA, Hanson RB. Differences in colonic tone and phasic response to a meal in the transverse and sigmoid human colon. *Gut* 1995;**37**:264–69.
18. Crowell MD, Bassotti G, Cheskin LJ, Schuster MM, Whitehead WE. Method for prolonged ambulatory monitoring of high-amplitude propagated contractions in the colon. *Am J Physiol* 1991;**261**:G263–G268.
19. Bassotti G, Gaburri M. Manometric investigation of high amplitude propagated contractile activity of the human colon. *Am J Physiol* 1988;**18**: G660–G664.
20. Di Lorenzo C, Flores AF, Hyman PE. Age-related changes in colon motility. *J Pediat* 1995;**127**:593–6.
21. Bassotti G, Gaburri M, Imbibo BP, Morelli A, Whitehead WE. Distention stimulated propagated contractions in the human colon. *Dig Dis Sci* 1996;**39**:1955–60.
22. Hardcastle JD, Mann CV. Study of large bowel peristalsis. *Gut* 1968;**9**:412–20.
23. Ritchie J. Mass peristalsis in the human colon after contact with oxyphenisation. *Gut* 1972;**13**:211–19.
24. Schang JC, Hemond M, Herbert M, Pilote M. Changes in colonic myoelectric spiking activity during stimulation by bisacodyl. *Can J Physiol Pharmacol* 1986;**65**:39–43.
25. Orkin BA, Hanson RB, Kelly KA. The rectal motor complex. *J Gastrointest Motil* 1989;**1**:5–8.
26. Kumar D, Williams NS, Waldron D, Wingate DL. Prolonged manometric recording of anorectal activity in ambulant human subjects: evidence of periodic activity. *Gut* 1989;**30**:1007–1111.
27. Kumar D, Thompson PD, Wingate DL. Absence of synchrony between human small intestinal migrating motor complex and rectal motor complex. *Am J Physiol* 1990;**258**:G171–2.
28. Prior A, Fearn VJ, Read NW. Intermittent rectal motor activity: a rectal motor complex? *Gut* 1991;**32**:1360–63.
29. Snape WJ Jr, Matarazzo GA, Cohen S. Effect of eating and gastrointestinal hormones on human colonic myoelectrical and motor activity. *Gastroenterology* 1978;**75**:373–8.

30. Snape WJ Jr, Wright SH, Battle WM, Cohen S. The gastrocolic response: evidence of a neural mechanism. *Gastroenterology* 1979;**77**:1235–40.
31. Daly J, Bergin A, Sun WM, Read NW. Effect of food and anti-cholinergic drugs on the pattern of rectosigmoid contractions. *Gut* 1993;**34**:799–802.
32. Chowdhury AR, Dinoso VP, Lorber SH. Characterization of a hyperactive segment at the rectosigmoid junction. *Gastroenterology* 1976;**71**:584–8.
33. Loening-Baucke V, Anuras S. Effect of a meal on the motility of the sigmoid colon and rectum in healthy adults. *Am J Gastroenterol* 1983;**78**: 393–7.
34. Moreno-Osset E, Bazzochi G, Lo S, *et al.* Association between post-prandial changes in colonic intraluminal pressure and transit. *Gastroenterology* 1990;**98**:686–93.
35. Misiewicz JJ, Connell AM, Pontes FA. Comparison of the effect of meals and prostigmine on the proximal and distal colon in patients with and without diarrhoea. *Gut* 1996;**7**:468–73.
36. Kerlin P, Zinsmeister A, Phillips S. Motor response to food of the ileum, proximal colon and distal colon of healthy humans. *Gastroenterology* 1983;**84**:762–70.
37. Bassotti G, Imbimbo BP, Gaburri M, Daniotti S, Morelli A. Transverse and sigmoid colon motility in healthy humans, effects of eating and of cimetropium bromide. *Digestion* 1987;**37**:59–64.
38. Wright SH, Snape WJ Jr, Battle W, Cohen S, London RL. Effect of dietary components on gastrocolonic response. *Am J Physiol* 1980;**238** (*Gastrointest Liver Physiol 1*): G228–G232.
39. Levinson S, Bhasker M, Gibbon TR, Morin R, Snape WJ Jr. Comparison of intraluminal and intravenous mediators of colonic response to eating. *Dig Dis Sci* 1985;**30**:33–9.
40. Ford MJ, Camilleri M, Wiste JA, Hanson RB. Differences in colonic tone and phasic response to a meal in the transverse and sigmoid human colon. *Gut* 1995;**37**:264–9.
41. Hammer J, Phillips SF. Fluid loading of the human colon: effects on segmental transit and stool composition. *Gastroenterology* 1993;**105**:988–98.
42. Steadman CJ, Phillips SF, Camilleri M, Haddad AC, Hanson RB. Variation of muscle tone in the human colon. *Gastronterology* 1991;**101**:373–81.
43. Cannon WB. The movement of the intestines: studies by means of the roentgen rays. *Am J Physiol* 1902;**6**:251–77.
44. Picon L, Lemann M, Flourie B, Rambaud J-C, Rain J-D, Jian R. Right and left colonic transit after eating assessed by a dual isotopic technique in healthy humans. *Gastroenterology* 1992;**103**:80–85.
45. Krevsky B, Malmud LS, D'Ercole F, Maurer AH, Fisher RS. Colonic transit scintigraphy, a physiologic approach to the quantitative measurement of colonic transit in humans. *Gastroenterology* 1986;**91**:1102–1112.
46. Roarty TP, Suratt PM, Hellmann P, McCallum RW. Colonic motor activity in women during sleep. *Sleep* 1998;**21**:285–8.
47. Rao SS, Beaty J, Chamberlain M, Lambert PG, Gisolfi C. Effects of acute graded exercise on human colonic motility. *Am J Physiol* 1999;**276**:G221–G226.
48. Sesboue B, Arhan P, Devroede G, *et al.* Colonic transit in soccer players. *J Clin Gastro* 1995;**20**:211–14.
49. Liu F, Kondo T, Toda Y. Brief physical inactivity prolongs colonic transit time in elderly active men. *Int J Sports Med* 1993;**14**:465–7.
50. Roberston G, Meshkinpour H, Vandenberg K, James N, Cohen A, Wilson A. Effects of exercise on total and segmental colon transit. *J Clin Gastro* 1993;**16**:300–303.
51. Rao SS, Hatfield RA, Suls JM, Chamberlain MJ. Psychological and physical stress induce different effects on human colonic motility. *Am J Gastroenterol* 1998;**93**:985–90.
52. Maleki D, Camilleri M, Zinsmeister AR, Rizza RA. Effect of acute hyperglycemia on colorectal motor and sensory function in humans. *Am J Physiol* 1997;**273** (*Gastrointest Liver Physiol* 36): G859–G864.
53. Von Der Ohe MR, Hanson RB, Camilleri M. Comparison of simultaneous recordings of human colonic contractions by manometry and barostat. *Neurogastroenterol Motil* 1994;**6**:213–22.
54. Cummins JH. Fermentation in the human large intestine; evidence and implications for health. *Lancet* 1983;**1**:1206–1209.
55. Hammer HF. Colonic hydrogen absorption: quantification of its effect on hydrogen accumulation caused by bacterial fermentation of carbohydrates. *Gut* 1993;**34**:818–22.
56. Spiller RC, Brown ML, Phillips SF. Decreased fluid tolerance, accelerated transit and abnormal motility of the human colon induced by oleic acid. *Gastroenterology* 1986;**91**:100–107.
57. Steadman CJ, Phillips SF, Camilleri M, Talley NJ, Haddad A, Hanson R. Control of muscle tone in the human colon. *Gut* 1992;**33**:541–6.
58. Lagier E, Delvaux M, Vellas B, *et al.* Influence of age on rectal tone and sensitivity to distention in healthy humans subjects. *Neurogastroenterol Motil* 1999;**11**:101–107.
59. Hinton JM, Lennard-Jones JE, Young AC. A new method for studying gut transit times using radiopaque markers. *Gut* 1969;**10**:842–7.
60. Waller S. Differential measurement of small and large bowel transit times in constipation and diarrhea: a new approach. *Gut* 1975;**16**:372–8.
61. Arhan P, Devroede G, Jehannin B, *et al.* Segmental colonic transit time. *Dis Colon Rectum* 1981;**24**:625–9.
62. Metcalf AM, Phillips SF, Zinsmeister AR, MacCarty RL, Beart RW, Wolff BG. Simplified assessment of segmental colonic transit. *Gastroenterology* 1987;**92**:40–47.
63. Camilleri M, Colemont LJ, Phillips SF, *et al.* Human gastric emptying and colonic filling of solids characterized by a new method. *Am J Physiol* 1989;**257** (*Gastrointest Liver Physiol*): G284–G290.
64. Proano M, Camilleri M, Phillips SF, Brown ML, Thomforde GM. Transit of solids through the human colon: regional quantification in the unprepared bowel. *Am J Physiol* 1990;**258** (*Gastrointest Liver Physiol* 21): G856–G862.
65. Proano M, Camilleri M, Phillips SF, Thomforde GM, Brown ML, Tucker R. The unprepared human colon does not discriminate between solids and liquids. *Am J Physiol* 1991;**260**:G13–G16.
66. Lampe JW, Fredstrom SB, Slavin JL, Potter JD. Sex differences in colonic function: a randomised trial. *Gut* 1993;**34**:531–6.

67. Degen LP, Phillips SF. Variability of gastrointestinal transit in healthy women and men. *Gut* 1996;**39**:299–305.
68. Hinds JP, Stoney B, Wald A. Does gender or the menstrual cycle affect colonic transit? *Am J Gastroenterol* 1989;**84**:123–6.
69. O'Donnell LJD, Virjee J, Heaton KW. Detection of pseudodiarrhoea by simple clinical assessment of intestinal transit rate. *BMJ* 1990;**300**:439–40.
70. Degen LP, Phillips SF. How well does stool form reflect colonic transit? *Gut* 1996;**39**:109–113.
71. Price JM, Davis SS, Wilding IR. Characterisation of colonic transit of disintegrating tablets in healthy subjects. *Dig Dis Sci* 1993;**38**:1015–1021.
72. Phillips SF, Giller J. The contribution of the colon to electrolyte and water conservation in man. *J Lab Clin Med* 1973;**81**:733–46.
73. Debongie JC, Phillips SF. Capacity of the human colon to absorb fluid. *Gastroenterology* 1978;**74**:698–703.
74. Kamath PS, Phillips SF, O'Connor MK, Brown ML, Zimsmeister AR. Colonic capacitance and transit in man; modulation by luminal contents and drugs. *Gut* 1990;**31**:443–9.
75. Steed KP, Bohemen EK, Lamont GM, Evans DF, Wilson CG, Spiller RC. Proximal colonic response and gastrointestinal transit after high and low fat meals. *Dig Dis Sci* 1993;**38**:1793–800.
76. Lubowski DZ, Meagher AP, Smart RC, Butler SP. Scintigraphic assessment of colonic function during defecation. *Int J Colorectal Dis* 1995;**10**:91–3.
77. Herbst TF, Kamm MA, Morris GP, Britton K, Woloszko J, Nicholls RJ. Gastrointestinal transit and prolonged ambulatory colonic motility in health and faecal incontinence. *Gut* 1997;**41**:381–9.
78. Bassotti G, Germani U, Morelli A. Flatus-related colorectal and anal motor events. *Dig Dis Sci* 1996;**41**:335–8.
79. Kumar D, Waldron D, Williams NS, Browning C, Hutton MRE, Wingate DL. Prolonged anorectal manometry and external anal sphincter electromyography in ambulant human subjects. *Dig Dis Sci* 1990;**35**:641–8.
80. Cohen S, Harris LD, Levitan R. Manometric characteristics of the human ileocecal junctional zone. *Gastroenterology* 1968;**54**:72–5.
81. Quigley EMM, Borody TJ, Phillips SF, Wienbeck M, Tucker RL, Haddad A. Motility of the terminal ileum and ileocecal sphincter in healthy humans. *Gastroenterology* 1984;**87**:857–66.
82. Nasmyth DG, Williams NS. Pressure characteristics of the human ileocecal region; a key to its function. *Gastroenterology* 1985;**89**:345–51.
83. Corazziari E, Barberani F, Tosoni M, Torsoli A. Perendoscopic manometry of the distal ileum and ileocecal junction in humans. *Gastroenterology* 1991;**101**:1314–19.
84. Dinning PG, Bampton PA, Kennedy MI, *et al.* Basal pressure patterns and reflexive motor responses in the human ileocolonic junction. *Am J Physiol* 1999;276 (*Gastrointest Liver Physiol* **39**) G331–G340.
85. Faussone Pellegrini MS, Ibba Manneschi L. The caecocolonic junction in humans has a sphincteric anatomy and function. *Gut* 1995;**37**:493–8.
86. Kumar D, Phillips SF. The contribution of external ligamentous attachments to function of the ileocecal junction. *Dis Colon Rectum* 1987;**30**:410–416.
87. Hammer J, Camilleri M, Phillips SF, Aggarwal A, Haddad AM. Does the ileocolonic junction differentiate between solids and liquids? *Gut* 1993;**34**:222–6.
88. Spiller RC, Brown ML, Phillips SF. Emptying of the terminal ileum in intact humans: influence of meal residue and ileal motility. *Gastroenterology* 1987;**92**:724–9.
89. Kamath PS, Phillips SF, Zimsmeister AR. Short-chain fatty acids stimulate ileal motility in humans. *Gastroenterology* 1988;**95**:1996–1502.
90. Jian R, Najean Y, Bernier JJ. Measurement of intestinal progression of a meal and its residues in normal subjects and patients with functional diarrhoea by a dual isotope technique. *Gut* 1984;**25**:728–31.
91. Coffin B, Lemann M, Flourie B, Picon L, Rambaud J-C, Jian R. Ileal tone in humans: effects of locoregional distentions and eating. *Am J Physiol* 1994;**267**:G569–G574.

Chapter 8

The central control of the pelvic floor

Gert Holstege, Judith A M L Sie

INTRODUCTION

The pelvic floor consists of many different muscles, which include the striated sphincters of the bladder and anus. It forms the lowest part of the abdominal cavity and can be considered as the bottom of the abdominal wall. The striated muscles of the pelvic floor are innervated by the pudendal nerve, the motor fibers of which originate from motoneurones in the ventral horn of the upper sacral or, in a few species, lower lumbar cord.

PELVIC FLOOR MOTONEURONES

In most vertebrates the pelvic floor motoneurones are located in one particular nucleus, called the nucleus of Onuf (ON), after Onufrowicz who described this nucleus in 1899. At that time, he thought that the nucleus was particularly involved in sexual activity and not in continence for feces and urine.[1] However, until 30 years ago, the nucleus was not yet identified as containing pelvic floor motoneurones, and was called group Y.[2] In the rat,[3,4] the ON consists of two nuclei, but in species like the hamster,[5] cat,[6–8] dog,[7] monkey,[9] and human,[10] it is one nucleus on the ventrolateral border of the ventral horn in the upper sacral cord. In the species in which the ON is one nucleus, the motoneurones innervating the anal sphincter are located dorsomedially to those innervating the bladder sphincter (Fig. 8.1). In the pig[11] and Mongolian gerbil[12] anal sphincter motoneurones are located in a competely different location, dorsal and dorsolateral to the central canal, in the area of the intermediomedial nucleus (see below).

In non-experimental sections, the ON can be recognized by its wealth of longitudinally oriented dendrites,[13] indicating that the motoneurones have many connections within the nucleus itself. In the rat, in the dorsolateral nucleus, containing motoneurones innervating the ischiocavernosus muscle and the external urethral sphincter, as well as in the spinal nucleus of the bulbocavernosus so called gap junctions have been demonstrated,[14]. The number of these gap junctions is influenced by testosterone levels.[15] Such gap junctions do not seem to be present in the ON of the cat,[16] but perhaps further research is necessary, to determine whether there really is a difference between rat and cat in this respect. There are also strong dendritic connections with the intermediolateral, and as far as the external anal sphincter is concerned, with the intermediomedial cell groups.[17] Furthermore, ON motoneurones are smaller than those of the neighboring motoneurones, innervating limb muscles or tail. Moreover, ON motoneurones, although they innervate striated musculature, have more or less the appearance of autonomic motoneurones, similar to the parasympathetic motoneurones in the sacral intermediolateral cell

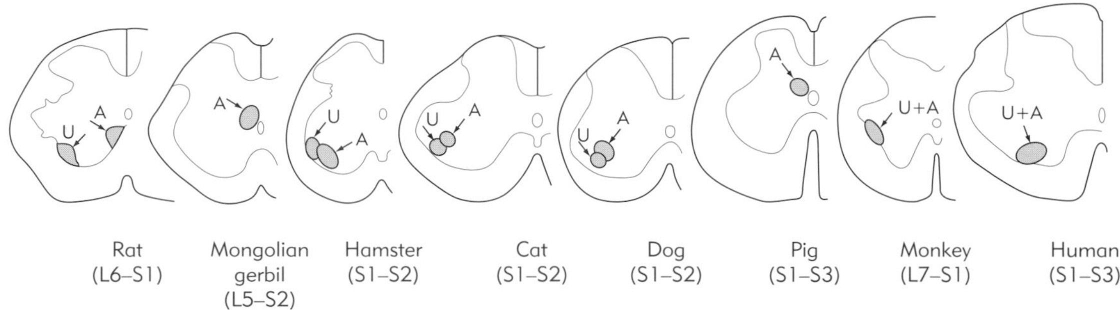

Figure 8.1 Schematic overview of the pelvic floor motoneurones in various mammalian species. A: external anal sphincter. U: external urethral sphincter.

column, innervating the detrusor muscle of the bladder or the distal part of the colon, sigmoid and rectum.

Another peculiar phenomenon is that ON motoneurons, unlike all other somatic motoneurons in the spinal cord, seem to be unaffected by amyotrophic lateral sclerosis (ALS), or affected only in the very latest stages of the disease. In ALS all the somatic, but not the autonomic motoneurons are affected and finally disappear. On the other hand, similar to autonomic motoneurons, but unlike somatic motoneurons, ON motoneurons are affected in Shy-Dräger disease.[18,19] Thus, ON motoneurons innervate striated musculature, but behave differently from the other somatic motoneurons in the spinal cord. The most likely reason for this difference is that their function is closely linked with the function of parasympathetically innervated bladder and distal alimentary tract.

SPINAL INFLUENCE ON NUCLEUS OF ONUF MOTONEURONS

For most somatic motoneurons, there exists a well organized spinal system of local interneurons, the so-called propiospinal pathways, in which interneurons in the intermediate zone connect strongly with the somatic motoneurons (see Ref. 20 for review). However, such a propiospinal system does not exist for ON motoneurons. For example, an injection of the anterograde tracer ^{3}H-leucine in the intermediate zone of the L7 segment resulted in strong fiber labeling in the various limb or proximal muscle motoneuronal cell groups at the S1–S2 levels, but not in the ON (Fig. 8.2). Within the spinal cord, most interneurons projecting to the ON are located in the sacral dorsal gray commissure or intermediomedial cell group.[21,22] Many of these cells contain GABA[23] or glycine[24] and have an inhibitory effect on ON motoneurons.[25,26]

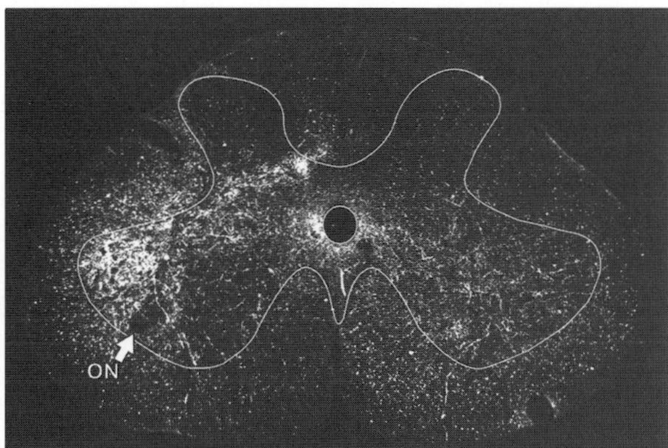

Figure 8.2 Darkfield photomicrograph of a transverse section of the S1 segment of the cat. An injection of ^{3}H-leucine in the L7 intermediate zone resulted in strong fiber labeling in the somatic motoneuronal cell groups, but not in ON (arrow).

Another site which also contains some interneurons projecting to the ON is the sacral intermediolateral cell group, with parasympathetic motoneurons innervating bladder, distal colon, sigmoid and rectum. It has been demonstrated that these motoneurons and the interneurons projecting to the ON are not the same.[22] There are no reports of other spinal cord interneurons projecting to the ON.

SUPRASPINAL PROJECTIONS

In contrast to the relatively sparse projections from spinal levels, there exist several specific projections to the ON from supraspinal levels, i.e. brainstem and diencephalon. Some of these projections take part in descending brainstem systems projecting to all spinal cord motoneurons, but others represent much more specific descending systems. Especially with regard to the last kind of projections, the ON differs from other spinal motoneuronal cell groups. Examples of the first kind of projections are those originating in the ventromedial medullary tegmentum including the caudal raphe nuclei and the locus coeruleus and/or the nucleus subcoeruleus. Examples of specific supraspinal-ON projections are the nucleus retroambiguus, the pontine lateral tegmental cell group called the L-region, and the paraventricular nucleus of the hypothalamus. The pontine micturition center does not project directly to the ON motoneurons, but reaches them via the sacral dorsal gray commissure.

THE VENTROMEDIAL MEDULLARY TEGMENTAL FIELD

This region of the medulla does not project specifically to the motoneurons of ON but to all somatic and autonomic motoneurons in the spinal cord and, to a certain extent, in the caudal brainstem. Therefore, this projection to the ON seems to be part of a very diffuse projection system of which one neuron projects to a very large number of inter- and motoneuronal cell groups at many different levels of the spinal cord, e.g. to cell groups in the cervical as well as the lumbosacral cord.[27–29] It is thought that this diffuse system has a very global and general effect on motoneurons and does not represent a system controlling one particular function of the body. Neurons in the ventromedial medullary tegmentum are known to contain neurotransmitters such as serotonin and GABA, as well as neuropeptides such as substance P, leucine-enkephalin, thyrotropin releasing hormone, methionine, somatostatin, vasoactive intestinal peptide and cholecystokinin (see Ref. 20 for review). It has been demonstrated that there are terminals with these substances on the ON motoneurons.[30–32] Their function is not yet known, although one might assume that they have a similar modulatory effect as on all other spinal motoneurons.

LOCUS COERULEUS; NUCLEUS SUBCOERULEUS

The locus coeruleus and, especially in the cat, the nucleus subcoeruleus, contain a large number of cells containing noradrenaline (norepinephrine). Similar to the cells in the ventromedial medulla, these noradrenergic neurons project to all cells in the spinal cord, including the ON. Similar to the projection from the ventromedial medullary tegmentum, it is unlikely that this diffuse noradrenergic pathway represents a specific control of the ON, but, in all likelihood, has a very general probably excitatory effect on all motoneurons, somatic as well as autonomic.

NUCLEUS RETROAMBIGUUS

The nucleus retroambiguus (NRA) is located laterally in the most caudal medulla, between the obex and spinal cord. It was defined for the first time as a separate nucleus in the human in 1954 by Olszewski and Baxter.[33] In 1970 the NRA was demonstrated to be involved in respiration, its caudal part in expiration, and its rostral part in both expiration and inspiration.[34–39] Holstege and Kuypers (1982)[28] were the first to show that the NRA maintains direct projections to the area of the abdominal and intercostal muscle motoneurons, and these projections were recently demonstrated to be excitatory.[40] Holstege and Tan (1987)[41] were the first to demonstrate that the NRA also has a direct projection to the ON. Holstege (1989)[42] demonstrated that the NRA received specific projections from the periaqueductal gray (PAG) and that the NRA sends direct projections to the dorsal group of the nucleus ambiguus, containing motoneurons of soft palate, pharynx and larynx. Combining these pathways led to the concept that the PAG-NRA-motoneuronal pathway is involved in vocalization (Fig. 8.3). The reason for this idea was that stimulation in the same area of the PAG that projected to the NRA elicited vocalization in at least 10 species (see Ref. 42 for review). Later studies corroborated this concept, because lesioning the NRA interrupted vocalization elicited by PAG stimulation.[43,44] The NRA is also known to be involved in the central control of vomiting.[45] Apparently, all functions in which an increased abdominal pressure is necessary, i.e. expiration, vocalization, vomiting and probably also defecation and parturition, make use of the neurons in the NRA. In this respect it is important to realize that the pelvic floor forms the bottom of the abdominal cavity and, therefore, is also involved in increasing abdominal pressure. Recently it

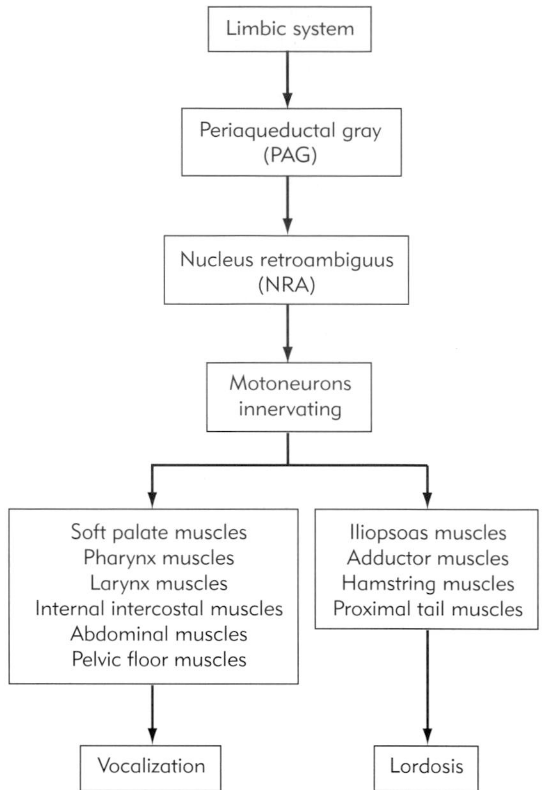

Figure 8.3 Schematic representation of the involvement of the NRA in vocalization and mating behavior in the cat.

has been shown that the NRA is also involved in eliciting the mating posture in female cats, because of its projections to a distinct set of hip and limb muscle motoneurons in the lumbosacral cord (Fig. 8.3).[46,47] Interestingly, these NRA projections are rather weak in non-estrus cats but very strong in estrus cats, and the NRA fibers appear to 'grow' when the cat is in estrus.[48] This growth process was demonstrated by the presence of growth cones in estrus cats and the absence in non-estrus cats. It remains to be elucidated whether the pelvic floor muscles also play a role in this mating posture. Perhaps an investigation whether or not there are growth cones in the ON in estrus cats might give further insight.

INDIRECT PROJECTION FROM THE PONTINE MICTURITION CENTER

It is well known that micturition is regulated by a relatively small compact nucleus in the dorsal pontine tegmentum called Barrington's nucleus,[49] M-region,[50] or pontine micturition center (PMC). Ultrastructural evidence indicates that the PMC cells make a direct excitatory connection with the parasympathetic autonomic motoneurons in the sacral intermediolateral cell group innervating the bladder.[51] Stimulation of the PMC, therefore, elicits bladder contraction.[50] Although the PMC does not project to the ON, it is also involved in micturition, because during voiding, the bladder sphincter has to be relaxed. The PMC inhibits ON motoneurons by way of a direct excitatory projection to the GABA-ergic and glycinergic neurons in the intermediomedial cell group of the sacral cord.[23,24] These cells (see above), in turn project to the ON where they have a strong inhibitory effect.[25,26] Via this relay the PMC inhibits the bladder sphincter motoneurons and produces sphincter relaxation together with bladder contraction. Possibly, the PMC, within the intermediomedial cell group, exclusively projects to interneurons, inhibiting the bladder sphincter motoneurons in the ON and not to the interneurons inhibiting the anal sphincter motoneurons in ON, but there are no data to confirm this assumption.

In order to start micturition, the PMC has to be aware of the situation concerning bladder filling but also of the circumstances of the individual with respect to the safety of the environment. With respect to bladder filling, stretch receptors in the bladder wall relay information to the dorsal horn and lateral intermediate zone of the upper sacral cord,[52] where many cells are located that project to the PAG. Direct sacral cord projections to the PMC do not exist in the cat,[53] although in the rat such projections have been demonstrated.[54,55] The PAG, according to the concept of Holstege and co-workers, being informed about the level of bladder filling, but also under enormous influence of major parts of the limbic system and orbitofrontal cortex, 'decides' whether or not to start micturition. For this reason it has a direct connection with the PMC.[56]

The PMC, apart from the PAG, also receives afferents from a distinct part of the preoptic region.[57] It has been suggested that this pathway might be inhibitory, but there are no data to confirm this. The precise function of the preoptic-PMC pathway, therefore, is not yet clear, but one might speculate that it plays a role in mating behavior, during which micturition is obviously not appropriate.

Although the direct supraspinal control of micturition seems to be rather well elucidated (Fig. 8.4), this is not the case for defecation. It is suggested that defecation, in contrast to micturition, is more or less regulated by the spinal cord, although there are supraspinal influences (see L-region). Perhaps some of the afferents from the distal colon, sigmoid and rectum have a direct connection with the inhibitory interneurons of the anal sphincter motoneurons in the ON.

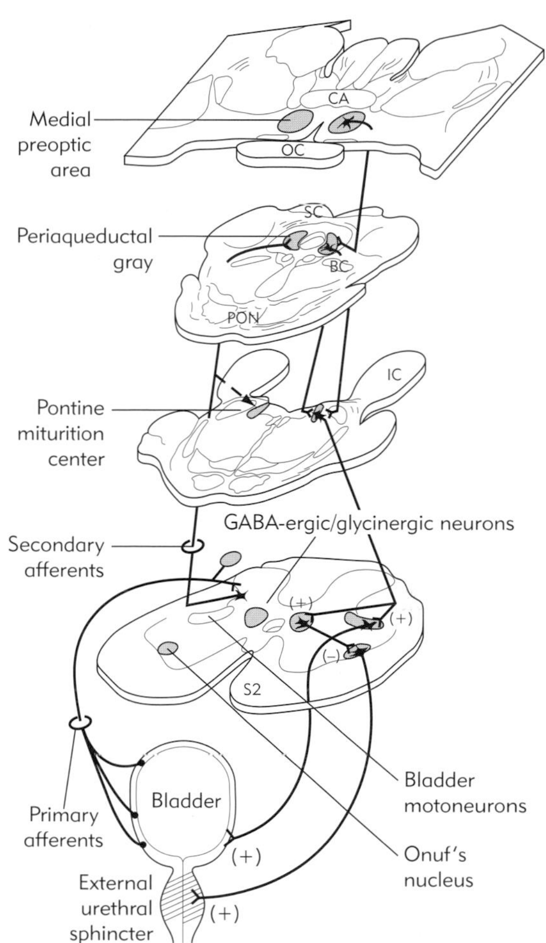

Figure 8.4 Schematic overview of the micturition pathways with the ascending and descending components in the cat.

L-REGION

In 1979, Holstege *et al.* had demonstrated a direct pathway from an area laterally in the pontine tegmentum, slightly ventral to the lateral parabrachial nuclei, to the ON.[27] At that time its function was completely obscure. In the meantime it has been shown in the cat that stimulation of a cell group, lateral in the pontine tegmentum called the L-region (L = lateral) elicits contraction of the pelvic floor,[50] and bilaterally lesioning the L-region results in an extreme form of urge-incontinence.[58] Apparently, the L-region has a continuous excitatory effect on ON motoneurons (both bladder and anal sphincter motoneurons and possibly the motoneurons of the other pelvic floor muscles as well). This idea is corroborated by the ultrastructural finding that there is a direct connection from the L-region with the bladder sphincter motoneurons (Fig. 8.5). All these results suggest that the L-region might be considered as a 'continence' center, which has a steady excitatory control of the pelvic floor. A still unresolved and very important question is what, in turn, controls this L-region. Its location close to the parabrachial nuclei

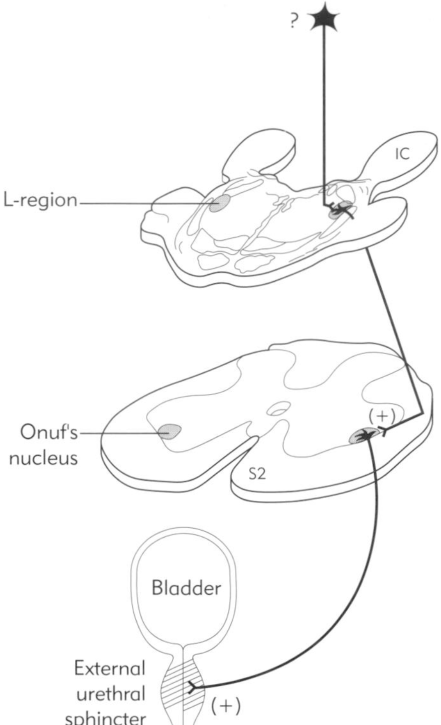

Figure 8.5 Schematic overview of the projections of the L-region or continence center in the cat.

makes this a question difficult to resolve. Possible candidates for supplying such afferents are the PAG, receiving afferents from the sacral cord, as well as parts of the limbic system that control motor activities related to the pelvic floor.

THE PARAVENTRICULAR NUCLEUS OF THE HYPOTHALAMUS (PVN)

Holstege (1987)[57] was the first to reveal that the PVN has a direct connection with the sacral parasympathetic autonomic motoneurons in the intermediolateral cell colums as well as with ON motoneurons (Fig. 8.6). The function of this pathway is not known. In addition to the ON and the sacral intermediolateral cell group, the PVN projects to virtually all other autonomic motoneurons (sympathetic and parasympathetic) in the caudal brainstem and spinal cord.[57] Furthermore, the PVN, albeit other cells, projects to the hypophysis, where they stimulate the production of ACTH, oxytocin and vasopressin. Perhaps the PVN projection to the ON plays a role in a more general system in which the PVN produces its effects on 'autonomic' functions via fiber connections in the central nervous system, as well as via hormones via the hypophysis and bloodstream.

PET-SCAN RESULTS OF MICTURITION CONTROL IN HUMANS

In three separate studies, Blok and Holstege have demonstrated that with respect to pelvic floor activities during micturition in men and women,[59,60] as well as in voluntary contraction,[61] the supraspinal control systems

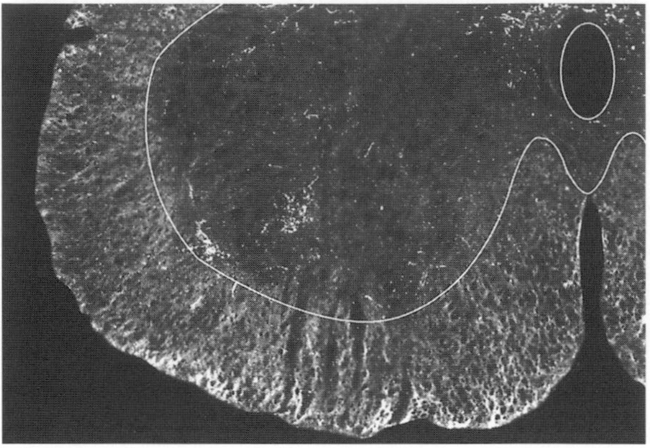

a

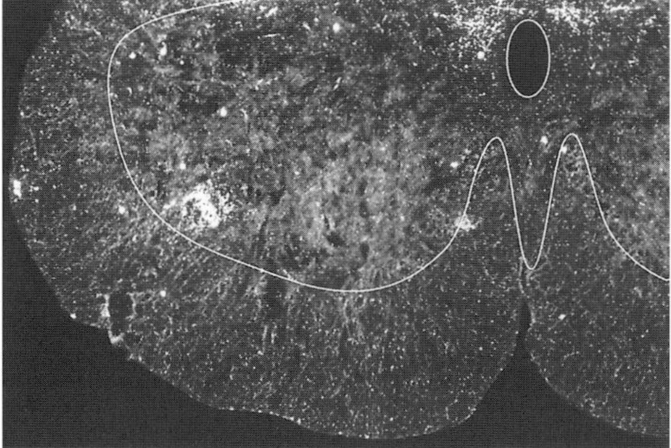

b

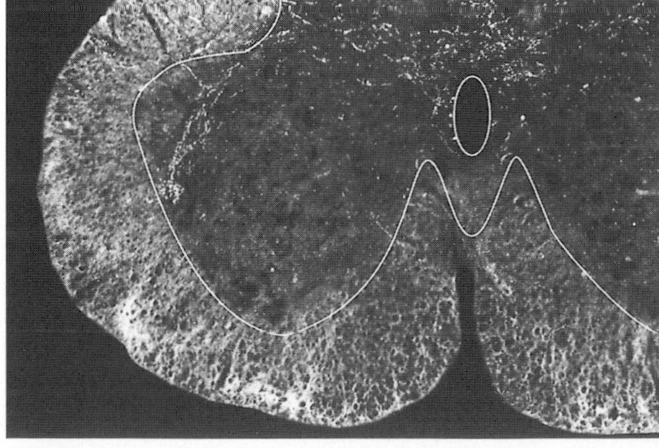

c

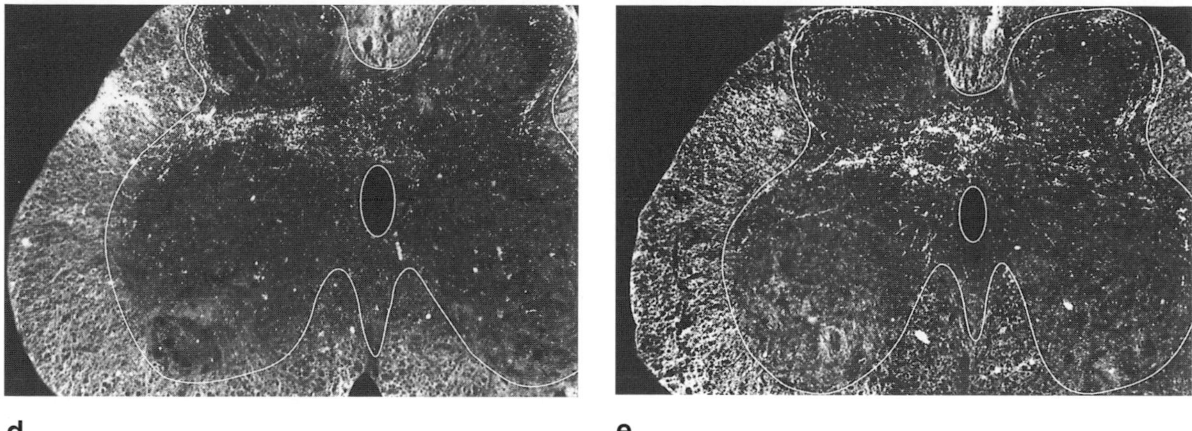

Figure 8.6 Darkfield photomicrographs of the labeled fibers in the ON in the first and second sacral segment of the cat after injection of ^{3}H-leucine in the paraventricular hypothalamic nucleus (PVN). Note in (a) the PVN projection to the most rostral ON, split into two parts. In (b) ON is complete and in (c) there is a PVN projection to the most rostral intermediolateral cell group (IML) and the dendrites in between. Note in (d) and (e) the heavy PVN projection to the IML as well as the intermediomedial cell group.

seem to be very similarly organized in humans and in cats. Of the volunteers that were asked to micturate while lying with their heads in the PET-scan, half of them could satisfactorily perform the task. In this group the same regions as observed in the cat to be involved in micturition, were found to be active in humans, i.e. an area in the dorsal pontine tegmentum, probably representing the PMC (Fig. 8.7, left), an area in the PAG and one in the hypothalamus or preoptic region. The other group of volunteers, who were willing to micturate, but for emotional reasons could not perform, tightly contracted their pelvic floor. Surprisingly, the PET-scan results in these volunteers revealed an area in the ventrolateral pontine tegmentum, which might represent

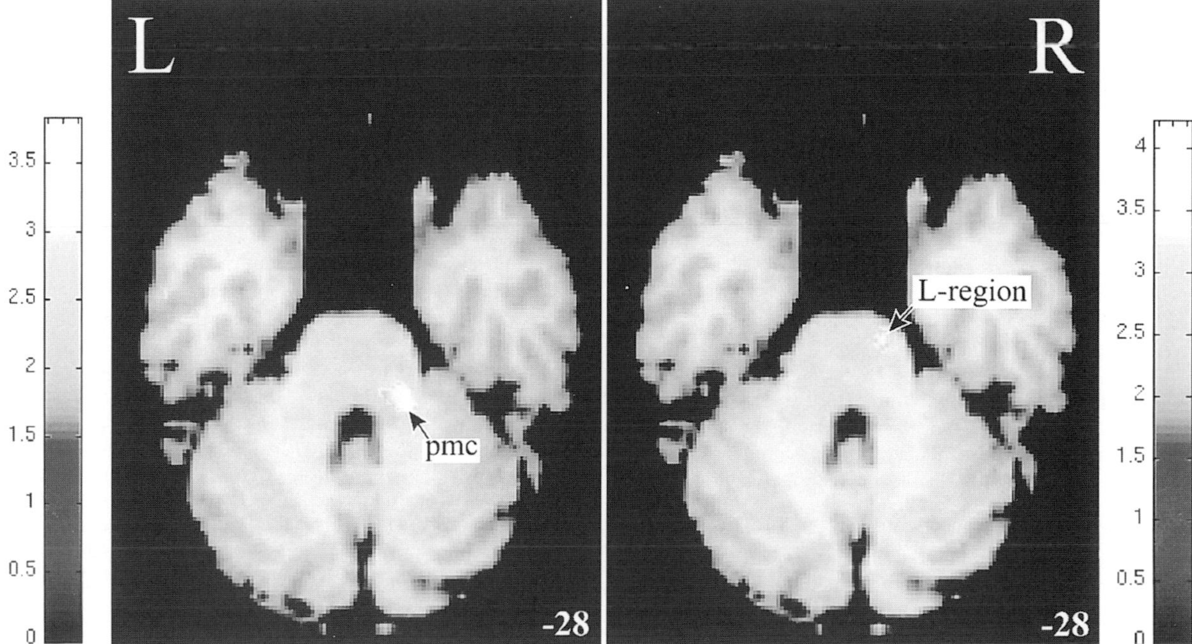

Figure 8.7 PET-scan results during micturition (left) and emotional contraction (right) of the pelvic floor in women.

the L-region or continence center (Fig. 8.7, right). These results suggest that micturition control in cats and humans is, at least at the brainstem level, similarly organized. With respect to the voluntary contraction of the pelvic floor it was found that none of the micturition control regions were active, but only the motor cortical regions that were directly involved in voluntary pelvic floor contraction.[61] It also suggests that the motor cortical system is completely separate from the basic micturition control system that takes part in the emotional motor system.[62]

REFERENCES

1. Onufrowicz B. Notes on the arrangement and function of the cell groups in the sacral region of the spinal cord. *J Nerv Mental Dis* 1899;**26**:498–504.
2. Romanes GJ. The motor cell columns of the lumbosacral spinal cord of the cat. *J Comp Neurol* 1951;**94**:313–63.
3. Schrøder HD Organization of the motoneurons innervating the pelvic muscles of the male rat. *J Comp Neurol* 1980;**192**:567–87.
4. McKenna KE, Nadelhaft I. The organization of the pudendal nerve in the male and female rat. *J Comp Neurol* 1986;**248**:532–49.
5. Gerrits PO, Sie JAML, Holstege G. Motoneuronal location of the external urethral and anal sphincters: a single and double labeling study in the male and female golden hamster. *Neurosci Lett* 1997; **226**:191–4.
6. Sato M, Mizuno N, Konishi A. Localization of motoneurons innervating perineal muscles: a HRP study in cat. *Brain Res* 1978;**140**:149–54.
7. Kuzuhara S, Kanazawa I, Nakanishi T. Topographical localization of the Onuf's nuclear neurons innervating the rectal and vesical striated sphincter muscles: a retrograde fluorescent double labeling in cat and dog. *Neurosci Lett* 1980;**16**:125–30.
8. Ueyama T, Mizuno N, Nomura S, Konishi A, Itoh K, Arakawa H. Central distribution of afferent and efferent components of the pudendal nerve in cat. *J Comp Neurol* 1984;**222**:38–46.
9. Roppolo JR, Nadelhaft I, de Groat WC. The organization of pudendal motoneurons and primary afferent projections in the spinal cord of the rhesus monkey revealed by horseradish peroxidase. *J Comp Neurol* 1985;**234**:475–88.
10. Schrøder HD. Onuf's nucleus X: a morphological study of a human spinal nucleus. *Anat Embryol* 1981;**162**:443–53.
11. Blok BFM, Roukema G, Geerdes B, Holstege G. Location of external anal sphincter motoneurons in the sacral cord of the female domestic pig. *Neurosci Lett* 1996;**216**:203–6.
12. Ulibarri C, Popper P, Micevych PE. Motoneurons dorsolateral to the central canal innervate perineal muscles in the Mongolian gerbil. *J Comp Neurol* 1995;**356**:225–37.
13. Dekker JJ, Lawrence DG, Kuypers HGJM. The location of longitudinally running dendrites in the ventral horn of cat spinal cord. *Brain Res* 1973;**51**:319–25.
14. Matsumoto A, Arnold AP, Micevych PE. Gap junctions between lateral spinal motoneurons in the rat. *Brain Res* 1989;**495**:362–5.
15. Matsumoto A, Armold AP, Zampighi GA, Micevych PE. Androgenic regulation of gap junctions between motoneurons in the rat spinal cord. *J Neurosci* 1988;**8**:4177–83.
16. Takahashi K, Yamamoto T. Ultrastructure of the cell group X of Onuf in the cat sacral spinal cord. *Z Mikrosk Anat Forsch* 1979;**93**:244–56.
17. Sasaki M. Morphological analysis of external urethral and external anal sphincter motoneurons of cat. *J Comp Neurol* 1994;**349**:269–87.
18. Sung JH, Mastri AR, Segal E. Pathology of Shy–Dräger syndrome. *J Neuropathol Exp Neurol* 1979;**38**:353–68.
19. Chalmers D, Swash M. Selective vulnerability of urinary Onuf motoneurons in Shy–Dräger syndrome. *J Neurol* 1987;**234**:259–60.
20. Holstege G. Descending motor pathways and the spinal motor system: limbic and non-limbic components. *Prog Brain Res* 1991;**87**:307–421.
21. Konishi A, Itoh K, Sugimoto T, Yasui Y, Kaneko T, Takada M, Mizuno N. Leucine-enkephalin-like immunoreactive afferent fibers to pudendal motoneurons in the cat. *Neurosci Lett* 1985;**61**:109–113.
22. Nadelhaft I, Vera PL. Neurons in the rat brain and spinal cord labeled after pseudorabies virus injected into the external urethral sphincter. *J Comp Neurol* 1996;**375(3)**:502–17.
23. Blok BFM, de Weerd H, Holstege G. The pontine micturition center projects to sacral cord GABA immunoreactive neurons in the cat. *Neurosci Lett* 1997;**233**:109–12.
24. Sie JAML, De Weerd H, Blok BFM. Ultrastructural evidence for direct pontine micturition center projections to sacral glycinergic neurons in the cat. *Soc Neurosci Abs* 1999;**25**:1170 (473.5).
25. Blok BFM, van Maarseveen JTPW, Holstege G. Electrical stimulation of the sacral dorsal gray commissure evokes relaxation of the external urethral sphincter in the cat. *Neurosci Lett* 1998; **249**:68–70.
26. Grill WM, Bhadra N, Wang B. Bladder and urethral pressures evoked by microstimulation of the sacral spinal cord in cats. *Brain Res* 1999;**836**:19–30.
27. Holstege G, Kuypers HGJM, Boer RC. Anatomical evidence for direct brain stem projections to the somatic motoneuronal cell groups and autonomic preganglionic cell groups in cat spinal cord. *Brain Res* 1979;**171**:329–33.
28. Holstege G, Kuypers HGJM. The anatomy of brain stem pathways to the spinal cord in cat. A labeled amino acid tracing study. *Prog Brain Res* 1982;**57**:145–75.
29. Huisman AM, Kuypers HGJM, Verburgh CA. Differences in collateralization of the descending spinal pathways from red nucleus and other brain stem cell groups in cat and monkey. *Prog Brain Res* 1982;**57**:185–217.
30. Ramirez-Léon V, Ulfhake B, Arvidsson U, Verhofstad AA, Visser TJ, Hökfelt T. Serotoninergic, peptidergic and GABAergic innervation of the ventrolateral and dorsolateral motor nuclei in the cat S1/S2 segments: an immunofluorescence study. *J Chem Neuroanat* 1994;**7**:87–103.
31. Ramirez-Léon V, Hökfelt T, Cuello AC, Visser TJ, Ulfhake B. Enkephalin-, thyrotropin-releasing hormone- and substance P-immunoreactive axonal innervation of the ventrolateral dendritic bundle in the cat sacral spinal cord: an ultrastructural study. *J Chem Neuroanat* 1994;**7**:203–15.

32. Holstege JC, Van-Dijken H, Buijs RM, Goedknegt H, Gosens T, Bongers CM. Distribution of dopamine immunoreactivity in the rat, cat and monkey spinal cord. *J Comp Neurol* 1996;**376**:631–52.
33. Olszewski J, Baxter D. Cytoarchitecture of the human brainstem. Switzerland: J.B. Lippincott, 1954.
34. Merrill EG. The lateral respiratory neurons of the medulla: their associations with nucleus ambiguus, nucleus retroambigualis, the spinal accessory nucleus and the spinal cord. *Brain Res* 1970; **24**:11–28.
35. Kirkwood PA, Sears TA. Proceedings: monosynaptic excitation of thoracic expiratory motoneurons from lateral respiratory neurons in the medulla of the cat. *J Physiol* 1973;**234**:87P–89P.
36. Davies JG, Kirkwood PA, Sears TA. The detection of monosynaptic connexions from inspiratory bulbospinal neurons to inspiratory motoneurons in the cat. *J Physiol* 1985;**368**:33–62.
37. Feldman JL, Loewy AD, Speck DF. Projections from the ventral respiratory group to phrenic and intercostal motoneurons in cat: an autoradiographic study. *J Neurosci* 1985;**5**:1993–2000.
38. Merrill EG, Lipski J. Inputs to intercostal motoneurons from ventrolateral medullary respiratory neurons in the cat. *J Neurophysiol* 1987;**57**:1837–53.
39. Zhang SP, Davis PJ, Carrive P, Bandler R. Vocalization and marked pressor effect evoked from the region of the nucleus retroambigualis in the caudal ventrolateral medulla of the cat. *Neurosci Lett* 1992;**140**:103–7.
40. Boers J, Holstege G. Evidence for direct projections from the nucleus retroambiguus to the motoneurons of the external oblique in the female cat. *Soc Neurosci Abs* 1999;**25**:117 (51.3).
41. Holstege G, Tan J. Supraspinal control of motoneurons innervating the striated muscles of the pelvic floor including urethral and anal sphincters in the cat. *Brain* 1987;**110**:1323–44.
42. Holstege G. Anatomical study of the final common pathway for vocalization in the cat. *J Comp Neurol* 1989;**284**:242–52.
43. Zhang SP, Bandler R, Davis PJ. Brain stem integration of vocalization: role of the nucleus retroambigualis. *J Neurophysiol* 1995;**74**:2500–12.
44. Davis PJ, Zhang SP, Bandler R. Midbrain and medullary regulation of respiration and vocalization. *Prog Brain Res* 1996;**107**:315–25.
45. Miller AD, Tan LK, Suzuki I. Control of abdominal and expiratory intercostal muscle activity during vomiting: role of ventral respiratory group expiratory neurons. *J Neurophysiol* 1987;**57**:1854–66.
46. VanderHorst VGJM, Holstege G. Caudal medullary pathways to lumbosacral motoneuronal cell groups in the cat: evidence for direct projections possibly representing the final common pathway for lordosis. *J Comp Neurol* 1995;**359**:457–75.
47. VanderHorst VGJM, de Weerd H, Holstege G. Evidence for monosynaptic projections from the nucleus retroambiguus to hindlimb motoneurons in the cat. *Neurosci Lett* 1997;**224**:33–6.
48. VanderHorst VGJM, Holstege G. Estrogen induces axonal outgrowth in the nucleus retroambiguus-lumbosacral motoneuronal pathway in the adult female cat. *J Neurosci* 1997;**17**:1122–36.
49. Barrington FJF. The effects of lesions of the hind- and mid-brain on micturition in the cat. *Quart J Exp Physiol Cogn Med* 1925;**15**:81–102.
50. Holstege G, Griffiths D, de Wall H, Dalm E. Anatomical and physiological observations on supraspinal control of bladder and urethral sphincter muscles in the cat. *J Comp Neurol* 1986;**250**:449–61.
51. Blok BFM, Holstege G. Ultrastructural evidence for a direct pathway from the pontine micturition center to the parasympathetic preganglionic motoneurons of the bladder of the cat. *Neurosci Lett* 1997;**222**:195–8.
52. Nadelhaft I, Vera PL, Card JP, Miselis RR. Central nervous system neurons labelled following the injection of pseudorabies virus into the rat urinary bladder. *Neurosci Lett* 1992;**143**:271–4.
53. Blok BFM, De Weerd H, Holstege G. Ultrastructural evidence for a paucity of projections from the lumbosacral cord to the pontine micturition center or M-region in the cat: a new concept for the organization of the micturition reflex with the periaqueductal gray as central relay. *J Comp Neurol* 1995;**359**:300–9.
54. Ding YQ, Zheng HX, Gong LW, Lu Y, Zhao H, Qin BZ. Direct projections from the lumbosacral spinal cord to Barrington's nucleus in the rat: a special reference to micturition reflex. *J Comp Neurol* 1997;**389**:149–60.
55. Blok BFM, Holstege G. The pontine micturition center in rat receives direct lumbosacral input. An ultrastructural study. *Neurosci Lett* 2000;**282**:29–32.
56. Blok BFM, Holstege G. Direct projections from the periaqueductal gray to the pontine micturition center (M-region). An anterograde and retrograde tracing study in the cat. *Neurosci Lett* 1994; **166**:93–6.
57. Holstege G. Some anatomical observations on the projections from the hypothalamus to brainstem and spinal cord: an HRP and autoradiographic tracing study in the cat. *J Comp Neurol* 1987;**260**:98–126.
58. Griffiths D, Holstege G, De Wall H, Dalm E. Control and coordination of bladder and urethral function in the brainstem of the cat. *Neurourol Urodyn* 1990;**9**:63–82.
59. Blok BFM, Willemsen AT, Holstege G. A PET study on brain control of micturition in humans. *Brain* 1997;**120**:111–21.
60. Blok BFM, Sturms LM, Holstege G. Brain activation during micturition in women. *Brain* 1998; **121**:2033–42.
61. Blok BFM, Sturms LM, Holstege G. A PET study on cortical and subcortical control of pelvic floor musculature in women. *J Comp Neurol* 1997;**389**:535–44.
62. Holstege G. The emotional motor system in relation to the supraspinal control of micturition and mating behavior. *Behav Brain Res* 1998;**92**:103–9.

SECTION 3

Investigation of pelvic floor dysfunction

Chapter 9

Investigation of pelvic floor dysfunction: anterior pelvic floor; clinical features

Philip Toozs-Hobson, Linda Cardozo

INTRODUCTION

Prolapse is a generic term derived from the Latin 'to fall', and is used in the context of the anterior female pelvis to describe descent of the pelvic organs and sometimes the small bowel through a defect in the supporting tissues. The term pelvic relaxation is also sometimes used to describe conditions where the supporting tissues can no longer maintain the pelvic viscera.

Prolapse is estimated to occur in up to 50% of parous women. On its own, prolapse does not always cause symptoms and treatment is not always required. Prolapse occurs as a result of evolutionary changes in function of the pelvic floor, with the adoption of a biped posture. This has resulted in a change in the pelvis from primarily a urogenital function to one of support of the pelvic and abdominal viscera.

The term cystocele is commonly applied to the displacement of the anterior vaginal wall. This term itself is strictly incorrect as what it represents is a displacement of the anterior vaginal wall. A cystocele refers to a prolapse of the bladder and a urethrocele to urethral and bladder displacement, which can occur as a separate prolapse or together with a cystourethrocele.

Management of anterior vaginal wall prolapse is based mainly on surgery and as long ago as 1909 cystocele was quoted as being the last unsolved problem in plastic gynecology.[1] Since this time the management of female genital prolapse has remained largely unchanged. The advent of modern imaging modalities such as MRI are now facilitating re-opening the debate on the management of anterior vaginal wall prolapse. Recent advances in the thinking and investigation of vaginal prolapse will be discussed in this chapter together with the clinical symptoms and signs of this condition.

ANATOMY

The anterior compartment of the pelvis is composed of the anterior vaginal wall, and the structures ventral to it, including the pelvic fascia, separating the urethra and bladder from the vagina. The anterior vaginal wall is suspended between two condensations of connective tissue which form ligaments called the arcus tendinieus fasciae pelvis. These structures run between the ischial spine dorsolaterally passing ventromedially to the lower edge of the pubic symphysis. The arcus tendinieus fascia pelvis represents the line of insertion of the muscles making up the side walls of the pelvis. On the superior border is the insertion of obturator internis running laterally to insert on the obturator membrane covering the obturator foramen; and inferiorly is the origin of the levator; complex of puborectalis (pubovaginalis), pubococcygeus and iliococcygeus which merge with their contralateral counterparts. Suspended between the two arcus tendinious fasciae pelvis ligaments is a sheet of connective tissue known as the pubocervical fascia. This fascia blends into the cardinal ligament at the cervix at its dorsal end and with the pubic symphysis at its ventral end.

The advantage of the anterior vaginal wall being suspended between the two ATFP (arcus tendineous fasciae pelvis) is in its ability to respond to dynamic circumstances. This allows changes in the shape of the anterior compartment of the pelvis in response to different conditions. Traditionally anatomy has looked at static function and it is only recently that the dynamic changes have begun to be appreciated by DeLancey leading to a new idea of pelvic floor function.[2] He proposed a hammock theory whereby contraction of the pelvic floor musculature alters the position of the ATFP. The change in this position results in elevation of the pubocervical fascia and hence compresses the urethra against the pubic bone. There has been much debate over the presence or absence of compressor urethrae muscle fibers and the importance of active and passive responses to raised intra-abdominal pressure. DeLancey's model also allows for pelvic floor relaxation reducing the extrinsic compression on the urethra as part of the complexly coordinated action of voiding. It also explains why some women may be able to void by pelvic floor relaxation alone.

The pelvic floor musculature itself is also important in maintaining the pelvic viscera in their normal position. Since adopting a vertical posture the transmission of forces has been such that the pelvic floor is now responsible for maintaining the pelvic and abdominal viscera within the abdomino-pelvic cavity. The normal resting position of the vagina is overlying the levator plate. An increase in the size of the 'defect' within the pelvis has been shown to be associated with an increased risk of prolapse.[3] The major risk factor for this increase appears to be childbirth[4] as prolapse is uncommon in nulliparous women.

HISTORY

SYMPTOMS OF ANTERIOR VAGINAL WALL PROLAPSE

The most common complaint resulting from vaginal prolapse is of vaginal discomfort and the sensation of something coming down. This discomfort may be as a direct result of the prolapse or secondary to urogenital atrophy from prolonged hypoestrogenism. However anterior compartment prolapse can result in loss of normal bladder function. Most commonly this manifests as stress incontinence due to displacement of the bladder neck and urethra from their normal position. This displacement leads to a loss of pressure transmission and the development of the so-called type one stress urinary incontinence (hypermobility). Alternatively displacement of the bladder with a lesser degree of urethral mobility may lead to an element of voiding dysfunction, due to kinking of the proximal urethra and relative bladder neck obstruction. This possible bladder neck obstruction is an indication for urodynamics with a ring pessary to reduce the prolapse.[5] The reduction of the prolapse in these circumstances will exclude or confirm occult genuine stress incontinence and may alter the management of the patient. Less commonly women will describe disruption of normal vaginal function and either soreness or discomfort during intercourse.

THE ROLE OF CHILDBIRTH IN VAGINAL PROLAPSE

The most commonly quoted precipitating factor for anterior vaginal prolapse is pregnancy and childbirth. Several studies have investigated which of these factors are associated with the development of incontinence and prolapse.

Instrumental delivery is commonly quoted in textbooks as a risk factor. In England the assisted delivery rate among primiparous women varies from 10–24%.[6] In 1993 the UK forceps delivery rate was 6.6% and ventouse extraction 3.5%.[7] Given the relatively frequent use of these instruments there is a paucity of objective evidence to support the claim of their involvement in the etiology of stress incontinence or subsequent prolapse. Our Medline search found one postal study showing a ten-fold increase in stress incontinence (68% vs. 6.8%)[8] with instrumental delivery. This publication however stands virtually alone in suggesting an increase in the incidence of incontinence after instrumental delivery. Dimpfl *et al.*[9] showed that vaginal delivery and maternal age over 30 increased the incidence of stress incontinence. They found associations with ventouse and forceps, but these were not statistically significant; none of these studies mentioned prolapse.

The difficulty with assessing the role of pregnancy and childbirth on the development of urogenital prolapse is that prolapse may develop over time. Most research is conducted over a relatively short period of time and therefore prolapse is not an easy end-point. Longer term studies will be needed to fully investigate the exact effect of different aspects of parturition.

Cesarean section is thought to protect against damage and pelvic floor dysfunction. In a recent survey[10] 31% of female obstetricians described cesarean section as their personal preferred method of delivery, with 80% citing fear of pelvic floor damage as the reason. Wilson *et al.*[11] reported that cesarean section reduced the prevalence of urinary incontinence from 27% in women delivering vaginally to 5% after cesarean section. There was little difference in this study between elective and emergency cesareans. The protective effect seemed to lessen with subsequent operative deliveries and three cesarean sections conferred no advantage over vaginal births. Conversely Iosif and Ingermarsson[12] found significant symptoms when they retrospectively analysed results from 204 women undergoing elective cesarean section over a 5-year period. They concluded that stress incontinence results from a combination of hereditary predisposition, changes as a result of pregnancy and damage from delivery.

Problematic stress incontinence prior to pregnancy has been reported[13] to be associated with a decrease in mature collagen. This results in less cross-linking of the collagen strands, the effect of which is to reduce tensile strength of the connective tissue. These findings have also been reported in parous women who have developed genitourinary prolapse in later life.[14]

Peptide hormones such as relaxin may also play a role in connective tissue metabolism during pregnancy.[15]

This hormone, produced mainly by the placenta, attains highest plasma levels during pregnancy and has been shown to induce collagen remodeling and consequent softening of the tissues of the birth canal.[16] To date no studies have examined the degree of recovery of these tissues after pregnancy or postulated on the accumulative effect of subsequent pregnancies. Urinary incontinence certainly occurs most with the first pregnancy and delivery with a much smaller increase after subsequent pregnancies. Since prolapse usually presents later in life, it is difficult to say when it occurs and which of the potential insults actually precipitate it.

In a recent study[4] we have demonstrated that vaginal delivery is associated with an increase in the dimensions of the levator hiatus compared with the antenatal period, whilst cesarean section showed a decrease in this area, suggesting that pregnancy itself either directly through pressure or indirectly through hormonal changes results in increased levator hiatus area. These findings have been confirmed by another study in the United States.[17] Weak collagen has been shown to be associated with an increased risk of incontinence and prolapse from observational studies, looking at Elhers–Danlos syndrome and women with joint hypermobility. The evidence for defective collagen is strengthened by epidemiological data from Musshkat *ct al.*[18] who interviewed first-degree relatives of 257 women with stress incontinence and compared them with first-degree relatives of 165 matched controls. More direct evidence has been demonstrated by Falconer *et al.* who demonstrated a decrease in collagen content in the connective tissue of stress-incontinent women.[19] Jackson *et al.*[20] also found a decrease in collagen content to be associated with prolapse; this was in conjunction with an increase in immature cross-linking reducing the tensile strength of the tissue. The same group have subsequently demonstrated that estrogen may have a beneficial effect stimulating collagen synthesis and increasing cross-linking.[21] It has yet to be shown whether long-term prophylactic treatment prevents (or reverses) prolapse formation. A small unpublished series from our unit has also suggested that pelvic floor exercises may lead to a decrease in the levator hiatus area. Whether or not these can be used in treatment or as a prophylactic measure has yet to be studied.

The effect of estrogen on collagen and the lower urinary tract has recently also centered on how estrogen may act on the pelvic floor through steroid receptor expression. This has been demonstrated in the levator anterior muscle,[22] throughout the lower urinary tract and vagina.[23] Estrogen has also been demonstrated to have a significant effect on cell cycle activity.[24] Whether this translates to an improvement of clinical outcome is still debated. Byck *et al.*[25] have suggested that it improved the outcome of colposuspension and Mikkelson *et al.*[26] suggested that estrogen therapy has no effect on the recurrence rate of prolapse. However, the study was small and only used the topical estradiol preoperatively for 3 weeks. The authors themselves concluded that long-term treatment may be necessary.

PREVIOUS SURGERY

Surgery disrupts the normal anatomy of the pelvis and consequently has an effect on the support of the pelvic organs. The effects may be two-fold; the disruption of the supporting structures and the development of scar tissue altering the properties of the remaining tissues. The success rate of continence surgery is certainly compromised by previous surgery[27] and it is logical that this can be extended to prolapse surgery.

Hysterectomy in particular may precipitate pelvic floor relaxation and vault prolapse occurs in 0.4–43% of women after hysterectomy.[28] Although 50% of these will have had a vaginal hysterectomy usually involving an element of prolapse, the other 50% have undergone an abdominal hysterectomy without significant prolapse.

CHANGES TO THE ANTERIOR VAGINAL SUPPORTS RESULTING IN PROLAPSE

Changes or damage to the anterior compartment occur in response to normal physiology and endocrinology as a part of normal phases of life including puberty, pregnancy, childbirth and the menopause. As previously mentioned one of the important factors is the quality of the connective tissue and in particular collagen.

Traditionally anterior wall prolapse has been thought to occur as a result of stretching of the endopelvic fascia and is described as a pulsion type of anterior wall prolapse. The term pulsion suggests an etiology from increased 'pressure' pushing through a weakened or stretched pubocervical fascia and the classic method of repair has been a vaginal approach. This has been quoted as being associated with up to a 50% failure rate.[29] This high failure rate led to increased questioning of the validity of the traditional thinking about prolapse and led Richardson[30] to describe a series of 'fascial defects' said to be caused by damage to the pubocervical fascia or arcus tendinious fasciae pelvis.

He proposed that damage to the ATFP would cause displacement of the anterior vagina from its normal position and he described this as traction prolapse. This description of traction is applied to the prolapse to suggest that the prolapse results as a consequence of a traction or pulling injury. The resulting displacement will depend on where on the ATFP the defect has occurred. Unbeknown to Richardson, a similar description of these was made in 1909 by White.[1] Unfortunately White died at a young age before he was able to establish his theories in practice.

Richardson[29] described four types of defect. Firstly a paravaginal defect occurring at the arcus tendinious fasciae pelvis. Secondly, a posterior transverse defect caused by a disruption of the pubocervical fascia from the cervix. Thirdly, a midline defect and, fourthly, an anterior transverse defect at the level of the urethra where the urogenital diaphragm becomes disrupted.

DeLancey has also published on normal vaginal support[2,31] and classified the level of vaginal support into three levels:

- Level I: the cephalic 2–3 cm of the vagina.
- Level II: located between levels I and III.
- Level III: extending from the hymenal ring cranially for 2–3 cm.

Again, particular attention was paid to the identification of paravaginal tears.

Subsequent studies have subsequently demonstrated these changes in the vaginal support with MRI scanning.[32] The classification on MRI showed that the upper third of the vagina (level I) demonstrated the 'chevron sign,' whereas the middle third of the vagina (level II) displayed the 'saddlebags sign,' and the lower scans of bilateral fascial defects at the upper third of the vagina (level III) displayed the 'moustache sign.' This study also demonstrated the changes that occur as a result of hysterectomy exaggerating the effect of any defect. These images however are static pictures obtained in the supine position and have not been able to demonstrate the effect of posture or Valsalva.

CLINICAL ASSESSMENT OF DEFECTS

Examination of urogenital prolapse should start with a general examination and always involve an abdominal examination for abdomino-pelvic masses which can cause a displacement of the pelvic viscera. Pelvic examination is traditionally carried out in the left lateral position using a Simms speculum to retract the posterior vaginal wall allowing good visualization of the anterior vaginal wall. A sponge forceps may be employed to push back the anterior wall if assessment of the upper vagina is required.

Clinically these different types of traction prolapses are said to be identifiable with a simple clinical examination. Two tongue spatulas are placed within the vagina and elevated. Paravaginal defects are corrected when these spatulas (or spatula unilaterally) are elevated and the cystocele is contained on straining. If the cystocele is still present then a midline defect is present. A transverse defect will be evident when the defect comes from beyond the retraction aids.

Other features of the defects are also said to be present. The posterior transverse defect is said to result in a bullfrog type of cystocele, not associated with increased bladder neck movement and therefore not associated with a high incidence of urinary incontinence. The vaginal rugae are said to be retained and the cystocele will remain, despite attempts to reduce it manually in the office setting.

Paravaginal defects may be unilateral, more commonly on the right side or bilateral. These are associated with a loss of the normal vaginal rugae and can be replaced by pressure in the lateral vaginal fornix on the side of the defect. Bilateral defects will need both vaginal sulci to be elevated to reduce the prolapse. These defects will result in a loss of support of the bladder along the whole of one edge of the vagina and consequently are thought to be associated with an increase in the bladder neck mobility. Paravaginal defects are thought to correlate with a loss of squeeze on the affected side which is detectable during a formal pelvic floor assessment.

Anterior transverse or distal defects are thought to be relatively uncommon and associated with little prolapse, but troublesome urinary incontinence is associated with disruption of the proximal female urethral continence mechanisms.

The difficulty with this theory is the inability to demonstrate a fascial defect reliably to repair in all but the paravaginal defects and also the lack of published control data against published series.[33]

CLASSIFICATION AND QUANTIFICATION OF ANTERIOR WALL PROLAPSE

There are three different methods of quantifying prolapse. The first two are 'eyeball' methods and the third, most recent, is an objective assessment as part of a quantification of the whole vagina and its mobility.

STATIC ASSESSMENT OF ANTERIOR WALL PROLAPSE

- Grade I: anterior wall descends from its normal position towards, but not to the introitus.
- Grade II: the anterior wall prolapse descends to the introitus.
- Grade III: the anterior vaginal wall is everted past the introitus.

ACTIVE ASSESSMENT OF ANTERIOR VAGINAL WALL PROLAPSE

- Grade I: descent of the anterior vaginal wall towards the introitus on Valsalva.
- Grade II: descent of the anterior vaginal wall to the introitus on Valsalva.
- Grade III: descent of the anterior vaginal wall past the introitus on Valsalva.

- Grade IV: extrusion of the anterior vaginal wall through the introitus at rest.

QUANTIFICATION OF PELVIC ORGAN PROLAPSE

More recently the International Continence Society has introduced a quantification of pelvic organ prolapse[34] which assesses the objective displacement of the anterior and posterior vaginal walls as well as the cervix. This assessment includes the genital hiatus and perineal body which recognizes the importance of these structures in supporting the pelvic viscera.[35] This system has the added advantages of being highly reproducible[36,37] and therefore allows reliable comparisons between different physicians in assessing prolapse. It also quantifies changes to the other compartments of the pelvis which may be relevant in deciding which operation or treatment options to pursue.

Q TIP TEST

The Q tip test is a test of urethral hypermobility. The test involves inserting a standard Q-tip cotton wool bud into the urethra and measuring the change in the angle of the shaft of the Q-tip in response to the patient performing a Valsalva maneuver. The American literature has embraced this theory and the most commonly used classification of stress incontinence quantifies the degree of hypermobility to define the type of stress incontinence.[38] Consequently investigations such as the Q-tip test to assess urethral hypermobility have become popular. The Q-tip test has never gained widespread acceptance in Europe and has actually been shown to be a poor marker of bladder neck hypermobility.[39]

IMAGING OF THE ANTERIOR COMPARTMENT

Until the advent of transvaginal ultrasound and MRI there were no useful imaging modalities for assessing pelvic floor dysfunction. Ultrasound has now become established as a reliable technique for assessing bladder neck movement comparing favourably with lateral bead chain cystography[40] in assessing the urethrovesical angle. Descent of the urethrovesical junction of greater than 1 cm has been shown in one study to be 91% specific at detecting urinary stress incontinence.[41] Various routes have been tried for assessing the bladder neck. The accuracy of the transvaginal route has been questioned due to potential probe compression of the urethra.[42] This has led to greater use of the transperineal approach which can be performed easily with minimal discomfort to the woman. Mayer *et al.*[43] investigated the effect of childbirth on hypermobility in 214 women, 74 of whom were nulliparous, 29 had had one delivery, 64 had had two or more vaginal deliveries and 16 forceps. They also examined 32 women who complained of stress incontinence. This study found a significant increase in bladder neck movement on Valsalva in both the incontinent and forceps groups supporting the idea of hypermobility with incontinence and also a relationship with vaginal birth. Whilst MRI has increased our understanding of the static anatomy, at present there are few MRI machines fast enough to capture a true Valsalva or cough as an ultrasound machine can.

To date only one study using MRI has looked longitudinally at changes in the pelvis due to childbirth.[44] This did not show any significant changes. This is almost certainly because they were unable to investigate dynamic changes such as those described using perineal ultrasound above. The development of faster MRI is now allowing the dynamic assessment of the pelvic floor[45] and may yet supersede ultrasound in the dynamic assessment of the pelvic floor.

THE FUTURE

There is an increasing demand to attend to quality of life as well as longevity of life. Over recent years medicine has increasingly focused on this. Several quality of life tools have now been developed and validated to assess the effect of lower urinary tract dysfunction. Similar tools are being developed for vaginal prolapse and it is possible that these will become a routine part of the assessment of prolapse in the future, individualizing management

CONCLUSIONS

As medical care progresses, increased life expectancy coupled with more focus on quality of life will lead to an increasing emphasis on chronic conditions such as prolapse.

At the present time our understanding of the anterior pelvic floor is expanding with improved imaging techniques. To date we have not accurately fully demonstrated the full dynamics of normal pelvic floor function, and it is therefore not surprising that further work is required on the etiology and pathology of prolapse. Greater awareness of problems coupled with detailed clinical assessment will hopefully lead to accurate diagnosis and greater awareness of occult pathology. This may include greater assessment of trauma to the pelvic floor as a result of pregnancy and childbirth, intrinsic collagen type and estrogen status.

With improved understanding of the pathology of prolapse, our strategies for treatment will come under greater scrutiny which can only lead to an improvement in the management of this difficult problem.

REFERENCES

1. White GR. Cystocele. A radical cure by suturing lateral sulci of vagina to white line of pelvic fascia. *JAMA* 1909;**53**:1707–10.
2. DeLancey JOL. Structural aspects of the extrinsic continence mechanism. *Obstet Gynecol* 1988;**72**:296–301.
3. Athanasiou S, Boos K, Khullar V, Anders K, Cardozo L. Pathogenesis of genuine stress incontinence and urogenital prolapse *Obstet Gynecol* 1996;**15(4)**:339–40.
4. Toozs-Hobson P, Athanasiou S, Khullar V, Boos K, Hextall A, Cardozo L. Does vaginal delivery damage the pelvic floor? *Neurourol Urodyn* 1997;
5. Hextall A, Boos K, Cardozo L, Toozs-Hobson P, Anders K, Khullar V. Videocystourethrography with a ring pessary *in situ*. A clinically useful preoperative investigation for continent women with urogenital prolapse? *Int Urogynecol J* 1998;**9**:205–209.
6. Drife JO, Choice and instrumental delivery. *Br J Obstet Gynaecol* 1996;**103**:608–611.
7. Meinru GI. An analysis of recent trends in vacuum extraction and forceps delivery in the United Kingdom. *Br J Obstet Gynaecol* 1996;**103**:168–70.
8. Chiarelli P, Campbell E. Incontinence during pregnancy. Prevalence and opportunities for continence promotion. *Aust N Z J Obstet Gynaecol* 1997;**37(1)**:66–73.
9. Dimpfl T, Hesses U, Schussler B. Incidence and cause of postpartum stress incontinence. *Eur J Obstet Gynecol Reprod Biol* 1992;**43(1)**:29–33.
10. Al-Mufti R, McCarthy A, Fisk NN. Obstetricians personal choice and mode of delivery. *Lancet* 1996;**347**:544.
11. Wilson PD, Herbison RM, Herbison GP. Obstetric practice and the prevalence of urinary incontinence three months after delivery. *Br J Obstet Gynaecol* 1996;**103(2)**:154–61.
12. Iosif CS, Ingermarsson I. Prevalence of stress incontinence among women delivered by elective caesarean section. *Int J Gynaecol Obstet* 1982;**20(2)**:87–9.
13. Keane DP, Sims TJ, Abrams P, Bailey AJ. Analysis of collagen status in premenopausal nulliparous women with genuine stress incontinence. *Br J Obstet Gynaecol* 1997;**104(9)**:994–8.
14. Jackson S, Avery N, Eckford S, Sheperd A, Bailey A. Connective tissue analysis in genitourinary prolapse. *Neurourol Urodyn* 1995;**14(5)**:412–4.
15. Bell RJ, Eddie LW, Lester AR, Wood EC, Johnston PD, Niall HD. Relaxin in human pregnancy serum measured with an homologous radioimmunoassay. *Obstet Gynecol* 1987;**69**:585–9.
16. Bani D. Relaxin: A pleiotropic hormone. *Gen Pharmacol* 1997;**28**:13–22.
17. DeLancey JO, Hurd WW. Size of the urogenital hiatus in the levator hiatus muscles in normal women and women with pelvic organ prolapse. *Obstet Gynecol* 1998;**91(3)**:354–8.
18. Mushkat Y, Bukovsky I, Langer R. Female urinary stress incontinence – does it have familial prevalence? *Am J Obstet Gynecol* 1996;**174(2)**:617–9.
19. Falconer C, Ekman G, Malstrom A, Ulmsten U. Decreased collagen in stress incontinent women. *Obstet Gynecol* 1994;**84(4)**:583–6.
20. Jackson S, Avery N, Tarlton JF, Ecford S, Abrams P, Bailey A. Changes in metabolism of collagen in genitourinary prolapse. *Lancet* 1996;**347(9016)**:1658–61.
21. Jackson S, Avery N, Shepherd A, Abrams P, Bailey A. The effect of oestradiol on vaginal collagen in postmenopausal women with stress urinary incontinence. *Neurourol Urodyn* 1996;**15(4)**:327–8.
22. Smith P, Heimer G, Norgren A, Ulmsten U. Localisation of steroid receptors in the pelvic muscles. *Eur J Obstet Gynecol Reprod Biol* 1993;**50(1)**:83–5.
23. Blakeman P, Hilton P, Bulmer JN. Mapping oestrogen and progesterone receptors throughout the female urinary tract. *Neurourol Urodyn* 1996;**15(4)**:324–5.
24. Blakeman PJ, Hilton P, Bulmer JN. Oestrogen status and cell cycle activity in the female lower urinary tract. 1996;**15(4)**:325–6.
25. Byck DB, Varner RE, Clough C. Urinary complaints after modified Burch urethropexy: an analysis. *Am J Obstet Gynecol* 1994;**171(6)**:460–2.

26 Mikkelson AL, Felding C, Clausen HV. Clinical effects of preoperative oestradiol treatment before vaginal repair operation. A double blind randomised trial. *Obstet Gynecol Invest* 1995;**40**(2):125–8.

27 Menachem A, Monga A, Stanton S. Burch colposuspension: a 10–20 year follow up. *Br J Obstet Gynaecol* 1995;**102**(9):740–45.

28 Cruickshank SH. Sacrospinous ligament fixation – should this be performed at the time of vaginal hysterectomy? *Am J Obstet Gynecol* 1991;**164**:1072–76.

29 Richardson AC. Cystocele paravaginal repair. In: Benson JT (ed.) *Female pelvic disorders. Investigation and management*, Chapter 12A:280–87. Norton Medical Books, ISBN0-393-71013-0.

30 Richardson AC, Lyon JB, Williams NL. A new look at pelvic relaxation *Am J Obstet Gynecol* 1976;**126**:568.

31 DeLancey JOL Structural aspects of the extrinsic continence mechanism. *Obstet Gynecol* 1988;**72**: 296–301.

32 Huddleston HT, Dunnihoo DR, Huddleston PM, Meyers PC. Magnetic resonance imaging of defects in DeLancey's vaginal support levels I, II, and III. *Am J Obstet Gynecol* 1995;**172**(6):1778–82.

33 Taylor PW. Comment on Richardson AC, Lyon JB, Williams NL. A new look at pelvic relaxation. *Am J Obstet Gynecol* 1976;**126**:572.

34 The standardisation of terminology of female pelvic organ prolapse and pelvic floor dysfunction final draft. International Continence Society, August 1994.

35 Bump RC, Mattiasson A, Bo K, *et al.* The standardisation of terminology of female pelvic organ prolapse and pelvic floor dysfunction. *Am J Obstet Gynecol* 1996;**175**(1):10–7.

36 Athanasiou S. Hill S, Gleeson C, *et al.* Validation of the ICS proposed pelvic organ descriptive system. *Neurourol Urodyn* 1995;**14**(5):414–5.

37 Schussler B, Peschers U. Standardisation of terminology of female genital prolapse according to the new ICS criteria: Inter-examiner reproducibility. *Neurourol Urodyn* 1995;**14**(5):437–8.

38 Blavis JG. Classification of stress urinary incontinence. *Neururol Urodyn* 1983;**2**:103.

39 Caputo RM, Benson JT. The Q tip test and urethrovesical junction mobility. *Obstet Gynecol* 1993;**82**(6):892–6.

40 Bergman A, McKenzie CJ, Richmond J, *et al.* Transrectal ultrasound versus cystography in the evaluation of anatomical stress urinary incontinence. *Br J Urol* 1988;**62**(3):228–34.

41 Bergman A, Ballard CA, Platt LD. Ultrasonic evaluation of urethrovesical junction in women with stress urinary incontinence. *J Clin Ultrasound* 1988;**16**(5):295–300.

42 Wise B, Burton G, Cutner A, Cardozo L. Effect of vaginal ultrasound probe on lower urinary tract function. *Br J Urol* 1992;**70**:12–16.

43 Meyer S, De Grandi P, Schreyer A, Caccia G. The assessment of bladder neck position and mobility in continent women using perineal ultrasound: a future office procedure. *Int Urogynecol J Pelvic Floor Dysfunct* 1996; **7**(3):138–46.

44 Hayat SK, Thorp JM, Kullar JA, Brown BD, Semelka RC. Magnetic resonance imaging of the pelvic floor in the postpartum patient. *Int Urogynecol J Pelvic Floor Dysfunct* 1996;**7**(6):321–4.

45 Bo K, Lilleas F, Talseth T. Dynamic MRI of the pelvic floor and coccygeal movement during pelvic floor contraction and straining. *Neurourol Urodyn* 1997;**16**(5):409–10.

Chapter 10

Voiding studies

John M Reynard

In clinical practice voiding studies have two principal uses – diagnosis and prediction of outcome of treatment. They are most often used for diagnosis of voiding dysfunction in men presenting with lower urinary tract symptoms (LUTS), particularly those associated with benign prostatic enlargement (BPE) due to benign prostatic hyperplasia (BPH). As a consequence, this chapter principally concerns the diagnostic and prognostic value of voiding studies in men with LUTS presumed to be secondary to BPE or bladder outlet obstruction (BOO). Symptoms during voiding (as opposed to storage symptoms such as frequency or urgency) are less common in women than in men. As a consequence voiding studies have a more restricted role to play in the assessment of women with LUTS. The use of voiding studies in children is beyond the scope of this chapter.

Three types of voiding study are in common use – uroflowmetry, pressure–flow studies and measurement of postvoid residual urine volume (PVR). PVR measurement is not strictly a *voiding* study, but because the volume of urine remaining in the bladder at the end of a void is so closely related to the act of micturition and is thus a reflection of voiding function, PVR estimation is included in the subsequent discussion. Videourodynamics, the combination of pressure–flow studies with radiographic screening of the bladder and urethra during voiding, is discussed in Chapter 11, but their use in diagnosis of lower urinary tract problems in women is discussed in this chapter. Micturitional urethral pressure profilometry (MUPP) is used in a few interested centers in the United States and Europe and the principals and application of this technique to diagnosis of lower urinary tract dysfunction are briefly discussed.

UROFLOWMETRY

INTRODUCTION

Drake (1948) developed the first uroflowmeter allowing urine flow rate to be simultaneously plotted against time.[1] von Garrelts (1956) introduced the electronic flowmeter.[2] Modern flowmeters are direct descendants of those developed by von Garrelts and allow urine flow rates to be measured with ease and accuracy. They are computerized and produce a print-out of flow pattern plotted against time, together with computer generated

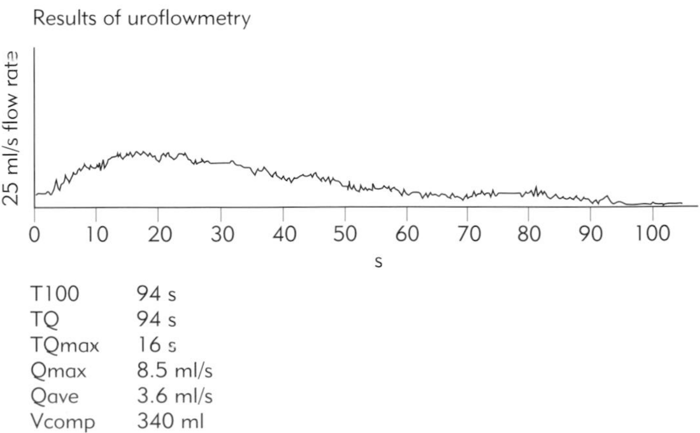

Figure 10.1 A uroflow trace showing the computerized print-out and machine derived parameters of Qmax and voided volume. From Ref. 128, with permission.

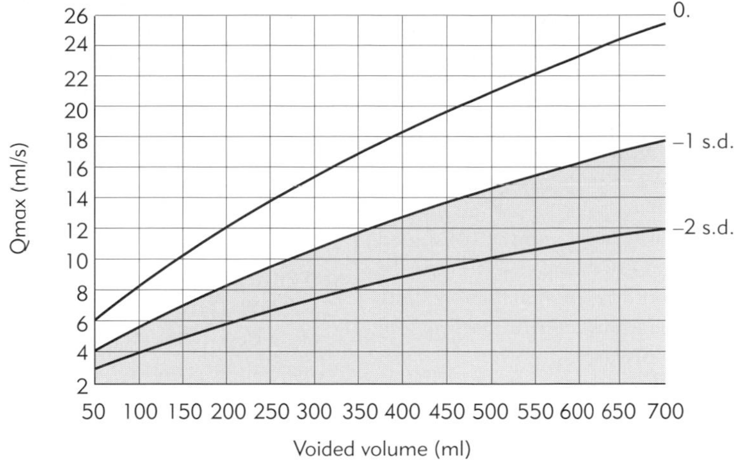

Figure 10.2 The Bristol flow rate nomogram. From Ref. 128, with permission.

values for maximum flow rate (Qmax), average flow rate and voided volume (Fig. 10.1). Other variables are also measured such as total voiding time (T100) and time to maximum flow rate (TQmax). However, in practice Qmax is the most useful parameter derived from uroflowmetry. A recent survey reported that urologists also regard voided volume and flow curve pattern as important in the interpretation of uroflow traces.[3]

QMAX (MAXIMUM FLOWRATE)

Qmax is dependent on voided volume, but the relationship between Qmax and voided volume is non-linear, so it is difficult to define a normal flow rate in the absence of information about voided volume. For this reason a number of flow-rate nomograms have been developed to relate Qmax to voided volume. The Siroky nomogram was developed from flow measurements in asymptomatic men aged less than 50.[4] Two Liverpool nomograms have been constructed, one for normal men below the age of 50 and one for men aged over 50.[5] The Bristol nomogram (Fig. 10.2) was based on flow recordings from asymptomatic men aged more than 50.[6] These nomograms allow an individual flow rate to be related to a normal reference range depending on the voided volume. Flow rate nomograms in women are discussed below.

Other factors which influence Qmax include voiding position and age. Riehmann (1998) has shown that in normal men and male nursing home residents urinary flow rate is significantly lower in the recumbent compared with the standing position.[7] In normal individuals there was no difference in postvoid residual urine volume measured after recumbent and standing voids and though in the nursing home residents PVR in the standing position was lower than after voiding in the recumbent position, this difference was small and only just reached statistical significance. Interesting though these observations are, positional effects on Qmax are unlikely to be important in terms of the interpretation of uroflowmetry as most flow studies tend to be performed in the standing position.

Qmax has been shown to fall with increasing age. In a community based study of 2113 randomly selected men, median Qmax in those aged 40–44 years was 20.5 ml/s and in those aged 75–79 it was 11.5 ml/s.[8] These findings have been confirmed in other studies of asymptomatic subjects.[5,9] More recently, Homma (1994) reported a decline in both maximum detrusor pressure and flow rate in both men and women with increasing age.[10] Interestingly in this study the decline was more marked in women.

QMAX AND VOIDED VOLUME

Voided volumes <150 ml are traditionally thought of as being uninterpretable. This is based on Drach's observation[11] that the good correlation between Qmax and voided volume above voided volumes of 150 ml disappears at voided volumes below 150 ml,[12] though this was not the experience reported by Haylen in the development of the Liverpool flow nomogram in men, where Qmax could be correlated with voided volume even below 150 ml.[5]

In an attempt to increase the percentage of men voiding more than 150 ml during uroflowmetry, urine flow rate clinics have been established in some urology departments. In these clinics between two and four flows are obtained and residual urine volume can be estimated after each flow. Such clinics have been shown to increase the proportion of men voiding over 150 ml. In one such clinic the percentage of patients who voided less than 150 ml fell from from 59% to 21%.[13]

Reynard and Abrams have re-examined the value of low volume voids and have suggested that they do provide useful diagnostic information.[14] Using a cut-off value of Qmax of 10 ml/s to indicate the presence of bladder outlet obstruction (BOO) they found that voids of less than 150 ml had a positive predictive value for the presence of BOO of 83% compared with a positive predictive value of 79% for voids greater than 150 ml. In a more recent study of 1271 men with LUTS those voiding <150 ml were found to have a 72% chance of BOO (overall prevalence of BOO 60%) and the likelihood of BOO in those voiding over 150 ml was 56%.[15] On the basis of these studies it would seem that low volume voids can provide useful diagnostic information and they should probably not be discarded.

INTERPRETATION OF FLOW STUDIES – ARTIFACTS

Some care with interpretation of flow recordings is necessary. Artifacts of machine-read traces, when compared with visual readings, have been reported. Grino (1993) performed over 23 000 flow recordings in 1645 men and compared the estimate of Qmax from simple visualization of the flow trace with the machine's computerized print out.[16] A difference between the machine-read and observer-read flow rate of > 2 ml/s occurred in 20% of the recordings and a difference of > 3 ml/s was found in 9% of cases. Such differences are often due to the presence of the so-called wag artifact. Here a slight variation in the direction of flow can result in the patient voiding directly into the center of the uroflowmeter (Fig. 10.3). A summation of flows occurs, resulting in an artifactually high flow rate. Sudden, rapid rises in flow rate on the flow curve tracing should thus be interpreted with caution. Witjes (1998) has designed a computer program to detect artifacts such as these on uroflow traces and has tested this system against traces manually read by independent observers.[17] There was a considerable degree of inter-observer variability in the assessment of Qmax. About 50% of the maximum flow values assessed by two observers varied by >1 ml/s. The computer 'corrected' traces showed less variability in the value for Qmax than did the values given by the observers.

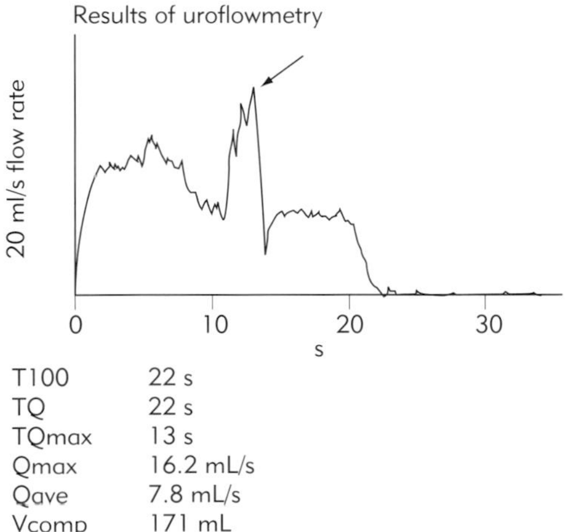

Figure 10.3 A 'wag' artifact producing a spuriously high computer derived interpretation of Qmax. The 'real' value of Qmax is approximately 12 ml/s. From Ref. 128, with permission.

INTER-OBSERVER VARIATION IN INTERPRETATION OF FLOW STUDIES

Van de Beek (1997) has studied inter-observer and intra-observer agreement in the interpretation of uroflow curve patterns.[3] Of 58 urologists who were questioned, 77% felt that visual inspection of flow curve traces was relevant for interpretation. Inter-observer agreement (expressed as kappa for 'normalcy' and kappa for 'most likely diagnosis') was moderate for normalcy (kappa 0.46) and poor (kappa 0.3) for most likely diagnosis. In terms of intra-observer agreement, in 29% of cases different values were chosen for normalcy and in 41% of cases another diagnosis was given on second, later inspection of the same uroflow trace. This variability in interpretation of individual flow traces casts doubt on the diagnostic value of flow curve patterns. Unambiguous definitions of terminal dribbling and intermittency on flow curve patterns have been developed.[18,19] If applied correctly they are not subject to inter or intra-observer error. As discussed later, such flow patterns can be useful for the diagnosis of BOO.

REPRODUCIBILITY OF QMAX

Several studies have addressed the variability and reproducibility of measurements of Qmax. Over the short term Reynard (1996) reported a significant increase in Qmax in patients who voided three or four times over the space of a single morning (all flow traces were visually read by a single observer).[20] In patients voiding four times, Qmax increased from 10.2 ml/s on void 1 to 14.9 ml/s on void 4. This increase in Qmax occurred in the absence of a significant increase in voided volume across the four voids. In men with LUTS reinvestigated over a longer time period (2 weeks) Barry (1995) found that the mean difference in Qmax was just 0.1 ml/s.[21] In the placebo arm of a 'BPH' drug trial Jepsen (1998) noted a statistically significant increase in Qmax from 8.6 to 9.4 ml/s in flows recorded over a 4-week period, though the clinical significance of such a small increase is questionable.[22]

Thus, when several flow studies are performed on the same day there does appear to be a learning effect in elderly men with later recorded flows being higher, but over a longer time frame single flow measurements appear to be reproducible. The 4th International

Consultation on BPH has recently recommended that because of intra-individual variability of peak flow rate, at least two flow rate recordings should be obtained prior to making any treatment decisions.[23]

NEW METHODS FOR DETERMINATION OF QMAX

Since some patients may be inhibited by the environment of the flow clinic, home uroflowmetry has been advocated as a way of obtaining flow rate measurements which are more likely to be representative of a patient's normal voiding pattern.[24] Golomb has found wide variation in measurement of Qmax performed at home in both normal individuals and those with LUTS (1992).[25] Thomas and Abrams (1998) compared home based measurement of Qmax and postvoid residual urine volume with those recorded in the flow clinic.[26] Home recorded residual volumes were recorded with a portable ultrasound scanner which the subjects were trained to use. Voided volumes did not vary significantly. Values for Qmax were higher at home than in the clinic when compared with the initial clinic flow, but not when compared with a second clinic flow. Home recorded PVR was significantly lower than the clinic recorded PVR (85 v. 117 ml), though in clinical terms such a difference is small.

Home uroflowmetry requires a considerable investment in time and additional equipment, all of which add to its expense. There is the further disadvantage that it does not lend itself easily to the measurement of postvoid residual urine volume. There may be a tendency for patients to over-perform in the clinic environment if they are instructed to void at abnormally high bladder volumes, while other patients may under-perform through anxiety. The large volumes of fluid consumed by patients in flow clinics may be partly responsible for the observation that the mean volume of clinic voids was 48 ml higher than that of home voids (determined from voiding diaries).[15]

PRESSURE–FLOW STUDIES

INTRODUCTION

Pressure–flow studies (PFS) involve the simultaneous recording of detrusor pressure and flow rate. The basic principles of performing this investigation remain essentially unchanged since von Garrelts described the methodology in 1956.[2] The measured parameters are intravesical pressure (Pves, recorded by a urethral or suprapubic catheter) and intra-abdominal pressure (Pabd, usually recorded intrarectally). From these pressures detrusor pressure (Pdet) is derived by subtraction of abdominal from intravesical pressure. All pressures are expressed in cmH_2O. In combination with these pressure measurements flow rate expressed in ml/s is also measured and the value for maximum flow rate, Qmax, can be obtained. The pressure measurements are recorded by fluid-filled catheters connected to external pressure transducers placed at the level of the superior border of the symphysis pubis and zeroed to atmospheric pressure. Alternatively, catheter-tip transducers can be used, though these are more expensive and once in position checking zero pressure is difficult if not impossible.

MEASURING PRESSURE AND FLOW

A computerized print-out of Pves, Pabd, Pdet and Qmax is produced by modern pressure–flow machines. Maximum flow rate and detrusor pressure at maximum flow, PdetQmax, are the most useful measurements derived from the pressure–flow plot. As with uroflowmeter derived free-flow traces, direct inspection of the raw pressure and flow data is important to identify artifacts. There is some degree of interobserver variation in the interpretation of pressure–flow traces. Abrams reported that when pressure–flow recordings were independently read by two observers, values for Qmax varied by an average of 0.8 ml/s and values for PdetQmax varied by an average of 2.5 cmH_2O. Values for Qmax differed by <2 ml/s in 93% of cases and those for PdetQmax by <15 cmH_2O in 92% of cases.[23]

Amongst factors with a potential influence on variables measured during pressure–flow studies, catheter size and position (urethral v. suprapubic) and urethral instrumentation have recently been studied. In a group of men with LUTS, Walker (1997) compared the suprapubic and transurethral methods of measuring intravesical pressure to determine whether the presence of a 10 Ch urethral catheter during the voiding phase affected the grading of BOO.[27] The commonly used grading systems for BOO were used (the Abrams–Griffiths number, linear passive urethral resistance ratio (linPURR) and the urethral resistance algorithm, URA). With transurethral pressure recording 26% of patients increased the linPURR class by one (i.e. were classified as more obstructed) and 6% by two classes. Using the Abrams–Griffiths nomogram, 17% moved from a classification of equivocal to obstructed and 3% from unobstructed to equivocal and using a value of URA >29 as indicating obstruction, 57% were obstructed using the suprapubic and 74% using the transurethral method. The transurethral studies clearly tended to indicate a greater degree of obstruction than that using suprapubic catheter derived pressure values. Walker concluded that the interpretation of urodynamic studies should take into account the technique used and that where the transurethral route is the method chosen, the smallest catheter available should be used. In this respect, in a study of men with BPE undergoing two PFS with and then without an 8 Ch urethral catheter in place, Reynard

(1996) found no significant difference in Qmax, but a slight reduction in PdetQmax once the catheter had been removed (from 80 v. 67 cmH_2O).[28] There was no significant difference in the value of URA with or without the 8 Ch urethral catheter in place and only five of 52 men moved from obstructed to non-obstructed voiding (using URA to categorize obstruction). Neal (1987) showed a fall in Qmax and a rise in voiding pressure when a 10 Ch urethral catheter was used during pressure measurement.[29] Thus, an 8 Ch filling urethral catheter seems to represent the threshold size above which catheter diameter influences pressure–flow classification.

EFFECT OF URETHRAL INSTRUMENTATION ON QMAX

It has been suggested that urethral instrumentation may influence pressure–flow variables recorded during urodynamic studies. Walker (1998) studied the effect of urethral instrumentation on pressure–flow variables by passing a 12 Ch urethral catheter followed by a 17 Ch cystoscope, after which pressure–flow flow studies were performed.[30] While there were statistically significant differences in the detrusor pressure at maximum flow and detrusor opening pressure between the uninstrumented and instrumented pressure–flow studies, there was no effect on the Abrams–Griffiths number or urethral resistance algorithm (URA) between studies.

REPRODUCIBILITY OF PRESSURE–FLOW STUDIES

The reasonably high reproducibility of PFS has been shown in several studies in both men and women. In a series of 90 men with LUTS undergoing two fill and void sequences during pressure–flow studies van de Beek (1992) found excellent test–retest reproducibility (coefficient of determination for URA of 0.91 between repeated measurements).[31] Using the CHESS classification system Tan (1995) found no significant differences in a variety of urodynamic parameters (both pressures and flow rates) when two consecutive pressure flow studies were performed in 128 men with symptoms suggestive of BPH.[32] Rosier (1995) studied 75 patients undergoing two consecutive pressure–flow studies.[33] About 87% of individuals showed intra-individual differences in Qmax of <2 ml/s and in 80% the two values of PdetQmax differed by <15 cmH_2O. Average PdetQmax for the whole group was slightly lower for the second void (71.4 v. 74.4 cmH_2O). These differences were seldom large enough to lead to a change in diagnosis or in the grade of obstruction determined by the Schäfer nomogram. More recently, Hansen (1997) found no difference in Qmax between first and second voids in 105 consecutive pressure–flow studies.[34] PdetQmax decreased by just 2.8 cmH_2O. Only 13 patients (12%) changed their classification on the Abrams–Griffiths nomogram and the majority of these (69%) shifted from a more to a less obstructed classification.

The reproducibility of pressure and flow recordings over the medium term (6 months) has been studied in the placebo arm of a clinical drug trial. The average change in Qmax was 2.3 ± 2.1 ml/s and the mean change in PdetQmax was 15.6 ±14.8 cmH_2O.[35] Such changes in flow and pressure parameters are not enough to result in a change in urodynamic classification.

ANALYSIS OF THE PRESSURE–FLOW RELATIONSHIP

The definition of BOO is to some extent dependent on the method of description of the pressure–flow relationship (the pressure–flow plot). The commonly used methods are the Abrams–Griffiths nomogram, recently superseded by the 'ICS provisional nomogram', URA and Schäfer's linearized passive urethral resistance relationship (linPURR).

The Abrams–Griffiths nomogram was based on data from 117 patients and described three zones of classification, distinguished by an upper and lower line (Figure 10.4).[36] These boundary lines were arrived at 'by a combination of theoretical insight and clinical judgement'.[23] The 'ICS provisional nomogram' (Figure 10.5)[37] has superseded the Abrams–Griffiths nomogram. The upper boundary of this new nomogram is identical to that of the Abrams–Griffiths and Schäfer nomograms. The lower boundary is slightly higher than that of the Abrams–Griffiths nomogram, making the 'equivocal' zone somewhat smaller than in the Abrams–Griffiths nomogram. As a consequence fewer patients fall into the equivocal zone and more patients are classified as either clearly obstructed or clearly unobstructed.

The Schäfer method of classifying obstruction, based on the linear PURR concept, was later modified to a nomogram (Fig. 10.6).[38] Seven grades are described – 0 and I represent no obstruction, II represents mild obstruction and III–VI are increasing grades of obstruction. The

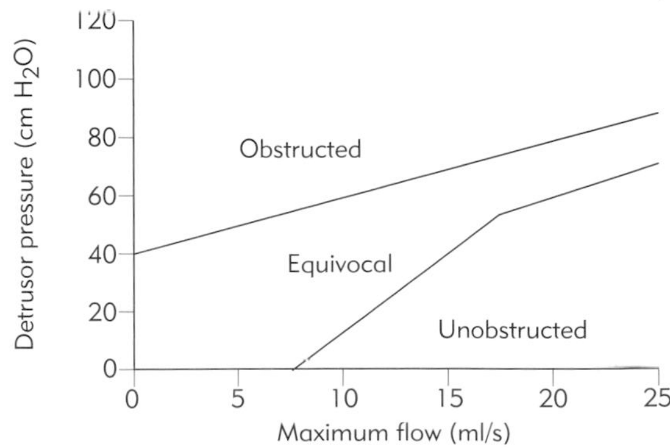

Figure 10.4 The Abrams–Griffiths nomogram. From Ref. 127, with permission.

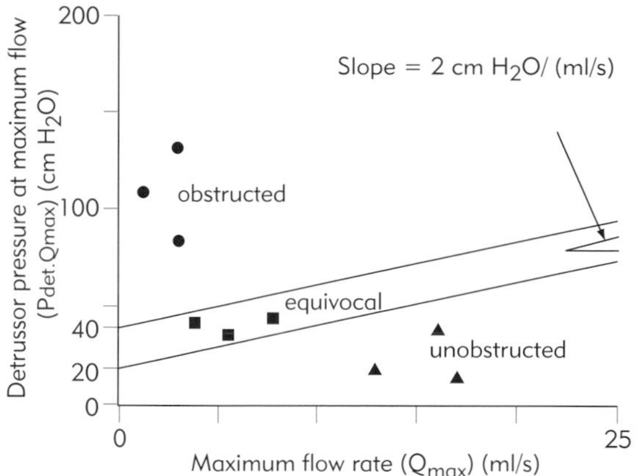

Figure 10.5 The 'ICS provisional nomogram'. From Ref. 37, with permission.

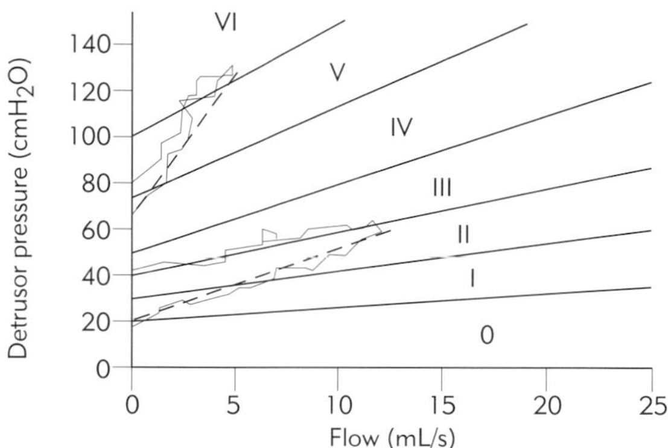

Figure 10.6 The Schäfer method of classifying obstruction. From Ref. 127, with permission.

size of the grades were chosen by test–retest data. Grade II (slightly obstructed) fulfils a similar function to the equivocal zone of the Abrams–Griffiths nomogram.

URA – the group-specific urethral resistance relationship – was based on statistical analysis of pressure–flow plots from 193 patients.[39] This system grades urethral resistance on a continuous scale and is represented by a series of parabolic curves on the pressure–flow graph. A curved boundary line was added separating obstructed from non-obstructed voiding. The position of maximum flow rate is plotted on the pressure–flow plot and the point of intersection with the pressure axis represents the value for URA (Fig. 10.7). Values above 29 cmH_2O indicate obstruction.

Newer methods of analysis of PF plots include Höfner's CHESS system,[40] Kranse and van Mastrigts' OBI method,[41] Spångberg's method,[42] DAMPF[43] and the Abrams–Griffiths number.[44] The OBI method is a computer based system which derives three parameters from lowest part of the pressure–flow plot and reduces these to

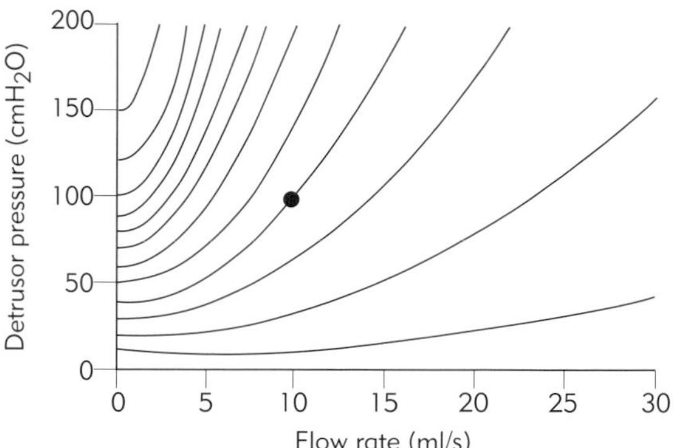

Figure 10.7 URA, the group-specific urethral resistance relationship. From Ref. 127, with permission.

a single index of obstruction. Schäfer's DAMPF (detrusor adjusted mean PURR factor) was specifically designed as a grading system for obstruction which is independent of detrusor function. This system integrates a line of standardized detrusor contraction power into the pressure–flow diagram (linPURR), without the need for a computer for the analysis. Using this system outflow conditions are classified using the seven band grading system of linPURR, but expanded to include a bladder contractility factor. The Abrams–Griffiths number (AG number) is calculated from a simple equation derived from the original Abrams–Griffiths nomogram: AG number = PdetQmax – 2Qmax). The AG number gives a continuous variable with the values 20 (< 20 being unobstructed) and 40 (40 being obstructed) corresponding to the boundaries of the ICS provisional nomogram.

Comments on Analysis

None of these methods are commonly used in day-to-day practice. The current recommendations of The 4th International Consultation on BPH are that one simple standard method of analysis is used so that the results from different centers can be compared. The method recommended is the ICS nomogram (the provisional ICS method for definition of obstruction). The advantages of the ICS nomogram lie in its simplicity of use, the fact that it does not need a computer for data analysis and the fact that it is the best clinically evaluated system. For the purpose of clinical trials, if the severity of obstruction is to be graded the Schäfer nomogram may be used.

How comparable are these different systems? Ding and Lieu (1998) compared the correlation between the AG number, DAMPF and URA.[45] The Pearson correlation coefficient for the AG number versus DAMPF was 0.94 and for the AG number versus URA it was 0.89. Ding and Lieu concluded that DAMPF and URA are highly correlated with the AG number. These findings are similar to those of Lim and Abrams (1995) who found a

Pearson correlation coefficient between the AG number and URA of 0.9.[46]

POSTVOID RESIDUAL URINE VOLUME

INTRODUCTION

Postvoid residual urine volume (PVR) is defined by the ICS as the volume of urine remaining in the bladder immediately following the completion of micturition.[47] Residual urine volume can be expressed as an absolute value (in ml) or as a percentage of bladder capacity, giving an estimation of voiding efficiency.[48] This latter method is not commonly used in practice.

TECHNIQUES OF MEASUREMENT

Various techniques of measurement of PVR are available. Catheterization is regarded as the gold-standard method. Technique is important since failure to completely empty the bladder can lead to underestimation of PVR. Stoller and Millard (1989) found incomplete bladder emptying occurred in 134 (26%) of 515 patients undergoing PVR estimation by catheterization by experienced urology nurses.[49]

Urethral catheterization is obviously invasive and unpleasant for the patient. Less invasive methods for estimating PVR volume have been described. Use of radioisotopes to determine PVR volume (by measurement of radioactivity over the bladder) has been reported, and though accurate when compared with catheterized PVR volume this method has not found a place in routine practice or indeed in research studies. Some studies have found estimation of PVR volume based on measurement of bladder area on postvoid films of IVUs to be inaccurate,[50] while others report a good correlation (5–10% error) between estimated and actual PVR.[51] Again, IVU estimation of PVR is not used in routine practice.

Ultrasound estimation of PVR volume has the advantage of being non-invasive and easy to measure. A variety of different formulae for calculation of PVR volume from measurement of bladder height, width and depth have been used and most report a correlation coefficient with catheter recorded volume of greater than 0.9.[23] For practical purposes the formula 0.52 × height × width × anteroposterior diameter (the volume of an ellipsoid) is sufficiently accurate for estimating postvoid residual urine volume from ultrasound derived bladder dimensions, with a correlation coefficient of 0.98 with catheter recorded volume.[52]

While Reynard (1996)[20] showed no significant change in residual volumes recorded over a period of 3 to 4 hours (values for mean PVR on four flows ranged between 128 and 136 ml), several studies, using both ultrasound and catheterization have shown considerable variability in residual volume in individuals measured on the same day.[53,54] In the elderly, Griffiths (1992) has reported that residual urine volume shows a diurnal variation, being as much as 40% larger in the morning compared with later in the day.[55] Thus, it is likely that single measurements of postvoid residual urine volume are of limited value.

More recently, Dunsmuir (1996) concluded that there is considerable variation in day-to-day measurements of PVR volume.[56] In this study the longer term test–retest reliability of PVR estimations was assessed by measurement of residual volume on six occasions over a 3-month period using abdominal ultrasound in men awaiting transurethral prostatectomy (TURP). Though one third of the men had residual volumes varying by <120 ml, two thirds had a variation between 150 and 670 ml!

RECOMMENDATIONS FOR MEASURING POSTVOID RESIDUAL URINE VOLUME

As a consequence of these studies the 4th International Consultation on BPH has recommended that several measurements of PVR volume should be made if the first measurement reveals a significant volume.[23]

WHAT IS 'NORMAL' POSTVOID RESIDUAL URINE VOLUME?

How should 'normal' postvoid residual volume be defined? 'Normality' can be expressed in absolute or relative terms. In absolute terms, Hinman (1967) defined normal PVR by postvoid catheterization in four 'normal' men (not defined) and found a mean PVR of 0.53 ml (range 0.09 to 2.24 ml).[57] Di Mare (1966) found that in 78% of 48 normal men (aged between 17 and 45) had residuals (measured by catheterization) less than 5 ml and 100% less than 12 ml.[58]

However, though Hinman and Di Mare have studied PVR in normal young individuals, exactly what represents an abnormal PVR in a healthy, aysmptomatic *elderly* man or woman is not clear. The presence of some residual urine volume in elderly individuals is common. Kolman (1999) measured PVR volume in 477 randomly selected men from Olmsted County, Minnesota aged between 40 and 79 years and with mild LUTS only.[59] PVR volume was highly skewed with a median value of 9.5 ml and 25th and 75th percentiles equal to 2.5 and 35.4 ml (the 95th centile was 141 ml). In regression analyses PVR volume was not related to age or Qmax.

In terms of what represents a normal PVR volume a specific value based on PVR volume in asymptomatic individuals may be of less clinical significance than a level of residual volume which has been shown to represent a threat to health or well-being. In theory, at least, residual urine can lead to urinary tract infection or back pressure on the kidneys resulting in hydronephrosis and renal failure. Rather than attempting to define a 'normal' postvoid residual urine volume in elderly men and women, the concept of a *safe* level of residual urine volume is probably clinically more useful as it will form the basis upon which decisions on treatment are made.

What volume of residual urine is safe? Abrams (1979)[36] and George (1983)[60] have identified a residual urine volume greater than 300 ml as a potential risk factor for upper tract dilatation and renal failure – the scenario of high pressure chronic retention. However, the proportion of elderly men and women in the general population having a PVR of > 300 ml and the proportion of these individuals who later develop hydronephrosis (and renal failure) is not known. Koch (1996) studied the results of ultrasound scanning, in relation to serum creatinine level, in 556 consecutive patients presenting with LUTS.[61] In those with a normal serum creatinine (less than 115 μmol/L), only four of 503 (0.8%) had pelvicalyceal dilatation on renal ultrasound. In those with a serum creatinine above 115 μmol/L renal dilatation was seen in 10 of 53 (19%). Koch concluded that serum creatinine was a good predictor of the presence of dilatation. Serum creatinine estimation might therefore be a more useful guide to the likelihood of upper tract dilatation. Koch suggested that renal ultrasound in men with LUTS thought to be due to benign prostatic enlargement is indicated only in patients with a serum creatinine above 130 μmol/L or with a creatinine of between 115 μmol/L and 130 μmol/L together with a postvoid residual urine volume of more than 150 ml.

CONSEQUENCES OF AN 'ABNORMAL' RESIDUAL VOLUME

The data available on the natural history of PVR suggest that residual volumes, even when moderately high, do not necessarily progress to higher residual volumes. In the placebo arm of a drug study, Witjes (1996)[62] has shown that residual urine volume actually *decreased* over a 6-month period from 48 to 34 ml. In a recently published study by Wasson (1995) in which over 500 men with moderate LUTS and a PVR < 350 ml were randomized to TURP or watchful waiting and followed over 3 years, most patients in the watchful waiting arm did not progress to TURP and did not show a rise in creatinine or of PVR.[63] Mean PVR volume was 113 ml in the watchful waiting group. Only eight of 276 (3%) in the watchful waiting group developed retention, 11 of 276 (4%) had a rise in residual (to > 350 ml) and only one of the 276 men developed a doubling over baseline of serum creatinine (compared with three of 280 in the TURP group). At 3 years of follow-up in the watchful waiting group mean PVR was 72 ml, a *decrease* of 41 ml from baseline. Qmax in the watchful waiting group *increased* from baseline by 0.4 ml/s. Wasson concluded that watchful waiting is a safe alternative for men with *moderate* LUTS. More recently, in a long-term follow-up study (mean follow-up 13 years) of men with voiding dysfunction and urodynamically proven BOO who had received no treatment, Thomas (1998) found no significant change in PVR (or indeed, of any other voiding parameter).[26]

In terms of the popular perception that elevated residual urine volumes predispose to urinary tract infection, Riehmann (1994) has recently reported that the presence of bacteriuria in 30 of 99 institutionalized men was not associated with residual urine volume (or for that matter age, previous diagnosis of BPH or LUTS).[64]

COMMENT

Until more data is available regarding the natural history of postvoid residual urine volume, a value of < 350 ml may represent a value above which individuals are at risk of upper tract dilatation. Whether residual urine volume represents a risk factor for development of urinary tract infections in men with LUTS remains to be established. Clearly long-term follow-up studies of the type published by Thomas (1998), with monitoring of serum creatinine and PVR, will be necessary to establish the progression, if any, of elevated residual urine volumes.[65]

MICTURITIONAL URETHRAL PRESSURE PROFILOMETRY (MUPP)

In this technique a triple lumen catheter which simultaneously measures bladder and urethral pressure is slowly withdrawn down the length of the urethra during micturition. The point of maximum pressure drop defines the site of maximum obstruction.[66,67] Good correlation between MUPP and BOO defined by Schäfer's linear PURR method and the Abrams–Griffiths nomogram (determined by conventional pressure–flow studies) has been shown in patients with LUTS.[68,69] This method is not widely used in the assessment of lower urinary tract function.

USE OF UROFLOWMETRY FOR DIAGNOSIS

The advantage of uroflowmetry as a diagnostic test for BOO lies in its ease of measurement and non-invasiveness.

A number of studies have investigated the relationship between Qmax and BOO. In 1271 men with LUTS who underwent both uroflowmetry and pressure–flow studies Reynard *et al.* (1988) found that Qmax was significantly lower in those with BOO (9.7 ml/s) than in those with no obstruction (12.6 ml/s).[15] The performance statistics for two thresholds of Qmax (10 and 15 ml/s)

Table 10.1 Performance statistics for two thresholds of Qmax (10 ml/s and 15 ml/s) for diagnosing bladder outlet obstruction

Threshold of Qmax	Specificity for BOO	Sensitivity for BOO	PPV for BOO	1-NPV
10 ml/s	70%	47%	70%	54%
15 ml/s	38%	82%	67%	42%

for BOO (defined as Schäfer category 3–6) are shown in Table 10.1.

About 60% of men in this series had BOO, so measurement of Qmax was able to achieve only a modest improvement in diagnostic power over no measurement at all. These findings are in broad agreement with those of other studies.

While generally speaking BOO is associated with low Qmax, low Qmax is not specific for BOO and high flow rates can occur in patients with obstruction. In a series of men with LUTS, Schäfer (1989) found that 25% were not obstructed.[70] Conversely, in Gerstenberg's series (1982),[71] 7% of men with a Qmax above 15 ml/s were obstructed by pressure–flow criteria and in Iversen's study (1983),[72] an even greater proportion (25%) of those with a Qmax above 15 ml/s had BOO. Clearly the fundamental problem in using uroflowmetry alone to diagnose BOO is its inability to distinguish low flow due to impaired detrusor contractility from that due to bladder outlet obstruction.[73]

Various attempts have been made to improve the diagnostic ability of uroflowmetry, in an attempt to avoid the need for pressure–flow studies. Schäfer has stated that 'the shape of the flow curve is often a more reliable indicator of obstruction than the peak flow and might even indicate the type and site of obstruction'.[74] As discussed above, inter-observer variability in the interpretation of uroflow traces is a potential limitation to diagnosis by analysis of flow pattern shape. Nonetheless, analysis of uroflow patterns by methods which are not subject to the vagaries of visual interpretation have been shown to improve the specificity and positive predictive value of uroflowmetry for BOO. In a series of men with LUTS the presence of terminal dribbling (a gradient from Qmax to the end of the flow of < 25%) or an intermittent flow pattern (stopping and starting of flow more than once) improved the positive predictive value of uroflowmetry for BOO to 88% and 92% respectively.[18,19] The presence of such flow patterns is easy to identify by simple visual inspection of the flow trace. No complex computer analysis is necessary.

Multiple flow studies increase the specificity and positive predictive value of Qmax for BOO.[20] For example, choosing a cut-off value of Qmax of 10 ml/s (a value below this indicating the presence of BOO), the specificity and PPV of Qmax for BOO were 71 and 79% respectively for a single flow study. However, a Qmax of less than 10 ml/s on all of four voids increased the specificity and PPV for BOO to 96 and 93%. The practical problems of obtaining this number of flows can be made easier by the establishment of a dedicated 'flow' clinic as discussed earlier. With such a system three or four flows can be obtained within as many hours. Time consuming though this might seem, by obviating the need for pressure–flow studies, multiple free flow studies have obvious potential for sparing the patient an unpleasant and invasive investigation, quite apart from their potential for financial savings.

In day-to-day practice, measurement of Qmax can provide a reasonable degree of accuracy for the diagnosis of BOO, particularly if more than one flow is obtained and if the flow pattern as well as the absolute values of Qmax are analysed. Depending on what cut-off value of Qmax is chosen a proportion of individuals with BOO who have a high Qmax will not be diagnosed correctly (as having BOO) and a proportion who have a low Qmax will be misdiagnosed as having BOO.

USE OF PRESSURE–FLOW STUDIES FOR DIAGNOSIS

It is generally agreed that pressure–flow studies are the best method of analysing voiding function quantitatively as they allow simultaneous recording of detrusor pressure and flow rate and so give the most complete description of voiding function in an individual.[37] Thus, they allow more precise diagnosis of pathophysiological conditions of the lower urinary tract. Their disadvantage lies in their invasiveness and expense. Their role in the diagnosis of BOO has been discussed above. Their place in predicting outcome of treatments for LUTS is discussed below.

USE OF POSTVOID RESIDUAL URINE VOLUME FOR DIAGNOSIS

An elevated residual urine volume has been regarded as a sign of BOO, but Abrams and Griffiths (1979)[36] found an elevated residual urine volume in 50% of men with no urodynamic evidence of outlet obstruction while others have reported an elevated residual volume to be a common finding in elderly women who have no BOO.[55]

Conversely, Griffiths and Castro (1970) found that 24% of patients in their series had a marked degree of obstruction, but had a PVR of less than 50 ml![75]

An elevated PVR probably more closely reflects diminished detrusor contractility (decreased detrusor reserve), of which BOO may be a cause, but not the only cause. Thus, a normal detrusor contraction at the start of micturition may fall before the end of micturition leaving residual urine in the bladder.[76] In elderly men and women without BOO Griffiths' work (1992) suggests that primary detrusor underactivity is the main factor leading to the development of residual urine.[55] Certainly bladder contractility has been shown to diminish with age in females,[77] and in males without BOO.[78]

Thus, residual urine should be regarded as a sign of detrusor hypocontractility rather than of BOO *per se*, though as stated above BOO may be an underlying cause of the residual urine if bladder contractility is sub-optimal. Evidence to support the association of detrusor hypocontractility with an elevated residual urine volume has recently been provided by Sullivan and Yalla (1996).[79] In a group of men with LUTS they measured potential detrusor reserve defined as maximum isometric contraction pressure minus maximum detrusor pressure during voiding. Potential detrusor reserve was significantly correlated with PVR volume, patients with a PVR of > 200 ml having a significantly lower detrusor reserve than those with smaller residual volumes.

USE OF UROFLOWMETRY FOR PREDICTING PROGNOSIS AND OUTCOME OF TREATMENT

A number of papers suggest that Qmax can predict out come of prostatectomy. Abrams (1977) found that treatment failures had a significantly higher preoperative Qmax (11.2 ml/s) than treatment successes (Qmax 8 ml/s).[80] In a further study Abrams (1979) again showed that Qmax could predict outcome.[81] The inclusion of Qmax in the preoperative assessment of these patients would have reduced the symptomatic failure rate from 28% to 12%. Similar results were reported by Jensen (1984) who found a favorable outcome after prostatectomy in 92% of patients with a flow rate <15 ml/s compared with only 71% in those with a preoperative flow rate of >15 ml/s.[82] Conversely, Dorflinger (1986) reported that men with a preoperative Qmax <7 ml/s did equally well after prostatectomy in terms of symptom reduction when compared with those with a flow rate >7 ml/s.[83] A more recent study supports this suggestion that Qmax cannot predict the likelihood of a favorable outcome after TURP. In the Department of Veterans Affairs randomized trial,[63] comparing TURP to watchful waiting in moderately symptomatic elderly men, Bruskewitz (1997) reported that no objective physiological parameter (Qmax or PVR estimation) made a clinically significant contribution towards predicting outcome.[84] Though men with a Qmax <10 ml/s did show a greater reduction in symptom score compared with those with a Qmax >15 ml/s (mean decrease 10.8 v. 8.6) and this difference was *statistically* significant, in *clinical* terms this represents a very small difference in symptom improvement between these two groups. Of more significance is the fact that the reduction in bother score did not differ between the low and high flow groups. There was no significant difference in failure rate between the low and high flow groups (failure being defined in various ways, but including worsening symptom score, new incontinence, or worsening PVR volume).

USE OF PRESSURE–FLOW STUDIES FOR PREDICTING PROGNOSIS AND OUTCOME OF TREATMENT

The ability of pressure–flow studies to predict the outcome of treatment for LUTS and BOO, particularly TURP, has been the subject of much debate over the last decade.

THE USE OF PRESSURE–FLOW STUDIES FOR PREDICTING THE OUTCOME OF TREATMENT WITH ALPHA BLOCKERS

The majority of men with LUTS thought to be due to BPO who opt for treatment rather than watchful waiting are managed initially by a trial of an alpha blocker and if these fail to adequately control their symptoms TURP or other invasive treatments such as TUMT are the next step in treatment. How useful are pressure–flow studies in predicting the response to alpha blockers? The published series suggest that there is an equivalent improvement in symptoms (and Qmax) irrespective of the presence or absence of urodynamically proven BOO (i.e. pressure–flow studies) in men receiving treatment with alpha blockers. Witjes (1996) found that both obstructed and non-obstructed men had equivalent improvement in symptoms and Qmax when treated with the alpha blocker terazosin.[62] Similarly in a study of men treated with doxazosin there was an almost identical decline in symptom scores in those with and those without urodynamic evidence of BOO.[85] Thus, urodynamic evaluation does not appear to be useful in predicting response to treatment with alpha blockers.

THE USE OF PRESSURE–FLOW STUDIES FOR PREDICTING THE OUTCOME OF TURP

Alpha blockers have little or no effect on Qmax or voiding pressure. Conversely, because TURP is designed specifically to relieve BOO and has been shown to be effective at doing so, one might expect that men with urodynamically proven BOO would be more likely to have a favorable symptomatic outcome after TURP than those with no BOO. This is an important issue since 20–30% of men have persistent, bothersome LUTS after TURP, and as a consequence urologists have been keen to find a preoperative test with predictive value for symptomatic outcome. Furthermore, if pressure–flow studies were able to identify those individuals unlikely to benefit from TURP substantial financial savings might result and potential morbidity associated with TURP might be avoided.

Abrams and Griffiths (1979) reported that obstructed men had a 93% chance of a favorable symptomatic outcome compared with only 78% of non-obstructed men.[36] Jensen (1989) reported a subjective improvement rate after prostatectomy of 78% in those without BOO compared with 93% in those with BOO.[86–87] In a smaller study Rollema and van Mastrigt (1992) reported the persistence of symptoms in 70% of unobstructed and 20% of obstructed patients.[39] In men selected for prostatectomy on the basis of symptoms and a Qmax <15 ml/s, Neal reported a poor outcome in 21% of those with BOO compared with 36% in those without BOO. However, most of those without obstruction did well and pressure–flow studies were unable to predict the likelihood of a poor outcome in *individual* cases.[88] More recently, Javlé (1998) has reported that urodynamic grading of BPO and detrusor contractility can reliably predict treatment outcome in individual cases.[89] Outcome was significantly better in men with unequivocal obstruction and normal detrusor contractility. About 80% of patients with equivocal obstruction and impaired detrusor contractility and all unobstructed patients had a poor symptomatic outcome from TURP. Pressure–flow analysis of voiding had a positive predictive value of 95% for predicting treatment outcome. In the context of urinary retention, Djavan (1997) found that those who failed to void after prostatectomy had a lower PdetQmax (24 v. 74 cmH_2O) compared with those who voided successfully.[90]

In contrast to these studies a number of reports suggest that preoperative pressure–flow studies are unable to predict outcome of prostatectomy.[91–94] Kaplan (1996) found that over the long term (12 years) in men with LUTS treated by prostatectomy the degree of symptomatic improvement and patient satisfaction did not correlate with pre-treatment urodynamic findings.[95]

Robertson (1993) measured detrusor contraction strength (the power factor or WF – derived from computerized analysis of pressure–flow traces) and reported that the presence of a weak detrusor is associated with persistence of LUTS after prostatectomy.[96] However, the overall subjective clinical outcome in individual patients was not strongly associated with WF. Romano (1998) has reported similar findings.[97]

Thus, there exist two polarized schools of thought with regard to the role of pressure–flow studies for predicting the outcome of TURP. While PFS probably do improve the prediction of outcome, the pressures on urodynamic services in most hospitals are such that most urologists do not use them in day-to-day practice.[98] It has been argued that the costs of performing pressure–flow studies in all patients being considered for TURP could be recouped by avoiding TURP in non-obstructed individuals.[99] However, most patients without BOO still have a good symptomatic outcome after TURP and it is debatable whether they should be denied the opportunity for symptom relief, when other treatments have failed, simply because they do not have urodynamic evidence of BOO.

THE USE OF PFS FOR PREDICTING THE OUTCOME OF TREATMENT WITH TUMT

Transurethral microwave thermotherapy (TUMT) offers a less invasive treatment for LUTS. For both low and high energy TUMT pressure–flow studies have been shown, at least in some studies, to be able to predict the chance of symptomatic improvement.

Though Tubaro (1995)[100] found that pressure–flow studies were not useful for predicting symptomatic outcome after low energy TUMT, Höfner (1998)[101] reported better symptomatic improvement after low energy TUMT (Prostatsoft version 2.0) in those with urodynamically confirmed BOO compared to those with no obstruction. Conversely, using the same low-energy TUMT system Walden (1998) found significantly better symptomatic improvement in patients with low to moderate obstruction compared with more marked obstruction and concluded that patients with a high obstruction index were probably unsuitable for TUMT (v 2.0).[102]

With the high energy, T3 Urologix thermotherapy device, Javlé (1996) reported that improvement in symptom score, flow rate and residual urine was significantly better in patients with marginal obstruction than in patients with unequivocal obstruction.[103] The presence of obstruction was also a determinant of improvement in Qmax and PdetQmax after HE-TUMT using Prostasoft version 2.5 (those with *higher* grades of obstruction – in contrast to Javle's study – being more likely to show an improvement in Qmax and PdetQmax), but it was not a determinant for improvement in symptoms (de la Rosette 1996).[104]

THE ROLE OF POSTVOID RESIDUAL URINE VOLUME FOR PREDICTING OUTCOME OF TREATMENT

Bruskewitz (1982) found that pre-operative residual volume was not related to a patient's subjective assessment of postoperative outcome (i.e. symptomatic outcome).[54] Though PVR volume estimation was useful to some extent for predicting outcome of men undergoing TURP in Jensen's study (1988) in that those men having a successful outcome were correctly identified, not one of the 14 patients who had an unsatisfactory outcome could be identified preoperatively.[86] More recently, in the Veterans Affairs trial of TURP versus watchful waiting Bruskewitz (1997) found that men with a PVR of 100 ml or less had no significant difference in symptom reduction after TURP compared with those with a PVR from 101–350 ml.[84] Somewhat surprisingly, despite the absence of any difference in symptom reduction, those men with lower PVR volumes had a significantly greater reduction in bother score!

While residual urine volume is of limited value for predicting outcome of TURP for symptoms, two recent studies have shown that in urinary retention, preoperative retention volume can predict postoperative ability to void. Djavan (1997) found that a retention volume >1500 ml was associated with failure to void or need for clean intermittent catheterization after prostatectomy.[90] In a review of 381 TURPs Reynard and Shearer (1999)[105] found that failure to void after catheter removal (usually removed 48 hours after operation) occurred in 10% of patients with acute retention (painful inability to void, retention volume <800 ml), 38% with chronic retention (maintenance of voiding, retention volume >500 ml) and in 44% with acute on chronic retention (painful retention, retention volume >800 ml). Ultimately, only 1% of patients were managed by long-term catheterization. This data is useful for warning patients undergoing TURP of the likelihood of temporary failure to void or of the potential need for long-term intermittent catheterization.

CONCLUSIONS

Voiding studies are used as diagnostic tests for men presenting with LUTS. Measurement of Qmax provides a simple, non-invasive means of investigating voiding function. While individual flow studies are of limited diagnostic value, multiple studies and analysis of uroflow patterns can improve the performance statistics of uroflowmetry for diagnosing BOO. Pressure–flow studies remain the most precise method for defining lower urinary tract function, but their invasive nature remains an obstacle for their widespread use. Residual urine volume estimation, by ultrasound, provides an indirect assessment of bladder function and may have an important role as a safety parameter.

While voiding studies are useful for diagnosing pathological conditions of the lower urinary tract, their ability to predict the outcome of treatment for these conditions is limited.[106] In the case of TURP this may be because the indications for this procedure have been broadened beyond the specific urodynamic condition of BOO. TURP is nowadays recognized as a treatment for LUTS, rather than specifically a treatment for LUTS due to BOO. We now know that there is at best a very weak relationship between LUTS and BOO. The absence of BOO in some patients with LUTS may explain why TURP does not always relieve their symptoms and why pressure–flow studies in such cases may have limited value for predicting outcome of treatment.

What then is the role of uroflowmetry, measurement of PVR volume or pressure–flow studies in predicting the outcome of TURP or other treatments for LUTS due to prostatic obstruction? In the case of TUMT pressure–flow studies do seem to be useful for predicting outcome. In general terms, uroflowmetry and PVR volume measurement are unable to accurately predict outcome of TURP. Opinions regarding the ability of pressure-flow studies to predict outcome of TURP are polarized. Some studies suggest that PFS can predict outcome while others suggest the opposite. In the United States the Agency for Health Care Policy and Research (McConnell 1994) has issued 'Clinical Practice Guidelines' stating that pressure–flow studies lack the ability to identify patients who will benefit from surgical treatment for LUTS and does not recommend their use in routine practice.[107,108] The Guidelines conclude that 'establishing a precise diagnosis is of minimal value if the information does not lead to a difference in clinical outcome.'[108] Conversely, in The 4th International Consultation on BPH the Urodynamics Sub-committee states that 'outcome from therapy is related to the pretreatment urodynamic findings, with obstructed patients faring better than those who are unobstructed' and 'performing preoperative urodynamics is cost effective, allowing treatment to be directed at those patients who are most likely to benefit.'[99] The members of the Urodynamics Sub-committee of The 4th International Consultation on BPH have stated that 'the clinician must decide, after proper consultation with the patient, whether the aims of therapy are to treat symptoms or to treat outlet obstruction.'[99]

There clearly exists a dichotomy of opinion regarding the use of voiding studies for predicting outcome of TURP. At the present time the role of voiding studies in the prediction of outcome of TURP remains an unresolved question.

The behavior of practising clinicians gives some idea of the perceived value of voiding studies for predicting outcome of various treatment modalities. In the United States the American Urological Association recently commissioned the Gallup Organization to conduct a study of urologists' practice patterns in the evaluation of men with LUTS thought to be due to BPH.[98] Of a random sample of 514 urologists who were questioned, 53% routinely used uroflowmetry, 71% routinely obtained an estimate of PVR volume, but only 11% of urologists routinely used PFS. This more than anything reflects the perception amongst urologists that PFS are of limited value in terms of predicting outcome from treatment and reflects the fact that many urologists regard pressure-flow studies as invasive and costly.

VOIDING STUDIES IN WOMEN

Voiding studies have a limited role to play in the assessment of women with LUTS since most symptoms in women relate to the storage phase (e.g. incontinence or 'irritative' symptoms occurring during bladder filling).[109] Intuitively, cystometry is likely to provide more information about the cause of storage symptoms than are voiding studies. Relatively few women complain of symptoms during the act of voiding. This may be because bladder outlet obstruction in women is relatively rare, with only 3–9% of women undergoing urodynamics for LUTS having BOO,[110–115] compared with approximately 60% of otherwise unselected men with LUTS.[15]

UROFLOWMETRY IN WOMEN

'NORMAL' QMAX IN WOMEN

Jorgensen (1996) states that 'in the normal uroflow in women Qmax reaches 20 to 36 ml',[116] but Qmax in women is volume dependent as shown by Drach (1979),[117] Gleason (1982)[118] and Haylen (1989),[5] and therefore normality can only be expressed along with voided volume. Haylen showed that women have a higher Qmax, for a given voided volume, than men.[5] In this study single flow recordings were obtained from 249 women volunteers who were deemed to be 'normal' on the basis of absence of both LUTS and any prior urological history. From this data set a nomogram – the 'Liverpool female nomogram' – relating voided volume to Qmax was obtained in centile form, giving a reference range for Qmax over a wide range of voided volumes.

Both Drach[117] and Haylen[5] noted that Qmax did not fall with increasing age – contrary to the decline in Qmax with age in men – though more recently Madersbacher (1998) reported a significant fall in Qmax with age in women, from a mean of 24 ml/s in those aged 40–50 years to 16 ml/s in those aged over 80.[110] However, this was interpreted as being due to a fall in voided volume with age along with reduced bladder contractility with the advancing years.

In terms of reproducibility of uroflowmetry in women, two flows performed over an interval of 2 months showed little variability in Qmax, the coefficient of variation between the two flows being only 18%.[119]

QMAX IN WOMEN WITH BOO

Massey and Abrams (1988) found a mean Qmax of 10 ml/s in 163 women with BOO.[115] This is comparable with Groutz's (2000)[112] study of Qmax in women with BOO (9 ml/s) and those with isolated sphincter weakness incontinence (25 ml/s) and also with Chassagne's study[120] comparing controls (mean Qmax 23 ml/s) with obstructed women (mean Qmax ~10 ml/s). Nitti (1999) also found significantly higher values for Qmax in unobstructed women (mean Qmax 20 ml/s) when compared with those with urodynamically confirmed BOO (mean Qmax 9 ml/s).[121]

Generally speaking, however, uroflowmetry is regarded as having insufficient diagnostic accuracy to be useful for the assessment of voiding dysfunction in women.[122] As in men Qmax cannot distinguish between BOO and impaired detrusor contractility and has not found widespread use in routine urological practice. Indeed, in a recent review of the investigation of women with LUTS (1997) Abrams made no reference to uroflowmetry amongst the various recommended tests.[123]

POSTVOID RESIDUAL URINE VOLUME MEASUREMENT IN WOMEN

NORMAL PVR VOLUME IN WOMEN

Whilst authors compare PVR volume in women with BOO and those with incontinence, it is difficult to find any studies that have measured PVR volume in asymptomatic women. What one can say is that women aged between 40 and 75 years with incontinence have a PVR volume ranging between 5 to 40 ml.[111,112,121] Madersbacher (1998) has recently reported that PVR volume in women increases slightly (by 4 ml per decade), as it does in men.[110]

THE RELATIONSHIP BETWEEN PVR VOLUME AND BOO IN WOMEN

Massey and Abrams reported an average PVR of 152 ml (range 10–440 ml) in women with BOO, though there was no comparison with age-matched, non-obstructed women.[115] Groutz (2000) noted a significant difference in PVR volume in women with BOO (86 ml) when compared with those with isolated sphincter weakness incontinence (40 ml).[112]

PRESSURE–FLOW STUDIES AND BOO IN WOMEN

There are no universally accepted urodynamic criteria for the diagnosis of BOO in women. Griffiths (1996)[124] has summarized the problem faced in the definition of obstruction in women – 'Although voiding pressure is elevated in women with genuine BOO, severe obstruction as seen in some men is very unusual and so the Abrams–Griffiths nomogram or the linPURR may not be the best methods of analysis. There currently is, however, little alternative to these or other methods designed for men'. Certainly, severe obstruction in women (or at least marked elevations in voiding pressures) are unusual in women, as shown by Chassagne's data (1998).[120] In this series PdetQmax ranged from 2.5 to 76 cmH_2O with a mean of approximately 45 cmH_2O and a mean Qmax of 10 ml/s – hardly the high voiding pressures and low flows seen in men with BOO.

The diagnosis of BOO in women relies on clinical suspicion – based on history and physical examiantion – supplemented by radiological and urodynamic investigations. There is no consensus on the urodynamic definition of obstruction in women.

URODYNAMIC DEFINITIONS OF BOO IN WOMEN

Farrar (1975) defined BOO in women principally on the basis of uroflowmetry, though bladder pressure was simultaneously measured.[114] A Qmax <15 ml/s with a voided volume of more than 200 ml was said to indicate the presence of BOO. Two populations of obstructed women were identified, those with a pressure > 50 cmH_2O and those with a pressure <50 cmH_2O. Clearly such a definition cannot distinguish low flow due to detrusor hypocontractility from that due to BOO. Massey and Abrams (1988) defined BOO as the presence of two or more of the following – a Qmax <12 ml/s, PdetQmax >50 cmH_2O, urethral resistance (P/F2) > 0.2 or the presence of 'significant' residual urine in association with a high voiding pressure.[115] Axelrod and Blaivas (1987)[125] and more recently Groutz (2000) defined bladder neck obstruction (one of several causes of BOO in women) as a sustained detrusor pressure of 20 cmH_2O or more with a Qmax of less than 12 ml/s, in the presence of radiographic evidence of obstruction at the bladder neck.[113]

Chassagne (1998) compared a group of control patients and patients with 'clinical' obstruction and derived receiver operating characteristic curves from a number of cut-off values for Qmax and PdetQmax.[120] Voiding cystography was used to confirm visually whether there was obstruction or not. The best combination of sensitivity (74%) and specificity (91%) was obtained using a cut-off value for Qmax of <15 ml/s and for PdetQmax of >20 cmH_2O. This value is comparable with the mean value for PdetQmax in Nitti's study (22 cmH_2O), which used a combination of radiographic and urodynamic criteria (see below) to define BOO.[121] While Chassagne concluded that 'the strict diagnosis of obstruction (in women) on the basis of pressure-flow cut-off values is not possible at the present time', the data does provide performance statistics for a number of cut-off values for pressure and flow (Table 10.2).[120]

Nitti (1999) used videourodynamics to define obstruction as 'radiographic evidence of obstruction between the bladder neck and distal urethra in the presence of a sustained detrusor contraction of any magnitude'.[121] This is usually associated with a low flow rate, though not always. The key features of this definition are *a focal* area of urethral narrowing in the presence of a *sustained* bladder contraction. Impaired detrusor contractility can be defined as an unsustained contraction or a contraction inadequate to produce a normal flow rate or complete bladder emptying in the absence of a visualized, focal area of obstruction in the urethra.

The use of videourodynamics to define obstruction rather than reliance on strict pressure and flow criteria overcomes the problem of categorizing cases in which an area of urethral narrowing during video screening can be clearly seen, but where voiding pressure and flow are normal. Webster (1975) concluded that women with obstruction show a greater degree of overlap of the parameters of flow and pressure, a suggestion supported by Nitti's data which show that Qmax and PdetQmax in obstructed and non-obstructed cases are similar.[126] In Nitti's study (1999) mean Qmax was 9 ml/s in obstructed and 20 ml/s in non-obstructed individuals, and PdetQmax was 43 cmH_2O in obstructed and 22 cmH_2O in non-obstructed individuals.[121] These small differences between obstructed and non-obstructed populations may reflect the fact that women have a much lower urethral resistance than men and that, as a consequence small degrees of obstruction may be enough to cause symptoms without at the same time resulting in a marked rise in voiding pressures.

The use of videourodynamics for the diagnosis of BOO in women has the added advantage of allowing identification of the numerous and varied causes of obstruction. These causes include previous anti-incontinence surgery, prolapse (cystocele, rectocele, uterine),

Table 10.2 Performance statistics for a variety of cut-off values for Qmax and PdetQmax (modified from Chassagne 1998)[122]

Threshold of Qmax (ml/s) and PdetQmax (cmH_2O)	Specificity for BOO	Sensitivity for BOO	PPV for BOO	NPV
Qmax ≤ 10, PdetQmax >10	94%	67%	75%	91%
Qmax ≤ 15, PdetQmax >20	91%	74%	70%	93%
Qmax ≤ 15, PdetQmax >15	83%	80%	57%	94%

dysfunctional voiding (a functional obstruction, with no demonstrable anatomical abnormality occurring in the neurologically normal), primary bladder neck obstruction, detrusor external sphincter dyssynergia, urethral stricture, and urethral diverticulum.

FINAL CONCLUSION

Contrary to the use of voiding studies in men, measurement of PVR volume and Qmax in women with LUTS are of limited value when compared with pressure–flow studies (in particular videocystourethrography). The latter clearly provides a more complete picture of lower urinary tract function. There is, at present, no agreement on the urodynamic definition of BOO in women, but given the greater number of causes of BOO in women it seems sensible to perform radiological screening simultaneously with measurement of voiding pressure and flow (i.e. videocystourethrography), to identify not only the presence of BOO, but also its cause.

REFERENCES

1. Drake WM. The uroflowmeter: an aid to the study of the lower urinary tract. *J Urol* 1948;**59**:650–8.
2. von Garrelts B. Analysis of micturition: a new method of recording the voiding of the bladder. *Acta Chir Scand* 1956;**112**:326–40.
3. van de Beek C, Stoevelaar HJ, McDonnell J, *et al.* Interpretation of uroflowmetry curves by urologists. *J Urol* 1997;**157**:164–8.
4. Siroky MB, Olsson CA, Krane RJ. The flow rate nomogram. I. Development. *J Urol* 1979;**122**:665–8.
5. Haylen BT, Ashby D, Sutherst JR, *et al.* Maximum and average flow rates in normal male and female populations – the Liverpool nomograms. *Br J Urol* 1989;**64**:30–38.
6. Kadow C, Howell S, Lewis P, *et al.* A flow rate nomogram for normal males over the age of 50. In: *Proceedings of the International Continence Society*, 15th Annual Meeting, London, 1985:138–9.
7. Riehmann M, Bayer WHB, Drinka PJ, *et al.* Position-related changes in voiding dynamics in men. *Urology* 1998;**52**:625–30.
8. Girman CJ, Panser LA, Chute CG, *et al.* Natural history of prostatism: urinary flow rates in a community-based study. *J Urol* 1993;**150**:887–92.
9. Jørgensen JB, Jensen KM-E, Bille-Brahe NE, *et al.* Uroflowmetry in asymptomatic elderly males. *Br J Urol* 1986;**58**:390–95.
10. Homma Y, Imajo C, Takahashi S, *et al.* Urinary symptoms and urodynamics in a normal elderly population. *Scand J Urol Nephrol* (Suppl.) 1994;**157**:27–30.
11. Drach GW, Layton TN, Binard WJ. Male peak urinary flow rate: relationship to volume voided and age. *J Urol* 1979;**122**:210–214.
12. Koyanagi T. Initial diagnostic evaluation of men with lower urinary tract symptoms. In: Denis L, Griffiths K, Khoury S, *et al.* (eds). *Proceedings of The 4th International Consultation on Benign Prostatic Hyperplasia.* Health Publication Ltd, 1998; p. 212.
13. Carter PG, Lewis P, Abrams P. Single versus multiple flows in the diagnosis of obstruction. *J Urol* 1991;**145**:397A.
14. Reynard J, Abrams P. Low volume uroflowmetry – useful or useless? *J Urol* 1996;**155**:394A.
15. Reynard JM, Yang Q, Donovan JL, *et al.* The ICS-'BPH' Study: uroflowmetry, lower urinary tract symptoms and bladder outlet obstruction. *Br J Urol* 1998;**82**:619–23.
16. Grino PB, Bruskewitz R, Blaivas JG, *et al.* Maximum urinary flow rate by uroflowmetry: automatic or visual interpretation. *J Urol* 1993;**149**:339–41.
17. Witjes WPJ, de la Rosette JJMCH, Zerbib M, *et al.* Computerised artifact detection and correction of uroflow curves: towards more consistent quantitative assessment of maximum flow. *Eur Urol* 1998;**33**:54–63.
18. Reynard J, Lim C, Abrams P. The significance of intermittency in men with lower urinary tract symptoms. *Urology* 1996;**47**:491–6.
19. Reynard J, Lim C, Peters T, *et al.* The significance of terminal dribbling in men with lower urinary tract symptoms. *Br J Urol* 1996;**77**:705–10.
20. Reynard J, Lim C, Peters T, *et al.* The value of multiple free-flow studies in men with BPH. *Br J Urol* 1996;**77**:813–18.
21. Barry MJ, Girman CJ, O'Leary MP, *et al.* The Benign Prostatic Hyperplasia Treatment Outcomes Study Group: using repeated measures of symptom score, uroflowmetry and prostate specific antigen in the clinical management of prostate disease. *J Urol* 1995;**153**:99–103.
22. Jepsen JV, Leverson G, Bruskewitz RC. Variability in urinary flow rate and prostate volume: an investigation using the placebo arm of a drug trial. *J Urol* 1998;**160**:1689–94.
23. Koyanagi T. Initial diagnostic evaluation of men with lower urinary tract symptoms. In: Denis L, Griffiths K, Khoury S, *et al.* (eds). Health Publication Ltd, *Proceedings of The 4th International Consultation on Benign Prostatic Hyperplasia*, 1998, p. 205.
24. de la Rosette JJMCH, Witjes WP, Debruyne FMJ. Improved reliability of uroflowmetry investigations: results of a portable home-based uroflowmetry study. *Br J Urol* 1996;**78**:385–90.
25. Golomb J, Linder A, Siegel Y, *et al.* Variability and circadian changes in home uroflowmetry in patients with benign prostatic hyperplasia compared to normal controls. *J Urol* 1992;**147**:1044–7.
26. Thomas AW, Abrams P. A comparison of home-based uroflowmetry and post-void residual values with outpatient flow clinic assessment. *Neurourol Urodyn* 1998;**17**:69–70.
27. Walker RMH, Di Pasquale B, Hubregtse M, *et al.* Pressure–flow studies in the diagnosis of bladder outlet obstruction: a study comparing suprapubic and transurethral techniques. *Br J Urol* 1997;**79**:693–7.
28. Reynard JM, Lim C, Swami S, Abrams P. The obstructive effect of a urethral catheter. *J Urol* 1996;**155**:901–903.
29. Neal DE, Rao CVS, Styles RA, *et al.* Effects of catheter size on urodynamics in men undergoing elective prostatectomy. *Br J Urol* 1987;**60**:64–8.
30. Walker RMH, Patel A, St Clair Carter S. Is there a clinically significant change in pressure–flow study values after ure-

thral instrumentation in patients with lower urinary tract symptoms? *Br J Urol* 1998;**81**:206–10.
31. van de Beek C, Rollema HJ, van Mastrigt R, *et al.* Objective analysis of intravesical obstruction and detrusor contractility; appraisal of the computer program Dx/CLIM and Schäfer nomogram. *Neurourol Urodyn* 1992;**11**:394–5.
32. Tan HK, Höfner K, Krah H, *et al.* Reporducibility of pressure–flow analysis in the diagnosis of BPH-obstruction. *J Urol* 1995;**153**:452A.
33. Rosier PFWM, de la Rosette JJMCM, Koldewijn EL, *et al.* Variability of pressure–flow analysis parameters in repeated cystometry in patients with benign prostatic hyperplasia. *J Urol* 1995;**153**:1520–25.
34. Hansen F, Olsen L, Atan A, *et al.* Pressure–flow studies, an evaluation of within testing reproducibility – validity of the measured parameters. *Neurourol Urodyn* 1997;**16**:521–32.
35. Witjes WPJ, de Wildt MJAM, Rosier PFWM, *et al.* Variability of clinical and pressure flow study variables after 6 months of watchful waiting in patients with lower urinary tract symptoms and benign prostatic enlargement. *J Urol* 1996;**156**:1026–34.
36. Abrams P, Griffiths DJ. The assessment of prostatic obstruction from urodynamic measurements and residual urine. *Br J Urol* 1979;**51**:129–34.
37. Griffiths D, Höfner K, van Mastrigt R *et al.* Standardisation of terminology of lower urinary tract function: pressure–flow studies of voiding, urethral resistance and urethral obstruction. *Neurourol Urodyn* 1997;**16**:1–18.
38. Schäfer W. Analysis of bladder-outlet function with the linearised passive urethral resistance relation, linPURR, and a disease-specific approach for grading obstruction: from complex to simple. *World J Urol* 1995;**13**:47–58.
39. Rollema HJ, van Mastrigt R. Improved indication and follow-up in transurethral resection of the prostate using the computer program CLIM: a prospective study. *J Urol* 1992;**148**:111–16.
40. Höfner K, Kramer AE, Tan HK, *et al.* CHESS classification of bladder-outflow obstruction. A consequence in the discussion of current concepts. *World J Urol* 1995;**13**:59–64.
41. Kranse M, van Mastrigt R. The derivation of an obstruction index from a three parameter model fitted to the lower part of the pressure flow plot. *J Urol* 1991;**145**:261A.
42. Spångberg A, Terio H, Ask P, *et al.* Pressure/flow studies preoperatively and postoperatively in patients with BPH: estimation of the urethra pressure/flow relation and urethral elasticity. *Neurourol Urodyn* 1991;**10**:139–67.
43. Schäfer W. A new concept for simple but specific grading of bladder outflow conditions independent from detrusor function. *J Urol* 1993;**149**:356A.
44. Lim CS, Reynard J, Cannon A, Abrams PH. The Abrams–Griffiths number: a simple way to quantify bladder outlet obstruction. *Neurourol Urodyn* 1994;**13**:475–6.
45. Ding YY, Lieu PK. Comparison of three methods of quantifying urethral resistance in men. *Urology* 1998;**52**:858–62.
46. Lim CS, Abrams P. The Abrams–Griffiths nomogram. *World J Urol* 1995;**13**:59–64.
47. Abrams P, Blaivas JG, Stanton SL, *et al.* Standardization of terminology of lower urinary tract function. *Neurourol Urodyn* 1988;**7**:403–427.
48. Rosier PFWM, de Wildt MJAM, de la Rosette JJMCH, *et al.* Analysis of maximum detrusor contraction power in relation to bladder emptying in patients with lower urinary tract symptoms and benign prostatic enlargement. *J Urol* 1995;**154**:2137–42.
49. Stoller ML, Millard RJ. The accuracy of a catheterized residual urine. *J Urol* 1989;**141**:15–16.
50. Bretland PM. Relationship of bladder shadow to bladder volume on excretion urography. *J Fac Radiol* 1958;**9**:152–3.
51. Dadfar H, Zinsser HH. Bladder volumes from cystogram films. *Invest Urol* 1972;**9**:363–4.
52. Roehrborn CG, Peters PC. Can transabdominal ultrasound estimation of post-void residual (PVR) replace catheterisation? *Urology* 1988;**31**:445–9.
53. Birch NC, Hurst G, Doyle PT. Serial residual volumes in men with prostatic hypertrophy. *Br J Urol* 1988;**62**:571–5.
54. Bruskewitz RC, Iversen P, Madsen PO. Value of post-void residual urine determination in evaluation of prostatism. *Urology* 1982;**20**:602–4.
55. Griffiths DJ, McCracken PN, Harrison GM, *et al.* Characteristics of urinary incontinence in elderly patients studies by 24-hour monitoring and urodynamic testing. *Age Ageing* 1992;**21**:195–201.
56. Dunsmuir WD, Feneley M, Corry DA, *et al.* The day-to-day variation (test–retest reliability) of residual urine measurement. *Br J Urol* 1996;**77**:192–93.
57. Hinman F, Cox CE. Residual urine volume in normal male subjects. *J Urol* 1967;**97**:641–5.
58. Di Mare JR, Fish S, Harper JM, *et al.* Residual urine in normal male subjects. *J Urol* 1966;**96**:180–81.
59. Kolman C, Girman CJ, Jacobsen SJ, Lieber MM. Distribution of post-void residual urine volume in randomly selected men. *J Urol* 1999;**161**:122–7.
60. George NJR, O'Reilly PH, Barnard RJ, *et al.* High pressure chronic retention. *Br Med J* 1983;**286**:1780–83.
61. Koch WFRM, El Din KE, de Wildt MJAM, *et al.* The outcome of renal ultrasound in the assessment of 556 consecutive patients with benign prostatic hyperplasia. *J Urol* 1996;**155**:186–9.
62. Witjes WPJ, Rosier PFWM, de Wildt JAM, *et al.* Urodynamic and clinical effects of terazosin therapy in patients with symptomatic benign prostatic hyperplasia. *J Urol* 1996;**155**:1317–23.
63. Wasson JH, Reda DJ, Bruskewitz RC, *et al.* A comparison of transurethral surgery with watchful waiting for moderate symptoms of benign prostatic hyperplasia. The Veterans Affairs Cooperative Study Group on Transurethral Resection of the Prostate. *N Engl J Med* 1995;**332**:75–9.
64. Riehmann M, Goetzman B, Langer E, *et al.* Risk factors for bacteriuria in men. *Urology* 1994;**43**:617–20.
65. Thomas AW, Cannon A, Bartlett E, *et al.* The natural history of voiding dysfunction in the male: the long term follow up of detrusor underactivity. *Neurourol Urodyn* 1998;**17**:366–7.
66. Yalla SV, Blute R, Bedford Waters W, *et al.* Urodynamic evaluation of prostatic enlargement with micturitional vesicourethral static pressure profiles. *J Urol* 1981;**125**:685–9.

67. Valla SV, Blute R, Snyder H, *et al.* Urodynamic localisation of isolated bladder neck obstruction in men: studies with micturitional vesicourethral static pressure profile. *J Urol* 1981;**125**:677–84.
68. Desmond AD, Ramaya GR. Comparison of pressure/flow studies with micturitional urethral pressure profiles in the diagnosis of urinary outflow obstruction. *Br J Urol* 1988;**61**:224-9.
69. Du Beau CE, Sullivan MP, *et al.* Correlation between micturitional urethral pressure profile and pressure–flow criteria in bladder outlet obstruction. *J Urol* 1995;**154**:498–503.
70. Schäfer W, Rubben H, Noppeney R, *et al.* Obstructed and unobstructed 'prostatic obstruction': a plea for objectivation of bladder outflow obstruction by urodynamics. *World J Urol* 1989;**6**:198–203.
71. Gerstenberg TC, Anderson JT, Klarskov P, *et al.* High flow infravesical obstruction in the male. *J Urol* 1982;**127**:943–5.
72. Iversen P, Bruskewitz RC, Jensen KM-E, *et al.* Transurethral prostatic resection in the treatment of prostatism with high urinary flow. *J Urol* 1983;**129**:995–7.
73. Chancellor MB, Blaivas JG, Kaplan SA, *et al.* Bladder outlet obstruction versus impaired detrusor contractility: the role of uroflow. *J Urol* 1991;**145**:810–12.
74. Schäfer W. Urethral resistance? Urodynamic concepts of physiological and pathological bladder outlet function during voiding. *Neurourol Urodyn* 1985;**4**:161–201.
75. Griffiths HJ, Castro J. An evaluation of the importance of residual urine. *Br J Radiol* 1970;**43**:409–413.
76. Rosier PFWM, de Wildt MJAM, Wijkstra H *et al.* Residual urine and the correlation with detrusor contractility in bladder outlet obstruction in symptomatic BPH. *J Urol* 1995;153 (Suppl.):452A.
77. Griffiths D, Constantinou CE, van Mastrigt R. Urinary bladder function and its control in normal females. *Am J Physiol* 1986;**251**:225–30.
78. van Mastrigt R. Age dependence of urinary bladder contractility. *Neurourol Urodyn* 1992;**11**:315–17.
79. Sullivan MP, Yalla SV. Detrusor contractility and compliance characteristics in adult male patients with obstructive and nonobstructive voiding dysfunction. *J Urol* 1996;**155**:1995–2000.
80. Abrams PH. Prostatism and prostatectomy: the value of urine flow rate measurement in the preoperative assessment for operation. *J Urol* 1977;**117**:70–1.
81. Abrams PH, Farrar DJ, Tumer-Warwick RT, *et al.* The results of prostatectomy: a symptomatic and urodynamic analysis of 152 patients. *J Urol* 1979;**121**:640–42.
82. Jensen KM-E, Bruskewitz RC, Iversen P, *et al.* Spontaneous uroflowmetry in prostatism. *Urology* 1984;**24**:403–9.
83. Dorflinger T, Bruskewitz RC, Jensen KME, *et al.* Predictive value of low maximum flow rate in benign prostatic hyperplasia. *Urology* 1986;**27**:569–73.
84. Bruskewitz RC, Reda DJ, Wasson JH, *et al.* Testing to predict outcome after transurethral resection of the prostate. *J Urol* 1997;**157**:1304–8.
85. Gerber GS, Kim JH, Contreras BA, *et al.* An observational urodynamic evaluation of men with lower urinary tract symptoms treated with doxazosin. *Urology* 1996;**47**:840–44.
86. Jensen KM-E, Jorgensen JB, Mogensen P. Urodynamics in prostatism. I. Prognostic value of medium-fill water cystometry; and II. Prognostic value of pressure/flow study combined with stop-flow test. *Scand J Urol Nephrol* 1988;(Suppl.) **114**:72–77 & 78–83.
87. Jensen KM-E, Jorgensen JB, Mogensen P. Long-term predictive role of urodynamics: an 8 year follow-up of prostatic surgery for lower urinary tract symptoms. *Br J Urol* 1996;**78**:213–18.
88. Neal DE, Ramsden PD, Sharples L, *et al.* Outcome of elective prostatectomy. *Br Med J* 1989;**299**:762–7.
89. Javlé P, Jenkins SA, Machin DG, *et al.* Grading of benign prostatic obstruction can predict the outcome of transurethral prostatectomy. *J Urol* 1998;**160**:1713–17.
90. Djavan B, Madersbacher S, Klingler C, *et al.* Urodynamic assessment of patients with acute urinary retention: is treatment failure after prostatectomy predictable? *J Urol* 1997;**158**:1829–33.
91. Bruskewitz R, Jensen KM-E, Iversen P, Madsen PO. The relevance of minimum urethral resistance in prostatism. *J Urol* 1983;**129**:769–71.
92. Jensen KM-E, Bruskewitz RC, Iversen P, *et al.* Predictive value of voiding pressures in benign prostatic hyperplasia. *Neurourol Urodyn* 1983;**2**:117–25.
93. Frimodt-Moller PC, Jensen KME, Iversen P, *et al.* Analysis of presenting symptoms in prostatism. *J Urol* 1984;**132**:272–6.
94. Bruskewitz RC, Larsen EH, Madsen PO, *et al.* 3-year follow-up of urinary symptoms after transurethral resection of the prostate. *J Urol* 1986;**136**:613–15.
95. Kaplan SA, Bowers DL, Te AE, *et al.* Differential diagnosis of prostatism: a 12-year retrospective analysis of symptoms, urodynamics and satisfaction with therapy. *J Urol* 1996;**155**:1303–1308.
96. Robertson AS, Airey R, Griffiths CJ, *et al.* Detrusor contraction strength in men undergoing prostatectomy. *Neurourol Urodyn* 1993;**12**:109–122.
97. Romano G, Carter S, Vicentini AC, *et al.* Clinical outcome of prostate surgery in patients with low detrusor contractility. *Neurourol Urodyn* 1998;**17**:396–97.
98. Gee WF, Holtgrewe HL, Albertsen PC, *et al.* Practice trends in the diagnosis and management of benign prostatic hyperplasia in the United States. *J Urol* 1995;**154**:205–206.
99. Abrams P. The urodynamic assessment of lower urinary tract symptoms. In: Denis L, Griffiths K, Khoury S, *et al.* (eds). *Proceedings of The 4th International Consultation on Benign Prostatic Hyperplasia.* Health Publication Ltd, 1998, 323–77.
100. Tubaro A, Carter S St, del a Rosette J, *et al.* The prediction of clinical outcome from transurethral microwave thermotherapy by pressure-flow analysis. A European multicentre study. *J Urol* 1995;**153**:1526–30.
101. Höfner K, Tubaro A, de la Rosette JJ, *et al.* Analysis of outcome after thermotherapy using different classifications of bladder outlet obstruction. *Neurourol Urodyn* 1998;**17**:109–120.
102. Walden M, Dahlstrand C, Schafer W, *et al.* How to select

patients suitable for transurethral microwave thermotherapy: a systematic evaluation of potentially predictive variables. *Br J Urol* 1998;**81**:817–22.

103. Javlé P, Blair M, Palmer M, *et al.* The role of an advanced thermotherapy device in prostatic voiding dysfunction. *Br J Urol* 1996;**78**:391–7.
104. de la Rosette JJ, de Wildt MJ, Hofner K, Carter SS, Debruyne FM, Tubaro A. Pressure-flow study analyses in patients treated with high energy thermotherapy. *J Uro.* 1996 Oct;**156**:1428-33.
105. Reynard JM, Shearer RJ. Failure to void after transurethral resection of the prostate and mode of presentation. *Urology* 1999;**53**:336–9.
106. Gerber GS. The role of urodynamic study in the evaluation and management of men with lower urinary tract symptoms secondary to benign prostatic hyperplasia. *Urology* 1996 Nov;**48**:668–75.
107. McConnell JD. Why pressure-flow studies should be optional and not mandatory studies for evaluating men with benign prostatic hyperplasia. *Urology* 1994;**44**:156–8.
108. McConnell JD, Barry MJ, Bruskewitz RC, *et al. Benign prostatic hyperplasia: diagnosis and treatment.* Rockville, Maryland: Agency for Health Care Policy and Research, Public Health Service, US Department of Health and Human Services, 1994.
109. Jackson S, Donovan J, Brookes S, *et al.* The Bristol female lower urianry tract symptoms questionnaire: development and psychometric testing. *Br J Urol* 1996;**77**:805–812.
110. Madersbascher S, Pycha A, Schatzl G, *et al.* The aging lower urinary tract: a comparative urodynamic study of men and women. *Urology* 1998;**51**:206–12.
111. Madersbascher S, Pycha A, Klingler CH, *et al.* The International Prostate Symptom Score in both sexes: a urodynamics-based comparison. *Neurourol Urodyn* 1999;**18**:173.
112. Groutz A, Blaivas JG, Fait G, *et al.* The significance of the American Urological Association symptom index in the evaluation of women with bladder outlet obstruction. *J Urol* 2000;**163**:207–211.
113. Rees DL, Whitfield HN, Islam AK, *et al.* Urodynamic findings in adult females with frequency and dysuria. *Br J Urol* 1975;**47**:853–60.
114. Farrar DJ, Osborne JL, Stephenson TP, *et al.* A urodynamic view of bladder outflow obstruction in the female: factors influencing the results of treatment. *Br J Urol* 1975;**47**:815–22.
115. Massey JA, Abrams PH. Obstructed voiding in the female. *Br J Urol* 1988;**61**:36–9.
116. Jorgensen JB, Jensen K-ME. Uroflowmetry. *Urol Clin N Am* 1996;**23**:237–42.
117. Drach GW, Ignatoff J, Layton T. Peak urinary flow rate: observations in female subjects and comparison to male subjects. *J Urol* 1979;**122**:215–19.
118. Gleason DM, Bottacini MR. Urodynamic norms in female voiding. II. The flow modulating zone and voiding dysfunction. *J Urol* 1982;**127**:495.
119. Sorensen S. Urodynamic investigations and their reproductibility in healthy postmenopausal females. *Scand J Urol Nephrol* 1988;**114**:(Suppl.)42–7.
120. Chassagne S, Bernier PA, Haab F, *et al.* Proposed cutoff values to define bladder outlet obstruction in women. *Urology* 1998;**51**:408–411.
121. Nitti VW, Mai Tu L, Gitlin J. Diagnosing bladder outlet obstruction in women. *J Urol* 1999;**161**:1535–40.
122. Carr LK, Webster GD. Bladder outlet obstruction in women. *Urol Clin N Am* 1996;**23**:385–91.
123. Abrams P. Lower urinary tract symptoms in women: who to investigate and how. *Br J Urol* 1997;**80** 1:43–8.
124. Griffiths DJ. Pressure flow studies of micturition. *Urol Clin N Am* 1996;**23**:279–97.
125. Axelrod SL, Blaivas JG. Bladder neck obstruction in women. *J Urol* 1987;**137**:497–9.
126. Webster JR. Combined video/pressure/flow cystourethrography in female patients with voiding disturbances. *Urology* 1975;**5**:209.
127. Reynard J, Abrams P. Clinical Evaluation of Bladder Outflow Obstruction. Textbook of Genitourinary Surgery, Blackwell. Science 1998, Eds HN Whitfield, WF Hendry, RS Kirby, JW Duckett, p480–496.

Chapter 11

Imaging of the bladder and urethra

Johnathan Sullivan, Paul Abrams

INTRODUCTION

Imaging of the urinary tract dates back to the development of radiography and the advent of modern cystoscopy at the end of the 19th century. The introduction of contrast media led to more comprehensive visualization of the bladder and urethra and the possibility of dynamic studies of the function of the lower urinary tract such as voiding cystourethrography. In the early 1950s cinefluoroscopy of the bladder stimulated a new understanding of the function of the lower urinary tract. Imaging of the bladder and urethra was later combined with measurement of pressure,[1,2] leading to the development of videourodynamics, which has rapidly become the central imaging investigation in the assessment of lower urinary tract dysfunction.

In the last three decades imaging has been revolutionized by the introduction of powerful new imaging modalities, particularly ultrasound (US), computed tomography (CT) and magnetic resonance imaging (MRI). The imaging of the pelvic floor is one of the last areas to be affected by this revolution, so that most of the research into the application of these new modalities to pelvic floor dysfunction has only taken place in the last few years. These newer imaging techniques are extending investigation to structures that have previously been inaccessible, such as the pelvic floor and the urethral sphincter, and providing a much wider range of dynamic imaging than previously available.

The investigation of incontinence has historically been limited to the measurement of pressure and the study of the position of various landmarks at rest and during dynamic maneuvers. Modern imaging techniques allow us to investigate the deep anatomical structure of the pelvis in a way that was previously impossible. Rather than working backwards from symptoms to try to deduce the anatomical cause of dysfunction, we can now study the incidence of anatomical defects and try to discover which individuals become symptomatic, and why. The new modalities of pelvic imaging therefore have the potential to bring about a major shift in our understanding and treatment of stress incontinence and genitourinary prolapse.

Since incontinence and other forms of dysfunction are multifactorial, anatomical studies will remain only one part of the investigation of pelvic floor dysfunction. The newer modalities of lower urinary tract imaging have not yet secured a place in the standard, routine assessment of pelvic floor dysfunction or incontinence, but there is no doubt that as research tools they are rapidly increasing our understanding of the mechanisms of dysfunction in these patients. This chapter reviews the imaging techniques currently available and attempts to clarify their position in the evaluation of patients with pelvic floor dysfunction and/or urinary incontinence. A detailed discussion of the role of imaging in the investigation of incontinence is available in the report of the 1st International Consultation on Incontinence.[3]

PLAIN RADIOGRAPHY

Plain abdominal radiography is of limited value in the evaluation of incontinence because it normally provides no information on the soft tissues of the pelvis, and cannot demonstrate urinary incontinence. A standard view covering the kidneys, ureters and bladder (KUB) is normally of use only for the identification of urinary tract stones. Excluding bladder stones as a cause of lower urinary tract symptoms may be useful in a small minority of patients, for example those where bladder outlet obstruction is suspected or those at high risk of stones (e.g. patients with previous enterocystoplasty). As other modalities such as ultrasound are able to demonstrate bladder stones, plain radiography is not normally indicated. In the presence of a history of hematuria or a past history of urinary tract stones plain abdominal radiography (in conjunction with upper urinary tract US) may be indicated.

INTRAVENOUS UROGRAPHY

Intravenous urography (IVU) does not generally yield useful information on the bladder or urethra with regard to pelvic floor function or incontinence. However, when extraurethral urinary incontinence due to ectopic ureter is suspected IVU is the first, and often the only, investigation required.[4] Delayed films and tomography are sometimes useful as the renal moiety associated with ureteric ectopia is often poorly functioning. If ureteric ectopia is still suspected as the likely cause of incontinence after a negative IVU, other imaging modalities may be useful, for example CT.[5]

IVU is also useful for the detection of ureterovaginal fistulae, which are typically related to pelvic surgery.[6] IVU or other forms of upper tract imaging are not routinely indicated in the evaluation of incontinence, but they may be very useful in evaluating and monitoring evidence of upper urinary tract damage in patients with incontinence related to neurogenic lower urinary tract dysfunction.[3]

CYSTOURETHROSCOPY

Historically, lower urinary tract endoscopy has been considered to be a useful part of the evaluation of incontinence by a number of authors, but the evidence suggests that it has a poor sensitivity and specificity in identifying defects of bladder support or intrinsic sphincter deficiency.[3] Cystoscopy may be used to observe the ability of the urethral sphincter to close, or to evaluate hypermobility or urethral closure dynamically during straining. However, cystourethroscopy identified only a small proportion of patients with maximum urethral closure pressure < 20 cmH_2O (indicative of intrinsic sphincter deficiency) in a study by Horbach and Ostergard.[7] Similarly Govier *et al.* found that cystourethroscopy underestimated the degree of sphincter deficiency in a high proportion of women when compared to grading by videourodynamic appearances.[8]

Cystourethroscopy is also not necessary for the routine evaluation of symptoms of stress and/or urge incontinence, as it has usually been found to have a low yield of abnormal findings which generally do not influence patient management.[3] However, where there is evidence of microscopic hematuria in conjunction with storage symptoms such as urge incontinence, cystourethroscopy should be performed as a routine investigation. Lower urinary tract endoscopy may also be useful in the evaluation of patients with extraurethral incontinence due, for example, to ureteral ectopia or vesicovaginal fistula.

CYSTOURETHROGRAPHY

Voiding cystourethrography (VCUG) is the simplest dynamic contrast radiological technique for the evaluation of lower urinary tract function. A technique using lateral projection was introduced by Mikulicz-Radecki as long ago as 1931.[9] Visualization of the urethrovesical junction is improved by the introduction of a bead chain into the urethra (lateral bead chain cystourethrography) and the addition of vaginal contrast (colpocystourethrography) helps in the delineation of the anatomy of the bladder base. VCUG provides images of many anatomical features such as the bladder shape and outline, and may demonstrate pathological features such as vesicoureteric reflux, bladder and urethral diverticula, urethral narrowing in bladder outlet obstruction and so on. The female bladder base is normally flat, sloping upwards and posteriorly with the internal urethral orifice located just above a line running horizontally from the lower border of the symphysis pubis, between the anterior and middle thirds of the bladder base. The urethra is normally straight, running downwards and forwards from the base of the bladder, and the vagina runs at the same angle around 1.5 cm posterior to the urethra.[3]

Defects of bladder support may be assessed by the measurement of various angles and distances from the films obtained. Parameters described include the posterior urethrovesical angle (the angle between a line drawn along the trigone and a line drawn along the axis of the urethra), and the symphysis-orifice (SO) distance (between the inferior border of the symphysis pubis and the internal urethral orifice). Funneling of the proximal urethra, flatness of the bladder base, and the position of the lowest part of the bladder base may all be assessed on films obtained during straining.

The principal advantages and disadvantages of cystourethrography are set out in Table 11.2. The reproducibility of cystourethrography is in the same region as that for other radiological examinations. There is general agreement that neither lateral bead chain cystourethrography nor voiding colpocystourethrography can discriminate between continence and stress incontinence, and it is not possible to distinguish patients with good or bad surgical outcomes on the basis of these tests.[3] The recent 1st International Consultation on Incontinence stated that cystourethrography 'cannot be recommended for the diagnosis or classification of incontinence'.[3]

Comparisons of cystourethrography and ultrasonography have shown good agreement between the findings of the tests,[10–12] with most authors in favor of ultrasound as the preferred method. Since ultrasound of the bladder base is apparently more or less equivalent to cystourethrography in measurement accuracy but does not require ionizing radiation, introduction of contrast medium, or access to a radiology department, cystourethrography is likely to diminish in importance in future. In neurological patients, where there is an increased incidence of pathology such as vesicoureteric reflux and bladder diverticula which may not be easily identified on ultrasound, cystourethrography will remain a useful investigation.

In centers where videourodynamics are not available cystourethrography may be useful, particularly if access to ultrasonography is limited. However, while it is possible to identify incontinence during cystourethrography, it is not possible to accurately differentiate between detrusor instability and genuine stress incontinence without information on detrusor pressure. If imaging of the bladder base and urethra is considered important for an individual patient, videourodynamics is probably the best single test available, because it combines both pressure measurement and imaging.

VIDEOURODYNAMICS

The introduction of synchronized lower urinary tract imaging and pressure measurement in the 1960s[1] provided a new method to investigate the structure and dynamics of bladder and urethral dysfunction. This method has subsequently developed into the modern technique of videourodynamics (VUDS). The role of VUDS in the routine investigation of incontinence is debatable, but there is no doubt that it is the investigation of choice in the more complex cases of lower urinary tract dysfunction, for example patients with probable neurogenic lower urinary tract dysfunction or those with persisting symptoms after incontinence surgery. Videourodynamics provides imaging of the anatomy of the lower urinary tract at rest, and also provides information on dynamic behavior during coughing, straining and voiding. The information which can be obtained includes:

- **During filling**: pressure changes due to detrusor overactivity or poor bladder compliance.
- **Full, at rest**: bladder capacity, shape and outline (diverticula, trabeculation, bladder neck opening), vesicoureteric reflux at rest.
- **Full, coughing or straining**: assessment of bladder base descent and bladder neck competence (see Fig. 11.1), diagnosis of genuine stress incontinence (see Fig. 11.2).
- **During voiding**: extent and speed of bladder neck opening, caliber of urethra, sites of obstruction or dilatation, urethral diverticula, vesicoureteric reflux.
- **'Stop Test'**: speed and completeness of urethral closure, 'milk back' of urine from the posterior urethra into the bladder, or trapping of urine in the urethra between the bladder neck and the sphincter.

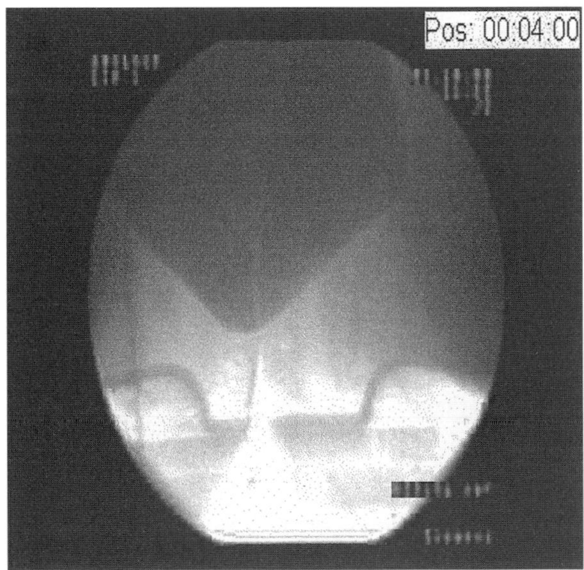

a

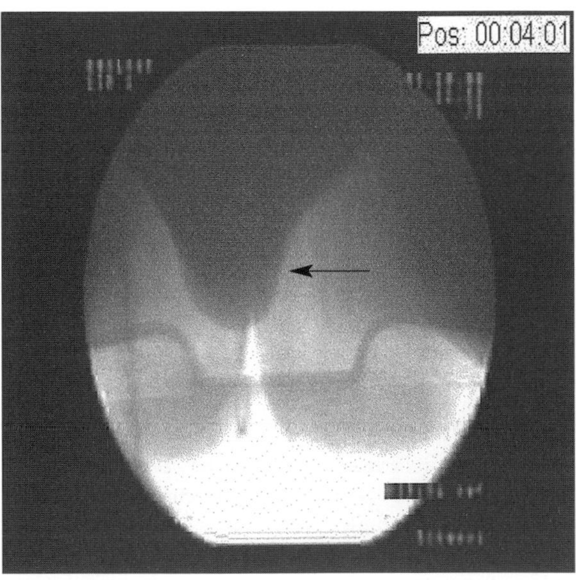

b

Figure 11.1 Videourodynamic images from a 64 year old woman with 5 years of stress incontinence, and a history of surgery for meningioma more than 10 years earlier, but denying frequency, urgency or urge incontinence.
a) Before Valsalva maneuver. The radiolucent commode seat is faintly visible below the bladder outline.
b) During Valsalva maneuver bladder neck descent and anterior vaginal wall prolapse are seen (arrow), but without leakage. VUDS confirmed genuine stress incontinence later in filling phase, and also significant detrusor overactivity with an accompanying sensation which patient then acknowledged occurred frequently under normal conditions. VUDS confirmed normal voiding. (Bristol Urological Institute)

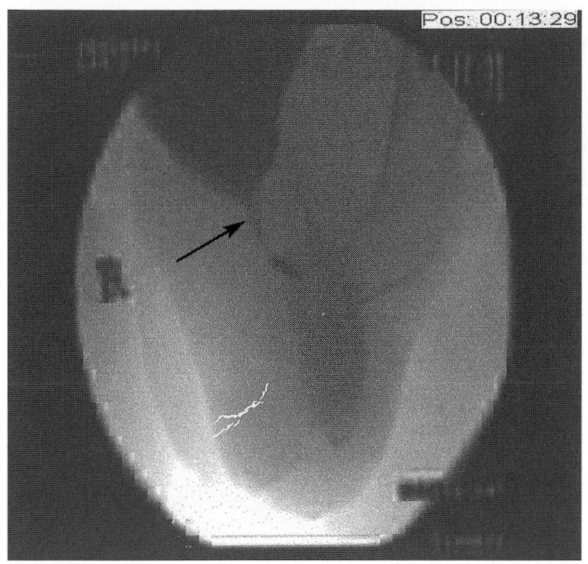

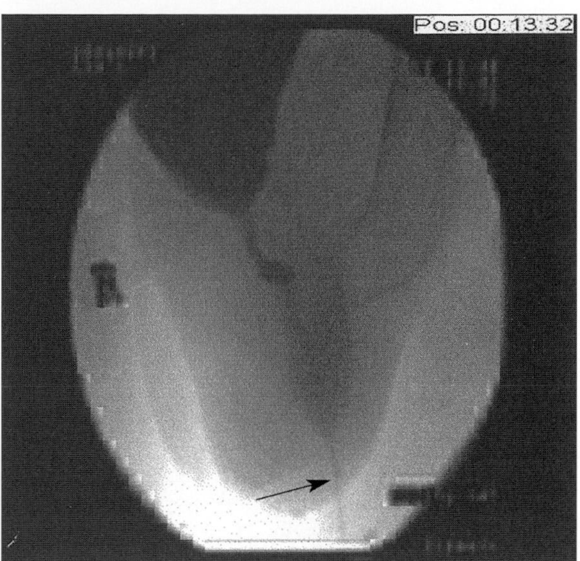

a b

Figure 11.2 Videourodynamic images from a 63 year old man with stress incontinence after cystoprostatectomy and formation of neobladder.
a) Small amount of contrast medium has leaked into membranous and bulbar urethra with previous coughs (arrow).
b) On repeat cough a large leak occurs, with a continuous stream of contrast visible along the entire length of the urethra (arrow).
VUDS confirmed genuine stress incontinence, and also demonstrated slightly low urethral pressure, normal compliance of neobladder, voiding by straining and good bladder emptying. (Bristol Urological Institute)

- **During voiding**: pressure–flow relationships, e.g. for the diagnosis of bladder outlet obstruction or detrusor underactivity.
- **After voiding**: size of bladder diverticula, degree of vesicoureteric reflux, residual urine (see Figure 11.3).

While the more complicated patients may have several pathologic features detectable only by VUDS, for many patients routine UDS without imaging will suffice, although some urodynamicists consider VUDS to be the investigation of choice for all women with incontinence.[13,14] In our view the routine use of VUDS for the investigation of all incontinent patients is unnecessary: firstly because the additional information gained is unlikely to significantly enhance the diagnostic power of the test, and secondly because there are small but well known risks associated with the use of ionizing radiation and contrast media. However, because symptoms are unreliable in the diagnosis of incontinence[15] less complicated cases of incontinence should certainly be evaluated with routine urodynamics.

The indications for VUDS in our unit are summarized in Table 11.1. The recent report of the 1st International Consultation on Incontinence similarly stated[16] that with regard to the investigation of incontinence videourodynamics is indicated:

- in patients with neurogenic lower urinary tract dysfunction;
- in other patients when the history and simpler urodynamic tests do not lead to a definitive diagnosis;
- in patients where initial therapy based on a less precise method of diagnosis has failed.

TECHNIQUE OF VIDEOURODYNAMICS

The pressure measurement technique of VUDS should follow the procedures recommended by the International Continence Society (ICS) standardization committee.[17] The techniques employed in our unit have been described in detail elsewhere.[18] Some specific points of technique are discussed below.

Although some authors consider the measurement of rectal pressure to be unnecessary[14] most urodynamicists consider the recording of rectal pressure and subtracted detrusor pressure to be mandatory. The use of subtracted detrusor pressure allows detection of subtle degrees of detrusor overactivity and provides important information on the quality of pressure transmission, for example at the start of the test or when testing for equal pressure transmission by asking the patient to cough.

Erect posture is well recognized as a provocation for detrusor overactivity, and since the large majority of our

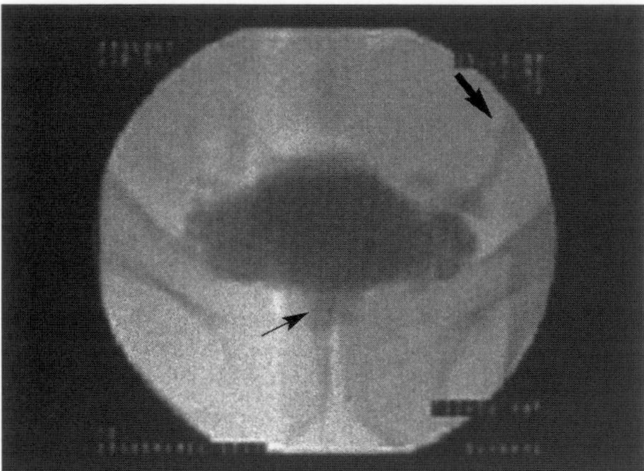

Figure 11.3 Videourodynamic image obtained at end of voiding in a 78 year old man with a history of previous bladder neck incision and urethral dilatation, and more recent frequency and urgency, and occasional left loin pain. Trabeculation and diverticula are seen around the bladder outline. The bladder neck (small arrow) is open, and left vesicoureteric reflux is also clearly seen (large arrow). There is a moderate amount of residual urine. VUDS also showed marked detrusor instability and small capacity, and showed clear bladder outlet obstruction. (Bristol Urological Institute).

Table 11.1 Indications for videourodynamics

1. Patients with probable neurological disease causing LUTD.
2. Women with problems after previous surgery to correct incontinence.
3. Men under 50 years with suspected bladder outlet obstruction.
4. Men with incontinence after lower urinary tract surgery.
5. Patients with LUTD and impaired renal function in the absence of intrinsic renal disease.
6. Children with LUTD.

patients experience most of their symptoms while standing or sitting (even if wheelchair-bound) it seems illogical to perform filling cystometry in the supine position, whether it is for standard urodynamics or for VUDS. Although it is possible for women to void in a standing position during VUDS with the help of a specially designed funnel, this is obviously a very abnormal form of voiding. Most authors therefore prefer the use of a radiolucent commode seat to allow female patients to void in the seated position. The bladder is filled with radiological contrast medium rather than saline, but most other aspects of technique are identical to those employed during routine urodynamics. Although there is a lack of good evidence, it is generally assumed that the higher viscosity, pH and osmolarity of contrast medium do not influence the results of VUDS. Recent (unpublished) research in Bristol suggests that any effect is probably small.

It is helpful to visualize the bladder neck in a lateral projection, although this increases the radiation dose as the X-ray beam has to penetrate the proximal femur and the pelvis. Most units perform VUDS in radiology departments, where the quality of image obtainable is higher, particularly for lateral projections. At Bristol we continue to use an image intensifier within the urodynamic department, which produces a less alien environment for the patient compared with a busy radiology department. We consider that the resulting gain in flexibility in the running of the department and the performance of the test outweighs the disadvantage of a slight reduction in image quality.

Modern urodynamic equipment can present pressure and flow information on the same screen as the VUDS image, which allows the simultaneous interpretation of all of the information available. Pressure and flow tracings may be displayed alongside the image or superimposed upon it. The video recordings obtained are useful for review of the findings of VUDS by others, although this is no substitute for the presence of a clinician during the test. We also find that review of these video images is a very useful teaching tool in our department.

NORMAL AND ABNORMAL APPEARANCES DURING VIDEOURODYNAMICS

During filling a normal bladder has a round shape and a relatively smooth outline, and the ureters are not seen. Typical cystometric bladder capacities are lower than the 'true' normal capacity by around 40%.[19] Trabeculation is visible as an irregularity of the outline of the bladder, and may often be accompanied by more obvious pools of contrast medium lying within bladder diverticula. Diverticula and minor degrees of vesicoureteric reflux may be obscured by the dense bladder outline, so that a change of projection to the left or right oblique position may be useful. A marked abnormality of the bladder outline may be seen in neuropathic patients, where a characteristic 'fir cone' shape is seen, with thickening of the bladder wall, severe trabeculation and diverticula.

The bladder neck is normally closed at rest, but in up to 50% of continent postmenopausal women the bladder neck opens on coughing. In men and in younger women opening of the bladder neck during stress or posture change is not normal. Such opening may be due to intrinsic incompetence of the bladder neck (e.g. in spina bifida patients), or opening in association with an unstable detrusor contraction. Leakage of contrast medium during stress or unstable detrusor contractions is abnormal in either sex. The position of the bladder neck at rest is assessed on an anterior view. The presence of a cystocele and the degree of bladder neck descent on coughing or straining are also assessed during filling (see Fig. 11.1), providing information as to the quality of support of the bladder and urethra. If a cystocele is present, it may easily obscure the bladder neck and urethra on an anteroposterior view, so that a lateral view of the bladder and urethra, or at least an oblique view, is essential. In the lateral view it is also possible to assess the angle between the axis of the urethra and the bladder base.

The principal advantage of VUDS as opposed to voiding cystourethrography is the additional information from the simultaneous measurement of pressure during filling and voiding. The measurement of pressure is, of course, essential for the identification of genuine stress incontinence (GSI) to exclude an unstable detrusor contraction triggered by stress maneuvers. We would agree with the spirit of McGuire's definition of detrusor instability as 'a bladder contraction that occurs without the owner's permission',[20] and therefore consider any obvious wave of increasing detrusor pressure (in practice at least 5 cmH_2O in amplitude) to be representative of detrusor instability, particularly if it is accompanied by urgency. Pressure measurement during filling also allows poor bladder compliance to be identified.

A number of authors emphasize the usefulness of the abdominal leak point pressure (ALPP).[14,20] This test can, of course, be performed during routine urodynamics by directly observing urinary leakage from the urethral orifice rather than imaging leakage of contrast on VUDS. There is still a need for standardization of the technique employed during the ALPP, as the bladder volume at the time of testing or the presence of a catheter may influence the likelihood of leakage.[21] There are a number of other potential pitfalls with the ALPP which must be taken into account, including the possibility of pelvic floor contraction during the maneuver and some patients having difficulty in understanding how to perform a Valsalva maneuver. For this reason imaging may be useful during the test to ensure that the manoeuvre is performed correctly.[20]

The normal events at the initiation of voiding are bladder base descent and a fall in urethral pressure, followed by opening of the bladder neck accompanied by detrusor pressure increase. Flow then progresses through a normal caliber urethra as the detrusor pressure rises to a maximum and then returns to baseline pressure (normally close to zero). Detrusor pressure may rise at the end of voiding, the so-called after-contraction – most available evidence suggests that these after-contractions are not related to detrusor instability, as previously thought.[19] At the end of flow, urethral pressure rises, flow stops and the bladder is normally empty, with no residual urine.

Urethral caliber on VUDS is dependent on the projection used, so that it may appear wider in an AP projection than in a lateral or oblique projection. For this reason the assessment of urethral caliber during voiding is more qualitative than quantitative. The urethra is normally relaxed throughout voiding; where the urethra is overactive there is a characteristic narrowing at the level of the distal urethral sphincter mechanism. Distention of the urethra proximal to the overactive sphincter due to the force of detrusor contraction may be seen, sometimes emphasizing the appearance of the bladder neck as a bar or ring. Urethral diverticula may also be visible during voiding as they fill with contrast.

If the flow of urine is voluntarily interrupted during voiding (the 'stop test') then the interruption occurs at the level of the pelvic floor. Urine in the proximal urethra is 'milked' back into the bladder, followed by elevation of the bladder base and closure of the bladder neck. This sudden interruption of the flow of urine produces a rise in the detrusor pressure (the isometric detrusor pressure, pdet.iso), the height of which is a reflection of detrusor contractility. The ability to voluntarily interrupt the urinary stream also provides some evidence as to the quality of pelvic floor function.

The bladder neck normally remains wide open during voiding, but may be narrow due to either a weak detrusor contraction (with a low detrusor pressure recorded during voiding) or a failure of relaxation (detrusor-bladder neck dyssynergia or bladder neck obstruction, with a high detrusor pressure). In the latter case 'trapping' of contrast in the proximal urethra may occur on attempting to stop the flow of urine. Bladder neck contracture secondary to previous prostatic surgery produces a similar appearance of narrowing at the bladder neck. Useful information on lower urinary tract function is also obtained from the pressure–flow relationship during voiding. Bladder outlet obstruction is characterized by a low flow in the presence of a high pressure voiding detrusor contraction. Detrusor underactivity may be identified from a weak detrusor contraction resulting in a slow flow and residual urine. Interruption of flow during voiding can provide information on detrusor contractility in the form of the pdet.iso, as discussed above. In women the bladder may empty with virtually no detectable detrusor contraction because of low outlet resistance, and it is in such cases that a stop test is most useful in order to assess detrusor contractility.

ADVANTAGES AND DISADVANTAGES OF VIDEOURODYNAMICS

Compared with other modalities of lower urinary tract imaging, videourodynamics has a number of advantages, but also several limitations (Table 11.2). Its particular advantage is the large amount of information that it provides from a single test, so that VUDS is likely to remain central to the investigation of lower urinary tract dysfunction for the foreseeable future. Modalities such

Table 11.2 Advantages and disadvantages of different techniques for imaging the bladder and urethra

	Cystourethrography	Videourodynamics	Ultrasound	MRI
Advantages				
Information on pressure changes	–	+	–	–
Soft-tissue imaging	–	–	+/–	++
Static imaging of bladder neck	+	+	+	+
Dynamic imaging of bladder neck	+	+	+	+/–
Disadvantages				
Cost	+	++	+	+++
Ionizing radiation	+	+	–	–
Invasiveness	+	+	+/–	–
Time consumed	+	++	+	++

as MRI and ultrasound can provide a good deal of information on other aspects of lower urinary tract function inaccessible to VUDS, particularly in providing images of the pelvic floor. They are therefore gradually establishing a place in the investigation of such patients, especially for research purposes. The rest of this chapter concentrates on these newer modalities and their role in the investigation of lower urinary tract dysfunction.

ULTRASONOGRAPHY

Ultrasound has rapidly established a place in the evaluation of a large range of clinical problems since it was first developed in the 1940s and 1950s. It has several clear advantages over conventional radiology, particularly in that it does not expose patients to ionizing radiation and allows imaging of a variety of different solid organs and soft tissues without the need for contrast media. Since the early 1980s there has been increasing interest in the use of ultrasound[22] as a substitute for established methods such as videourodynamics and lateral bead chain cystourethrography in the evaluation of incontinence. The principal advantages and disadvantages of ultrasound imaging are listed in Table 11.2.

The rapid development of lower urinary tract ultrasound by multiple different routes has led to some difficulties in the comparison of different studies, and there is still a clear need for standard procedures to be adopted. It has been recognized from experience with ultrasound as well as with other techniques, such as the ALPP[21] and the Q-tip test,[23] that various aspects of technique such as patient posture or bladder filling may alter the results of tests of lower urinary tract function. Steps have therefore recently been taken towards standardization of ultrasound technique by the German Association of Urogynaecology, whose recommendations were summarised in a report in 1996.[24] Further recommendations on ultrasound technique have recently been provided by the committee on imaging from the 1st International Consultation on Incontinence sponsored by the WHO in Monaco in 1998.[3] Useful summaries of recent research on ultrasound, and other modalities of imaging, may also be found elsewhere.[25–28]

ROUTE OF LOWER URINARY TRACT ULTRASOUND

Ultrasound of the lower urinary tract may be performed by several different routes:

1. External sonography: transabdominal, perineal and introital sonography.
2. Endosonography: transvaginal and transrectal sonography.
3. Endoluminal: intraurethral ultrasound.

The choice of the route of ultrasound depends to a great degree on the equipment available in individual units. Each route has potential advantages and disadvantages. Although transabdominal ultrasound is a very valuable investigation in many aspects of urological and gynecological practice, it is inferior to other methods of imaging of the bladder base and urethra because during stress the bladder neck and urethra may be obscured by the symphysis pubis.[22]

Introital and perineal sonography employ the same types of ultrasound probe as normally used in gynecological practice.[24] In perineal scanning a curved array linear probe (frequency of 3.5 to 5 MHz) is applied to the perineum, whereas in introital sonography a sectorial vaginal probe (5 to 7.5 MHz) is placed under the distal part of the urethra at the introitus. Vaginal and transrectal ultrasonography employ 5 to 7.5 MHz linear probes introduced into the cavity of the vagina or rectum.[3]

The quality of the images obtained by different routes of scanning depends partly on the proximity of the probe to the target area, so that endosonography, and particularly vaginal sonography, produce the clearest images. However, the placement of probes within the body has a number of disadvantages, not least in reducing the acceptability of the investigation to the patient. Other potential disadvantages include displacement of the bladder neck at rest or during stress, and compression of the urethra, which may be particularly important if pressures are measured concurrently with ultrasound imaging. The sensation caused by the probe can also alter lower urinary tract function, especially during dynamic studies such as transrectal voiding ultrasonography, leading to inhibition of normal voiding.[29] The choice of the route of ultrasound imaging therefore depends upon the precise information required, and often requires a compromise between the quality of image and the degree of interference in normal lower urinary tract function which is considered acceptable.

Few direct comparisons of different routes of ultrasound have been published, perhaps because most centers have developed a particular expertise based on the type of ultrasound probe already available to them. Hol *et al.* found no difference between the position of the bladder neck at rest or during stress when comparing transrectal and transvaginal US.[30] In a comparison of transrectal and perineal ultrasonography, Hong *et al.* found small but significant differences in the degree of measured bladder neck descent between the two routes, with transrectal US showing reduced bladder neck descent.[31] Pajoncini *et al.* compared US evaluation of women with stress incontinence and pelvic floor abnormalities by transrectal, transvaginal and perineal routes,[32] and found that all three approaches were able to visualize bladder neck position, funneling and mobility. Transrectal US gave good resolution and did not interfere with the degree of pelvic organ descent during stress but was more uncomfortable for the patient and suffered from reduced visualization when the rectum was filled with gas. Transvaginal US gave the best resolution of the urethra and was better tolerated, at the cost of significant interference with dynamic movements during stress maneuvers. Perineal US was the easiest to perform and the probe used is more widely available, but image resolution may be mediocre, especially during straining, and probe pressure tends to compress cystoceles and thus underestimate their size.

Another route of lower urinary tract ultrasound which has become available more recently is endourethral ultrasound. Endoluminal ultrasound in general evolved from early attempts at miniaturization of ultrasound transducers, and particularly from the development of fine ultrasound probes in the 1970s for the evaluation of vascular structures.[33] The probes come in the form of a 12.5 to 20 MHz ultrasound transducer mounted on a 6 to 9 Fr catheter.[34] This higher frequency of ultrasound produces better resolution (0.1–0.2 mm) at the expense of lower depth of penetration (20–25 mm),[35] so that these probes are useful in imaging structures very close to the urethral lumen. Unlike the sagittal section image typically used with other methods of lower urinary tract ultrasound, endoluminal ultrasound provides a 360° cross-sectional image, which is very useful for the examination of the intra-urethral striated sphincter and the periurethral tissues.

ULTRASOUND OF THE BLADDER

Clearly a review of all aspects of bladder ultrasound is beyond the scope of this chapter. For the imaging of the bladder *per se*, transabdominal ultrasound is normally the route of choice, since it is painless, simple, cheap and acceptable to the patient.

The methods typically employed for the measurement of residual urine volume after voiding are based on the assumption that the bladder is either spherical or ellipsoid in shape. The volume of the residual urine is calculated by measuring either three dimensions (height, breadth, length) or the length and the cross-sectional area, and multiplying the product of these dimensions by a constant, usually between 0.5 and 0.7.[36] The standard error of the estimation is generally around 20% when compared with the 'gold standard' of catheterization and drainage of the residual urine.[37]

Ultrasound estimation of bladder wall thickness has been described in both men and women, with contrasting conclusions. Khullar *et al.* used transvaginal ultrasound to measure bladder wall thickness in the empty bladder (i.e. containing < 50 ml), taking the mean of measurements at the thickest part of the trigone, the dome of the bladder, and the anterior bladder wall.[38] They found that 94% of women with a mean bladder wall thickness of > 5 mm had detrusor instability on either routine cystometry or ambulatory urodynamics, compared to 18% of women with a thickness of < 3.5 mm. Bladder wall thickness was therefore suggested as a useful screening test for detrusor instability. Patients with a mean bladder wall thickness between 3.5 and 5 mm did not undergo ambulatory urodynamics in this study, therefore the incidence of detrusor instability in this group is not clear. However, this test certainly seems to have some promise as a screening test for detrusor instability.

In contrast, Manieri *et al.* found that in men referred with lower urinary tract symptoms bladder wall thickness correlated with bladder outlet obstruction, but not with the presence of detrusor instability.[39] The method of bladder wall thickness estimation differed from the preceding study, in that the bladder was filled to 150 ml before scanning and that the transabdominal route was used for scanning. The study showed that 88% of men with a bladder wall thickness of > 5 mm had bladder outlet obstruction on pressure-flow studies compared to 63% of men with a thickness of < 5 mm. Bladder wall thickness correlated with multiple urodynamic indices including detrusor pressure at maximum flow ($r = 0.76$) and maximum flow rate ($r = 0.34$). The presence of detrusor instability 'did not influence bladder wall thickness'. However, detrusor instability was seen in only 12% of patients, which is lower than the rate normally seen in such patients. The relationship between ultrasound measured bladder wall thickness and detrusor instability is therefore still unclear, but further studies would be interesting.

ULTRASOUND OF THE BLADDER NECK AND URETHRA AND ASSESSMENT OF THE PELVIC FLOOR

Assessment technique

Lower urinary tract ultrasound can identify a variety of different structures, including the bladder wall and lumen, the bladder neck, the urethral wall and lumen, the pubic bone, the vagina, the rectum and the uterus. It is also possible to identify other pelvic structures such as the levator ani muscle. In the assessment of incontinence and pelvic floor dysfunction several variables have been measured by different authors. The sagittal plane is used to obtain a cross sectional view through the bladder and urethra. The long axis of the symphysis pubis and the lower border of the symphysis are normally used as the fixed landmarks. The position of the bladder neck, the angle of the urethra and the angle of the bladder base can then be assessed in relation to these points (and each other) at rest, and during Valsalva, coughing and pelvic floor contraction (Fig. 11.4).

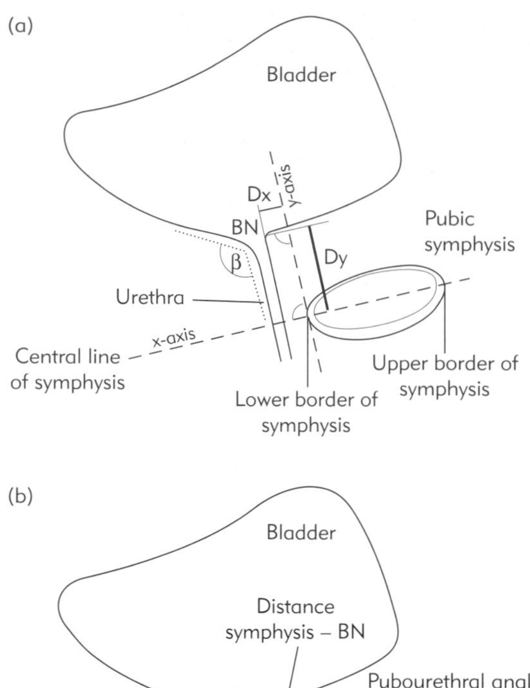

Figure 11.4 Measurement methods for bladder neck position and retrovesical angle β. The position of the bladder neck (BN) can be defined by either a) two distances or by b) a distance and an angle. From Ref. 24, with permission.

Correct identification of bladder neck funneling is a problem in ultrasonography,[40] particularly with external scanning techniques. Identification of the bladder neck may be enhanced by the insertion of a Q-tip to delineate the urethra,[11] or the use of Foley catheters, where the junction of the balloon and the catheter helps identify the bladder neck.[41,30] Unfortunately these methods may interfere with the static and dynamic measurements, and are again invasive. A 14 Fr Foley catheter shortens the distance between the bladder neck and the inferior border of the symphysis,[42] and causes an increase in the random variation of measurements compared with repeated measurement without catheter, but catheters have no effect on bladder neck rotational mobility. Schaer *et al.* have suggested that bladder neck position, bladder neck funneling and urinary leakage may be identified more easily with the use of ultrasound contrast medium.[40] Comparing ultrasound scans performed with the bladder filled with saline and then again with ultrasound contrast medium, they identified a much higher proportion of patients with bladder neck funneling during Valsalva maneuver with the use of contrast medium (Fig. 11.5). The instillation of contrast medium converts sonography into an invasive procedure, thus removing one of its principal advantages over lateral bead chain cystourethrography, but sonography still has the advantages of avoiding exposure to ionizing radiation and lower cost.

As with many other functional tests, several aspects of technique might affect the measurements made. Vierhout and Jansen studied the effect of posture change on the results of bladder neck ultrasound, finding significant alterations in the position of the bladder neck at rest, during straining and during pelvic floor contraction, when comparing sonography in supine and sitting positions.[43] They suggested that standardization of the technique is essential. Mouritsen and Bach studied the effect of posture, catheters and bladder volume on sonographic measurements of bladder neck mobility.[42] Moving to a more vertical posture increased the resting angle between the urethra and the axis of the symphysis pubis, but did not alter the magnitude of

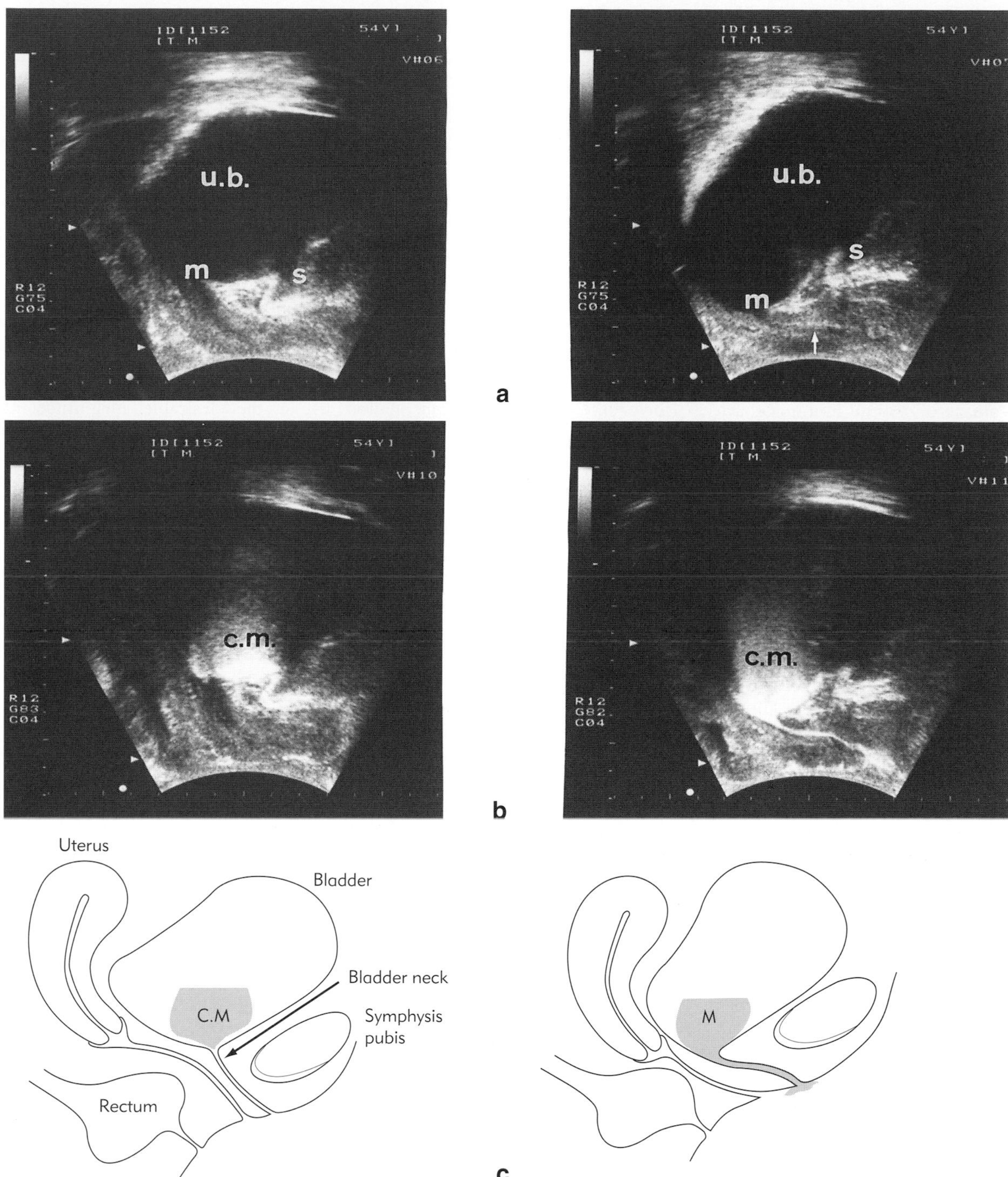

Figure 11.5 Perineal ultrasound in upright position in a woman with stress incontinence. Images on left – at rest; on right – during Valsalva maneuver.

a) Funneling of the bladder neck and 'urethral double line' during Valsalva (white arrow).

b) Similar examination, but with the addition of ultrasonographic contrast medium shows improved visualization of bladder neck funneling and delineation of bladder neck during Valsalva

c) Schematic line drawing of b). From Ref. 40, with permission.

u b urinary bladder   s pubic symphysis   m internal urethral meatus   c m contrast medium bladder neck mobility during Valsalva. The bladder neck was closer to the symphysis in the sitting position. A more recent analysis by Chen *et al.* similarly found that change of posture altered the resting position of the bladder neck, but did not significantly alter bladder neck mobility during straining.[44] In a detailed study of perineal ultrasound, Schaer *et al.* found that the sitting position resulted in a lower resting position of the bladder neck and much higher rates of detection of bladder neck funneling.[45]

An increase in bladder volume from 50–200 ml has a small (but significant) effect on some rotational measurements, but no effect on the distance between bladder neck and pubic symphysis.[42] Hol *et al.* found no difference in the position of the bladder neck at rest or on straining when comparing scans obtained at a bladder volume of 250 ml and at capacity.[30] However, Dietz *et al.* found that bladder filling influences the position and mobility of the bladder neck and the degree of funneling observed on transperineal ultrasound.[46] Schaer *et al.* considered that increasing bladder filling did not affect measurements made during perineal ultrasound, but did improve the rate of detection of bladder neck funneling. The best overall image quality was at 300 ml, which was subsequently recommended as the standard bladder volume to be used during lower urinary tract US by the German Association of Urogynecology.[24]

It has been suggested that the ultrasound probe can produce significant alterations in the anatomy and function of the lower urinary tract, particularly when endosonographic techniques are used.[25] However, the available evidence is contradictory. Bergman *et al.* stated that a probe did not alter the mobility of the bladder neck or the angle of a Q-tip placed in the urethra, although systematic data were not provided.[11] Hol *et al.* found that the presence of a vaginal probe did not significantly alter the position of a Q-tip in the urethra[30] in 20 women studied. However, Wise *et al.* studied the effect of a sectorial vaginal probe in more detail, and found sizeable differences in maximum urethral pressure and functional profile length on urethral pressure profilometry (UPP)[47] with the probe in place. They also showed that the probe elevated the bladder neck towards the symphysis pubis at rest, and restricted the descent of the bladder neck during stress when simultaneously visualizing the bladder neck by lateral bead chain cystourethrography. In contrast Beco *et al.* found no significant differences in UPP parameters with and without a linear array vaginal probe, but found an alteration in the Q-tip position at rest and a reduction in the Q-tip displacement on stress.[48] They attributed the lack of an effect on the UPP to the fact that under most circumstances linear array probes require no pressure by the examiner. Schaer *et al.* found that pressure on a perineal probe could cause distortion of measurements both at rest and during Valsalva.[45]

Overall, the evidence certainly suggests that there is always a potential for distortion of the anatomy when performing lower urinary tract sonography, and therefore the minimum pressure required to obtain a good image should be used at all times.[24] The maneuver used for measurements during stress should probably be standardized, as the degree of bladder neck descent is greater with increase in Valsalva.[30] Hol *et al.* chose a standardized intravesical pressure increase on Valsalva of 30 cmH_2O, which they found virtually all women could achieve.[30] During Valsalva the bladder neck lies lower and more dorsally than during coughing,[45] because the pelvic floor is usually relaxed during a Valsalva maneuver and contracted during a cough. The reports of the German Association of Urogynecology[24] and the 1st International Consultation on Incontinence[3] did not make a specific recommendation as to the desirable magnitude of pressure change during Valsalva. However, the German Association of Urogynecology report advocates dynamic testing by coughing, Valsalva and pelvic floor contraction in all patients.[24]

Reproducibility

The reproducibility of bladder neck US has been assessed by several authors. Using a Foley catheter with an inflated balloon to identify the bladder neck, Creighton *et al.* demonstrated the reproducibility of various measurements of bladder neck position made by a single observer in six patients.[41] Based on the findings of repeated perineal ultrasound in 10 patients, Caputo *et al.* similarly suggested that ultrasound assessment of bladder neck descent has good reproducibility.[49] In a larger study of perineal ultrasound (40 patients), Schaer *et al.* found that measurements of bladder neck position by different observers were reproducible with the exception of the posterior urethrovesical angle, which was not reproducible during Valsalva maneuver.[50] Hol *et al.* studied reproducibility of bladder neck displacement between two independent examiners using vaginal ultrasound in 20 patients, and found good agreement.[30] Mouritsen *et al.* studied the reproducibility of bladder neck position measurements by transvaginal ultrasonography when assessed by three observers of different levels of experience.[51] They found significant differences between the measurements made by the two more experienced observers and the inexperienced observer, and, perhaps predictably, also showed that the measurement variability was higher with a less experienced observer. None of these reproducibility studies used the most advanced analyses of measurement variability, which have been suggested to be more appropriate by others,[52] and the description of the blinding and statistics used is limited in several studies. Current evidence therefore suggests reasonable reproducibility of bladder neck US in general, but further studies are needed.

Sonography compared with other forms of assessment

In assessing the value of sonography in evaluation of the bladder neck and the urethra it is natural to compare it to the previous standard investigation, namely lateral bead chain cystourethrography. Bergman *et al.* compared transrectal sonography and lateral bead chain cystourethrography (LBCUG) and found similarly high sensitivity in the diagnosis of genuine stress incontinence, but did not formally assess the agreement between the two methods.[11] Gordon *et al.* compared perineal US using a catheter to delineate the urethra with LBCUG and found good correlation between bladder neck descent measured by the different methods (r = 0.86), although the perineal scan and LBCUG were performed in different postures.[10] Schaer *et al.* found some discrepancies between measurements of bladder neck mobility and particularly the posterior urethrovesical angle, when comparing perineal US and LBCUG.[50] These discrepancies may be due to several factors: LBCUG images are a projection through the whole bladder, including the bladder base lateral to the midline, with a potential for incorrect interpretation; the bead chain within the urethra may alter bladder neck mobility during the test; and the abdominal pressure during Valsalva maneuver was not standardized in either test.[50] LBCUG was more sensitive in identifying bladder neck funneling than perineal US. Voigt *et al.* also found good agreement between perineal sonography and LBCUG.[53] Interestingly, they considered that this form of sonography requires an investigator with a great deal of experience, in contrast to other authors who have stressed that lower urinary tract sonography is an easy technique to learn.[54,41]

Perineal US has also been compared with the Q-tip test by Caputo *et al.*[49] Although they found both methods to be reproducible, the Q-tip test was much less sensitive in identifying hypermobility of the bladder base. The study has been criticized because the two tests were performed in different postures (Q-tip lying, US sitting). However, Handa *et al.* found a lower proportion of positive Q-tip tests when performed in the standing position,[23] so the difference in postures is unlikely to fully explain the discrepancy.

Lower urinary tract ultrasound seems to be as good as lateral bead chain cystourethrography in the evaluation of bladder neck hypermobility, although it does not produce exactly equivalent quantitative measurements. Sonography is preferable to LBCUG in that it can be readily performed in any department which already owns an ultrasound scanner, it does not expose patients to radiation, it is less invasive, and it is more acceptable to the patient. Sonography appears to be more accurate than the Q-tip test, although it is obviously more expensive and requires a greater level of training to perform.

Diagnosis of genuine stress incontinence

The assessment of bladder neck mobility is well established in the evaluation of women with urinary incontinence, and in the selection of surgical procedures. It is well known that bladder neck position at rest or on straining is not diagnostic of genuine stress incontinence, a fact which is consistent with the multiple factors thought to be involved in the pathogenesis of this condition. Some authors have found that sonographic measurements of bladder neck mobility have a high sensitivity and specificity in the identification of genuine stress incontinence,[11,51] and advocate a cut-off of >1 cm of bladder neck descent on stress to indicate bladder neck hypermobility.[11] There are certainly significant differences between continent and stress incontinent patients in parameters such as the posterior urethrovesical angle,[53] the bladder neck to pubic symphysis distance[53] and magnitude of bladder descent on straining.[11] Hol *et al.* similarly found lower bladder neck position at rest and greater mobility during stress, but found a very large degree of overlap between the two groups, and suggested that sonographic assessment of bladder neck position and mobility cannot predict genuine stress incontinence. Recently Meyer *et al.* also found considerable overlap between bladder neck position and mobility between continent and stress incontinent patients.[54] In spite of this well documented overlap between continent and incontinent women all of these authors agree that sonographic evaluation of the bladder neck is a useful test in the preoperative evaluation of incontinent women.

Other ultrasonically measured variables have been evaluated in incontinent women, although they are likely to remain research tools only. For example, Boos *et al.* used transvaginal US to measure the dimensions of the urogenital hiatus in asymptomatic women and women with GSI but without prolapse.[55] The urogenital hiatus was significantly larger on both static and dynamic imaging in GSI patients compared with controls, and US imaging provided interesting insights into the dynamic changes in the shape of the urogenital hiatus during Valsalva. The blood supply to the trigone area can also be estimated by color Doppler ultrasound, using the position of the ureteric jet as a landmark. Women with genuine stress incontinence have been shown to have reduced peak and mean velocities of blood flow compared with women with detrusor instability, which may be related to the known effects of estrogens on blood flow to the urethra.[56] Three-dimensional ultrasound of the urethra has recently been used in women with GSI, showing that the volume of the urethral sphincter is smaller in women with GSI than in those without.[57]

The debate about the importance of different mechanisms in the pathogenesis of stress incontinence and the ideal clinical assessment of such patients is certainly not yet settled. In the recent recommendations of the 1st International Consultation on Incontinence, bladder neck and pelvic floor ultrasound were considered only as an investigational imaging technique in the evaluation of female incontinence and pelvic floor disorders, and not diagnostic of stress or urge incontinence.[3] However, it was felt that ultrasound may be helpful in diagnosing urethral hypermobility and is helpful to document pelvic floor anatomy.

Assessment of changes related to childbirth or treatment of incontinence

While sonography is not diagnostic of genuine stress incontinence, it is acceptable to patients, safe and relatively cheap. It is therefore well suited to the evaluation of the effect of treatment on lower urinary tract function, or of other changes over time, for example in relation to pregnancy and childbirth.

Peschers *et al.* used repeated perineal ultrasound to study changes in bladder neck mobility in women before and after vaginal delivery or cesarean section.[58] Scans were performed in late pregnancy, 3–7 days after delivery, and 5–10 weeks after delivery. They found that voluntary pelvic floor contraction power was reduced immediately after delivery but was rapidly re-established, whereas bladder neck passive mobility continued to increase even several weeks after delivery. However, using introital ultrasound Toozs-Hobson *et al.* were unable to demonstrate any significant change in bladder neck mobility or descent in relation to the development of incontinence symptoms after childbirth, but found a significant reduction in the diameter of the rhabdosphincter measured with 3-D ultrasound in women becoming symptomatic.[59] Toozs-Hobson *et al.* also found that amongst women with subjective incontinence antenatally, urethral sphincter volume was significantly lower in those with postnatal subjective incontinence than in those who no longer complained of incontinence.[60] Interestingly there was little difference between women delivered vaginally and by cesarean section, which may be a reflection of the fact that no distinction was drawn between women who had emergency rather than elective cesarean sections, or between those who had instrumental rather than normal vaginal deliveries. These and other studies have shown that sonography is well suited to research into pelvic floor function around the time of childbirth, although routine clinical application is not currently indicated.

Ultrasound has also been applied to investigation of the effects of pelvic floor exercises, both directly, in assessing the effect of PFEs on pelvic floor muscle thickness, and indirectly, to examine the effect on bladder neck mobility. Bernstein reported a detailed study of pelvic floor muscle thickness in several groups of women.[61] Using physiotherapists as healthy controls, muscle thickness was measured in the relaxed and contracted state using a perineal ultrasound probe placed lateral to the introitus. The muscle thickness increased on contraction from a median of 9.3 mm to a median of 11.4 mm. Inter-observer variation was found to be low, but the technique was not easy to perform. Women without significant incontinence recruited from the community showed a similar median thickness of 9.8 mm at rest and 11.2 mm during contraction. Amongst women referred with urinary incontinence the respective thicknesses were 9.2 mm and 10.2 mm, which were increased after a course of pelvic floor exercises to 9.7 and 11.2 mm. The increase in pelvic floor muscle thickness did not correlate with either the patient's subjective assessment of their improvement or with the reduction found in urinary leakage during a 1-hour pad test. Martan *et al.* used perineal ultrasound to examine the position and mobility of the bladder neck before and after PFEs in 20 incontinent and 10 continent women.[62] The study demonstrated significant improvements in both the position of the bladder neck at rest and the degree of descent during Valsalva, and it was concluded that perineal sonography is a valuable method in monitoring the effect of pelvic floor training.

During corrective surgery for genuine stress incontinence, assessing whether the operation has achieved the correct degree of bladder neck repositioning can be difficult. Ultrasound is potentially useful in assessing bladder neck mobility in this context. Richmond *et al.* found intraoperative transrectal ultrasound useful in the assessment of the effect of Pereyra suspension and Burch colposuspension, but found the technique a poor predictor of success in fascial sling procedures.[63] Yamada *et al.* found that intraoperative transrectal ultrasound was useful in assessing the effect of both Stamey bladder neck suspension[64] and suburethral sling procedures.[65]

Hol *et al.* studied women before and after Burch colposuspension using transvaginal US to evaluate the effect of surgery and the correlation with outcome.[66] The resting position and the mobility of the bladder neck were, as expected, improved after surgery, but it was also found that moderate bladder neck mobility after operation was still compatible with complete continence in a number of cases. Elia and Bergman used introital ultrasound at 3-month follow-up to evaluate the relation between the position of periurethral collagen implants and successful clinical outcome.[67] Collagen implants less than 7 mm from the bladder neck were associated with a positive outcome, and it was implied that US may be a useful way to evaluate the likelihood of success if repeat ultrasound is being considered. Clearly ultrasound lends itself well to both intraoperative use and to follow-up of incontinence surgery, but there is a lack of data to suggest that outcomes are improved as a result of its use.

COMBINED ULTRASOUND AND URODYNAMICS

Early in the development of sonography of the lower urinary tract it was realized that ultrasound might offer a realistic alternative to the use of X-rays in the imaging of the bladder and urethra during urodynamics. The particular appeals of this approach are that it does not require X-ray facilities for imaging, and that it does not require contrast medium or ionizing radiation, with all the associated risks. In 1982 Nishizawa *et al.* reported encouraging early experiences with transrectal ultrasonography combined with urodynamics.[68] Perkash and Friedland applied the technique in the evaluation of men with neurogenic lower urinary tract dysfunction, and were able to assess bladder neck and urethral opening, prostate size, and bladder emptying using transrectal US.[69] They also suggested that this imaging was useful in evaluation of treatment response and in biofeedback. Shabsigh *et al.* described the use of transrectal ultrasonography in spinal cord injured patients, with the patient supine or in lithotomy position, and found it to be similarly useful.[70] They identified two disadvantages to the approach. Firstly it is not possible to identify vesicoureteric reflux, and secondly the anterior urethra is not imaged. One of the obvious disadvantages with transrectal voiding ultrasonography that was not discussed was the inhibition of normal voiding which may result from the presence of an anal probe. Given the difficulties a number of patients already have with voiding in unfamiliar surroundings during urodynamics,[18] this is potentially a serious problem. However, in neurological patients without anal sensation this problem may well be diminished.

Nerstrøm *et al.* developed a technique of 3-dimensional transrectal voiding urodynamics and reported encouraging early experiences in 1991.[71] While the use of a chair-mounted ultrasound probe allowed the observer to remain distant from the patient during voiding, the need for men to sit during voiding with this technique might obviously be a significant problem unless they already void in the sitting position. Further studies in men have continued to appear in recent years, including evidence suggesting that the transrectal probe does indeed inhibit voiding,[29] as might be expected.

Schaer *et al.* recently described the use of a remote-controlled, chair-mounted ultrasound probe for the assessment of voiding in women.[72] Previous experience with perineal ultrasound of women during voiding had been limited in its success by the need for supine posture to allow fixation of the probe and to minimize pressure effects on the perineum. The new apparatus incorporated a commode and a pressure-controlled steering arm to allow adjustment of the pressure exerted by the probe, according to changes in the position of the perineum, while the patient voided in the sitting position. Of 30 women studied, 28 were able to void with or without the probe in place, and two were unable to void in either circumstance. The bladder base, bladder neck, and proximal urethra could be identified throughout voiding in all 28 women who voided. At present there is insufficient evidence as to whether or not the findings of urodynamics are significantly altered by the presence of a probe in contact with the perineum. Comparison of qualitative and quantitative urodynamic findings during voiding with and without a perineal probe in position will be required before this technique can be recommended as a substitute for videourodynamics. Voiding ultrasonography remains an interesting research tool at present, which may in time come to offer a serious alternative to VUDS if some of the current difficulties can be overcome.

ENDOLUMINAL ULTRASOUND

Endoluminal urethral ultrasound developed as an extension of a new technology originally designed for the evaluation of blood vessels. Early descriptions of the application of endoluminal ultrasound in urology tended to concentrate on evaluation of the ureter and renal pelvis, although imaging of the periurethral anatomy was described.[34] The application of endoluminal US specifically for the diagnostic imaging of the urethra was described by Klein *et al.* in 1993.[73] A correlation was found between grade of stress incontinence and the area of the urethral sphincter in women ($r = -0.41$), although it appears that incontinence was defined only clinically in this study, rather than by UDS. Some problems were experienced with imaging, with three out of 32 women excluded from analysis due to the poor quality of their US images, and incomplete delineation of the sphincter in a further 12 women.

Messelink *et al.* studied asymptomatic volunteers using endoluminal US, and found that the quality of sphincter imaging was higher than transvaginal ultrasound in the same subjects.[35] Discomfort was a significant problem, perhaps because the catheter on which the US transducer was mounted was designed for endovascular rather than endourethral use. Strasser *et al.* used endoluminal US to study the sphincter mechanism in men after radical prostatectomy, including eight men with postprostatectomy incontinence.[74] In addition to measuring the maximum urethral closure pressure (MUCP) during urethral pressure profile, the authors measured a new variable of sphincter function: the reduction in distance between the inner edge of the rhabdosphincter and the intraurethral US transducer on cross sectional images obtained during voluntary contraction of the pelvic floor. Mean values of both the MUCP and the rhabdosphincter-transducer distance were

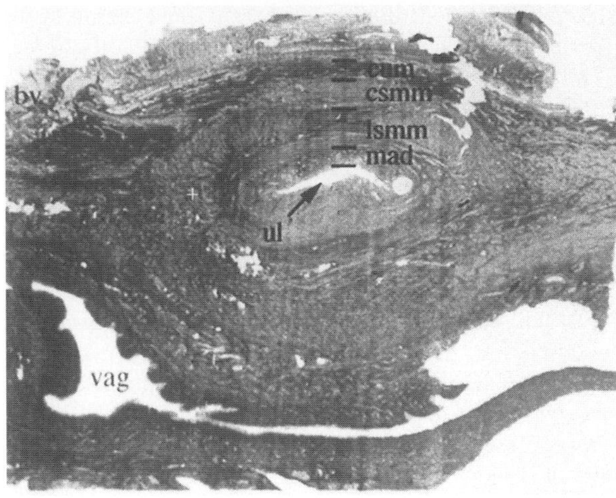

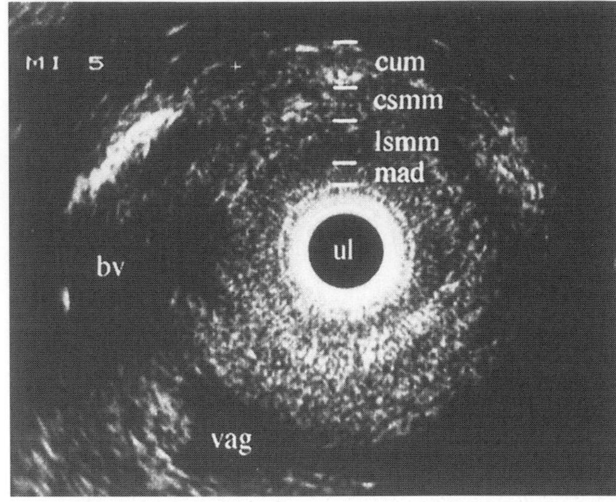

c

Figure 11.6 Comparison of histological sections (left side) and intraurethral ultrasound images (right side) of the urethra in the cadaver of a 55 year old female.
Cross sections taken at a) 15 mm, b) 20 mm, and c) 25 mm from internal meatus. Key: uL = urethral lumen; mad = mucosa and adventitia; lsmm = longitudinal smooth muscle; csmm = circular smooth muscle; ssm = striated sphincter muscle; cum = compressor urethrae and urethrovaginal muscle; vag = vaginal wall; bv = blood vessels. From Ref. 75, with permission.

reduced in the incontinent patients compared with those remaining continent after radical prostatectomy (ranges of values were not provided); the correlation of these measurements with the grade of incontinence was much higher for rhabdosphincter-transducer distance than MUCP. The authors suggested that the UPP and ALPP could be abandoned in favor of intraurethral US, although this assertion was criticized as premature in the accompanying editorial.

In order to correlate the different structures identified on endoluminal US with the true anatomy, Schaer *et al.* examined female cadavers by comparing serial transurethral US images with serial histological sections from the same patients.[75] This study demonstrated that the inner hypoechoic ring on US images is produced by the smooth muscle of the urethra, and that the outer hyperechoic ring is formed by the intraurethral striated muscle sphincter (Fig. 11.6). In contrast to these findings, a similar study of male cadavers by Strasser *et al.* found that the rhabdosphincter appeared as a hypoechoic structure separated from the smooth muscle of the membranous urethra by a hyperechoic sheet of connective tissue.[74] It is likely that this difference in interpretation reflects a difference between the sexes, as the sonographic appearances of the different layers should remain the same.[75] Further work may be needed in this area.

Chancellor *et al.* found intraurethral US useful in the evaluation of women undergoing operation for urethral diverticula,[76] in that ultrasound imaging could precisely define the position and shape of the diverticulum, identify other useful features such as periurethral inflammation and wall thickness, and provide confirmation of complete excision. Endoluminal US of the urethra has also been used to guide other urethral procedures such as periurethral collagen injections and deployment of intraprostatic and intrasphincteric stents.[77] Intraurethral ultrasound remains an interesting imaging option for research into urethral function and dysfunction, although on current evidence it seems unlikely that it will find a role in the routine investigation of incontinence.

COMPUTERIZED TOMOGRAPHY

Computerized tomography (CT) scanning has revolutionized a number of areas of medicine such as neurosurgery, and has a major role in investigation in many other areas. However, CT is of limited use in the evaluation of incontinence and pelvic floor dysfunction because it provides inferior resolution of soft tissue anatomy in comparison to MRI. It is also limited because the imaging is axial, so that all the images generated are normally in the transverse plane. Data from CT scans can be reconstructed to provide three dimensional images of the lower urinary tract (Fig. 11.7), and similar techniques can be applied to allow these images to be explored, a technique known as 'virtual reality' endoscopy. This technique has been used to image the lower urinary tract in patients after orthotopic reconstruction.[78] While the clarity of the images produced was impressive, it was recognized that the diagnostic yield of 3-D CT and virtual reality endoscopy as an accessory form of imaging was low, all pathological findings being

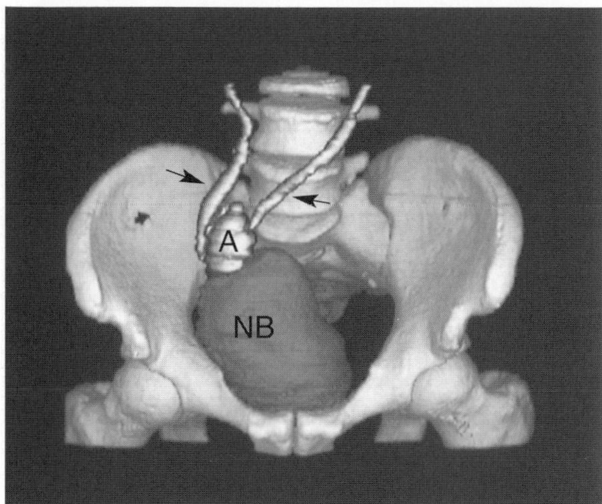

Figure 11.7 Reconstructed 3-dimensional CT image of the lower urinary tract after orthotopic ileal neobladder. The ureters (arrows), afferent limb (A), and neobladder (NB) are clearly demonstrated. The precise positions of the structures and anastomoses can be explored by manipulation of the images. (Image courtesy of Professor Arnulf Stenzl.)

visible on conventional CT images. The technique also requires a good deal of time (and therefore higher cost) for image processing. 3-D CT and virtual reality endoscopy may have a role in research, and they certainly produce beautiful pictures, but it seems unlikely they will find widespread use in imaging in pelvic floor dysfunction.

MAGNETIC RESONANCE IMAGING

Magnetic resonance imaging (MRI) has only recently become available as an imaging tool for evaluating the pelvic floor and lower urinary tract. Since the early report of Klutke *et al.*[79] advances in MRI technology have led to rapid improvements in the quality of imaging available. MRI provides high resolution images of the soft tissues of the pelvis in multiple planes, and is thus superior to other currently available imaging modalities in the evaluation of static pelvic anatomy in normal subjects or in patients with pelvic floor dysfunction (Fig. 11.8). Dynamic imaging is more problematic, because of the time required to obtain images, so that at present ultrasound or radiographic techniques are superior in assessing mobility of the bladder and urethra. The time and cost involved in performing and analysing MRI studies are clearly major obstacles to the widespread use of MRI in the evaluation of the lower urinary tract, and routine clinical application is therefore not likely for the foreseeable future.[80,81] However, as a research tool

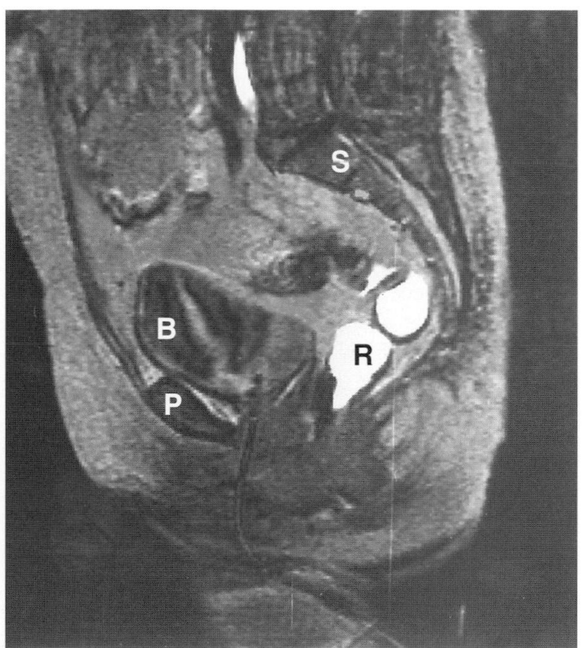

a

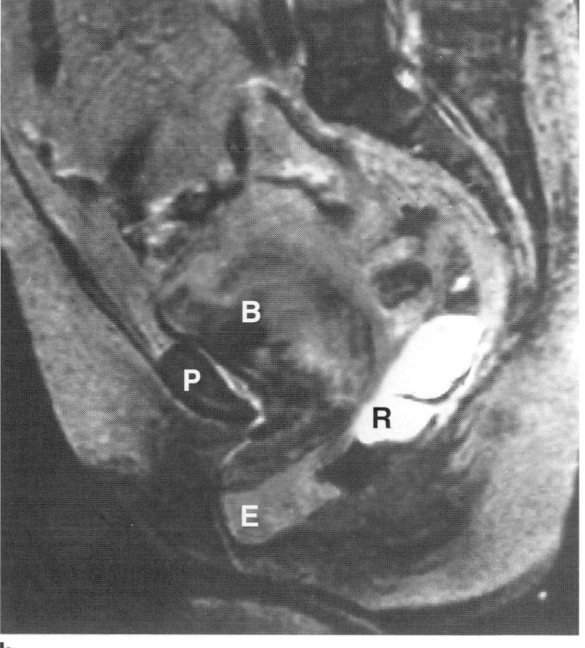

b

Figure 11.8 Sagittal MRI of female pelvis obtained at rest (a) and during sustained Valsalva maneuver (b). Past history of hysterectory and vaginal repair. P = symphysis pubis; S = sacrum; B = bladder. Note the use of gadolinium DTPA to improve definition of the rectum. During Valsalva maneuver, a prominent enterocele (E) and small rectocele (R) are demonstrated. From Ref. 106, with permission.

MRI has a huge potential to explore the mechanisms of urinary incontinence and/or genitourinary prolapse in individual patients, and to study changes in anatomy over time in relation to aging, childbirth or conservative or surgical treatment. The main advantages and disadvantages of MRI are summarized in Table 11.2.

TECHNIQUE OF MAGNETIC RESONANCE IMAGING

Detailed discussion of the principles of MRI is beyond the scope of this chapter. For brief discussions of aspects of MRI technique relevant to urogynecology the reader is referred to the study of Aronson *et al.*[82] and the review by Kirschner-Hermanns *et al.*[81] Standard MRI uses data obtained from the primary coil, the 'body' coil. For detailed evaluation of the soft tissues of the pelvis improved resolution is provided by the use of surface coils placed close to the area of interest. However, the improvement in resolution comes at the cost of increased depth sensitivity, i.e. there is a greater loss of signal strength with increasing distance from the coil. The recent introduction of endoluminal coils increases the image resolution which can be achieved in the pelvis, albeit within a limited distance from the coil (3.5 cm). In combination with an array of surface coils (the phased array multicoil technique), the distance at which good resolution can be obtained increases (6–8 cm),[82] allowing detailed visualization of structures around the endoluminal coil. In a comparison of MR images obtained with body coil to those obtained using an endovaginal coil, Tan *et al.* found that the endovaginal MRI technique was superior in demonstrating pelvic floor and urethral anatomy.[83]

While endoluminal coils increase the resolution of MRI images, as with vaginal US[47] there is a potential for interference with resting anatomy and mobility of pelvic structures. Although the coil is soft and pliable, expansion of the vaginal lumen around the probe may lead to concealment of anatomical defects lateral to the vagina, and the mass of the coil may act like a pessary to support the anterior vaginal wall.[82] As yet there are no data available on the magnitude of this effect. However, improvements in the resolution which can be obtained from standard MRI techniques may in future render the use of endoluminal coils unnecessary.

MRI of the pelvis is generally performed in three planes – axial, sagittal, and coronal – although customization of the image plane may be useful for imaging of specific structures.[80] Indeed, it is one of the unique advantages of MRI, that the plane of the image may be made perpendicular or parallel to the axis of any structure of interest. Older MRI scanning techniques required minutes rather than seconds to acquire data, so that movement artefact was a significant problem and dynamic studies of the pelvis were effectively impossible. More recently fast-spin echo (FSE) imaging has very

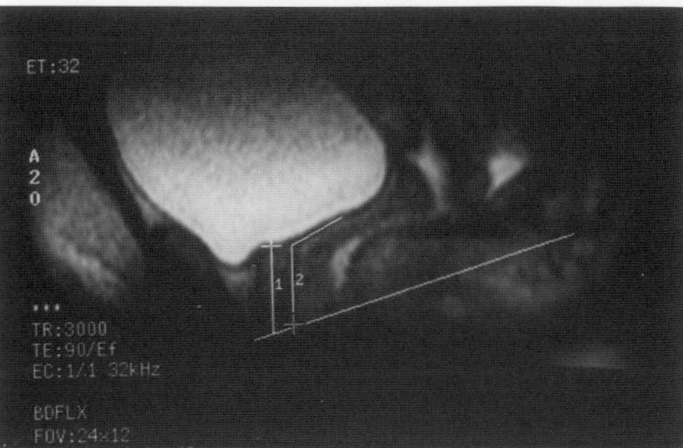

Figure 11.9 Sagittal T2 weighted MRI of female pelvis in sitting position shows high signal urine within the bladder. The distance between bladder neck and the pubococcygeal line (1) and the posterior urethrovesical angle (2) can be measured in the more physiological sitting position. From Ref. 84, with permission.

much reduced the time taken to obtain T2 weighted scans, reducing motion artefact considerably. Gradient echo (GRE) images can be obtained very rapidly (<1 s each), allowing dynamic imaging of the mobility of pelvic floor structures during Valsalva, but the lower signal to noise ratio of GRE compared with FSE prevents the delineation of small structures with GRE. Glucagon (or butylscopolamine) is normally administered to the patient to reduce artefact resulting from peristalsis of adjacent bowel.

In general MRI has been performed with the patient in the supine position. While this is perfectly adequate for most purposes, it is obviously not ideal for assessing the position and mobility of pelvic structures, where symptoms and signs are related to the posture and the effect of gravity. Recently an open-configuration magnet has become available, allowing imaging in seated and other positions, so that static and dynamic MRI studies can be performed in a more physiological upright posture[84] (Fig. 11.9). The image resolution which can be obtained with these scanners is inferior to that obtained by standard supine scans, so that at present the two techniques are complementary.

ASSESSMENT OF THE BLADDER NECK, URETHRA AND PELVIC FLOOR

The use of MRI for the investigation of lower urinary tract and pelvic floor dysfunction dates back only a decade, to the early study of Klutke *et al.* in 1990.[79] At this stage, scanning times were generally too long to record dynamic changes of the pelvic floor,[85] but it was clear that improvements in MRI technology would create major new opportunities for pelvic floor evaluation. MRI was able to confirm pelvic floor damage, and identify defects not suspected from clinical examination.[85] Early experience with imaging of the urethra was also encouraging, providing high-resolution images of the urethra and surrounding structures, including the use of dynamic images obtained during graduated abdominal straining.[86] Further evidence on the value of dynamic imaging in assessing pelvic floor descent came from the same authors in 1991, again using rapid acquisition of MRI images (6–12 s) during straining.[87] Pelvic organ descent was measured in relation to a line drawn from the inferior border of the symphysis pubis to the last coccygeal joint. The authors found that the resting position of the pelvic organs did not allow accurate prediction of the position at maximum prolapse during straining, suggesting that dynamic imaging is more helpful. The technique was able to image pelvic prolapse in all three compartments simultaneously, and was valuable in the identification of enteroceles or of defects in the rectovaginal septum, which could be visualized well. The authors pointed out that the simultaneous measurement of detrusor pressure might be useful.

Kirschner-Hermanns *et al.* used MRI to image the pelvis of stress incontinent patients and healthy volunteers with and without contrast medium.[88] MRI identified changes in the levator ani of the stress incontinent patients, such as a reduction in the dorsal angulation of the levator plate and a reduced signal intensity of the muscle suggestive of degeneration in the form of replacement of muscle by fatty and connective tissues. Traumatic defects in the levator ani due to childbirth, instrumentation or incontinence surgery could be clearly seen. Goodrich *et al.* again used conventional MRI and dynamic imaging to study pelvic floor descent during Valsalva in normal volunteers and in women with pelvic floor relaxation.[89] Static and dynamic MRI were reported to be more sensitive in assessing and grading pelvic floor relaxation than clinical pelvic examination. The authors considered MRI assessment of the posterior urethrovesical angle to be more accurate than that achieved by lateral bead chain cystourethrography because MRI does not interfere with anatomy (although the MRI scans were performed in the supine position). The authors also reported the use of a pseudokinematic cineloop to demonstrate pelvic floor descent using images from a series of increasingly strong, graduated Valsalva maneuvers. As MR image acquisition times fall with advancing technology, the possibility of showing the movement of the entire pelvis during increases in abdominal pressure in this way is very attractive.

As discussed previously, the use of an endovaginal coil combined with a pelvic phased array coil can enhance the image resolution obtained during pelvic MRI. Employing this technique, Aronson *et al.* found that the mean volume of the retropubic space was roughly twice as great in stress incontinent compared with continent nulliparous controls.[82] The technique allowed visualization of landmarks such as the paravaginal attachment of the endopelvic fascia to the arcus tendineus fascia pelvis, and the condensation of the posterior pubourethral ligament. Demonstration of the quality of such pelvic support structures might prove useful to surgeons in the selection of the correct operation for incontinence or pelvic organ prolapse. In a similar fashion, Tan *et al.* used fast-spin echo (FSE) endovaginal MRI in healthy nulliparous volunteers to examine in detail the normal anatomy of the female pelvic floor.[90] The pelvic diaphragm and urogenital diaphragm were seen clearly, but the endopelvic fascia was not convincingly demonstrated using this technique. Images were sufficiently detailed for the authors to identify two structures not previously described, termed the periurethral and paraurethral ligaments, which were also identified on MRI and dissection studies of cadavers.

Christensen et al studied pelvic floor contractions in normal volunteers using MRI, demonstrating the dynamic displacement of the pelvic organs during the maneuver.[91] The images were difficult to obtain because the authors used slower scanning techniques (about 90 seconds for each plane of section), and the position of the pelvic organs was thus dependent on the ability of the subjects to maintain pelvic floor contraction for an extended period. Bø *et al.* have recently demonstrated significant movement of the coccyx during pelvic floor contraction,[92] particularly in healthy volunteers, suggesting that the coccyx is perhaps not an ideal reference point for measuring pelvic floor descent during dynamic MRI studies. Bladder neck mobility during straining and pelvic floor contraction could be measured, as with ultrasound, with reduced elevation on pelvic floor contraction and larger descent on straining in incontinent patients compared with healthy volunteers.

A recent comparison of pelvic floor muscle morphology in asymptomatic women and women with urinary incontinence identified several characteristic features frequently found in incontinent women (Fig. 11.10), including loss of the hammock-like shape of the vagina on cross-sectional images, and higher signal intensity of the levator ani muscles.[93] However, urodynamic and functional parameters did not correlate with the changes in the pelvic floor muscles seen on MRI. It was acknowledged that measurement of the thickness of the levator ani muscle by MRI is prone to a number of methodological problems. Firstly, limitations in measurement accuracy are imposed by the spatial resolution of the scanning technique. More importantly, depending on the parameters used for MR imaging, the chemical-shift artefact occurring at the interface between tissues of different composition may exaggerate the thickness of the levator muscle on one side and underestimate the muscle thickness on the other.

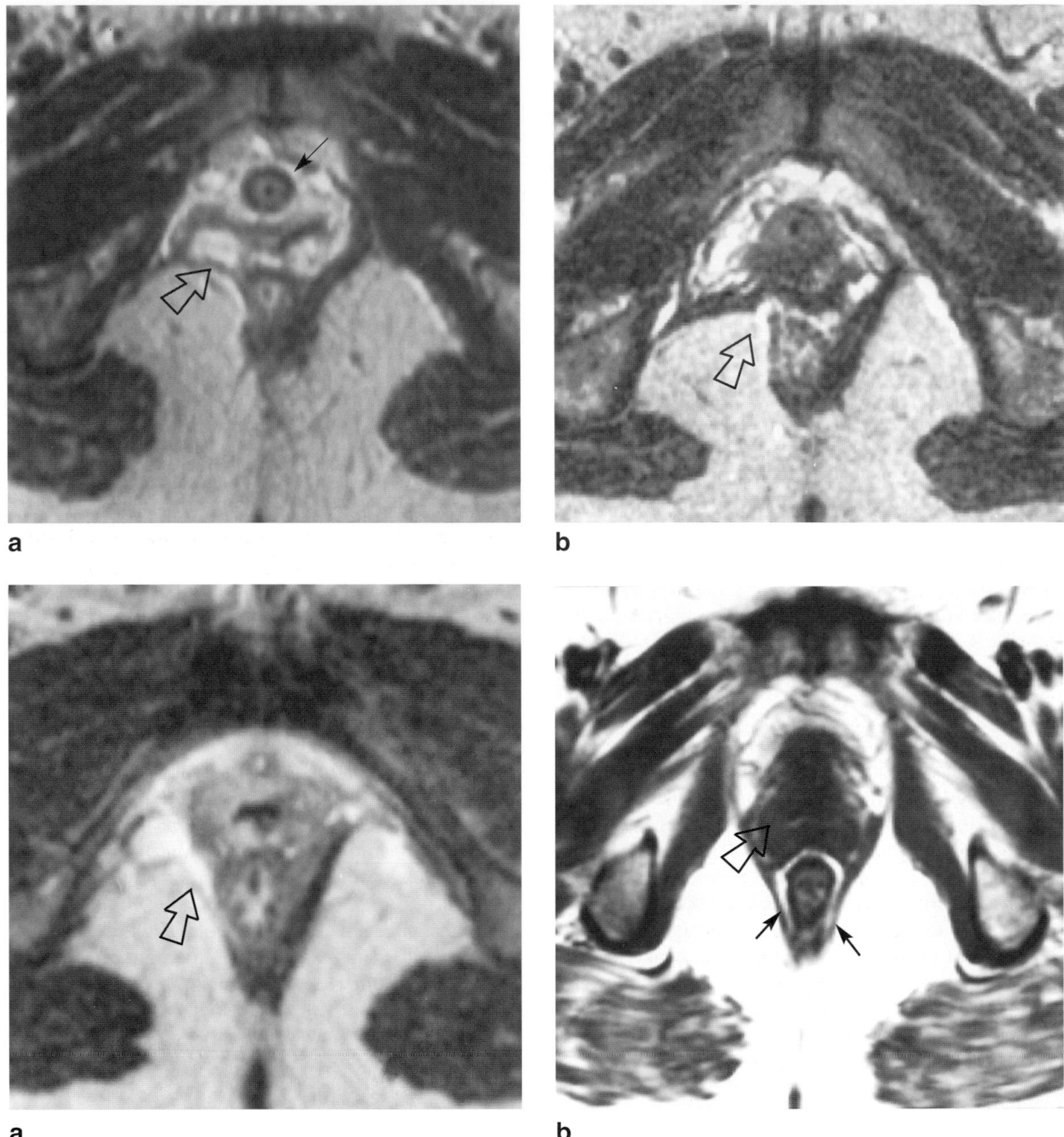

Figure 11.10 Transverse T1 weighted MRI sections (patient supine) showing some typical findings in women with pelvic floor dysfunction.

a) Increased signal intensity of the right levator muscle (large arrow) shows the 'chemical shift artefact'. Normal target-like appearance of the urethra (small arrow).

b) Normal left levator muscle, but no demonstration of pararectal (arrow) or paraurethral portions of levator muscle on right side.

c) No visible striated muscle of right levator (arrow) in a patient with previous forceps delivery.

d) Loss of the hammock-like configuration of the vagina (large arrow). Normal wine-glass shape (small arrows) of levator muscle, but thin levator and increased urethrosymphyseal distance. From Ref. 93, with permission.

Few comparisons have been made between MRI and other modalities of imaging the pelvic floor and lower urinary tract, partly because MRI has only very recently started to provide the sort of dynamic imaging readily achieved with other modalities. Vanbeckevoort *et al.* compared MRI of the pelvis to colpocystodefecography (CCD), and found that CCD was superior to MRI in the detection of genitourinary prolapse in all three compartments, and especially the anterior and middle compartments.[94] One reason for the superiority of CCD in detecting prolapse in this study may have been that it was carried out in the sitting position, whereas MRI was performed with the patient supine. In contrast to these findings, Gufler *et al.* compared dynamic MRI with either colpocystorectography or lateral bead chain cystourethrography and found that MRI was as good as or better than the other modalities in the detection of prolapse.[95] Clearly there are other advantages to the use of MRI, e.g. non-invasiveness and avoidance of ionizing radiation (see Table 11.2).

Early experience with the use of MRI for the evaluation of the male pelvic floor was reported recently by Mikuma *et al.*[96] Static MRI images in healthy volunteers showed the bulk of the intra-urethral striated sphincter muscle to be anterior and lateral to the urethra, and demonstrated the levator ani, including the pubourethral portion. Dynamic images obtained by FSE scanning during voluntary anal contraction demonstrated movement of the membranous urethra and bladder base towards the symphysis pubis, and also thinning of the intra-urethral striated sphincter muscle. It was unclear whether this thinning was a passive or active event. Myers *et al.* studied 15 men with MRI of the pelvis before they underwent radical prostatectomy, and found the images useful in clarifying pelvic anatomy.[97] They felt that MRI provided a better understanding of the anatomy of perineal and retropubic radical prostatectomy without any of the artefact caused by dissection in cadaver studies. It will be interesting to see what other insights can be gained into the mechanism of post-prostatectomy incontinence in future studies.

Hricak *et al.* found MRI useful in the evaluation of the urethra, demonstrating the characteristic 'target' appearance of the urethra on contrast enhanced T1 weighted images and unenhanced T2 weighted images.[98] The three circles of the target were considered to correspond to an outer layer of (smooth and striated) muscle, an inner layer of urethral mucosa, and the vascular submucosa between them. MRI was useful in the identification of urethral diverticula. Kirschner-Hermanns *et al.* also found that the urethra was well demonstrated after injection of contrast medium (intravenous gadolinium-DTPA), with a characteristic target appearance formed by an inner and an outer hypointense ring around a middle hyperintense ring.[88] They considered the middle hypointense ring to represent the smooth muscle layer, rather than submucosa. Comparison of urethral anatomy on MRI scans with the cross-sectional anatomy of the urethra in cadavers[90,99] confirmed that the MRI target appearance is produced by an outer ring representing the striated sphincter, a middle ring representing the smooth muscle layer, and an inner ring the submucosa and mucosa. Tunn *et al.* evaluated the proximal urethral diameter in women without and with urinary incontinence or genitourinary prolapse, and found no difference between the diameters in the two groups.[93] MRI is, however, useful in the detection of a wide range of abnormalities of the urethra and periurethral tissues, e.g. congenital abnormalities, fistulae, diverticula, and tumours.[100] It has also been suggested that MRI is superior to double-balloon catheter urethrography, often considered to be the gold standard investigation for urethral diverticula, and that it should now be the primary imaging modality for such patients.[101] MRI has been used in the evaluation of voiding in men, using fast snapshot images obtained with an echoplanar imaging (EPI) scanner.[102] Images obtained allowed non-invasive analysis of bladder emptying during voiding, albeit with the subjects lying on their side in a cradle. Whether this technique can be developed to a point where it is useful in research remains to be seen. Newer scanners allowing imaging in an upright position might provide a more physiological, and therefore perhaps more useful, technique.

ASSESSMENT OF CHANGES IN THE PELVIC FLOOR IN RELATION TO CHILDBIRTH OR SURGERY

As a non-invasive imaging technique which avoids the need for ionizing radiation, MRI lends itself well to research studies of the changes in the pelvic floor over time in relation to childbirth or surgery. Obviously US is preferable in terms of cost and availability, but MRI provides greater detail of pelvic organ support than ultrasound. Goodrich *et al.* put MRI to good use in evaluating the anatomical effects of surgery for prolapse by a vaginal approach in five women.[89] Interestingly, after surgery the levator hiatus tended to widen and the levator plate was more vertical than before surgery, but all of the women showed minimal movement of the levator plate on straining, similar to that of the healthy volunteers, and the prolapse was considered to be completely resolved. Carr *et al.* found MRI to be an excellent research tool in evaluating the fate of periurethral collagen injected for stress incontinence.[103] In a study of the position and volume of periurethral collagen after surgery in 32 women, neither the position nor the volume of injected collagen were predictive of clinical outcome. Further MRI studies into the relation between the anatomical effects of surgery and the ultimate clinical outcome may well contribute in future to a growing understanding of stress incontinence and pelvic organ prolapse, and perhaps allow the development of improved surgical techniques.

Changes in the pelvic floor after vaginal delivery were retrospectively analysed by Hayat *et al.* from serial scans of 14 women, originally obtained for a study of uterine involution using MRI.[104] They found minimal changes in a variety of anatomical parameters obtained from the scans and no correlation between these measurements and birthweight, although the very small number of patients followed serially (six subject) suggests that study size may have been insufficient to demonstrate any significant differences. Recovery of the levator ani muscle after vaginal delivery has been documented by Tunn *et al.* using MRI of the pelvis.[105] At one day after delivery the signal intensity of the levator ani muscle was reduced on T1 weighted images in most women, and increased on T2 weighted images, suggesting muscle damage, but these changes resolved in almost all women by 6 months. Both the levator hiatus and the urogenital hiatus were enlarged immediately after delivery, and returned to their normal size within 2 weeks, although the magnitude of the changes varied widely. Further studies of this type would be interesting, especially larger studies and studies with controls obtained from prenatal scans in the same patients, or matched groups of nulliparas. MRI is potentially a powerful tool for studying postpartum changes in pelvic floor anatomy and function, and future research will no doubt increase our understanding of the mechanisms of pelvic floor damage and dysfunction after childbirth.

SUMMARY

Imaging is potentially very useful in the evaluation of pelvic floor dysfunction and incontinence since it can identify anatomical abnormalities on static images and provide additional evidence of abnormalities of pelvic floor function during dynamic imaging. Each of the techniques has its own advantages and disadvantages (Table 11.2). Although a large number of anatomical defects associated with dysfunction have been identified, demonstrating abnormalities of structure is unlikely to fully explain the mechanism of dysfunction in individual patients because so many different factors are involved in pelvic floor dysfunction and incontinence. While our understanding of the precise detail of the mechanisms of genitourinary prolapse and stress incontinence remains limited, imaging will continue to play only an adjunctive role in the routine assessment of these patients. In the report of the 1st International Consultation on Incontinence, only residual urine measurement by transabdominal ultrasound was recommended as part of the routine initial evaluation of the incontinent patient, as a safety parameter and in the evaluation of treatment outcome.

The roles of the different imaging modalities will continue to change in future as new research clarifies the relative accuracy and repeatability of the different techniques. Advances in imaging technology may well increase the role of some modalities, particularly MRI, where shorter scanning times, new scanner configurations, and higher resolution will increase the power of the technique. Imaging of the anatomy of the soft tissues of the pelvis by MRI or ultrasound, previously inaccessible except at operation, may allow much more precise understanding of anatomical defects in individual patients. It will be interesting to see whether the greater depth of anatomical information available before surgery using modern imaging will influence the anatomical or clinical outcome after surgery.

For now, imaging remains a very useful tool in selected patients with pelvic floor dysfunction and incontinence. The use of modern imaging modalities in research will no doubt contribute to a rapid advance in our understanding of pelvic floor function and dysfunction in the future.

REFERENCES

1. Enhorning G, Miller ER, Hinman F. Urethral closure studied with cineroentgenography and simultaneous bladder-urethra pressure recording. *Surg Gynecol Obstet* 1964;**118**:507–16.
2. Bates CP, Whiteside CG, Turner-Warwick R. Synchronous cine/pressure/flow/cystourethrography with special reference to stress and urge incontinence. *Br J Urol* 1970;**42**:714–23.
3. Artibani W, Andersen JT, Ostergard DR, *et al.* Imaging and other investigations. In: *Incontinence. Report of the 1st International Consultation on Incontinence*, Monaco, 1998.
4. Carrico C, Lebowitz RL. Incontinence due to an infrasphincteric ectopic ureter: why the delay in diagnosis and what the radiologist can do about it. *Pediat Radiol* 1998;**28**(12):942–9.
5. Braverman RM, Lebowitz RL. Occult ectopic ureter in girls with urinary incontinence: diagnosis using CT. *Am J Roentgen* 1991;**156**:365.
6. Mandal AK, Sharma SK, Vaidyanathan S, Goswami AK. Ureterovaginal fistula: summary of 18 years' experience. *Br J Urol* 1990;**65**:453–6.
7. Horbach NS, Ostergard DR. Predicting intrinsic sphincter dysfunction in women with stress urinary incontinence. *Obstet Gynecol* 1994;**84**:188–92.
8. Govier FE, Pritchett TR, Kornman JD. Correlation of the cystoscopic appearance and functional integrity of the female urethral sphincteric mechanism. *Urology* 1994;**44**:250.
9. Mikulicz-Radecki F. Röntgenologische studien zur ätiologie der urethralen inkontinenz. *Zbl Gynak* 1931;**55**:7.
10. Gordon D, Pearce M, Norton P, *et al.* Comparison of ultrasound and lateral chain urethrocystography in the determination of bladder neck descent. *Am J Obstet Gynecol* 1989;**160**(1):182–5.

11. Bergman A, McKenzie CJ, Richmond J, *et al.* Transrectal ultrasound versus cystography in the evaluation of anatomical stress urinary incontinence. *Br J Urol* 1988;**62**:228–34.
12. Dietz HP, Wilson PD. Anatomical assessment of the bladder outlet and proximal urethra using ultrasound and video-cystourethrography. *Int Urogyn J* 1998;**9**(6):365–9.
13. Barnick CG, Cardozo LD, Benness C. Use of routine video-cystourethrography in the evaluation of female lower urinary tract dysfunction. *Neurourol Urodyn* 1989;**8**:447–9.
14. McGuire EJ, Cespedes RD, Cross CA, *et al.* Videourodynamic studies. *Urol Clin North Am* 1996;**23**(2): 309–21.
15. Sand PK, Hill RC, Ostergard DR. Incontinence history as a predictor of detrusor stability. *Obstet Gynecol* 1988;**71**(2):257–60.
16. Homma Y, Batista JE, Bauer SB, *et al.* Urodynamics. In: *Incontinence. Report of the 1st International Consultation on Incontinence*, Monaco, 1998.
17. Abrams P, Blaivas J, Stanton SL, *et al.* The standardisation of terminology of lower urinary tract function. *Scand J Urol Nephrol* 1988;(Suppl.)**114**:5–19.
18. Abrams P. *Urodynamics*, 2nd edn. London: Springer-Verlag, 1997.
19. Massey A, Abrams P. Urodynamics of the female lower urinary tract. *Urol Clin North Am* 1985;**12**(2):231–46.
20. Dupont MC, Albo ME, Raz S. Diagnosis of stress urinary incontinence. An overview. *Urol Clin N Am* 1996;**23**(3):407–15.
21. Faerber GJ, Vashi AR. Variations in valsalva leak point pressure with increasing vesical volume. *J Urol* 1998;**159**(6):1909–11.
22. White RD, McQuown D, McCarthy TA, *et al.* Real time ultrasonography in the evaluation of urinary stress incontinence. *Am J Obstet Gynecol* 1980;**138**:235–7.
23. Handa VL, Jensen JK, Ostergard DR. The effect of patient position on proximal urethral mobility. *Obstet Gynecol* 1995;**86**(2):273–6.
24. Schaer G, Koelbl H, Voigt R, *et al.* Recommendations of the German Association of Urogynecology on functional sonography of the lower female urinary tract. *Int Urogynecol J* 1996;**7**:105–8.
25. Koelbl H, Hanzal E. Imaging of the lower urinary tract. *Curr Opin Obstet Gynecol* 1995;**7**:382–5.
26. Khullar V, Cardozo L. Imaging in urogynaecology. *Br J Obstet Gynaecol* 1996;**103**:1061–7.
27. Schaer GN. Ultrasonography of the lower urinary tract. *Curr Opin Obstet Gynecol* 1997;**9**:313–6.
28. Weidner AC, Low VH. Imaging studies of the pelvic floor. *Obstet Gynecol Clin North Am* 1998;**25**(4):825–48.
29. Tosaka A, Fujii Y, Oka K. Evaluation of transrectal voiding ultrasonography in men with micturition difficulties without apparent organic obstruction of the lower urinary tract. *Eur Urol* 1997;**32**:420–4.
30. Hol M, van Bolhuis C, Vierhout ME. Vaginal ultrasound studies of bladder neck mobility. *Br J Obstet Gynaecol* 1995;**102**:47–53.
31. Hong JY, Lee YS, Lee KS. A comparative study of perineal and transrectal ultrasonography in patients with genuine stress incontinence (abstract). *Proceedings of the 23rd Annual Meeting of the International Continence Society*, Rome, 1993.
32. Pajoncini C, Rosi P, Morcellini R, *et al.* SUI and pelvic floor disease: the best ultrasound scanning approach (abstract). *Neurourol Urodyn* 1998;**17**(4):371–2.
33. Bom N, Lancee CT, van Egmond FC. An ultrasonic intra-cardiac scanner. *Ultrasonics* 1972;**10**:72–6.
34. Goldberg BB, Liu J-B. Endoluminal urologic ultrasound. *Scand J Urol Nephrol* 1991;(Suppl.)**137**:147–54.
35. Messelink EJ, Dabhoiwala NF, Vrij V, *et al.* A pilot study of endoluminal urethral ultrasound – a new modality for cross sectional imaging of the urethra? (abstract). *Proceedings of the 25th Annual Meeting of the International Continence Society*, Sydney, Australia, 1995:431–2.
36. Roehrborn CG, Kurth KH, Leriche A, *et al.* Diagnostic recommendations for clinical practice. In: Cockett ATK, Khoury S, Aso Y, *et al* (eds) Chapter 8. *Proceedings of the 2nd International Consultation on Benign Prostatic Hyperplasia.* Jersey: Scientific Communications International, 1993.
37. Birch NC, Hurst G, Doyle PT. Serial residual urine volumes in men with prostatic hypertrophy. *Br J Urol* 1988;**62**:571–5.
38. Khullar V, Cardozo L, Salvatore S, *et al.* Ultrasound: a non-invasive screening test for detrusor instability. *Br J Obstet Gynaecol* 1996;**103**:904–8.
39. Manieri C, Carter SSC, Romano G, *et al.* The diagnosis of bladder outlet obstruction in men by ultrasound measurement of bladder wall thickness. *J Urol* 1998;**159**:761–5.
40. Schaer GN, Koechli OR, Schuessler B, *et al.* Improvement of perineal sonographic bladder neck imaging with ultrasound contrast medium. *Obstet Gynecol* 1995;**86**(6):950–4.
41. Creighton SM, Pearce JM, Stanton SL. Perineal video-ultrasonography in the assessment of vaginal prolapse: early observations. *Br J Obstet Gynaecol* 1992;**99**:310–3.
42. Mouritsen L, Bach P. Ultrasonic evaluation of bladder neck position and mobility: the influence of urethral catheter, bladder volume, and body position. *Neurourol Urodyn* 1994;**13**:637–46.
43. Vierhout ME, Jansen H. Supine and sitting rectal ultrasound of the bladder neck during relaxation, straining and squeezing. *Int Urogynecol J* 1991;**2**:141–3.
44. Chen GD, Lin LY, Gardner JD, *et al.* Dynamic displacement changes of the bladder neck with the patient supine and standing. *J Urol* 1998;**159**:754–7.
45. Schaer GN, Koechli CR, Schuessler B, *et al.* Perineal ultrasound: determination of reliable examination procedures. *Ultrasound Obstet Gynecol* 1996;**7**(5):347–52.
46. Dietz HP, Wilson PD. The influence of bladder volume on the position and mobility of the urethrovesical junction. *Int Urogyn J* 1999;**10**(1):3–6.
47. Wise BG, Burton G, Cutner A, *et al.* Effect of vaginal ultrasound probe on lower urinary tract function. *Br J Urol* 1992;**70**:12–16.
48. Beco J, Léonard D, Lambotte R. Study of the artefacts induced by linear array transvaginal ultrasound scanning in urodynamics. *World J Urol* 1994;**12**:329–32.
49. Caputo RM, Benson JT. The Q-tip test and urethrovesical junction mobility. *Obstet Gynecol* 1993;**82**(6):892–6.

50. Schaer GN, Koechli OR, Schuessler B, *et al.* Perineal ultrasound for evaluating the bladder neck in urinary stress incontinence. *Obstet Gynecol* 1995;**85**(2):220–4.
51. Mouritsen L, Rasmussen A. Bladder neck mobility evaluated by vaginal ultrasonography. *Br J Urol* 1993;**71**:166–71.
52. Khan KS, Chien PFW, Honest MR *et al.* Evaluating measurement variability in clinical investigations: the case of ultrasonic estimation of urinary bladder volume. *Br J Obstet Gynaecol* 1997;**104**:1036–42.
53. Voigt R, Halaska M, Michels W, *et al.* Examination of the urethrovesical junction using perineal sonography compared to urethrocystography using a bead chain. *Int Urogynecol J* 1994;**5**:212–4.
54. Meyer S, De Grandi P, Schreyer A, *et al.* The assessment of bladder neck position and mobility in continent nullipara, multipara, forceps-delivered and incontinent women using perineal ultrasound: a future office procedure? *Int Urogynecol J* 1996;**7**:138–46.
55. Boos KPW, Hextall A, Toozs-Hobson P, *et al.* The dynamics of urinary incontinence (abstract). *Int Urogynecol J* 1997;**8**(1):S61.
56. Khullar V, Cardozo LD, Kelleher CJ, *et al.* Blood flow in the lower urinary tract in women with genuine stress incontinence and detrusor instability (abstract). *Ultra Obstet Gynecol* 1993;**3**(Suppl. 2):105.
57. Athanasiou S, Khullar V, Boos K, *et al.* Imaging the urethral sphincter with three-dimensional ultrasound. *Obstet Gynecol* 1999;**94**(2):295–301.
58. Peschers U, Schär G, Anthuber C, *et al.* Postpartal pelvic floor damage – is connective tissue impairment more important than neuromuscular changes? (abstract) *Neurourol Urodyn* 1994;**13**:376–7.
59. Toozs-Hobson P, Athanasiou S, Khullar V, *et al.* Why do women develop incontinence after childbirth? (abstract) *Neurourol Urodyn* 1997;**16**:384–5.
60. Toozs-Hobson P, Khullar V, Cardozo L, *et al.* Predicting incontinence six months after childbirth. Does urethral sphincter volume help? (abstract). *Neurourol Urodyn* 1998;**17**(4):369–70.
61. Bernstein IT. The pelvic floor muscles: muscle thickness in healthy and urinary-incontinent women measured by perineal ultrasonography with reference to the effect of pelvic floor training. Estrogen receptor studies. *Neurourol Urodyn* 1997;**16**:237–75.
62. Martan A, Halaška M, Drbohlav P, *et al.* Bladder neck ultrasound: changes with pelvic floor exercises. *Proceedings of the 23rd Annual Meeting of the International Continence Society*, Rome, 1993:207–8.
63. Richmond DH, Murray A. Intra-operative transrectal ultrasound for prediction of surgical outcome in female patients with urinary incontinence (abstract). *Proceedings of the 18th Annual Meeting of the International Continence Society*, Oslo, 1988:208–9.
64. Yamada T, Kawakami S, Mizuo T, *et al.* Bladder neck suspension for stress urinary incontinence by ultrasonically monitored procedure (abstract). *Proceedings of the 22nd Annual Meeting of the International Continence Society*, Halifax, 1992:V1.
65. Yamada T, Nagahama K, Arai G, *et al.* Application of ultrasonography in suburethral sling procedure for stress urinary incontinence (abstract). *Proceedings of the 26th Annual Meeting of the International Continence Society*, Athens, 1996, 131.
66. Hol M, van Bolhuis C, Vierhout ME. Standardized vaginal ultrasound in stress incontinent women before and after Burch colposuspension (abstract). *Proceedings of the 22nd Annual Meeting of the International Continence Society*, Halifax, 1992:180.
67. Elia G, Bergman A. Ultrasound follow-up of periurethral collagen implant. *Proceedings of the 26th Annual Meeting of the International Continence Society*, Athens, 1996:77–8.
68. Nishizawa O, Takada H, Morita T, *et al.* Combined ultrasonotomographic and urodynamic monitoring. *Proceedings of the 12th Annual Meeting of the International Continence Society*, Leiden, 1982:172–3.
69. Perkash I, Friedland GW. Transrectal sonographic urodynamics. *Proceedings of the 13th Annual Meeting of the International Continence Society*, Aachen, 1983:170–2.
70. Shabsigh R, Fishman IJ, Krebs M. Experience with transrectal ultrasonography in urodynamics. *Proceedings of the 16th Annual Meeting of the International Continence Society*, Boston, 1986.
71. Nerstrøm H, Holm HH, Christensen NEH, *et al.* 3-dimensional ultrasound based demonstration of the posterior urethra during voiding combined with urodynamics. *Scand J Urol Nephrol* 1991;(Suppl.)**137**:125–9.
72. Schaer GN, Siegwart R, Perucchini D, *et al.* Examination of voiding in seated women using a remote-controlled ultrasound probe. *Obstet Gynecol* 1998;**91**(2):297–301.
73. Klein H-M, Kirschner-Hermanns R, Lagunilla J, *et al.* Assessment of incontinence with intraurethral US: preliminary results. *Radiology* 1993;**187**:(1)141–3.
74. Strasser H, Frauscher F, Helweg G, *et al.* Transurethral ultrasound: evaluation of anatomy and function of the rhabdosphincter of the male urethra. *J Urol* 1998;**159**:100–5.
75. Schaer GN, Schmid T, Peschers U, *et al.* Intraurethral ultrasound correlated with urethral histology. *Obstet Gynecol* 1998;**91**(1):60–4.
76. Chancellor MB, Liu JB, Rivas DA, Karusick S, Bagley DH, Goldberg B. Intraoperative endoluminal ultrasound evaluation of urethral diverticula. *J Urol* 1995;**153**:72–5.
77. Liu JB, Goldberg BB. Endoluminal vascular and nonvascular sonography: past, present and future. *AJR* 1995;**165**:765–74.
78. Stenzl A, Frank R, Eder R, *et al.* 3-dimensional computerized tomography and virtual reality endoscopy of the reconstructed lower urinary tract. *J Urol* 1998;**159**:741–6.
79. Klutke C, Golomb J, Barbaric Z, *et al.* The anatomy of stress incontinence: magnetic resonance imaging of the female bladder neck and urethra. *J Urol* 1990;**143**:563–6.
80. Strohbehn K, Ellis JH, Strohbehn JA, *et al.* Magnetic resonance imaging of the levator ani with anatomic correlation. *Obstet Gynecol* 1996;**87**(2):277–85.
81. Kirschner-Hermanns R, Fielding JR, Versi E, *et al.* Magnetic resonance imaging of the lower urinary tract. *Curr Opin Obstet Gynecol* 1997;**9**:317–9.
82. Aronson MP, Bates S, Jacoby AF, *et al.* Periurethral and paravaginal anatomy: an endovaginal magnetic resonance imaging study. *Am J Obstet Gynecol* 1995;**173**(6):1702–8.

83. Tan IL, Stoker J, Lameris JS. Magnetic resonance imaging of the female pelvic floor and urethra: body coil versus endovaginal coil. *Magma* 1997;**5**(1):59–63.
84. Fielding JR, Versi E, Mulkern RV, *et al.* MR imaging of the female pelvic floor in the supine and upright positions. *J Magn Reson Imaging* 1996;**6**:961–3.
85. Debus-Thiede G, Hesse U, Mayr B, *et al.* NMRI of the pelvic floor – a preliminary report (abstract). *Neurourol Urodyn* 1990;**9**:392.
86. Yang A, Mostwin J, Zerhouni E. Magnetic resonance imaging of the female urethra. (abstract) *Neurourol Urodyn* 1990;**9**:393.
87. Yang A, Mostwin JL, Rosenshein NB, *et al.* Pelvic floor descent in women: dynamic evaluation with fast MR imaging and cinematic display. *Radiology* 1991;**179**(1):25–33.
88. Kirschner-Hermanns R, Wein B, Niehaus S, *et al.* The contribution of magnetic resonance imaging of the pelvic floor to the understanding of urinary incontinence. *Br J Urol* 1993;**72**:715–8.
89. Goodrich MA, Webb MJ, King BF, *et al.* Magnetic resonance imaging of pelvic floor relaxation: dynamic analysis and evaluation of patients before and after surgical repair. *Obstet Gynecol* 1993;**82**(6):883–91.
90. Tan IL, Stoker J, Zwamborn AW, *et al.* Female pelvic floor: endovaginal MR imaging of normal anatomy. *Radiology* 1998;**206**(3):777–83.
91. Christensen LL, Djurhuus JC, Lewis MT, *et al.* MRI of voluntary pelvic floor contractions in healthy female volunteers. *Int Urogynecol J* 1995;**6**:138–52.
92. Bø K, Lilleas F, Talseth T. Dynamic MRI of pelvic floor and coccygeal movement during pelvic floor muscle contraction and straining (abstract). *Neurourol Urodyn* 1997;**16**:409–10.
93. Tunn R, Paris S, Fischer W, *et al.* Static magnetic resonance imaging of the pelvic floor muscle morphology in women with stress urinary incontinence and pelvic prolapse. *Neurourol Urodyn* 1998;**17**:579–89.
94. Vanbeckevoort D, Van Hoe L, Oyen R, *et al.* Pelvic floor descent in females: comparative study of colpocystodefecography and dynamic fast MR imaging. *J Magn Reson Imaging* 1999;**9**(3):373–7.
95. Gufler H, Laubenberger J, DeGregorio G, *et al.* Pelvic floor descent: dynamic MR imaging using a half-Fourier RARE sequence. *J Magn Reson Imaging* 1999;**9**(3):378–83.
96. Mikuma N, Tamagawa M, Morita K, *et al.* Magnetic resonance imaging of the male pelvic floor: the anatomical configuration and dynamic movement in healthy men. *Neurourol Urodyn* 1998;**17**:591–7.
97. Myers RP, Cahill DR, Devine RM, *et al.* Anatomy of radical prostatectomy as defined by magnetic resonance imaging. *J Urol* 1998;**159**(6):2148–58.
98. Hricak H, Secaf E, Buckley DW, *et al.* Female urethra: MR imaging. *Radiology* 1991;**178**:527–35.
99. Strohbehn K, Quint LE, Prince MR, *et al.* Magnetic resonance imaging anatomy of the female urethra: a direct histologic comparison. *Obstet Gynecol* 1996;**88**(5):750–6.
100. Siegelman ES, Banner MP, Ramchandani P, *et al.* Multicoil MR imaging of symptomatic female urethral and periurethral disease. *Radiographics* 1997;**17**(2):349–65.
101. Neitlich JD, Foster HE, Glickman MG, *et al.* Detection of urethral diverticula in women: comparison of a high resolution fast spin echo technique with double balloon urethrography. *J Urol* 1998;**159**:408–10.
102. Craggs M, Mundy A, Bellringer J, *et al.* Ultra-fast snapshot magnetic resonance imaging during micturition. *Proceedings of the 25th Annual Meeting of the International Continence Society*, Sydney, 1995:149–50.
103. Carr LK, Herschorn S, Leonhardt C. Magnetic resonance imaging after intraurethral collagen injected for stress urinary incontinence. *J Urol* 1996;**155**:1253–5.
104. Hayat SK, Thorp Jr JM, Kuller JA, *et al.* Magnetic resonance imaging of the pelvic floor in the postpartum patient. *Int Urogynecol J* 1996;**7**:321–4.
105. Tunn R, DeLancey JOL, Howard D, *et al.* Levator ani muscle recovery following vaginal birth: MR imaging analysis. *Neurourol Urodyn* 1998;**17**(4):433–4.
106. Tunn R, Paris S, Taupitz M, Hamm B, Fischer W. MR Imaging in posthysterectomy vaginal prolapse. *Int Urogynecol J* 2000;**11**:87–92.

Chapter 12

Electrophysiology of the anterior pelvic floor and urinary sphincter

Simon Podnar, David B Vodušek, Clare J Fowler

INTRODUCTION

The pelvic floor is, for practical reasons, often divided by a sagittal plane along the superficial transverse perineal muscle, splitting the perineal body. In front of the superficial transverse perineal muscle lies the anterior part of the pelvic floor with the genital and urinary tracts, posteriorly the terminal part of the gastrointestinal tract. This division of the pelvic floor follows the traditional division of the pelvic floor among the different surgical disciplines, the anterior part being the domain of gynecologists and urologists, and the posterior part of proctologists.

As a consequence of this arbitrary division, the anterior part of the pelvic floor is mostly concerned with urological and gynecological issues related to the lower urinary tract and sexual function. Table 12.1 presents anterior pelvic floor structures accessible to electrophysiologic tests.

Table 12.1 Anterior pelvic floor structures and their innervation accessible to electrophysiological investigation

Muscles	Bulbocavernosus muscle Urethral sphincter Levator ani
Somatic nerves	Sacral spinal roots Direct sacral plexus branches Pudendal nerve Dorsal penile/clitoral nerves
Vegetative fibers	Sympathetic skin innervation
Central nervous	Sacral spinal cord motor nuclei
System	Corticospinal tracts Motor cortex Dorsal column tracts Brain somatosensory tracts

CLASSIFICATION OF ELECTROPHYSIOLOGICAL TESTS FOR ASSESSMENT OF THE ANTERIOR PELVIC FLOOR AND URINARY SPHINCTERS

Within the pelvic floor, only striated muscles and their associated nerves can be, strictly speaking, electrophysiologically assessed. Testing of the somatosensory and autonomic innervation of the same spinal segments is however also important in evaluation of pelvic floor dysfunction. Hence reference will be made to all electrophysiological tests.

Various classifications of electrophysiological tests are possible. For classification of these tests we have used a functional anatomic approach, as this enables correlation between individual tests and particular nerve or muscle elements (Fig. 12.1). For the purposes of this classification, the nervous system is divided into two motor systems (the somatic and the autonomic), and the (somato) sensory system. Each subsystem comprises central and peripheral parts. An integrative, interneuronal system exists at various levels of the central nervous system.

The motor system comprises an upper motor neuron (i.e. all neurons involved in supraspinal motor control), a lower motor neuron (motor neurons in the spinal cord) and muscle. The somatosensory system can be subdivided into a peripheral part (receptors and the sensory input into the spinal cord) and a central part (ascending pathways in the spinal cord and the brain). Sensory fibers from skin and muscle are called somatic afferents, while those accompanying autonomic (parasympathetic or sympathetic) fibers are referred to as visceral afferents.

This simplified model of the sacral neuromuscular system enables functional grouping of the electrophysiological tests of the anterior pelvic floor and urinary sphincters (Fig. 12.1):

(a) Tests evaluating the somatic motor system (electromyography – EMG, terminal motor latency measurements, and motor evoked potentials – MEP).
(b) Tests evaluating the sensory system (sensory neurography, somatosensory evoked potentials – SEP).
(c) Methods assessing reflexes (i.e. evaluating in its entirety the respective part of the somatic or visceral sensory system, the central integrative processes, and motor pathways); described in Chapter 17.
(d) Tests assessing the autonomic nervous system functioning of sympathetic or parasympathetic fibers.

Such a classification allows a more logical delineation of tests, which is preferable to a random description of tests by terms given to them by the authors who introduced them.

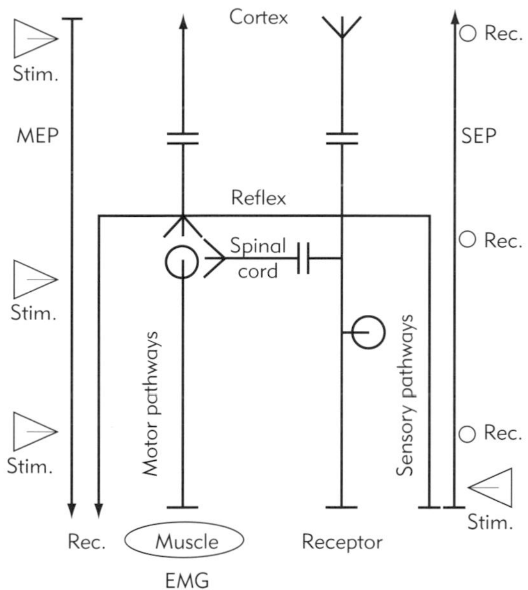

Figure 12.1 Components of the somatic sensory and motor systems and the electrophysiological tests that evaluate them. Arrows on the motor (left) side indicate different stimulation sites (from above) of motor cortex, spinal roots and peripheral nerves (terminal motor latency test). Small circles on the sensory (right) side indicate different recording sites (from below) from peripheral nerve (sensory nerve action potenial – SNAP), spinal roots/cord, somatosensory cortex. (Note that for SNAP recording either distal stimulation and proximal recording[57] or reverse[58] could be employed.) In addition, concentric needle electromyography (CNEMG) and single fiber electromyography (SFEMG) assess the lower motor neuron and muscle. Kinesiological EMG evaluates the integrity of upper motor neuron and neurocontrol reflex arcs.

SOMATIC MOTOR SYSTEM TESTS

Electromyography (EMG)

The term 'EMG' is used without consistent qualifiers for several different diagnostic procedures, all of which record the bioelectrical activity from muscle.

The EMG most practically indicates the activity in a particular muscle during the test period. If urodynamic parameters (such as bladder pressure and uroflow) are recorded simultaneously, and the findings correlated, important information can be obtained on the lower urinary tract function (particularly bladder/sphincter coordination). This has been termed a 'kinesiological' EMG to distinguish it from other types of diagnostic EMG procedures.[1] The kinesiological EMG signal can be recorded by various types of surface or intramuscular (needle or wire) electrodes.

Several types of analysis of specifically recorded EMG assist in the differentiation of normal, denervated/reinnervated and myopathic muscle. This has been called a 'motor unit' EMG (as distinct from 'kinesiological'), and it is performed using needle (concentric or single fiber) electrodes.

The EMG can be used to show muscle has been activated through its motor nerve, either by stimulation of motor (M wave, MEP) or of sensory pathways (reflex response). For these purposes both surface and intramuscular electrodes may be used.

EMG with surface electrodes

For non-invasive EMG recordings from the anterior pelvic floor and urethral sphincter various surface-type electrodes have been devised. Small skin-surface electrodes can be applied to the perineal skin. For intravaginal recording a disposable electrode mounted on a foam pad or other custom-built devices are available.[2] Catheter-mounted ring electrodes enable recording from the urethral sphincter.[3] Surface-type electrode recordings are however prone to artefact (which may be difficult to identify), to contamination of the signal from other muscles and the amplitude of muscle activity recorded by surface electrodes is usually low.

EMG with intramuscular electrodes

Recordings with intramuscular electrodes are selective and artefacts can be readily recognized. However, the procedure is invasive and the recordings may not represent the state of the whole large pelvic floor muscles. Bioelectrical activity is typically sampled from one intramuscular detection site in kinesiological EMG, and by recordings of M waves, MEP or reflex responses. Generally, several sites from one or more skin penetrations on each side of a particular muscle are sampled in a concentric needle EMG (CNEMG) and single fiber EMG (SFEMG). The audio output from the electromyographic system's loudspeaker allows assessment of the 'quality of recording' and recognition of the electrophysiologic phenomena.

The female urethral sphincter, which is anatomically separate from the pelvic floor musculature,[4] can be approached either from the perineum (transmucosally), with a needle insertion 0.5 cm lateral to the urethral orifice, or transvaginally, with the aid of a speculum. Transperineal approach is slightly more painful, but provides more muscle tissue for EMG analysis.[5] Some authors recommend the use of a local anesthetic if the perineal approach to the urethral sphincter is employed. This however has no effect on the pain on needle movement within the muscle, and may affect concurrent reflex studies. Few authors recommend cutaneous anesthesia for other muscles, while most laboratories do not use local anesthetic at all. The male urethral sphincter is reached by inserting the needle transcutaneously from the perineum, about 4 cm anterior to the anus, then advancing it towards the fingertip palpating the apex of the prostate. The levator ani muscle can be located by transrectal or transvaginal palpation and reached transcutaneously from the perineum or transvaginally with the needle electrode. The bulbocavernosus muscle, which in the female is a very thin muscle, is reached by needle insertion transcutaneously from the perineum lateral to the labia majora, to a depth of about 1–2 cm. In males the bulbocavernosus muscle is easy to locate, the needle being advanced transcutaneously paramedially in the perineum to a similar depth as in the female.

Kinesiological EMG

The normal (kinesiological) sphincter EMG shows some continuous activity of low threshold motor unit potentials (MUPs) at rest. Such activity has been recorded for up to 2 hours[6] and during sleep.[7] However, only some recording sites in the levator ani muscle show such activity.[8] Higher threshold motor units (MUs) may be recruited voluntarily or reflexly. Voluntary activation of the urethral sphincter and the pubococcygei can only usually be maintained for about 1 minute.[8]

Normally all EMG activity in the urethral sphincter disappears on voiding. However, lesions between the lower sacral segments and the upper pons result in increased sphincter EMG activity instead of inhibition preceding detrusor contractions (detrusor sphincter dyssynergia).[9] On the basis of the temporal relationship between urethral sphincter and detrusor contractions, three types of dyssynergia have been described.[10] Sphincter contraction (or failure of relaxation) during involuntary detrusor contractions have also been reported in patients with Parkinson's disease.[11] This neurogenic, uncoordinated sphincter action must be distinguished from 'voluntary' contractions that may occur in poorly compliant patients. The pelvic floor muscle contractions seen in non-neuropathic voiding dyssynergia may be a learned abnormal behavior,[12] and may be encountered in women with dysfunctional voiding,[13] which is treatable by bio-feedback.[14]

In the normal female the pubococcygeus shows similar activity patterns to the urethral sphincters at most test sites, i.e. continuous activity at rest, usually some increase of activity during bladder filling, and reflex increase in activity during any activation maneuver performed by the subject (talking, deep breathing, coughing). The pubococcygeus relaxes during voiding; the muscles on either side act together.[8] In stress-incontinence, the activation patterns and the coordination between the two sides may be lost.[15] Abnormal activation of the pubococcygeus was found in a subgroup of women with urinary retention.[14,15]

Little is known about the normal activity patterns of different anterior pelvic floor muscles (urethral sphincter, urethrovaginal sphincter, etc.). It is generally assumed that they all act in a coordinated fashion ('as one muscle'), but differences have been demonstrated even between the intra- and peri-urethral sphincter in normal females.[16] Coordination is frequently lost in pathological states, as is seen also with the urethral sphincter.[17]

The demonstration of voluntary and reflex activation of pelvic floor muscles is indirect proof of the integrity of the respective neural pathways and should be a part of the CNEMG examination (which is performed primarily to diagnose a 'lower motor neuron' lesion).

Concentric needle EMG

The concentric needle electrode consists of a central insulated platinum wire, which is inserted through a steel cannula, with the tip ground to give an elliptical area of 580 × 150 μm. The commonly used amplifier filter settings for CNEMG are 5–10 000 Hz; these need to be defined if MUP parameters are to be measured.[18]

CNEMG can provide information on insertion activity, normal and abnormal spontaneous activity, MUPs, and interference pattern. This type of electrode is able to record electromyographic activity mostly to a distance of 2.5 mm.[19] The number and characteristics of MUs recorded depend both upon the local arrangement of muscle fibers within the MU and the extent of muscle contraction.

In normal muscle, needle movement elicits a short burst of 'insertion activity,' which is due to mechanical stimulation of excitable muscle fiber membranes. This is recorded at a gain setting of 50 μV per division or cm (sweep speed 5–10 ms/division), which is also used to record spontaneous activity (Fig. 12.2). Spontaneous activity can be described according to its density (slight: +, moderate: ++, profuse: +++), or by counting the number of sites (out of 10) at which it is present.

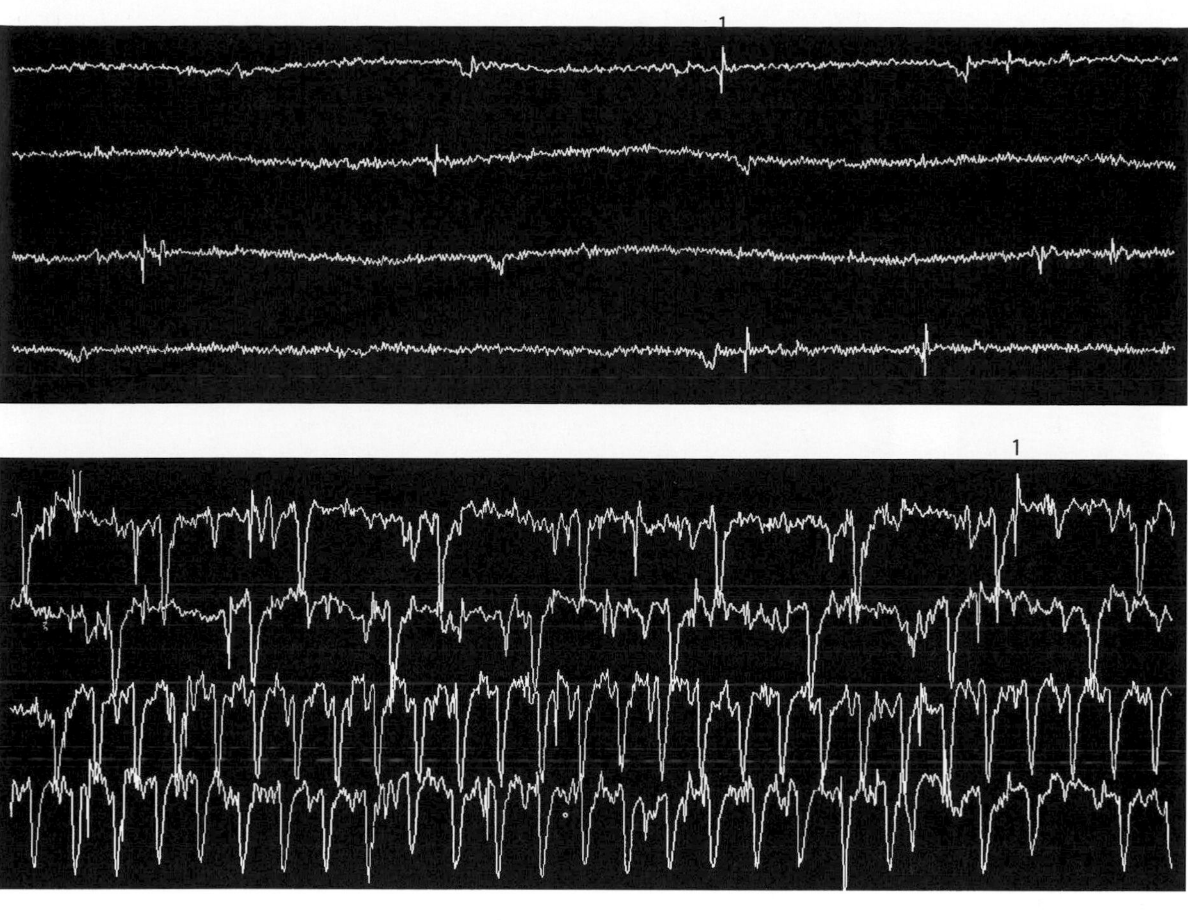

Figure 12.2 Denervation activity in the urethral sphincter muscle (above) and bulbocavernosus muscle (below). (73-year-old female 4 months after cauda equina compression by a postoperative epidural hematoma.) Note abnormal spontaneous activity in the form of short biphasic spikes (fibrillation potentials – 1), biphasic potentials with prominent positive deflections (positive sharp waves – 2), pairs of positive sharp waves (3) and a simple repetitive discharge (lower two lines). Spontaneous activity is more prominent in the bulbocavernosus muscle (+++) than in the urethral sphincter muscle (+).

Continuous firing of low threshold MUPs is the only normal activity recorded with a resting electrode in sphincter muscles in a relaxed subject. (But in the bulbocavernosus and in parts of the pubococcygeal muscle 'electrical silence' is present in relaxation, as in limb muscles.) This 'spontaneous' or 'tonic' low threshold MUP activity has not yet been quantified. Although possible, counting of MUPs is unreliable and impractical. Methods for quantification of the interference pattern (turns/amplitude analysis) are technically not adapted for such a low level of activity.

Additional MUPs are activated reflexly or voluntarily (Fig. 12.3). There are different methods for analysing the bioelectrical activity of MUs, either by analysis of individual MUPs or of the overall activity of intermingled MUPs (the 'interference pattern'). From the practical point of view, some new computer-assisted methods of quantitative EMG ('Multi-MUP') are theoretically preferable to less sophisticated, 'manual' techniques, because of their speed, accuracy, lack of bias and the array of different measures they provide for quantification of MUP.[20,21] Additionally, with the aid of these new techniques it is possible to sample up to 6 MUPs from a single recording site (Fig. 12.3), which is crucial for tiny muscles such as the urethral sphincter. However, no studies using these methods for anterior pelvic floor muscles and the urethral sphincter have yet been published.

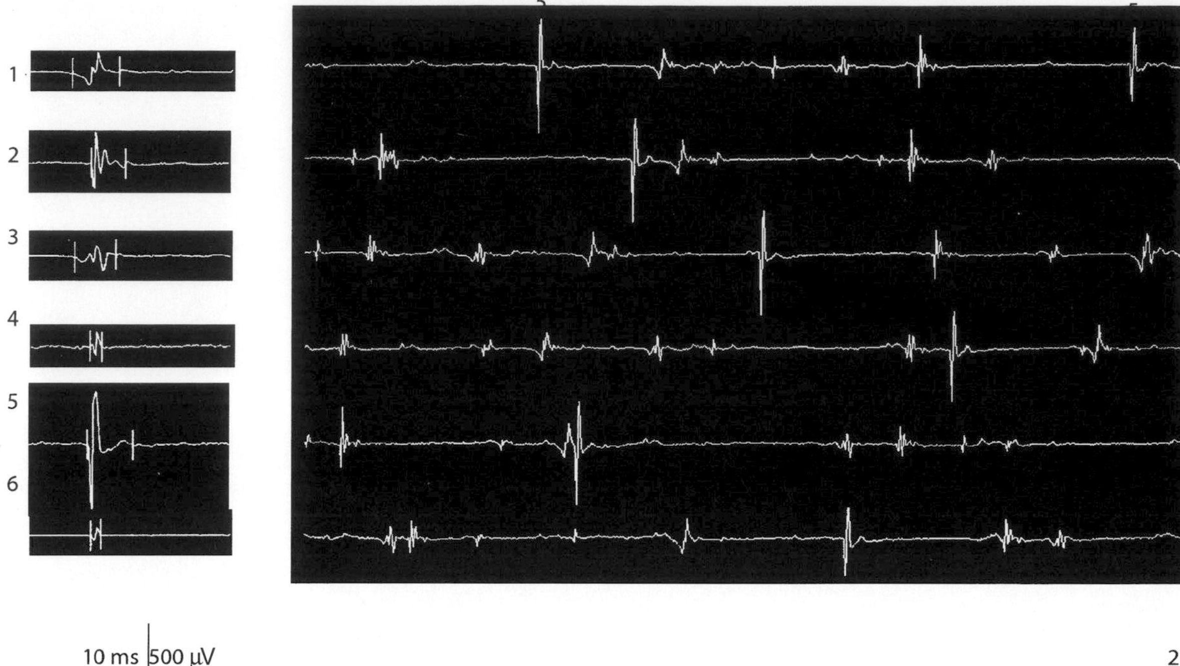

Figure 12.3 Slight voluntary contraction of the left urethral sphincter muscle. (51-year-old female 10 years after cauda equina compression by a herniated intervertebral disk.) Right part of the figure: original recording. At this level of activity computer-assisted ('Multi-MUP') analysis collected six motor unit potentials (MUPs, in the left column). Altogether 15 MUPs were collected in the left half of the muscle (mean amplitude 405 μV, duration 6.6 ms, area 438 μVms, and 33% MUP polyphasicity). (Compare mean duration to 'cut-off' value [47]) Different sweep speeds are used in MUP sample (left column) and original signal.

With manual MUP analysis the MUPs should be analysed at constant settings for amplification (50–500, usually 200 μV/division) and time scale (5–20, usually 10 ms/division), which need to be defined. It has been suggested that only those MUPs which are 'in focus', i.e. with a rise time of the positive-negative slope of the MUP below 0.5 ms, should be analysed.[22] If MUPs are sampled automatically, care should be taken that whole MUPs are displayed on the screen.

Several MUP parameters have proven empirically useful in examining limb muscles in the diagnosis of neuromuscular disease. Traditionally, amplitude, duration, and the number of phases have been measured. If computer analysis is available, other parameters (number of turns, area, rise time of negative peak, spike duration, area of negative peak, thickness, size index) can also be employed.[23,24] Size index was shown in a limb muscle to be particularly useful in differentiating normal from reinnervated MUPs,[24] and it is also potentially useful in pelvic floor muscles.

Several controversies still exist regarding MUP analysis. 'Satellite' potentials are defined as components of MUPs that begin more than 3 ms after the end of the main component.[25] Most authors would not include 'satellite' potentials[25] in MUP duration, but especially on manual MUP analysis this may prove less clear in the laboratory setting than in theory. MUPs with 'satellite' potentials are in themselves a sign of neuromuscular pathology. Their number should be counted and reported, as this may be particularly helpful in the diagnosis of sphincter abnormalities in multiple system atrophy (MSA) patients. Another controversy concerns MUP 'phases'. They are defined as the 'number of the potential baseline crossings plus one'.[18] Some define as polyphasic MUPs that have four or more phases,[26] while others only those which have more than four,[27] or even more than five phases.[28] Some of the MUPs from normal MUs had five phases in simulation experiments.[29] However, it has been shown that the pattern of abnormalities did not change when either four or five phases were taken as polyphasic,[29] but each criterion should be consistently applied.

On manual MUP analysis each MUP can be included in the sample only if it repeatedly appears in a prolonged recording of EMG activity (Fig. 12.3). Individual MUPs need to be recorded at least three times to ensure individuality. Using a trigger and delay line and, most importantly, automated computer methods facilitates identification of MUPs (including their late components). Identification of MUPs becomes less reliable on stronger activation of muscle.

In the urethral sphincter muscle ten different MUPs must be recorded; sampling of 20 MUPs is preferable (as is the case in other muscles).[26] This will probably become feasible with the introduction of newer computer-assisted methods (Fig. 12.3).

The amplitude of MUPs is mostly below 1 mV and certainly below 2 mV in the normal urethral sphincter. Most are less than 7 ms in duration, and few (less than 15%) are above 10 ms. Most are bi- and tri-phasic, but up to 15–33% may have four or more phases (polyphasic). However, potentials with more than six phases are practically never encountered in healthy subjects. Normal MUPs are stable – their shape does not change on repetitive recording. Because of differences in technique and lack of common standards, it is not realistic to provide more precise 'normative' data, but individual studies can be referred to.[16,28,30–32]

By voluntary and reflex activation higher threshold MUPs are recruited. The number of these recruitable MUs is estimated. Normally, MUPs should intermingle to produce an 'interference' pattern on the oscilloscope when muscle is well contracted, and during a strong cough. At such levels of activity instead of MUP analysis, automatic quantitative analysis of the interference pattern using the turns/amplitude plot could be employed, but this has not yet been used in the anterior pelvic floor muscles. Several parameters have been described in the interference pattern analysis as well: number of turns/second, amplitude/turn,[33] activity, number of short segments and envelope.[34] The sensitivity and specificity of different EMG parameters in revealing denervation, and reinnervation, have not been adequately investigated and no relevant studies exist for the anterior pelvic floor muscles or the urethral sphincter. A study of limb muscles has shown superior sensitivity, and similar specificity for reinnervation, of automated interference pattern analysis, as compared with quantitative MUP duration assessment, when the final neurological diagnosis was taken as the 'gold standard'.[35] In addition, such automated interference pattern analysis is even faster and easier to apply than the latest quantitative MUP analysis techniques. Parameters analysed in the interference pattern also allow identification of changes in MU architecture.

Although EMG abnormalities are detected as a result of a host of different lesions and diseases, there are in principle only two standard manifestations which can occur: (i) disease of the muscle fibers themselves; and (ii) changes in their innervation.

CONCENTRIC NEEDLE EMG FINDINGS DUE TO DENERVATION

Complete denervation results in cessation of all MU activity. Complete electrical silence is noted in the first days following denervation. The diagnosis of complete denervation also requires electrical stimulation of the relevant motor nerve to demonstrate the absence of muscle response. Motor axons take some days to degenerate after injury, so diagnosis is not available for up to 5–7 days after a denervation injury. This is however rarely required in the acute stage because the clinical condition is usually obvious. Approximately 10–20 days after denervation, the 'insertion activity' becomes prolonged and abnormal spontaneous activity appears (Fig. 12.2) in the form of short biphasic spikes (fibrillation potentials) and biphasic potentials with prominent positive deflections (positive sharp waves). (This abnormal activity is derived from denervated single muscle fibers. It gradually decreases and disappears with either reinnervation or complete muscle atrophy.) With axonal reinnervation, MUPs appear again; initially they are short, bi- and tri-phasic, followed shortly by polyphasic, serrated MUPs with a prolonged duration.[27]

In the anterior pelvic floor muscles, complete denervation can be seen after traumatic lesions of the lumbosacral spine or particularly of the pelvis. Most lesions however result in partial denervation.

In partially denervated muscle, some MUPs remain and are eventually intermingled with abnormal spontaneous activity, which appears after 10–20 days. The bulbocavernosus muscle, in which continuously firing MUPs are not seen, is therefore very useful in the assessment of partially denervated muscle (Fig. 12.2). In degenerative conditions, the described changes probably occur during the phase of subclinical sphincter involvement. As the MUPs in sphincter muscles are also short and mostly bi- or tri-phasic, as is pathological spontaneous activity, differentiation of these patterns requires experience.

Chronically partially denervated muscle shows peculiar abnormal insertion and spontaneous activity, which is referred to as 'simple' (Fig. 12.2) or 'complex' repetitive discharges. It is made up of repetitively firing groups of potentials with so little 'jitter' between the potentials that it is deduced that the activity must be due to direct transmission of impulses between muscle fibers.[36] This activity may be provoked by needle movement, muscle contraction, etc., or may occur spontaneously. Such activity may also be found in subjects without any other evidence of neuromuscular disease or lower urinary tract disorder (in such cases it is usually not marked). Abundant repetitive discharges have been proposed to cause impaired relaxation of the urinary sphincter muscle, resulting in urinary retention in some young women (Fowler's syndrome). This pathological spontaneous activity has also been called 'decelerating bursts and complex repetitive discharges'.[37]

In partially denervated sphincter muscle there is, by definition, a loss of MUs. This is difficult to establish, however, as the recruitment of MUs is dependent on patient cooperation. In women this is often more difficult to achieve. The parameters of (i) a reduced number of activated MUs and of (ii) activation of MUs at increased firing rates (as assessed in limb muscles) have been poorly studied (but see Ref. 38). The main barrier to assessment of these parameters is a lack of simultaneous measurement of force (level of contraction), which the electromyographer always assesses in limb muscles.

Collateral reinnervation is shown by prolongation of the waveform of the MUP, which may have small, late components ('satellite potentials'). MUPs show 'instability' ('jitter' and 'blocking' of individual components in a complex potential) due to insecure transmission in newly formed axon sprouts and end-plates. This is not being assessed in routine sphincter EMG, as demonstrated by published reports. Nonetheless, it can be a helpful parameter, which can be evaluated both by SFEMG, as originally described,[39] and by CNEMG, if a low frequency cut-off filter of 0.5 (up to 2) kHz is used along with a trigger-delay unit.[40] In skeletal muscle, providing there is no further deterioration in innervation, the reinnervating axonal sprouts increase in diameter, with a resultant increase in their conduction velocity, so that activation of all parts of the reinnervated MU becomes more synchronous. Thus the amplitude increases and the duration of the MUPs decreases towards normal as measured with CNEMG (Fig. 12.3). In sphincter muscles however, long duration MUs remain a prominent feature of reinnervated MUs, at least in degenerative disease.[41]

CNEMG CHANGES IN PRIMARY MUSCLE DISEASE

There are only a few reports of pelvic floor muscle EMG in generalized myopathy. In skeletal muscle, the typical features of myopathy are small, low amplitude polyphasic units recruited at mild effort. Such changes have not been reported in the anterior pelvic floor even in patients known to have generalized myopathy.[42] Histological involvement of the pelvic floor muscle in limb-girdle muscular dystrophy in a nulliparous female has been reported, but concentric needle EMG of her urethral sphincter was reported as normal.[43] Myopathic involvement has been reported in the puborectalis in patients with myotonic dystrophy.[44]

Single fiber EMG

The SFEMG has been used almost exclusively in the posterior pelvic floor to assess changes due to reinnervation in chronic denervation of the anal sphincter and is dealt with in Chapter 16. It was utilized for assessment of the urethral sphincter and the bulbocavernosus muscle in the late 1970s (when SFEMG was introduced for pelvic floor muscles in Ljubljana), but the examination requires more 'searching for potentials' than CNEMG, and is thus more painful in the female urethral sphincter than CNEMG, and more cumbersome in the deep-lying male sphincter than CNEMG. In the bulbocavernosus muscle (which lacks 'tonic' firing of MU) it is difficult to achieve the prolonged regular activation needed for fiber density measurements. Thus, fiber density measurements in these muscles have been abandoned, while they continued to be employed in the anal sphincter muscle.[45] The possibility of SFEMG to very selectively record the activity of single alpha motor neurons has been applied to study physiological characteristics of the bulbocavernosus reflex responses.[46]

EMG abnormalities in disease states

FINDINGS IN TRAUMATIC AND DEGENERATIVE CONDITIONS

In several conditions gross changes of reinnervation may be detected in MUs of the anterior part of the pelvic floor and the urethral sphincter. A cauda equina lesion results in prolongation and polyphasic MUPs (Fig. 12.3).[28] Similar changes are seen in patients with lumbosacral meningomyelocele. Definite 'neuropathic' changes can be recorded in sphincter muscles of patients with MSA. This entity, which now includes patients previously diagnosed as Shy–Drager syndrome,[41,47] is a progressive neurodegenerative disease, which is often, particularly in its early stages, mistaken for Parkinson's disease. Urinary incontinence occurs early in this condition, often some years before the onset of obvious neurological abnormalities.[48] Urethral sphincter EMG aids in differentiating idiopathic Parkinson's disease from MSA,[41,47] but diagnostic differences may be absent in the early phase of disease.[11]

A study addressing the value of urethral sphincter CNEMG as a means of distinguishing patients with MSA from those with Parkinson's disease found a sensitivity of 0.62 and specificity of 0.92, taking the clinical diagnosis as the 'gold standard'. (The authors rightly point out that these values will depend on the 'cut off' values; they took a mean MUP duration of greater than 6.5 ms and 20% or more MUPs longer than 10.5 ms.)[47]

In general, CNEMG (detection of pathologic spontaneous activity) has good sensitivity and specificity to reveal moderate and severe partial denervation, and complete denervation, of pelvic floor muscles 3 weeks or more after injury. CNEMG (MUP and interference pattern analysis) has good sensitivity to reveal changes due to reinnervation, which appear months after injury and in chronically progressive conditions. Few comparative studies have been carried out, but CNEMG and SFEMG seem to have, in principle, comparable sensitivity for MU changes due to collateral reinnervation.[45,49] As mentioned, SFEMG has not been systematically employed in the anterior pelvic floor. The use of recently introduced MUP and interference pattern analysis parameters could help to further improve the power of CNEMG. Mostly neurogenic conditions have been studied so far. The specificity of neurogenic versus myogenic changes is not known.

EMG CHANGES IN WOMEN WITH LOWER URINARY TRACT DYSFUNCTION OF POORLY DEFINED CAUSE

Pelvic floor muscle denervation has been suspected to be important in the genesis of genuine stress incontinence (GSI). A relationship between stress incontinence, genito-urinary prolapse and partial denervation of the pelvic floor has been demonstrated, and it was concluded that the pubococcygeus is partially denervated and then reinnervated in women with stress incontinence and/or genital prolapse.[50] CNEMG examination of the pubococcygeus following childbirth shows a significant increase in duration of individual MUPs following labor and vaginal delivery.[51] These changes were most marked in women who had urinary incontinence 8 weeks after delivery, with a history of prolonged second stage and who had given birth to larger babies. In a more recent study significantly more fibrillation potentials, fewer MUPs, a higher percentage of polyphasia, and less maximum voluntary electrical activity were found on a urethral sphincter CNEMG in women with GSI, compared with controls. On muscle biopsy the patient group had lower skeletal muscle, but higher connective tissue content.[52]

CNEMG, which detects both changes of denervation and reinnervation (as occur with peripheral neuromuscular conditions), and abnormal ('idiopathic') spontaneous activity (associated with retention in Fowler's syndrome),[37,53] is recommended in women with unexplained urinary retention.[13–14,53]

Other electrophysiological tests of the somatic motor system

Pudendal nerve conduction tests

Measurement of motor conduction velocity is the standard method of functional evaluation for a motor nerve, but it requires stimulation of the nerve at two well-separated points and measurement of the distance between them. It is especially useful in myelin damage (nerve compression, generalized myelinopathies, etc.) occurring between stimulation points. Two-point stimulation cannot be carried out in the pelvis. The alternative electrophysiological parameter to evaluate a peripheral motor nerve function is the measurement of the terminal motor latency of a muscle response, which requires stimulation of the nerve at only one point.[25] The muscle response is the compound muscle action potential or M-wave.[25] This is supposed to show damage to terminal motor nerve branches as a result of traction to nerves innervating the pelvic floor (during childbirth, chronic constipation, etc). However, it is not a direct measure of denervation or reinnervation of these muscles; the functional relevance of minor latency delays is questionable.

In the anterior pelvic floor terminal motor latency of the pudendal nerve can be measured by recording with a concentric needle electrode from the bulbocavernosus, and the urethral sphincter muscles in response to bipolar surface stimulation placed perianally or perineally.[30] Transrectal stimulation is most frequently utilized, with a specially constructed surface electrode assembly on a gloved finger.[54] Transvaginal stimulation can also be employed. Responses recorded with concentric needle have been reported, but mostly a catheter-mounted electrode has been used for recording EMG responses from the urethral sphincter. Amplitudes of muscle responses have not been evaluated as yet.

Studies have shown that the (perineal) terminal motor latency is significantly prolonged in the group of patients with urinary stress incontinence compared with controls.[50,55] The pudendal terminal latency is prolonged in women with pelvic floor prolapse.[50,56] This is further prolonged following vaginal dissection for repair or suspension procedures.[56]

Motor nerve fibers can also be depolarized (by electrical or magnetic stimulation) within the cauda equina, as can be motor tracts and the motor cortex. These tests are discussed in Chapter 16.

SENSORY SYSTEM TESTS

In addition to clinical (neurological) testing of skin sensation in the perineal region (touch, pinprick) and testing of sensation during cystometry, sensory nerve pathway function is also tested by clinical electrophysiological tests (Fig. 12.1): peripheral sensory pathways are tested by sensory neurography, and the pathways within the central nervous system by somatosensory evoked potentials (SEP).

Sensory neurography

By placing a pair of stimulating electrodes across the glans and a pair of recording electrodes across the base of the penis, a compound nerve action potential can be recorded (with an amplitude of c. 10 μV).[57] It can also be recorded by stimulating transrectally[58] or transperineally (Fig. 12.4). In principle, the method would help to differentiate between sensory and motor fiber involvement (i.e. diagnosis of sensory neuropathy), and between a supra- and infra-ganglionary lesion in a patient with penile sensory loss (giving a normal (Fig. 12.4) or absent compound nerve action potential, respectively). Limited clinical experience with the test has been reported in a few articles.[58]

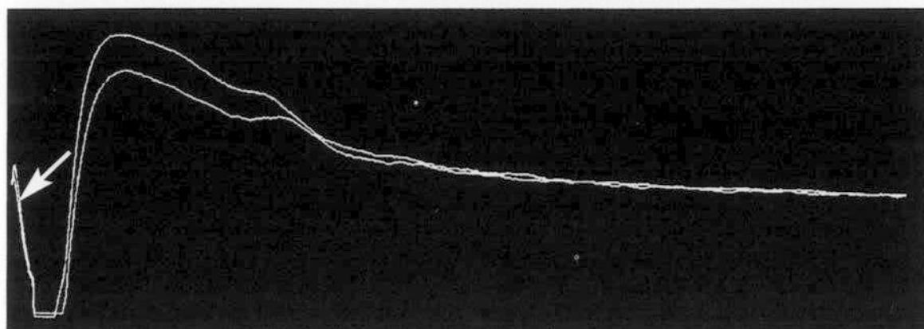

Figure 12.4 Compound sensory nerve action potential (SNAP) recorded with ring electrodes from the penis in a 24-year-old male. He sustained polytrauma due to a traffic accident (including a fracture of the L1 vertebrae and pelvic fracture with urethral injury), one year previously. The patient had paresthesiae in lower limbs; a sensory loss in the saddle area, and particularly the penis (with erectile and ejaculatory difficulties) remained. Arrow points to beginning of two consecutive recordings of 16 averaged SNAPs of the dorsal penile nerve on electrical stimulation of pudendal nerve. A conventional bipolar surface electrode ('pushed' into the perineum 2 cm anteriorly to the anus) was used for stimulation. The patient had abnormal findings on concentric needle electromyography (CNEMG) of the anal sphincter muscle compatible with reinnervation. No reflex response could be obtained on the penile stimulation with the same ring electrodes used for recording. The finding was interpreted as demonstrating a lesion of sensory nerve fibers proximal to the spinal ganglia. A major lesion of pudendal nerve could be excluded.

Neurography of dorsal sacral roots

Compound sensory root action potentials may be directly recorded on stimulation of the dorsal penile and clitoral nerves after exposure of the sacral roots.[59] This enables preservation of roots necessary for perineal sensation in spastic children undergoing dorsal rhyzotomy and decreases the incidence of postoperative voiding dysfunction.[59] In a study using epidural electrodes for recording, root potentials could be obtained in four out of 11 subjects[60] on stimulation of the dorsal penile nerves.

Somatosensory evoked potentials (SEP)

Pudendal SEP

SPINAL SEP

Postsynaptic segmental spinal cord activity (the spinal SEP)[61–64] is revealed by stimulation of the dorsal penile nerve and recording with surface electrodes at the level of the Th12–L2 vertebrae (and the S1, Th6 or iliac spine as reference). Unfortunately, this spinal SEP may be difficult to record in healthy obese male subjects and in women.[61,62] For this reason, such recordings are not in routine use. Stimulation of the dorsal penile nerves, even with epidural electrodes, elicited sacral root potentials in only 13, and cord potentials in nine of 22 subjects.[60] Latencies of these spinal SEPs were about 12 ms,[60] substantiating the results obtained by surface recording.[61–63]

CEREBRAL SEP

On electrical stimulation of the dorsal penile or clitoral nerve, a cerebral SEP can be recorded.[61–63] This SEP is, as a rule, of maximum amplitude at the central recording site (Cz – 2 cm: Fz of the International 10–20 EEG System)[65] and is highly reproducible. Using a stimulus, which is two to four times the sensory threshold current strength,[63] the first positive peak at about 40 ms (called P1 or P40) is usually clearly defined in healthy subjects (compare Fig. 12.5). Later negative (at about 55 ms) and then positive waves show variability in amplitude and expression between individuals.[61,62]

Mechanical stimulation of the distal penis by a custom-designed electromechanical hammer triggered by an oscilloscope has elicited cerebral SEP comparable to standard electrical stimulation in male children (Fig. 12.4).[66] Painless mechanical stimulation is obviously preferable to electrical stimulation when investigating children.

Pudendal SEPs have been advocated in patients with neurogenic bladder dysfunction, e.g. in multiple sclerosis. However, even in patients with multiple sclerosis and bladder symptoms, the tibial cerebral SEP is more often abnormal than the pudendal SEP. Only rarely are the pudendal SEPs abnormal but the tibial SEPs normal, pointing to isolated conus involvement.[32] The pudendal SEP has been found to be of lesser value than a clinical examination looking for signs of spinal cord disease in the lower limbs, i.e. lower limb hyperreflexia and extensor plantar responses in the investigation of urogenital symptoms for detecting relevant neurological disease.[67] Cerebral SEP on penile/clitoral stimulation has been reported as possibly a valuable intraoperative monitoring method in patients whose cauda equina or conus is at risk during a surgical procedure.[68]

CEREBRAL SEP ON ELECTRICAL STIMULATION OF URETHRA AND BLADDER

Cerebral SEP can also be obtained by stimulation of the bladder mucosa.[69] However, it is crucial to use bipolar stimulation since otherwise, somatic afferents are depolarized.[70] These cerebral SEPs have been shown to have a maximum amplitude over the midline (Cz – 2 cm: Fz).[70] As the potential is of low amplitude (1 μV and less) and has a variable configuration, it may be difficult to identify in some control subjects.[64,70] The typical latency of the most prominent negative potential (N1) has been reported to be about 100 ms, but data are variable.[64,70]

These visceral SEPs are claimed to be more relevant in neurogenic bladder dysfunction than the pudendal SEP, as the Aδ sensory (visceral) afferents from the

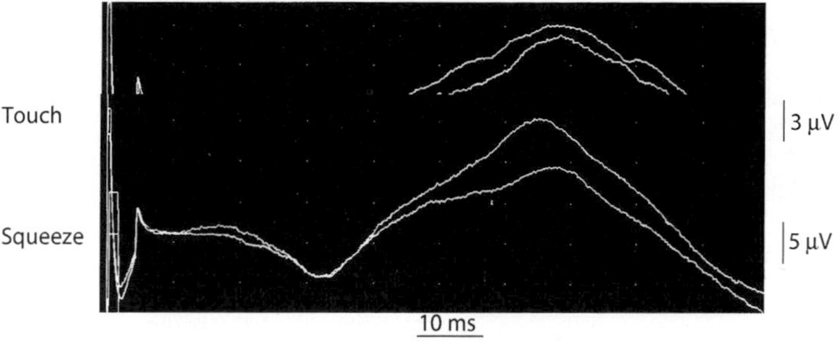

Figure 12.5 Cerebral pudendal somatosensory evoked potential (SEP) on mechanical stimulation of penis in a healthy young male. Upper trace was obtained by electromechanical hammer 'touching' the penile shaft and glans, whereas in the ower trace it was obtained by 'squeezing' them (100 responses averaged twice). Arrows point to peak of wave P40 (P1). The latency decreases and amplitude increases by increasing stimulus strength. Note different amplifications and prominent artefact of electromechanical hammer at the beginning of both recordings.

bladder and proximal urethra accompany the autonomic fibers in the pelvic nerves.[70]

SACRAL REFLEXES

These are presented in Chapter 17.

AUTONOMIC NERVOUS SYSTEM TESTS

All the uro-neurophysiological methods discussed so far only assess the thicker myelinated fibers, whereas it is the autonomic nervous system (especially the parasympathetic system) which is most important for urinary and sexual functions. Information on parasympathetic bladder innervation can to some extent be obtained by cystometry (Chapter 10). Methods by which the parasympathetic and sympathetic nervous system innervating the pelvic viscera could be assessed directly are needed.

In cases of suspected generalized autonomic dysfunction, tests of cardiovascular innervation may be useful. If a general involvement of thin fibers is expected, an indirect way to examine autonomic fibers is to assess thin visceral sensory fiber function by stimulating the proximal urethra or bladder, and by recording sacral reflex responses or cerebral SEP (described in Chapter 17 and above, respectively).

Sympathetic skin respone (SSR)

The sympathetic nervous system mediates sweat gland activity in the skin. Changes in sweat gland activity lead to changes in skin resistance. On 'stressful stimulation,' a potential shift can be recorded with surface electrodes from the skin of the palms and the soles. This has been reported to be a useful parameter in assessment of neuropathy involving unmyelinated nerve fibers.[71] The response, known as the sympathetic skin response (SSR), can also be recorded from perineal skin and the penis.[72-74] The SSR is a reflex; its arc consists of myelinated sensory fibers, a complex central integrative mechanism and a sympathetic efferent limb with postganglionic unmyelinated C fibers. The stimulus used in clinical practice is usually an electric pulse delivered to an upper or lower limb (to mixed nerves), but the genital organs can also be stimulated.[73] The latencies of SSR on the penis following stimulation of a median nerve at the wrist have been reported between 1.5[73,75] and 2.3 s[74] and could be obtained in all normal subjects, with a large variability. The responses are easily habituated, and depend on a number of endogenous and exogenous factors including skin temperature, which should be above 28°C. Amplitudes (but not latencies) were reported reduced in older subjects.[72] It is commonly suggested that only an absent SSR can be taken as abnormal.

ROLE OF ELECTROPHYSIOLOGICAL EXAMINATION OF THE POSTERIOR PELVIC FLOOR IN EVALUATION OF URINARY AND SEXUAL DYSFUNCTION

It should be pointed out that, because of similar innervation and functional characteristics of the pelvic floor, electrophysiological assessment of posterior pelvic floor structures is often performed for evaluation of anterior pelvic floor (urinary and sexual) dysfunction. This is probably reasonable when overall involvement of sacral spinal nuclei (as in multiple system atrophy), or very proximal disturbances or injuries are suspected (located in conus of the spinal cord, cauda equina, or injury to proximal parts of the pudendal nerves or direct sacral root branches). In all these instances neural elements innervating the whole pelvic floor are not expected to be selectively affected. As a consequence it is assumed that findings in the posterior pelvic floor will be a good approximation for the anterior pelvic floor situation. Muscles in the posterior part are of larger bulk, it is easier to approach them, and examination is less unpleasant.

There are, however, situations in which this approach will not suffice. Only direct examination of anterior pelvic floor structures will reveal selective dysfunction; the typical example is the young female with urinary retention.

CONCLUSION

Several electrophysiological tests have been proposed for evaluation of the (anterior) pelvic floor, the urinary sphincter muscle and their motor and sensory innervation. Although all tests mentioned in this chapter continue to be of research interest, it is particularly the concentric needle EMG which is, in the opinion of the authors, of definite usefulness in everyday routine diagnostic evaluation of selected groups of patients. These patient groups are defined more by the fact that they have known or suspected nervous system involvement than any particular form or degree of sacral dysfunction. In particular, CNEMG is suggested as helpful in patients with atypical parkinsonism, and those with traumatic lesions. Probably the only group of patients in whom the type of sacral dysfunction per se should be considered an indication for CNEMG are young females with urinary retention.

It is expected that new computer-assisted methods of analysis of CNEMG will improve the usefulness of the test as a diagnostic method to reveal neurogenic pelvic floor muscle involvement.

Further research into and experience with the neurophysiological tests discussed will reveal their contribution to clinical assessment of individual patients, which is presently very limited.

REFERENCES

1. Vodušek DB. Electrophysiology. In: Schübler B, Laycock J, Norton P, *et al.* (eds). *Pelvic floor re-education, principles and practice.* London: Springer-Verlag, 1994:83–97.
2. Smith A, Hosker G, Warrell D. The role of pudendal nerve damage in the aetiology of genuine stress incontinence in women. *Br J Obstet Gynaecol* 1989;**96**:29–32.
3. Nordling J, Meyhoff H, Walter S, *et al.* Urethral electromyography using a new ring electrode. *J Urol* 1978;**120**:571–3.
4. Gosling JA. Anatomy. In: Stanton SL (ed.) *Clinical gynecologic urology.* St. Louis: Mosby, 1984:3–12.
5. Olsen AL, Benson JT, McClellan E. Urethral sphincter needle electromyography in women: comparison of periurethral and transvaginal approaches. *Neurourol Urodyn* 1998;**17**:531–5.
6. Chantraine A, Leval J, Onkelinx A. Motor conduction velocity in the internal pudendal nerves. In: Desmedt JE (ed.) *New developments in electromyography and clinical neurophysiology*, Vol. 2. Basel: Karger, 1973:433–8.
7. Jesel M, Isch-Treussard C, Isch F. Electromyography of striated muscle of anal and urethral sphincters. In: Desmedt JE (eds). *New developments in electromyography and clinical neurophysiology*, Vol. 2. Basel: Karger, 1973:406–20.
8. Deindl FM, Vodušek DB, Hesse U, *et al.* Activity patterns of pubococcygeal muscles in nulliparous continent women. *Br J Urol* 1993;**72**:46–51.
9. Blaivas JG, Sinha HP, Zayed AAH, *et al.* Detrusor-external sphincter dyssynergia. *J Urol* 1981;**125**:542–4.
10. Chancellor MB, Kaplan SA, Blaivas JG. Detrusor-external sphincter dyssynergia. In: Bock G, Whelan J (eds). *Neurobiology of incontinence.* Ciba Foundation Symposium 151. Chichester: John Wiley, 1990:195–206.
11. Stocchi F, Carbone A, Inghilleri M, *et al.* Urodynamic and neurophysiological evaluation in Parkinson's disease and multiple system atrophy. *J Neurol Neurosurg Psychiat* 1997;**62**:507–11.
12. Rudy DC, Woodside JR. Non-neurogenic neurogenic bladder: The relationship between intravesical pressure and the external sphincter electromyogram. *Neurourol Urodynam* 1991;**10**:169–76.
13. Deindl FM, Vodušek DB, Bischof Ch, *et al.* Zwei verschiedene Formen von Miktionsstörungen bei jungen Frauen: Dyssynerges Verhalten im Beckenboden oder Pseudomyotonie im externen urethralen Sphinkter? *Akt Urol* 1997;**28**:88–94.
14. Deindl FM, Vodušek DB, Bischoff C, *et al.* Dysfunctional voiding in women: which muscles are responsible? *Br J Urol* 1998;**82**:814–9.
15. Deindl F, Vodušek DB, Hesse U, *et al.* Pelvic floor activity patterns: comparison of nulliparous continent and parous urinary stress incontinent women. A kinesiological EMG study. *Br J Urol* 1994;**73**:413–7.
16. Chantraine A, De Leval J, Depireux P. Adult female intra- and peri-urethral sphincter-electromyographic study. *Neurourol Urodynam* 1990;**9**:139–144.
17. Vereecken RL, Verduyn H. The electrical activity of the paraurethral and perineal muscles in normal and pathological conditions. *Br J Urol* 1970;**42**:457–63.
18. Stålberg E, Andreassen S, Falck B, *et al.* Quantitative analysis of individual motor unit potentials: A proposition for standardized terminology and criteria for measurement. *J Clin Neurophysiol* 1986;**3**:313–48.
19. Nandedkar S, Sanders D, Stålberg E, *et al.* Simulation of concentric needle EMG motor unit action potentials. *Muscle Nerve* 1988;**11**:151–9.
20. Bischoff C, Stålberg E, Falck B, *et al.* Reference values of motor unit action potentials obtained with Multi-MUAP analysis. *Muscle Nerve* 1994;**17**:842–51.
21. Stålberg E, Falck B, Sonoo M, *et al.* Multi-MUP EMG analysis – a two year experience in daily clinical work. *Electroenceph Clin Neurophysiol* 1995;**97**:145–54.
22. International Federation of Societies for Electroencephalography and Clinical Neurophysiology. *Recommendations for Practice of Clinical Neurophysiology.* Amsterdam: Elsevier, 1983.
23. Nandedkar S, Barkhaus P, Sanders D, *et al.* Analysis of the amplitude and area of the concentric needle EMG motor

unit action potentials. *Electroenceph Clin Neurophysiol* 1988;**69**:561–7.

24. Sonoo M, Stålberg E. The ability of MUP parameters to discriminate between normal and neurogenic MUPs in concentric EMG: analysis of the MUP 'thickness' and the proposal of 'size index'. *Electroenceph Clin Neurophysiol* 1993;**89**:291–303.
25. AAEE glossary of terms used in clinical electromyography. *Muscle Nerve* 1987;**10**:G1–G60.
26. Ludin H-P. *Praktische Elektromyographie.* Stuttgart: Ferdinand Enke Verlag, 1976;53–63.
27. Brown FW. *The physiological and technical basis of electromyography.* London: Butterworth, 1984;287–338.
28. Fowler CJ, Kirby RS, Harrison MJG, *et al.* Individual motor unit analysis in the diagnosis of disorders of urethral sphincter innervation. *J Neurol Neurosurg Psychiat* 1984;**47**:637–41.
29. Nandedkar SD, Sanders DB. Simulation of myopathic motor unit action potentials. *Muscle Nerve* 1989;**12**:197–202.
30. Vodušek DB, Light JK. The motor nerve supply of the external urethral sphincter muscles. *Neurourol Urodynam* 1983;**2**:193–200.
31. Fanciullaci F, Kokodoko A, Garavaglia PF, *et al.* Comparative study of the motor unit potentials of the external urethral sphincter, anal sphincter, and bulbocavernosus muscle in normal men. *Neurourol Urodynam* 1987;**6**:65–9.
32. Rodi Z, Vodušek DB, Denišlič M. Clinical uro-neurophysiological investigation in multiple sclerosis. *Eur J Neurol* 1996;**3**:574–80.
33. Nandedkar SD, Sanders DB, Stålberg EV. Simulation and analysis of the electromyographic interference pattern in normal muscle. Part I: Turns and amplitude measurements. *Muscle Nerve* 1986;**9**:423–30.
34. Nandedkar SD, Sanders DB, Stålberg EV. Automatic analysis of the electromyographic interference pattern. Part I: Development of quantitative features. *Muscle Nerve* 1986;**9**:431–9.
35. Nirkko AC, Rösler KM, Hess KW. Sensitivity and specificity of needle electromyography: a prospective study comparing automated interference pattern analysis with single motor unit potential analysis. *Electroenceph Clin Neurophysiol* 1995;**97**:1–10.
36. Trontelj J, Stålberg E. Bizarre repetitive discharges recorded with single fibre EMG. *J Neurol Neurosurg Psychiat* 1983;**46**:310–6.
37. Fowler CJ, Kirby RS, Harrison MJG. Decelerating bursts and complex repetitive discharges in the striated muscle of the urethral sphincter associated with urinary retention in women. *J Neurol Neurosurg Psychiat* 1985;**48**:1004–9.
38. Siroky MB. Electromyography of the perineal floor. In: Boone TB (ed.) *Urodynamics I.* The Urologic Clinics of North America. Philadelphia: WB Saunders, 1996;299–307.
39. Stålberg E, Trontelj JV. *Single fiber electromyography: studies in healthy and diseased muscle*, 2nd edn. New York: Raven Press, 1994;45–82.
40. Vodušek DB. Individual motor unit analysis in the diagnosis of urethral sphincter innervation. *J Neurol Neurosurg Psychiat* 1989;**52**:812–3.
41. Palace J, Chandiramani VA, Fowler CJ. Value of sphincter EMG in the diagnosis of Multiple system atrophy. *Muscle Nerve* 1997;**20**:1396–1403.
42. Caress J, Kothari M, Bauer S, *et al.* Urinary dysfunction in Duchenne muscular dystrophy. *Muscle Nerve* 1996;**19**:819–22.
43. Dixon PJ, Christmas TJ, Chapple CR. Stress incontinence due to pelvic floor muscle involvement in limb-girdle muscular dystrophy. *Br J Urol* 1990;**65**:653–60.
44. Herbaut AG, Nogueira MC, Panzer JM, *et al.* Anorectal incontinence in myotonic dystrophy: a myopathic involvement of pelvic floor muscles. *Muscle Nerve* 1992;**5**:1210–1.
45. Vodušek DB, Janko M, Lokar J. EMG, single fiber EMG and sacral reflexes in assessment of sacral nervous system lesions. *J Neurol Neurosurg Psychiat* 1982;**45**:1064–6.
46. Vodušek DB, Janko M: The bulbocavernosus reflex: a single motor neuron study. *Brain* 1990;**113**:813–20.
47. Eardley I, Quinn NP, Fowler CJ, *et al.* The value of urethral sphincter electromyography in the differential diagnosis of parkinsonism. *Br J Urol* 1989;**64**:360–2.
48. Beck RO, Betts CD, Fowler CJ. Genitourinary dysfunction in multiple system atrophy: clinical features and treatment in 62 cases. *J Urol* 1994;**151**:1336–41.
49. Rodi Z, Vodušek DB, Denišlič M. External anal sphincter electromyography in the differential diagnosis of parkinsonism. *J Neurol Neurosurg Psychiat* 1996;**60**:460–1.
50. Smith ARB, Hosker GL, Warrell DW. The role of partial denervation of the pelvic floor in aetiology of genitourinary prolapse and stress incontinence of urine. A neurophysiology study. *Br J Obstet Gynaecol* 1989;**96**:24–8.
51. Allen R, Hosker G, Smith A, *et al.* Pelvic floor damage and childbirth: a neurophysiological study. *Br J Obstet Gynaecol* 1990;**97**:770–9.
52. Hale DS, Benson JT, Brubaker L, *et al.* Histologic analysis of needle biopsy of urethral sphincter from women with normal and stress incontinence with comparison of electromyographic findings. *Am J Obstet Gynecol* 1999;**180**:342–8.
53. Fowler CJ, Kirby RS. Electromyography of the urethral sphincter in women with urinary retention. *Lancet* 1986;**1(8496)**:1455–6.
54. Kiff ES, Swash M. Normal proximal and delayed distal conduction in the pudendal nerves of patients with idiopathic (neurogenic) faecal incontinence. *J Neurol Neurosurg Psychiat* 1984;**47**:820–3.
55. Snooks SJ, Badenoch DF, Tiptaft RC, *et al.* Perineal nerve damage in genuine stress incontinence. *Br J Urol* 1985;**57**:422–6.
56. Benson T, McClellan E. The effect of vaginal dissection on the pudendal nerve. *Obstet Gynecol* 1993;**82**:387–9.
57. Bradley WE, Lin JTY, Johnson B. Measurement of the conduction velocity of the dorsal nerve of the penis. *J Urol* 1984;**131**:1127–9.
58. Amarenco G, Kerdraon J. Pudendal nerve terminal sensitive latency: technique and normal values. *J Urol* 1999;**161**:103–6.
59. Deletis V, Vodušek DB, Abbott R, *et al.* Intraoperative monitoring of dorsal sacral roots: minimizing the risk of iatrogenic micturition disorders. *Neurosurgery* 1992;**30**:72–5.

60. Ertekin C, Mungan B. Sacral spinal cord and root potentials evoked by the stimulation of the dorsal nerve of penis and cord conduction delay for the bulbocavernosus reflex. *Neurourol Urodynam* 1993;**12**:9–22.
61. Haldeman S, Bradley WE, Bhatia N. Evoked responses from the pudendal nerve. *J Urol* 1982;**128**:974–80.
62. Opsomer RJ, Caramia MD, Zarola F, *et al.* Neurophysiological evaluation of central-peripheral sensory and motor pudendal fibres. *Electroenceph Clin Neurophysiol* 1989;**74**:260–70.
63. Vodušek DB. Pudendal somatosensory evoked potential and bulbocavernosus reflex in women. *Electroenceph Clin Neurophysiol* 1990;**77**:134–6.
64. Gänzer H, Madersbacher H, Rumpl E. Cortical evoked potentials by stimulation of the vesicourethral junction: clinical value and neurophysiological considerations. *J Urol* 1991;**146**:118–23.
65. Guérit JM, Opsomer RJ. Bit-mapped imagine of somatosensory evoked potentials after stimulation of the posterior tibial nerves and dorsal nerve of the penis/clitoris. *Electroenceph Clin Neurophysiol* 1991;**80**:228–37.
66. Podnar S, Vodušek D, Tršinar B, *et al.* A method of uroneurophysiological investigation in children. *Electroenceph Clin Neurophysiol* 1997;**104**:389–92.
67. Delodovici ML, Fowler CJ. Clinical value of the pudendal somatosensory evoked potential. *Electroenceph Clin Neurophysiol* 1995;**96**:509–15.
68. Vodušek DB, Deletis V, Abbott R, *et al.* Prevention of iatrogenic micturition disorders through intraoperative monitoring. *Neurourol Urodynam* 1990;**9**:444–5.
69. Badr GG, Carlsson CA, Fall M, *et al.* Cortical evoked potentials following the stimulation of the urinary bladder in man. *Electroenceph Clin Neurophysiol* 1982;**54**:494–8.
70. Hansen MV, Ertekin C, Larsson LE. Cerebral evoked potentials after stimulation of the posterior urethra in man. *Electroenceph Clin Neurophysiol* 1990;**77**:52–8.
71. Shahani BT, Halperin JJ, Boulu P, *et al.* Sympathetic skin response – a method of assessing unmyelinated axon dysfunction in peripheral neuropathies. *J Neurol Neurosurg Psychiat* 1984;**47**:536–42.
72. Ertekin C, Ertekin N, Mutlu S, *et al.* Skin potentials (SP) recorded from the extremities and genital regions in normal and impotent subjects. *Acta Neurol Scand* 1987;**76**:28–36.
73. Opsomer RJ, Pesce Fr, Abi Aad A, *et al.* Electrophysiologic testing of motor sympathetic pathways: normative data and clinical contribution in neurourological disorders. *Neurourol Urodynam* 1993;**12**:336–8.
74. Daffertshofer M, Linden D, Syren M, *et al.* Assessment of local sympathetic function in patients with erectile dysfunction. *Int J Impotence Res* 1994;**6**:213–25.
75. Opsomer RJ, Boccasena P, Traversa R, *et al.* Sympathetic skin responses from the limbs and the genitalia: normative study and contribution to the evaluation of neurourological disorders. *Electroenceph Clin Neurophysiol* 1996;**101**:25–31.

Chapter 13

Clinical features of posterior pelvic floor dysfunction

John H Pemberton

The evaluation and management of *constipation* and *pelvic floor dysfunction* is a matter of increasing interest, perhaps because understanding of the underlying pathophysiology is improved, which in turn facilitates a more rational approach to treatment. Constipation and pelvic floor dysfunction are complex conditions with multiple causes. Manifestations vary from mild to incapacitating. Constipation is a subjective complaint, which may reflect various diseases and mechanisms; the term connotes both infrequent defecation as well as difficulty with defecation.

DEFINITIONS

It is important that the treatment of constipation be based on the varied etiologies of constipation. The 'extracolonic' causes of constipation are listed in Table 13.1 while Table 13.2 divides the 'colonic' causes into problems of colonic dysmotility or disordered defecation. Although such an extensive classification of extracolonic causes is intimidating, it is none the less important to have it available.

CLINICAL FEATURES

The history, of course, is key to understanding the underlying abnormality. What gives the patient the most problems are: *frequency of stools*, *straining*, *hard stools*, *incomplete evacuation* or other problems such as *anal pain* and *bloating*. If the patient relates that pain and bloating are the most distressing symptom, then there is likely underlying IBS (irritable bowel syndrome).[1,2]

Patients with pelvic floor dysfunction relate a typical history and have a typical physical examination. Prolonged and excessive straining is a key problem; sometimes, even soft stools and enema fluid cannot be evacuated. If the patient uses perineal or vaginal wall counter pressure in order to facilitate defecation, or more importantly, if the finger is used to pull stools out, it is important to determine if pelvic floor dysfunction

Table 13.1 Extracolonic causes of constipation

Endocrine and metabolic disorders
Carcinomatosis
Diabetes mellitus
Glucagonoma
Hypercalcemia
Hyperparathyroidism
Hypokalemia
Hypopituitarism
Hypothyroidism
Milk-alkali syndrome
Pheochromocytoma
Porphyria
Pregnancy
Uremia
Neurologic disorders
Peripheral
Autonomic neuropathy
Chagas' disease
Hirschsprung's disease
Hypoganglionosis
Intestinal pseudoobstruction (myopathy, neuropathy)
Multiple endocrine neoplasia, type IIB
Von Recklinghausen's disease
Central
Cauda equina syndrome
Cerebrovascular accident
Ischemia
Meningocele
Multiple sclerosis
Paraplegia
Parkinson's disease
Shy–Drager syndrome (multiple system atrophy)
Tabes dorsalis
Trauma to nervi erigentes
Tumors
Collagen vascular and muscle disorders
Amyloidosis
Dermatomyositis
Myotonic dystrophy
Scleroderma

Table 13.2 Causes of chronic severe constipation in adults

Colonic dysmotility
Slow transit
Constipation-predominant irritable bowel syndrome
Disordered defecation
Anismus
Descending perineum syndrome
Hirschprung's disease
Disturbed rectal sensation
Occult rectal prolapse
Procidentia (complete prolapse)
Rectocele
Posterior rectal hernia

Table 13.3 Anorectal and pelvic floor function tests

Balloon expulsion test
Defecation proctography
Ano-rectal manometry
Perineometry
Pudendal nerve terminal motor latency
Sphincter, puborectalis electromyogram
Measurement of recto-anal angle
Ultrasonography
Scintigraphic expulsion of artificial stool
Rectal sensation: mechanical, electrical

exists early in the evaluation as it does not respond well to standard laxative programs.

The answer to the following questions should be sought: does the patient have a 'call to stool?' Does the patient answer the call? What laxatives are being used, how often, and at what dosage and are suppositories or enemas used? What is the bowel frequency and what is the stool consistency?

The perineal and anal examination are key.

1. In the left lateral decubitus position, one notes descent/elevation of the perineum during simulated evacuation and retention squeeze. Evidence of fecal soilage should be sought and the anal reflex tested by a light pinprick.
2. The anal verge should be observed during straining to determine if it becomes patulous and/or if a prolapse exists.
3. Digital examination of the anal canal evaluates resting tone and squeeze increments. The puborectalis muscle should be palpated and any localized discomfort suggests levator spasm (puborectalis spasm syndrome). Finally, the patient should be instructed to expel the examining finger.
4. A vaginal speculum can then be used, in the lithotomy position, to look for a rectocele.

At the conclusion of the initial clinical evaluation, it should be possible to determine if the patient has pelvic floor dysfunction. Most patients will now require structural (flexible sigmoidoscopy plus barium enema or a colonoscopy) and functional studies (Table 13.3).

Complaints which suggest pelvic floor dysfunction include:[3] inability to evacuate the rectum, feeling of persistent rectal fullness, rectal pain, pelvic floor descent, and straining. Thus, symptoms such as the need to extract stool from the rectum digitally, application of pressure on the posterior wall of the vagina, or support of the perineum during straining imply pelvic floor dysfunction.

Before testing, an integral part of the assessment of patients with clinically suspected obstructed defecation is review by a psychologist: patients with eating disorders may have constipation. Psychologists also provide relaxation training for these patients and help identify depression that may have been missed. Constipation associated with features of obstructed defecation should be investigated using available techniques such as defecography, anal manometry, and balloon expulsion.

Importantly, defecography reveals abnormalities in as many as 50% of asymptomatic *healthy* persons. Others have shown a broad range of movements of the anorectal angle and pelvic floor in a study of 47 healthy young volunteers: these data overlap with pathologic states.[4] Most symptoms associated with difficult defecation can be treated medically by increasing dietary fiber. In only a few patients are significant anatomic defects associated with intractable constipation and which in turn might respond to surgical treatment. These defects include rectal prolapse and large rectoceles, which on defecography are filled preferentially with barium during attempts at defecation. Most commonly, outlet obstruction results from a non-relaxing pelvic floor, which impedes rectal emptying. There are many tests of anorectal and pelvic floor function.

A history suggesting abnormal defecation, such as excessive straining, finger disimpaction and an abnormal balloon expulsion are highly suggestive of pelvic floor dysfunction. A simple test to document a non-relaxing pelvic floor is to have the patient strain to expel the examining finger. Alternatively, movement of the puborectalis posteriorly during straining indicates proper coordination of the pelvic floor muscles.

Measuring perineal descent can be performed by either watching the perineum descend appropriately while straining, balloon outward (signifying descending perineum syndrome) or not move at all – signifying a non-relaxing pelvic floor).

One of the most useful tests at this juncture is balloon expulsion.[5] The overall defecatory process and relaxation of the puborectalis muscle is assessed by using this technique; failure to expel the balloon is commonly associated with pelvic floor dysfunction, anatomic defects of the rectum, or anismus.

At this point, if the balloon expulsion test is abnormal, patients should be assessed by a psychologist. The psychologist may identify concomitant eating disorder or depression, for which constipation is a predominant symptom. Further tests may be indicated in some patients, such as defecography or anal endosonography to detect surgically correctable anatomic defects as prolapse or rectal wall defects, or rarely puborectalis electromyogram to assess spasm or denervation.

In patients with severe constipation and a *megarectum*, sensory perception of the rectal vault to distention may be impaired simply from enlargement. This may be documented using manometric techniques to determine earliest sensation using an air-inflated balloon or the maximal tolerable rectal volume before the urge to defecate.[3,6]

CLINICAL FEATURES OF ANATOMIC DEFECTS CAUSING PELVIC FLOOR DYSFUNCTION

HIRSCHSPRUNG'S DISEASE

Despite the reports of 1978[7] and 1987,[8] congenital aganglionosis is an extremely rare cause of adult constipation. None the less, it does occur and should be suspected when symptoms have been present 'since childhood' and barium enema shows a widened rectal vault above the level of the ano-rectal ring. Absence of the recto-anal inhibitory response and ganglion cells confirm the diagnosis. The biggest problem in diagnosing adult Hirschsprung's disease is the wide variation in the density of ganglion cells at the level of anorectal junction in perfectly healthy people.[9,10]

Once diagnosed, surgery is indicated. The surgical principle to be achieved is to bypass or excise completely the aganglionic segment. The Swenson,[11] Duhamel[12] and Soave[13] operations have been devised for this purpose. Of the three, Duhamel's operation appears to be the most effective in adults.[14]

DESCENDING PERINEUM SYNDROME

The cause of abnormal perineal descent is believed to be related to injury to the sacral nerves and/or pudendal nerves or to damage to the muscles themselves during childbirth or chronic straining at stool. An abnormal degree of perineal descent occurs in a high percentage of patients with constipation and chronic straining at stool[15] and conversely, most patients with perineal descent give a history of excessive straining to achieve a bowel movement.[16] Fecal incontinence may occur later in the natural history of abnormal perineal descent. At our institution, patients with profound perineal descent and obstructed defecation undergo pelvic floor retraining but with only fair to poor results. If perineal descent occurs with occult intussusception, anterior resection may cure the prolapse, but the perineal descent, with its symptoms, usually persists.

RECTOCELE

Patients with functionally significant rectoceles on defecating proctogram undergo operative repair only after medical options have been exhausted. Low and mid-level rectoceles, within 7–8 cm of the sphincter, are best treated by transanal repair.[17–21] Strengthening and shortening the lower end of the defect, based on the technique of Sullivan, Leaverton and Hardwick,[17] restores the normal relationship between the sphincter and the perineal body, smoothes out the rectal 'funnel' and allows normal passage of stool. This technique renders patients asymptomatic, or considerably improved, nearly 90% of the time.[18,19] Block[20] described a simplified approach of transrectal repair of mid-level rectoceles using obliterative sutures in 60 patients, 14 of whom were symptomatic. The rectocele was corrected in all patients, with $1\frac{1}{2}$–4 years of follow-up, and all 14 patients who were symptomatic before surgery remained free of symptoms. On the other hand, patients who have high rectoceles should be repaired transvaginally using a posterior colporrhaphy because a rectal approach provides inadequate exposure.[17,18]

RECTAL PROLAPSE

Anterior mucosal prolapse, internal rectal intussusception, solitary rectal ulcer syndrome and abnormal perineal descent are frequently seen in patients with obstructed defecation.[21] Patients presenting with anterior mucosal prolapse and perineal descent have a 30% chance of becoming incontinent over the subsequent 5 years and a 20% chance of developing complete rectal prolapse.[22] A high proportion of patients with complete rectal prolapse suffer from chronic constipation, but a role for this symptom in the genesis of rectal prolapse has not been established conclusively. Moreover, a cause and effect relationship between pelvic floor weakness and rectal prolapse has not been proven.

It seems likely that without repair of the prolapse, incontinence would eventually develop as repeated traction on the pudendal nerves during prolapse and descent of the perineum leads to permanent neurapraxia.[23,24] Repeated dilatation of the anus by the intussusceptus also damages the anal sphincter muscles.

Complete rectal prolapse is the condition for which operative treatment is most clearly indicated. The multitude of techniques for repair of rectal prolapse, which proliferated over the past few decades, have mostly faded. Two general approaches give satisfactory results.

The majority of patients are best served by an abdominal approach, whereby the rectum is completely mobilized and either resected[25] or fixed to the sacrum.[26] The need to perform a concurrent sigmoid resection is controversial, but is advised if the anastomosis is performed in the peritonealized portion of the completely mobilized rectum.[25] Sigmoid resection enhances fixation and anecdotally reduces the frequency of postoperative constipation.

In frail or debilitated patients, a perineal approach results in fewer systemic complications, while still having an acceptable chance of success. The procedures of Delorme[27] and Altemeier[28] both yield reasonable results.

Approximately one-half of the patients with complete full thickness rectal prolapse who are incontinent preoperatively will continue to be incontinent for more than 6 months after rectopexy.[29] Of central note is the fact that none of the procedures available for treating rectal prolapse deal with any of the potential underlying factors; indeed, constipation is a common preoperative symptom which often becomes more severe after rectopexy.[30] This is probably the reason that rectopexy alone fails to alleviate the symptoms of obstructed defecation associated with occult rectal prolapse.

The management of occult rectal prolapse remains a challenging problem. Bowel retraining, with avoidance of straining, and biofeedback techniques have been used with some success in some patients (J.H. Pemberton, unpublished observation). Bulk laxatives are unhelpful. The role of surgical procedures is controversial. Ihre and Seligson[31] performed Ripstein repairs on 40 patients. Those who were incontinent preoperatively appeared to benefit; 20 of 26 regained continence. Those who had symptoms of outlet obstruction, however, did poorly, none of 14 being the same or worse after operation. Nicholls and Simson[32] used anteroposterior rectopexy to treat 14 patients with solitary rectal ulcer due to presumed internal prolapse. Twelve were improved 2–48 months after surgery. However, Bartolo[33] reported less satisfactory results, noting relief of symptoms in only 25% of patients. A fully satisfactory approach to the management of symptomatic internal rectal prolapse has yet to be devised.

REFERENCES

1. Drossman DA (ed). *The functional gastrointestinal disorders.* Boston: Little, Brown, 1994, Chapter 4:115–73.
2. Mertz H, Naliboff B, Mayer E. Physiology of refractory constipation. *Am J Gastroenterol,* 1999;**94**:609–615.
3. Pemberton JH. Anorectal and pelvic disorders: putting physiology into practice. *J Gastroenterol Hepatol* 1990;**5**:127–43.
4. Shorvon PJ, McHugh S, Diamant NE, Somers S, Stevenson GW. Defecography in normal volunteers: results and implications. *Gut* 1989;**30**:1737–49.
5. Fleshman JW, Dreznik Z, Cohen E, Fry RD, Kodner IJ. Balloon expulsion test facilitates diagnosis of pelvic floor outlet obstruction due to nonrelaxing puborectalis muscle. *Dis Colon Rectum* 1992;**35**:1019–25.
6. Pezim ME, Pemberton JH, Levin KE, Litchy WJ, Phillips SF. Parameters of anorectal and colonic motility in health and in severe constipation. *Dis Colon Rectum* 1993;**36**:484–91.
7. Martelli H, Devroede G, Ahran P, Duguay C. Mechanisms of idiopathic constipation: outlet obstruction. *Gastroenterology* 1978;**75**:623–31.
8. Yoshioka K, Keighley MRB. Anorectal myectomy for outlet obstruction. *Br J Surg* 1987;**74**:373–6.
9. Aldridge RT, Campbell PE. Ganglion cell distribution in the normal rectum and anal canal: a basis for the diagnosis of Hirschsprung's disease by anorectal biopsy. *J Pediat Surg* 1968;**3**:475–90.
10. Weinberg AS. The anorectal myenteric plexus: its relationship to hyperganglionosis of the colon. *Am J Clin Pathol* 1970;**54**:637–42.
11. Swenson O, Bill AH Jr. Resection of rectum and rectosigmoid with preservation of sphincter for benign spastic lesions producing megacolon: experimental study. *Surgery* 1948;**24**:212–20.
12. Duhamel B. A new operation for the treatment of Hirschsprung's disease. *Arch Dis Child* 1960;**35**:38–9.
13. Soave F. Hirschsprung's disease: a new surgical technique. *Arch Dis Child* 1964;**39**:116–24.
14. Elliot MS, Todd IP. Adult Hirschsprung's disease: Results with Duhamel procedure. *Br J Surg* 1985;**72**:884–5.
15. Kiff ES, Swash M. Slowed conduction in the pudendal nerve in idiopathic (neurogenic) faecal incontinence. *Br J Surg* 1984;**71**:614–16.
16. Parks AG, Porter NH, Hardcastle J. The syndrome of the descending perineum. *Proc Roy Soc Med* 1966;**59**:477–82.
17. Sullivan ES, Leaverton GH, Hardwick CE. Transrectal perineal repair: an adjunct to improved function after anorectal surgery. *Dis Colon Rectum* 1968;**11**:106–114.
18. Capps WF Jr. Rectoplasty and perineoplasty for the symptomatic rectocele: a report of fifty cases. *Dis Colon Rectum* 1975;**18**:237–43.
19. Sehapayak S. Transrectal repair of rectocele: an extended armamentarium of colorectal surgeons. A report of 355 cases. *Dis Colon Rectum* 1985;**28**:422–33.
20. Block IR. Transrectal repair of rectocele using obliterative suture. *Dis Colon Rect* 1986;**29**:707–711.
21. Bartolo DCC, Roe AM, Virjee J, Mortenson NJ. Evacuation proctography in obstructed defaecation and rectal intussusception. *Br J Surg* (Suppl.) 1985;**72**:111–16.
22. Allen-Mersch TG, Henry MM, Nicholls RJ. Natural history of anterior mucosal prolapse. *Br J Surg* 1987;**74**:679–82.
23. Neill ME, Parks AG, Swash M. Physiological studies of the anal sphincter musculature in faecal incontinence and rectal prolapse. *Br J Surg* 1981;**68**:531–6.
24. Kiff ES, Barnes PRH, Swash M. Evidence of pudendal neuropathy in patients with perineal descent and chronic straining at stool. *Gut* 1984;**25**:1279–82.
25. Schlinkert RT, Beart RW Jr, Wolff BG, Pemberton JH. Anterior resection for complete rectal prolapse. *Dis Colon Rectum* 1985;**28**:409–412.
26. Ripstein CB, Lauter B. Etiology and surgical therapy of massive prolapse of the rectum. *Ann Surg* 1963;**157**:259–64.

27. Delorme M. Communication sur le traitement des prolapsus du rectum totaux, par l'excision de la mugueuse rectale ou rectocolique. Bell *et al.*, *Mem De Chir De Paris* **26**:499–518. (Translation: McGill N. *Dis Colon Rectum* 1985;**28**:544–53.
28. Altemeier WA, Culbertson WR. Technique for perineal repair of rectal prolapse. *Surgery* 1965;**58**:758–64.
29. Schoetz DJ Jr, Veidenheimer MC. Rectal prolapse: pathogenesis and clinical features. In: Henry MM, Swash M (eds). *Coloproctology and the Pelvic Floor*. London: Butterworths, 1985:303–307.
30. Mann CV, Hoffman C. Complete rectal prolapse: the anatomical and functional results of treatment by an extended abdominal rectopexy. *Br J Surg* 1988;**75**:34–7.
31. Ihre T, Seligson U. Intussusception of the rectum – internal procidentia: treatment and results in 90 patients. *Dis Colon Rectum* 1975;**18**:391–6.
32. Nicholls RJ, Simson JNL. Anteroposterior rectopexy with the treatment of solitary rectal ulcer syndrome without overt rectal prolapse. *Br J Surg* 1986;**73**:222–4.
33. Bartolo DCC. Pelvic floor disorders: diarrhoea, constipation, and obstructed defecation. *Perspect Colon Rectal Surg* 1988;**1**:(1).

Chapter 14

Colonic and ano-rectal motility studies

R W Hagger, Davinder Kumar

INTRODUCTION

Colonic and ano-rectal motility can be considered in terms of the electrical activity of the muscle layers, intraluminal pressure fluctuations produced by contractions of the muscle layers, and the resultant displacement of the intraluminal contents. Each reflects different aspects of motor activity, but are complimentary in the evaluation of colonic and anorectal motility. Investigation of motility is therefore based on electrophysiological, manometric and transit studies. The anorectum is easily accessible for evaluation; function in health and disease is well documented, and assessment of anorectal motility is common in clinical practice. The patterns of motility of the colon in health and in disease are still relatively poorly understood. This is in part due to the inaccessibility of the organ, the regional variations in motor activity and the intermittent and sporadic nature of colonic activity. Only transit studies are routinely used in the clinical evaluation of patients with functional disorders of the colon. Electrophysiological and manometric studies of colonic motility are still mainly research based, or are only available at specialist centers.

COLONIC MOTILITY

COLONIC ELECTRICAL ACTIVITY

Human colonic electrical activity is produced by ionic fluxes across the cell membrane, which occur during pacemaking and contractile activity. It is characterized by two distinct patterns: slow waves, which are rhythmic oscillations of the membrane potential, and spike potentials. Superimposition of spike potentials on slow waves signifies contractile activity. Electrical activity of the human colon has been assessed by both *in vitro* and *in vivo* studies.

In vitro studies allow the individual muscle layers to be assessed in isolation and for co-ordinated activity between the muscle layers to be evaluated. In the human circular muscle layer the slow wave frequency is variable, and lies within the range of 4–60 cpm,[1,2] but is most commonly found to lie within one of two frequency ranges: 4.5–12 cpm or 14–28 cpm.[1,3] The frequency and amplitude are both variable and change with stimulation: periods of electrical quiescence are apparent.[1] Contractions occur with either high amplitude depolarizations, or more usually with spiking activity.[1] The variable slow wave frequency suggests that multiple pacemakers exist. In the human longitudinal muscle layer electrical oscillations are observed in a narrow frequency range with superimposition of spiking activity. The frequency of electrical oscillations is constant within an individual muscle strip,[1] and lies within the range of 24–36 cpm.[1,3] Electrical activity is interspersed with periods of quiescence or low amplitude oscillations.[1] The electrical activity of human colonic muscle is highly dependent on physical and chemical stimuli. Stretch is excitatory,[1] as are cholinergic stimuli.[4] Adrenergic stimuli are inhibitory.[4]

In vivo studies record electrical activity from the circular and longitudinal muscle layers simultaneously, the recording therefore reflects activity of both muscle groups. In principle, *in vivo* studies should provide a more physiological description of electrical activity, however this is confounded by technical difficulties which arise during this type of study: other extra colonic sources of electrical activity may be detected, loss of contact between electrode and colonic wall may result in loss of signal, which may be difficult to interpret due to the intrinsic variation in both frequency and amplitude of the electrical waveforms, and the different activities of the longitudinal and circular muscle layers have to be studied in unison.[5]

Electrical activity of the human colon has been recorded *in vivo* using serosal electrodes implanted perioperatively, bipolar mucosal suction needle electrodes, bipolar clip electrodes and intraluminal monopolar or bipolar ring electrodes. Despite the differences in methodologies employed the patterns of electrical activity observed are similar between studies. Monopolar techniques employ an electrode within the gut and an electrode at an indifferent reference point (such as the skin). Bipolar electrodes record potential differences between two closely spaced electrodes. The bipolar technique is less likely to detect movement, respiratory or cardiac artefacts than the monopolar technique. Implanted serosal electrodes have the advantages that electrode displacement is unlikely, positioning of the electrodes is accurate, and the method allows study of the electrical communications between longitudinal and circular muscle layers. However, implanted electrodes require a laparotomy; postoperative recordings can not be seen as reflective of normal motor activity, and this method would not be acceptable for the routine study of patients. Probe mounted needle electrodes (attached by suction) and clip electrodes (which requires repeated endoscopy for placement of multiple pairs of electrodes) allow study of both slow wave and spiking activity. Intraluminal electrodes with no fixed attachment to the mucosa only reliably record spiking activity. Many of the studies to date have only evaluated the distal colon, and cannot be considered representative of the whole colon which shows regional variations in motility.

The description of patterns of electrical activity is confused by the different nomenclature used by individual authors. Slow waves have been referred to as electrical control activity.[6] Short duration spiking activity on individual slow waves has been termed: short spike bursts, discrete electrical response activity, or rhythmic spike potentials.[7–9] Longer duration spiking activity has been referred to as: long spike bursts, continuous electrical response activity, and sporadic spike potentials.[7–9] Longer duration spiking activity which propagates has been described as migrating long spike bursts, and the contractile electrical complex.[7,8]

Slow wave activity has been recorded from all regions of the colon, it is highly variable in both frequency and amplitude. Two rhythms with different frequency ranges have been reported; a lower frequency range of 2–9 cpm and a higher frequency range 6–13 cpm are described.[6–8,10] If the two slow wave frequency ranges are considered separately then no gradient in frequency is apparent along the longitudinal axis of the colon.[6] Regional differences are apparent only when the overall dominant frequency is considered; in the right and left colon the overall dominant frequency is in the lower frequency range, but in the transverse colon the overall dominant frequency is in the higher frequency range.[6]

Spike activity is either of short or long duration. Short spike bursts of 1.5–4.5 second duration are associated with individual slow waves, and occur at a frequency of 0.2–12/min.[7,8,11,12] Short spike burst activity shows no regional differences.[11] Long spike bursts are electrical oscillations in the frequency range 25–40 cpm; long spike bursts are unrelated to and are superimposed on background slow wave activity.[8] The duration of long spike bursts ranges mainly between 10–70 seconds.[7,8,11–13] The frequency of long spike bursts is 0.3–2/minute.[8] Duration and frequency of long spike bursts show regional variation.[8,11] Long spike bursts may propagate orad, aborad or remain stationary.[7,8,11] Short spike bursts, long spike bursts and migrating long spike bursts correlate with colonic contractile activity,[12,14] and displacement of intraluminal contents.[14]

The frequency of long spike bursts shows diurnal variation: long spike bursts decrease during sleep.[13] However, in this study short spike burst activity was found to be constant throughout the day and did not show diurnal variation.[13]

Short spike burst activity does not show a response to food.[11,13] The frequency of long spike bursts shows a postprandial response; long spike bursts increase following a meal.[11,13] The duration of the postprandial response shows regional variation. In the right colon the increase in long spike burst activity returns to basal levels after 20 minutes, in the left and sigmoid colon the increased long spike burst activity persists for over 100 minutes.[11] The fat component of a meal stimulates sigmoid colonic spiking activity, whereas the protein component of a meal, especially pure amino acids, has an inhibitory effect.[15]

COLONIC MANOMETRY

Manometric studies in the colon have mainly been performed using static perfused tube assemblies or ambulatory catheters with solid state pressure microtransducers. Multilumen perfused catheters have enabled the study of colonic events; including the interaction of motor events, propagated activities and regional variations.[16] Much of the data on which understanding of patterns of colonic motility are based used perfused tube manometry. This equipment consists of a low compliance pneumohydraulic perfusion system. Water is perfused at a constant rate through the multilumen catheters. Two theories account for the ability to detect intraluminal pressure fluctuations. The first proposes that pressure changes alter the rate of flow of fluid through the catheters, which is measured: the second theory proposes that the water column within the catheter acts as a manometer. The bulky extracorporal apparatus precludes its use for ambulatory studies, requiring the subject to remain sedentary and be placed in the abnormal environment of the laboratory. The results from these studies may not reflect the normal physiological pattern. Technological advances, with the introduction of solid state pressure transducers and portable battery powered solid state digital data loggers have led to the use of ambulatory manometry to study gut motility. These systems allow the subjects to be studied in their own environment whilst performing their usual activities. This has led to a greater understanding of the normal patterns of motility in the colon and rectum and the pathophysiological basis of colorectal motor disorders.

Telemetry

Ambulant colonic motor activity can also be recorded using radiotelemetry. It is well tolerated,[17] but has many disadvantages. There is little control over the location of the capsule, the position can be detected but not altered as necessary. The capsule moves ahead of the motor activity it is measuring. When used singly, the capsule only detects pressure changes at one site and so can not detect propagation of waveforms. A maximum of three capsules have been used in combination,[18] which compares unfavorably with the number of transducers on a direct recording probe.

Computer-aided analysis

The pressure waveforms obtained from manometry recordings can be analysed qualitatively by reviewing the analogue trace on the screen. Computer software programs have been developed to analyse data quantitatively,[19,20] saving a great deal of time compared with labor intensive manual analysis. Various parameters of motility may be examined, including the mean amplitude of waveforms, the percentage duration of activity, the motility index and the activity index. The *motility index* is calculated as the product of mean amplitude and percentage duration of activity in each epoch; *the activity index* is the total area beneath the waveform/time curve.[20] This activity index would perhaps give the best indication of colonic work.[21] With such calculations it is important to define at what threshold pressure peaks are recorded.[20] The software programs are available commercially. It is proposed that if such software was used routinely and widely for research purposes then it would form a basis for better comparison of investigations.[20]

Effect of manometric technique on motility data

Manometric profiles of gastrointestinal motor activity are, however, influenced by the technique used; the gold standard is the use of serosal strain gauges, but this would be impractical for routine study of the human colon, as laparotomy is required for placement. Perfused tube manometry has been shown to accurately reflect motor activity of a hollow viscus,[22] and may be superior to tube mounted strain gauge systems,[22,23] recording a greater proportion of phasic and tonic contractions than tube mounted strain gauge systems.[23] The accuracy of perfused tube manometry is, however, subject to greater regional and/or anatomic variation than tube mounted strain gauges.[22] The main disadvantage of tube mounted strain gauge systems, though, is misrepresentation of contractile events: discrepancies occur with polarity, in which contractile events may be represented by a negative deflection, and with frequency, in which bifid or biphasic waveforms may erroneously indicate a waveform of higher frequency.[23] It has been suggested, however, that a tube strain gauge system is a more reliable method for measuring colonic pressure, than an open tip perfused tube system, when the viscosity of intraluminal contents is taken into account.[24] Any blockage of the catheter lumen by kinking of the catheter or obstruction of the side port by intestinal contents can lead to inaccurate measurements. The method of introduction of the manometric probes may also influence the recordings of colonic activity. A bowel preparation is often used, and colonoscopic placement causes air insufflation and intraluminal distention of the bowel. Bowel preparation affects motor activity,[25,26] with a trend for motor activity to be increased in the cleansed bowel, especially with regard to stimulation of high amplitude propagated contractions (HAPC).[26] Distention of the colon by air insufflation may also affect motility. Each method therefore has advantages and disadvantages in comparison with the other. The principle benefit of tube mounted strain gauge systems, however, is that ambulatory studies can be performed, something which cannot be done by perfused tube manometry at present.

Manometry can be used to detect motor events in the colorectum, although not all types of activity are detected. Manometers may detect contractions of the colonic wall, but variations in colonic wall tone may not be recorded. Barostats are used to study tonic changes, and in both the colon and rectum dual barostat–manometer assemblies have been shown to record changes in colonic and rectal tone which are not associated with changes of intraluminal pressure as recorded by manometers.[27,28]

Prolonged pancolonic studies of the colon using multilumen perfused catheters have allowed the colon to be studied at many levels so that the interaction of motor events, propagated activities and regional variations can be described. The use of a thick catheter to make the recordings in a sedentary patient, and the need for bowel preparation, sedation and colonoscopy with air insufflation of the colon to place the catheter makes these studies less 'physiological' than desired.

Colonic motor activity

Most colonic motor activity consists of ill defined, low amplitude motor complexes (Fig. 14.1). Periods of complete quiescence alternate with periods of motor activity.[16,26,29] The contractions are of low amplitude (<60 mmHg),[16] occurring sporadically or sometimes as bursts,[16] with a frequency of between 3–8 cpm.[16,26,29] Regional differences in motor patterns exist: the ascending colon has a predominant rhythm of 6 cpm, the distal colon has a rhythm of between 2.5–3.5 cpm.[30] Duration

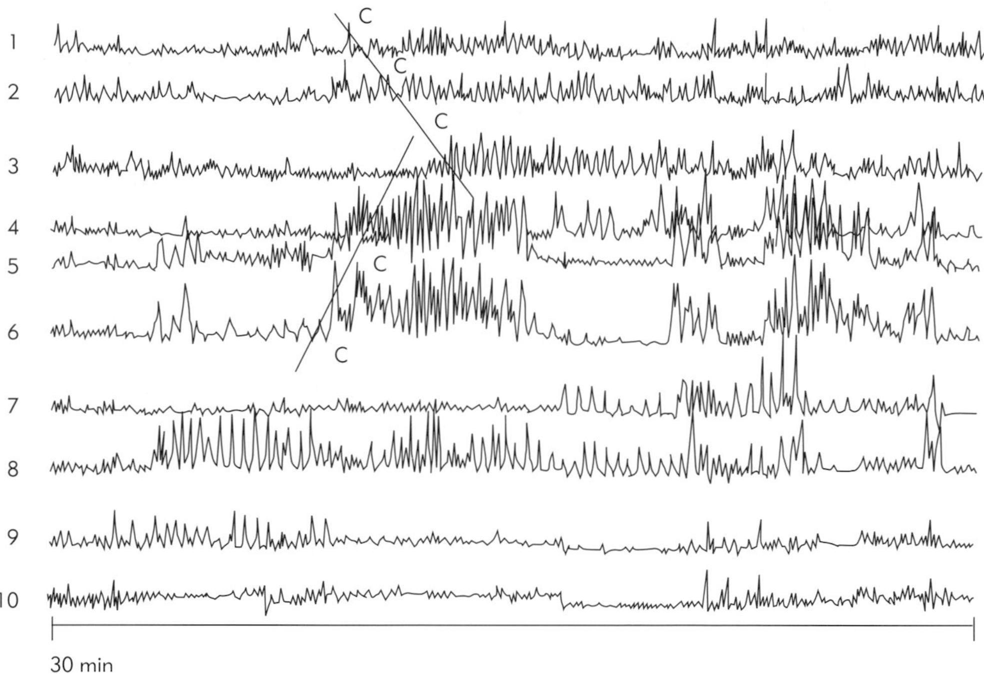

Figure 14.1 Low amplitude motor complexes in the colon (C), in recording leads 1–6 propagating oradly and aboradly in the colon. Time bar denotes 30 minutes. Reproduced with permission.

of such activity ranges between 1–30 minutes.[26] Occasional orad or aborad propagation of low amplitude complexes over short distances has been described,[16] but most low amplitude activity is regarded as segmental and non-propulsive.

High amplitude propagated contraction (HAPC)

High amplitude propagated contractions are occasional, but powerful contractions which may represent the equivalent of the mass movements (Fig. 14.2). The frequency (mean 6.2/24 h) and speed of propagation (mean 1.24 cm/s) are similar in both ambulatory and static perfusion studies.[31,32] However, the amplitude of the contraction is greater, and duration of contraction shorter in ambulant subjects.[31] The origin of HAPC in the human colon requires clarification; HAPC have been reported to originate in the cecum or ascending colon (or are first seen at the most proximal pressure transducer), and propagate to the sigmoid colon.[26] Another study reports that HAPC arise in the transverse colon or descending colon.[16] HAPC identified in the sigmoid colon propagate in orad as well as aborad directions,[31] and therefore HAPC cannot solely arise in the proximal colon. Parameters of HAPC show regional variation, with mean amplitude and propagation velocity being greater in the distal colon.[26]

HAPC occur more frequently preceding defecation.[31] HAPC preceding a bowel movement tend to be higher in amplitude and longer in duration; multiple closely spaced HAPC are seen in association with defecation.[31] HAPC are frequently associated with a mild abdominal discomfort and an urge to defecate.[16] Intraluminal distention is probably not the stimulus for HAPC generation.[33]

Age effects

Age related changes in colonic motility have been described, the frequency of HAPC decreases and the frequency of non-HAPC contractions increases during postnatal maturation of the colon.[34]

Diurnal variation

Diurnal variation of motor activity is present,[29] with the colon quiescent at night and activity increasing on waking (Fig. 14.3),[16] which contrasts with the electrophysiological findings of Frexinos *et al.* that short spike burst activity did not show diurnal variation.[13] Sleep has a profound inhibitory effect on both propagating and non-propagating colonic motor activity which is related to the sleep stage.[35] REM sleep, arousal and waking have an immediate stimulatory action on colonic motility.[35] Colonic tone is also reduced during sleep.[27]

Diurnal variation in the frequency of HAPC has been demonstrated, with a reduction during late afternoon and during sleep,[32] and an increased frequency on waking,[16,31,32] when HAPC are frequently grouped.[32]

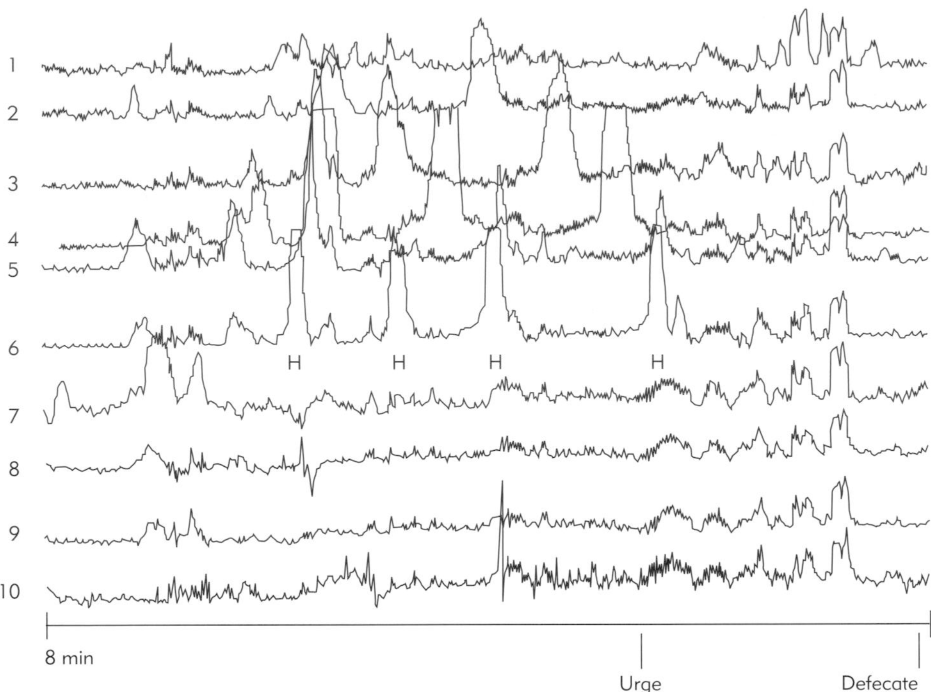

Figure 14.2 A cluster of HAPC in the colon (H) prior to defecation. The HAPC are seen in recording leads 2–6, occur prior to the sensation of an urge to defecate followed by defecation. Time bar denotes 8 minutes. Reproduced with permission.

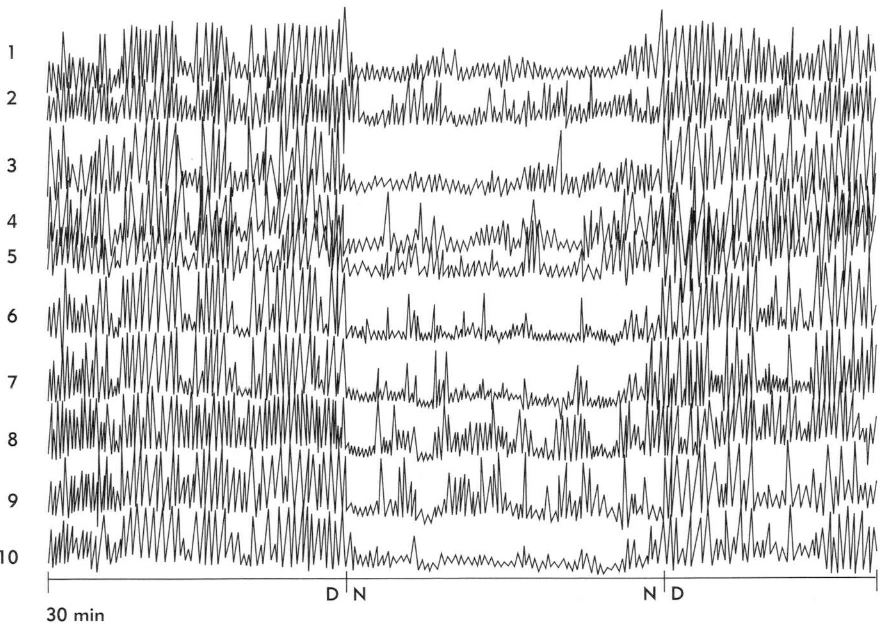

Figure 14.3 Diurnal variation of colorectal motor activity. There is a marked reduction of motor activity at night (N) in comparison to daytime (D). Time bar 19.5 hours. Reproduced with permission.

Effect of eating

The frequency and duration of low amplitude activity is increased after eating, the response to eating is bimodal with an early phase (peaking within 10–40 minutes) and a later phase occurring after 1–2 hours.[16,36] The postprandial response shows regional variation; the increase of non-propagating motor activity is greater in the descending colon in comparison to the transverse and sigmoid colon, intraluminal contents at the splenic flexure are displaced in both orad and aborad directions.[37] Colonic compliance and postprandial increase in tone is greater in the transverse colon than the sigmoid colon. However, pre- and postprandial phasic activity is greater in the sigmoid colon.[36] This quantitatively different but qualitatively similar tonic and phasic response to a meal in the transverse and sigmoid colon may reflect the different viscoelastic properties and luminal dimensions of the segments.[36] The fat component of the diet is the major stimulus to increased sigmoid colonic motor activity, whereas amino acids have an inhibitory action; this parallels the electrical spiking activity in the sigmoid colon.[15] HAPC activity is stimulated by a high fat meal, and HAPC are also grouped after meals.[31]

Ambulatory studies show that physical stressors enhance distal colonic motor activity.[38] However, acute exercise may decrease colonic motor activity and decreased colonic contractions may offer less resistance to flow, hence enhancing colonic transit.[39]

COLONIC MOTOR DISORDERS

Electrophysiological and manometric studies of the colon and rectum have provided insights into the pathophysiology of diseases in which dysmotility is a component. Abnormalities of electrical rhythm, motor frequencies, HAPC, and responses to stimuli have been identified. There are, however, a number of problems with these studies and many of the observations have not been confirmed. The studies themselves often involve only small numbers of patients. Despite the availability of consensus definitions of the functional bowel disorders one must accept that each major grouping comprises a heterogeneous group of patients; this makes consistent selection of patients for study difficult and comparison of such patients even within study groups impractical. The studies differ with regard to: type of apparatus used, bowel preparation, region of the colon studied (often only the distal colon), definition of the parameters measured and data analysis; again making comparison of data obtained from these studies difficult. Often a significant difference in a single parameter of motility is highlighted, even though the role of such an abnormality in the pathophysiology of the disorder is hard to reconcile. The deficiencies of these studies therefore decrease their value, especially if a clinical use is proposed.

CHRONIC IDIOPATHIC CONSTIPATION

The frequency of the slower slow wave rhythm has been shown to be significantly greater in the sigmoid colon of constipated patients in comparison with controls. It was suggested that this may lead to an increase in segmenting contractions and a slowing of colonic transit.[40] The significance of this observation is debatable, however, as no differences in spiking activity or motor activity were identified.[40] In a second study the frequency of short spike bursts was significantly increased in the constipated group,[7] perhaps acting as a brake to movement of intraluminal contents. However a relative lack of propagating spike activity has been observed in colonic inertia.[41] An unconfirmed study reports two distinctly abnormal patterns of electrical activity in the rectum: *bradyrectia* and *tachyrectia*. Bradyrectia is seen in patients with slow transit type constipation, slow wave activity is infrequent, although other parameters of slow wave activity are not significantly different from normal.[41] Tachyrectia is observed in obstructive constipation; regular and reproducible slow waves were recorded which had a significantly greater frequency and velocity than in normal subjects.[42]

In patients with chronic idiopathic constipation, the number of HAPC per 24 hours is significantly reduced as is the duration of the waveform.[43] The amplitude of the waveform is reduced, but not significantly; the velocity of propagation is unaltered.[43] Diurnal variation in HAPC frequency is maintained, but the burst of activity following waking is reduced.[43]

The motor response to a meal has been shown to be abnormal in chronic constipation with no increase in motor activity in the transverse and descending colon, but a reduced increase in motor activity persisted in the sigmoid colon.[44] The normal pressure gradient observed after a meal between the descending colon and the transverse and sigmoid colons is lost.[44]

Exercise may reduce colonic motility, but this effect was less marked in patients with constipation than those with a normal bowel habit.[45]

A hyperactive segment at the rectosigmoid junction has been described, whether this was in patients who had chronic constipation alone, associated with diverticular disease, or constipation-predominant irritable bowel syndrome.[46]

FUNCTIONAL DIARRHEA

An absence of short spike bursts and a significant reduction in the frequency of long spike bursts has been reported in patients with functional diarrhea. A complete lack of short spike bursts, which may be the electrical equivalent of segmenting contractions, may lead to a lack of braking motor activity and increased rate of transit of intraluminal colonic contents.[7]

IRRITABLE BOWEL SYNDROME

A significant increase in the proportion of slow waves having a frequency of 3 cpm has been reported;[47,48] however this has not been confirmed in later studies.[49–51] An increase in spiking activity in those with irritable bowel syndrome has been described.[52] The number and duration of contractions at the rectosigmoid junction was significantly greater amongst patients with irritable bowel syndrome.[50]

HAPC were virtually non-existent in constipation-predominant irritable bowel syndrome.[44,53] The postprandial increase in motor activity was significantly reduced, but normal orad and aborad movement of intraluminal contents persisted.[44]

An abnormal colonic motor response to eating has been reported with irritable bowel syndrome. Instead of two transient increases in motor activity observed in healthy controls there is a sustained increase in activity in the postprandial period.[54]

High amplitude, propagated contractions in diarrhea-predominant irritable bowel syndrome have a similar frequency, duration and propagation velocity to normal controls.[55]

HIRSCHSPRUNG'S DISEASE

An *in vitro* investigation of aganglionic muscle strips revealed that the longitudinal muscle layer was electrically quiescent, and the circular muscle layer was mainly quiescent with occasional low frequency action potentials, indicating an aperistaltic obstruction of the colon.[2] This abnormality of slow wave generation is reflected in the irregular slow waves of low potential recorded *in vivo* in patients with Hirschsprung's disease.[56]

POSTOPERATIVE COLONIC ACTIVITY

In the postoperative period colonic motility commenced with short spike bursts and long spike bursts on the third postoperative day,[57] first in the right then in the left colon.[58] Normalization of electrical activity occurred on the sixth postoperative day.[57,58]

The character of distal colonic motility in the postoperative period has been studied with strain gauge manometers. The effect of a colonic anastomosis[59] and the prokinetic agent cisapride have been evaluated.[60] It was concluded that a colonic anastomosis has an inhibitory affect on distal colonic motility, and although cisapride does increase some indices of colonic motility this was unlikely to be clinically relevant.[59,60]

DIVERTICULAR DISEASE

The motor activity of the sigmoid colon, with respect to the motility index and amplitude of contractions was increased pre- and postprandially in patients with diverticular disease.[61]

CHRONIC IDIOPATHIC INTESTINAL PSEUDO-OBSTRUCTION

Perfusion manometry has been used to investigate children with chronic idiopathic intestinal pseudo-obstruction, a diagnosis of the myopathic or neuropathic form of the disease having been made on the basis of small bowel biopsy and/or antroduodenal manometry. Two abnormal motor patterns were described. In the myopathic form of the disease there is an absence of contractile activity, and in the neuropathic form of the disease there is an absence of the response to eating and significantly reduced numbers of HAPC were seen.[62]

ANO-RECTAL MOTILITY

The ano-rectum is the continuation of the colon. The muscle layer comprises an inner circular muscle layer and an outer longitudinal muscle layer. The circular muscle layer is in continuity with the internal anal sphincter, formed from smooth muscle. The external anal sphincter is formed from striated muscle and is under voluntary control. The external anal sphincter is subdivided into deep, superficial and subcutaneous bands. The longitudinal muscle layer of the rectum splits to pass on either side of the external anal sphincter to insert into the subcutaneous tissues of the skin.

ANO-RECTAL ELECTRICAL ACTIVITY

In vitro and *in vivo* studies of anal electrical motor activity have been performed. Ambulatory electromyography (EMG), using cutaneous electrodes to monitor external anal sphincter activity,[63] and also with implantable fine wire electrodes to record internal anal sphincter, external and sphincter and puborectalis activity,[64] can be combined with ambulatory manometry.

ANO-RECTAL MANOMETRY

Rectal manometry can be performed using the same techniques as used in the assessment of the colon. Static anal manometry has been performed using microballoon systems, sleeve catheters and also with multilumen perfusion catheters. Microballoon systems are reliable for measuring resting and voluntary contraction anal canal pressure. Microballoon systems are generally fluid filled, although air filled systems are proposed to be as equally useful.[65] A single balloon transducer using a continuous or station pull-through technique can measure both of these parameters and anal canal length. Balloon systems are multidirectional and can detect contractions from any sector of the sphincter. Measurement periods are, however, short and do not show periodic events. The usual method has the patient in the left lateral position which may not accurately reflect erect anal and rectal pressures, as both have been shown to be posture dependent.[66] Multilumen perfusion catheters allow pressure recordings at many levels, but are also laboratory based. Again the patient is in the left lateral position and the leakage of fluid from the catheters may disturb reflex activity in the ano-rectum. Depending on the catheter assembly the manometers may be unidirectional or multidirectional. Localized defects in the external anal sphincter have been identified by anal pressure vectography.[67] Sleeve catheter assemblies have a fluid-filled sleeve mounted over a catheter which spans the sphincter complex. Fluid is constantly perfused; ano-rectal contractions obstruct fluid perfusion and are recorded. The sleeve catheter however cannot distinguish at which level of the anal canal the contraction occurred.

Probe-mounted, solid-state pressure transducers allow ambulatory manometric studies of ano-rectal motility to be performed. The probe should have as a minimum two transducers, one in the rectum and one in the mid-anal canal; an additional transducer in the upper anal canal adds more valuable information. Simultaneous recordings from more than one level enable assessment of interactive events in the ano-rectum.

The main advantages of ambulatory monitoring are that prolonged periods of study can be performed outside the laboratory under more normal physiological conditions. This permits examination of ano-rectum during micturition, passing flatus, defecation, sleeping and in the postprandial period. Anal canal pressures are posture dependent,[66] therefore the data collected from studies with subjects in more natural positions such as standing, sitting or lying is likely to be more relevant. Even so, results have shown that motor activity is disturbed for the first hour after beginning ambulatory recordings,[68] indicating that there is a period of accommodation to instrumentation before normal activity resumes. Therefore, a minimum recording period of one hour is recommended. This finding further suggests that prolonged ambulatory recording is required to provide representative data.

Ambulatory recording is technically demanding. Probe displacement after the subject has left the laboratory may occur. Most investigators have relied on adhesive tape at the anal margin to secure the probe.[61,69] A silicone mould in the shape of the natal cleft has been used as a means for maintaining probe position, and also to facilitate accurate and reproducible positioning after displacement.[70] It has been shown that the radial orientation of the pressure transducer influences the recorded pressure value.[71] This therefore has to be considered and controlled when positioning the probe, since a standard orientation should be made to allow intersubject comparison. Use of a single direction of orientation may provide an incomplete assessment of the sphincter.

The assessment of ano-rectal motility is complemented by imaging in the form of endoanal ultrasound, isotope defecography and cinedefecography.

Rectal motor activity

The rectum has been shown to exhibit periodic motor activity,[72] which has diurnal variation. The rectal motor complex (Fig. 14.4) describes clusters of sustained, regular activity in the rectum, and runs of powerful (greater than 50 mmHg) contractions with a dominant frequency of three cycles per minute and sustained for three to ten minutes, with a periodicity of about 92 minutes during the day and 56 minutes at night.[72] In addition to the rectal motor complex there are isolated prolonged contractions, mainly occurring during the day, and post prandial clusters of contractions.[72] Periodic rectal motor activity (PRMA) has been associated temporally with more proximal colonic motor activity, suggesting that PRMA is triggered by the arrival of stool or gas from the colon, and may serve as a braking mechanism to prevent untimely flow of colonic contents.[73]

Electrical activity in the internal anal sphincter comprises irregular slow wave activity, with a contraction frequency of 15–25 cpm.[74–76] This is reflected in the findings of manometric studies; the predominant pattern of motor activity in the anal canal are slow waves at 10–20 cpm,[74,76] and amplitude 5–25 cmH_2O.[69] Ultraslow waves (0.5–2 cycles per minute) have also been identified in normal subjects.[68,77] Ambulatory resting anal pressures in healthy subjects have a median value of 94 cmH_2O.[77,78] The frequency of contraction of the internal anal sphincter shows a linear relationship with resting anal canal pressure. The internal anal sphincter accounts for approximately 85% of resting anal canal pressure;[79] the remaining 15% is provided by the anal cushions.[80] The external anal sphincter (EAS) is continuously active, responds to stimuli and is under voluntary control.[81] Contraction of the external anal sphincter can increase basal pressures by 175–250%; however the muscle is fatigable and this response is not prolonged.

Recto-anal inhibitory reflex

The recto-anal inhibitory reflex describes the relaxation of the internal anal sphincter in response to distention of the rectum. Anal pressure returns after continuous or submaximal rectal distention. The internal anal sphincter remains relaxed though with maximal rectal distention. Slow distention of the rectum may not cause a fall in anal canal pressure, became the internal anal sphincter can maintain continence during slow rectal filling.[82]

The anal sampling reflex

The sampling reflex describes a transient fall in anal canal pressure so that it is equal to or less than rectal pressure. It is a normal event, occurring about seven times each hour in health.[69] The reflex may be associated with the awareness of flatus. The fall in anal canal pressure is mainly in the upper anal canal so that rectal pressure does not exceed mid-anal canal pressure in normal subjects.[78] There is a diurnal variation in the number of sampling reflexes per hour; the frequency is significantly reduced (mean 1.7/h) during sleep.[63] They are termed sampling reflexes as it is thought the equalization of

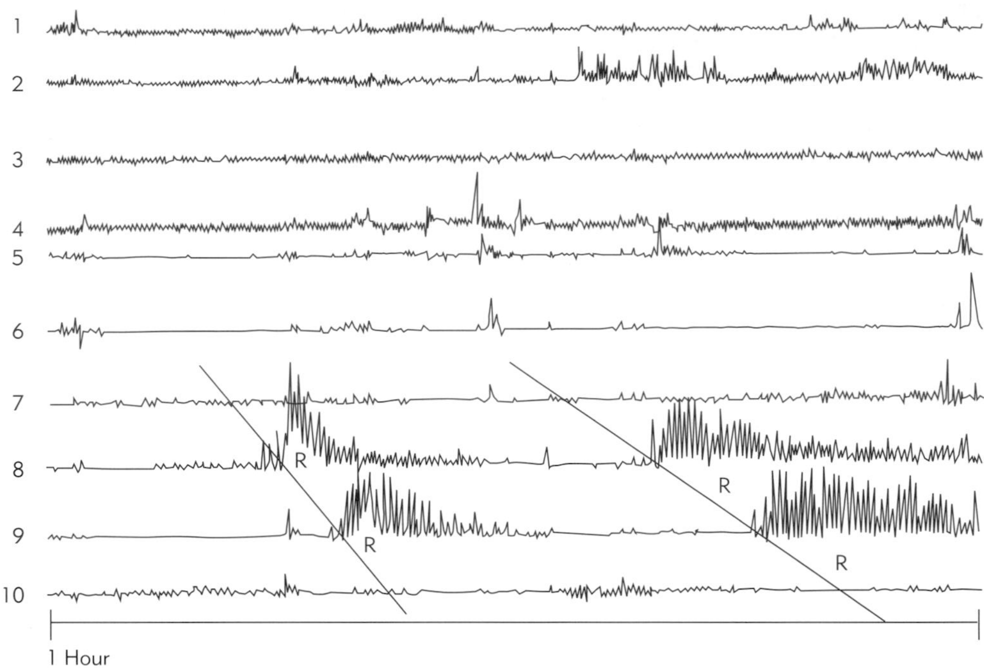

Figure 14.4 Rectal motor complexes (R) in recording leads 8 and 9 propagating aborally. Time bar denotes one hour. Reproduced with permission.

rectal and upper anal canal pressure allows rectal contents to come into contact with the sensitive anal canal mucosa allowing discrimination of rectal contents.

The passage of flatus has been associated with no change in anal canal pressures, an increase in anal canal pressure, or a transient relaxation of anal canal pressure followed by contraction.[63] Another group report a fall in anal canal pressure with a relatively small rise in rectal pressure, events not statistically different from those noted with awareness of flatus.[83]

During micturition, anal canal pressure increases. This has been correlated with an increase in activity of the external anal sphincter,[63] and may protect against the relaxation of the internal anal sphincter that has been described to occur during micturition.[78] There is a postprandial change in the pattern of motor activity of the anal canal, with an increase in the number of sampling reflex episodes per hour (mean 9.2/h).[63] This may be a consequence of the increased rectal activity.

During sleep it has been noted that sampling reflex activity decreases, and the resting anal canal pressure also falls, to about 25% of daytime basal values.[76]

RECTAL MOTOR DISORDERS

FECAL INCONTINENCE

The pathophysiology underlying fecal incontinence has been much studied. In neurogenic fecal incontinence the resting pressure in the anal canal is reduced (median 54 cmH_2O), and this is associated with a decrease in the internal anal sphincter electromyographical frequency.[68] The number of transient relaxations of the internal anal sphincter per hour is increased.[68,84,85] During these transient relaxations the fall in the mid anal pressure is greater than normal such that rectal pressure may exceed mid anal canal pressure. This does not occur in normal subjects.[68] External anal sphincter recruitment during these episodes is poor,[68,85] and the duration of anal canal relaxation is longer.[84] The recto-anal inhibitory reflex is increased in amplitude. The sampling reflex is abnormal in incontinent patients.[86] All these factors may predispose to episodes of incontinence. An electromechanical dissociation of the internal anal sphincter has been described, although its contribution to the disorder is unclear.[78] External sphincter weakness has been associated with fecal incontinence, especially in those patients with a hypersensitive rectum.[82] In urge fecal incontinence contributory events in the rectum have been identified, Large rectal pressure waves with no compensatory increase in anal tone precede episodes of incontinence, Resting anal canal pressures in these patients is normal.[88] External anal sphincter dysfunction is reported in urge incontinence.[89] Instability of the internal anal sphincter may play a role in the etiology of fecal incontinence in diabetes.[90]

CONSTIPATION

Patients with chronic idiopathic constipation exhibit reduced frequency of the anal sampling reflex (mean 2.4/h), perhaps reflecting decreased transit of feces from the colon into the rectum.[91] The motor activity in the rectum is abnormal with decreased amplitude (mean 42 mmHg) of the rectal motor complex.[91] It is suggested that a neuropathy involving the rectum may be a factor in the disease.

PRURITIS ANI

It is proposed that idiopathic pruritis ani may result from abnormal transient internal sphincter relaxation. Resting anal canal pressure and sampling reflex activity are similar to normal controls. However during the sampling reflex, the rise in rectal pressure, the fall in anal canal pressure and the duration of anal sphincter relaxation were significantly greater in those with pruritis ani, perhaps predisposing to minor fecal leakage and perianal soiling.[92]

CHRONIC ANAL FISSURE

Ambulatory studies have confirmed anal sphincter hypertonia (median anal resting pressure of 132 cmH_2O) as a factor in the etiology of some chronic anal fissures,[77] associated with a reduction in the number of sampling episodes per hour. Following surgical intervention and healing of the fissure, resting anal canal pressure fell significantly so that it was similar to normal controls, and the frequency of the sampling reflex increased.[77] These findings could form the basis of a test to check efficacy of surgery in reducing anal canal pressure if healing did not follow intervention. Postpartum anal fissures, however, are associated with reduced anal canal pressures. Surgical interference should therefore be avoided.[93]

RECTAL PROLAPSE

Patients with rectal prolapse have reduced resting anal canal pressures, with sustained high pressure rectal contractions which coincide with a decrease in anal canal pressure, leading to a desire to defecate or an episode of incontinence.[94] The high pressure rectal contractions are absent following resection rectopexy,[64,94] and probably reflect the presence of the intersusscepting organ in the rectum, rather than a causative factor.

HEMORRHOIDS

In the presence of hemorrhoids, there is normal rectal motor activity,[95] increased or normal rates of anal sampling,[95,96] and increased resting anal canal pressure (median value of 116 cmH_2O).[77] It has been suggested that increased vascular pressure in the anal cushions is the cause for the raised resting anal canal pressure[97] and not hypertrophy of the internal anal sphincter.[94] Ultraslow wave and giant ultraslow wave activity were seen more frequently in those with hemorrhoids.[98] External anal sphincter overactivity has been described in patients with hemorrhoids.[98]

POUCH FORMATION

Restorative proctocolectomy with ileal pouch formation and ileoanal anastomosis is used in the management of ulcerative colitis and familial adenomatous polyposis. Ambulatory pouch and anal manometry has given valuable insights into the post operative physiology, indicating why some surgical techniques may give better functional results. Internal anal sphincter electromyographic activity and resting anal pressure are reduced following surgery with incomplete recovery at 18 months.[99] Giant contraction waves in the pouch, associated with increased stool frequency, are more frequent if the pouch is less than 300 mL in capacity.[100] Nocturnal incontinence has been associated with increased frequency of pouch contractions.[101] The value of performing a mucosal proctectomy and endoanal anastomosis rather than preservation of the entire anal canal and stapled ileoanal anastomosis without mucosectomy has been debated. In comparative studies it has been found that those who did not undergo mucosectomy showed basal motor activity in the internal sphincter and a normal rate of anal sampling, whereas the mucosal proctectomy group exhibited basal motor activity and the rate of rectal sampling was much lower.[102] Higher resting anal pressures have been reported with a stapled ileoanal anastomosis.[103] It has been concluded that the internal anal sphincter was damaged during mucosal proctectomy, perhaps accounting for the poorer results in terms of fecal leakage.[102] It may be expected that patients with low resting anal pressures before pouch surgery would do badly. However, it has been shown that in such patients a deleterious decrease in pressure does not occur but actually improves postoperatively,[104] so they should not be denied this surgical option.

LOW ANTERIOR RESECTION OF THE RECTUM

The effect of low anterior resection has been investigated. The adverse clinical outcomes such as urge and frequency of defecation are associated with significantly higher neorectal pressures and lower resting anal pressures.[105] It was suggested that to achieve better functional results the capacity of the neorectum should be increased.

HIRSCHSPRUNG'S DISEASE

The recto-anal inhibitory reflex is absent, ano-rectal manometry can be used to diagnose the disease in the newborn period.[106]

PROCTALGIA FUGAX

Paroxysmal hyperkinesis of the anus (high amplitude, high frequency myoelectrical activity of the anal sphincter) has been observed in proctalgia fugax.[107] This observation was made in a single patient with paraplegia so can not be regarded as conclusive evidence for the etiology of the condition.

CONCLUSIONS

Assessment of the ano-rectum is common in clinical practice. Electrophysiological and manometric studies of the large bowel have given insights into gut motility in health and disease, but the complete pattern of colorectal motor activity is still to be fully defined. Ambulant manometry, using fully portable pressure measuring and recording systems, and commercially available analysis packages should make studies performed in a normal environment with measurements made during daily physiological activities an achievable target in the short term.

Pancolonic studies with suitable spacing of pressure transducers are needed to determine regional variations in colonic motility. Once the normal patterns have been defined then colonic motor abnormalities can be assessed in disease states. Ambulant manometry has the advantage of allowing study under more physiological conditions, and will probably become the gold standard in the assessment of colonic and ano-rectal motor activity.

Ambulant manometry may also have a role in the evaluation of therapeutic interventions, and patient selection prior to surgical intervention, and may be complementary to the use of transit study assessment of colonic motility. Further advances in technology and wider availability of reliable measurement systems will enable the transition of colorectal motility measurements, whether manometric or electrophysiological, from the research laboratory to the clinical arena.

REFERENCES

1. Huizinga JD, Stern HS, Chow E, *et al.* Electrophysiologic control of motility in the human colon. *Gastroenterology* 1985;**88**:500–11.
2. Kubota M, Ito Y, Ikeda K. Membrane properties and innervation of smooth muscle cells in Hirschsprung's disease. *Am J Physiol* 1983;**252**: C215–C224.
3. Gill RC, Cote KR, Bowes KL, *et al.* Human colonic smooth muscle: electrical and contractile activity *in vitro*. *Gut* 1986;**27**:293–9.
4. Huizinga JD, Stern HS, Chow E, *et al.* Electrical basis of excitation and inhibition of human colonic smooth muscle. *Gastroenterology* 1986;**90**:1197–204.
5. Huizinga JD. Electrophysiology of human colon motility in health and disease. *Clin Gastroenterol* 1986;**15**:879–901.
6. Sarna SK, Bardakjian BL, Waterfall WE, *et al.* Human colonic electrical control activity (ECA). *Gastroenterology* 1980;**78**:1526–36.
7. Bueno L, Fioramonti J, Ruckebusch Y, *et al.* Evaluation of colonic myoelectrical activity in health and functional disorders. *Gut*, 1980;**21**:480–5.
8. Sarna SK, Waterfall WE, Bardakjian BL, *et al.* Types of human colonic electrical activities recorded postoperatively. *Gastroenterology* 1981;**81**:61–70.
9. Schang JC, Devroede G. Fasting and postprandial myoelectric spiking activity in the human sigmoid colon. *Gastroenterology* 1983;**85**:1048–53.
10. Taylor I, Duthie HL, Smallwood R, *et al.* Large bowel myoelectrical activity in man. *Gut* 1975;**16**:808–14.
11. Dapoigny M, Trolese JF, Bommelaer G, *et al.* Myoelectric spiking activity of right colon, left colon, and rectosigmoid of healthy humans. *Dig Dis Sci* 1988;**33**:1007–12.
12. Sarna SK, Latimer P, Campbell D, *et al.* Electrical and contractile activities of the human rectosigmoid. *Gut* 1982;**23**:698–705.
13. Frexinos J, Bueno L, Fioramonti J. Diurnal changes in myoelectric spiking activity of the human colon. *Gastroenterology* 1985;**88**:1104–10.
14. Schang JC, Hemond M, Hebert M, *et al.* Myoelectrical activity and intraluminal flow in human sigmoid colon. *Digest Dis Sci* 1986;**31**:1331–7.
15. Wright SH, Snape WJ, Jr. Battle W, *et al.* Effect of dietary components on gastrocolonic response. *Am J Physiol* 1980;**238**:G228–32.
16. Narducci F, Bassotti G, Gaburri M, *et al.* Twenty four hour manometric recording of colonic motor activity in healthy man. *Gut* 1987;**28**:17–25.
17. Reynolds JR, Clark AG, Evans DF, *et al.* Investigation of the daily variation of colonic motor activity in man using a portable pressure recording system. *Digest Dis Sci* 1986;**31**:414–15.
18. Morris DL, Clark AG, Evans DF, *et al.* Triple radioelectric pill study of postoperative ileus. *Digest Surg* 1987;**4**:160–63.
19. Parker R, Whitehead WE, Schuster MM. Pattern-recognition program for analysis of colon myoelectric and pressure data. *Digest Dis Sci* 1987;**32**: 953–61.
20. Rogers J, Misiewicz JJ. Fully automated computor analysis of intracolonic pressures. *Gut* 1989;**30**:642–9.
21. Nordgren S, Abrahamson H. Methods for the investigation of colonic motility. *Eur J Surg* 1991;Suppl.**564**:63–71.
22. Valori RM, Collins SM, Daniel EE, *et al.* Comparison of methodologies for the measurement of antroduodenal motor activity in the dog. *Gastroenterology* 1986;**91**: 546–53.
23. Cook IJ, Reddy SN, Collins SM, *et al.* Influence of recording techniques on measurement of canine colonic motility. *Dig Dis Sci* 1988;**33**:999–1006.
24. Sasaki Y, Munakata A. High viscous luminal content causes different manometric outcomes between methodologies. *Gastroenterology* 1995;**108**:A683.
25. Dinoso VP, Murphy SNS, Goldstein J, *et al.* Basal motor activity of the distal colon, a reappraisal. *Gastroenterology* 1983;**85**:637–42.
26. Lemann M, Flourie B, Picon L, *et al.* Motor activity recorded in the unprepared colon of healthy humans [see comments]. *Gut* 1995;**37**:649–53.
27. Steadman CJ, Phillips SF, Camilleri M, *et al.* Variation of muscle tone in the human colon. *Gastroenterology* 1991;**101**:373–81.

28. Bell AM, Pemberton JH, Hanson RB, *et al.* Variations in muscle tone of the human rectum: recordings with an electromechanical barostat. *Am J Physiol* 1991;**260**:G17–25.
29. Soffer EE, Scalabrini P, Wingate DL. Prolonged ambulant monitoring of human colonic motility. *Am J Physiol* 1989;**257**:G601–G606.
30. Kerlin P, Zinsmeister A, Philips S, Motor responses to food of the ileum, proximal colon, and distal colon of healthy humans. *Gastroenterology* 1983;**84**:762–60.
31. Crowell MD, Bassotti G, Cheskin LJ, *et al.* Method for prolonged ambulatory monitoring of high-amplitude propagated contractions from colon. *Am J Physiol* 1991;**261**:G263–8.
32. Bassotti G, Gaburri M. Manometric investigation of high-amplitude propagated contractile activity of the human colon. *Am J Physiol* 1988;**255**:G660–4.
33. Bassotti G, Gaburri M, Imbimbo BP, *et al.* Distension-stimulated propagated contractions in human colon. *Dig Dis Sci* 1994;**39**:1955–60.
34. Di Lorenzo C, Flores AF, Hyman PE. Age-related changes in colon motility. *J Pediat* 1995;**127**:593–6.
35. Furukawa Y, Cook IJ, Panagopoulos V, *et al.* Relationship between sleep patterns and human colonic motor patterns [see comments]. *Gastroenterology*, 1994;**107**: 1372–81.
36. Ford MJ, Camilleri M, Wiste JA, *et al.* Differences in colonic tone and phasic response to a meal in the transverse and sigmoid human colon. *Gut* 1995;**37**:264–9.
37. Moreno-Osset E, Bazzocchi G, Lo S, *et al.* Association between postprandial changes in colonic intraluminal pressure and transit. *Gastroenterology* 1989; **96**:1265–73.
38. Rao SSC, Suls J, Hatfield R, *et al.* Effects of psychological and physical stress on human colonic motor activity. *Gastroenterology* 1995;**108**:A674.
39. Rao SSC, Chamberlain M, Leistikow J, *et al.* Effects of acute graded exercise on human colonic motility. *Gastroenterology* 1997;**112**:A810.
40. Frieri G, Parisi P, Corazziari E, *et al.* Colonic electromyography in chronic constipation. *Gastroenterology* 1983;**84**:737–40.
41. Schang JC, Devroede G, Duguay C, *et al.* Constipation caused by colonic inertia and distal obstruction: electromyographic study. *Gastroenterol Clin Biol* 1985;**9**:480–5.
42. Shafik A. Electrorectography in chronic constipation. *World J Surg* 1995;**19**:772–5.
43. Bassotti G, Gaburri M, Imbimbo BP, *et al.* Colonic mass movements in idiopathic chronic constipation. *Gut*, 1988;**29**:1173–9.
44. Bazzocchi G, Ellis J, Villanueva-Meyer J, *et al.* Postprandial colonic transit and motor activity in chronic constipation. *Gastroenterology* 1990;**98**:686–93.
45. Rao SSC, Chamberlain M, Leistikow J, *et al.* Does exercise stimulate colonic motility in constipation? *Gastroenterology* 1997;**112**:A809.
46. Chowdhury AR, Dinoso VP, Lorber SH. Characterization of a hyperactive segment at the rectosigmoid junction. *Gastroenterology* 1976;**71**:584–8.
47. Snape WJ, Jr, Carlson GM, Cohen S. Colonic myoelectric activity in the irritable bowel syndrome. *Gastroenterology* 1976;**70**:326–30.
48. Taylor I, Darby C, Hammond P, *et al.* Is there a myoelectrical abnormality in the irritable colon syndrome? *Gut* 1978;**19**:391–5.
49. Katschinski M, Lederer P, Ellermann A, *et al.* Myoelectric and manometric patterns of human rectosigmoid colon in irritable bowel syndrome and diverticulosis. *Scand J Gastroenterol* 1990;**25**:761–8.
50. Latimer P, Sarna S, Campbell D, *et al.* Colonic motor and myoelectrical activity: a comparative study of normal subjects, psychoneurotic patients, and patients with irritable bowel syndrome. *Gastroenterology* 1981;**80**:893–901.
51. Welgan P, Meshkinpour H, Hoehler F. The effect of stress on colon motor and electrical activity in irritable bowel syndrome. *Psychosomat Med* 1985;**47**:139–49.
52. Welgan P, Meshkinpour H, Beeler M. Effect of anger on colon motor and myoelectric activity in irritable bowel syndrome. *Gastroenterology* 1988;**94**:1150–6.
53. Crowell MD, Whitehead WE, Cheskin LJ, *et al.* Twenty four hour ambulatory monitoring of peristaltic activity from the colon in normals and constipation prodominant IBS patients. *Gastroenterology* 1989;**96**:A103.
54. Narducci F, Bassotti G, Granata MT, *et al.* Colonic motility and gastric emptying in patients with irritable bowel syndrome. Effect of pretreatment with octylonium bromide. *Digest Dis Sci* 1986;**31**:241–6.
55. Crowell MD, Whitehead WE, Pelli MA, *et al.* Colonic mass movements in diarrhea-predominant IBS patients. *Gastroenterology* 1990;**98**:A326.
56. Marin AM, Rivarola A, Garcia H. Electromyography of the rectum and colon in Hirschsprung's disease. *J Pediat Surg* 1976;**11**:547–52.
57. Giorgio I, Abbattista N, Tritto G, *et al.* [Reorganization of the electrical activity of the transverse colon after cholecystectomy. Study in humans with implanted electrodes]. *Pathol Biol* 1987;**35**:367–74.
58. Condon RE, Cowles VE, Ferraz AA, *et al.* Human colonic smooth muscle electrical activity during and after recovery from postoperative ileus. *Am J Physiol* 1995;**269**:G408–17.
59. Roberts JP, Benson MJ, Rogers J, *et al.* Characterization of distal colonic motility in early postoperative period and effect of colonic anastomosis. *Digest Dis Sci* 1994;**39**:1961–7.
60. Roberts JP, Benson MJ, Rogers J, *et al.* Effect of cisapride on distal colonic motility in the early postoperative period following left colonic anastomosis. *Dis Colon Rectum* 1995;**38**:139–45.
61. Trotman IF, Misiewicz JJ. Sigmoid motility in diverticular disease and the irritable bowel syndrome. *Gut* 1988;**29**:218–22.
62. Di Lorenzo C, Flores AF, Reddy SN *et al.* Colonic manometry in children with chronic intestinal pseudo-obstruction. *Gut* 1993;**34**:803–7.
63. Kumar D, Waldron D, Williams NS, *et al.* Prolonged anorectal manometry and external anal sphincter electromyography in ambulant human subjects. *Dig Dis Sci* 1990;**35**:641–8.
64. Farouk R, Duthie GS, Bartolo DC, *et al.* Restoration of continence following rectopexy for rectal prolapse and recovery of the internal anal sphincter electromyogram. *Br J Surg* 1992;**79**:439–40.

65. Miller R, Bartolo DC, James D, *et al.* Air-filled microballoon manometry for use in anorectal physiology. *Br J Surg* 1989;**76**:72–5.
66. Johnson GP, Pemberton JH, Ness J, *et al.* Transducer manometry and the effect of body position on anal canal pressures. *Dis Colon Rectum* 1990;**33**: 469–75.
67. Perry RE, Blatchford GJ, Christensen MA, *et al.* Manometric diagnosis of anal sphincter injuries. *Am J Surg* 1990;**159**:112–6; discussion 116–7.
68. Farouk R, Duthie GS, Pryde A, *et al.* Internal anal sphincter dysfunction in neurogenic faecal incontinence. *Br J Surg* 1993;**80**:259–61.
69. Miller R, Lewis GT, Bartolo DC, *et al.* Sensory discrimination and dynamic activity in the anorectum: evidence using a new ambulatory technique. *Br J Surg* 1988;**75**:1003–1007.
70. Auwerda JJ, Schouten WR. New device for adequate fixation of recording instruments in ambulant anorectal manometry. *Dis Colon Rectum* 1994;**37**:383–5.
71. Miller R, Bartolo DC, Roe AM, *et al.* Assessment of microtransducers in anorectal manometry. *Br J Surg* 1988;**75**:40–3.
72. Kumar D, Williams NS, Waldron D, *et al.* Prolonged manometric recordings of anorectal motor activity in ambulant human subjects: evidence of periodic activity. *Gut* 1989;**30**:1007–1011.
73. Rao SSC, Welcher K. Periodic rectal motor activity: The intrinsic colonic gatekeeper? *Am J Gastroenterol* 1996;**91**:890–97.
74. Wankling WJ, Brown BH, Collins CD, *et al.* Basal electrical activity in the anal canal in man. *Gut* 1968;**9**:457–60.
75. Monges H, Salducci J, Naudi B. Electrical activity of internal anal sphincter. A comparative study in man and cat. In: Christensen JM (ed.) *Gastrointestinal motility*. New York: Raven Press, 1980;495–502.
76. Kerremans R. Electrical activity and motility of the internal anal sphincter: an *in vivo* electrophysiological study in man. *Acta Gastroenterol Belg* 1968;**31**:465–82.
77. Farouk R, Duthie GS, MacGregor AB, *et al.* Sustained internal sphincter hypertonia in patients with chronic anal fissure. *Dis Colon Rectum* 1994;**37**:424–9.
78. Farouk R, Duthie GS, MacGregor AB, *et al.* Evidence of electromechanical dissociation of the internal anal sphincter in idiopathic fecal incontinence. *Dis Colon Rectum* 1994;**37**:595–601.
79. Frenckner B, von Euler C. Influence of pudendal nerve block on the function of the anal sphincters. *Gut* 1975;**16**:482–9.
80. Lestar B, Penninckx F, Kerremans R. The composition of anal basal pressure. An *in-vivo* and *in-vitro* study in man. *Internat J Colorectal Dis* 1989;**4**:118–22.
81. Floyd W, Walls E. Electromyography of the sphincter ani externus in man. *J Physiol* 1953;**16**:638–44.
82. Sun WM, Read NW, Prior A, *et al.* Sensory and motor responses to rectal distention vary according to rate and pattern of balloon inflation. *Gastroenterology* 1990;**99**:1008–15.
83. Miller R, Bartolo DCC, Cervero F, *et al.* Ambulatory anorectal manometry: a new technique for the investigation of anorectal function. *Br J Surg* 1988;**75**:605.
84. Kumar D, Waldron D, Williams NS. Anorectal motility and external sphincter electromyography in idiopathic fecal incontinence: an ambulant assessment. *Gastrenterology* 1989;**96**:A277.
85. Sun WM, Read NW, Miner PB, *et al.* The role of transient internal sphincter relaxation in faecal incontinence? *Internat J Colorect Dis* 1990;**5**:31–6.
86. Miller R, Bartolo DC, Cervero F, *et al.* Anorectal sampling: a comparison of normal and incontinent patients. *Br J Surg* 1988;**75**:44–7.
87. Sun WM, Donnelly TC, Read NW. Utility of a combined test of anorectal manometry, electromyography, and sensation in determining the mechanism of 'idiopathic' faecal incontinence. *Gut* 1992;**33**:807–13.
88. Roberts JP, Williams NS. The role and technique of ambulatory anal manometry. *Baillière's Clin Gastroenterol* 1992;**6**:163–78.
89. Gee AS, Durdey P. Urge incontinence of faeces is a marker of severe external anal sphincter dysfunction. *Br J Surg* 1995;**82**:1179–82.
90. Sun WM, Katsinelos P, Horowitz M, *et al.* Disturbances in anorectal function in patients with diabetes mellitus and faecal incontinence. *Eur J Gastroenterol Hepatol* 1996;**8**:1007–12.
91. Waldron DJ, Kumar D, Hallan RI, *et al.* Evidence for motor neuropathy and reduced filling of the rectum in chronic intractable constipation. *Gut* 1990;**31**:1284–8.
92. Farouk R, Duthie GS, Pryde A, *et al.* Abnormal transient internal sphincter relaxation in idiopathic pruritus ani: physiological evidence from ambulatory monitoring. *Br J Surg* 1994;**81**:603–6.
93. Corby H, Donnelly VS, *et al.* Anal canal pressures are low in women with postpartum anal fissure. *Br J Surg* 1997;**84**:86–8.
94. Farouk R, Duthie GS, MacGregor AB, *et al.* Rectoanal inhibition and incontinence in patients with rectal prolapse. *Br J Surg* 1994;**81**:743–6.
95. Waldron DJ, Kumar D, Hallan RI, *et al.* Prolonged ambulant assessment of anorectal function in patients with prolapsing hemorrhoids. *Dis Colon Rectum* 1989;**32**:968–74.
96. Sun WM, Peck RJ, Shorthouse AJ, *et al.* Haemorrhoids are associated not with hypertrophy of the internal anal sphincter, but with hypertension of the anal cushions. *Br J Surg* 1992;**79**:592–4.
97. Sun WM, Read NW, Shorthouse AJ. Hypertensive anal cushions as a cause of the high anal canal pressures in patients with haemorrhoids. *Br J Surg* 1990;**77**:458–62.
98. Waldron DJ, Kumar D, Hallan RI, *et al.* Prolonged ambulant assessment of anorectal function in patients with prolapsing hemorrhoids. *Dis Colon Rectum* 1998;**32**:968–74.
99. Farouk R, Duthie GS, Bartolo DC. Recovery of the internal anal sphincter and continence after restorative proctocolectomy. *Br J Surg* 1994;**81**:1065–8.
100. Kumar D, Waldron D, Nicholls RJ, *et al.* Motor function of the ileal reservoir following restorative proctocolectomy. *Gastroenterology* 1989;**96**:A276.
101. Miller R, Orrom WJ, Duthie G, *et al.* Ambulatory anorectal physiology in patients following restorative proctocolectomy for ulcerative colitis: comparison with normal controls. *Br J Surg* 1990;**77**:895–7.

102. Holdsworth PJ, Sagar PM, Lewis WG, *et al.* Internal anal sphincter activity after restorative proctocolectomy for ulcerative colitis: a study using continuous ambulatory manometry. *Dis Colon Rectum* 1994;**37**:32–6.
103. Reilly WT, Pemberton JH, Wolff BG, *et al.* Randomized prospective trial comparing ileal pouch-anal anastomosis performed by excising the anal mucosa to ileal pouch-anal anastomosis performed by preserving the anal mucosa. *Ann Surg* 1997;**225**:666–6; discussion 676–7.
104. Takao Y, Weiss EG, Nogueras JJ, *et al.* Should ileoanal pouch surgery be denied to patients with low resting pressures? *Am Surg* 1997;**63**:726–31.
105. Williamson ME, Lewis WG, Holdsworth PJ, *et al.* Decrease in the anorectal pressure gradient after low anterior resection of the rectum. A study using continuous ambulatory manometry. *Dis Colon Rectum* 1994;**37**:1228–31.
106. Lopez-Alonso M, Ribas J, Hernandez A, *et al.* Efficiency of the anorectal manometry for the diagnosis of Hirschsprung's disease in the newborn period. *Eur J Pediat Surg* 1995;**5**:160–3.
107. Rao SS, Hatfield RA. Paroxysmal anal hyperkinesis: a characteristic feature of proctalgia fugax. *Gut* 1996;**39**:609–12.

Chapter 15

Coloproctology and the pelvic floor – Imaging

Clive I Bartram, Steve Halligan

INTRODUCTION

Imaging has a central role in the investigation of pelvic floor disorders, crossing barriers between urogynecology and coloproctology. Both the structure and function of the ano-rectum can be imaged in detail, and a global view of pelvic floor changes obtained during rectal evacuation. The modalities involved include fluoroscopy, endosonography and MRI.

COLONIC TRANSIT STUDIES

Colonic function may be measured directly with ambulatory pressure recording techniques[1], but for routine clinical use these are too complex, and indirect assessment of function from colonic transit more practical. These vary in complexity, and may be divided into scintigraphic techniques that image the passage of radio-isotope labeled material through the large bowel, or the use of plain films to assess the transit of radio-opaque markers.

Scintigraphic techniques are commonly based on the administration of resin microspheres labeled with radioactive indium in a pancake with the patient scanned at regular intervals over the next day or so. The 'center of mass' or COM[2] is the point in the colon that lies 50% ahead of the radioisotope mass, and may be used to indicate transport through the colon. A simplified protocol based on three scans may be used to determine segmental transit.[3] Scintigraphy has shown that the percentage segmental evacuation during defecation was 20% for the right colon, 32% for the left and 66% for the rectum,[4] confirming the interaction between colonic function and rectal evacuation during physiological defecation.

Stool transit through the colon may also be estimated with radio-opaque markers. Patient irradiation may be avoided by X-raying collected stool, but this method is only really applicable for research purposes to establish normal transit times.[5] The simplest practical transit study is to give a known number of small radio-opaque markers with abdominal X-ray taken 120 hours later, when 80% of the markers should have been cleared.[6] A refinement of this is to use three different geometric shapes, so that these may be counted separately. Twenty markers are given at 0 h, 24 h and 48 h with a film at 120 h, when less than four, six and 12 markers respectively should remain. In effect this gives three different estimations on one film. The advantage is that if the patient has only one bowel action at the beginning of the study, this will not invalidate the examination. If only one set of markers is used, these could all be passed, suggesting normal stool frequency. With three sets of markers, the first set might be normal, but the others abnormal so that the diagnosis of slow transit would still be established.

Radio-opaque markers have been used to estimate segmental transit, giving multiple markers with either a film on one,[7,8] or multiple days.[9,10] To estimate segmental transit the colon is divided into three segments (Fig. 15.1). A steady state is assumed and the number of markers in each segment counted, and multiplied by 1.2 (24 h divided by the number of markers – 20). The 'center of mass' of markers has been compared with radio-isotope estimation.[2] The markers tended to be ahead of the isotope, with a mean difference never more than one segment. The calculation of diffusion coefficients for the compartments may reveal abnormalities even when the overall transit is normal.[11] Although there is evidence to suggest there may be several abnormal segmental transit patterns in constipation,[12] and subtotal colectomy advocated on the basis of these,[13] there is no consensus on the value of estimating segmental transit. For routine assessment the three markers with a single film method would seem adequate.

EVACUATION PROCTOGRAPHY

Evacuation proctography[14] (EP) is the fluoroscopic imaging of voiding a barium paste enema. Radiological studies of rectal evacuation have been performed for nearly 50 years,[15] but found general acceptance only when a practical technique and system for interpretation was introduced by Mahieu *et al.* in 1984.[16,17]

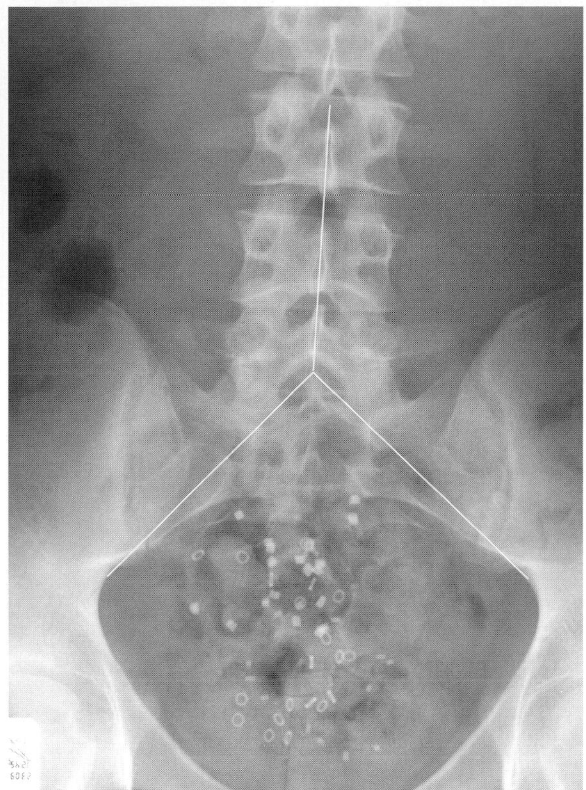

Figure 15.1 Transit study showing retention of markers in the rectosigmoid. The film has been marked to show the right and left colons, and the rectosigmoid (Arhan et al, 1981).

Although EP is now well established, it remains confined to specialist centers. Furthermore, its role is still controversial despite many years of clinical use. The examination has been termed defecography,[16] but during the procedure none of the colonic reflexes are invoked that normally accompany defecation,[18] so that this is not physiological defecation, only a test of voluntary rectal evacuation.

Difficulty in defecation is the main indication for EP. Some authors have suggested a role in the investigation of incontinence,[19] to categorize the degree of incontinence, and based on finding an obtuse ano-rectal angle to identify patients who might benefit from postanal repair, should the anal sphincters be normal. The involuntary loss of barium may be sufficient for diagnosis of fecal incontinence,[20] and unless rectal prolapse is suspected, the role of EP is limited in this scenario.

TECHNIQUE

Evacuation proctography is a rapid and simple technique to perform. The rectum may be emptied prior to EP, either by administration of glycerine suppositories or an enema, and a fixed volume of contrast agent administered. Although this is not physiological, it does standardize the examination so that comparisons of evacuation time and completeness, either on follow-up, or in comparisons with normal subjects may be made. The passage of stool during the examination may inhibit complete evacuation, and a prepared rectum is more acceptable both to patients and staff. Contrast consistency should approximate to feces. Mixing barium suspension with potato starch or methylcellulose creates a suitable consistency, or commercial barium pastes may be used. The total volume used is variable; some investigators instil contrast until a strong urge to evacuate is provoked, whereas others use a fixed volume for the reasons given above. The high viscosity paste is usually syringed (Fig. 15.2) into the rectum with the patient in the left-lateral position on the fluoroscopy table, and injection continued during withdrawal to mark the anal canal and verge. The table is brought upright and a commode (Fig. 15.3) placed on the footrest. The commode must incorporate some filtration[21] (equivalent to 4 mm copper) to prevent screen flare.

If a commode is unavailable, or the patient grossly incontinent, the examination may be carried out with the patient supine on the table, lying on their left side[22] with absorbent padding around the anus. Static values

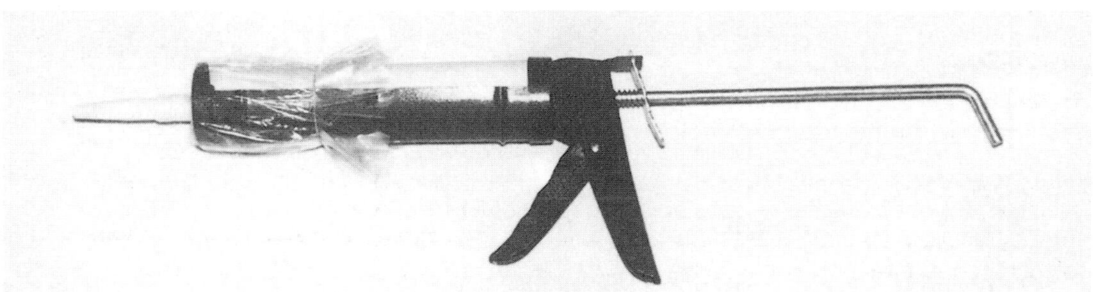

Figure 15.2 Pistol injector used for defecography.

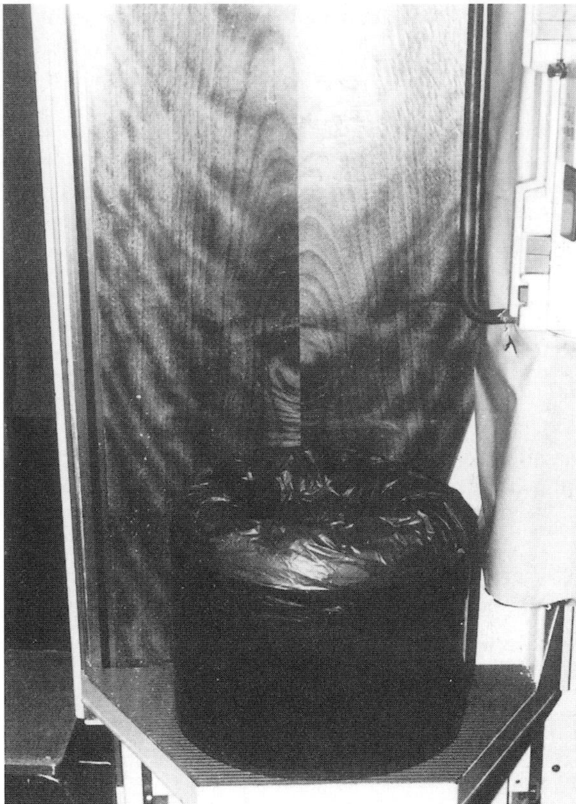

Figure 15.3 Commode designed by Mahieu for defecography.

Figure 15.4 Normal evacuation proctogram. (A) At rest the anal canal is outlined by barium and the posterior impression of the puborectalis is visible (arrow). The rectal outline is smooth and the anterior wall convex. The ano-rectal junction lies above the inferior plane of the ischial tuberosities. (B) Evacuation has commenced, the anterior wall of the rectum is concave, there has been pelvic floor descent and the anal canal is widely open. There is no residual impression from the puborectalis. (C,D) Progressive emptying of the rectum. (E) The rectum is almost completely emptied. (F) The patient stops straining; the pelvic floor elevates so that the anorectal junction is above the plane of the ischial tuberosities, the anal canal closes and the puborectalis impression returns with restoration of the normal resting anorectal angle.

for pelvic floor position will be higher in the supine position as the pelvic floor is not subject to the weight of the abdominal contents.[23]

It is essential to obtain continuous or rapid recording of rectal evacuation, either by spot filming (Fig. 15.4A–F) (conventional or digital) or videofluoroscopy. Although spot filming will provide the best spatial resolution, the ability of videofluoroscopy to playback the entire examination at normal speed, or part in slow motion, may be invaluable to diagnose subtle findings. Patient dose is lowest with videofluoroscopy, but may be significantly reduced using digital films at 1 per second with a low dose protocol.[24] A compromise is to videotape the examination with spot films taken at key events, and to screen only intermittently if voiding takes >30 s.

MODIFICATIONS TO THE BASIC TECHNIQUE

The technique described above will image rectal configuration during voiding and determine the rate and completeness of evacuation. It is well recognized that middle and anterior compartment pelvic floor weakness often accompanies posterior weakness, and the standard proctographic examination may be modified to take this into account.

The commonest addition is dilute oral barium suspension approximately 1–2 hours prior to the procedure, to opacify the distal small bowel so that enteroceles may be visualized directly.[25] Vaginal opacification (Fig. 15.5) will demonstrate rectovaginal separation during evacuation, and vaginal prolapse. Barium gel is preferable to a tampon, as the latter may splint the vagina.[26] Liquid barium suspension may be injected prior to the paste to fill the sigmoid colon and detect any sigmoidocele.[27]

Dynamic cystoproctography[28] involves opacification of the bladder, as well as the vagina, small bowel and rectum. Bladder catheterization is necessary.[29,30] Some investigators have also injected water-soluble contrast directly into the peritoneal cavity to image the pelvic peritoneal recesses during voiding.[31] The level of information required by the referring clinician will govern modifications to the standard EP. The combination of rectal and small bowel opacification is now routine for coloproctology, with dynamic cystoproctography more the province of the urogynecologist.

THE NORMAL EXAMINATION

Based on the findings in 56 asymptomatic patients. Mahieu[16] defined five criteria for normal evacuation (Fig. 15.4A–F):

- an increase in ano-rectal angulation
- obliteration of the puborectalis impression
- wide anal canal opening
- total evacuation of contrast
- normal pelvic floor resistance.

Several subsequent studies of asymptomatic volunteers have revealed a wide range of normal values.[14,33]

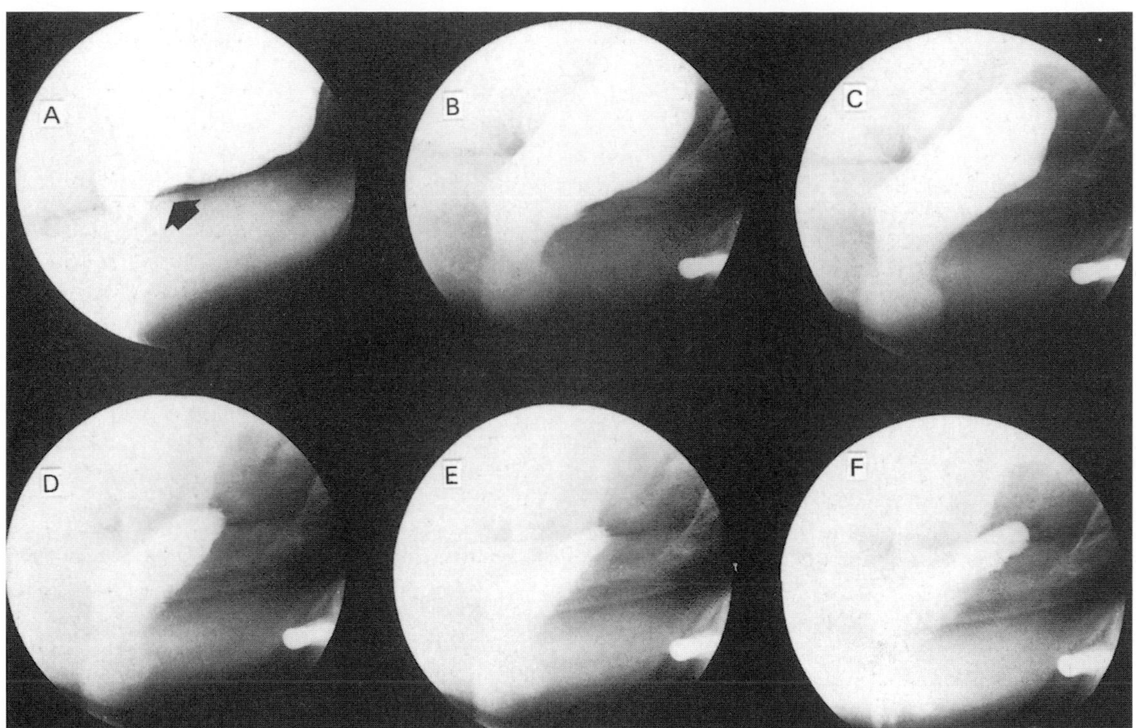

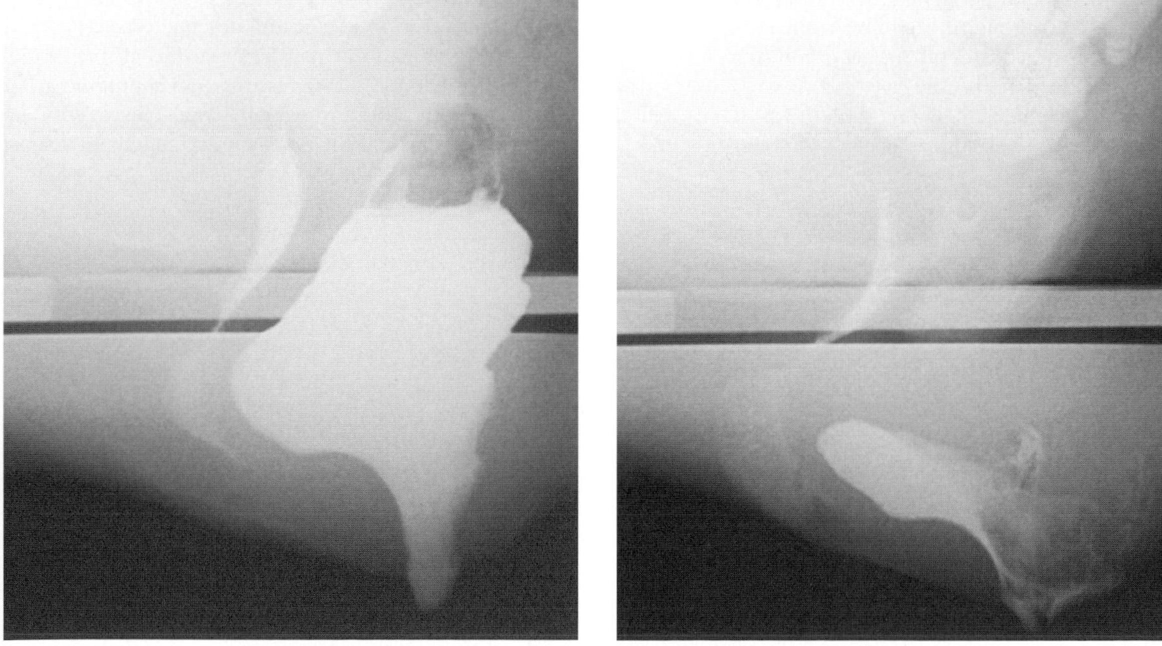

Figure 15.5 (a) vaginal opacification using ultrasound gel mixed with barium powder. Note the close proximity of the vagina to the rectum. (b) at the end of evacuation there is separation of the vagina from the rectum with a small enterocele. Note also the small anterior rectocele and intra-anal intussusception.

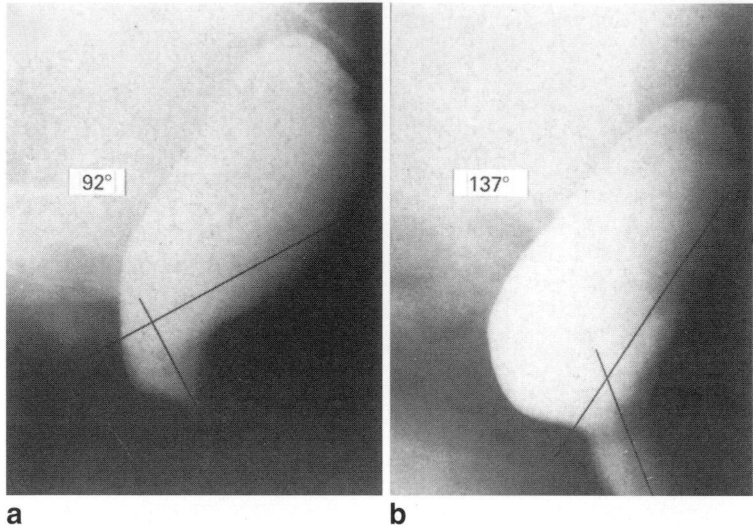

Figure 15.6 (a) Ano-rectal angle at rest and (b) during defecation, measured along the posterior wall of the rectum. From Ref. 17, with permission.

Nevertheless, there is a consensus of opinion broadly agreeing with Mahieu's original description.

The examination may be considered in three stages: *pre-evacuation*, *evacuation* and *post-evacuation*. The initial lateral view records pre-evacuation ano-rectal configuration and pelvic floor position. The ano-rectal angle (ARA) is thought to be important for maintaining continence and considerable attention has been devoted to its measurement. The ARA is usually measured between the anal canal axis and the posterior rectal wall (Fig. 15.6a&b), although variability in this makes assessment unreliable. The junction between the rectal ampulla and anal canal, the ano-rectal junction (ARJ), is easy to appreciate at rest. The pubococcygeal line (Fig. 15.7) is the standard definition for the level of the pelvic floor, but may be difficult to place accurately with a limited fluoroscopic field of view. Instead the pelvic floor position at rest and descent during evacuation may be related to the inferior surface of the ischial tuberosities (Fig. 15.8). At rest the ARJ should be at, or just above this plane, the anal canal closed with no contrast leakage, and the ARA approximately 90°. Some

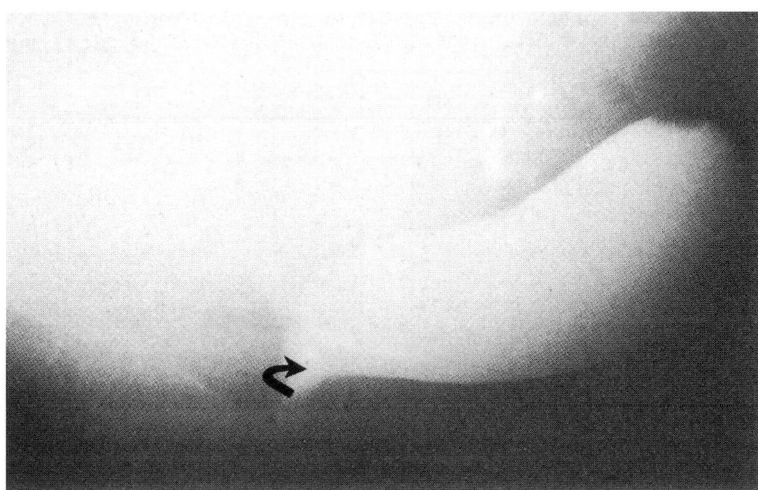

Figure 15.7 Normal position of the pelvic floor at rest with the patient sitting. The anorectal junction (arrow) is 1.8 cm below the pubococcygeal line

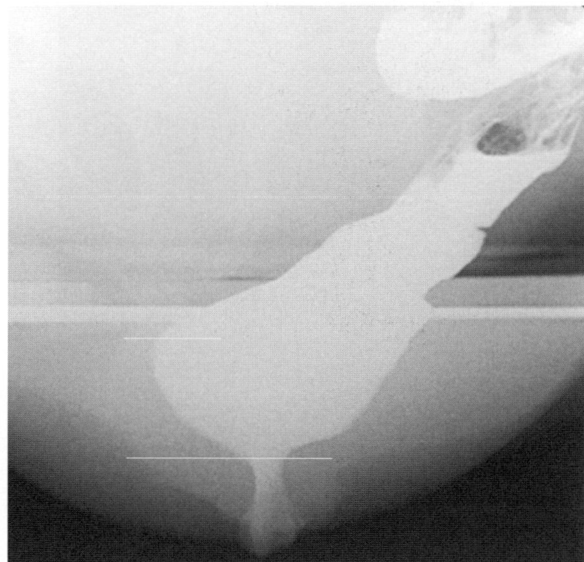

Figure 15.8 The upper white line marks the level of the ischial tuberosities, the lower the ARJ, to show pelvic floor descent at the initiation of evacuation.

investigators then advocate squeeze views to evaluate the activity of voluntary pelvic floor musculature, with cough views to stress the continence mechanism. The patient may also be asked to strain down without actually evacuating, to assess pelvic floor descent. However, the ARA may paradoxically increase during this maneuver as patients contract their pelvic floor to ensure continence.

The patient is then asked to empty their rectum as rapidly and completely as possible during imaging. This sequence is central to the examination because it provides a functional assessment of rectal evacuation and visualizes ano-rectal configuration during this. Evacuation should be rapidly initiated and is first evidenced by pelvic floor descent. The puborectal impression is lost as the ARA becomes more obtuse by approximately 20°, and the anal canal opens widely and shortens. After evacuation the anal canal closes and the ARJ and ARA return to their original positions. Patients who utilize digital maneuvers to aid emptying should be instructed to do so, so that their effect can be evaluated. It may be relevant to examine the patient in the frontal position, after rectal emptying, to reveal coronal rectal configuration, which may diagnose intussusception not apparent on lateral views.[34] If the patient has not emptied the rectum, it may be necessary to send them to the toilet and then re-screen when the rectum is empty. Enteroceles and intussusception only become apparent as the rectum empties. If the bladder has been opacified, this should be examined before the rectum is filled, as a large cystocele may inhibit enterocele formation.[28]

ABNORMAL FINDINGS

Abnormalities may be considered as either structural or functional. Although many measurements are possible, few have any diagnostic value and diagnosis depends on the recognition of certain specific patterns.

Structural abnormalities

Rectocele

A rectocele describes a bulge on the anterior wall of the rectum, usually developing during evacuation. The depth of a rectocele may be measured from the anterior border of the anal canal to the most anterior part of the rectocele (Fig. 15.9). A depth of < 2 cm is considered a normal variant in women. Large rectoceles of > 4 cm have been considered a cause of difficult defecation, although the presence and size of a rectocele has not been shown to effect evacuation time of paste or a small balloon.[35] Trapping of barium within a rectocele that does not collapse completely at the end of evacuation does appear to be significant (Fig. 15.10A–F). A marked pressure drop with the rectocele has been associated with this phenomenon.[36] Digitation with pressure applied to the perineum or posterior vaginal wall (Fig. 15.11A–C) is commonly necessary to complete rectal emptying.[37,38] Anismus may be an additional problem. Proctography may be used after surgical repair of a rectocele to determine technical success should the patient remain symptomatic.[39]

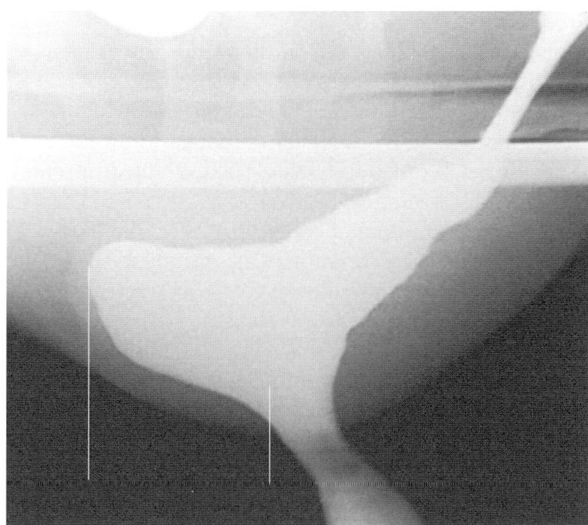

Figure 15.9 Depth of an anterior rectocele measured (between the two vertical white lines) from its outer edge to the anterior aspect of the anal canal.

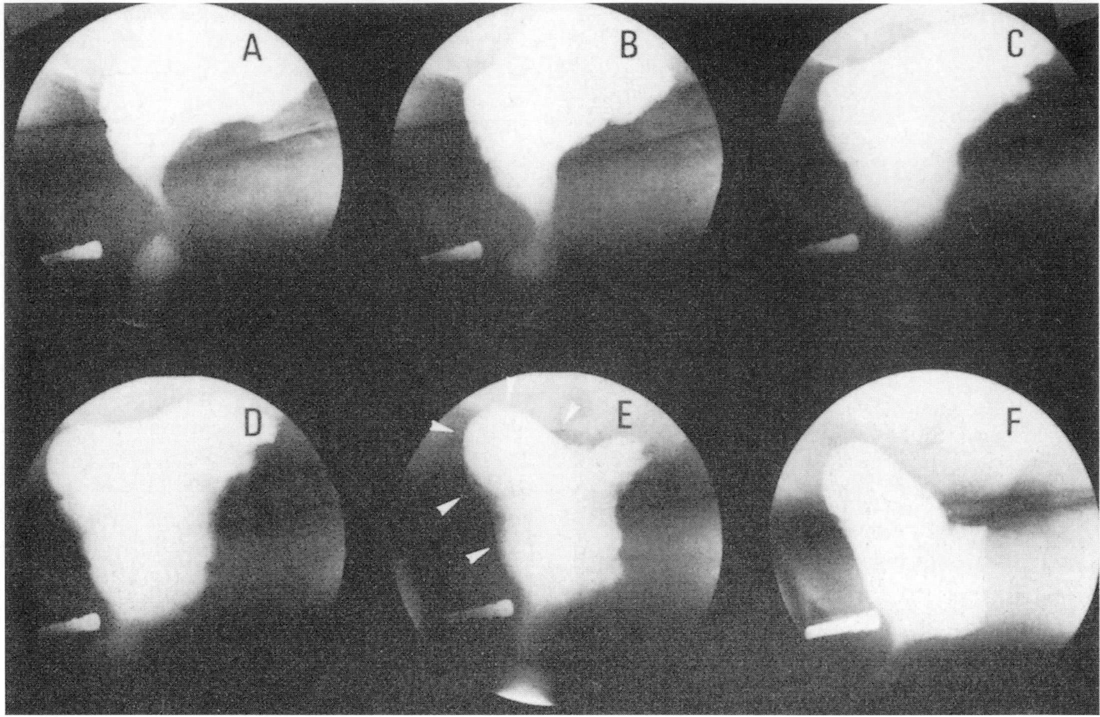

Figure 15.10 There is a large anterior rectocele (arrowheads, E) with trapping of barium at the end of evacuation (F).

Rectoceles may also be posterior (Fig. 15.12a&b), where they are perhaps more correctly termed posterior perineal hernias[40] because the defect occurs laterally, through the levator plate, rather than in the midline.

Prolapse

Intussusception may be intra-rectal, intra-anal or external to form a complete rectal prolapse. Anterior mucosal prolapse[41] has not been associated with a diagnostic feature on EP. Internal intussusception has been graded on a seven-point scale,[33] and divided into high or low grades, supposedly reflecting severity. There is considerable confusion regarding the diagnosis of intussusception, based on imaging entirely in the lateral plane. As the rectum collapses it folds over under the influence of the valves of Houston. This pattern is apparent in the AP plane (Fig. 15.13a&b), but in the lateral plane the rectum is flattened out against the levators, so that the folds are not seen.[34] However, the angulation of the rectum may produce appearances that simulate intussusception, particularly as the anterior wall of the rectum inverts as it collapses over the anal canal (Fig. 15.13a). There is no clear definition on proctography of a purely intra-rectal intussusception. It is likely that all internal intussusception rapidly extends down into the anal canal, so that the intra-rectal component is transitory. Intra-anal intussusception is seen in the lateral plane as an infolding of the distal rectal wall >3 mm thick that extends down into the anal canal (Fig. 15.14). It may be on either the anterior or posterior wall, but is often circular (Fig. 15.15). In the AP plane the intussusception is seen as one of the rectal wall folds prolapsing down into the anal canal and splaying it apart (Fig. 15.16).[34]

The concept of defecation block dates back to Wallden.[15] Internal intussusception may be thought to obstruct rectal emptying, but really occurs only at the end of evacuation. The ampullary segment of the rectum below the main fold is the part of the rectum that is emptied during the voluntary evacuation at proctography. Significant obstruction to emptying is unusual.

Enterocele

An enterocele is present if small bowel enters the rectogenital space, passing below the proximal one third of the vagina in women. Enteroceles are almost the norm posthysterectomy. All proctographic studies have shown a higher detection rate for enteroceles compared with clinical examination.[25,29,30,42] The potential space in the rectogenital area may be filled by a cystocele, sigmoidocele, prolapsing uterus or large

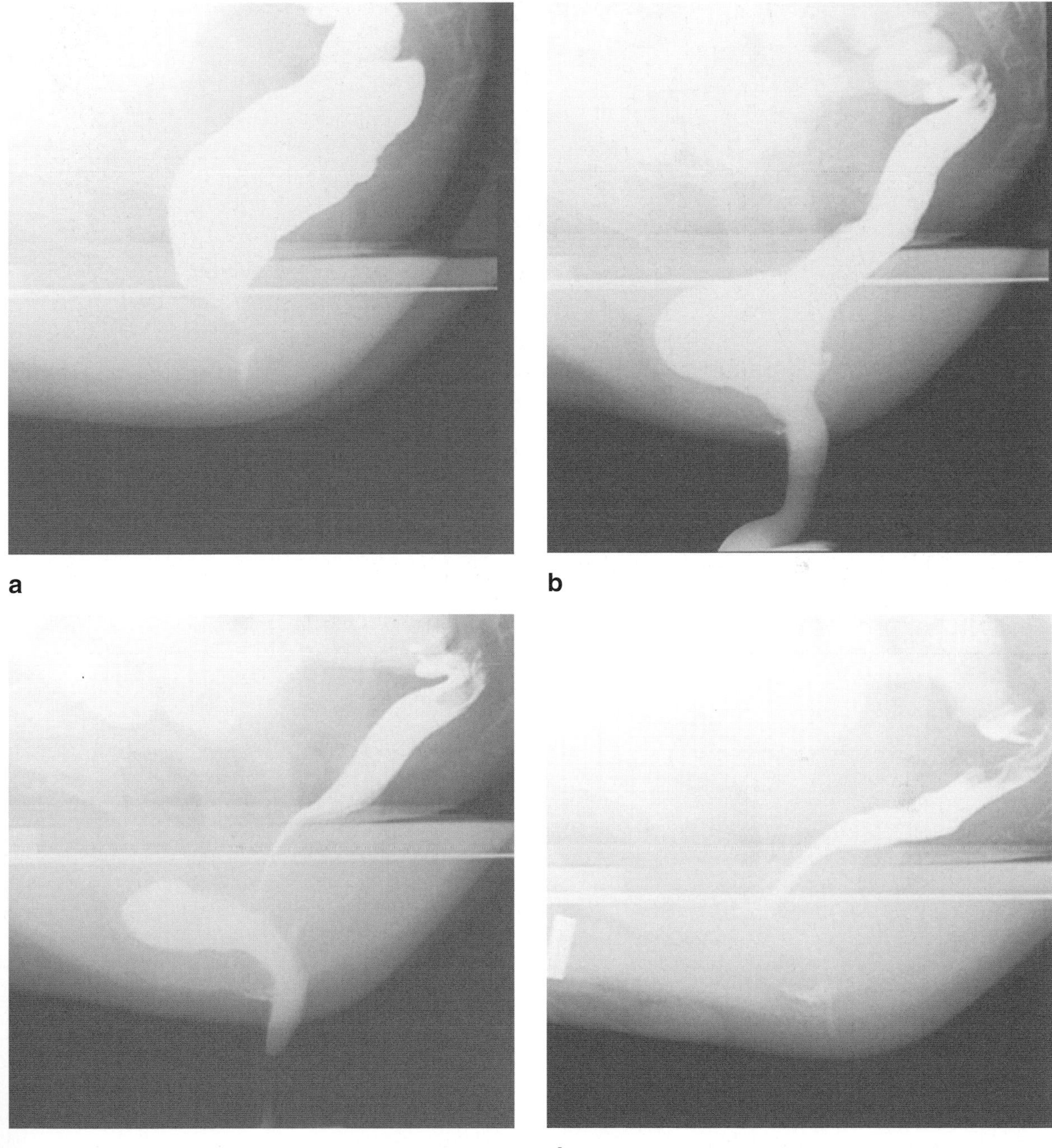

Figure 15.11 During evacuation an anterior rectocele develops (a&b). At the end of evacuation there is significant trapping in the rectocele (c) that the patient empties (d) by pressing on the perineum (ring on finger visible).

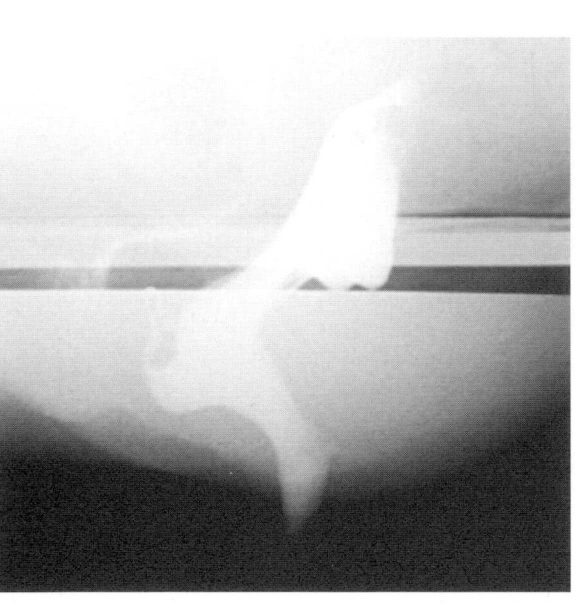

a

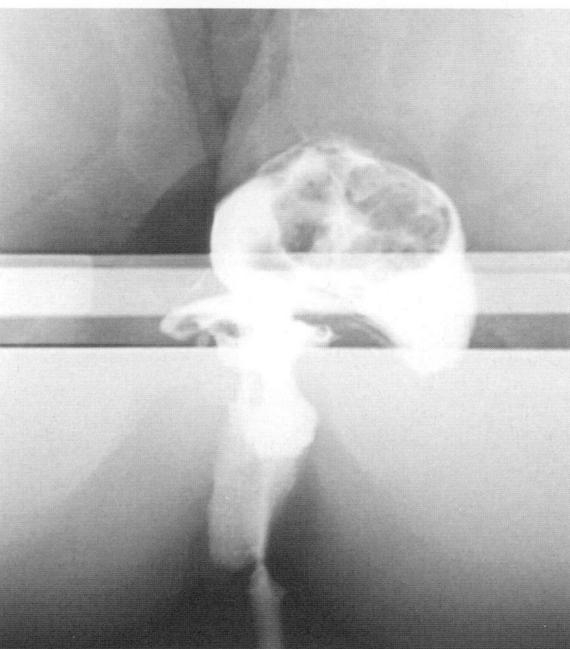

b

Figure 15.12 (a) The lateral view shows a pronounced posterior bulge, which on the AP view (B) is seen to be due to a left sided herniation of the rectum. MRI confirmed a levator defect at this site.

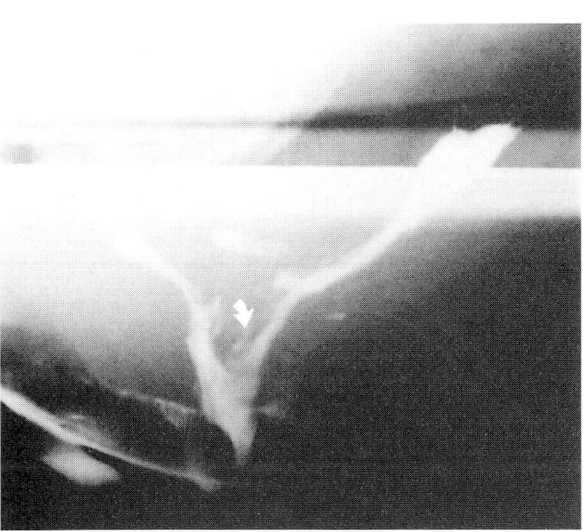

a

Figure 15.13 (a) Anterior wall inversion (arrow) creating a broad fold at the end of evacuation. Small anterior rectocele. There is no intussusception (see also Fig. 15.13b).

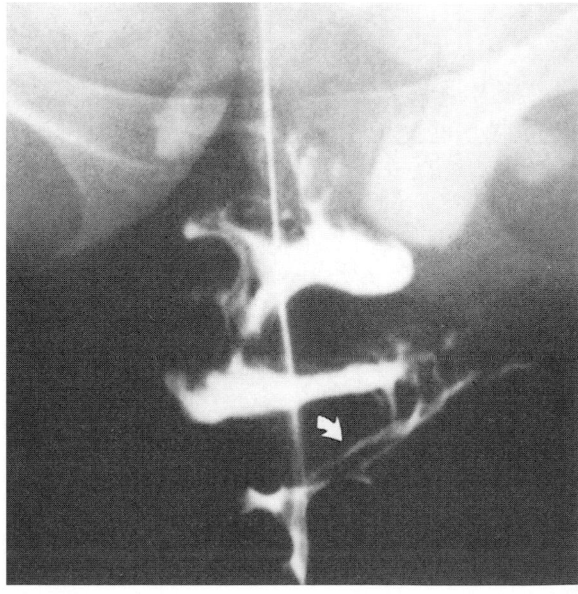

b

Figure 15.13 (b) Anteroposterior view of the same patient shown in Fig. 15.13(a) illustrating the rectum folds over towards the end of evacuation, creating the appearance of folds and anterior wall inversion (arrow) as the walls appose laterally. Note that there is no intussusception of any fold.

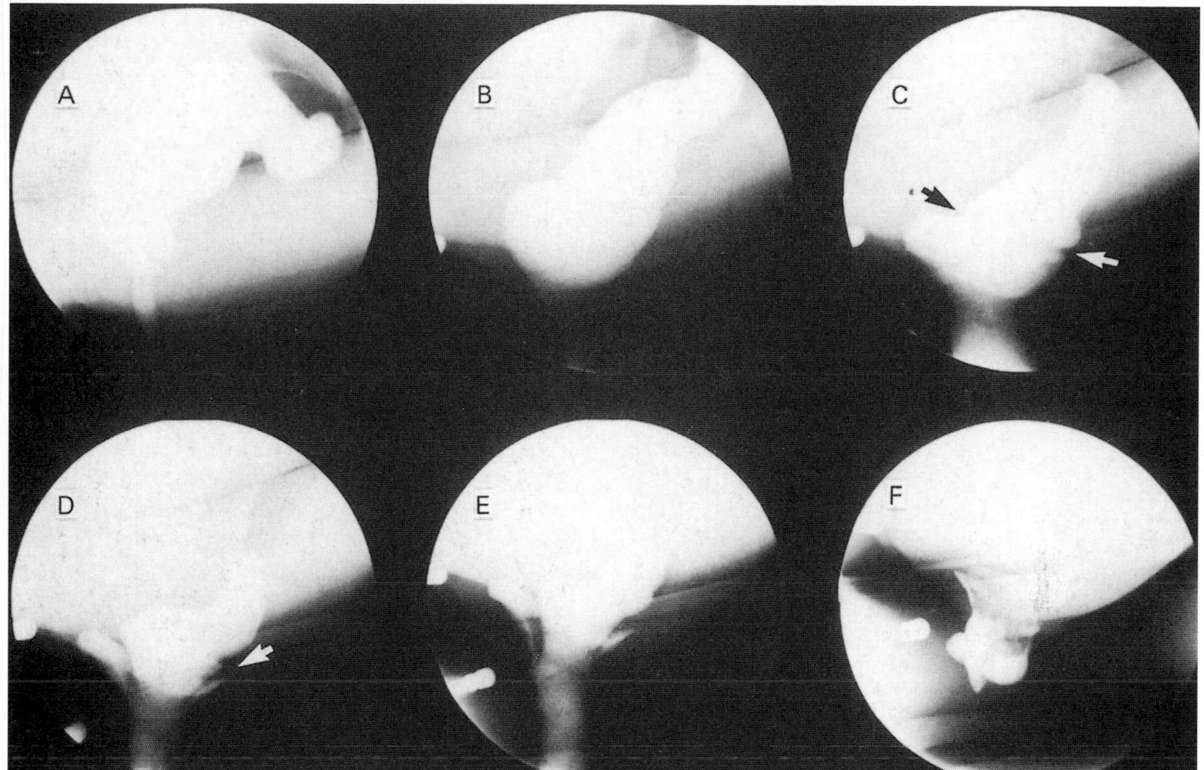

Figure 15.14 Intra-anal intussusception. (A) Slight pelvic floor descent at rest. Rectum normal in outline. At the start of evacuation. (B) Small annular folds (arrowheads in C) develop and invaginate (E) into the anal canal (F).

rectocele, which will then prevent an enterocele forming. The bladder and rectum must be empty, and the patient strain maximally to demonstrate an enterocele (Figs 15.17a–c, 15.18). If rectal emptying is not complete at the end of proctography, the patient should be sent to the toilet and reviewed after further attempts to evacuate. A sigmoidocele may be recognized by gas in fecal residue (Fig. 15.19) if it has not been opacified by barium.

Pelvic floor descent

Parks described a syndrome characterized by excessive pelvic floor descent, which was attributed to pudendal neuropathy.[43] EP allows a more accurate estimate of pelvic floor descent than clinical methods, as straining is maximal to the point of anal canal opening. The anorectal junction may be measured at rest and at the initiation of evacuation, so that pelvic floor descent at rest and during evacuation may be assessed. Descent during evacuation is normally less than 3.0 cm. In patients who strain chronically or are incontinent, the degree of descent during evacuation may be reduced, but the position of the pelvic floor at rest is lower.[44]

Functional abnormality

Some constipated patients find it difficult to empty the rectum, irrespective of the volume or consistency of its content, a phenomenon that may be disclosed clinically by inability to evacuate a rectal balloon.[45] Evacuation failure may be associated with involuntary contraction of striated pelvic floor musculature (Fig. 15.20), a syndrome termed anismus[46] or inappropriate puborectalis contraction (Fig. 15.21). The relevance of this finding is uncertain because it can be demonstrated in both normal and incontinent patients[47] and may become absent if recordings are taken away from the hospital environment.[48] Nevertheless, there is a clear association with difficult rectal evacuation and the success of biofeedback therapy in a significant proportion of patients suggests that diagnosis is worthwhile.[49] The pelvic floor and recto-anal coordination required to facilitate defecation is complex and involves both conscious and unconscious pathways. It is probably an over-simplification to suggest that anismus is confined to excessive puborectal contraction; it is likely that the entire pelvic floor is involved to some degree and the condition may be better termed pelvic floor incoordina-

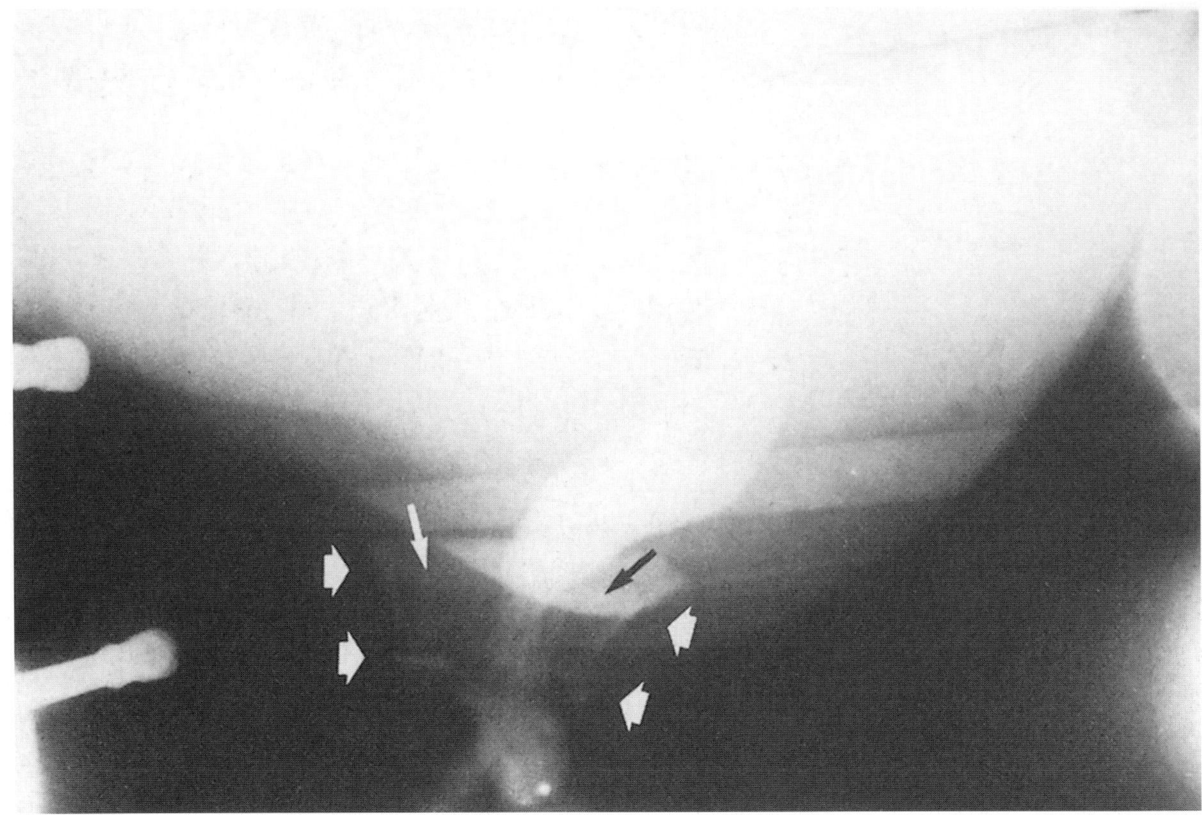

Figure 15.15 Intra-anal intussusception. The head of the intussusception (black arrow) lies within the anal canal (white arrows). Note the transverse fold (between black arrows) that the invagination of the intussusception creates in the rectal wall.

tion.[50] For example, some patients may fail to raise intra-rectal pressure adequately.[35]

The proctographic diagnosis of anismus has usually concentrated on inappropriate puborectal contraction, intuitively suggesting a prominent puborectal impression during voiding coupled with failure of the ano-rectal angle to open, both frequently cited EP signs of anismus. However, there is little evidence that these findings are specific; simultaneous EP and puborectal electromyography (Fig. 15.20) reveal no correlation between puborectal activity and ano-rectal junction configuration.[52] Instead, it is more appropriate to base a proctographic diagnosis on failure to void contrast adequately. Normal subjects void rapidly and completely in contrast to those with a functional disorder, whose evacuation is prolonged and incomplete (Fig. 2.22),[53] a difference that can be quantified by EP.[54] A proctographic study of 24 patients in whom a diagnosis of anismus had been established by multiple clinical and physiological criteria found that puborectal morphology and ano-rectal angulation did not differ from controls, but prolonged and incomplete contrast voiding (Fig. 15.23) was highly specific.[55] The time taken to initiate anal canal opening and void are more relevant than the percentage of contrast evacuated, as most patients will eventually empty their rectum if given enough time to do so.

CLINICAL RELEVANCE

Although EP has been widely practised for several years, debate concerning its clinical relevance continues. Much of this derives from the excessive attention that has been devoted to the various anatomical measurements and findings provided by EP. Any rectal configuration during emptying, other than that of a symmetrically collapsing tube, has been considered abnormal, although varying rectal configurations can be demonstrated in asymptomatic patients who have no evidence of impaired voiding. Shorvon and co-workers

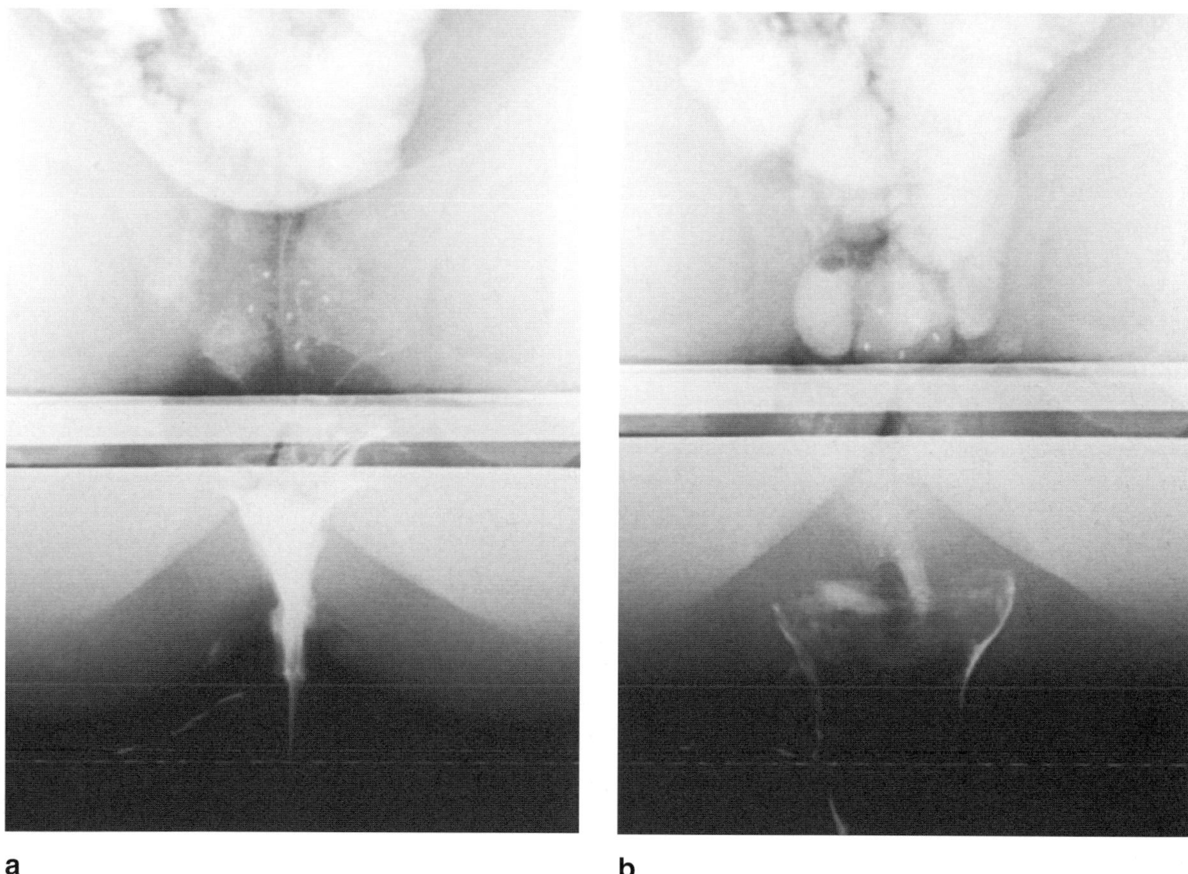

Figure 15.16 (a) AP view at rest. (b) during evacuation the infolding of the distal rectum wall can be seen splaying the anal canal apart.

demonstrated low-grade intussusception in 80% of men and 81% of women,[33] suggesting the finding was of little relevance. In contrast, high-grade intussusception is likely to be abnormal; there is a clear association with difficult evacuation and the solitary rectal ulcer syndrome,[56] and surgical repair can ameliorate symptoms.[57] However, this does not mean that it is the primary cause of difficult evacuation. Some studies of patients whose symptoms were attributed to intussusception have found that these may persist after surgical repair,[58,59] suggesting that intussusception is merely a secondary phenomenon. It is easy to imagine how this may occur if an underlying functional disorder results in chronic straining.

Similarly, chronic straining may engender rectoceles and enteroceles, both of which are found in association with functional disorders; a study of 41 patients with difficult evacuation ascribed to rectocele found anismus in 29 (71%).[60] Furthermore, a proctographic study of 58 constipated patients found that the only significant difference from controls was a prolongation of evacuation time and failure to fully empty the rectum, clearly suggesting that functional measurements of emptying are more important than changes in rectal configuration.[21] There are also perceptual differences between patients. Some have heightened rectal awareness, which may lead to sensations of incomplete evacuation ignored by others. Also, some may experience sensations of rectal fullness, perceiving this due to incomplete evacuation, despite evidence that the rectum is empty. For example, it is believed that enteroceles compress the rectum, preventing evacuation, an opinion derived from proctographic appearances suggesting rectal blockade,[15] but formal studies of rectal evacuation in these subjects are usually normal.[37] This may be because afferent pathways for rectal distention actually lie within the surrounding musculature,[61] allowing them to be triggered by the enterocele sac, raising the possibility that symptoms are due to the sac itself rather than any secondary effect on rectal emptying.

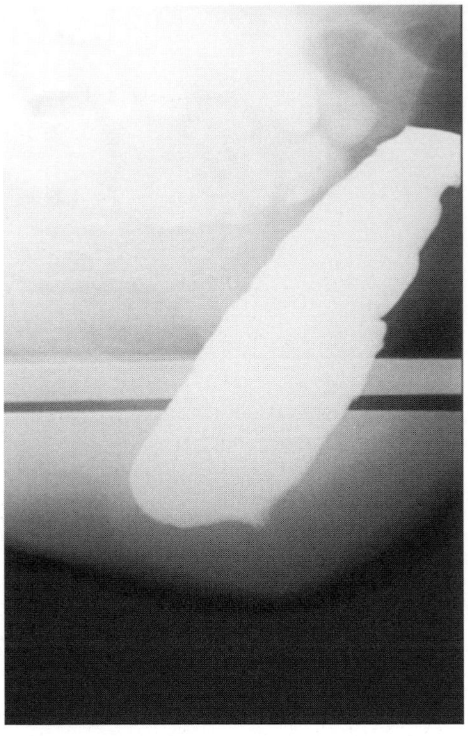

a

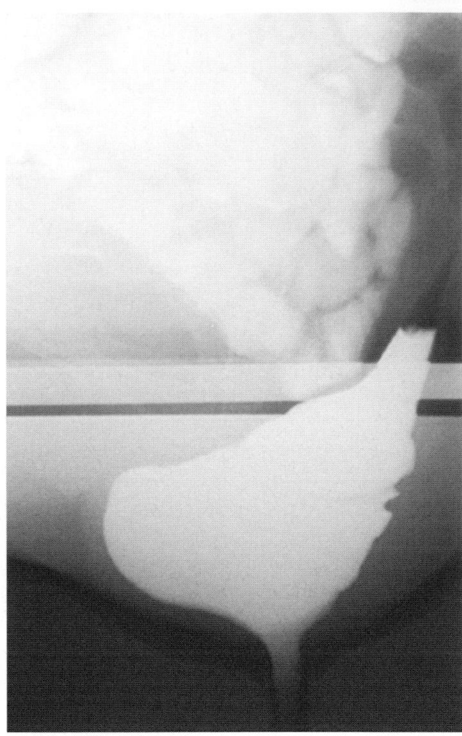

b

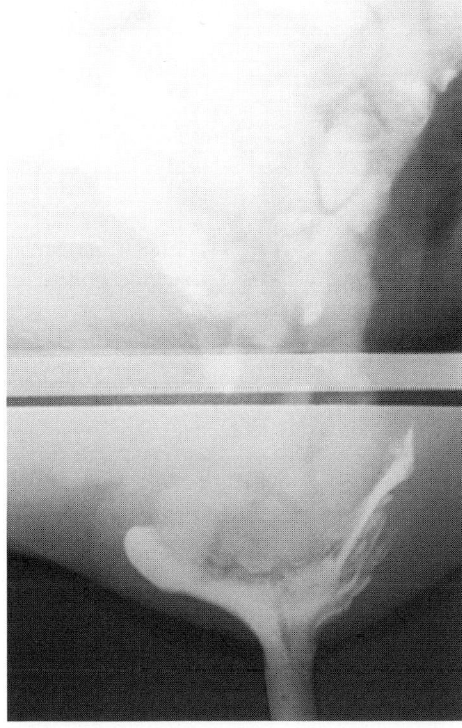

c

Figure 15.17 (a–c) The enterocele develops only as the rectum empties.

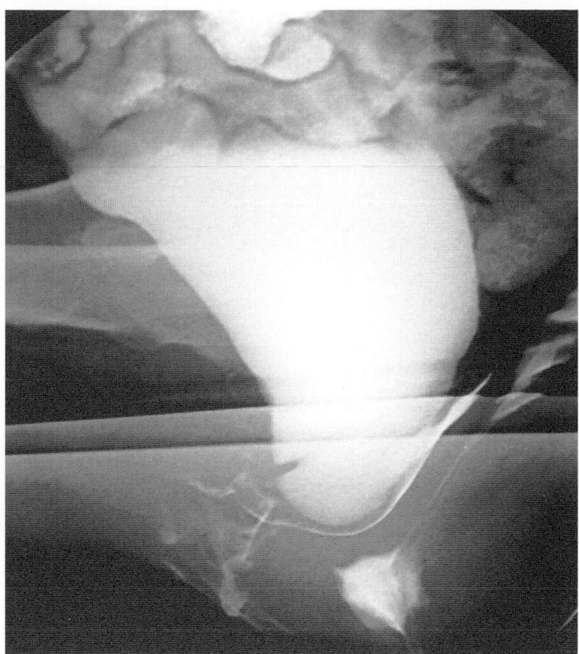

Figure 15.18 The large cystocele occupies the entire pelvic cavity, and can be seen pressing down on the anterior wall of the opacified vagina. The enterocele became apparent only when the bladder emptied, and space became available for the small bowel to descend.

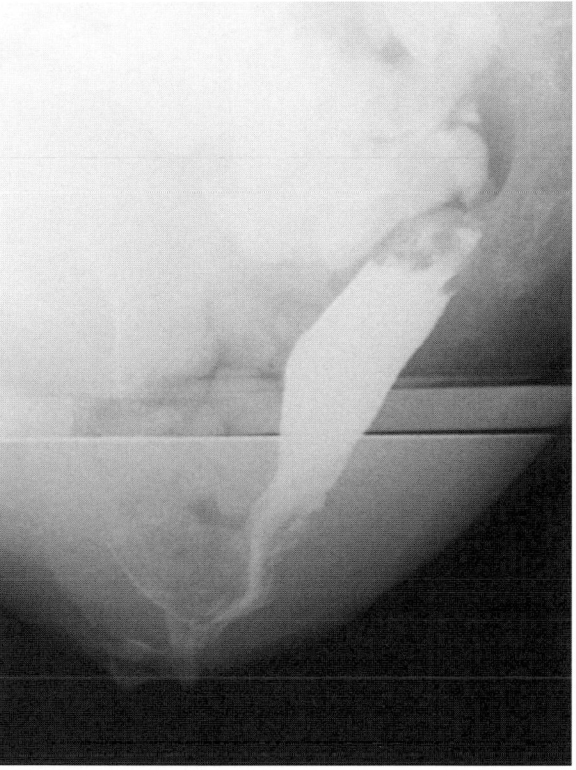

Figure 15.19 Sigmoidocele extending down to the perineum revealed by the presence of gas within fecal matter.

The significance of excessive pelvic floor descent is also uncertain. Some studies show significant differences between constipated patients and controls,[62] whereas others show no difference between incontinent and constipated patients.[44] Interestingly, although chronic straining is believed to result in pudendal neuropathy there is no correlation between neuropathy and pelvic floor descent as assessed by EP.[63]

The main value of EP relates to its ability to simultaneously diagnose both structural and functional abnormalities, and determine which is most likely to be relevant.[64] Generally, impaired evacuation suggests that functional abnormality may underpin symptoms. In this scenario, the possibility that any apparent abnormalities of rectal configuration are secondary should be considered. For example, a study of patients undergoing rectopexy for solitary rectal ulcer syndrome found that persistent postoperative symptoms were related to impaired evacuation on preoperative EP, rather than the presence of any prolapse.[65] This approach will direct patients towards biofeedback therapy rather than surgery, since the latter is unlikely to treat the underlying disorder. Furthermore, biofeedback is less invasive, cheaper and does not preclude a surgical option in the future. It has been argued that EP should be the initial test performed in all patients with severe constipation, including those with slow colonic transit, because this may be a secondary physiological response to an inability to evacuate. This approach ensures that treatment aimed at improving rectal evacuation, such as biofeedback, precedes all other measures.[66]

Much of the uncertainty related to the benefits or otherwise of EP has been generated by studies where the possibilities for functional diagnoses have been ignored, or where benefit has been assessed by outcome, an approach which inevitably includes assessment of any treatment.[67,68] In contrast, studies which have directly addressed the value of proctography in the clinical decision making process have found it to be overwhelmingly useful: a study of 50 consecutive referrals found that the proctographic result significantly increased diagnostic confidence, with over 90% of clinicians generally finding the test useful.[69]

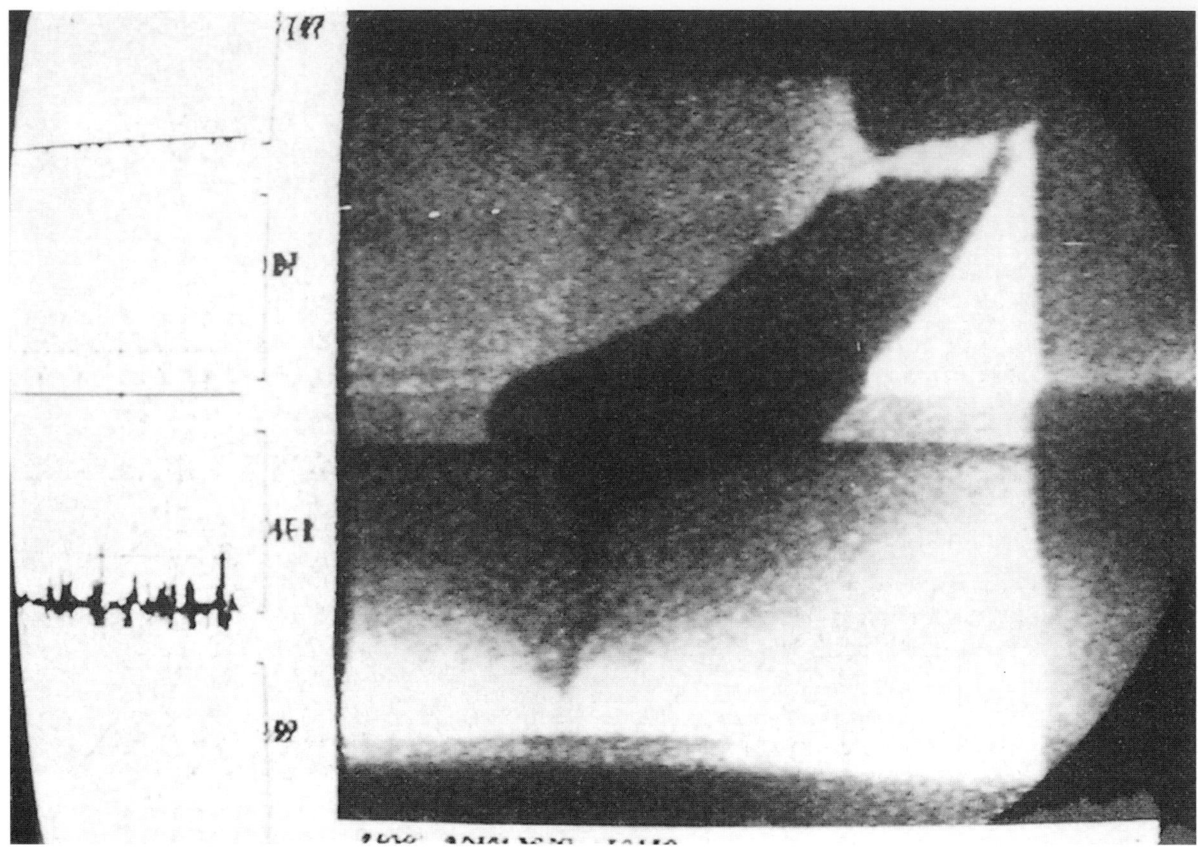

Figure 15.20 Integrated proctography showing typical 'sphincter dysfunction' with delayed evacuation, a 'V'-shaped narrow canal associated with a paradoxical increase in EMG activity from a needle in the puborectalis, shown in the bottom left hand channel.

FUTURE POSSIBILITIES – MRI

The standard EP, which now incorporates small bowel opacification, is rapid and easy to perform, whereas the modifications necessary to image the bladder are time-consuming and invasive. The demographics of severe constipation mean that most of the subjects studied are young women in their childbearing years, so that EP exposes them to pelvic irradiation. Furthermore, the musculature of the pelvic floor itself is not visualized. MRI has the ability to image the bladder, vagina, uterus and bowel without opacification, as well as the musculature of the pelvic floor directly. Initial studies just with rest/stress maneuvers have been promising,[70,71] and direct comparison made with proctography.[72] Although patients must be examined supine in a standard magnet, this need not preclude rectal evacuation. If the patient is examined with a full bladder, the vagina and rectum opacified with ultrasound gel, the entire dynamics of the pelvic floor and associated structures may be examined directly during bladder and rectal voiding (Fig. 15.24a–c).[73] Evacuation in the sitting position is possible in an open bore magnet,[74,75] though such machines are rare at present. The spatial resolution, tissue contrast and safety of this modality make it likely to be at the forefront of proctographic imaging research in the foreseeable future.

'SPHINCTEROLOGY' – THE ANAL SPHINCTER

Endosonography provides a relatively simple method for obtaining detailed information as to the thickness and integrity of the components of the anal sphincter. In common with all sonography the examination is more difficult to interpret than to perform. Cross sectional imaging, using CT or MRI, will outline the sphincters, but does not provide sufficient detail unless an endocoil is used with MR.

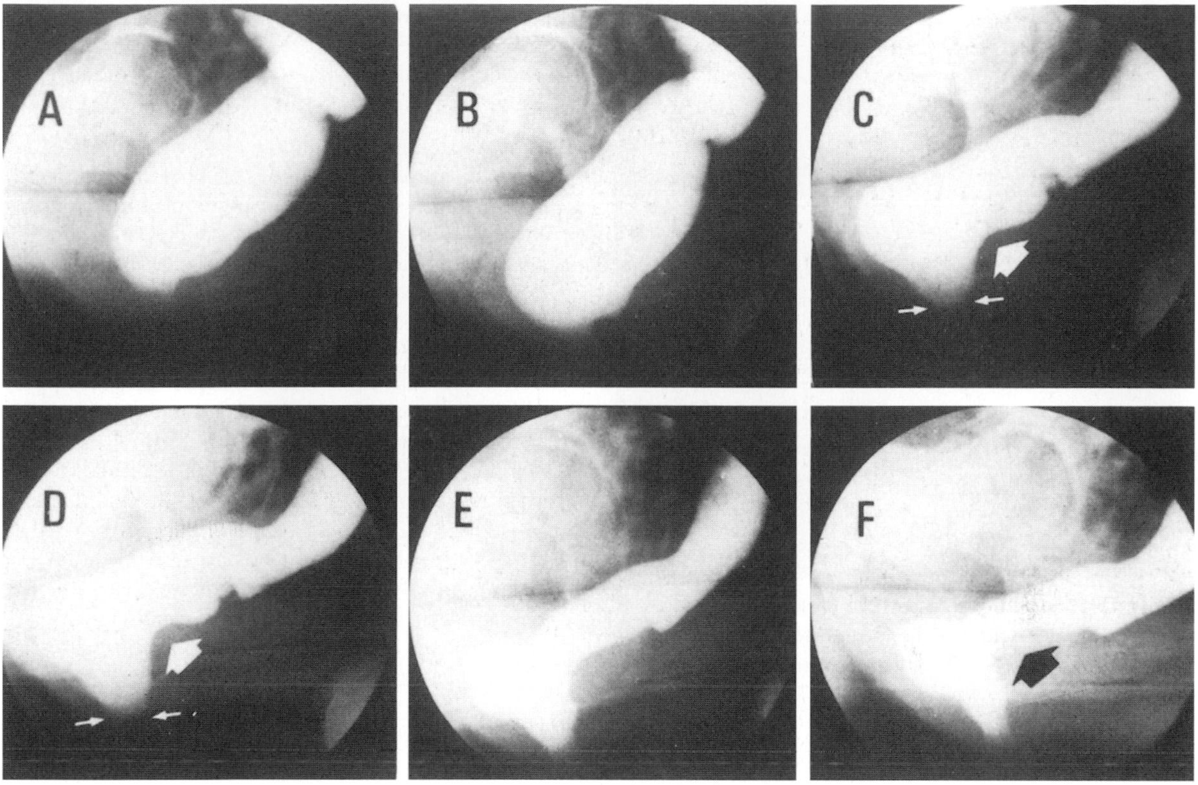

Figure15.21 Paradoxical contraction of the puborectalis. At rest (A) and during the initiation of evacuation (B) the outline of the rectum is normal, but during evacuation (C) there is a sudden increase in the tone of the puborectalis (arrow), with the formation of an anterior rectocele (F). In spite of repeated straining, evacuation is incomplete and the impression from the puborectalis has become more pronounced. From Ref. 17, with permission.

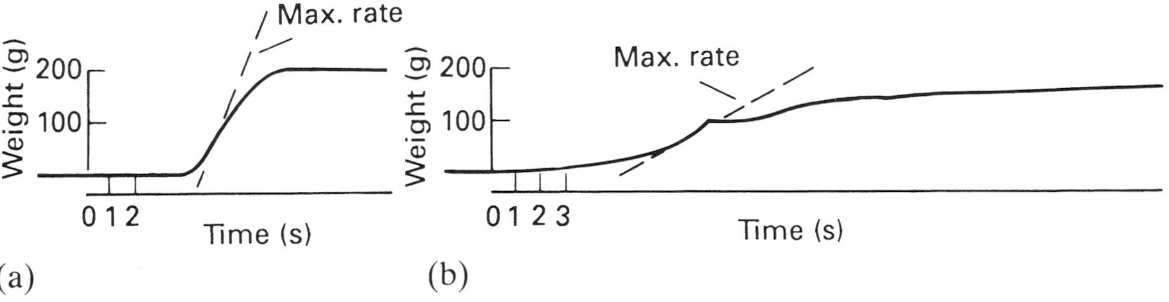

Figure 15.22 (a) Tracing from a normal subject showing rapid (4 s) and complete (100%) evacuation. (b) Tracing from a patient with constipation showing a slow maximum rate of emptying with incomplete evacuation (83%) over a prolonged period (33 s). From Ref. 53, with permission.

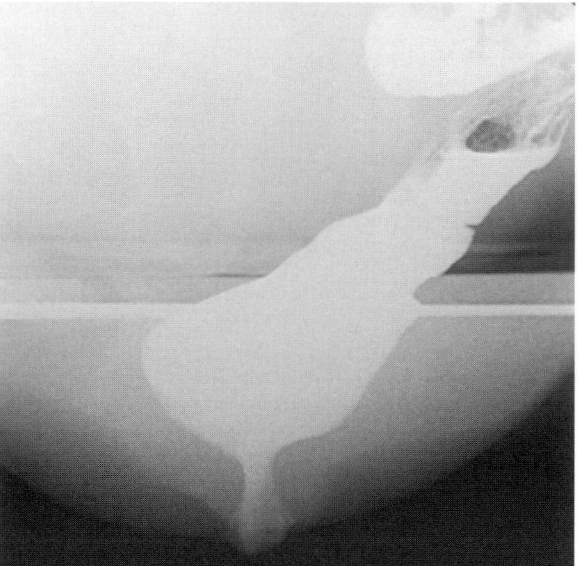

Figure 15.23 Anismus with pelvic floor descent and a concave anterior border to the rectum indicating that the patient is straining, but there is poor opening of the anal canal with delayed emptying at 30 s.

ANAL ENDOSONOGRAPHY

Several manufacturers have equipment suitable for these examinations. B&K Medical (B&K Medical A/S, Sandtoften 9, DK-2820 Gentofte, Denmark) have a dedicated endoprobe for ano-rectal endosonography. This consists of a 10 MHz mechanical rotated transducer. The water filled balloon system for rectal examination may be exchanged for a hard plastic cap to examine the anal canal (Fig. 15.25).

Technique

The cone is filled with degassed (boiled) water and the cone protected with a condom that has been liberally covered with ultrasound gel, both inside and outside, to prevent any air interface and ensure good acoustic contact. Patients, especially females, should be examined prone as the left lateral position results in some deformity of the anterior structures. The probe should be inserted gently into the rectum, and rotated so that the rectovaginal septum or prostate is uppermost. The image will then be in the standard orientation. The probe is slowly withdrawn with images recorded at different levels.

Anatomy

A sonographic image is formed from reflections at acoustic interfaces, and the level of reflectivity most appropriately describes the acoustic quality of a tissue layer.

The cross sectional image shows alternating bands of reflectivity creating a basic four-layer pattern (Fig. 15.26):

1. *submucosa* – just outside the two bright interface reflections from the cone this layer is of moderate reflectivity. It may contain well defined rounded areas of low reflectivity due to venous channels.
2. *Internal sphincter* – this is a clearly defined landmark presenting as a circular band of low reflectivity about 2 mm thick.
3. *Longitudinal muscle* – bundles of low reflective muscles may be seen higher up amongst more reflective fibroelastic tissue. Fat in the plane between the longitudinal layer and the external sphincter often causes a prominent interface reflection, demarcating the surgical 'intersphincteric plane'.
4. *External sphincter* – the deep part fuses with the puborectalis. In both sexes this shows the characteristic appearance of striated muscle with a fibrillated texture due to acoustic reflections from the perimysium. In females the superficial part has a more uniform higher reflectivity, whereas in males it is of lower reflectivity. The clarity with which the outer border of the external sphincter is defined varies.

The canal may be divided into three levels (Fig. 15.27a–c):

- HIGH at the level of the puborectalis that forms a 'U' sling around the vagina, perineum and anus.
- MID where in females the external sphincter has formed a complete ring anteriorly and the internal sphincter is still present.
- LOW at the level of the subcutaneous part of the external sphincter, just below the termination of the internal sphincter.

The external sphincter is a complex structure in the female, being shorter anteriorly than posteriorly. High in the canal there does not appear to be any anterior external sphincter. The perineum at this level is relatively amorphous sonographically and blends in with the paravaginal muscle. In the mid canal the sides of the external sphincter are cut across as they slope down to form a complete anterior ring (Fig. 15.28a&b).

INTERNAL ANAL SPHINCTER

Increased fibroelastic tissue in the aging sphincter makes it thicker with age, measuring < 1 mm in neonates, 1–2 mm in young adults, 2–3 mm in middle age and 3–4 mm in the elderly. The sphincter is not completely symmetric, either in thickness or termina-

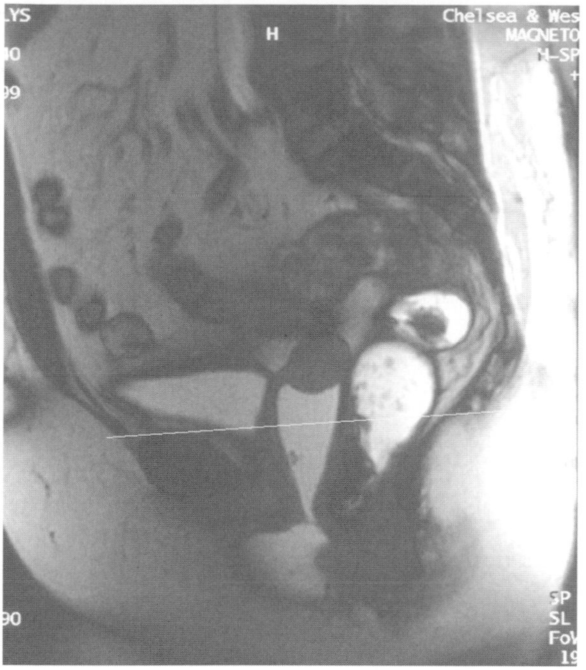

a

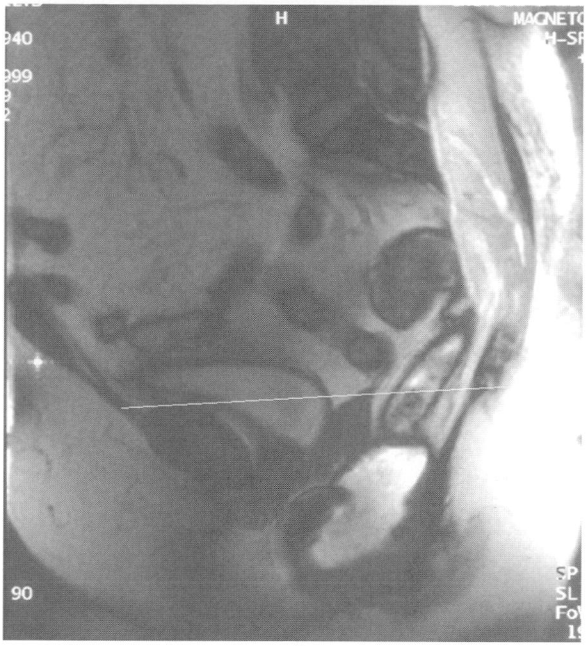

b

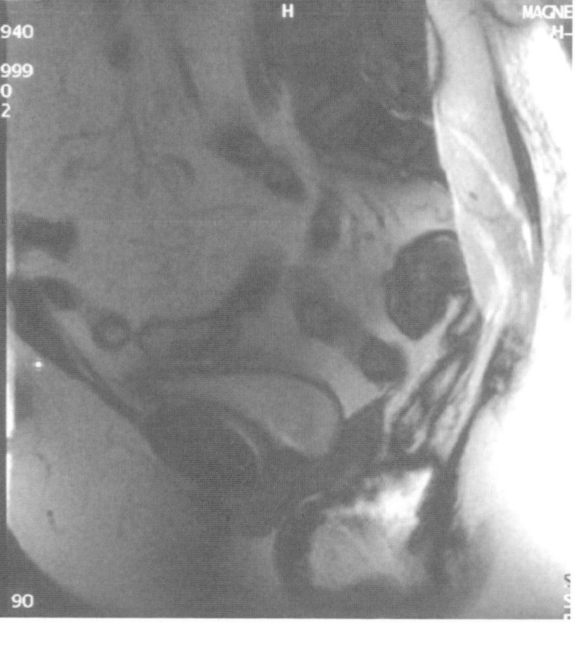

c

Figure 15.24 Dynamic MRI with the vagina and rectum opacified with ultrasound gel, and the bladder filled normally. (a) The white line indicates the plane of the pelvis. During evacuation (b) a cystocele and vaginal vault prolapse are seen, with trapping at the end of evacuation in an anterior rectocele (c).

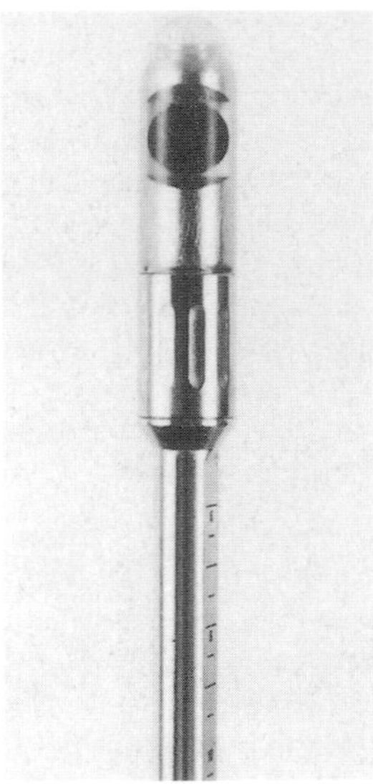

Figure 15.25 Brüel and Kjær 7 MHz anal transducer with 1.7 cm plastic cone filled with degassed water.

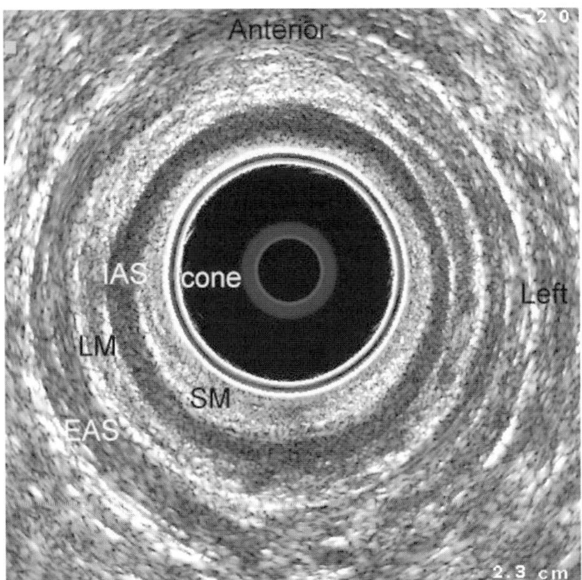

Figure 15.26 Normal axial scan in mid canal in a male. The orientation of the image is seen with anterior uppermost. The cone creates two bright interface reflections. The submucosa (SM) and longitudinal muscle (LM) are of moderate reflectivity, the internal (IAS) and external (EAS) sphincters of relatively low reflectivity.

tion. Measurements should be taken at 3 or 6 o'clock in the thickest part. At a given age the sphincter may be either too thick or too thin.

A thick sphincter, usually in the 3–4 mm range in a young adult is invariably associated with SRUS (Fig. 15.29) and rectal intussusception,[76] whereas sphincters > 4 mm may be due to hereditary internal sphincter myopathy (Fig. 15.30), a rare condition presenting with proctalgia fugax.[77] A thin sphincter (< 2 mm in a patients > 50 years) may be associated with passive fecal incontinence.[78] The cause of primary internal sphincter degeneration (Fig. 15.31) is unknown, but it may be a significant cause of faecal incontinence in the elderly.

Disruption of the sphincter is easy to appreciate from the loss of continuity of the low reflective ring. Anal stretch procedures may disrupt or fragment (Fig. 15.32) the sphincter.[79] Lateral sphincterotomy may extend too high and involve the entire sphincter, particularly in the female where this sphincter is rather short (Fig. 15.33).[80] An incomplete sphincterotomy increases the likelihood of recurrence,[81] but the length of the sphincterotomy relates to the incidence of incontinence.[82] Patients who become incontinent after hemorrhoidectomy may be found to have damage to the internal sphincter. After a low anterior resection 18% may have damage to the internal sphincter.[83] Other causes of trauma, notably vaginal delivery, cause more damage to the external than the internal sphincter.

EXTERNAL ANAL SPHINCTER

When the external sphincter is torn, the separated muscle fibres heal with granulation tissue and fibrosis. The resulting scar is relatively homogeneous and sonographically of low reflectivity (Fig. 15.34). The commonest cause of external sphincter damage is vaginal delivery.[84] Tears affect the anterior part of the sphincter and the perineum (Fig. 15.35), often on the other side to an episiotomy (Fig. 15.36).[85] Although large tears may be diagnosed clinically, neither visual inspection of the perineum,[85] nor digital examination[86] is sufficiently accurate to exclude a tear.

The incidence of sphincter damage during the first vaginal delivery may be up to 35%,[87] and as high as 80% following forceps assisted delivery.[88] Initially it was thought that internal sphincter damage could occur in isolation. With improved resolution this is now thought to be unlikely, and all patients have an external sphincter tear. When there is concomitant internal sphincter injury, the defects are usually adjacent, but are always anteriorly placed. A posterior internal sphincter defect is never obstetric in origin.

Sphincter repair should oppose (Fig. 15.37), or preferably overlap (Fig. 15.38) the margins of the normal sphincter, so that a complete ring is restored.[89] A successful outcome also requires good function in the remaining sphincter muscle. External sphincter atrophy has been described using MR with an endocoil

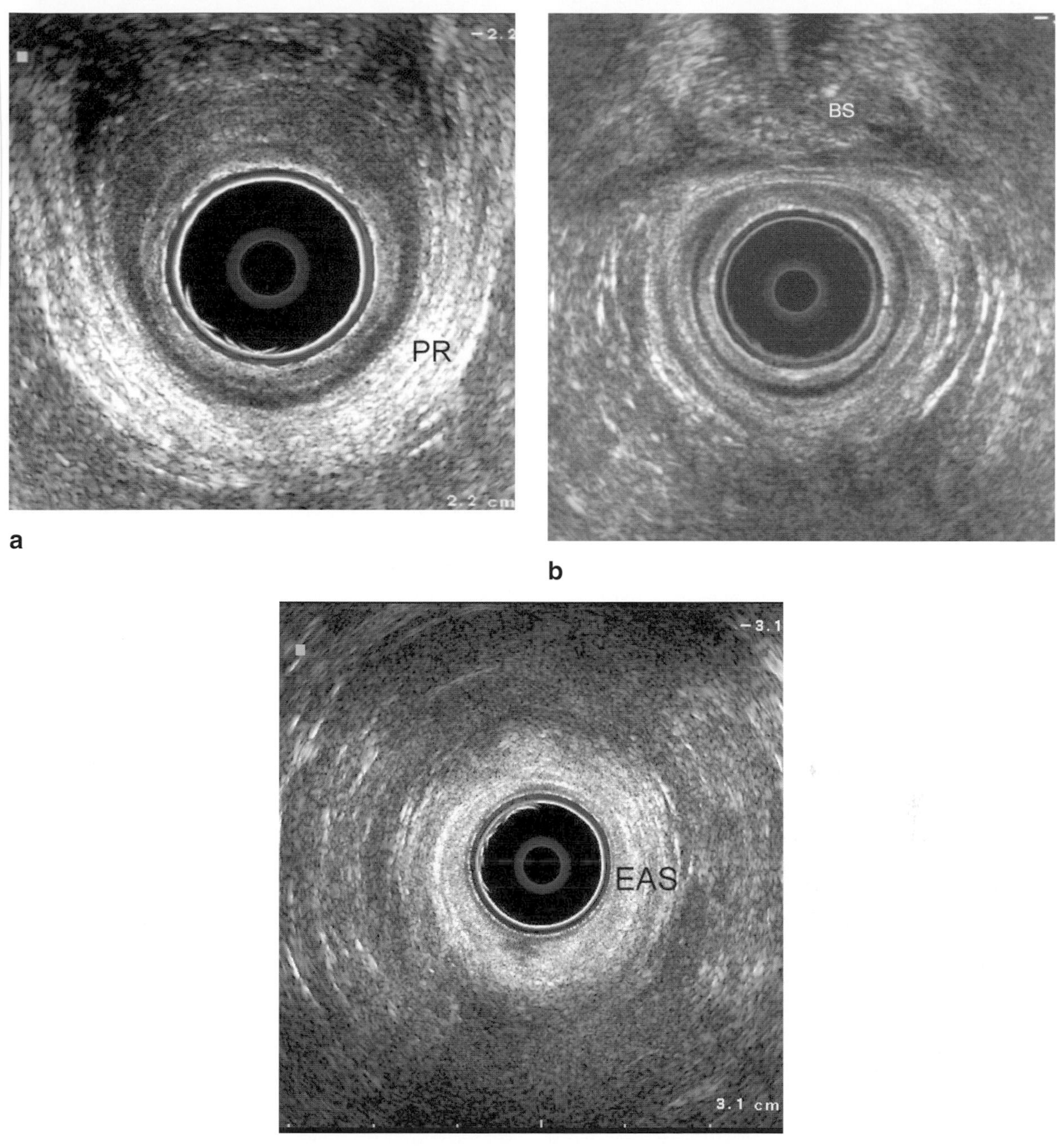

Figure 15.27 Canal levels in a female. (a) High level at the puborectalis (PR). (b) Mid level with the anterior ring of the external sphincter intact. The bulbospongiosus (BS) is seen anteriorly and the internal sphincter clearly defined. (c) Low level below the termination of the internal sphincter with the subcutaneous external sphincter (EAS).

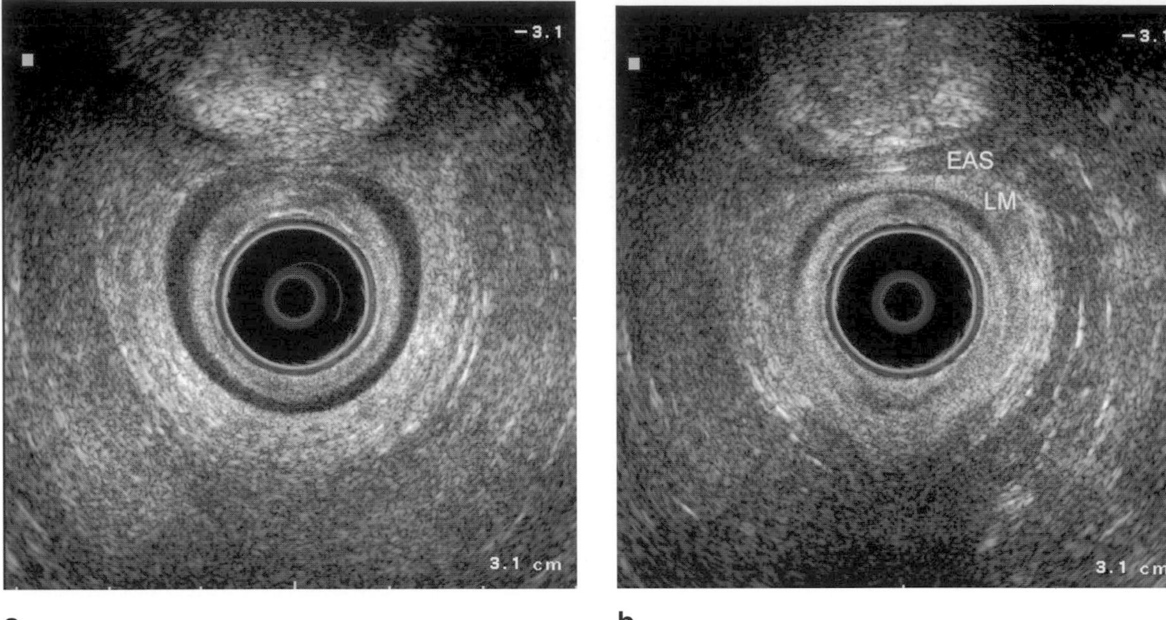

Figure 15.28 Formation of the anterior external sphincter ring in the female. (a) The sloping ends of the sphincter are cut through, whereas just below this level (b) the ring is intact.

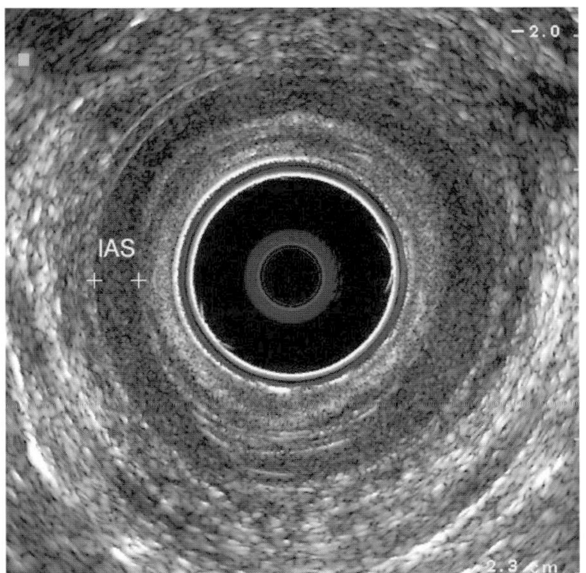

Figure 15.29 Thick internal sphincter (3.3 mm) in a young patient with solitary rectal ulcer syndrome and intra-anal prolapse.

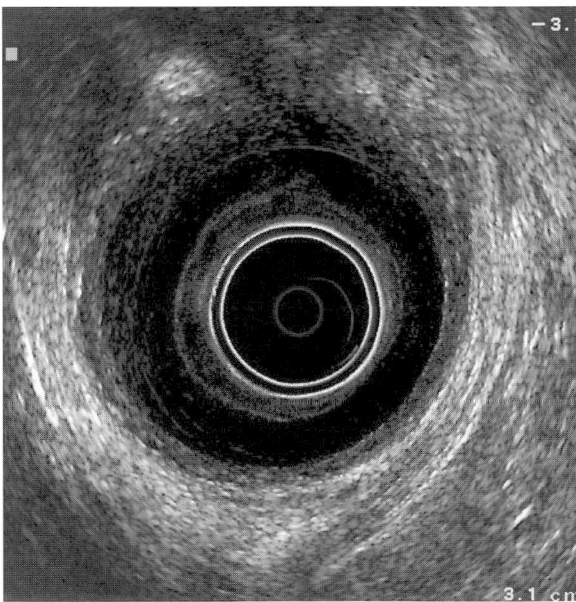

Figure 15.30 Grossly thickened internal sphincter in hereditary internal sphincter myopathy.

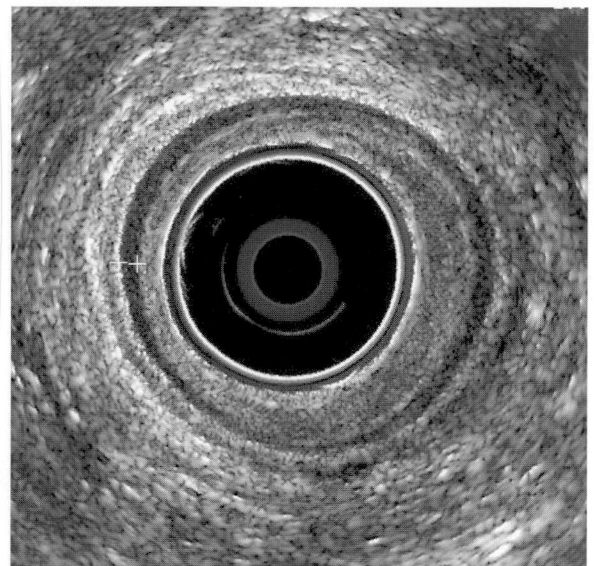

Figure 15.31 Thin internal sphincter (1.3 mm) in a 60-year-old patient with passive fecal incontinence.

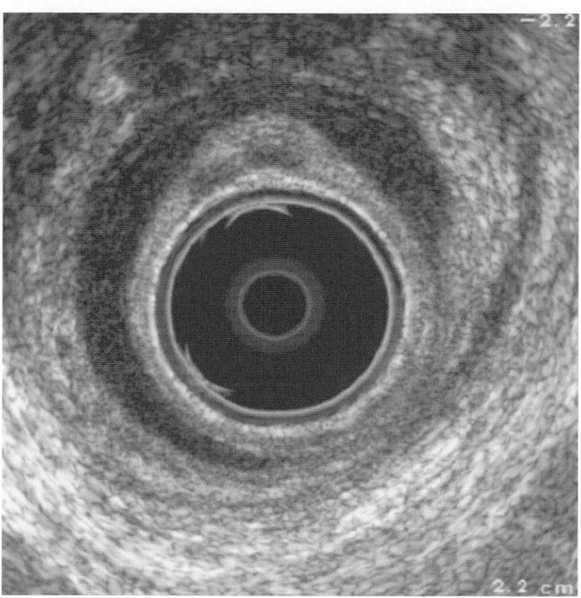

Figure 15.33 Lateral internal sphincterotomy. The sphincter defect is seen extending up into the high level of the canal indicating complete separation of the sphincter.

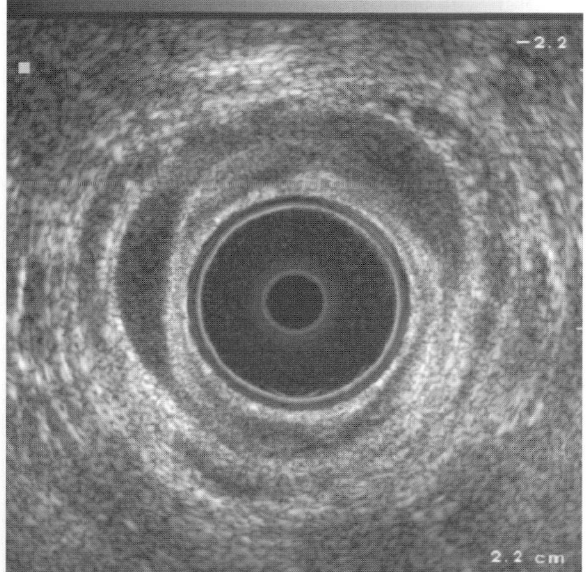

Figure 15.32 Fragmentation of the internal sphincter following anal dilatation.

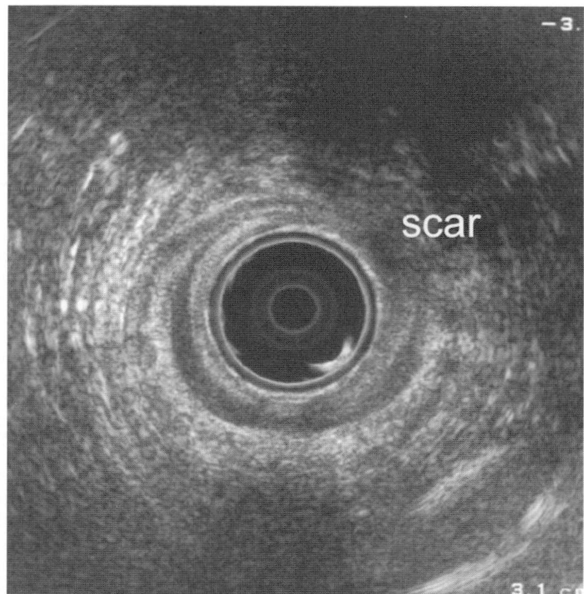

Figure 15.34 Scar tissue between 12–3 following obstetric trauma.

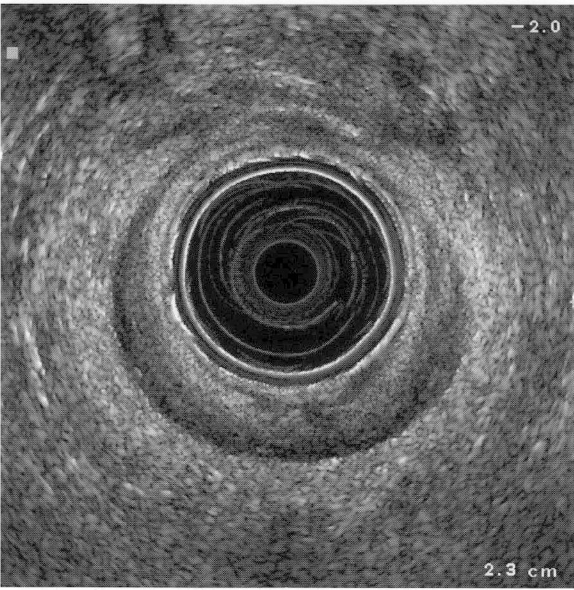

Figure 15.35 Typical obstetric trauma with anterior tear to the external and internal sphincters between 11–2.

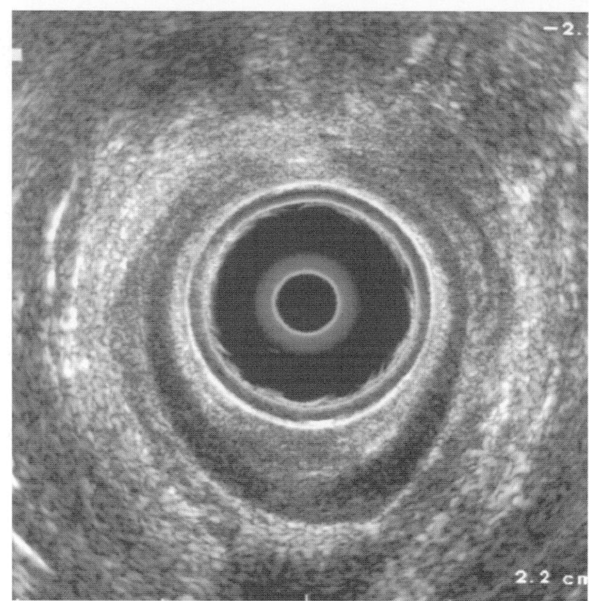

Figure 15.36 Obstetric trauma with a tear in the internal sphincter anteriorly between 11–1, and in the external sphincter between 1–2. The episiotomy was right sided.

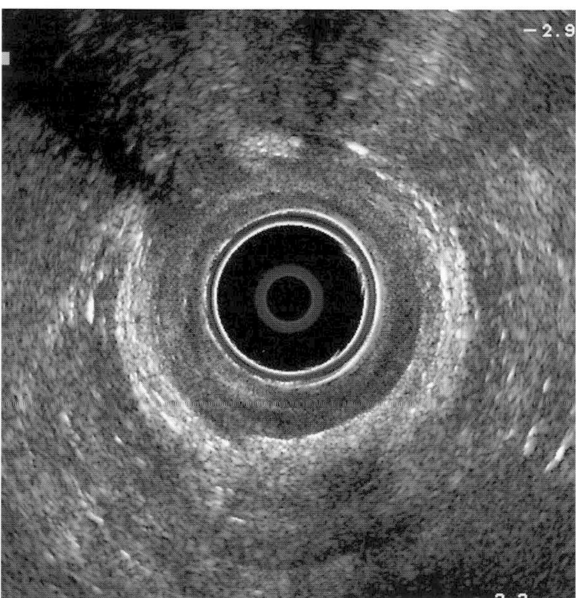

Figure 15.37 Incomplete repair of an obstetric tear with a persisting defect between 10–1.

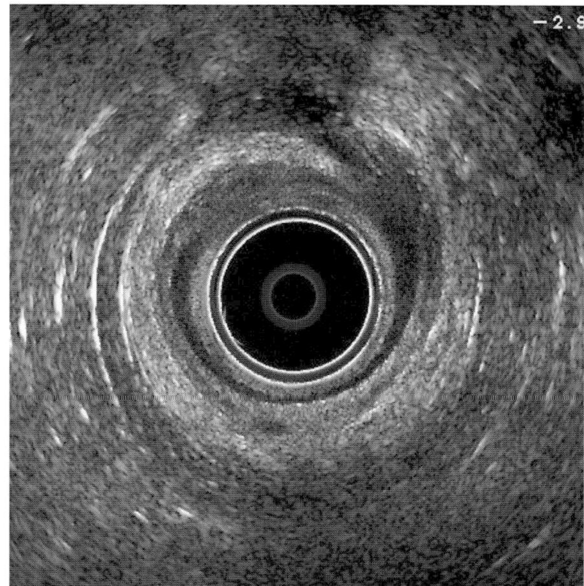

Figure 15.38 An overlapping repair at 1–2.

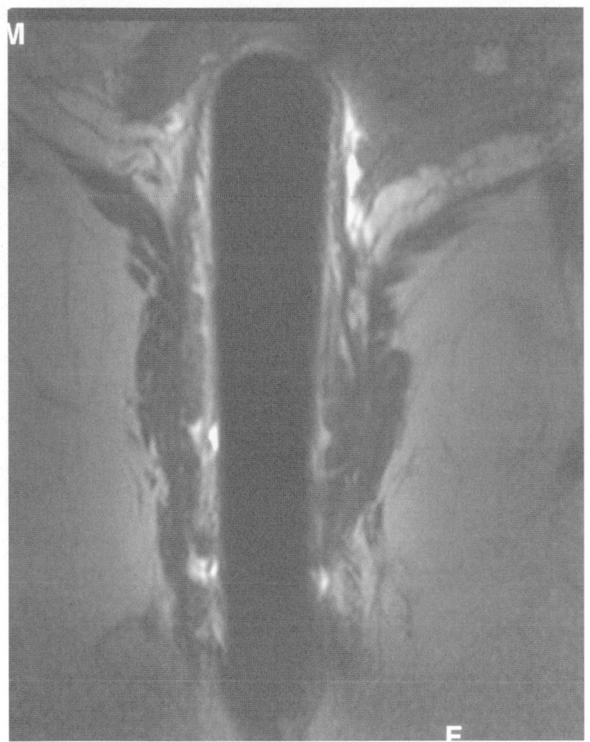

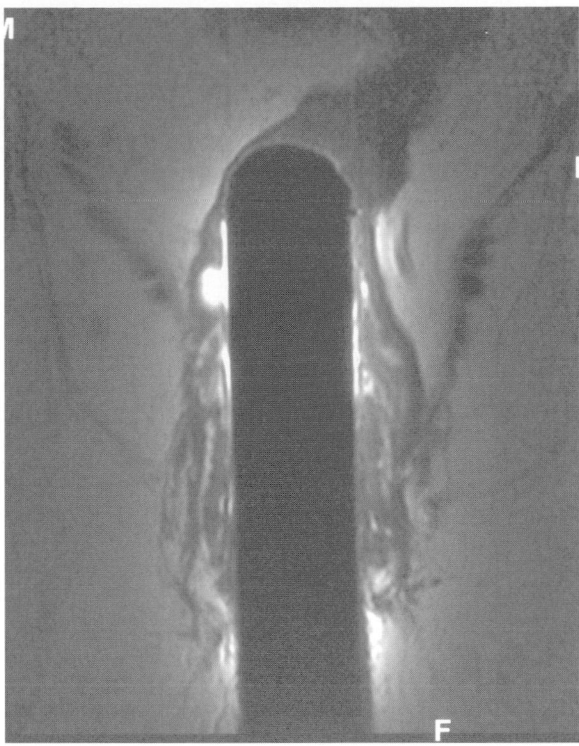

Figure 15.39 External sphincter atrophy. Extensive generalized loss of external sphincter bulk is seen in this coronal MRI endocoil view (a) compared with a normal sphincter (b).

(Fig. 15.39a and b).[90] This technique shows striated muscle as a low signal band clearly defined against the high signal from the fat in the ischio-anal fossa, and has been considered superior to endosonography.[91] However, the signal from scar tissue is difficult to differentiate from muscle, and the internal sphincter less clearly demonstrated. Both techniques have their relative merits, and as so often with ultrasound, once other modalities clarify some anatomical complex this may then be recognized on ultrasound. At the time of writing MR endocoils for the anus are currently available from only one manufacturer (Picker, Stevenage, UK).

REFERENCES

1. Herbst F, Kamm MA, Morris GP, Britton K, Woloszko J, Nicholls RJ. Gastrointestinal transit and prolonged ambulatory colonic motility in health and faecal incontinence. *Gut* 1997;**41**:381–9.
2. van der Sijp JR, Kamm MA, Nightingale JM, *et al.* Radioisotope determination of regional colonic transit in severe constipation: comparison with radio opaque markers [see comments]. *Gut* 1993;**34**:402–408.
3. Notghi A, Hutchinson R, Kumar D, Smith NB, Harding LK. Simplified method for the measurement of segmental colonic transit time. *Gut* 1994;**35**:976–81.
4. Lubowski DZ, Meagher AP, Smart RC, Butler SP. Scintigraphic assessment of colonic function during defaecation. *Internat J Colorectal Dis* 1995;**10**:91–3.
5. Evans RC, Kamm MA, Hinton JM, Lennard-Jones JE. The normal range and a simple diagram for recording whole gut transit time. *Int J Colorect Dis* 1992;**7**:15–17.
6. Hinton JM, Lennard-Jones JE, Young AC. A new method for studying gut transit times using radio-opapue markers. *Gut* 1969;**10**:842–7.
7. Metcalf AM, Phillips SF, Zinsmeister AR, MacCarty RL, Beart RW, Wolff BG. Simplified assessment of segmental colonic transit. *Gastroenterology* 1987;**92**:40–47.
8. Bouchoucha M, Devroede G, Arhan P, *et al.* What is the meaning of colorectal transit time measurement? *Dis Colon Rectum* 1992;**35**:773–82.
9. Arhan P, Devroede G, Jehannin B, *et al.* Segmental colonic transit time. *Dis Colon Rectum* 1981;**24**:625–9.
10. Chaussade S, Khyari A, Roche H, *et al.* Determination of total and segmental colonic transit time in constipated patients. Results in 91 patients with a new simplified method. *Dig Dis Sci* 1989;**34**:1168–72.
11. Bouchoucha M, Devroede G, Renard P, Arhan P, Barbier JP, Cugnenc PH. Compartmental analysis of colonic transit reveals abnormalities in constipated patients with normal transit. *Clin Sci (Colch)* 1995;**89**:129–35.

12. Krevsky B, Maurer AH, Fisher RS. Patterns of colonic transit in chronic idiopathic constipation. *Am J Gastroenterol* 1989;**84**:127–32.
13. de Graaf EJ, Gilberts EC, Schouten WR. Role of segmental colonic transit time studies to select patients with slow transit constipation for partial left-sided or subtotal colectomy. *Br J Surg* 1996;**83**:648–51.
14. Bartram CI, Turnbull GK, Lennard-Jones JE. Evacuation proctography: an investigation of rectal expulsion in 20 subjects without defecatory disturbance. *Gastrointest Radiol* 1988;**13**:72–80.
15. Wallden L. Roentgen examination of the deep rectogenital pouch. *Acta Radiol* 1953;**39**:105–116.
16. Mahieu PH, Pringot J, Bodart P. Defecography: 1. Description of a new procedure and results in normal patients. *Gastrointest Radiol* 1984;**9**:247–51.
17. Mahieu PH, Pringot J, Bodart P. Defecography: 2. Contribution to the diagnosis of defecation disorders. *Gastrointest Radiol* 1984;**9**:253–61.
18. Kamm MA, van der Sijp JR, Lennard-Jones JE. Observations on the characteristics of stimulated defaecation in severe idiopathic constipation. *Int J Colorectal Dis* 1992;**7**:197–201.
19. Piloni V, Ascoli G, Marmorale C. Contribution of defaecography to the diagnosis of faecal incontinence. *Coloproctology* 1988;**10**:297–301.
20. Alstrup N, Ronholt C, Fu C, Rasmussen O, Sorensen M, Christiansen J. Viscous fluid expulsion in the evaluation of the constipated patient. *Dis Colon Rectum* 1997;**40**:580–84.
21. Turnbull GK, Bartram CI, Lennard-Jones JE. Radiologic studies of rectal evacuation in adults with idiopathic constipation. *Dis Colon Rectum* 1988;**31**:190–97.
22. Poon FW, Lauder JC, Finlay IG. Technical report: evacuating proctography – a simplified technique. *Clin Radiol* 1991;**44**:113–16.
23. Jorge JM, Ger GC, Gonzalez L, Wexner SD. Patient position during cinedefecography. Influence on perineal descent and other measurements. *Dis Colon Rectum* 1994;**37**:927–31.
24. Hare C, Bartram CI, Halligan S. Dose reduction in evacuation proctography. *Eur Radiol* 2001;**11**:432–4.
25. Kelvin FM, Maglinte DD, Hornback JA, Benson JT. Pelvic prolapse: assessment with evacuation proctography (defecography). *Radiology* 1992;**184**:547–51.
26. Archer BD, Somers S, Stevenson GW. Contrast medium gel for marking vaginal position during defecography. *Radiology* 1992;**182**:278–9.
27. Jorge JM, Yang YK, Wexner SD. Incidence and clinical significance of sigmoidoceles as determined by a new classification system. *Dis Colon Rectum* 1994;**37**:1112–17.
28. Maglinte DD, Kelvin FM, Hale DS, Benson JT. Dynamic Cystoproctography: a unifying diagnostic approach to pelvic floor and anorectal dysfunction. *Am J Roentgenol* 1999;**169**:759–67.
29. Hock D, Lombard R, Jehaes C, *et al.* Colpocystodefecography. *Dis Colon Rectum* 1993;**36**:1015–21.
30. Kelvin FM, Maglinte DD, Benson JT, Brubaker LP, Smith C. Dynamic cystoproctography: a technique for assessing disorders of the pelvic floor in women. *Am J Roentgenol* 1994;**163**:368–70.
31. Bremmer S, Ahlback SO, Uden R, Mellgren A. Simultaneous defecography and peritoneography in defecation disorders. *Dis Colon Rectum* 1995;**38**:969–73.
32. Halligan MS, Bartram CI. Evacuation proctography combined with positive contrast peritoneography to demonstrate pelvic floor hernias. *Abdom Imaging* 1995;**20**:442–5.
33. Shorvon PJ, McHugh S, Diamant NE, Somers S, Stevenson GW. Defecography in normal volunteers: results and implications. *Gut* 1989;**30**:1737–49.
34. McGee SG, Bartram CI. Intra-anal intussusception: diagnosis by posteroanterior stress proctography. *Abdom Imaging* 1993;**18**:136–40.
35. Halligan SH, Thomas J, Bartram CI. Intrarectal pressures and balloon expulsion related to evacuation proctography. *Gut* 1995;**37**:100–4.
36. Halligan S, Bartram CI. Is barium trapping in rectoceles significant? *Dis Colon Rectum* 1995;**38**:764–8.
37. Halligan S, Bartram CI. Is digitation associated with proctographic abnormality? *Internat J Colorect Dis* 1996;**11**:167–71.
38. Siproudhis L, Dautreme S, Ropert A, *et al.* Dyschezia and rectocele – a marriage of convenience? Physiologic evaluation of the rectocele in a group of 52 women complaining of difficulty in evacuation. *Dis Colon Rectum* 1993;**36**:1030–36.
39. Watson SJ, Loder PB, Halligan S, Bartram CI, Kamm MA, Phillips RK. Transperineal repair of symptomatic rectocele with Marlex mesh: a clinical, physiological and radiologic assessment of treatment. *J Am Col Surg* 1996;**183**:257–61.
40. Poon FW, Lauder JC, Finlay IG. Perineal herniation. *Clin Radiol* 1993;**47**:49–51.
41. Allen-Mersh TG, Henry MM, Nicholls RJ. Natural history of anterior mucosal prolapse. *Br J Surg* 1987;**74**:679–82.
42. Kelvin FM, Maglinte DD. Dynamic cystoproctography of female pelvic floor defects and their interrelationships. *Am J Roentgenol* 1997;**169**:769–74.
43. Parks AG, Hardcastle JD, Hardcastle JD. The syndrome of the descending perineum. *Proc R Soc Med* 1966;**59**:477–82.
44. Skomorowska E, Hegedus V, Christiansen J. Evaluation of perineal descent by defaecography. *Int J Colorectal Dis* 1988;**3**:191–4.
45. Barnes PR, Lennard-Jones JE. Balloon expulsion from the rectum in constipation of different types. *Gut* 1985;**26**:1049–52.
46. Preston DM, Lennard-Jones JE. Anismus in chronic constipation. *Dig Dis Sci* 1985;**5**:413–18.
47. Jones PN, Lubowski DZ, Swash M, Henry MM. Is paradoxical contraction of the puborectalis muscle of functional importance? *Dis Colon Rectum* 1987;**30**:667–70.
48. Bartolo DC, Duthie GS. Pelvic floor incoordination. In: Kamm MA, Lennard-Jones JE (eds). *Constipation* Petersfield, UK: Wrightson Biomedical Publishing Ltd, 1994:77–85.
49. Bleijenberg G, Kuijpers HC. Biofeedback treatment of constipation: a comparison of two methods. *Am J Gastroenterol* 1994;**89**:1021–6.
50. Halligan S, Bartram C. Proctographic diagnosis of anismus [letter]. *Dis Colon Rectum* 1998;**41**:1070–71.
52. Thorpe AC, Williams NS, Badenoch DF, Blandy JP, Grahn MF. Simultaneous dynamic electromyographic proctography and cystometrography. *Br J Surg* 1993;**80**:115–20.

53. Kamm MA, Bartram CI, Lennard-Jones JE. Rectodynamics – quantifying rectal evacuation. *Int J Colorectal Dis* 1989;**4**:161–3.
54. Halligan S, McGee S, Bartram CI. Quantification of evacuation proctography. *Dis Colon Rectum* 1994;**37**:1151–4.
55. Halligan S, Bartram CI, Park HJ, Kamm MA. Proctographic features of anismus. *Radiology* 1995;**197**:679–82.
56. Halligan S, Nicholls RJ, Bartram CI. Evacuation proctography in patients with solitary rectal ulcer syndrome: anatomic abnormalities and frequency of impaired emptying and prolapse. *Am J Roentgenol* 1995;**164**:91–5.
57. van Tets WF, Kuijpers JH. Internal rectal intussusception – fact or fancy? *Dis Colon Rectum* 1995;**38**:1080–83.
58. Christiansen J, Zhu BW, Rasmussen OO, Sorensen M. Internal rectal intussusception: results of surgical repair. *Dis Colon Rectum* 1992;**35**:1026–8.
59. Orrom WJ, Bartolo DC, Miller R, Mortensen NJ, Roe AM. Rectopexy is an ineffective treatment for obstructed defecation. *Dis Colon Rectum* 1991;**34**:41–6.
60. Johansson C, Nilsson BY, Mellgren A, Dolk A, Holmstrom B. Paradoxical sphincter reaction and associated colorectal disorders. *Int J Colorectal Dis* 1992;**7**:89–94.
61. Lubowski DZ, King DW, Finlay IG. Electromyography of the pubococcygeus muscles in patients with obstructed defaecation. *Int J Colorectal Dis* 1992;**7**:184–7.
62. Pinho M, Yoshioka K, Ortiz J, Oya M, Keighley MR. The effect of age on pelvic floor dynamics. *Int J Colorectal Dis* 1990;**5**:207–208.
63. Jorge JM, Wexner SD, Ehrenpreis ED, Nogueras JJ, Jagelman DG. Does perineal descent correlate with pudendal neuropathy? *Dis Colon Rectum* 1993;**36**:475–83.
64. Halligan S, Bartram CI. The radiological investigation of constipation. *Clin Radiol* 1995;**50**:429–35.
65. Halligan S, Nicholls RJ, Bartram CI. Proctographic changes after rectopexy for solitary rectal ulcer syndrome and preoperative predictive factors for a successful outcome. *Br J Surg* 1995;**82**:314–17.
66. Karlbom U, Pahlman L, Nilsson S, Graf W. Relationships between defecographic findings, rectal emptying, and colonic transit time in constipated patients. *Gut* 1995;**36**:907–12.
67. Hiltunen KM, Kolehmainen H, Matikainen M. Does defecography help in diagnosis and clinical decision-making in defecation disorders? *Abdom Imaging* 1994;**19**:355–8.
68. Ott DJ, Donati DL, Kerr RM, Chen MY. Defecography: results in 55 patients and impact on clinical management. *Abdom Imaging* 1994;**19**:349–54.
69. Harvey CJ, Halligan S, Bartram CI, Hollings N, Sahdev A, Kingston K. Evacuation proctography: a prospective study of diagnostic and therapeutic effects. *Radiology* 1999;**211**:223–7.
70. Healy JC, Halligan S, Reznek RH, *et al.* Magnetic resonance imaging of the pelvic floor in patients with obstructed defaecation. *Br J Surg* 1997;**84**:1555–8.
71. Healy JC, Halligan S, Reznek RH, Watson S, Phillips RK, Armstrong P. Patterns of prolapse in women with symptoms of pelvic floor weakness: assessment with MR imaging. *Radiology* 1997;**203**:77–81.
72. Healy JC, Halligan S, Reznek RH, *et al.* Dynamic MR imaging compared with evacuation proctography when evaluating anorectal configuration and pelvic floor movement. *Am J Roentgenol* 1997;**169**:775–9.
73. Lienemann A, Anthuber C, Baron A, Kohz P, Reiser M. Dynamic MR colpocystorectography assessing pelvic-floor descent. *Eur Radiol* 1997;**7**:1309–1317.
74. Hilfiker PR, Debatin JF, Schwizer W, Schoenenberger AW, Fried M, Marincek B. MR defecography: depiction of anorectal anatomy and pathology. *J Comput Assist Tomogr* 1998;**22**:749–55.
75. Schoenenberger AW, Debatin JF, Guldenschuh I, Hany TF, Steiner P, Krestin GP. Dynamic MR defecography with a superconducting, open-configuration MR system. *Radiology* 1998;**206**:641–6.
76. Halligan S, Sultan A, Rottenberg G, Bartram CI. Endosonography of the anal sphincters in solitary rectal ulcer syndrome. *Int J Colorectal Dis* 1995;**10**:79–82.
77. Kamm MA, Hoyle CH, Burleigh DE, *et al.* Hereditary internal anal sphincter myopathy causing proctalgia fugax and constipation. A newly identified condition. *Gastroenterology* 1991;**100**:805–10.
78. Vaizey CJ, Kamm MA, Bartram CI. Primary degeneration of the internal anal sphincter as a cause of passive faecal incontinence. *Lancet* 1997;**349**:612–15.
79. Speakman CT, Burnett SJ, Kamm MA, Bartram CI. Sphincter injury after anal dilatation demonstrated by anal endosonography. *Br J Surg* 1991;**78**:1429–30.
80. Sultan AH, Kamm MA, Nicholls RJ, Bartram CI. Prospective study of the extent of internal anal sphincter division during lateral sphincterotomy. *Dis Colon Rectum* 1994;**37**:1031–33.
81. Garcia-Granero E, Sanahuja A, Garcia-Armengol J, *et al.* Anal endosonographic evaluation after closed lateral subcutaneous sphincterotomy. *Dis Colon Rectum* 1998;**41**:598–601.
82. Garcia-Aguilar J, Belmonte MC, Perez JJ, *et al.* Incontinence after lateral internal sphincterotomy: anatomic and functional evaluation. *Dis Colon Rectum* 1998;**41**:423–7.
83. Farouk R, Duthie GS, Lee PW, Monson JR. Endosonographic evidence of injury to the internal anal sphincter after low anterior resection: long-term follow-up. *Dis Colon Rectum* 1998;**41**:888–91.
84. Kamm MA. Obstetric damage and faecal incontinence. *Lancet* 1994;**344**:730–33.
85. Frudinger A, Bartram CI, Spencer JA, Kamm MA. Perineal examination as a predictor of underlying external anal sphincter damage. *Br J Obstet Gynaecol* 1997;**104**:1009–1013.
86. Sultan AH, Kamm MA, Talbot IC, Nicholls RJ, Bartram CI. Anal endosonography for identifying external sphincter defects confirmed histologically. *Br J Surg* 1994;**81**:463–5.
87. Sultan AH, Kamm MA, Hudson CN, Thomas JM, Bartram CI. Anal-sphincter disruption during vaginal delivery. *N Engl J Med* 1993;**329**:1905–1911.
88. Sultan AH, Kamm MA, Bartram CI, Hudson CN. Anal sphincter trauma during instrumental delivery. *Int J Gynaecol Obstet* 1993;**43**:263–70.
89. Engel AF, Kamm MA, Sultan AH, Bartram CL, Nicholls RJ. Anterior anal sphincter repair in patients with obstetric trauma. *Br J Surg* 1994;**81**:1231–4.

90. deSouza NM, Puni R, Gilderdale DJ, Bydder GM. Magnetic resonance imaging of the anal sphincter using an internal coil. *Magn Reson Q* 1995;11:45–56.

91. Stoker J, Hussain SM, Lameris JS. Endoanal magnetic resonance imaging versus endosonography. *Radiol Med (Torino)* 1996;92:738–41.

Chapter 16

Electrophysiological investigation of the posterior pelvic floor musculature

Michael Swash

INTRODUCTION

Continence, representing continued storage of urine and feces, and voiding of urine or defecation, is a complex function that requires coordinated responses in the pelvic floor sphincter muscles and in the bladder detrusor and ano-rectal and abdominal muscles.[1–4] The rectum and the anal canal are normally empty of feces. Rectal filling, produced by increased colonic peristaltic activity, like bladder filling in the urinary system, is one of the factors that triggers evacuation by defecation. The rectum itself is situated above the pelvic floor and the anal canal lies below this level. The ano-rectal junction thus lies at the level of the levator ani muscles and, at this point, there is normally a sharp angulation, called the ano-rectal angulation.[2] The ano-rectal angulation (Fig. 16.1), together with resting tonic contraction of the internal and external anal sphincter muscles, are three important factors in the maintenance of continence. Parks suggested that the normal ano-rectal angulation, maintained by the pull of the muscular sling formed in this region by the puborectalis muscles,[1,5,6] was particularly important in normal anal continence.[2,7,8] The puborectalis muscles are situated at the apex of the funnel-like muscular floor of the pelvis formed by the paired levator ani muscles (Figs 16.1 and 16.2). Since Parks' ideas, however, it has become apparent that the pull of the puborectalis muscles is only one of several important forces that maintain both urinary and fecal continence (see this book).

The paired puborectalis muscles form a sling originating from the pubis on each side and passing backward to the posterior wall of the ano-rectal junction (Fig. 16.1). They are composed of two parts.[9] These are the puboanalis sling, consisting of fibers of the puboanalis muscle which decussate behind the anal canal to form a sling, and the puboanal sphincteric sling, situated slightly caudally, in the region of the external anal sphincter muscle. The latter consists of deep superficial and cutaneous parts. The upper portion of the external anal sphincter muscle is histologically similar to the puborectalis muscle[6,10] and shows marked histological differences from the levator ani muscle, suggesting that the former two muscles form a functional unit separate from the levator ani itself. The circular external anal sphincter muscle has often been regarded as playing only a minor role in the maintenance of fecal continence,[1,6,11] but this view is probably an oversimplification.[12] The internal anal sphincter muscle is particularly important in controlling continence to flatus, but in normal subjects it is probably of little importance in the maintenance of fecal continence itself.[13]

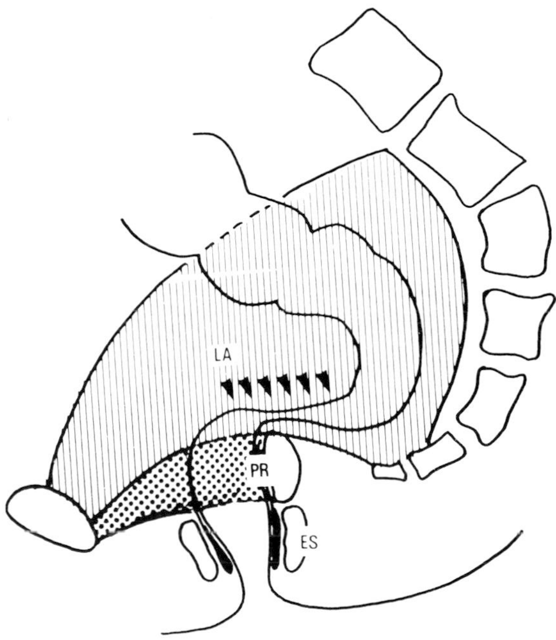

Figure 16.1 The flap-valve mechanism of the anorectal angle. The valve is closed by the intra-abdominal pressure (arrowheads) acting against the pull of the puborectalis (PR) muscles. ES, external sphincter; LA, levator ani.

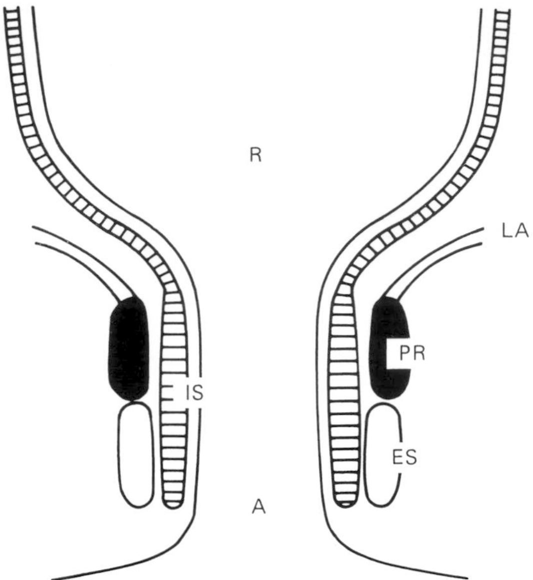

Figure 16.2 The muscles of the funnel-like pelvic floor. IS, internal sphincter; ES, external sphincter; LA, levator ani; PR, puborectalis; R, rectum; A, anal canal.

INNERVATION OF THE PELVIC FLOOR MUSCULATURE

The nerve supply of the pelvic floor muscles is derived from two distinct sources; the pudendal nerve, and a direct branch from the S3 and S4 motor roots. The pudendal nerve arises from the anterior primary rami of the second, third and fourth sacral nerves. Its inferior rectal branches cross the ischiorectal fossa to reach the external anal sphincter muscles, and its perineal branches pass forwards to innervate the periurethral striated sphincter muscle and thus to control urinary continence. Other branches of the third and fourth sacral roots reach the pelvic floor via its visceral surface.[9,14,15] The standard textbook descriptions of the motor innervation of the pelvic floor suggest that the pudendal nerve is the more important of these two innervations, and that the direct branch from S3 and S4 usually supplies only the more peripheral parts of the pelvic floor musculature. The direct branch of S3 and S4 also carries sensory fibers originating in the posterior urethra and in the anal canal. The motor supply to the puborectalis, the most important muscle for the maintenance of fecal continence, has been considered in these accounts to travel with the pudendal nerve.

Our histological studies of patients with anal incontinence (see below) suggested that this standard description of the innervation of these muscles was incorrect. In an electrophysiological study of the motor nerve supply to these muscles, we found that the puborectalis was innervated by a branch of the sacral nerve (S3 and S4) which lies above the pelvic floor. The pudendal nerve supplied the ipsilateral external anal sphincter muscle, but not the puborectalis muscle.[16,17] The puborectalis and the external anal sphincter muscles are thus innervated by different motor nerves, although both originate in the same spinal cord segments. Cross-innervation from side to side has not been studied in the puborectalis, but in the external anal sphincter muscles an experimental study in the monkey[18] showed substantial overlap in the pudendal innervation on the two sides. This is related to interdigitations of muscle fascicles across the midline anteriorly in this circular muscle. This functionally overlapping innervation enables reinnervation to be partially accomplished from the opposite side when there is pudendal nerve damage, an important aspect of the histological features of the muscle in incontinent patients.

The internal anal sphincter muscles are smooth muscles which receive autonomic innervation through the pelvic plexus. This consists not only of cholinergic nerve terminals but of catecholaminergic nerve terminals. The functional interrelationships of the different types of autonomic innervation in this muscle, and their physiological interaction with the somatic innervation of the puborectalis and external anal sphincter muscles, have not yet been fully studied.

HISTOLOGY OF THE PELVIC FLOOR MUSCLES IN ANO-RECTAL INCONTINENCE

It is important to understand the histological abnormalities likely to be present in muscles that are studied by electrophysiological methods. Histological abnormalities are a feature of patients with idiopathic incontinence, although they vary in degree from case to case.[10,19–21] The external anal sphincter is the most abnormal of the three muscles and the levator ani is usually the least affected; in some cases, the levator ani muscle appears normal. The abnormalities found in the external anal sphincter muscle differ slightly from those found in the puborectalis muscle. In particular, muscle fiber hypertrophy is much more marked in the puborectalis muscles than in the external anal sphincter or levator ani muscles (Table 16.1).

EXTERNAL ANAL SPHINCTER AND PUBORECTALIS MUSCLES

In the most abnormal of the external anal sphincter and puborectalis muscles, the biopsy contains only a few scattered striated muscle fibers embedded in fibrous and adipose tissue (Fig. 16.3), situated adjacent to the smooth muscle fibers of the internal anal sphincter muscle (see Fig. 16.4). In some biopsies there is a fibrous

Table 16.1 Summary of histometric abnormalities in pelvic floor muscles in fecal incontinence

Muscle	Muscle fiber type	Increase in diameter in incontinent patients (%)	Type 1 fiber predominance (%) Control	Incontinence
External anal sphincter	Type 1	36	78	85
	Type 2	54		
Puborectalis	Type 1	132	75	82
	Type 2	135		
Levator ani	Type 1	21	69	68
	Type 2	61		

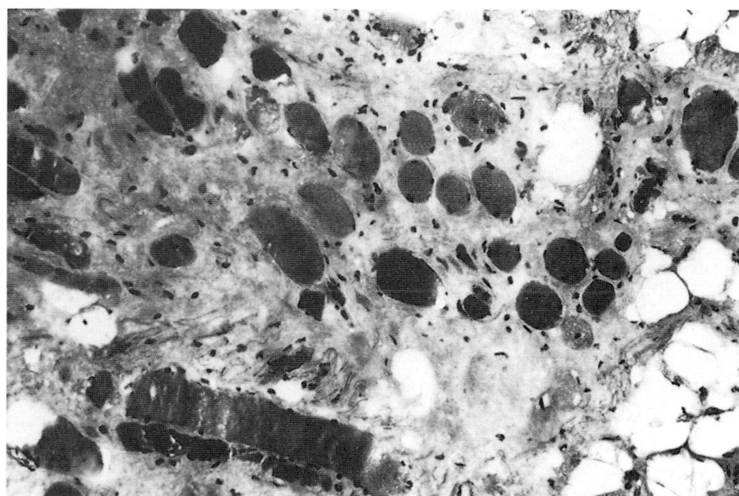

Figure 16.3 External anal sphincter. Hematoxylin and eosin, × 140. Incontinence. There is marked fibrosis and fat replacement. The few remaining muscle fibers are markedly hypertrophied. Scattered tiny atrophic fibers are present.

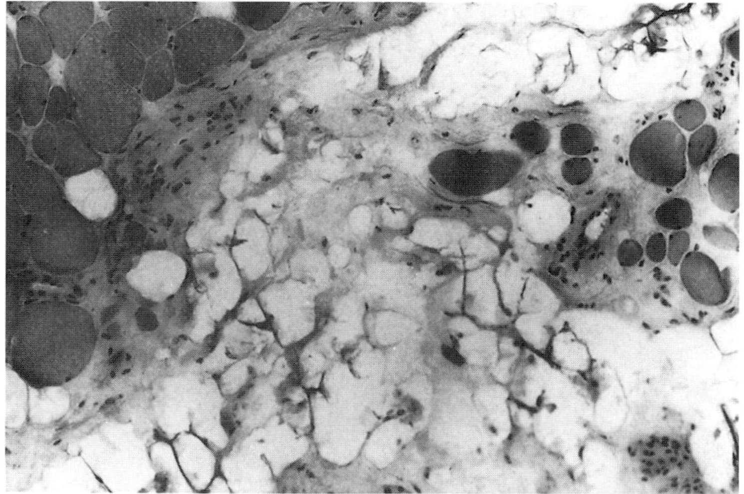

Figure 16.4 Puborectalis. Hematoxylin and eosin, ×200. Incontinence. Groups of fibers are relatively isolated from each other. In several regions there are groups of small atrophic fibers consistent with denervation atrophy.

scar replacing the muscle tissue. In less abnormal biopsies the muscle fibers are arranged in groups of 10–60 fibers of approximately uniform size, separated from each other by bands of fibrous or adipose tissue (Figs 16.4 and 16.5. These groups of fibers are of uniform histochemical type (Fig. 16.6), indicating that reinnervation had occurred, resulting in fiber-type grouping. Fiber-type grouping is also a feature in muscles in which less marked destructive changes had occurred (Fig. 16.7). Minor degrees of reorganization of the normal mosaic distribution of type 1 and type 2 fibers may be the only abnormality in these muscles in patients with less severe incontinence (Fig. 16.8). Small atrophic fibers are found scattered in the biopsies, consistent with denervation atrophy (Fig. 16.9). In the most severely abnormal biopsies, such extensive muscle destruction may have occurred that it is not possible to recognize histological features of reinnervation.

Two other features were noted in these muscles. First, there was marked hypertrophy of the remaining fibers, an abnormality which was found in both type 1 and type 2 fibers (compare Figs. 16.3–16.9 with Figs 16.10 and 16.11). This was especially marked in the puborectalis biopsies. Secondly, secondary myopathic

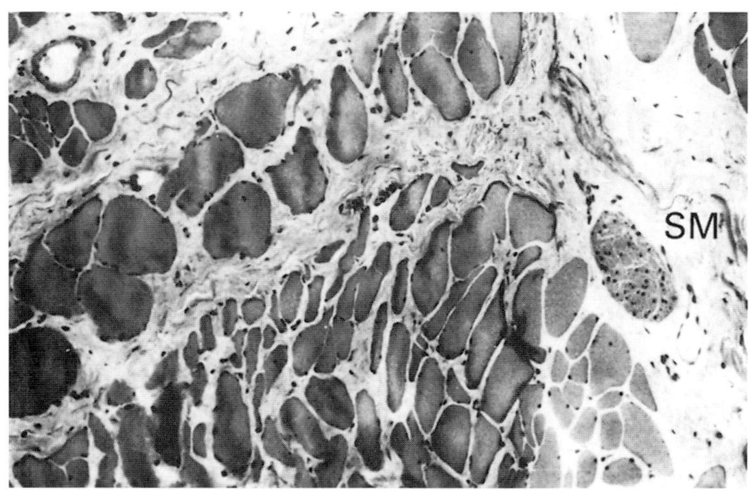

Figure 16.5 External anal sphincter. Hematoxylin and eosin (paraffin embedded), ×140. Incontinence. Groups of fibers of varying size are separated by fibrous tissue. Marked fiber-type hypertrophy is present, but fibers in individual groups tend to be of similar size. A part of the non-striated internal sphincter is included in the biopsy. SM, smooth muscle.

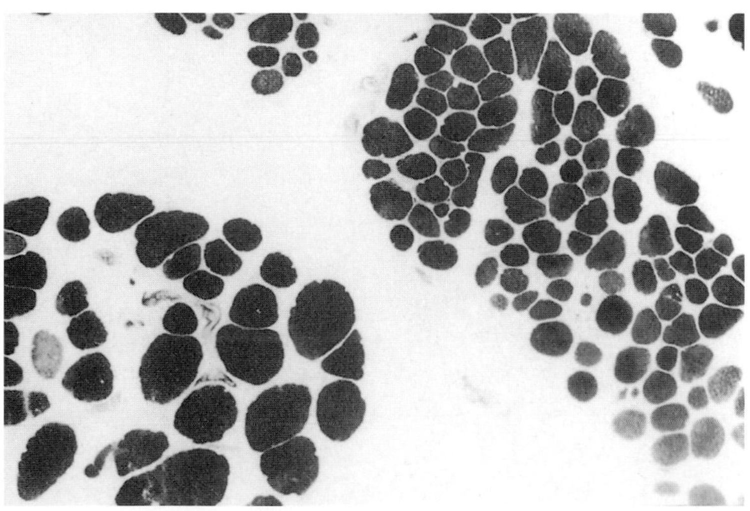

Figure 16.6 Puborectalis. ATPase, pH 4.3, × 140. Incontinence. The groups of fibers consist almost exclusively of type 1 fibers. Fiber hypertrophy is evident.

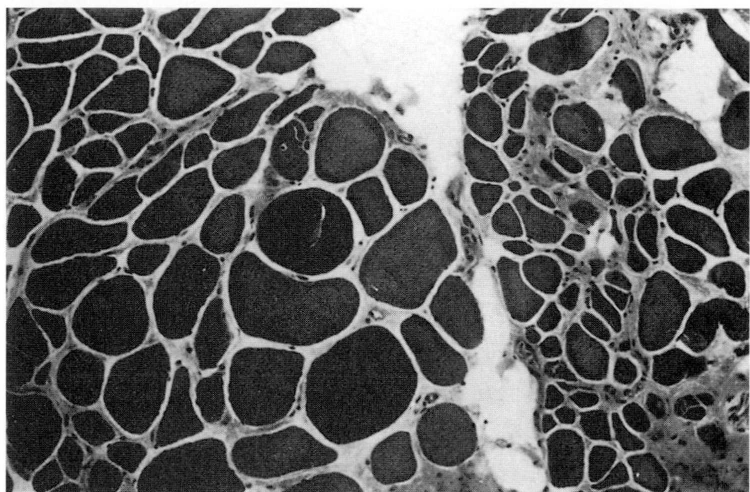

Figure 16.7 Puborectalis. ATPase, pH 4.3, ×140. Incontinence. There is fiber hypertrophy with both type 1 and type 2 fiber grouping.

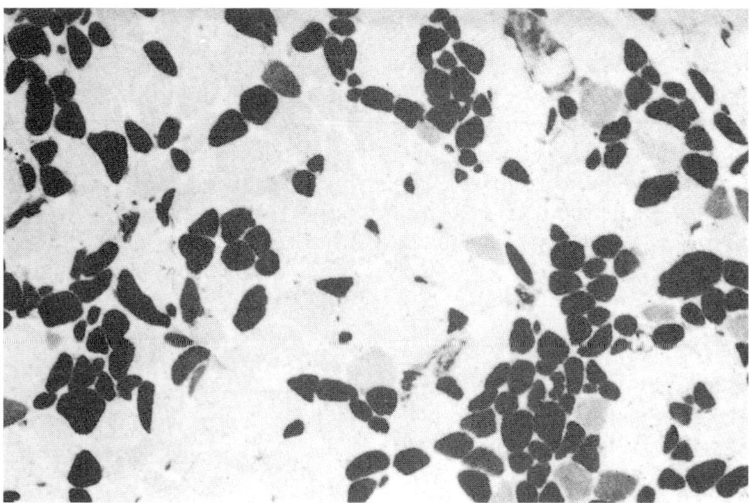

Figure 16.8 External anal sphincter. ATPase, pH 4.3, ×140. Incontinence. There is some hypertrophy of both fiber types, most marked in type 2 fibers, and reorganization of the fiber-type mosaic has begun, but fiber-type grouping is not yet well developed. There are a few scattered atrophic type 1 fibers.

changes were prominent in some biopsies, with fibrosis and fatty replacement of muscle fibers, marked variability in fiber size, prominent centrally located nuclei, with splitting or fragmentation of individual muscle fibers.[22]

LEVATOR ANI MUSCLE

Levator ani muscles usually show only mild abnormalities such as disseminated neurogenic atrophy. Grouped denervation atrophy is found in some cases. Fiber hypertrophy is not as prominent as in the puborectalis and external anal sphincter muscles. Myopathic abnormalities are rarely found.

OTHER FEATURES

Muscle spindles are found occasionally in each of the three muscles. They usually appear normal, but in the external anal sphincter and puborectalis muscles some fibrosis of their periaxial spaces and capsules may be evident (Fig. 16.12), an abnormality consistent with, but not diagnostic of, denervation.[23]

Figure 16.9 External anal sphincter, ATPase, pH 4.3. × 140. Incontinence. There is fiber hypertrophy, and atrophy, with marked type 1 and type 2 fiber grouping.

INNERVATION

Small intramuscular nerve bundles[19] in the external anal sphincter and puborectalis muscles contain reduced numbers of nerve fibres and show fibrosis. Small nerve bundles in the levator ani biopsies are normal. In three patients, biopsies taken from small nerves supplying the external anal sphincter muscles showed a marked reduction in the number of myelinated nerve fibres, with proliferation of Schwann cells. Segmental or paranodal demyelination was not found, and the unmyelinated nerve fibers were normal. The interstitial collagen was unusually prominent (Fig. 16.13).

HISTOMETRIC OBSERVATIONS

The mean diameters of type 1 and type 2 muscle fibers in the three pelvic floor muscles in patients with fecal incontinence, and in normal subjects, are shown in Fig. 16.14.[10] In the external anal sphincter and puborectalis muscles of control subjects, type 2 fibers are slightly larger than type 1 fibers. Type 2 fibers are generally larger in men than in women, as in other human skeletal muscles,[24] but fibers of both histochemical types are much smaller in these two muscles in normal subjects than in other striated muscles.[25] However, in the levator ani muscle of adult female control subjects, type 1 fibers are markedly larger than type 2 fibers.

The reversal of type 1 and type 2 fiber diameters in the levator ani muscle in women might be a hormone-dependent phenomenon. In the female rat, the levator ani muscles, homologous to the external anal sphincter of primates, undergo involution during puberty.[26] In women with fecal incontinence, the mean diameters of both type 1 and type 2 fibers were increased in all the pelvic floor muscles studied. This fiber hypertrophy was not prominent in the puborectalis and affected type 2 fibers more than type 1 fibers, both in this muscle and in the external anal sphincter muscle. In the levator ani muscle, both fiber types were slightly hypertrophied, but in women with ano-rectal incontinence, hypertrophy of type 1 fibers was less marked in this muscle. Fiber hypertrophy in the external anal sphincter and puborectalis muscles was accompanied by increased variability in fiber diameter, shown by increased interquartile range of fiber diameter in the incontinent patients.[10]

OTHER PELVIC FLOOR DISORDERS

Perineal descent and rectal prolapse are associated features of many patients with the syndrome of idiopathic ano-rectal incontinence.

PERINEAL DESCENT

In perineal descent,[8] the perineum 'balloons' downward during a cough or strain. The position of the ano-rectal angle with respect to the bony pelvis is changed, so that it lies at a lower level than in the normal. This syndrome, or physical sign, is often associated with painful discomfort in the perineum, sometimes due to mucosal prolapse. There may be a sensation of inadequate defecation, leading to persistent straining at stool. Some degree of fecal incontinence occurs in about half the patients with this syndrome, and abnormal descent of the perineum during straining is observed in nearly all patients with idiopathic fecal incontinence. An extreme form of the disorder occurs in cauda equina lesions, in which the perineal musculature is denervated.[27] In a

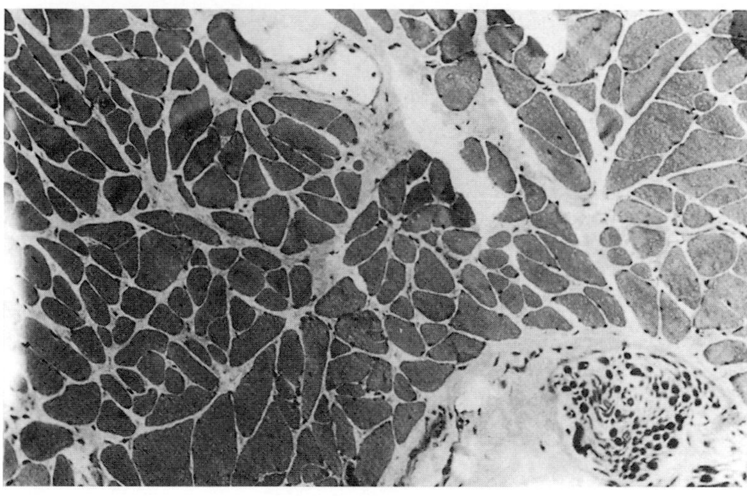

a

Figure 16.10 (a) External anal sphincter. Normal subject. Hematoxylin and eosin, ×140. The muscle fibers are small, closely packed and arranged in fascicles.

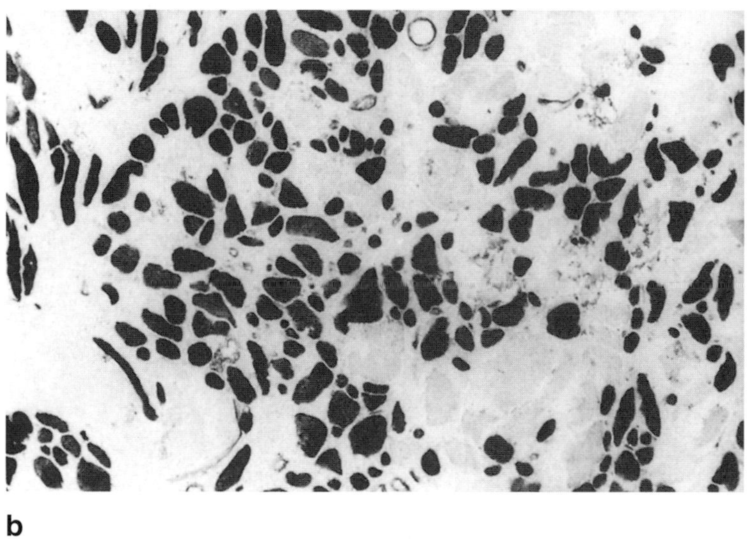

b

Figure 16.10 (b) ATPase, pH 4.3, ×140. A mosaic of type 1 and type 2 fibers is present, with type 1 fiber predominance.

series of patients with perineal descent, we found that there was hypertrophy of both type 1 and type 2 fibers in the external anal sphincter muscle to a similar degree to that found in patients with incontinence.[28] However, features of denervation of this muscle were not prominent in those patients, in whom fecal incontinence was not a symptom. These investigations suggested that the descending perineum syndrome is a symptom complex which may precede the development of frank incontinence, and that it may lead to damage to the nerve supply to the anal sphincter musculature.[28]

RECTAL PROLAPSE

A similar series of investigations, both histological and physiological, has been carried out in patients with rectal prolapse, a disorder which is sometimes also associated with descent of the perineum and with incontinence.[29] In these studies, two groups of patients with

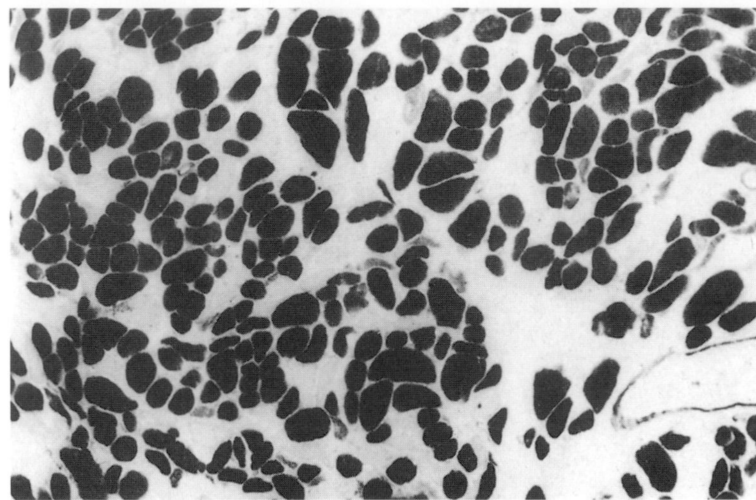

Figure 16.11 Puborectalis. ATPase, ×140. Normal subject. This muscle closely resembles the external anal sphincter

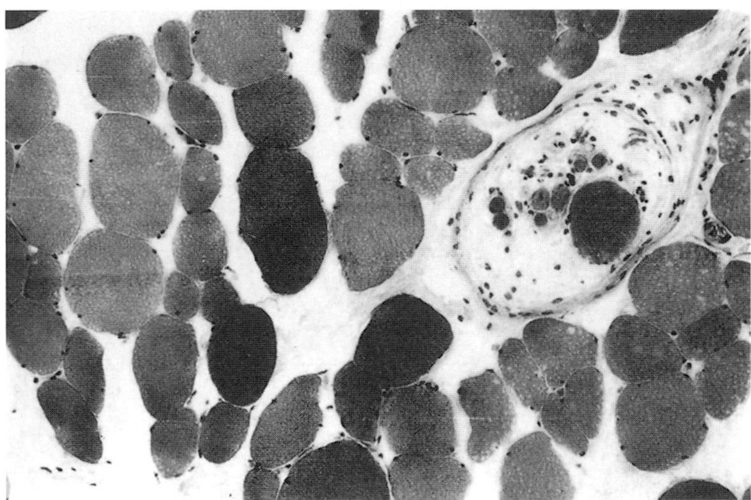

Figure 16.12 Puborectalis. Hematoxylin and eosin, ×350. Incontinence. A muscle spindle, with fibrosis and increased capsular lamellation; neighboring extrafusal muscle fibers are hypertrophied and rounded.

rectal prolapse were identified. In one group, in which rectal prolapse was associated with incontinence, there was electromyographic (EMG) evidence of denervation of the external anal sphincter and puborectalis muscles. In the second group, in which rectal prolapse was not associated with incontinence, no EMG or histological abnormality was found in these muscles.

HEMORRHOIDS

Teramoto, Parks and Swash (1981)[30] found a marked degree of hypertrophy of both type 1 and type 2 fibers in the external anal sphincter muscles in patients with hemorrhoids (see Chapter 25). In addition, these muscles showed increased type 1 fiber predominance. These histological studies did not reveal evidence of reinnervation or denervation of this muscle in this disorder. The findings were interpreted as evidence for an increased workload of the external anal sphincter in these patients. This is consistent with the high anal resting pressure found in patients with this disorder, and there is evidence that this might be due to reflex contraction of the external anal sphincter muscle complex induced by the stimulus of the presence of a hemorrhoidal bolus within the anal canal. Bruck *et al.* (1988),[31] in a physio-

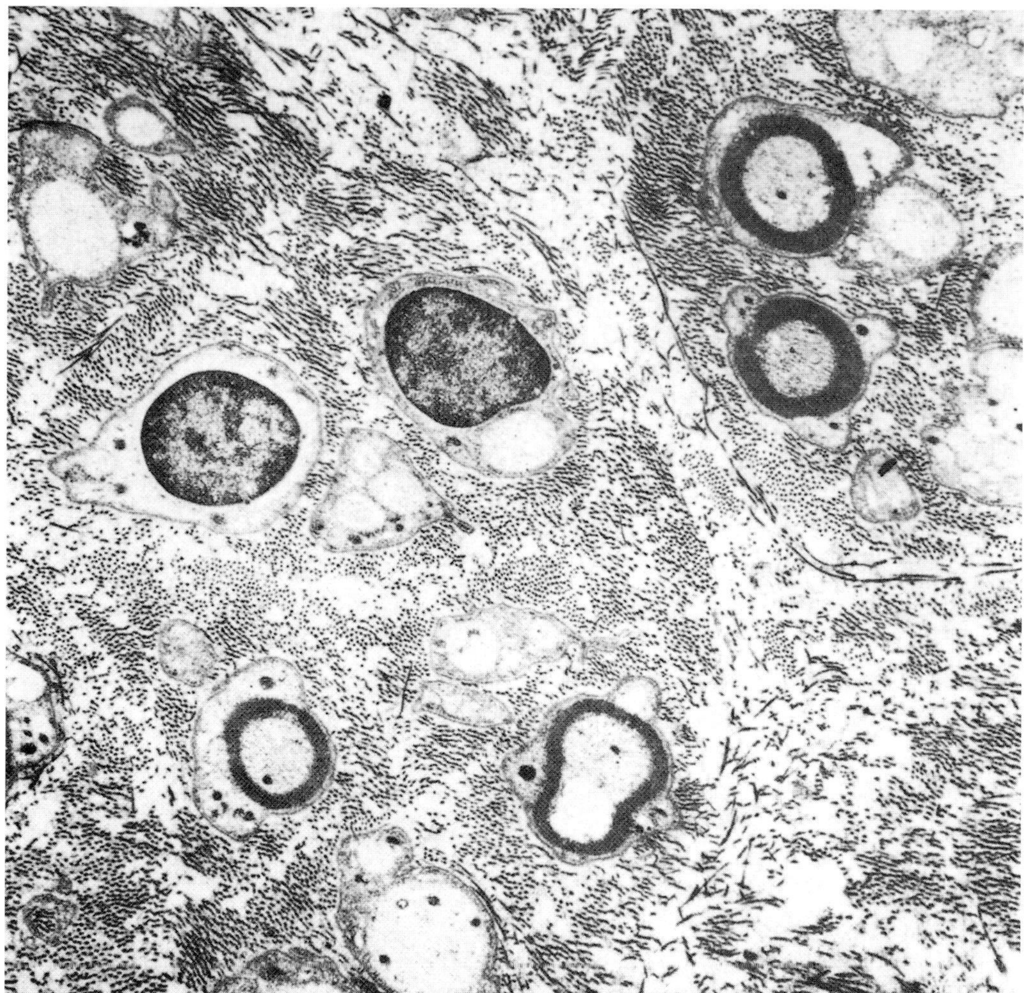

Figure 16.13 Nerve supplying external anal sphincter taken from a patient with incontinence (electron micrograph). There is an increase in interstitial collagen and a reduced number of myelinated nerve fibers. Magnification ×16 000.

logical study, found that patients with hemorrhoids were more likely to have pudendal neuropathy, with neurogenic changes in electromyographic studies of the external anal sphincter when there were clinical features of abnormal perineal descent on straining.

URINARY INCONTINENCE

Although stress urinary incontinence has been much investigated clinically, there are no detailed histological studies of the anterior perineal muscles comparable with those available for the posterior perineum. However electromyographic studies suggest that similar neurogenic changes occur in these muscles in stress urinary incontinence to those found in the striated ano-rectal musculature in idiopathic fecal incontinence.[32]

ELECTROMYOGRAPHY OF THE PELVIC FLOOR

Electromyography (EMG) is a powerful investigative technique which is much used in neurological and orthopedic practice in the investigation of patients with neuromuscular diseases, particularly in the evaluation of disorders in which the nerve supply of muscles is damaged, whether from diseases of the spinal cord, spinal nerve roots or peripheral nerves.[33] The technique depends on the recording of electrical activity arising in muscle fibers during voluntary contraction and at rest. A number of different methods for quantification of this electrical activity are available, but these are not all applicable to the EMG analysis of the pelvic floor musculature. As with most measurement techniques in medicine, it is important to recognize the advantages and limitations of the different methods.

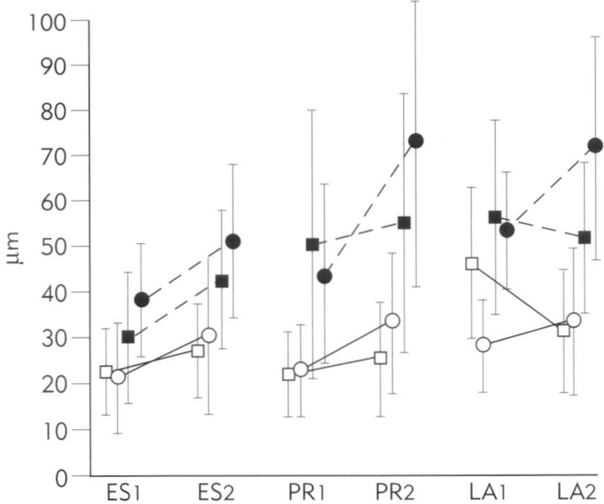

Figure 16.14 Means and standard deviations of fiber diameter in type 1 and type 2 fibers in external anal sphincter, puborectalis and levator ani muscles of normal subjects and incontinent patients of either sex. See text for discussion. Filled symbols, incontinent patients; open symbols, normal subjects. Square symbols, male; round symbols, female. ES1, external sphincter, type 1 fibers; ES2, external sphincter, type 2 fibers; PR, puborectalis; LA, levator ani.

EMG can provide useful clinical information about the function of the pelvic floor musculature, particularly the external anal sphincter and puborectalis muscles.[6,29,34–36] The levator ani is not readily accessible for EMG exploration. The more anteriorly situated perineal muscles, particularly the periurethral striated musculature, can be studied by EMG.[37]

EMG can be used as a functional test of muscle activity. For example, quantitative measurements of electrical activity in the external anal sphincter or puborectalis muscles during rest and straining have been applied to the investigation of patients with incontinence, rectal prolapse and solitary rectal ulcer syndrome (Figs 16.15 and 16.16). Measurements of the amplitude, duration and number of phases of motor unit action potentials provide quantitative data about the innervation and functional state of individual motor units within the muscle. Electrical activity in muscle fibers can be recorded using surface electrodes, monopolar electrodes, concentric needle electrodes or single fiber EMG electrodes. These techniques will be discussed separately in this chapter.

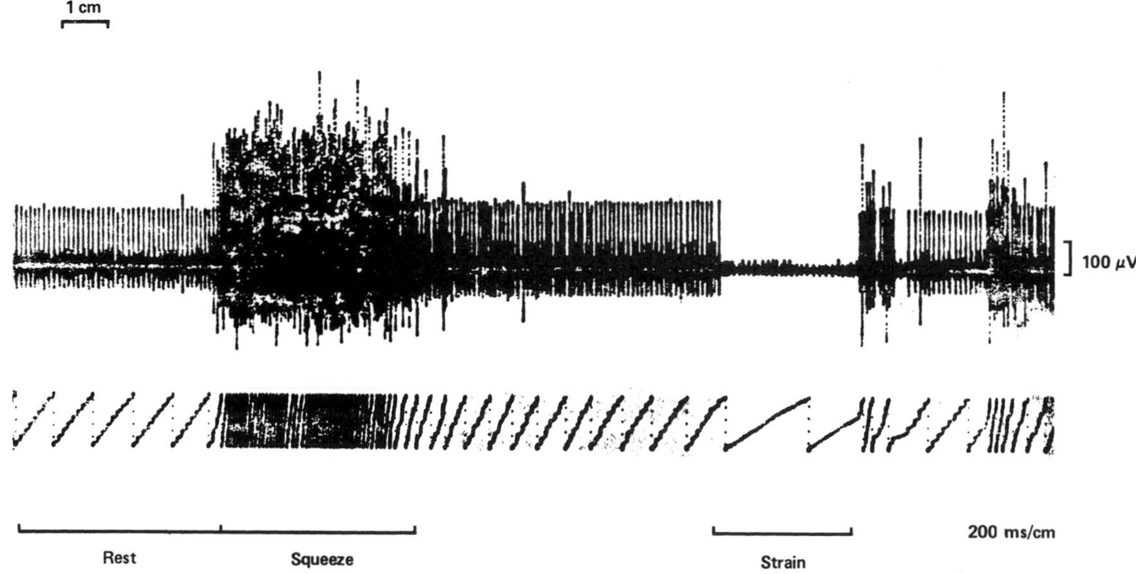

Figure 16.15 Puborectalis muscle. Concentric needle electromyography (EMG), 200 ms/cm. The upper trace shows EMG activity in this muscle. The lower trace shows the summated rectified EMG activity expressed in volt-seconds. The trace rises with the acquisition of potentials until 1 V has been stored, so that the quantitative activity in the muscle is represented by counting the number of accessions during a period of 1 s (or less). At rest there is some ongoing basal activity. The amount of EMG activity, and of muscle contraction, increases during voluntary squeezing of the anal sphincter muscle. This gradually relaxes after cessation of voluntary activity. During an attempted strain, as if in defecation, the puborectalis muscle relaxes and EMG activity in this muscle decreases. Basal activity is resumed at the end of the voluntary strain, and increases during a cough, seen at the end of the recording

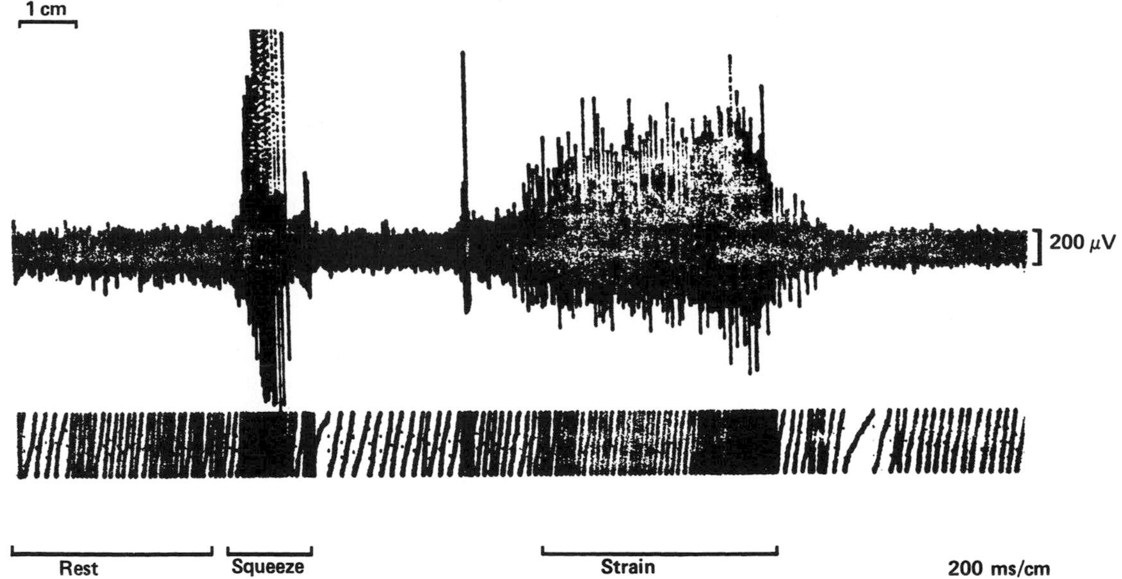

Figure 16.16 Solitary rectal ulcer syndrome. Puborectalis muscle. Concentric needle electromyography, 200 ms/cm. The recording resembles Figure 16.15. Basal activity is rather more evident. During straining, there is a paradoxical increase in activity in the puborectalis muscles. Similar abnormalities are found in the same patients with constipation (anismus: see Chapter 22).

BASIC CONCEPTS OF EMG

All electromyographic techniques depend on the recording of electrical activity generated in muscle fibers during voluntary contraction, or occurring in abnormally innervated muscle fibers at rest. The electrical activity of contracting muscle was first recorded with a string galvanometer from the human forearm flexor muscles by Piper (1908),[38] but the technique did not come into clinical use until the advent of the coaxial (concentric) needle electrode devised by Adrian and Bronck (1929).[39] In normal muscle, depolarization of the muscle fiber membrane, leading to the generation of the muscle action potential, which is propagated along the length of the muscle fiber at a velocity of about 3 m/s, is initiated by depolarization at the specialized motor end-plate zone. This is caused by the arrival of quanta of acetylcholine released from the presynaptic motor nerve terminal by the nerve impulse.

When the muscle fiber membrane becomes depolarized, the process of excitation/contraction coupling is initiated, resulting in shortening of the actin–myosin bands by sliding of one filament inside the other in each sarcomere. This is an energy-dependent process. Individual muscle fibers show specialization into fibers adapted for continuous contraction (tonic fibers) and those adapted for brief forceful contractions (phasic fibers). These physiological characteristics can be correlated with the type I and type II enzyme histochemical types determined by light microscopy.[33]

THE MOTOR UNIT

Our concept of the organization of the innervation of muscle fibers within individual muscles derives from the work of Sherrington, who recognized that individual muscles contained more muscle fibers than the number of large, heavily myelinated motor nerve fibers innervating these muscles. The term 'motor unit', which he introduced, refers to the anterior horn cell, its axon, and the axonal branches, motor end-plates and muscle fibers innervated by this cell. In some muscles, for example the intrinsic muscles of the hand, there are relatively small numbers of muscle fibers innervated by individual axons, perhaps only 6–10 muscle fibers, whereas in other muscles, for example the hip flexor muscles, much larger numbers of muscle fibers (for example 100–200) are innervated by an individual axon. The motor unit is thus smaller in the intrinsic hand muscles that in the hip flexor muscles. The former are specialized for fine and carefully controlled movements, and the latter for movements requiring considerable force.

Electromyography allows the recording of action potentials derived from motor units within a contracting muscle. The muscle fibers making up individual motor units are scattered quasi-randomly through the cross-sectional area of individual muscles in such a way that a mosaic pattern of muscle fibers representing interlocking motor units can be demonstrated. In pathological studies of human skeletal muscles, it is possible to recognize the mosaic pattern of type I, type IIa and type IIb fibers, an appearance resembling a chequerboard. During voluntary contraction of individual units, the individual muscle fiber action potentials derived from the contracting unit summate to form the motor unit action potential, a potential of larger amplitude and longer duration than that derived from single muscle fibers. Because of the small size and brief duration of individual muscle fiber action potentials, single muscle fiber potentials can only be recorded when the recording electrode is in close proximity to the fiber undergoing contraction, but motor unit action potentials, representing the activity of several or most fibers within a motor unit, can be recorded at a greater distance.

CHANGES IN DISEASE

There are two broad classes of neuromuscular disease: the myopathies and the neurogenic disorders. These can be distinguished in EMG recordings by the different patterns of electrical activity recorded. However, EMG of the pelvic floor musculature is not usually applied to this kind of investigative problem, which is better approached by EMG of limb muscles. In pelvic floor disorders, the major indications for EMG are to assess the functional activity of the pelvic floor muscles during voluntary contraction, e.g. straining at stool or in reflexly controlled contractions, as in the cough reflex or the rectoanal sphincteric reflex, or in order to assess the presence of damage to the innervation of these muscles. The latter application has become of increasing importance in clinical practice in coloproctology.

CHANGES IN EMG ACTIVITY RELATED TO NEUROGENIC DISTURBANCES

When the nerve supply of a muscle is damaged, some or all of the muscle fibers become denervated. This loss of functional innervation of muscle fibers leads to loss of responsiveness of those muscle fibers to nerve fiber activity, and to atrophy of the affected fibers. This can be recognized pathologically by the presence of scattered atrophic muscle fibers (see Chapter 12). If the process is incomplete, and reinnervation occurs either by regrowth of the damaged axons from the site of damage in the nerve itself, or by sprouting of nearby unaffected axons within the muscle so as to take on the innervation of neighboring denervated fibers, effective reinnervation may occur. This process begins within a few days of nerve injury and may result in effective recovery during a period of a few days to several weeks, depending on the site of the injury.

Sprouting of axons within the damaged muscle leads to a change in the distribution of muscle fibers within motor units, so that there is a tendency for these fibers not to retain their random distribution within the muscle, but to be clustered together in small groups of fibers innervated by branches of a single axon. This process is called fiber-type grouping. This change in the spatial distribution of muscle fibers within motor units results in a change in the amplitude and duration of motor unit action potentials recorded by EMG. It is important to recognize that denervated muscle fibers cannot contract in response to voluntary activity and that the EMG changes during slight voluntary activity thus reflect the process of reinnervation rather than the process of denervation. Denervated muscle fibers may show spontaneous activity at rest (fibrillations, fasciculations and positive sharp waves; see Swash and Schwartz, 1990[22] for descriptive details) but, while these are relatively easy to recognize in limb muscles, they are difficult to find in sphincter muscles.

SPECIAL CHARACTERISTICS OF PELVIC FLOOR AND ANAL SPHINCTER MUSCLES

The muscles of the pelvic floor differ from most striated muscles both anatomically and physiologically. The pelvic floor muscle fibers are generally smaller than striated muscle fibers and contain a higher proportion of type I, tonic muscle fibers than do the limb muscles. The external anal sphincter muscle, puborectalis muscle and periurethral striated musculature particularly show these differences. The external anal sphincter muscle is also unusual in that it consists of two deep parts and a superficial part. The latter inserts into skin and the former portions insert not into tendons or fascia, but into the endomysium of the muscle itself, since it occupies a circular position around the anal orifice. However, the muscle fibers in these muscles, like all other striated muscles in the body with the exception of the external ocular muscles, are each innervated by single motor end-plates. Muscle spindles, the stretch sensitive receptors of striated muscles, have been identified in the levator ani, puborectalis and external anal sphincter muscles[4] and they presumably also exist in the periurethral striated sphincter muscle. These muscles might therefore be expected to respond to stretch by reflex contraction generated by a reflex arc dependent on the anterior horn cells in the spinal cord.

Because the muscle fibers in the external anal sphincter and puborectalis muscles are smaller than those in other striated human muscles, the amplitude of action potentials derived from individual fibers, and therefore of the motor unit action potentials themselves, might be expected to be somewhat smaller than in other striated muscles. This point is of particular importance in single fiber electromyography and in quantitative concentric needle EMG techniques.

Recording of spontaneous activity, that is, activity not generated by voluntary contraction, in these muscles is difficult to evaluate, since the external anal sphincter muscle, and probably the puborectalis muscle, are in mild continuous tonic contraction.[40] The periurethral sphincter muscle also exhibits slow continuous electrical activity. This activity varies from moment to moment, but is present even during sleep. This observation illustrates the importance of these muscles in the maintenance of continence. During defecation or micturition, the activity of the sphincter ceases.

EMG RECORDING TECHNIQUES

EMG equipment consists of a recording electrode, a preamplifier, amplifier and loudspeaker, and an oscilloscope for display of electrical activity. Modern commercial EMG equipment provides variable amplitude and timebase duration controls within a range suitable for electromyography, together with low pass and high pass filter options suitable for the recording techniques in common use. A number of computer-assisted methods for data analysis are available, and these can be applied to sphincter EMG.

SURFACE ELECTRODES

Electrical activity recorded with surface electrodes is difficult to analyse because the recording electrode is at some distance from the contracting muscle, so that the intervening tissue acts as a filter excluding low frequency activity, and modulating the action potentials recorded. In addition, it is difficult to be sure that the activity recorded is actually generated within the muscle close to the electrode. Adjacent muscles, which might also be in contraction, will also contribute to the activity recorded by the surface electrodes. Surface electrodes are usually mounted in pairs on a muscle to be assessed, with a ground electrode at a distance. Despite these technical problems, O'Donnell *et al.* (1988)[41] obtained adequate motor unit potentials from the external anal sphincter muscle using a surface electrode recording technique, and this method is useful in dynamic recordings designed to assess the timing of muscle activity. Surface electrode recording techniques are particularly applicable to motor nerve conduction velocity and terminal motor latency measurements in which muscle activity is initiated by direct electrical stimulation of the nerve supply of the muscle under test. These techniques are much used in clinical EMG and have been applied to pelvic floor disorders.

Surface electrode recording techniques, using plate electrodes within the anal canal to record the external anal sphincter activity, have also been applied in biofeedback therapy as a form of conditioning, particularly in the treatment of patients with weak pelvic floor muscles, or incontinence, and in attempts to improve the function of sphincter muscle activity in patients with hyperactive sphincter muscles, for example in patients with anal pain. The amplified electrical activity of the sphincter muscle is recorded with a telephone-jack-type electrode in the anal canal and is amplified through a loudspeaker so that the patient is made aware of the state of contraction of the muscle. With appropriate education, some improvement in function can often be obtained.

MONOPOLAR ELECTRODES

Monopolar electrodes, that is, electrodes with a single leading-off surface, consisting of a solid steel electrode insulated to the tip with a resin coat, are used in some centres for EMG recordings. The reference electrode is placed on the skin at a distance from the muscle under test and a separate ground electrode is used. The use of such a monopolar recording system allows activity to be recorded at some distance from the tip of the recording electrode. The method is particularly useful when looking for fibrillations and fasciculations, that is, spontaneous activity in denervated muscle, in limb muscles, but it is not generally applicable to sphincter EMG. The results obtained vary according to the diameter of the tip of the recording electrode.

CONCENTRIC NEEDLE ELECTRODES

The concentric needle electrode introduced by Adrian and Bronk (1929)[29] consists of a steel wire 0.1 mm in diameter contained within a thin-pointed cannula resembling a hypodermic needle. The central wire electrode is separated from the cannula (needle) by insulating resin. The recording surface consists of the oval bare tip of the wire electrode, and the reference electrode is the edge of the cannula itself. Thinner electrodes are available. Most clinical EMG work on limb muscles is carried out with electrodes of this type. The uptake area of the electrode is relatively small, probably including the territory of parts of several motor units in normal muscle. Needle electrodes generally offer the possibility of selective recordings from individual muscles. Since the uptake area of the electrode tip is relatively small, any electrical activity recorded is derived from the muscle into which the needle electrode is inserted. Quantitative methods were applied to concentric needle EMG by Buchthal and Rosenfalck and their colleagues in Copenhagen,[42] and in subsequent work by Stalberg and colleagues.[43] These can be applied not only to limb muscles but also to the external anal sphincter muscle (Figs 16.15 and 16.16).

MOTOR UNIT POTENTIAL ANALYSIS

The important parameters in the study of motor unit action potentials (MUP) are *amplitude*, *duration*, *number of phases* and *firing rate*. Because needle electrodes have a limited uptake area, dependent on the size of their leading-off surface and on volume conduction within the muscle,[44] these measures will vary according to the position of the electrode within the territory of individual motor units. For measurements of amplitude, duration and phase, the recording electrode should be in close proximity to the active muscle fibers because volume conduction effects will themselves modify these parameters when recordings are made at a distance. The two major criteria for determining the proximity of a recording electrode to an active muscle fiber are a fast rise time of the action potential and an adequate amplitude (greater than about 150 μV). In children, motor unit action potentials are smaller and of shorter duration than in adults.

MUP analysis – phases

A potential with more than four phases is termed a polyphasic motor unit potential. Buchthal (1977)[45] has defined a phase as that part of the motor unit potential which lies between two crossings of the baseline. Those parts of the potential between the onset and the first crossing and at the end of the potential are also considered as separate phases. EMG recordings from normal limb muscles contain up to 12% polyphasic motor unit action potentials.[46] However, in some muscles a larger proportion of polyphasic motor unit action potentials have been recorded. The number of phases in individual motor unit action potentials is best assessed during a continuous tonic voluntary contraction, with a trigger delay line (Fig. 16.17). The trigger delay line consists of an electronic circuit that enables the isolation of individual potentials by triggering on a potential at a preset amplitude level and displaying the motor unit potential (MUP) after a short delay, so that the earliest parts of the triggered potential can be displayed (Fig. 16.17). A storage oscilloscope, now available on all EMG machines, is useful so that the trace can be kept and displayed during the acquisition of additional potentials.

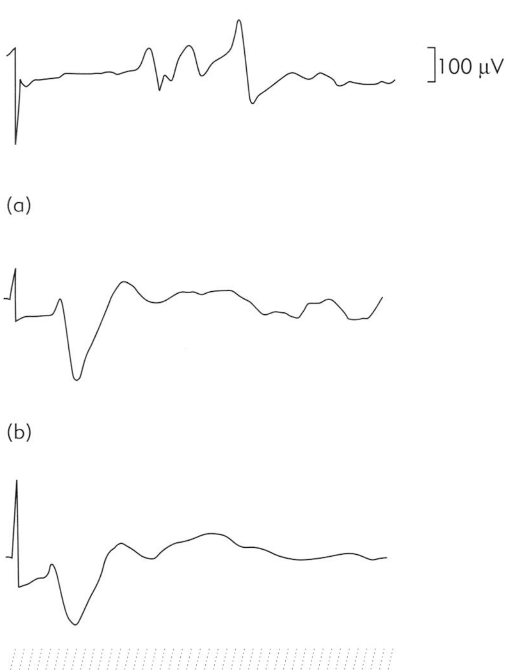

Figure 16.17 External anal sphincter muscle. Concentric needle electromyography. Upper trace: normal subject. The motor unit potential is biphasic and of short duration (<2 ms). The trigger delay line has been used to display the potential in the centre of the oscilloscope screen. Distant basal activity is visible to the right of the screen. Lower trace: incontinent subject. The motor unit potential is complex (4 phases) and of longer duration (4 ms)

Type I units are the first to be activated during voluntary contraction, but during the successive recruitment of additional units during increasingly forceful contraction, other units appear and the latest appearing units are likely to be type II units. Type I units are tonic units, and type II units are twitch units. Henneman's size principle is also important in recruitment of motor units in normal muscles. The smaller units are recruited first, and larger units are recruited only during more vigorous contraction. The full electrical activity of maximally contracting muscle, recorded with a concentric needle electrode, is called the full *interference pattern* (see Figs 16.15 and 16.16). This activity should exceed 2 mV in amplitude in the external anal sphincter (see Swash and Schwartz, 1997, for discussion).[33]

MUP analysis – shape

The shape of the motor unit action potential recorded during concentric needle EMG is dependent on the size (number of muscle fibers) of the motor unit and, especially, on the filtering characteristics of the amplifier. For most purposes, it is conventional to use filter settings of 100 Hz for the low pass and 10 Hz for the high pass filter with sweep speeds varying from 2 to 20 ms. Increasing the level of the low pass cut-off through 500 Hz or 1000 Hz results in sharpening of the action potential configuration, but in the loss of low frequency components. However, changing the filter characteristics in this manner does allow recognition of the contribution of individual muscle fiber action potentials in high amplitude, complex, motor unit action potentials of increased duration. This is best investigated using the technique of single fiber EMG.

MUP analysis – duration

The duration of the MUP is a function of a number of factors. The most important of these is the presence of smaller muscle fibers in the MUP. Smaller muscle fibers have slower propagated conduction velocities than large muscle fibers; the propagated conduction velocity of a muscle fiber is proportional to the square of the diameter of the fiber. Slower conducting muscle fibers will cause the MUP to be of increased duration. A less important factor is enlargement and dispersion of the motor unit territory through the muscle, so that some muscle fibers are a larger than normal distance from the recording electrode. Changes in volume conduction in the tissue, due to fibrosis, will also lead to increased MUP duration. Enlargement of the motor point has only a slight effect.

MUP analysis – amplitude

MUP amplitude is dependent on the size (number of muscle fibers) in the motor unit. Increased synchronicity of muscle fiber recruitment, dependent on the converse of those factors leading to increased duration, will also lead to increased amplitude. Increased MUP amplitude is therefore found in reinnervated motor units, and decreased amplitude when there has been loss of muscle fibers for a motor unit, as in denervation without compensatory reinnervation, and primary myopathies in which individual muscle fibers are diseased.

MUP analysis – turns and amplitude relationships

In concentric needle EMG studies of limb muscles the relation between turns, that is the number of times in a MUP that the EMG trace changes the direction of its polarity, and the amplitude of the MUP, has been developed as an on-line approach to automatic analysis of the EMG signal. This derivative gives information about the extent of abnormality that correlates with neurogenic and myopathic disorder in limb muscles. In the anal sphincter these methods can be applied to needle or surface recordings to give quantitative measures of EMG activity.[33,47]

SINGLE FIBER EMG

With concentric needle electrodes, individual muscle fiber action potentials cannot be recognized reliably within the motor unit action potential. Single muscle fiber action potentials can be recorded extracellularly by using an electrode with a small leading-off surface. The electrode, as commercially available, consists of a needle electrode of slightly narrower diameter than the conventional concentric needle electrode filled with resin. The recording surface consists of a central wire which opens at the mid-shaft of the electrode in a small circular leading-off surface of 25 μm diameter. Recordings are made using the cannula of the electrode as a reference electrode, with a separate surface ground electrode. An amplifier with a 500 Hz low frequency filter setting and a trigger delay line are required and most recordings are made with the time base of the amplifier set at 2–5 ms per division. The uptake radius of the electrode is about 270 square micrometers.

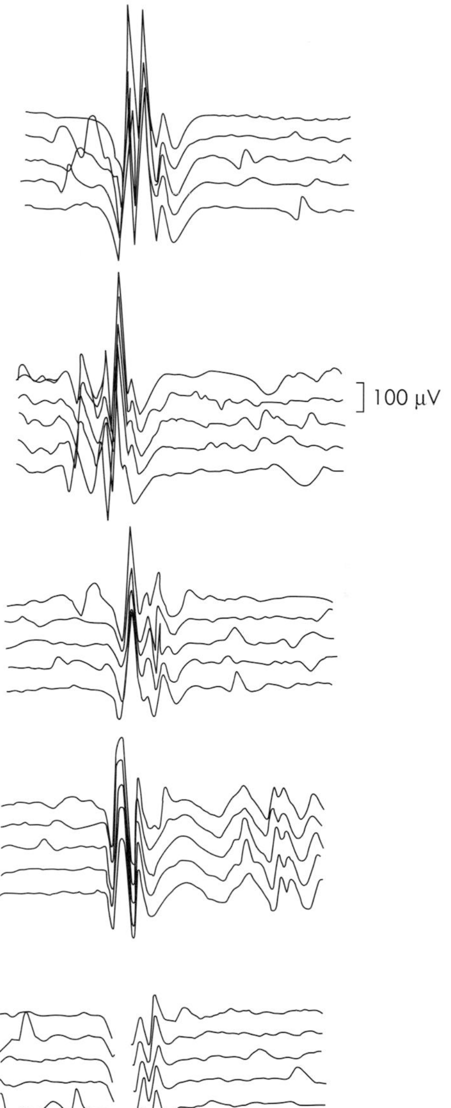

Figure 16.18 External anal sphincter muscle. Single fibre electromyography. Fecal incontinence. Five consecutively recorded traces of five different motor units in the muscle, displayed as part of the calculation of the fiber density. In the first motor unit potential there are three components, in the second four components, etc. The mean number of components in 20 such potentials is the fiber density. In the fourth recording, the cluster of late components proved, on analysis of additional recordings of this unit, to belong to a separate, unrelated motor unit potential.

Using this technique, single muscle fiber activity within motor units can be recorded. The method is particularly useful because the restriction in the active uptake area of the electrode surface 'focuses' the electrode to record from a restricted volume of the muscle. In normal muscles, this results in recordings of motor units in which one or two single muscle fiber action potentials can be identified within the uptake area of the electrode (Fig. 16.18). Because the recordings are made with a trigger delay line, it can be seen that these single muscle fiber potentials belong to the same motor unit. The mean duration of motor unit action potentials consisting of more than one component recorded by this method is less than 8 ms. In the normal extensor digitorum communis muscle of the forearm, the motor unit potential duration recorded by single fiber EMG did not exceed 4 ms in 95% of recordings.[48]

Fiber density

The technique of single fiber EMG lends itself to quantification in two respects. First, the fiber density (FD) can be calculated. The FD consists of the mean number of single muscle fiber action potentials recorded within the uptake area of the single fiber EMG electrode in 20 different positions within the muscle.[49] This usually implies four skin insertions of the electrode, with small adjustments of the position of the electrode within the individual insertions during the process of the recording. In normal subjects, the FD in most muscles is less than two,[48] although after the age of 60 years this value increases slightly.[50] In the external anal sphincter muscle, the normal FD is 1.5 ± 0.16.[35] The calculation of FD is dependent on the acquisition of recordings of sufficient clarity to allow the measurement. By convention, in limb muscles, components used for triggering must be greater than 150 μV in amplitude but, because of the smaller size of the muscle fibers in the pelvic sphincter muscles, potentials of greater than 100 μV are accepted. During the process of reinnervation and fiber-type grouping, with increasing compaction of the muscle fibers within individual motor units, the FD will increase because there are more fibers within the uptake area of the electrode innervated by an individual axon or its branches. Measurement of the FD is therefore useful assessing reinnervation (Fig. 16.18). Further, it lends itself to sequential studies during the natural history of a disease. It is important to recognize that the observer must be scrupulous in technique. *All potentials in which any one component is greater than 100 μV must be included in the calculation of the mean derived from the 20 recordings.* Thus, all single phase potentials must be included. It is tempting during the recording to discard single phase recordings in favor of the more visually exciting multiple-phase action potentials but this will give a falsely high value for the fiber density calculation. All the potentials recorded during the EMG should be stored and used for the calculation of fiber density. A repeatability study between different observers showed very low interobserver variability in EMG studies of the pelvic floor musculature.[51]

Neuromuscular jitter

The variability in the time interval between the triggering potential and the other potential or potentials belonging to the same motor unit recorded in the uptake area of the single fibre EMG electrode is called the neuromuscular jitter.[48,52] This jitter is mainly due to variation in the time of onset of the action potential generated by the end-plate potential and thus reflects variabilities in the onset of threshold for depolarization of the muscle fibers with respect to each other. It is thus mainly a measure of end-plate function. It has been much used in the study of neuromuscular diseases, particularly in neurogenic disorders, in limb muscles. In neurogenic disorders affecting limb muscles, the neuromuscular jitter is characteristically increased and there may be blocking of transmission at high rates of motor unit firing at individual motor end-plates. These two aspects of single fiber EMG, i.e. fiber density and jitter measurements, lend themselves to computer-based quantification,[53] and this is incorporated in all modern EMG machines for on-line analysis.

PRACTICAL APPLICATIONS OF PELVIC FLOOR EMG

EMG recordings of pelvic floor muscles, particularly of the striated anal and urinary sphincter musculature, can provide information relevant to the diagnosis and management of patients with fecal incontinence, urinary incontinence or double incontinence. It is also useful in the investigation of patients with other disorders of the pelvic floor, particularly rectal prolapse, solitary rectal ulcer syndrome[54,55] and anal pain in adults. In infancy, EMG of the anal sphincter has a particular value in mapping the position of the anal sphincter in congenital atresia of the ano-rectum prior to reparative surgery.[56] Similarly, in adults, sphincter mapping procedures are used when surgical attempts to reconstruct the anal canal are planned after trauma or, in some patients, after cancer surgery. However, ultrasound imaging has proved especially useful for this purpose and has largely supplanted EMG.[57,58] Nonetheless, only EMG can discern whether the muscle is capable of active voluntary contraction. EMG techniques have also been used in the assessment of retention of urine in women by Fowler and her colleagues (see this volume).

NORMAL EMG OF THE EXTERNAL ANAL SPHINCTER MUSCLE

The EMG activity of the striated anal sphincter was recorded by Beck (1930),[59] Floyd and Walls (1953),[40] Kawakami (1954),[60] Taverner and Smiddy (1959),[61] Ruskin and Davis (1969),[62] Chantraine (1966)[63] and Jesel *et al.* (1973),[34] using conventional concentric needle EMG techniques. These studies have revealed that the external anal sphincter shows continuous low frequency activity at rest, and even during sleep.[40] This activity consists of contraction of individual motor unit potentials at low firing rates, and of low amplitude (<500 μV). Distention of the rectum, or of the bladder, increases the basal activity in the anal sphincter muscle. Resting activity is also increased by changes in position, and by coughing (the cough reflex). During attempts at defecation, electrical silence occurs in the anal sphincter muscle and similar switching off of EMG activity occurs in the external urinary sphincter during the several seconds prior to detrusor contraction during micturition.[64] There is thus a degree of co-contraction, or reciprocal innervation, between the voluntary vesical and ano-rectal sphincter musculature.

Voluntary activity of the external anal sphincter muscle, as when asking the patient to squeeze the sphincter tight, produces an interference pattern comparable with that found during maximal voluntary contraction of a limb muscle. Summation of individual motor unit action potentials occurs so that the oscilloscope screen is filled with activity (see Fig. 16.17). The motor unit potentials reach 2 or 3 mV in amplitude, although the mean amplitude is somewhat lower (200–600 μV).[34] Normative data on the interference pattern in the external anal sphincter muscle has been collected,[65–67] but in these studies, appropriately, more emphasis was placed on MUP analysis than on conventional subjective decision-making about the interference pattern.

The mean duration of motor unit potentials during voluntary activity in the striated urinary and anal sphincter muscles is 5–7.5 ms.[62,68] Bartolo, Jarratt and Read (1983)[36] found that in normal subjects there was a wide variation in motor unit potential duration, and that this increased slightly with age, from a mean value of 5 ms at age 20 years to a mean of 6.5 ms at age 80 years (see Fig. 16.20). This observation, together with the finding in several of the studies discussed above that polyphasic units are more common in elderly subjects than in young adults, is consistent with our findings using single fiber EMG[29,32,35,69] that the fiber density in single fiber EMG recordings increases after the age of about 60 years. In 34 subjects less than 30 years old, the fiber density in the external anal sphincter was 1.37 ± 0.09,[70] but in people aged up to about 65 years it is 1.5 ± 0.16 (Percy *et al.*, 1982). At the age of 75 years, the upper limit of normal is 1.75.[32,69]

Podnar and Vodusek have addressed the factors in recordings leading to variability in the results of quantitative analysis, and especially pointed out that baseline instability is an important variable that must be controlled. They also noted that different firing rates recruited different types of motor unit, and that this would change the results. They recommended a low firing rate for this analysis, but it must be recognized that this limits the interpretation to a selected group of motor units[71–74]

REFLEX ACTIVITY

EMG activity increases in the anal sphincter muscle during coughing (the cough reflex), in response to scratching the anal skin (the anal reflex) or by eliciting the bulbocavernosus reflex. Further, stretching the anal sphincter by digital examination would itself result in activity in the external anal sphincter muscle. We used the latter method to increase anal sphincter activity during the acquisition of motor unit potentials for analysis during both conventional needle EMG and single fiber EMG in our early recordings.[36]

CLINICAL APPLICATIONS

The patient lies on an electrically insulated mat in the left lateral position on a couch in a warm room. The ground electrode is strapped to the right thigh. Where possible, the sphincter ring is palpated, the perianal skin cleaned and dried and, having warned the patient, the electrode is inserted 12 cm posterior to the anal verge at an angle of 30–45 degrees to the skin.[72] By inserting the needle nearly to its hilt, its tip enters the puborectalis, a position that can be ascertained by controlling the position of the tip of the needle with a finger in the rectum. More superficial needle placement records activity in the external anal sphincter muscle. A few minutes rest must be allowed to elapse after needle or patient movement, for the muscle activity to settle to a steady resting state. The patient is asked to squeeze the anus as hard as possible in order to record maximal voluntary contraction. Activity during straining can also be recorded, the patient being asked to strain as though having his bowels open. EMG activity gradually increases during this maneuver during a period of 5–10 s.

For single fiber EMG recordings, increased activity in the external anal sphincter and puborectalis muscles can be induced by the insertion of a balloon into the rectum, a 150 g weight tension being applied to this by allowing a string ending in the weight to dangle over the edge of the couch. This is sufficient to induce continuous low-grade activity suitable for recording individual motor unit potentials for single fiber EMG and quantitative concentric EMG analysis.[29,36]

ANAL MAPPING

This is performed by inserting a concentric needle electrode into the external anal sphincter muscle in the four quadrants of the muscle. Posterior insertion usually produces copious EMG activity, but anterior insertion in women is painful and the muscle is very thin at this site, even in normal subjects. Using this technique, by repeated adjustments in needle placement with the necessity of further skin insertions, the distribution of muscle fibers within the external anal sphincter can be accurately mapped and, in the case of patients with sphincter division,[75] and in infants with imperforate anus,[37,76] the position of the muscle, or the remaining fibres of the muscle, can be accurately mapped so that appropriate surgery can be planned.[77]

We used a simple quantitative method in concentric needle EMG recordings in carrying out sphincter mapping analysis by measuring the amount of EMG activity (voltage) occurring during 1 s periods. This requires the use of rectified EMG activity during successive 1 s activation periods.

INCONTINENCE

In patients with idiopathic neurogenic anorectal incontinence, characteristic EMG abnormalities are found in the external anal sphincter and puborectalis muscles. In the most severely affected patients, EMG activity is decreased and zones of the sphincter muscles may be electrically silent. The potentials recorded are of larger amplitude and longer duration than normal and show multiple phases when examined with a trigger delay line, both in concentric needle (Bartolo *et al.* 1983; and single fiber EMG recordings. The fiber density, therefore, is increased.[29,35,55,70] In less severely affected patients, the maximal amplitude during voluntary contraction is increased and the major abnormality consists of the polyphasic motor unit potentials and the increased fiber density. There may be an increased neuromuscular jitter between components of these polyphasic potentials, indicating an instability of innervation. Similar abnormalities are found in the puborectalis as in the external sphincter muscle.[78,79] In patients with rectal prolapse, the EMG activity in these two muscles is abnormal only if there is associated incontinence.[21]

EMG recordings of the external anal sphincter have been used to monitor activity in the external urinary sphincter in patients with urinary incontinence, and an increase in fiber density has been described in the external anal sphincter muscle in such patients,[80] implying that a similar abnormality has occurred in both muscles in urinary incontinence without fecal incontinence. Smith *et al.* (1989)[81] showed that women with stress incontinence of urine, or genitourinary prolapse, had a significant increase in fiber density in striated pelvic floor muscles compared with age-matched controls, and that older women with normal continence showed a slight increase in fiber density. Vereecken *et al.* (1981)[82] found abnormalities in concentric needle EMG in these muscles in 78% of women with stress incontinence. In patients with double incontinence, neurogenic abnormalities are found in the external anal and external urinary sphincter muscles.[70] EMG gives important information that can be obtained only by this method.

The neuromuscular jitter in the external anal sphincter muscle is increased when there is instability of reinnervation. In these patients the fiber density is increased and there are abnormalities in concentric needle EMG parameters consistent with reinnervation. Gee and Durdey (1997)[83] found that increased jitter in women with fecal incontinence was associated with a poor outcome following surgical repair to the pelvic floor. Jitter measurements require more prolonged EMG recordings of single motor units and are not well tolerated by most patients.

These findings, particularly the single fibre EMG feature of an increased fiber density, the increased motor unit potential duration, presence of polyphasic potentials, and increased amplitude in concentric needle electrode recordings, with increased jitter between individual components, are consistent with a neurogenic abnormality, that is with denervation and reinnervation of muscle fibers, in patients with incontinence. This EMG abnormality is also consistent with the histological features found in biopsies of the external anal sphincter and puborectalis muscles in patients with incontinence, and it is this combination of histological and EMG abnormalities that has led to electrophysiological investigation of the innervation of the pelvic floor muscles using the techniques of pudendal nerve terminal motor latency measurement. Latency measurements may also be made from spinal stimulation in the cauda equina.

MONITORING DURING NEUROSURGERY

EMG of the anal sphincter has been used as a monitoring technique during neurosurgical procedures in which the conus medullaris and sacral nerve roots are vulnerable.[84]

NERVE CONDUCTION STUDIES IN PELVIC FLOOR DISORDERS

Neurophysiological examination of the pelvic innervation requires special techniques. Studies of the conduction characteristics of pelvic nerves in disorders of the pelvic floor are complementary to EMG studies and should not be considered as a substitute for EMG examination. Nerve conduction studies evaluate the conduction time and efficiency in the peripheral nerve; they cannot evaluate denervation and reinnervation in the muscles innervated by these nerves. Both motor and sensory studies are possible, and both proximal and distal conduction can be evaluated, but the pudendal nerve terminal motor latency, a relatively simple technique, has proven especially useful in clinical practice, since it is not uncomfortable, and can be repeated during the course of management of a patient with a pelvic floor disorder, especially in fecal incontinence.

PUDENDAL AND PERINEAL NERVE STIMULATION

Pudendal and perineal nerve stimulation techniques assess the distal motor innervation of the pelvic floor musculature; i.e. the innervation of the external anal sphincter and periurethral striated sphincter muscles.

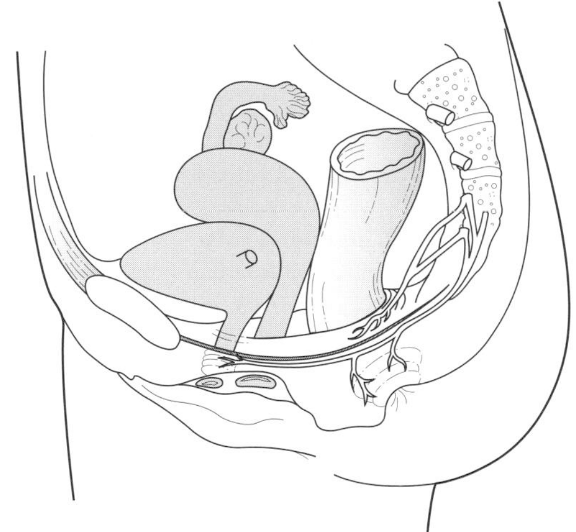

Figure 16.19 Pudendal nerve innervation of the external anal sphincter and periurethral striated sphincter muscles. The sacral motor innervation of the puborectalis is also shown.

The pudendal nerve consists of inferior rectal branches that innervate the external anal sphincter muscle and perineal branches that innervate the perineal striated sphincter musculature (Fig. 16.19). By selective recording from these two muscles following pudendal nerve stimulation, conduction in their motor innervation can be assessed separately.

Pudendal nerve terminal motor latency

Pudendal nerve stimulation is achieved using an intrarectal technique, with a pair of stimulating electrodes mounted on a fixed array on the tip of the index finger. The recording electrodes in this St Mark's pudendal electrode (Dantec) are mounted on the same array at the base of the finger, so that they come to lie in close apposition to the external anal sphincter muscle when the index finger is inserted into the anal canal and rectum as in a conventional clinical rectal examination. This technique was developed from the electroejaculation method introduced by Brindley (1981)[85] in order to obtain sperm from men with paraplegia. The recording electrodes are mounted 3 cm from the stimulating electrodes, and the cathode of the stimulating electrode is made smaller than the anode on order to improve localization of the stimulus current. The patient is grounded with a large thigh ground electrode, while the patient lies for the recording procedure in the left lateral position, for the right handed examiner.

The index finger bearing the electrode array is inserted into the anal canal and the ischial spine on one side is sought with the tip of the finger. Square wave stimuli of 0.1 ms duration and 50 V are applied via the tip-mounted stimulating electrodes at 1 s intervals. By slowly directing the tip of the finger the best position for stimulation and recording (from the base of the finger) is found and the potentials with the highest amplitude and fastest rise time are taken as the optimal compound muscle action potential (CMAP) from pudendal stimulation (Fig. 16.20). This procedure is performed on both sides of the pelvis in order to compare the findings from the two sides. The CMAP on the two sides is of opposite polarity since the direction of the electrode array is reversed on the two sides. Standard nerve conduction recording filter settings are used in the EMG amplifier.

The latency of the response is the time from stimulus onset to CMAP onset; this is the terminal motor latency in the pudendal nerve (PNTML). The normal range for

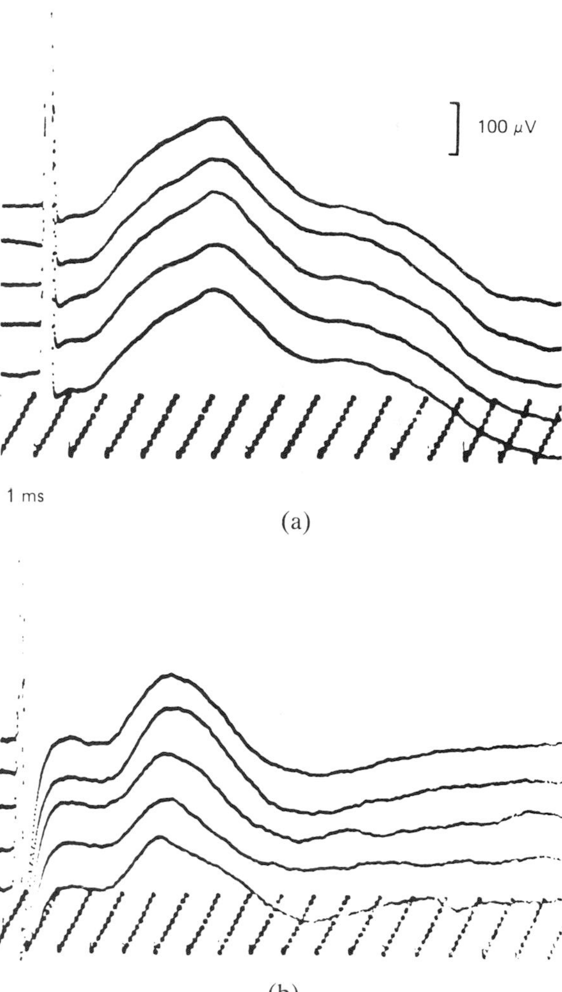

Figure 16.20 Pudendal (a) and perineal (b) evoked responses in the external anal sphincter and the periurethral striated sphincter muscles, respectively, in a normal subject.

Table 16.2 Distal nerve latencies – control subjects*

Nerve	No.	Mean age (years)	Age range (years)	Terminal nerve motor latency (ms)
Pudendal	40	50	25–75	2.1 ± 0.2
Perineal	20	42	25–60	2.4 ± 0.2

*All subjects female.

this PNTML is shown in Table 16.1. With aging the PNTML is slightly increased, especially in subjects older than about 50 years.[32] Parous women have longer PNTML values than nulliparous women.[70]

Perineal nerve terminal motor latency

Stimulation of the pudendal nerve is performed in the same fashion, but recordings are made from the peri-urethral striated sphincter muscle, using a surface electrode array mounted on an indwelling urinary catheter (Dantec 21L11). This intraurethral recording electrode array consists of two platinum recording surfaces each of 5 mm diameter mounted 3 mm apart. The CMAP responses resemble those of the external anal sphincter, but have a slightly longer latency (Fig. 16.20). The normal latencies are shown in Table 16.2. The perNTML increases with increasing age, after the age of 50 years.[32]

Relation of PNTML and perNTML

In normal subjects there is a linear relation between the terminal motor latencies in these two innervations, which form part of a single nerve (Fig. 16.19). The perNTML has a longer latency than the PNTML, indicating that this branch of the pudendal nerve is slightly longer than the inferior rectal branch. The curving course of the pudendal nerve and its branches in the pelvis does not follow the course of the examiner's index finger, and it is not possible to measure its length. The conduction velocity in this nerve cannot therefore be simply calculated, and comparison of the directly measured latencies is used for clinical assessment. Since this measurement has a very small variance this is a useful measure.[55,70,86–90]

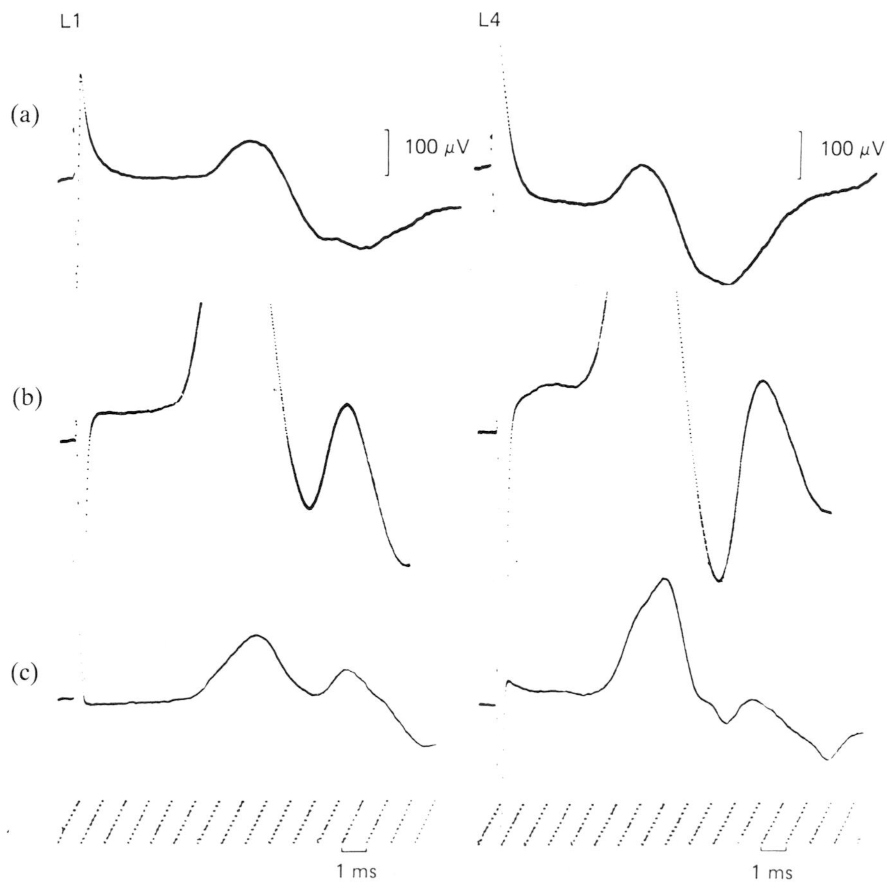

Figure 16.21 Transcutaneous translumbar spinal stimulation evoked responses in the external anal sphincter (a), puborectalis (b) and the urethral striated sphincter musculature (c) in a normal subject.

CAUDA EQUINA STIMULATION

It is also possible to stimulate the cauda equina nerve roots using magnetic stimulation. This was first done with an electrical stimulator, and different latencies from T12/L1 and L4/5 stimulation sites, recording from the anal sphincter, were obtained (Fig. 16.21). This enabled conduction velocity across the cauda equina nerve roots to be derived, or for the latencies to be directly compared as a ratio of the two latencies.[89] The advent of MR imaging of the lumbosacral spinal canal has rendered this electrophysiological technique largely obsolete.[91]

CERVICAL AND CORTICAL STIMULATION

Magnetic stimulation of the cortex, and of the cervical cord is also possible, and latencies to the anal sphincter and to other pelvic floor muscles can be obtained (Fig. 16.22). In addition the threshold for cortical stimulation can be assessed, and a map of the cortical representation of the pelvic floor muscles can be derived. This is abnormal after acute stroke. Cortical maps for the anal sphincter are probably also abnormal after spinal cord injury, when the cortex is disconnected from the anal sphincter muscle, but systematic studies of this and other neurological lesions have not yet been published. In multiple sclerosis there is an increased latency from cortical stimulation to activation of the anal sphincter muscle. This is of interest in functional studies, but it is not a phenomenon unique to multiple sclerosis, and is not therefore of practical use in diagnosis of this disorder.[92]

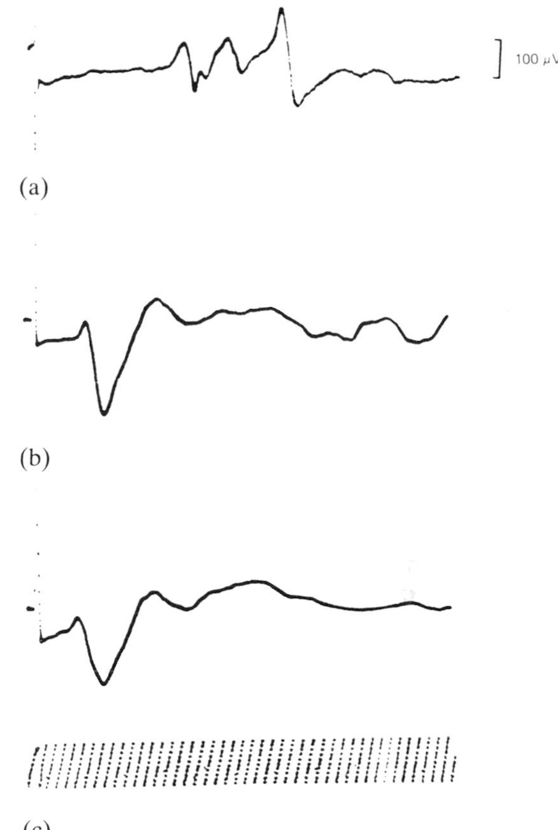

Figure 16.22 Transcutaneous cervicolumbar spinal stimulation evoked responses in the puborectalis muscle in a normal subject from (a) C6, (b) L1 and (c) L4. Time base calibration 1 ms.

CLINICAL APPLICATIONS

In ano-rectal incontinence there is slowed conduction in the pudendal nerves innervating the anal sphincter muscle, causing an increased PNTML.[70,86] This was found in 80% of women with idiopathic ano-rectal incontinence. Similarly, women with ano-rectal incontinence associated with rectal prolapse have increased PNTMLs, but those with rectal prolapse that is not associated with ano-rectal incontinence have a normal PNTML.[79,93] These abnormalities in PNTML are often asymmetrical,[94,95] a finding that has more recently been correlated with the prognosis for surgical repair of the sphincter muscles, and with cortical activation patterns in the two hemispheres (see this book). The majority of patients with idiopathic ano-rectal incontinence have distal neuropathy in their pudendal nerves; that is increased PNTML,[87] but in some, about 20%, there is also slowing of conduction across the cauda equina, between the T12/L1 and L4/5 stimulation sites.[89]

Patients with double incontinence have slowing of conduction in their perineal innervation, shown by increased perNTML, in addition to increased PNTML.[70] This is consistent with the finding, discussed above, that there is evidence of reinnervation in the periurethral striated sphincter muscle in women with stress urinary incontinence. Nonetheless, in this form of urinary incontinence there are other factors leading to sphincter dysfunction, and neurogenic weakness of the sphincter appears to be only one possible causative factor in this complex functional disorder (see this volume).

SENSORY STUDIES

Sensory thresholds are reduced in anorectal incontinence, as shown by measurement of temperature threshold in the anal canal,[96] by rectal distention appreciation studies[97] and by electrical threshold determination using constant current stimulation. Lubowski and Nicholls (1988)[98] found that reduced sensation could be a contributory cause of ano-rectal incontinence. These findings are consistent with the pudendal nerve abnormalities found in the motor latency studies.

Evaluation of pudendal nerve cortical evoked potentials has proved more difficult in clinical practice.

Loening-Baucke *et al.* (1991, 1994)[99,100] were able to record evoked potentials from the cerebral cortex after rectal stimulation, but others[101] found these were unreliable in practice. Since the defect of function is in the peripheral nervous system, a technique such as the measurement of cerebral sensory evoked potentials is unlikely to show great sensitivity to change. The technique involves repeated stimulation of the rectal mucosa, or of the pudendal nerve at the dorsal nerve of the clitoris or penis, and is uncomfortable and difficult to carry out as a routine procedure.

CONCLUSIONS

These EMG and nerve conduction methods provide useful clinical information in the investigation of patients with pelvic floor disorders, particularly incontinence. The finding of an increased fiber density, or of abnormalities in quantitative concentric needle EMG studies, suggests that there has been damage to the innervation of the pelvic floor muscles. Taken together with pudendal terminal motor latency measurements, and with the clinical data, this information can be used in planning treatment and management.

Since pelvic floor weakness is likely to be a progressive disorder, these investigations carry the practical advantage that they may be repeated during the natural history of the disorder without harm to the patient. More advanced neurophysiological techniques may prove useful in studying the central nervous system in the investigation of incontinence in certain patients.

REFERENCES

1. Duthie HL. Progress report: anal continence. *Gut* 1971;**12**:844–52.
2. Parks AG. Anorectal incontinence. *Proc Roy Soc Med* 1975;**68**:681–90.
3. Swash M. Idiopathic faecal incontinence: histopathological evidence on pathogenesis. In: Wright R (ed.) *Recent advances in gastrointestinal pathology.* London: W.B. Saunders, 1980:71–89.
4. Swash M. The neuropathology of idiopathic faecal incontinence. In: Cavanagh B, Thomas Smith W (eds). *Recent advances in neuropathology*, vol. 2. Edinburgh: Churchill Livingstone, 1982:243–71.
5. Thompson P. *The myology of the pelvic floor.* Newton, MA: McCorquodale, 1899.
6. Kerremans R. *Morphological and physiological aspects of anal continence and defaecation.* Brussels: Editions Arscia, 1969.
7. Parks AG, Porter NH, Melzack J. Experimenta; study of the reflex mechanism controlling the muscles of the pelvic floor. *Dis Colon Rectum* 1962;**5**:407–414.
8. Parks AG, Porter NH, Hardcastle J. The syndrome of the descending perineum. *Proc Roy Soc Med* 1966;**69**:477–82.
9. Lawson JON. Pelvic anatomy (i) pelvic floor muscles (ii) anal canal and associated sphincters. *Ann Roy Coll Surg* 1974;**54**:244–52, 288–300.
10. Beersiek F, Parks AG, Swash M. Pathogenesis of ano-rectal incontinence: a histometric study of the anal sphincter musculature. *J Neurol Sci* 1979;**42**:111–27.
11. Schuster MM. The riddle of the sphincters. *Gastroenterology* 1975;**69**:249–62.
12. Sultan AH, Kamm MA, Hudson CN. Pudendal nerve damage during labour; prospective study before and after childbirth. *Br J Obstet Gynaecol* 1994;**101**:22–30.
13. Bennett RC, Duthie HL. The functional importance of the internal anal sphincter. *Br J Surg* 1964;**51**:355–7.
14. Stelzner F. Uber die Anatomie des analen Sphincterorgans, wie sie der Chirurg Sieht. *Zeitschr Anat Entwicklungsges* 1960;**121**:525–35.
15. Williams PL, Warwick R. *Functional neuroanatomy of man.* Edinburgh: Churchill Livingstone, 1973.
16. Percy JP, Neill ME, Swash M, Parks AG. Electrophysiological study of the motor nerve supply of pelvic floor. *Lancet* 1981;**i**:16–17 (see also *Lancet* 1981;**I**:999–1000.
17. Snooks SJ, Swash M. Innervation of the muscles of continence. *Ann Roy Coll Surg Engl* 1986;**18**:45–9.
18. Wunderlich M, Swash M. The overlapping innervation of the two sides of the external anal sphincter by the pudendal nerve. *J Neurol Sci* 1983;**59**:91–109.
19. Parks AG, Swash M, Urich H. Sphincter denervation in anorectal incontinence and rectal prolapse. *Gut* 1977;**18**:656–65.
20. Parks AG, Swash M. Denervation of the anal sphincter causing idiopathic ano-rectal incontinence and rectal prolapse. *J Roy Coll Surg Edin* 1979;**24**:94–6.
21. Neill ME, Parks AG, Swash M. Physiological studies of the anal sphincter musculature in faecal incontinence and rectal prolapse. *Br J Surg* 1981;**68**:531–6.
22. Swash M, Schwartz MS. *Biopsy pathology of muscle*, 2nd edn. London: Chapman and Hall, 1990.
23. Swash M, Fox KP. The pathology of the muscle spindle: effect of denervation. *J Neurol Sci* 1974;**22**:1–24.
24. Dubowitz V, Brooke MH. *Muscle biopsy – A modern approach.* London: W.B. Saunders, 1973.
25. Polgar J, Johnson MA, Weightman D, Appleton D. Data on fibre size in thirty-six human muscles: an autopsy study. *J Neurol Sci* 1973;**19**:307–318.
26. Cihak R, Guttmann E, Hanzlikova V. Involution and hormone-induced persistence of the M sphincter (levator) ani in female rats. *Anat* 1970;**106**:93–101.
27. Butler ECB. Complete rectal prolapse following rEMGval of tumours of the cauda equina. *Proc Roy Soc Med* 1954;**47**:521–2.
28. Henry MM, Parks AG, Swash M. Electrophysiological and histological studies of the pelvic floor in the descending perineum syndrome. *Br J Surg* 1982;**69**:470–72.
29. Neill ME, Parks AG, Swash M. Physiological studies of the anal sphincter musculature in faecal incontinence and rectal prolapse. *Br J Surg* 1981;**68**:531–6.
30. Teramoto T, Parks AG, Swash M. Hypertrophy of the external anal sphincter in haemorrhoids. *Gut* 1981;**22**:45–8.
31. Bruck CE, Lubowski DZ, King DW. Do patients with haemorrhoids have pelvic floor denervation? *Internat J Colorect Dis* 1988;**3**:210–214.

32. Laurberg S, Swash M, Snooks SJ, Henry MM. Neuro logic cause of idiopathic incontinence. *Arch Neurol* 1988;**45**:1250–53.
33. Swash M, Schwartz MS. *Neuromuscular diseases: a practical approach to diagnosis and management*, 3rd edn. London: Springer-Verlag, 1997.
34. Jesel M, Isch-Treussard C, Isch F. Electromyography of striated muscles of anal and urethral sphincters. In: Desmedt JE (ed.) *New developments in electromyography and clinical neurophysiology*, vol. 2. Basle: Karger, 1973:406–420.
35. Neill ME, Swash M. Increased motor unit fibre density in the external sphincter muscle in anorectal incontinence: a single fibre EMG study. *J Neurol Neurosurg Psychiat* 1980;**43**:343–7.
36. Bartolo DCC, Jarrett JA, Read NW. The use of conventional electromyography to assess external sphincter neuropathy in man. *J Neurol Neurosurg Psychiat* 1983;**46**:1115–18.
37. Chantraine A. EMG examination of the anal and urethral sphincters. In: Desmedt JE (ed.) *New developments in electromyography and clinical neurophysiology*, vol. 2. Basle: Karger, 1973:421–32.
38. Piper H. Uber die Leitungsgeschwindigkeit in den markhaltigen, menslichen Nerven. *Pflug Arch Gesamte Physiol Mensch Tiere* 1908;**124**:591–600.
39. Adrian ED, Bronck DW. The discharge of impulses in motor nerve fibres. *J Physiol* 1929;**67**:119–51.
40. Floyd WF, Walls EW. Electromyography of the sphincter ani externus in man. *J Physiol* 1953;**122**:500–609.
41. O'Donnell P, Beck C, Doyle R, Eubanks C. Surface electrodes in perineal electromyography. *Urology*. 1988;**32**:375–9
42. Rosenfalck P. *Electromyography: sensory and motor conductions. Findings in normal subjects* Copenhagen: Rikshospitalet Laboratory of Clinical Neurophysiology, 1975.
43. Stalberg E, Nandedkar SD, Sanders DB, Falck B. Quantitative motor unit potential analysis. *J Clin Neurophysiol* 1996;**13**:401–422.
44. Rosenfalck P. Intra and extra cellular potential fields of active nerve and muscle fibres. *Acta Physiol Scand* 1969;(Suppl.)**321**:1–168.
45. Buchthal F. Diagnostic significance of the myopathic EMG. In: Rowland EP (ed.) *Pathogenesis of human muscular dystrophies*. Amersterdam: Excerpta Medica International Congress Series 404, 1977:205–218.
46. Caruso C, Buchthal F. Refractory period of muscle and EMG findings in relatives of patients with muscular dystrophy. *Brain* 1965;**88**:29–50.
47. Nandedkar SD, Sanders DB, Stalberg EV. Automatic analysis of the electromyographic interference. Part II: Findings in control subjects and in some neuromuscular diseases. *Muscle Nerve* 1986;**9(6)**:491–500.
48. Stalberg ES, Trontelj V. *Single fibre electromyography*. Old working: Mirvalle Press, 1979.
49. Stalberg E, Thiele B. Motor unit fibre density in the extensor digitorum communis muscle. *J Neurol Neurosurg Psychiat* 1975;**38**:874–80.
50. Laurberg S, Swash M. Effects of ageing on the anorectal sphincters and their innervation. *Dis Colon Rectum* 1989;**32**:734–42.
51. Rogers J, Laurberg S, Misiewicz JJ, *et al.* Anorectal physiology validated: a repeatability study of the motor and sensory tests of the motor and sensory tests of anorectal function. *Br J Surg* 1989;**76**:607–609.
52. Ekstedt J. Human single muscle fiber action potentials. *Acta Physiol Scand* 1964;**61**:(Suppl. 226):1–98.
53. Davis GR, Brown IT, Schwartz MS, Swash M. A dedicated microcomputer-based instrument for internal analysis of multi-component waveforms in single fibre EMG. *Electroencephalogr Clin Neurophysiol* 1983;**56**:110–13.
54. Rutter KRP, Riddell RH. The solitary rectal ulcer syndrome. *Clin Gastroenterol* 1975;**4**:505–530.
55. Snooks SJ, Badenoch D, Tiptaft R, Swash M. Perineal nerve damage in genuine stress urinary incontinence: an electrophysiological study. *Br J Urol* 1985;**57**:422–6.
56. Boyd SG, Kiely EM, Swash M. Use of electrophysiological studies of puborectalis and external and sphincter in incontinent children with corrected high anorectal anomalies. *Pediat Surg Internat* 1987;**2**:110–112.
57. Burnett SJ, Speakman CT, Kamm MA, *et al.* Confirmation of endoscopic detection of external anal sphincter defects by simultaneus electromyographic mapping. *Br J Surg* 1991;**78**:448.
58. Falk PM, Blatchford GJ, Cali RL, *et al.* Transanal ultrasound and manometry in the evaluation of fecal incontinence. *Dis Colon Rectum* 1994;**37**:468–71.
59. Beck A. Electromyographische Untersuchungen am Sphinkter ani. *Arch Physiol* 1930;**224**:278–92.
60. Kawakami M. Electromyographic investigation of the human external sphincter muscle of anus. *Jap J Physiol* 1954;**4**:1961.
61. Taverner D, Smiddy FG. An electromyographic study of the normal function of the external anal sphincter and pelvic diaphragm. *Dis Colon Rectum* 1959;**2**:153–60.
62. Ruskin AP, Davis JE. Anal sphincter electromyography. *Electroencephalogr Clin Neurophysiol* 1969;**27**:713.
63. Chantraine A. Electromyographie de sphincters striés ure'-tral et anal humains: étude descriptive et analytique. *Rev Neurol* 1966;**115**:396–403.
64. Hutch JA, Elliott HW. Electromyographic study of electrical activity in the paraurethral muscles prior to and during voiding. *J Urol* 1968;**99**:759–65.
65. Aanestad O, Flink R, Haggman M, Norlen BJ. Interference pattern in the urethral sphincter: a quantitative electromyographic study in patients before and after radical retropubic prostatectomy. Scand J Urol Nephrol. 1998;**32**:378–82.
66. Weidner AC, Sanders DB, Massey JM, Bump RC. Quantitative electromyographic analysis of levator ani and external anal sphincter muscles of nulliparous women. *Neurourol Urodynam* 1999;**18**:285–6.
67. Gilad R, Giladi N, Sadeh M. Quantitative EMG of sphincter ani in normal individuals and multiple system atrophy. *Clin Neurophysiol* 1999;**110**:S94–S95.
68. Petersen I, Franksson EE. Electromyographic study of the striated muscles of the male urethra. *Br J Urol* 1955;**27**:148–53.
69. Percy JP, Neill ME, Kandiah TK, Swash M. A neurogenic factor in faecal incontinence in the elderly. *Age Ageing* 1982;**11**:175–9.

70. Snooks SJ, Barnes PRH, Swash M. Abnormalities of the innervation of the voluntary anal and urethral sphincters in incontinence: an electrophysiological study. *J Neurol Neurosurg Psychiat* 1984;**47**:1269–73.
71. Podnar S, Rodi Z, Lukanovic A, *et al.* Standardisation of anal sphincter EMG: technique of needle examination. *Muscle Nerve* 1999;**22**:400–403.
72. Podnar S, Vodusek DB. Standardisation of anal sphincter EMG: low and high threshold motor units. *Clin Neurophysiol* 1999;**110**:1488–91.
73. Podnar S, Vodusek DB. Standardisation of anal sphincter electromyography: uniformity of the muscle. *Muscle Nerve* 2000;**23**:122–5.
74. Podnar S, Vodusek DB, Stalberg E. Standardization of anal sphincter electromyography: normative data. *Clin Neurophysiol* 2000;**111**:220–2207.
75. Kiff ES. The clinical use of anorectal physiology studies. *Ann Roy Coll Surg Engl* (Sir Alan Parks Symposium) 1983:27–9.
76. Archibald KC, Goldsmith EJ. Sphincteric electromyography. *Arch Phys Med Rehab* 1967;**48**:2349–52.
77. Kiff ES, Barnes P, Swash M. Evidence of pudendal neuropathy in patients with perineal descent and chronic straining at stool. *Gut* 1984;**25**:1279–82.
78. Bartolo DCC, Jarratt JA, Read MG, *et al.* The role of partial denervation of the puborectalis in idiopathic faecal incontinence. *Br J Surg* 1983;**70**:664–7.
79. Snooks SJ, Henry MM, Swash M. Anorectal incontinence and rectal prolapse: differential assessment of the innervation of the puborectalis and external anal sphincter muscle. *Gut* 1985;**26**:470–76.
80. Anderson RS. Increased motor unit fibre density in the external anal sphincter in genuine stress incontinence: a single fibre EMG study. anorectal function. *Neurol Urodynam* 1983;**2**:45–50.
81. Smith ARB, Hosker GL, Warrell DW. The role of partial denervation of the pelvic floor in the aetiology of genitourinary prolapse and stress incontinence of urine: a neurophysiological study. *Br J Obstet Gynaecol* 1989;**96**:24–8.
82. Vereecken RL, de Meirsman G, Puers B. Sphincter EMG in female incontinence. In: *Advances in diagnostic urology.* Berlin: Springer Verlag, 1981:314–18.
83. Gee AS, Durdey P. Preoperative increase in nueromuscular jitter and outcome following surgery for faecal incontinence. *Br J Surgery* 1997;**84**:1264–8.
84. James HE, Mulcahy JJ, Walsh JW, Palpan GW. Use of anal sphincter EMG during operations on the conus medullaris and sacral nerve roots. *Neurosurgery* 1979;**4**:821–3.
85. Brindley GA. Electroejaculation: its technique, neurological implications and uses. *J Neurol Neurosurg Psychiat* 1981;**44**:9–18.
86. Kiff ES, Swash M. Slowed conduction in the pudendal nerves in idiopathic (neurogenic) faecal incontinence. *Br J Surg* 1984;**71**:614–16.
87. Kiff ES, Swash M. Normal proximal and slowed distal onduction in the pudendal nerves of patients with idiopathic (neurogenic) faecal incontinence. *J Neurol Neurosurg Psychiat* 1984;**47**:820–23.
88. Snooks SJ, Swash M. Perineal nerve and transcutaneous spinal stimulation: new methods for investigation of the urethral striated sphincter musculature. *Br J Urol* 1984; **56**:406–409.
89. Snooks SJ, Swash M. Abnormalities of the urethral striated sphincter musculature in incontinence. *Br J Urol* 1984;**56**:401–405.
90. Snooks SJ, Setchell M, Swash M, Henry MM. Injury to the innervation of the pelvic floor musculature in childbirth. *Lancet* 1984;**2**:546–50.
91. Chokroverty S, Sachdeo R, Dilullo J, Duvoisin RC. Magnetic stimulation in the diagnosis of lumbosacral radiculopathy. *J Neurol Neurosurg Psychiat* 1989;**52**:767–72.
92. Mathers SE, Ingram DA, Swash M. Electrophysiology of motor pathways for sphincter control in multiple sclerosis. *J Neurol Neurosurg Psychiat* 1990;**53**:955–60.
93. Snooks SJ, Nicholls RJ, Henry MM, Swash M. Electrophysiological and manometric assessment of the pelvic floor in the solitary rectal ulcer syndrome. *Br J Surg* 1985;**72**:131–3.
94. Lubowski DZ, Jones PN, Swash M, Henry MM. Increase in pudendal nerve terminal motor latency with defaecation straining. *Br J Surg* 1988;**75**:1095–7.
95. Lubowski DZ, Jones PN, Swash M, Henry MM. Asymetrical pudendal nerve damage in pelvic floor disorders. *Int J Colerectal Dis* 1988;**3**:158–60.
96. Miller R, Bartolo DC, Cervero F, Mortensen NJ. Anorectal temperature sensation: a comparison of normal and incontinent patients. *Br J Surg* 1987;**74**:511–14.
97. Ferguson GH, Redford J, Barrett JA, Kiff ES. The appreciation of rectal distension in fecal incontinence. *Dis Colon Rectum* 1989;**32**:964–8.
98. Lubowski DZ, Nicholls RJ. Faecal incontinence associated with reduced pelvic sensation. *Br J Surg* 1988;**75**:1086–9.
99. Loening-Baucke V, Read NW, Yamada T. Cerebral evoked potentials after rectal stimulation. *Electroenceph Clin Neurophysiol* 1991;**80**:490–98.
100. Loening-Baucke V, Read NW, Yamada T, Barker AT. Evaluation of tehmotor and sensory components of the pudendal nerve. *Electroenceph Clin Neurophysiol* 1993;**34**:71–8.
101. Speakman CT, Kamm MA, Swash M. Rectal sensory evoked potentials: an assessment of their clinical value. *Int J Colorectal Dis* 1993;**8**:23–8.

Chapter 17

Sacral reflexes

David B Vodušek

INTRODUCTION

The integrity of the neural and muscular structures of the sacral segments S2 to S4 is tested clinically by eliciting the bulbocavernosus and anal reflex, in addition to evaluating the tone and contractile force of sphincter/pelvic floor muscles and skin sensation in the perineum. The stimulus for the bulbocavernosus reflex is a brisk squeeze of the glans, and the bulbocavernosus or anal sphincter muscle is palpated to check for the response.[1,2] Pricking the anal mucosa or the perianal skin leads to contraction of the anal sphincter, which was described by Rossolimo[3] as the anal reflex.

By the 1950s the recording of the reflex muscle response by electromyography (EMG) had been introduced,[4] and the palpatory or visual observation of contraction was complemented by recording muscle bioelectric activity. Such recordings were found to be more sensitive for demonstrating the presence of the bulbocavernosus reflex response (BCR) in healthy males, and particularly females, compared with clinical testing.[5] These studies still used, however, the standard clinical method to elicit the reflex. It was Rushworth[6] who introduced electrical current delivered to the penis as a means of defining the stimulus more precisely; thus he was able to measure the latency of the response as recorded by EMG. A similar principle was applied to demonstrate the different possible pelvic floor muscle responses to intramuscular electric stimulation; the latency measurements were rendered even more precise by recording with a single muscle fiber EMG needle. The recorded responses were characterized both by absolute latency values, and by latency variability measures, and were found to be direct, recurrent, and reflex in nature.[7] In a more diagnostically oriented study, Ertekin and Reel[8] measured BCR latencies in a group of 14 healthy males, and demonstrated abnormally delayed responses in patients with involvement of the sacral neuromuscular system. Thus a new measure was introduced; the reflex responses were no longer just 'present' or 'absent', but could be present, but pathological (delayed). The electrophysiological correlate of BCR was taken up by several authors who were eager to improve the diagnostic accuracy and sensitivity in patients with presumed neurogenic disorders of 'sacral functions' (lower urinary tract and erectile function, in particular), and further early reports were published.[9–11]

The electrophysiological correlate of the anal reflex was described by Pedersen *et al.*,[12] but early on some controversy existed as to the correct latency of the response.[13] Later studies confirmed that on perianal electrical stimulation both short and long-latency muscle responses were obtained from the anal sphincter.[14,15] It was suggested that the short latency responses (below 10 ms) were direct muscle responses (M waves), and only the later responses of 50 and more milliseconds reflex; some uncertainty exists as to the nature of intermediate latency responses of 13–15 ms.[14,15] The anal reflex as recorded electrophysiologically proved more variable in latency among the control population compared with the BCR, and only elicitable on strong stimulation.[15] Thus it appeared less helpful in ascertaining pathology in the lower sacral reflex arc; it has not been much applied in further studies or clinical practice.

After the publications in the late 1970s and early 1980s, electrophysiological recordings of pelvic floor/perineal muscle reflexes became quite popular, and many reports on electrical stimulation appeared;[15–19] mechanical,[20] and magnetic[21] stimulation were also introduced. Whereas the latter two modalities have only been applied to the penis and clitoris, electrical stimulation can be applied at various sites, including the dorsal penile nerve,[6,8,9,15,22,24] the dorsal clitoral nerve,[16,17,18,19] perineal,[12,15] and at the bladder neck/proximal urethra – using a catheter-mounted ring.[25,26] The latter reflexes have often been referred to as 'vesicourethral' and 'vesicoanal',[27] depending from which muscle the reflex responses were recorded. The pudendal nerve itself may be stimulated transrectally, transvaginally[28] or by applying needle electrodes transperineally.[29]

TERMINOLOGY

A large variety of techniques, but also a plethora of names for the recorded responses emerged in the 1980s.

The time honored term 'bulbocavernosus reflex' (BCR) was used by several authors to encompass different electrophysiologically elicited reflexes, or it was altogether abandoned for newly coined names. The term as such has been criticized as imprecise; it was suggested that 'glandipudendal' is better describing the reflex.[30] To avoid confusion it seemed practical to use the term 'sacral reflex' in electrophysiology (with further specification of stimulation and detection site). As an effort of standardization, the International Continence Society proposed that 'reflex contractions of pelvic floor in response to stimuli applied either to the perineum, the genitalia, or the mucosa of the lower urinary tract be referred to as the sacral reflexes.'[31] However, terminological variability continues to this day. In particular, the terms bulbocavernosus and anal reflex are bound to persist, as they are well known clinically elicited reflexes. It would seem logical that these terms can also be used in electrophysiology, but only for those responses (methods) testing anatomically identical reflex arcs as the clinical reflexes, and not for reflex tests with different anatomical arcs. It should be stressed that clinically either the bulbocavernosus/ischiocavernosus muscles or the anal sphincter are palpated to assess the presence of BCR. The efferent pathways are in both cases minimally different, but both responses are called BCR. It is practical – for the sake of simplicity – if the same term is used for their electrophysiologic correlates; thus, the term 'pudendoanal' reflex for the response recorded from the anal sphincter on stimulation of the dorsal nerve of penis/clitoris[32] seems to be superfluous.

It is a terminological paradox that reflexes were originally named for the muscle, but it turned out that responses (as characterized by latency, habituation etc.) are defined more by the site of stimulation than by the site of detection (i.e. muscle). Thus, on electrical stimulation of the penis, or the perianal skin, EMG responses with quite different latencies are recorded in the anal sphincter: in the first case with a typical latency of 33 ms, in the second case 55 ms! Therefore, to call both responses 'anal reflex' (because recorded in the same muscle) would be misleading. (The same holds for the bulbocavernosus muscle.)[15] Similarly on electrical stimulation in distal or proximal urethra, responses with quite different latencies are recorded in one and the same muscle (either anal sphincter or bulbocavernosus).[33]

THE SACRAL REFLEX ON STIMULATION OF PENIS/CLITORIS – THE BULBOCAVERNOSUS REFLEX

ANATOMY AND PHYSIOLOGY

The afferent limb of this reflex constitutes afferents from glans and penile receptors. Receptor density in the glans is higher than in any other area of the body.[34] In glans mucosa and penile skin there are non-specific nerve endings, constituting 80 to 90% of afferent terminations; the remainder are encapsulated endings. These are mucocutaneous endorgans (genital corpuscles), which are probably a variant of Meissner corpuscles.[35] In the deeper layers of skin – particularly on dorsum penis – there are a few Paccini corpuscles. The glans receptors were characterized as androgen dependent mechanoreceptors; some rapidly adapting to weak stimuli, others slowly adapting.[34] The cat dorsal penile nerve is said to contain 15% of myelinated fibers of group II, others belonging to group III. Temperature and erectile state may modulate the sensitivity of penile afferents.[36]

The efferent limb constitutes the axons of motoneurons, which innervate pelvic floor/perineal muscles. It has been demonstrated that on penile stimulation responses can be obtained in the bulbocavernosus, anal, and urethral sphincter, and in levator ani muscle.[15] The sphincter muscles in particular have smaller motoneurons as typical limb muscles (and they differ also in some further morphological characteristics as well as in their sensitivity to different pathological–degenerative processes).

The spinal integration of the BCR is complex and not entirely clarified. Animal experiments have demonstrated that androgens modulate the synaptic efficacy of transmission within the BCR.[37] The EMG recordings in humans often reveal two components, as in the blink reflex[15,23,38] (Fig. 17.1[39]). This may not always be obvious in the examinees, as the second component in most (but not all) has a higher threshold.[20] Its pathway probably involves more interneurons, but also it may include nociceptive afferents. The thresholds of the two components may be influenced by many factors and the ratio of thresholds of both components may not be the same in all different pelvic floor muscles. This may explain the unreproduced report that different latencies of reflexes were observed in bulbocavernosus and ischiocavernosus muscle on penile stimulation.[40] The threshold of the second component is low in upper motor neuron lesions – or the motoneurons are facilitated to fire repetitively – and more than two components of the reflex are often obtained in such patients.

BCR as such was thought to be polysynaptic, but a study of the latency variability of single motoneuron responses (measured on consecutive firing) within the early part of the first component gave similar values as for the first component of the blink reflex, which was shown to be oligosynaptic. Later responses, and particularly those within the second component of the reflex, had values typical for polysynaptic responses, as for instance the flexor reflexes in lower limb muscles[38] (Fig. 17.2). Measurements of BCR and H reflex latencies, and latencies of motor and sensory latencies from epidural

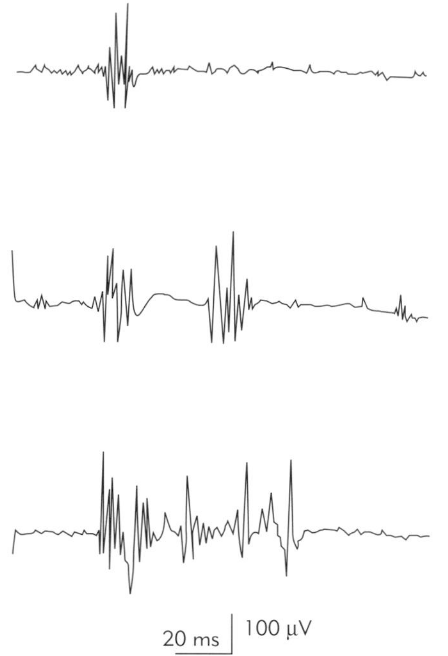

Figure 17.1 Concentric needle recording from the bulbocavernosus muscle on stimulation of dorsal penile nerve (with surface electrodes) in a 67-year-old healthy man. Upper beam shows the sacral reflex on just suprathreshold stimulation, the middle beam on stimulation increased by 30%, and lower beam on maximal tolerable stimulation (in this case 60% suprathreshold). Observe the early component of the sacral reflex being joined by the second component at stronger stimulation; the division in two components is blurred at very strong stimulation. Observe also the slight shortening of latency of the first component at stronger stimulation in comparison with just suprathreshold stimulation (from Ref. 39, with permission).

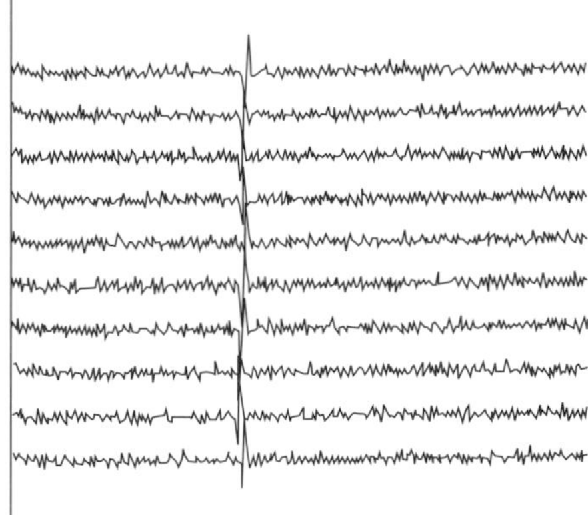

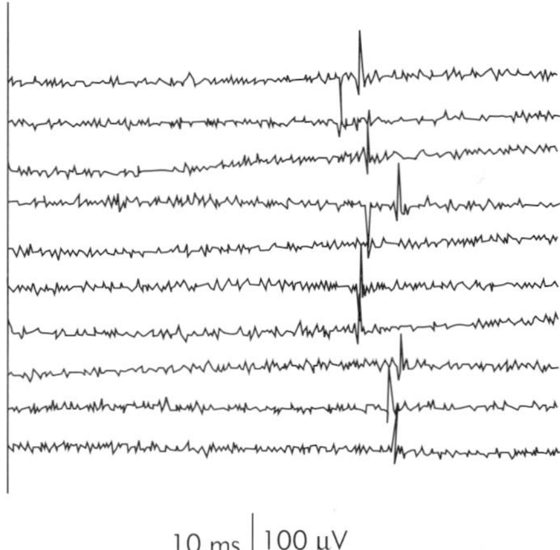

Figure 17.2 Typical variability of latencies of consecutive reflex responses of single motor units (recorded as latencies of single muscle fiber recorded with a single fiber EMG electrode) in a healthy volunteer. Above: 10 consecutive responses from within the latency range of the first components of BCR. Below: 10 consecutive responses from within the latency range of the second component of the BCR are shown. (Electrical stimulation on dorsal penile nerve; single fiber EMG recording from the bulbocavernosus muscle; healthy male volunteer – from Ref. 20.)

recordings made it possible to calculate intraspinal delay, which was 8.2 ms for BCR, and 1.1 ms for the H reflex. The authors concluded that 5–6 synapses are involved in the first component of BCR, although they did not exclude the possibility of some faster oligosynaptic linkage.[41]

As the stimulus for the reflex is given to penis (clitoris), and the response clinically observed as the contraction of the circular anal sphincter, the question of the laterality of the reflex never arose in clinical work. Although of course there are two dorsal nerves, and the perineal muscles have unilateral innervation, even the early electrophysiological reports did not address this issue. The response can be detected bilaterally by the usual method of electrical stimulation; it was claimed that such is also the case on unilateral penile stimulation.[23] Actually, on carefully increasing the strength of a unilateral stimulus, ipsilateral responses can be obtained in healthy volunteers with low threshold (Fig. 17.3), and contralateral responses only appear at higher strength of stimulus.[20] Unilateral responses have been described for the 'tonic reflex' elicited by vibration of glans, if one of the dorsal nerves was anesthetized.[30] This may be physiologically interesting; clinically it is not relevant as unilateral stimulation on the penis is technically questionable due to the spread of stimulus; this would be even more important in patients with partial denervation, in whom higher strengths of stimuli would have to be used. Unilateral stimulation is feasible if applied

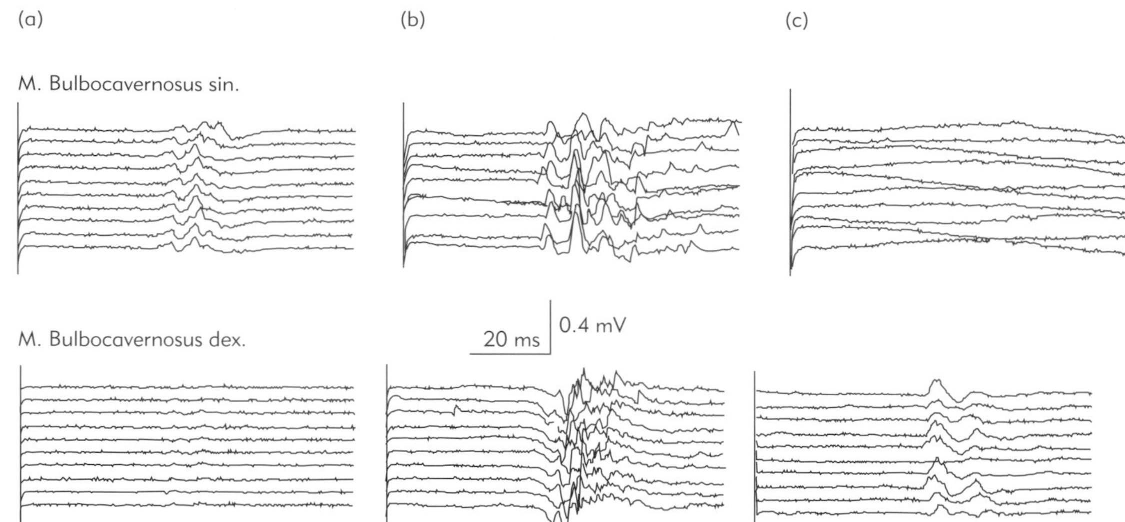

Figure 17.3 Sacral reflex responses in the bulbocavernosus muscle on unilateral electrical stimulation of penis in a healthy volunteer. Upper row: recordings from the left, and lower row: recordings from the right bulbocavernosus muscle. (a) Electrical stimulation on the left. (b) Electrical stimulation on dorsum. (c) Electrical stimulation on right side of penis. Electrical stimulus: rectangular pulse, 0.2 ms, just suprathreshold strength for stimulation on the lateral side of penis. It can be seen that the same strength of stimulus is much more effective in eliciting a reflex when applied to the dorsum of penis. When applied unilaterally, a unilateral reflex can be obtained. (Simultaneous bilateral recording from both bulbocavernosus muscles with a concentric needle EMG electrode in a healthy male volunteer – from Ref. 20).

directly to the pudendal nerve in the perineum (but this afferent limb contains a different set of fibers).

Consecutive elicitation of BCR facilitates the response. Testing with double electrical stimuli with interstimulus intervals from 2 to 1900 ms (the first stimulus being subthreshold) in five healthy young male volunteers revealed consistent facilitation at all intervals between 2 and 1000 ms, being most pronounced for intervals of 2–10 ms (increases in response surface up to 400%). Testing with 110% threshold stimuli pairs revealed similar results for interstimulus intervals from 20 to 1900 ms (i.e. facilitation for intervals 20–1000 ms, particularly pronounced for intervals 20–100 ms; Fig. 17.4). Facilitation was also revealed for concomitant (slight) voluntary activation of pelvic floor muscles, but not for the Jendrassik maneuver, and not during mental stress (arithmetic). Apart from increases in amplitude (surface) of responses on facilitatory maneuvers, shortening of latency was also observed.[20] Experience with strong facilitatory effect of double pulse stimulation led to the use of such stimulation in routine diagnostics; it was shown that preservation of the sacral reflex arc can be demonstrated using stimulation with two consecutive electrical pulses (interstimulus interval 3 ms) in patients with partial lesions, in whom stimulation with the standard single electrical pulse was inefficient even at maximum output of the available commercial stimulator unit.[42]

Testing with a prolonged series of regular repetitive stimuli at frequencies of 0.1 to 1 Hz, and suprathreshold strength (50–500 BCRs, recorded with surface electrodes) revealed little habituation of the first component (Fig. 17.5), and marked habituation of the second component. Spontaneous variability (of first component's amplitudes/surfaces) within the series decreased with increasing the strength of the suprathreshold stimulus. At frequencies of 2 to 10 Hz, sensitization of responses could be observed in series up to 60 consecutive BCRs. Indeed, as testing for the threshold strength revealed, any consecutive elicitation of BCR with frequencies above 0.1–10 Hz was eventually facilitatory if compared with single stimulation with prolonged interstimulation resting periods.[20] These findings are compatible with animal experiments revealing the absence of Renshaw inhibition for sphincter motoneurons.[43] Experience with BCR behavior on prolonged regular repetitive stimulation led to the proposal of this test for electrophysiological intraoperative monitoring.[44]

METHOD

The electrophysiological correlate of the BCR is the EMG recorded response from perineal/pelvic floor muscles on stimulation of the dorsal nerve of penis or clitoris. In the strict sense all other reflex responses (even those obtained on stimulation of the pudendal nerve, where it

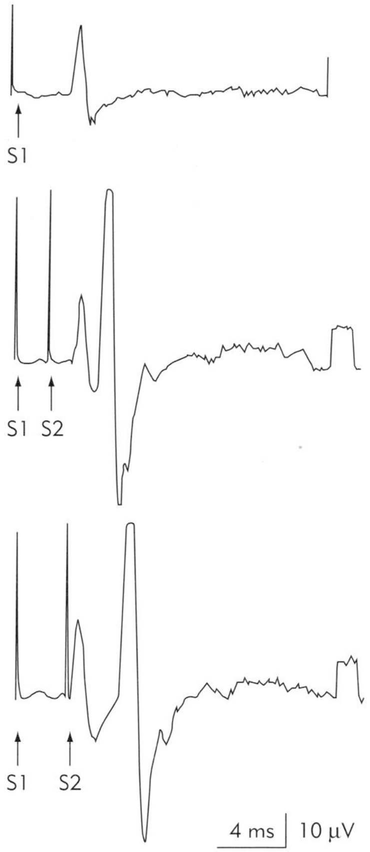

Figure 17.4 Facilitation of the bulbocavernosus reflex response in a double electrical pulse stimulation paradigm. Stimulation: rectangular electrical pulse, 0.2 ms duration, 10% suprathreshold for eliciting the bulbocavernosus reflex in the bulbocavernosus muscle (recorded with surface electrodes in a healthy volunteer). Upper row: the reflex response on single pulse (S1) stimulation; middle row: two pulses (S1 and S2) of the same strength are given at an interpulse interval of 20 ms; lower row: two pulses of the same strength are given at an interpulse interval of 30 ms. On double pulse stimulation, the second reflex response is significantly facilitated, although S2 is of the same strength as S1 (from Ref. 20).

already contains other afferent fibers) is not a BCR. The techniques will be described accordingly.

The authors used a different type of surface stimulating electrode, which does not seem to influence greatly the quality of the response. In males, we have found ring electrodes too cumbersome to apply, and prefer Velcro attached bipolar electrodes, or a custom-made 'clamp' electrode. EEG ear-clip electrodes are practical to apply in females.[19] Hand-held bipolar surface electrodes can be used in both sexes. All electrodes have to be detachable from cables to be easily cleansed and sterilized. As a rule single electrical pulses, 0.1 to 0.5 ms long, were used to elicit responses, and this has been successful in all normal subjects.[15,18] It has been demonstrated that double pulse stimulation (with an interstimulus interval of 3 ms) can elicit a response in patients, when single pulse stimulation was inefficient.[42] Recordings of EMG responses can be obtained by different types of surface or intramuscular electrodes from perineal muscles, and with intramuscular electrodes from the levator ani. Surface electrodes were shown to be not as sensitive in recording responses.[19] Different protocols have been advocated for establishing the latency of the response, which is somewhat variable and depends on the strength of stimulation (shortest values are only obtained on strong stimulation). Stimulation is started with weak stimuli, and the sensory threshold for the applied pulse is determined first (if used for nothing else it is at least a good way to make the examinee familiar with the sensation). Then the strength is increased to approximately three times threshold value, which can be tolerated by most patients. As a rule several responses need to be recorded to demonstrate their reproducibility. Some authors advocate averaging responses (up to 100), others advise recording consecutive individual responses. True shortest latency responses can be measured by recording a series of consecutive responses, but this is true for the bulbocavernosus muscle, where there is no interference from ongoing ('tonic') motor unit activity. The latter occasionally makes averaging in the sphincter muscles necessary. As the BCR is a very obvious robust response in most examinees it is usually adequate to record – after several reflexes have already been elicited to establish the strength of stimulus etc., so there has been some 'facilitation' of the response – a series of 10 consecutive responses at a stimulation of 1 or 0.5 Hz, and determine the shortest latency. If no response is obtained, stimulation with double pulse is performed. If the response is small (after the recording is technically checked), averaging is considered. If recordings are troubled by abundant motor unit activity in an anxious patient, randomly triggered pulses may be given, and averaging is an additional option.

The reports of sacral reflexes obtained on electrical stimulation of the dorsal penile or clitoral nerve are consistent in giving mean latencies (of onset of response; data given for different perineal muscles) between 31 ms and 38.5 ms, with standard deviations of about 5 ms.[6,8,9,15–19,23,24] Responses with latencies above 45 ms are regarded as pathologically delayed by most authors, but laboratories are expected to acquire their own normative data, as the above results from different laboratories were obtained using methods with at least slight technical differences. Standardization of technique would be desirable, but has not yet been achieved.

Mechanical stimulation can be applied by a soft blow to the penis by a reflex hammer with an integrated

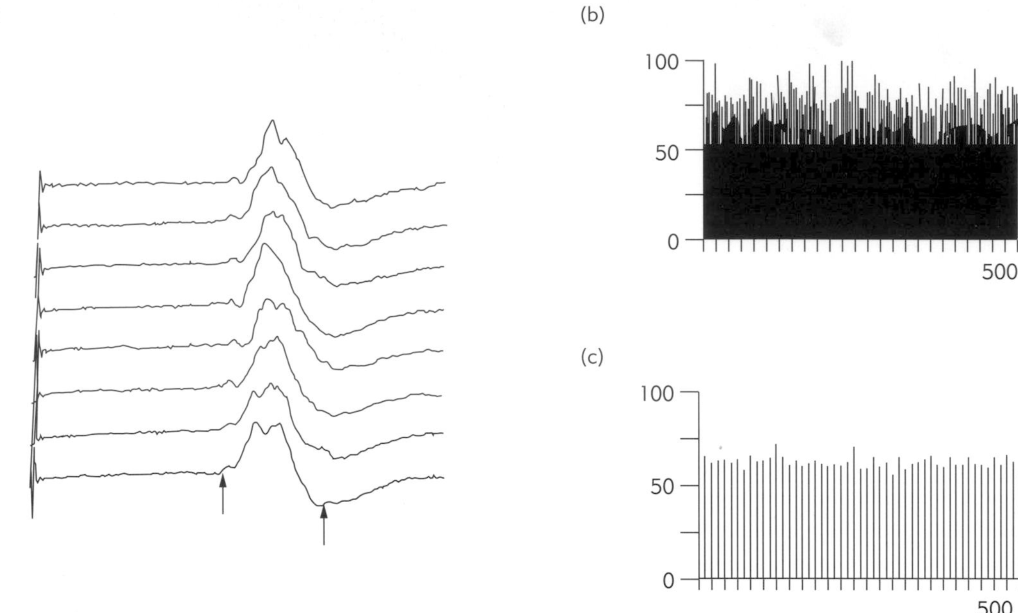

Figure 17.5 Variability of consecutively elicited bulbocavernosus reflex responses. Stimulation: rectangular electrical pulse, 0.2 ms duration, 50% suprathreshold strength, delivered at 1 Hz. Recorded with surface electrodes from the bulbocavernosus muscle in a healthy volunteer. Arbitrary units are used for calculation of the surface of responses. (a) Actual recording of consecutive bulbocavernosus reflexes. (a) Surface of the reflex response calculated between the two markers indicated in (a). The values of single reflex responses in arbitrary units are given as lines in (a), indicating a variability of consecutive responses. No trend can be seen in the whole series of 500 consecutive responses, i.e. no habituation of the reflex response. In (C) the same series of reflex responses is represented as averages of each 10 consecutive bulbocavernosus reflex responses (from Ref. 20).

electronic switch,[20] or by an air driven 'squeezer' (electromechanical device).[45] The latency of responses on mechanical stimulation of distal penis was reported as either shorter,[20] or longer[45] than on standard electrical stimulation, depending on the stimulator used.

Magnetic stimulation can be used as well; reflex latencies on such stimulation were reported as longer,[21] again at least in part related to technical aspects of the stimulator used.

OTHER SACRAL REFLEXES

'Modified BCR', as obtained by stimulation of one pudendal nerve transvaginally, transrectally or with needle electrodes transperineally have expectedly shorter latencies than responses obtained on stimulation of the dorsal nerve in the same subject. The potential benefit of these techniques is the demonstration of a unilateral afferent lesion, but they do not seem to be routinely applied.

Sacral reflex responses obtained on perianal stimulation have mean latencies between c. 50 and 65 ms SD.[12,15] Sacral reflex on perianal stimulation was called 'anal reflex' (as it is the electrophysiological correlate of the clinically examined reflex) and was elicited by single or double pulses, or a train of pulses applied to the perianal skin. Such stimulation is typically used to elicit flexor reflexes in lower limbs, and is often reported as bothersome by examinees. (In comparison, BCR is elicited at lower strength of stimuli, if the same pattern of stimuli is applied.) 'Anal reflex' studies were typically reported from the anal sphincter,[12,46] but could also be recorded from other perineal muscles, always with very similar latencies.[15] Their latencies are about 200 ms at threshold stimulation and decrease on stronger stimulation; the latencies are, however, never as short as the shortest reflex response obtained in the same muscle on penile/clitoral stimulation. With stronger stimulation the response becomes longer in duration and may show some repetitions of 'clusters' of motor units, particularly in patients with suprasacral cord lesions, who otherwise have same shortest latency of response as normal subjects.[12] The 'anal reflex' (i.e. the sacral reflex on strong stimulation of the perianal region) probably has thinner myelinated fibers in its afferent limb (in comparison with BCR) as it is produced by a nociceptive stimulus. On perianal electrical stimulation, a short latency compound muscle potential can also be recorded, as a result of depolarization of motor branches to the anal sphincter.[15,16]

Sacral reflex responses can be obtained in perineal muscles on distal urethral stimulation (these have same latency as the BCR,[47] and on proximal urethra/bladder neck stimulation, when their shortest latency is close to the latency of sacral reflex responses on perianal stimulation. Urethral stimulation is performed with catheter mounted electrodes, and using – as a rule – a train of stimuli. The principle was introduced (under the name of 'electromyelography') by Bradley,[25] and then studied by others.[18,24,26,48] The sacral reflex obtained on bladder neck/proximal urethral stimulation has a different afferent limb than BCR (i.e. thin visceral afferent fibers accompanying autonomic nerve fibers). These fibers would be expected to be involved in some strategically placed lesions, which would not affect the pudendal nerve. Recording of these sacral reflexes was reported as useful in investigating 'bladder function'.[49] In principle the discussed electrophysiological method should test the same reflex arc as the clinically used 'modified' BCR, where perineal muscle contraction is observed after tugging on an indwelling Foley catheter. In this reflex, which should really not be called BCR, there is some uncertainty as to which receptors are activated – it probably is more than one group, i.e. both bladder neck/urethral receptors, but also those in pelvic floor muscles supporting the mentioned structures. The visceral afferent fibers from bladder neck/proximal urethra accompany pelvic nerves, are thinly myelinated, and have a slower conduction velocity than the thicker pudendal afferents. Even when using electrical stimulation at the level of bladder neck/proximal urethra there is some uncertainty as to which afferents are depolarized. It is conceivable – and personal experience speaks in favor of such a hypothesis – that stronger stimulation used in patients with some sensory deficit spreads to depolarize afferents in pelvic floor muscles or the pudendal nerve branches, thus eliciting reflexes with shorter latencies (i.e. providing for false positive results of testing).

Reflex responses in sphincter muscles can also be obtained by electrical (and other) stimulation in the lower limbs, as in studies on flexor reflexes in lower limb muscles.[50]

All of the mentioned reflexes in perineal/pelvic floor muscles have been muscle contractions, although indeed there is reflex relaxation of these muscles also (during involuntary but integrated bladder and bowel emptying). Polygraphic recordings of lower urinary tract and anorectal function can determine the presence or absence of this reflex relaxation.

SACRAL REFLEX ON MECHANICAL STIMULATION

The stimulus used clinically to elicit the bulbocavernosus and anal reflexes is of course mechanical. A firm but non-painful squeeze suffices for eliciting the BCR, but nociceptive pricking or scratching of perianal skin is necessary to demonstrate the presence of the anal reflex. Judging from experience with needle EMG recordings from pelvic floor muscles, very slight mechanical stimulation of any part of the perineum causes an increase in firing of motor units (and recruitment of motor units), thus demonstrating the integrity of the reflex arc. Only the insensitivity of the means of observation (i.e. being dependent on feeling or seeing the contraction) makes it necessary to use relatively strong activation maneuvers to demonstrate the presence of reflex responses clinically. Partial nerve lesions may extinguish the clinically assessed reflex, whereas the partial preservation of the reflex arc can still be demonstrated electrophysiologically. In addition, stronger mechanical stimulation is more efficient in eliciting some response (as recorded electromyographically) in severe partial nerve lesions than the single electrical stimulus, although in these cases no latency can be measured (personal observation).

Furthermore, a more sophisticated mechanical stimulation paradigm with devices triggering the oscilloscope ray has been used to elicit BCR in both sexes[51] and found to be a robust technique.[20] Either a commercially available electrophysiological reflex hammer or a customized electromechanical hammer can be used.[45] Such stimulation is painless, and can be used in children or patients with pacemakers in whom electrical stimulation is contraindicated. The latency of the BCR elicited mechanically is comparable with the electrically elicited reflex in the same patients, but may be either slightly shorter[20] or longer[45] because of particular electromechanical device used.

TONIC SACRAL REFLEXES

Continuous vibratory stimulation of the glans penis was shown to elicit non-decaying reflex contraction of the perineal muscles. The tonic contraction increased with time in most subjects, was not influenced by the Jendrassik maneuver or by mental stress, and could not be voluntarily inhibited. It was present in spinal cord injury patients with lesions above the sacral cord. The reflex was called the tonic 'glandipudendal' reflex.[30] The continuous contraction (of bulbocavernosus muscle) is similar to the tonic vibratory reflex obtained in a limb muscle on vibration of its muscle tendon. Similar 'continuous reflex contraction' of the bulbocavernosus muscle can be obtained by repetitive electrical stimulation of penis/clitoris as described above, given the fact that the first component of BCR demonstrates no or little habituation.[20]

Apart from the vibration-induced reflex, all other previously discussed reflexes – both clinically or electrophysiologically evaluated – are 'phasic' muscle contractions. In addition to this phasic (time limited and synchronized) reflex muscle response to short (single, double or short train of stimuli) there also is – as a rule – a 'tonic' response. It consists of a prolonged increase in the firing rate of (already previously spontaneously active) motor units, and some prolonged firing of motor units recruited first during the 'phasic' reflex response. Such prolonged (reflex) increase of motor unit activity may perhaps also be called a 'tonic reflex'. This 'tonic reflex' is different from the vibratory response, as there is no ongoing stimulation; it is a prolonged response to phasic stimulation. Of course, it might be just another manifestation of the sensitization of sacral reflex activity, already discussed. (It may, however, be difficult to separate reflex activation from 'deteriorated' relaxation in a tense examinee.) Such 'tonic reflex activation' is pronounced in sphincters but is only just demonstrable in the bulbocavernosus muscle, which normally does not display any 'tonic activity' of motor units on relaxation). No quantification of such 'tonic' reflex has been tried so far.

AUTONOMIC REFLEXES RELEVANT FOR SACRAL FUNCTIONS

The neurophysiologically tested reflex responses discussed so far assess the thicker myelinated somatic motor fibers, whereas it is the autonomic nervous system (the parasympathetic part in particular) which is most relevant for sacral functions. It has been argued that local involvement of the sacral nervous system (such as trauma, compression etc.) will usually involve somatic and autonomic fibers simultaneously. However, there are some localized and several generalized pathological conditions, as a consequence of which purely isolated lesions can occur. Methods by which the parasympathetic and sympathetic nervous system innervating the pelvic viscera could be assessed directly would be very helpful. Information on parasympathetic bladder innervation can to some extent be obtained by cystometry (which may be said to test a parasympathetic reflex). Apart from 'activation' of detrusor (demonstrating the micturition reflex) reflex inhibition of the detrusor can also be demonstrated on electrical stimulation of pudendal nerves.[52] From a clinical neurophysiological point of view, direct electrophysiological testing of sacral autonomic reflex arcs would be desirable, but has not been as yet convincingly introduced. Thin visceral sensory fibers are tested by stimulating the proximal urethra or bladder, and by recording sacral reflex responses, or cerebral SEP. The only electrophysiological autonomic test directly relevant for urogenitoanal dysfunction (also being reflex in nature – although not a 'sacral reflex' in the narrow sense) is the sympathetic skin response,[53] which can be recorded in the perineum, and can also be elicited by electrical stimulation of penis/clitoris.

SACRAL REFLEXES – CLINICAL USES AND INTERPRETATION OF RESULTS

Generally speaking evaluation of reflex responses is important to help assess nervous system involvement, and to determine the level of the lesion.

Although all of the described electrophysiological sacral reflexes have been claimed to be of use in assessment of patients, only the reflex responses on stimulation of the dorsal penile and clitoral nerve (the BCR) are used more widely. EMG recording of the bulbocavernosus reflex has been shown to be more sensitive than the clinically assessed reflex response in males and particularly in females.[5] The recording of reflex latency should increase the sensitivity of recording abnormalities, but true sensitivity and specificity of the test are not known.

Testing BCR has been proposed to be valuable in patients with lower motor neuron lesions.[8,54] Pathological responses have been described in patients with presumed neurogenic erectile dysfunction,[22] in patients with neurogenic fecal incontinence,[18] women with retention of urine,[55] women with idiopathic intractable constipation,[56] and patients with dysraphism.[57,58] Detection of sacral reflex responses correlated with the existence of reflex detrusor activity, but was not a reliable indicator of detrusor function in patients after spinal cord injury.[59] The presence of BCR was found to be moderately sensitive in predicting the return of spontaneous voiding.[60]

Generally speaking, absent or delayed sacral reflexes (BCR and others) have been published in many reports on patients with known or presumed neurogenic sacral dysfunction, and are proposed to be valuable indicators of lesions of the S2–S4 reflex arc. As the reports usually included reasonable control groups, and data from different laboratories are quite comparable, such findings are indeed signifying some disturbance in the tested nervous system. However, there are several caveats. These seem to be best known for the BCR, which is the most explored sacral reflex and can probably be regarded as the only 'established' response in the clinical neurophysiological armamentarium.[61] As described, the BCR often demonstrates two components; these may behave somewhat differently in control subjects and in patients. In patients with partially denervated pelvic floor muscles, the first reflex component sometimes cannot be obtained with single stimuli, but on strong stimulation the later reflex component does occur. This may cause confusion, as a very 'delayed' reflex response may be recorded in a patient (implying 'pathological conduction'), not recognizing the possibility that it is not a delayed first component but an isolated second component of the reflex. The situation can be clarified by using double stimuli, which facilitate the reflex response and may reveal in such a patient the first component, which was not obvious on stimulation with single stimuli.[42] This is not to say that absence of response or a very delayed response obtained on standard stimulation should not be interpreted as abnormal; but simplified statements about 'slowed conduction' and 'complete lesions' should not be made. Complete reflex arc lesion should not be inferred by absence of response if only single pulse is used for stimulation. It should be noted that a reflex may not be absent in partial lesions, and neither is latency measurement sensitive to partial axonal nerve lesions. Some remaining fast conducting axons suffice to give a 'normal' result in the presence of a significant loss of axons, and neurological deficit. Demyelinative lesions may have, on the other hand, little direct functional consequences, although conduction may be significantly pathological. Thus abnormal responses do not necessarily imply abnormality of sacral function: patients with hereditary motor and sensory demyelinating neuropathy with normal bladder and sexual function have been found to have much delayed sacral reflex responses.[62] No correlation was found between the BCR and erectile dysfunction in MS patients.[63] In diabetic impotent patients the BCR latency was a poorer indicator of neuropathy than limb nerve conduction studies.[64,65] Also, latency of the reflex is not just dependent on conduction through peripheral pathways, but also on transmission through the spinal cord interneuronal system, thus influenced by several factors, which may not be controlled or controllable. No data are available on reflex amplitude as a test parameter.

Most reports deal with abnormally prolonged sacral reflex latencies, but it has been suggested that a very short reflex latency raises the possibility of the tethered cord syndrome.[66] In that instance, the short latency has been attributed to the low location of the conus. Shorter latencies of sacral reflexes in patients with suprasacral cord lesions have also been reported.[17]

Sacral reflex responses can be used as an indicator of spinal integrative function. Comparing BCR parameters (threshold, latency, elicitability) during different physiologic conditions or between different groups of patients (with central lesions or dysfunctional neurocontrol) may reveal information on spinal cord processing. Persistence of BCR during micturition was found to be an indicator of suprasacral upper motor neuron involvement (BCR tends to disappear during voiding in subjects without such a lesion).[67,68] A decreased BCR elicitability was demonstrated in enuretic as compared with normal boys, arguing for a disturbed balance of neurocontrol in enuretic children.[69]

Continuous intraoperative recording of BCR is feasible if double pulses[15,70] or a train of pulses are used.

CONCLUSION

When electrophysiologically tested sacral reflexes were first applied, it was expected that by their introduction neurogenic sacral dysfunction would be diagnosed with more confidence. But the correlation of reflex presence/absence and its latency to a particular lower urinary tract, ano-rectal or sexual dysfunction in an individual patient is too 'indirect' and complex to be unequivocally interpretable. Strictly speaking the tests as diagnostic tools can only be regarded as valid in the narrow sense (i.e. demonstrating preservation of reflex arc, normal or pathological conduction through this arc etc). It should also be stressed that nerves and muscles are composed of large populations of biological units (axons, motor units ...), and the test results only reflect the function of a sample. This has to be taken into account when interpreting findings of an individual test.

In conclusion, lower urinary tract, ano-rectal and sexual function rely on neurocontrol, the integrity of which is tested by clinical examination and several diagnostic methods, among them clinical neurophysiological tests. These include electrophysiologically tested sacral reflexes, such as the bulbocavernosus and anal reflexes (which represent correlates to the clinically elicited reflexes), and several other reflexes, which are defined by the applied stimulus (at a particular anatomical location), and recording (from a particular effector). In the author's opinion, clinical neurophysiological testing should be considered as a direct extension of the clinical examination in selected patients, particularly in those with suspected or known involvement of the peripheral neuromuscular system.

REFERENCES

1. Bors E, French JD. Management of paroxysmal hypertension following injuries to cervical and upper thoracic segments of spinal cord. *AMA Arch Surg* 1952;**64**:803–12.
2. Lapides J, Bobbit JM. Diagnostic value of bulbocavernosus reflex. *JAMA* 1956;**162**: 971–2.
3. Rossolimo G. Der Analreflex, seine Physiologie und Pathologie. *Neurol Zentralblatt* 1891;**10**:257–9.
4. Rattner WH, Gerlaugh RL, Murphy JJ, Erdman WJ. The bulbocavernosus reflex: I. Electromyographic study of normal patients. *J Urol* 1958;**80**:140–1.
5. Blaivas JG, Zayed AAH, Labib KB. The bulbocavernosus reflex in urology: a prospective study of 299 patients. *J Urol* 1981;**126**:197–9.
6. Rushworth G. Diagnostic value of the electromyographic study of reflex activity in man. *Electroenceph Clin Neurophysiol* 1967:(Suppl. **25**:)65–73.

7. Trontelj JV, Janko M, Godec C, Rakovec S, Trontelj M. Electrical stimulation for urinary incontinence. *Urol Internat* 1974;**29**:213–20.
8. Ertekin C, Reel F. Bulbocavernosus reflex in normal men and patients with neurogenic bladder and/or impotence. *J Neurol Sci* 1976;**28**:1–15.
9. Vacek J & Lachman M. The bulbocavernosus reflex in diabetics with erectile dysfunction: a clinical and EMG study. *Cas Lek Cesk* 1977;**33**:1014–7 (in Czech).
10. Siroky MB, Sax DS, Krane RJ. Sacral signal tracing: the electrophysiology of the bulbocavernosus reflex. *J Urol* 1979;**122**:661–4.
11. Vodusek DB, Lokar J, Janko M. Neurophysiological tests in erectile dysfunction. *Zdrav Vestn* 1981;**50**:703–7(in Slovene).
12. Pedersen E, Harving H, Klemar B, *et al.* Human anal reflexes. *J Neurol Neurosurg Psychiat* 1978;**41**:813–8.
13. Henry MM, Swash M. Assessment of pelvic floor disorders and incontinence by electrophysiological recording of the anal reflex. *Lancet* 1978;**i**:1290–1.
14. Pedersen E, Klemar B, Schroder HD, Torring J. Anal sphincter responses after perineal electrical stimulation. *J Neurol Neurosurg Psychiat* 1982;**45**:770–3.
15. Vodusek DB, Janko M, Lokar J. Direct and reflex responses in perineal muscles on electrical stimulation. *J Neurol Neurosurg Psychiat* 1983;**46**:67–71.
16. Bartolo DCC, Jarratt JA, Read NW. The cutaneo-anal reflex: a useful index of neuropathy? *Br J Surg* 1983;**70**:660–3.
17. Bilkey WJ, Awad EA, Smith AD. Clinical application of sacral reflex latency. *J Urol* 1983;**129**:1187–9.
18. Varma JS, Smith AN, McInnes A. Electrophysiological observations on the human pudendo-anal reflex. *J Neurol* 1986;**49**:1411–6.
19. Vodusek DB. Pudendal somatosensory evoked potential and bulbocavernosus reflex in women. *Electroenceph Clin Neurophysiol* 1990;**77**:134–6.
20. Vodusek DB. *Neurophysiological study of bulbocavernosus reflex in man.* D.Sc. Thesis, University of Ljubljana, 1988:1–129 (in Slovene).
21. Loening-Baucke V, Read NW, Yamada T, Barker AT. Evaluation of the motor and sensory components of the pudendal nerve. *Electroenceph Clin Neurophysiol* 1994;**93**:35–65.
22. Vodusek DB, Janko M, Lokar J. EMG, single fibre EMG and sacral reflexes in assessment of sacral nervous system lesions. *J Neurol Neurosurg Psychiat* 1982;**45**:1064–6.
23. Krane RJ, Siroky MB. Studies on sacral evoked potentials. *J Urol* 1980;**124**:872–6.
24. Vereecken RI, De Meirsman J, Puers B, *et al.* Electrophysiological exploration of the sacral conus. *J Neurol* 1982;**227**:135–44.
25. Bradley WE. Urethral electromyelography. *J Urol* 1972;**108**:563–4.
26. Sarica Y, Karacan I. Bulbocavernosus reflex to somatic and visceral nerve stimulation in normal subjects and in diabetics with erectile impotence. *J Urol* 1986;**138**:55–8.
27. Fowler CJ, Betts CD. Clinical value of electrophysiological investigations of patients with urinary symptoms. In: Mundy AR, Stephenson TP, Wein AJ (eds). *Urodynamics: principles, practice and application*, 2nd edn. Edinburgh: Churchill Livingstone, 1994:165–81.
28. Contreras Ortiz O, Bertotti AC, Rodriguez Nuñez JD. Pudendal reflexes in women with pelvic floor disorders. *Zentralbl Gynäkol* 1994;**116**:561–5.
29. Vodusek DB, Plevnik S, Janez J, Vrtacnik P. Detrusor inhibition on selective pudendal nerve stimulation in the perineum. *Neurourol Urodynam* 1988;**6**:389–93.
30. Brindley GS, Gillan P. Men and women who do not have orgasms. *Br J Psychiat* 1982;**140**:351–6.
31. Abrams P, Blaivas JG, Stanton SL, *et al.* Sixth report on the standardisation of terminology of lower urinary tract function. Procedures related to neurophysiological investigations: electromyography, nerve conduction studies, reflex latencies, evoked potentials and sensory testing. *Br J Urol* 1987;**59**:300–4.
32. Smith AN, Varma JS. The latency of the pudendo-anal reflex in man. *J Physiol* 1984; **360**:49P.
33. Flink R. Clinical neurophysiological methods for investigating the lower urinary tract in patients with micturition disorders. *Acta Obstet Gynecol Scand* 1997;(Suppl. 166):**76**: 50–8.
34. de Groat WC, Booth AM. Neural control of penile erection. In: Maggi CA (ed.) *The autonomic nervous system, Vol 3. Nervous control of the urogenital system.* London: Harwood Academic Publishers, 1993:465–522.
35. Winkelman R. Sensory receptors of the skin. In: Yaksh TL (ed.) *Spinal afferent processing.* New York: Plenum Press, 1986:19–57.
36. de Groat WC. Neurophysiology of the pelvic organs. In: Rushton DN (ed.) *Handbook of neuro-urology.* New York: Marcel Dekker, 1994:55–93.
37. Tanaka J, Arnold AP. Androgenic modulation of the activity of lumbar neurons involved in the rat bulbocavernosus reflex. *Exp Brain Res* 1993;**94**(2):301–7.
38. Vodusek DB, Janko M. The bulbocavernosus reflex – a single motor neuron study. *Brain* 1990;**113**(III):813–20.
39. Vodusek DB. Evoked potential testing. (Urodynamics II). *Urol Clin North Am* 1996; **23**(3):427–46.
40. Lavoisier P, Proulx J, Courtois F. Reflex contractions of the ischiocavernosus muscles following electrical and pressure stimulations. *J Urol* 1988;**139**:396–9.
41. Ertekin C, Mungan B. Sacral spinal cord and root potentials evoked by the stimulation of the dorsal nerve of penis and cord conduction delay for the bulbocavernosus reflex. *Neurourol Urodynam* 1993;**12**:9–22.
42. Rodi Z, Vodusek DB. The sacral reflex studies: single versus double pulse stimulation. *Neurourol Urodynam* 1995;**14**:496–7.
43. Mackel R. Segmental and descending control of the external urethral and anal sphincters in the cat. *J Physiol* 1979;**294**:105–22.
44. Vodusek DB, Deletis V, Kiprovski K. Intraoperative bulbocavernosus reflex monitoring: Decreasing the risk of postoperative sacral dysfunction. *Neurourol Urodyn* 1993;**12**: 425–7.
45. Podnar S, Vodusek D, Trsinar B, Rodi Z. A method of uroneurophysiological investigation in children. *Electroenceph Clin Neurophysiol* 1997;**104**:389 92.
46. Swash M. Early and late components in the human anal reflex. *J Neurol Neurosurg Psychiat* 1982;**45**:767–9.
47. Yang CC, Bradley WE. Innervation of the human anterior urethra by the dorsal nerve of the penis. *Muscle Nerve* 1998;**21**(4):514–18.

48. Bemelmans BLH, Meuleman EJH, Anten BWM, *et al.* Penile sensory disorders in erectile dysfunction: results of a comprehensive neuro-urophysiological diagnostic evaluation in 123 patients. *J Urol* 1991;**146**:777–82.
49. Fidas A, Galloway NTM, McInnes A, Chisholm GD. Neurophysiological measurements in primary adult enuretics. *Br J Urol* 1985;**57**:635–40.
50. Mai J, Pedersen E. Central effect of bladder filling and voiding. *J Neurol Neurosurg Psychiat* 1976;**39**:171–7.
51. Dystra D, Sidi A, Cameron J, *et al.* The use of mechanical stimulation to obtain the sacral reflex latency: a new technique. *J Urol* 1987;**137**:77–9.
52. Vodusek DB, Light JK, Libby JM. Detrusor inhibition induced by stimulation of pudendal nerve afferents. *Neurourol Urodynam* 1986;**5**:381–9.
53. Ertekin C, Ertekin N, Mutlu S, *et al.* Skin potentials (SP) recorded from the extremities and genital regions in normal and impotent subjects. *Acta Neurol Scand* 1987;**76**:28–36.
54. Ziemann U, Reimers CD. Anal sphincter electromyography, bulbocavernosus reflex and pudendal somatosensory evoked potentials in diagnosis of neurogenic lumbosacral lesions with disorders of bladder and large intestine emptying and erectile dysfunctions. *Nervenarzt* 1996;**67**(2):140–6.
55. Fidas A, Galloway NTM, Varma JS, *et al.* Sacral reflex latency in acute urinary retention in female patients. *Br J Urol* 1987;**59**:311–3.
56. Varma JS, Smith AN. Neurophysiological dysfunction in young women with intractable constipation. *Gut* 1988;**29**:963–8.
57. Galloway NTM, Tanish J. Minor defects of the sacrum and neurogenic bladder dysfunction. *Br J Urol* 1985;**57**:154–5.
58. Fidas A, MacDonald HL, Elton RA, *et al.* Prevalence of spina bifida occulta in patients with functional disorders of the lower urinary tract and its relation to urodynamic and neurophysiological measurements. *Br Med J* 1989;**298**:357–9.
59. Koldewijn EL, van Kerrebroeck PhEV, Bemelmans BLH, *et al.* Use of sacral reflex latency measurements in the evaluation of neural function of spinal cord injury patients: a comparison of neuro-urophysiological testing and urodynamic investigations. *J Urol* 1994;**152**:463–7.
60. Shenot PJ, Rivas DA, Watanabe T, Chancellor MB. Early predictors of bladder recovery and urodynamics after spinal cord injury. *Neurourol Urodynam* 1998;**17**:25–9.
61. Vodusek DB. Electromyogram, evoked sensory and motor potentials in neurourology. *Neurophysiol Clin* 1997;**27**:204–10.
62. Vodusek DB, Zidar J. Pudendal nerve involvement in patients with hereditary motor and sensory neuropathy. *Acta Neurol Scand* 1987;**76**:457–60.
63. Ghezzi A, Malvestiti GM, Baldini S, Zaffaroni M, Zibetti A. Erectile impotence in multiple sclerosis: a neurophysiological study. *J Neurol* 1995;**242**(6):123–6.
64. Vodusek DB, Ravnik-Oblak M, Oblak C. Pudendal versus limb nerve electrophysiological abnormalities in diabetics with erectile dysfunction. *Int J Impotence Res* 1993;**5**(1):37–42.
65. Espino P. Neurogenic impotence: diagnostic value of nerve conduction studies, bulbocavernosus reflex, and heart rate variability. *Electromyogr Clin Neurophysiol* 1994; **34**(6):373–6.
66. Hanson Ph, Rigaux P, Gilliard C, Bisset E. Sacral reflex latencies in tethered cord syndrome. *Am J Phys Med Rehabil* 1993;**72**:39–43.
67. Sethi RK, Bauer SB, Dyro FM, *et al.* Modulation of the bulbocavernosus reflex during voiding: loss of inhibition in upper motor neuron lesions. *Muscle Nerve* 1989;**12**: 892–7.
68. Amarenco G, Kerdraon J, Adba MA, *et al.* Persistance du réflexe bulbo-caverneux permictionnel dans les hyperactivities vésicales d'origine neurologique centrale. *Progrès Urol* 1994;**4**:959–65.
69. Podnar S, Trsinar B, Vodusek DB. A neurophysiological study of primary nocturnal enuresis. *Neurourol Urodynam* 1998;**17**(4):358–9.
70. Deletis V, Vodusek DB. Intraoperative recording of the bulbocavernosus reflex. *Neurosurgery* 1997;**40**(1):88–92.

SECTION 4

Pathophysiology and management of pelvic floor disorders

Chapter 18

Urogenital prolapse

Patrick Hogston

INTRODUCTION

The word 'prolapse' is derived from the Latin word 'to slip' or 'fall' and occurs when pelvic organs descend into or through the vagina. Although studied for several hundred years, adequate scientific data on the epidemiology, natural history, and pathophysiology of urogenital prolapse is lacking. Similarly, data on which to make evidence-based decisions on the management of this complex condition is urgently required, particularly as women are living longer and attending more often with pelvic organ prolapse. This chapter assesses our knowledge of the pathophysiology and management of this condition.

TERMINOLOGY

Most descriptions of prolapse refer to the organ that is prolapsing i.e. urethrocele, cystocele, uterovaginal prolapse, enterocele and rectocele. Only the term 'deficient perineum' indicates possible etiology. Severity is variously described in a subjective manner such as mild, moderate or severe or first, second or third degree. The term procidentia is wrongly used to signify complete uterine prolapse as it is just another word for prolapse. Following hysterectomy the term 'vault prolapse' is often used interchangeably with enterocele although the two conditions are different and may occur in isolation or together. In more recent years an attempt to use a definition of the causal defect rather than the effect of the prolapse has gained some acceptance, particularly in the United States.

EPIDEMIOLOGY AND PATHOPHYSIOLOGY

INCIDENCE AND PREVALENCE

The true incidence and prevalence of urogenital prolapse is unknown. This is largely because many women do not have symptoms or present to a doctor. Most women after childbirth have some degree of pelvic floor laxity and asymptomatic prolapse is common. Prolapse is more likely to cause symptoms when the descending part is through the introitus and hence the condition often is only recognized relatively late in its natural history. Some women appear to progress rapidly to advanced prolapse whereas the majority that progress do so over many years. More than a third of patients with urinary incontinence have evidence of 'significant' prolapse which may not cause any symptoms.

A prevalence study of prolapse in a Swedish urban setting of 11 000 revealed 641 women aged between 20 and 59 years.[1] Based on examination of 487 women (76%) the prevalence of urogenital prolapse of any degree was 31%. However only 2% had a prolapse that reached the introitus and none had prolapse outside the vagina. Since many women with prolapse present after the age of 60, the true prevalence is likely to be have been underestimated in this study by a considerable degree. On the other hand most patients had only minor degrees of prolapse and were asymptomatic, and only 55% of the women were parous. Prevalence studies in institutions have suggested that 25% of women over 60 have urogenital prolapse whilst less than 10% are incontinent and hence further studies are required.[2]

Incidence data are only feasible for patients undergoing surgery, and the lifetime risk of surgery for prolapse or incontinence is approximately 11%.[3] This retrospective cohort study of 149 554 women over 20 years of age effectively included all women who underwent surgery for prolapse in 1995 from an estimated population of two million predominantly white Americans.

An English study, The Oxford Family Planning Study, recruited 17 032 women aged between 25 and 39 years between 1968 and 1974 to assess the effects of oral contraception on health.[4] On review in 1994 the incidence of hospital admission for prolapse was 2.04 per 1000 person years of observation. These data will significantly underestimate the true risk as many women who smoked heavily or were overweight were excluded. Furthermore the risk will continue to increase.

In England at least 20% of women on gynecology waiting lists are waiting for prolapse surgery. In 1993–94, 37 961 operations for urogenital prolapse were performed, a 20% increase from 1988–89.[5]

ETIOLOGY

Childbirth and parity

Prolapse is the result of damage to the pelvic support system. Weakness of the pelvic diaphragm may be due to direct injury or denervation. Along with damage to the perineal body this results in widening of the levator hiatus. This results in tension being placed on all fascial supports. These fascial supports may also be broken and this cascade of damage is most commonly due to childbirth. Vaginal delivery seems to carry the greatest risk which may be eliminated by elective but not emergency cesarean section. The Oxford study has clearly shown the effect of parity calculating that a woman with two children has 8.4 times the risk of surgery for prolapse compared with a nulliparous woman. The risk with more than two children only rises by a factor of 1.3 compared with two children.

Evidence of pelvic floor damage has been shown by both nerve conduction studies and electromyography (EMG). Other studies have relied on reinnervation as evidence of damage which may be an adequate compensatory mechanism. Recovery is common and there is a lack of direct association between neurophysiological results and pelvic floor function. Despite evidence of denervation and muscle damage from some centers, a group from Switzerland has shown no significant decrease in the strength of the pelvic floor 2 months after vaginal birth. It thus remains uncertain whether muscle damage or neuropathy is the primary mechanism for the development of urogenital prolapse.[6]

Connective tissue disorder

The endopelvic fascia has a major role in pelvic organ support. Defects and deficiencies can therefore contribute to urogenital prolapse. An observation that women with prolapse had a high incidence of joint hypermobility and abdominal striae supports this concept. Most biochemical studies have investigated incontinent women and the issue of cause or effect is still to be settled. However a study of pubocervical fascia in women undergoing prolapse surgery has shown a decrease in the number of fibroblasts and an increase in abnormal collagen.[6] Similarly a controlled study of collagen in a periurethral vaginal biopsy in incontinent nulliparous women showed quantitative and qualitative defects. Analysis of pubocervical fascia in the women undergoing surgery showed an increase in abnormal collagen compared with women having surgery for other reasons.[7] Norton has also shown an increase in weaker collagen III in women with urogenital prolapse.[6]

Congenital

Although the collagen changes discussed above may be congenital, conditions such as bladder exstrophy have an incidence of urogenital prolapse between 10 and 50%. Conditions affecting the spinal cord and pelvic nerve roots (e.g. muscular dystrophy, meningomyelocele) resulting in flaccid paralysis of the pelvic floor cause prolapse.

Increased intra-abdominal pressure and trauma

Chronic and repetitive increases in intra-abdominal pressure are etiological factors in urogenital prolapse. Indirect evidence of increased intravesical pressure in obese women (raised body mass index) which reduces with weight loss has been shown, although weight on its own is also a factor. Smoking causes an increased incidence of stress incontinence, but has not been shown to increase the risk of prolapse. It is postulated that constipation is a major factor in prolapse with 95% of women with prolapse being constipated at presentation, with two thirds straining long before they developed prolapse.[8] Such patients have been shown to have pudendal nerve damage. The risk of surgery for prolapse is also raised in women involved in heavy lifting, as shown in a review of 1.6 million women.

Davis reports pelvic floor defects and urinary stress incontinence in six nulliparous airborne infantry trainees. These women undergo repeated high-impact aerobics, but could date their problems to impact after parachute jumping when they suffered sudden lower quadrant pain. Paravaginal defects were identified and confirmed at surgery.[9]

Age and menopause

It is difficult to separate the effects of age from estrogen deficiency. Progressive deterioration in the quality and quantity of collagen in the skin has been shown to occur after the menopause. This was reversed by estrogen therapy which can improve urethral function in postmenopausal women.[6]

Ethnic origin

Racial variations have been discussed by Nichols.[10] Prolapse in African and Chinese women is rare. This is likely to be due to behavioral differences as parity in Bantus is high and birthweight is comparable with Europeans. The incidence of prolapse in Chinese women in Hong Kong is similar to Caucasians, suggesting aspects of Western lifestyle are responsible.[11]

Previous pelvic surgery

The importance of previous hysterectomy in the development of urogenital prolapse was examined in the Oxford study.[4] The cumulative risk rises from 1% three years after a hysterectomy, to 5% 15 years after. The risk of prolapse following hysterectomy is 5.5 times higher in women whose initial operation was for prolapse.

There is a significant risk of prolapse after fixation of the anterior vagina in the treatment of urinary stress incontinence. A figure of 27% is reported by Wiskind.[12] Conversely posterior fixation of the vagina by sacrospinous fixation may predispose to anterior segment descent.[13] Although rates of up to 90% are quoted in unreported series, these studies do not assess the likelihood of such prolapse in women with already weak pelvic support. Smilen reported a retrospective controlled study of 322 patients with anterior defects and 73 without. He then compared these women depending on whether sacrospinous fixation of the vaginal vault was also required.[14] He found an incidence of 11.7% recurrent cystocele in women undergoing sacrospinous fixation compared with 9.4% among patients who did not require fixation. In the small group without anterior prolapse, a similar number of *de novo* anterior defects occurred in those in whom sacrospinous fixation was performed as in those in whom it was not. Whether sacrospinous vault fixation independently increases the risk of subsequent anterior vaginal defects is thus uncertain.

PREVENTION

EPISIOTOMY

For many years it has been standard teaching on both sides of the Atlantic that episiotomy will prevent more extensive pelvic floor damage than would otherwise occur. When this hypothesis was formally tested it became clear that the opposite was more likely to be the case. The North American Randomized Controlled Trial of liberal versus restricted use of episiotomy performed a secondary cohort analysis of 697 women.[15] They showed that both primiparous and multiparous women with an intact perineum had the strongest pelvic floor at 3 months. Those with an episiotomy, particularly if it extended into the anal sphincter, fared worse than spontaneous tears. The odds ratio of anal sphincter damage with episiotomy versus no episiotomy was +22.08. The authors conclude that episiotomy is more likely to be the cause of pelvic floor damage than to protect against it.

PELVIC FLOOR EXERCISES

Antepartum and postpartum pelvic floor exercises are widely advocated in order to prevent pelvic floor dysfunction. There is limited evidence on their efficacy, although they may give some protection against urinary incontinence. In a prospective controlled study Morkved and Bo evaluated the effect of antepartum exercises on pelvic floor strength.[16] They found a significant improvement in the group undergoing exercises at 8 and 16 weeks, even though the control group had stronger contractions to start with. The significance of this in the long term has not been evaluated.

CESAREAN SECTION

Labor and delivery are significant factors in the development of urogenital prolapse and urinary stress incontinence. It is clear that cesarean section gives some protection against pelvic floor damage, even if carried out in the second stage. However much still needs to be understood about the interaction of the various risk factors leading to significant incontinence and prolapse after vaginal delivery.

As not all women with prolapse require treatment it is essential that one end point of studies is the need for treatment as well as the presence of prolapse. The risk of emotional problems due to failing to give birth naturally also needs recognition.

A prenatal scoring system of joint hypermobility, family history and other factors is being investigated. Currently, only pregnant women with prior surgically treated prolapse or incontinence need to be considered for cesarean delivery.[17]

AVOIDING GYNECOLOGICAL SURGERY

The chance of a woman having a hysterectomy by the age of 55 in the UK is estimated at one in five, and in the USA one in four. This equates to over 72 000 hysterectomies in the UK and 592 000 in the USA in 1994.[18]

The rate of hysterectomy for dysfunctional bleeding however may be falling as other less invasive treatments become available. Improved patient education, acceptance of medical treatment, intra-uterine devices containing Levonorgestrol, and endometrial ablative techniques may reduce the need for hysterectomy for both dysfunctional uterine bleeding and fibroids which account for approximately 70% of operations.

This is likely to be of benefit to the pelvic floor in view of the association of hysterectomy with prolapse discussed above. Although other types of gynecological surgery such as colposuspension predispose to prolapse, other etiological factors are common to both the operation and its indication, i.e. stress incontinence. Further research is required into this association and its management.

CLINICAL FEATURES AND ASSESSMENT

A history of a lump or swelling in the vagina, typically worse at the end of the day is almost universal. Bleeding from local trauma may occur with severe prolapse which may also need to be pushed back to urinate or defecate. Frequency and urgency occur with cystocele, as does incomplete emptying and double voiding. Stress incontinence may be present, but is often masked in more severe cases by urethral kinking (occult stress incontinence). Posterior wall prolapse is associated with constipation, incomplete emptying and the need for digital splinting. Other colorectal symptoms can cause these symptoms and the relationship to the prolapse needs careful assessment. Fecal incontinence is also associated with urogenital prolapse, the likelihood increasing with the severity of the prolapse. Sexual problems may be present, although these may be due to causes other than prolapse. Weber found the prevalence of sexual problems no different when prolapse was present, even when severe.[19] It is important to discuss the likely impact of any therapy on future sexual function.

On pelvic examination the diagnosis is usually obvious although vaginal cysts, urethral mucosal prolapse, urethral diverticulae and uterine inversion may confuse the inexperienced. The degree of prolapse can be assessed adequately in the dorsal position with the patient performing maximum Valsalva. Further information is not usually obtained by examination in the standing position.[20]

Attempts to record pelvic examination findings in a reproducible manner to allow communication and comparison have not been successful. Numerous systems of grading of prolapse have been proposed, the latest being one adopted by the International Continence Society, the American Urogynecology Society and the Society of Gynecologic Surgeons in 1996, namely, the pelvic organ prolapse quantitation (POP-Q) system.[21] It does not use terms such as cystocele or rectocele and is often perceived as complex. However it has been shown to be easy to learn and reliable.[22] The system refers to points on the vagina (not the organs that lie behind) with reference to the hymen (Table 18.1). The genital hiatus, perineal body and vagina are measured and recorded on a grid (Fig. 18.1). Stages 0–4 are than assigned and classified by which part of the prolapse is most dependent (Table 18.2). The system does not identify the defect responsible for the prolapse (e.g. central or paravaginal) and does not indicate what treatment is required. However it has gained acceptance as a method of description of prolapse, particularly in reports of surgical treatment.

Table 18.1 Points of reference for quantitative pelvic organ prolapse examination (POP-Q)

Point A Three cm above the hymen on anterior vaginal wall (Aa) or posterior vaginal wall (Ap). Point Aa roughly corresponds with the urethrovesical junction. These points can range from −3 cm (no prolapse) to +3 cm (maximal prolapse.

Point B The lowest extent of the segment of vagina between point A and the apex of the vagina. Unlike points A they are not fixed but will be the same as A if point A is the most protruding point. In maximal prolapse it will be the same as point C.

Point C The most distal part of the cervix or vaginal vault.

Point D The posterior fornix, which is thus omitted in women with prior hysterectomy.

Genital hiatus From midline external urethral meatus to inferior hymenal ring.

Perineal body From inferior hymenal ring to middle of anal orifice.

Vaginal length This should be measured without undue stretching of the vagina.

A	B	C
Genital hiatus	Perineal body	Vaginal length
A	B	D

Figure 18.1 Grid for recording prolapse measurements from POP-Q examination.

INVESTIGATIONS

Although unusual, upper urinary tract problems such as hydronephrosis, and even renal failure, have been described with complete prolapse and hence renal assessment by biochemistry and ultrasound will need to be considered in such patients.

Post micturition residual urine measurement by ultrasound or catheterization will identify patients in chronic retention who may also have voiding difficulty after surgery. Additional investigations such as cystometry will be required if incontinence is present, but occult stress incontinence is increasingly recognized as a potential problem. The incidence of occult stress incontinence is variously reported between 28 and 83%[23] and occult detrusor instability can also occur. It is not clear whether all patients require investigations and local availability will be relevant. Urodynamics with a pessary

Table 18.2 Staging of pelvic organ prolapse based on POP-Q examination

Stage 0	No prolapse.
Stage I	Most distal prolapse more than 1 cm above hymenal ring.
Stage II	Most distal point is 1 cm or less above hymenal ring.
Stage III	Most distal point is more than 1 cm below the hymenal ring but not further than 2 cm less the total vaginal length i.e. > +1 cm but < + (TVL-2) cm.
Stage IV	Complete vaginal eversion.

in situ may be helpful to determine which patients would benefit from a bladder neck procedure.[24]

Investigations such as dynamic fluoroscopy or ultrasound can demonstrate the presence or absence of enterocele which may save tedious dissection in the operating theatre.

If there is doubt whether a patient's symptoms are due to prolapse, a pessary can be used as a diagnostic test. This is particularly useful if isolated symptoms such as backache are the only presenting feature of an otherwise asymptomatic prolapse.

CONSERVATIVE MANAGEMENT OF UROGENITAL PROLAPSE

Any prolapse can be asymptomatic, especially rectocele, and it is rare for surgical treatment to be required in such patients. No active treatment (other than reassurance) is also an option for many patients, particularly if further childbearing is desired or the woman is elderly, frail and immobile. Postmenopausal women usually benefit from local estrogen to improve tissue quality and relieve dryness and itching. There is no evidence that pelvic floor physiotherapy improves prolapse, although it may prevent mild symptoms getting worse. Many women will live with their prolapse reasonably satisfactorily without surgical treatment.

Prolapse in neonates is usually effectively treated with digital reduction and pessaries, although surgery has been described.

INTRAVAGINAL PESSARIES

Hippocrates described conservative treatment with pessaries of a half pomegranate soaked in wine. Inorganic pessaries have been in use for hundreds of years and a wide variety are in use world-wide.

It is generally believed that pessaries are second-line treatment for prolapse, although formal studies to compare surgical with pessary treatment have not been carried out. In a survey of American Urogynecology Society members, most tailored the type of pessary to the support defect. In the UK, ring and shelf pessaries are the most widely used. Some ring pessaries are rigid and painful to fit, and a large uterine prolapse may still protrude through the ring. However soft pessaries can be removed by the woman to allow coitus. Complications include discharge, granulations and ulceration, erosion and very rarely malignancy. The frequency of changing is not established and the need may vary from person to person. Concomitant estrogen cream may reduce complications. Pessaries are effective, but are discontinued by 20% of women even if they do not wish surgery.

SURGICAL MANAGEMENT OF UROGENITAL PROLAPSE

HISTORY

Langenbeck is generally credited with the first documented vaginal hysterectomy, a procedure that was done for cancer in a woman with prolapse. Various operations to constrict the capacity of the vagina and introitus were described by European surgeons in the 1800s and Le Fort described vaginal occlusion in 1877. In France in 1859 Hugvier suggested amputating the cervix, and in the USA Kelly described repair of the anterior and posterior vaginal walls. Donald in Manchester put all three operations together to describe what is usually called the Manchester–Fothergill procedure in 1908. Victor Bonney elucidated the principles underlying surgery for prolapse in 1934. These have since been consolidated by cadaver dissection and magnetic resonance imaging.

Since Kelly's description of bladder neck support for stress incontinence many papers on the surgical treatment of prolapse have come from the USA. Heaney reported 565 vaginal hysterectomies for prolapse in 1934 and his technique is largely still in use. McCall's method of vaginal vault support is only altered by suture choice and Nichols popularized sacrospinous ligament fixation in the 1970s, previously described in the German literature. The concept of fascial defects and their repair was introduced in the late 1960s by Baden and Walker and further elucidated by Cullen Richardson. It is this concept that dominates surgical debate on pelvic floor reconstruction today.

PREPARATION FOR SURGERY

The decision to operate is taken jointly between surgeon and patient. However it is unlikely that surgery will improve an asymptomatic prolapse. It is the author's opinion that all postmenopausal women with prolapse should use preoperative estrogen, either local or systemic. The condition of the tissues improves and this management accelerates cutaneous healing by increasing local growth factors.[25]

With an increasingly elderly population it is important to fully assess general medical health prior to surgery. However the risk of surgery is more related to reduced organ reserve and medical disease than to age alone.[26]

US Medicare data for incontinence surgery published in 1997 showed a death rate of 3.3/1000 under 85 rising sharply to 16/1000 over 85.[27] Avoidance of unnecessary dehydration by prolonged preoperative starving prevents renal problems and avoiding hypothermia reduces cardiac morbidity. Elderly patients are more prone to infection, a problem that is exacerbated by prolonged preoperative admission. Assessment should thus be completed as an outpatient and admission to surgery time should be as short as feasible. Similarly, preoperative shaving should not be performed, and prophylactic antibiotics are recommended by most authorities. A policy for anti-thrombotic measures should also be in place.

PRINCIPLES OF SURGERY FOR PROLAPSE

The aim of surgical treatment for urogenital prolapse is to restore vaginal support and function. The emphasis is on reconstruction, hence the use of the term pelvic floor reconstruction when describing such surgery. This is invariably achieved by the operation of 'vaginal hysterectomy and pelvic floor repair' in primary cases. This poorly describes the procedure since hysterectomy achieves nothing other than removing the uterus and does not signify which part of the pelvic floor is repaired. Ideally the surgeon should identify the site, etiology and extent of damage in order to select the correct procedure.

The vagina is surrounded by a layer of fascia which is attached laterally to the arcus tendineus, superiorly via the uterosacral ligaments to the sacrum and inferiorly to the perineal body (Fig. 18.2). Bonney, in 1914, described three levels of damage to pelvic supports that should be considered[28] although his suggestion of the round and broad ligaments as being particularly important is no longer accepted. De Lancey has further clarified the fascial support with cadaver dissection and magnetic resonance imaging. He defines level I support at the apex through the cardinal-uterosacral ligaments. Level II represents the fascial support of the midvagina and level III is the support offered by fusion of the vagina to the perineal body and urogenital diaphragm. Loss of level I support causes cervical or vault prolapse, loss of level II cystocele or rectocele and level III low rectocele and deficient perineum. Loss of all three levels of support results in total vaginal eversion.[29]

It has been assumed that these fascial supports are stretched or atrophied in women with prolapse and that shortening and plication will restore the necessary support. However, Goff histologically examined the anterior vaginal wall in women with prolapse and could not find a stretched or thinned fascia. He thus concluded that the etiology was not stretching and was a subject for future research. Baden and Walker identified a 30% failure rate of surgery and after cadaver dissections proposed that *breaks* in the fascia, rather than stretching could account for all defects. They further proposed that these breaks should be identified and repaired individually when treating prolapse surgically.[30] This particularly applied to anterior and posterior wall defects where fascia could be torn either laterally from the arcus tendineus, centrally or both (Fig. 18.3). Similarly, in uterine prolapse the uterosacral ligaments may be detached from the cervix or torn near their sacral attachment (Fig. 18.4). If one accepts the above argument then the surgical challenge is to find these defects during surgery; this will radically change the way prolapse surgery is performed.

(a)

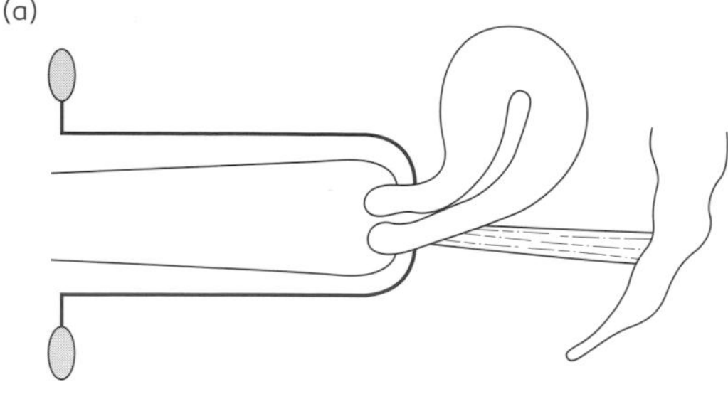

(b)

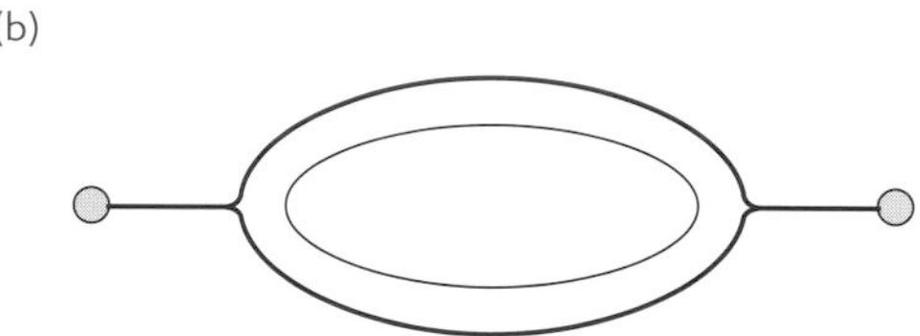

Figure 18.2 Fascial supporting layer of the vagina. (a) Longitudinal view; (b) transverse view at level of ischial spines.

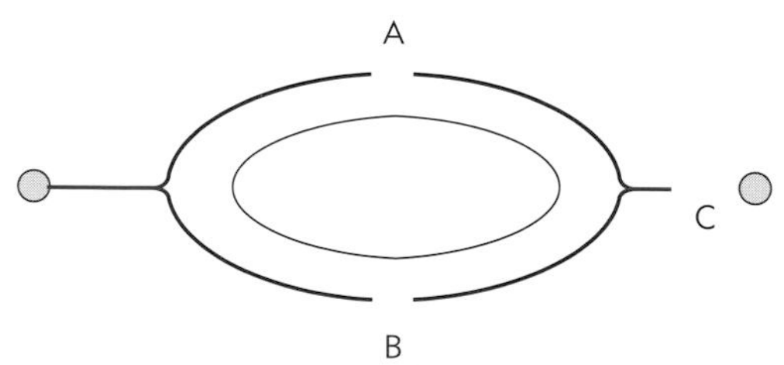

Figure 18.3 Cross-section of vagina at level of ischial spines to illustrate breaks in fascia. A: Central anterior defect. B: Central posterior defect. C: Lateral detachment at arcus tendineus.

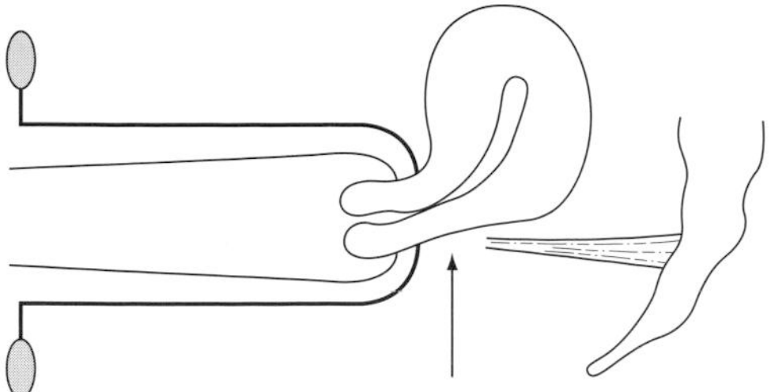

Figure 18.4 Diagram of uterovaginal prolapse with detachment of uterosacral ligament from the cervix (arrowed).

Another important surgical principle is the maintenance of vaginal length. If, after removal of the uterus the vagina is otherwise well supported and sits on an intact levator plate, intra-abdominal pressure applied to the vagina will be countered by pressure from the pelvic floor. The vagina will thus be compressed between the two and remain in place. If the vagina is shortened, it may telescope upon itself as intra-abdominal pressure is directed in the axis of the vagina. Preserving vaginal depth is thus an important feature of all genital surgery. In a woman with prolapse the vagina is displaced, not lengthened; hence it is erroneous to believe that there is excess vaginal skin, except in the most severe cases.

SUTURES

Little attention is given to suture selection in pelvic reconstructive surgery, perhaps for historical reasons when only catgut and silk were available. Neither should now be used, as superior synthetic sutures are available. Fascia holds sutures well but heals slowly. At 21 days catgut has lost all its strength and polyglycollic acid (PGA) 80% of its strength; however both will still act as a foreign body. These sutures are therefore not suitable for reconstructive surgery. As polyglactin and PGA handle well with good knot security, they are useful for pedicle tying at hysterectomy. If one uses an analogy with repair of inguinal hernia then permanent monofilament sutures such as Dermalon or polyester should be used as they maintain 80% strength at 2 years. However large knot size and protrusion into the vagina, bladder or rectum make them less than ideal for vaginal reconstruction. Delayed absorbable polydioxanone or polyglyconate are a reasonable compromise particularly for a first operation.[31]

Two types of permanent suture have been used in pelvic floor reconstructive surgery, namely, polytetrafluoroethylene (PTFE) and braided polyester. PTFE is a monofilament porous suture which is incorporated into adjacent structures by connective tissue ingrowth during healing whereas all other sutures are encapsulated. Although easy to tie the knots tend to slip and seven or eight throws are required. Because of the compression afforded by its porous structure, the total knot size is the same for three or four throws. Polyester is strong and available in fine sizes. However being braided it must be removed when there is infection. The size of the suture should not be too large, so as to avoid unnecessary foreign material, but not too thin to cut through the tissues. Smaller sizes are required for skin than fascia.

The other consideration is needle size and type. Cutting needles are not advised and needle punctures should be kept to a minimum. All sutures except PTFE are narrower than the needle and thus do not fill the hole made by the needle resulting in bleeding. As PTFE is 52% air, it is compressed at the junction with the needle and immediately expands to its designated size. Suture selection will be further discussed below but long-term data on the use of permanent sutures in the vagina are lacking.

SURGICAL TECHNIQUES FOR PROLAPSE REPAIR

Cervical amputation (Manchester–Fothergill procedure)

This operation was popularized by Donald in the UK in the early 20th century. After securing the uterosacral ligament the cervix is amputated and the ligament reattached to the cervix and vagina. Repair of the anterior and posterior vaginal wall is part of the procedure. It is important to reconstruct the cervix to avoid cervical stenosis and hematometra. The delayed presentation of intrauterine pathology is a major concern of this operation. The reported success rate was good and it was said to be useful in women wishing further children. However, It is probable that many women did not achieve this desire and today women would be encouraged to finish their childbearing before having reconstructive surgery. If this is not feasible, other operations such as abdominal hysterosacropexy or sacrospinous fixation would be more appropriate.

It would now be accepted practice to prefer vaginal hysterectomy as a more reliable way of mobilizing the supporting tissues of the cervix and upper vagina adequately for vault reconstruction. This also avoids future uterine pathology requiring hysterectomy. However occasionally where a women refuses hysterectomy, has an obliterated cul-de-sac or a very large uterus with an elongated cervix, the Manchester operation may be indicated. It will not succeed with severe prolapse as identification of the cardinal uterosacral ligament complex will be impossible.

Vaginal hysterectomy

Simple removal of the uterus does not support the vaginal apex. Successful support relies on shortening and re-attaching the uterosacral-cardinal ligament complex to the vagina. It is important to use a strong part of the ligament and if this has already been severed as the cause of the uterine prolapse it is important to find an adequate tissue support. Concern is often voiced in these situations about the position of the ureter. However De Lancey has shown increasing separation between the cervix and ureter with increasing uterine prolapse descent.[32] This means that patients with the largest prolapse can safely undergo the necessary shortening sometimes up to 15 cm. Whether this shortening is in fact finding the detached caudal end of the ligament previously torn as the cause of the prolapse may be academic. Following vaginal hysterectomy the vault should be supported by one of the techniques described below.

Support of the vaginal apex

Reconstructive techniques at hysterectomy

The support of the vaginal apex depends on the pericervical ring of fascia formed by fusion of pubocervical, rectovaginal and cardinal-uterosacral ligaments (Fig. 18.3).

Many techniques of vault support are described in the literature, most using the pedicle sutures themselves to resuspend the vault. McCall described his technique of culdeplasty in 1957, later modified by Nichols. After excising any enterocele sac a separate suture is placed through the full thickness of the vaginal vault (to include the rectovaginal septum) at a point selected to become the highest point of the reconstructed vault. The suture then picks up peritoneum and uterosacral ligament at the level to which the vault will be fixed. The suture then takes the same tissue on the other side and returns through the vaginal skin to be tied. McCall originally used silk, but a delayed absorbable material such as polyglactin or polyglycolic acid will cause fewer problems with suture erosion and granulation tissue. Evaluation of this method suggests an 85% success rate at 9 years.[33] Information from the Mayo clinic in a series of 693 patients with posthysterectomy vault prolapse identified only 47 (6.8%) patients with a previous vault repair after vaginal hysterectomy by this technique.

There is no evidence that sacrospinous fixation at the time of primary vaginal hysterectomy and repair offers any advantage. It may increase the complication rate.[34]

Posthysterectomy reconstruction

(I) CULDEPLASTY

Posthysterectomy vault prolapse is typically associated with enterocele formation. However enteroceles can occur alone without prolapse, when there is a break in the pericervical fascial ring. This defect can be repaired after ligating the enterocele sac by the McCalls technique described above. This method can also be used for posthysterectomy vault repair providing the ligaments can be identified.

The Mayo clinic reporting the use of culdoplasty in 693 patients with posthysterectomy prolapse[33] revealed that complications such as infection and bladder or rectal damage were infrequent (3%) and that there were no long-term sequelae. A postal survey of 660 patients operated on between 1976 and 1987 produced an 80% response. Only 36 (5.2%) patients had a major second operation; 493 (71%) patients, after a mean of 8.8 years had not had a further operation. Data on 164 (23.7%) were incomplete. Therefore culdoplasty is a very successful low morbidity procedure that should still be considered an operation of first choice.

An alternative method in posthysterectomy patients is to use the laparoscope to identify and tag the uterosacral ligaments at their attachment to the sacrum.[35] The enterocele is then opened vaginally and excised. The original sutures are retrieved and used to support the vaginal vault and the pericervical ring reconstructed. These authors[35] used 2-0 braided polyester, but did have some problems with suture erosions.

Identification of the cardinal-uterosacral ligaments is often difficult as they retract close to their origin at the sacrum. This is particularly true in total vaginal eversion when other techniques are usually indicated.

(II) SACROSPINOUS LIGAMENT FIXATION

Nichols popularized sacrospinous ligament fixation for posthysterectomy vaginal vault eversion. After opening the posterior vaginal wall and excising any enterocele sac the right rectal pillar is incised. The sacrospinous ligament is identified by a combination of blunt and sharp dissection. Two sutures are placed through the ligament two finger-breadths medial to the ischial spine. These two sutures are attached to the vaginal mucosa and held until the vagina is two-thirds closed. The sutures are then tied, thus firmly attaching the vaginal apex to the surface of the sacrospinous ligament without a suture bridge. Unilateral fixation is usually sufficient, but bilateral fixation can be considered in severe cases. It seems logical to use a non-absorbable suture, even though Nichols' original results used a combination of rapid and delayed absorbable sutures. Prolene, PTFE and Ethibond have all been used with attempts to bury the knots under the vaginal mucosa.

Over 1200 cases of sacrospinous fixation are reported in the literature, but follow-up times are often not specified, or are less than 1 year. The number of procedures performed in the UK is estimated to be between 2000 and 3500 per year (Cory Bros, personal communication) but the success rate and complications have been reported in the literature for less than 100 patients. The overall success rate in published series is between 77 and 92%, but early reports used absorbable sutures.

Specific complications of the procedure include buttock pain in approximately 3% due to damage to a small nerve running through the sacrospinous ligament. This settles spontaneously by 6 weeks. Gluteal pain and lumbar plexus neuropathy require immediate removal of sutures that have been incorrectly placed.

Cystocele is frequently reported as a long-term problem but only Smilen and colleagues have compared long-term results of similar patients undergoing pelvic floor repair with and without sacrospinous fixation (see above).[14] They found recurrent cystocele in similar numbers suggesting that other factors than the sacrospinous fixation determine subsequent cystocele. Subsequent stress incontinence is rare.

Although infrequent, more serious complications have been reported. With the more widespread use of the technique the overall complication rate may be under-reported. Life-threatening hemorrhage from laceration of the hypogastric venous plexus or inferior gluteal artery resulting in death has been reported. Anatomical variation means that the inferior gluteal artery may sometimes arise from the posterior division of the internal iliac artery. In this case, ligation of the hypogastric artery may increase pulse pressure and worsen hemorrhage. Vascular clips, packing or embolization are suggested in these difficult situations and involvement of other colleagues may be helpful.

(III) ILIOCOCCYGEAL SUSPENSION

Iliococcygeal fixation avoids the inherent risks of sacrospinous fixation because critical structures such as the gluteal vessels are not adjacent to the operative site. It also avoids acute posterior vaginal deflexion, but as the ischial spines are more inferior to the normal position of the apex the vagina is likely to be shorter. Partial vaginectomy seems to have been performed concomitantly in some reports which is itself a treatment, but will also result in a short vagina.

Obliterative techniques

There is still a limited indication for obliterative procedures in the very elderly woman by either partial or total colpocleisis. The partial operation described by Le Fort can even be performed under local infiltration. Total colpocleisis effectively excises most vaginal skin but can lead to stress incontinence.

Abdominal approaches to posthysterectomy reconstruction

The disadvantage of laparotomy is clear particularly in the elderly with more complications and a longer recovery time. However there are many reports of an abdominal approach to vault prolapse whereby mesh is interposed between the vagina and sacrum, an operation termed sacrocolpopexy. Positioning the mesh retroperitoneally involves careful dissection to avoid the ureter, middle sacral vessels, common iliac vein and mesocolon. Non-absorbable sutures are used to attach the mesh to vagina and sacrum with careful assessment of length to avoid overcorrection. Synthetic mesh is commonly Marlex, Mersilence or GoreTex and success rates in excess of 90% at 5 years are reported. A concomitant colposuspension can be performed if genuine stress incontinence is present, but any rectocele or deficient perineum will still require a vaginal repair.

A combined abdomino-perineal operation is described by Zacharin whereby the vagina is sutured to the levator plate after the levators are themselves sutured together. The abdominal surgeon retracts the ureters and places the most cephalad sutures. In a comparison by Creighton sacrocolpopexy was superior.[36]

Serious operative complications from sacrocolpopexy have been infrequently reported and are probably under-reported. Severe hemorrhage and death has occurred from presacral veins and the surgeon needs to be aware of the options including thumbtacks and magnetic applicators. Postoperative intestinal obstruction can occur if the mesh is not buried and graft extrusion and vaginal rupture can occur due to poor vascularity of the vaginal cuff itself.

The abdominal procedures have been performed via laparoscopy as opposed to laparotomy. Operating time is longer, but the risks of surgery seem similar in experienced hands. Initial success seems acceptable, but longer term results are awaited.

POSTHYSTERECTOMY VAULT PROLAPSE – WHICH OPERATION?

When the uterosacral ligaments are readily palpable McCall's culdoplasty with closure and excision of any enterocele is the first choice. When this is not possible or fails, then the choice is mainly between vaginal sacrospinous ligament fixation and abdominal sacrocolpopexy.

Experienced operators report high success rates with both procedures but vaginal operations have less morbidity. In younger women with concomitant urinary stress incontinence the abdominal approach is likely to be more appropriate, since colposuspension would be the operation of choice for stress incontinence.

In the absence of incontinence or cystocele, however, success rates are similar for both operations and the major difference is in the complications. For elderly patients it is clear that vaginal surgery carries less risk, lower morbidity, shorter hospital stay and faster return to normal activities. A comparative study from Canada reports a large personal series of 130 vaginal sacrospinous fixations and 80 abdominal sacrocolpopexies over 6 years. It is not clear why one operation was chosen over the other although 59 of the abdominal group (74%) had a colposuspension as well. The failure rate over a mean of 3 years was 2% in both groups perhaps highlighting good case selection for the procedures.

Benson[37] has reported the only randomized study of vaginal versus abdominal surgery for uterovaginal prolapse. Of 101 patients randomized 88 completed the study and half the patients in each group had complete pelvic organ prolapse (POP-Q Grade 4). Hysterectomy was performed in equal numbers in both groups and 35% of the abdominal group underwent Burch colposuspension. However other procedures such as Parks levatorplasty were also performed in 40% of patients. This is not widely practised by gynecologists and raises questions as to the relevance of this study to a general gynecologist's practice.

The effectiveness of surgical outcome in the vaginal group was classified as optimal in 29%, satisfactory 38% and unsatisfactory 33%. In the abdominal group surgical outcome was optimal in 58%, satisfactory 26% and unsatisfactory 16%. Abdominal sacrocolpopexy showed a higher success rate and the need for fewer subsequent operations. The relative risk of optimal effectiveness by the abdominal route was 2.03 and the relative risk of unsatisfactory outcome by the vaginal route was 2.11. The mixture of patients in each group makes it difficult to interpret the results, but the study shows that randomized surgical studies for vaginal prolapse are possible. Further studies are required to address these issues.

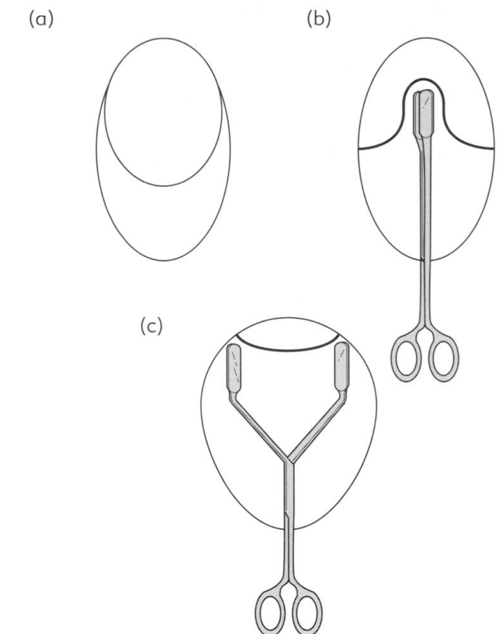

Figure 18.5 Clinical assessment of patient with large anterior wall prolapse due to a paravaginal defect. (a) Cystocele; (b) central support reveals lateral bulging; (c) lateral support reduces the cystocele.

Repair of anterior vaginal wall prolapse

Failure of anterior wall support results in prolapse of the bladder and/or urethra and sometimes stress incontinence. However if the anterior prolapse is severe stress incontinence may be masked by urethral kinking (occult stress incontinence).

Many surgical techniques for anterior wall prolapse are based on the presumption of the skin and fascia being stretched. These distention cystoceles usually have a smooth thin-walled appearance. After opening the vagina the fascia is plicated and the 'excess' vaginal skin excised. Kelly stitches plicate the bladder neck if stress incontinence is present. However defects in anterior vaginal wall support can occur laterally and superiorly as well as in the midline (Fig. 18.3). When hysterectomy is performed at the same time it is important to repair the fascia superiorly so that the pericervical ring is reconstituted. Failure to do so will result in a high cystocele. These displacement cystoceles retain the normal rugae of the vagina and thus often appear different to distention cystoceles.

Detachment of the fascia from the arcus tendineus results in a paravaginal defect which can be unilateral or bilateral and in conjunction with midline defects. Clinical examination with a modified sponge holder can usually distinguish the type of cystocele (Fig. 18.5). Midline support of the cystocele will still reveal lateral bulges with a paravaginal defect. Lateral support will reduce the cystocele if the defect is only at the arcus tendineus. However a central defect will still be revealed. It is uncertain how often these types of cystocele occur but lateral defects should be considered in recurrent cases.

Paravaginal defects have been repaired vaginally, abdominally and laparoscopically. The fascia is reattached to the white line although this structure can be difficult to see and weak and it may be necessary to place sutures into the obturator membrane and ischial periosteum.[38] Although high cure rates for cystocele are reported paravaginal repair is not adequate for stress incontinence. If stress incontinence is present an additional procedure to support the bladder neck or urethra is required (see below). In cases of two or more failed procedures, anterior repair with mesh is beneficial although erosion problems can occur.[39]

The reported success rate from anterior colporrhaphy for prolapse is 92% with up to 8-year follow-up. In the presence of stress incontinence, however, reported success rates are closer to 70%.[40] Furthermore, work from Austria has shown evidence of denervation of the urethra after vaginal surgery leading to a decrease in maximum closure pressure.[41] The surgeon is thus left with the decision as to whether to do an abdominal operation for incontinence in someone who would otherwise have a vaginal repair. In view of the increased morbidity of abdominal procedures we need to look carefully at what techniques are available for anterior prolapse in the presence of urinary stress incontinence.

By attention to technique and suture material, individual surgeons have produced good results from vaginal surgery. Beck described a vaginal retropubic urethropexy technique.[42] He reported a 94% success rate in 194 patients by (a) insertion of sutures close to the urethra at the level of the pubic bone to tighten and elevate the urethra; (b) using polyglycollic acid sutures rather than catgut; and (c) suprapubic catheter drainage. However this was an observational study with only 20 operations a year and was far from conclusive. Grody reported a technique of paraurethral fascial sling urethropexy and vaginal paravaginal repair in 75 patients using polytetrafluoroethylene sutures.[43] After opening the vagina two flaps of pubocervical fascia are fashioned and overlapped in a double-breasted fashion. Any paravaginal defect is repaired by re-attaching this flapped fascia to the obturator internus membrane and then any central cystocele repaired. At 2 years 92% of women were dry, but larger series using these techniques are required to confirm this encouraging result.

An alternative method is to create a weave of suture from one arcus tendineus to the other thus recreating the support to the urethra and bladder neck. Using PTFE a high rate of success in over 200 patients is possible with a low rate of complications (AD Clark, personal communication, 1999).

The surgeon is thus left with the hazard of a combined vaginal and abdominal operation with increased operating time and morbidity.

Treatment of occult genuine stress incontinence (GSI)

David Nichols addressed the issue of occult stress incontinence and advocated pubourethral ligament plication in massive prolapse in order to elevate the urethra and urethrovesical junction. Kelly's plication of the bladder neck is also necessary to eliminate funneling, but urethral plication is avoided as it narrows the lumen. Despite the appeal of this argument data to support his thesis have not been presented. Columbo addressed this issue in a randomized controlled trial of cystopexy alone versus cystopexy and pubourethral ligament plication in 102 continent patients undergoing surgery for prolapse.[44] At one year four patients in each arm (8%) had postoperative stress incontinence. They then investigated surgery in women undergoing surgery for prolapse and either stress incontinence or potential stress incontinence defined as 'positive stress test with repositioning' by randomizing 109 patients to either concomitant pubourethral ligament plication or Pereyra suspension.[45]

With a minimum 5 years follow-up, Pereyra suspension provided significantly better results for potential incontinence (100% v. 76% objective). However for incontinent patients the cure rate was only 57% and not significantly different in either arm. Complications were higher for the Pereyra group particularly reoperation. Veronikis proposes a sling urethropexy using Mersilene mesh or fascia lata for patients with total vaginal prolapse and a low pressure urethra with a 100% success at one year.[46]

It is possible that tension free vaginal tape could be used concomitantly with treatment of prolapse. In this technique a prolene tape is placed around the mid-urethra and relies on friction between the tape and the narrow canal formed by the introducer. However the patient needs to cough to test the tension and so that it can be adjusted if necessary and the operation is therefore usually done under local anesthesia. It is possible to do this prior to the introduction of a general anesthetic. The success rate is up to 86% with low failure rate.[47]

The optimum therapy for patients with urogenital prolapse and occult genuine stress incontinence remains to be determined.

Posterior vaginal wall repair

The indications for a posterior vaginal wall prolapse and rectocele are not always clear and need to be clarified with the patient. A decision to perform posterior repair should always be made preoperatively by examination of the unanesthetized patient. Posterior vaginal repair has been described for symptomatic prolapse, barium trapping, vaginal digitation during defecation, and as a prophylactic measure.[48] The latter is controversial since some surgeons advocate repair of all visible defects in all cases. However in the UK it is common not to repair small rectoceles when uterine prolapse predominates because they often cause little in the way of symptoms and posterior repairs are associated with vaginal stenosis and dyspareunia in a significant number of cases.

Repairing rectoceles for bowel symptoms needs careful consideration as other problems such as slow transit constipation or anal sphincter dysfunction may coexist. Constipation means different things to different patients and so the measure of success of surgery is equally difficult to quantify. It is important to remember that posterior vaginal wall repair may consist of three components – elimination of enterocele, repair of rectocele and perineorrhaphy.

Although most surgeons accept that rectoceles are due to defects in the rectovaginal septum, many textbooks on surgical technique do not describe posterior repair in terms of repairing this structure. Instead techniques such as suturing together of the levator ani muscles and excision of 'excess' skin is seen as paramount. However, this procedure brings the levator muscles into an abnormal position in front of the rectum thus leading to ridges and scarring. Similarly the excision of too much skin may result in vaginal narrowing. The high incidence of sexual problems after surgery may thus be explained by poor technique.

An alternative approach is to identify the defects in the rectovaginal septum and repair them. The problem lies in the fact that this septum is not always easy to define at surgery. Nichols showed that the rectovaginal septum is a distinct and relatively strong connective tissue layer 'always attached to the posterior aspect of the vaginal connective tissue but may be easily separated from it by blunt dissection'.[49] This adherence to the vaginal wall may partly explain why its existence has, at times, been denied. Surgeons may thus be working in the rectovaginal space whereas the defect of a mid-vaginal rectocele is on the vaginal side. A low rectocele is the result of detachment of the septum from the perineal body which must be reattached at the time of perineorrhaphy.

Data on the superiority of this technique are not easy to find as individual surgeons always believe their own technique is satisfactory. Follow-up data are not easy to collect and patients may not want to report adverse effects of surgery to the surgeon. Cundiff has reported on fascial repair of rectocele in 69 women.[50] At least half had other procedures, but perineorrhaphy was not performed. The fascial defects were repaired using 2–0 braided polyester, a permanent suture. He reports an improvement in symptoms of bulge in 87% at one year and a small decrease in dyspareunia. Splinting at defecation was eliminated in 69% and tenesmus resolved in 59%. Overall patient satisfaction was high. However this type of uncontrolled observational study assumes rather than proves that the repair is superior to other techniques and a randomized study is awaited.

Perineorrhaphy was not performed in the above study, yet is often necessary to draw the fascia of pubococcygeus closer to the perineal body and thus narrow the widened genital hiatus and lengthen the vagina. Stitches must not be placed in the belly of the muscle as this causes scarring and dyspareunia. The extent to which reconstruction of a loose outlet will improve coital satisfaction is overemphasized and other factors will be contributory.

With recurrent rectocele there is very little chance of effecting a simple fascial repair and a more radical approach is required. A rectovaginal examination will determine the defect and illustrate the amount of tissue available. A full dissection must be carried out to the lateral sidewalls and the full length of the vagina. If the vagina is shortened from previous surgery a zigzag vaginal wall incision later sutured longitudinally can give extra length. A ballooning rectum can be reduced by 2–0 polyglyconate or polydioxanone into the muscularis. Interrupted sutures should be placed transversely to rejoin torn rectovaginal septal fragments from each side. The rectum is depressed with the other hand, ensuring with each suture that the tissue is strong and will hold. Similarly sutures need to be strong and last and at least zero polyglyconate, polydioxanone or PTFE is required.[51]

A full perineorrhaphy is advised; this can add up to 5 cm of vaginal length. The base of the perineal body is restored by bringing adequate tissue from a relatively wide area to ensure insertion of bulbocavernosus and transverse perinei into their normal central attachments sites.

The biggest concern during this type of repeat repair is damage to the rectum. Full bowel preparation is rarely required and ensuring the lower bowel is empty by use of an enema is sufficient for most cases. If a perforation is made during the dissection copious lavage should be effected. However the dissection should be completed before attempting closure, particularly as the surgeon can now use the perforation as a guide to avoid other damage. Once completed the rectal wound is irrigated and repaired with 2–0 polyglyconate or polydioxanone. A stool softener should be used postoperatively.

POSTOPERATIVE CARE

Vaginal packing has advocates and opponents, but has never been subject to randomized studies. It is unlikely to be necessary in isolated vaginal hysterectomy or low rectocele repair but is widely used for more complex surgery. The aim is to use local compression to avoid blood loss from a large raw area and protect suture lines from sudden changes in intra-abdominal pressure in the early postoperative phase.

Suprapubic catheters are widely used after bladder neck surgery although indwelling catheterization followed by clean intermittent self-catheterization (CISC) is increasingly employed.

General care of the postoperative patient is standard, but aspects of nursing care are critical. This ranges from sitting patients up early to improve pulmonary ventilation, to ensuring spectacles and hearing aids are used as soon as possible to avoid sensory deprivation. Other aspects of nursing the often elderly patient include fluid balance and careful use of analgesics, since both narcotics and non-steroidal anti-inflammatory drugs have narrowed therapeutic ratios.

CONCLUSIONS

Urogenital prolapse is a common and apparently increasing problem in Western countries. Many issues relating to etiology and prevention still need to be resolved, particularly since they may affect obstetric care. Much is written on surgical techniques, but little scientific evaluation is available. Surgical trials are possible but remain difficult when so many variables are present. However with increasing emphasis on evidence-based medical and obstetric care the same criteria need to be addressed in surgical care.

REFERENCES

1. Samuelsson EC, Victor FT, Tibblin G, *et al.* Signs of genital prolapse in a Swedish population of women 20 to 59 years of age and possible related factors. *Am J Obstet Gynaecol* 1999;**180**:299–305.
2. Bump RC, Norton PA. Epidemiology and natural history of pelvic floor dysfunction. *Obstet Gynaecol Clin North America* 1998;**25**:723–46.
3. Olsen AL, Smith VJ, Bergstrom JO, *et al.* Epidemiology of surgically managed pelvic organ prolapse and urinary incontinence. *Obstet Gynaecol* 1997;**89**:501–506.
4. Mant J, Painter R, Vessey M. Epidemiology of genital prolapse: observations from the Oxford Family Planning Association study. *Br J Obstet Gynaecol* 1997;**104**:579–85.
5. Department of Health and Social Security Office of Population Censuses and Surveys. *Hospital In-Patient Enquiry Episode Statistics.* London: HMSO, 1996.
6. Gill EJ, Hurt WG. Pathophysiology of pelvic organ prolapse. *Obstet Gynaecol Clin North America* 1998;**25**:757–69.
7. Keane DP, Sims TJ, Abrams P, *et al.* Analysis of collagen status in premenopausal nulliparous women with genuine stress incontinence. *Br J Obstet Gynaecol* 1997;**104**:994–8.
8. Spence-Jones C, Kamm MA, Henry MM, *et al.* Bowel dysfunction: a pathogenic factor in uterovaginal prolapse and urinary stress incontinence. *Br J Obstet Gynaecol* 1994;**101**:147–52.
9. Davis GD, Goodman M. Stress urinary incontinence in nulliparous female soldiers in airborne infantry training. *J Pelvic Surg* 1996;**2**:68–71.
10. Nichols DH, Randall CL. Types of genital prolapse. In: *Vaginal surgery*, 4th edn. Baltimore: Williams & Wilkins, 1996:64–81.
11. Brieger GM, Yip SK, Fung YM, *et al.* Genital prolapse: a legacy of the west? *Aust NZ J Obstet Gynaecol* 1996;**36**:52–4.
12. Wiskind AK, Creighton SM, Stanton SL. The incidence of genital prolapse after the Burch colposuspension. *Am J Obstet Gynaecol* 1992; **167**:399–405.
13. Sze EH, Karram MM. Transvaginal repair of vault prolapse: a review. *Obstet Gynaecol* 1997;**89**:466–75.
14. Smilen SW, Saini J, Wallach SJ, *et al.* The risk of cystocele after sacrospinous ligament fixation. *Am J Obstet Gynaecol* 1998;**179**:1465–72.
15. Klein MC, Gauthier RJ, Robbins JM, *et al.* Relationship of episiotomy to perineal trauma and morbidity, sexual dysfunction, and pelvic floor relaxation. *Am J Obstet Gynaecol* 1994;**171**:591–8.
16. Morkved S, Bo S. The effect of postnatal exercises to strengthen the pelvic floor muscles. *Acta Obstet Gynaecol Scand* 1996;**75**:382–6.
17. Sultan AH, Stanton SL. Preserving the pelvic floor and perineum during childbirth – elective caesarean section? *Br J Obstet Gynaecol* 1996; **103**:731–4.
18. Vessey MP, Villard-Mackintosh L, McPherson K, *et al.* The epidemiology of hysterectomy; findings in a large cohort study. *Br J Obstet Gynaecol* 1992;**99**:402–7.
19. Weber AM, Walters MD, Schover LR, *et al.* Sexual function in women with uterovaginal prolapse and urinary incontinence. *Obstet Gynaecol* 1995;**85**:483–7.
20. Swift SE, Herring M. Comparison of pelvic organ prolapse in the dorsal lithotomy compared with the standing position. *Obstet Gynaecol* 1998;**91**:961–4.
21. Bump RC, Bo K, Brubaker L, *et al.* The standardisation of terminology of female pelvic organ prolapse and pelvic floor dysfunction. *Am J Obstet Gynaecol* 1996;**175**:10–17.
22. Steele A, Mallipeddi P, Welgoss J, *et al.* Teaching the pelvic organ prolapse quantitation system. *Am J Obstet Gynaecol* 1998;**179**:1458–64.
23. Rosenzweig BA, Pushkin S, Blumenfield D, *et al.* Prevalence of abnormal urodynamic test results in continent women with severe genitourinary prolapse. *Obstet Gynaecol* 1992;**79**:539–42.
24. Hextall A, Boos K, Cardozo L, *et al.* Videocystourethrography with a ring pessary *in situ*. A clinically useful preoperative investigation for continent women with urogenital prolapse. *Int Urogyn J Pelvic Floor Dysfunct* 1998;**9**:205–209.
25. Ashcroft GA, Dodsworth J, Van Boxtel E, *et al.* Estrogen accelerates cutaneous wound healing associated with an increase in TGF-B1 levels. *Nat Med* 1997;**3**:1209–1215.
26. Muller K. Operating on the elderly woman. *Curr Opinion Obstet Gynaecol* 1997;**3**:300–305.
27. Sultana CJ, Campbell JW, Pisanelli WS, *et al.* Morbidity and mortality of incontinence surgery in elderly women: an analysis of Medicare data. *Am J Obstet Gynaecol* 1997;**176**:344–8.
28. Bonney V. The principles that should underlie all operations for prolapse. *J Obstet Gynaecol Br Emp* 1934;**41**:669–83.
29. DeLancey JOL. Anatomic aspects of vaginal eversion after hysterectomy. *Am J Obstet Gynaecol* 1992;**166**:1719–24.
30. Baden WF, Walker T. *Surgical repair of vaginal defects.* Philadelphia: Lippincott, 1992.
31. Sanz LE. Sutures in gynaecologic surgery. *Contemp Obstet Gyn* 1998; **43**:57–72.
32. De Lancey JO, Strohbehn K, Aronson MP. Comparison of ureteral and cervical descents during vaginal hysterectomy for vaginal prolapse. *Am J Obstet Gynaecol* 1998;**179**:1405–1410.
33. Webb MJ, Aronson MP, Ferguson LK, *et al.* Posthysterectomy vaginal vault prolapse: primary repair in 693 patients. *Obstet Gynaecol* 1998;**92**: 281–5.
34. Colombo M, Milani R. Sacrospinous ligament fixation and modified McCall culdoplasty during vaginal hysterectomy for advanced vaginal prolapse. *Am J Obstet Gynaecol* 1998;**179**:13–20.
35. Miklos JR, Kohli N, Lucente V, *et al.* Site-specific fascial defects in the diagnosis and surgical management of enterocoele. *Am J Obstet Gynaecol* 1998;**179**:1418–23.
36. Creighton SM, Stanton SL. The surgical management of vaginal vault prolapse. *Br J Obstet Gynaecol* 1991;**98**:1150–54.
37. Benson JT, Lucente V, McClellan E. Vaginal versus abdominal reconstructive surgery for the treatment of pelvic support defects: a prospective randomised study with long

term outcome evaluation. *Am J Obstet Gynaecol* 1996;**175**:1418–22.

38. Scotti RJ, Garely AD, Greston WM, *et al.* Paravaginal repair of lateral vaginal wall defects by fixation to the ischial periosteum and obturator membrane. *Am J Obstet Gynaecol* 1998;**179**:1436–45.
39. Julian TM. The efficacy of Marlex mesh in the repair of severe, recurrent vaginal prolapse of the anterior midvaginal wall. *Am J Obstet Gynaecol* 1996;**175**:1472–5.
40. Weber AM, Walters MD. Anterior vaginal prolapse: review of anatomy and techniques of surgical repair. *Obstet Gynaecol* 1997;**89**:311–18.
41. Zivkovic F, Tamussino K, Ralph G, *et al.* Effect of vaginal surgery on the lower urinary tract. *Curr Opinion Obstet Gynaecol* 1997;**9**:329–31.
42. Beck RP, McCormick S, Nordstrom L. 25 year experience with 519 anterior colporrhaphy procedures. *Obstet Gynaecol* 1991;**78**:1011–18.
43. Grody MHT, Nyirjesy P, Kelley LM, *et al.* Paraurethral fascial sling urethropexy and vaginal paravaginal defects cystopexy in the correction of urethrovesical prolapse. *Int Urogyn J Pelvic Floor Dysfunct* 1995; **6**:80–85.
44. Columbo M, Maggioni A, Zanetta G, *et al.* Prevention of postoperative stress urinary incontinence after surgery for genitourinary prolapse. *Obstet Gynaecol* 1996;**87**:266–71.
45. Columbo M, Maggioni A, Scalambrino S, *et al.* Surgery for genitourinary prolapse and stress incontinence. A randomised trial of posterior pubourethral ligament plication and Pereyra suspension. *Am J Obstet Gynaecol* 1997;**176**:337–43.
46. Veronikis DK, Nichols DH, Wakamatsu MM. The incidence of low-pressure urethra as a function of prolapse-reducing technique in patients with massive pelvic organ prolapse (maximum descent at all vaginal sites). *Am J Obstet Gynaecol* 1997;**177**:1305–1314.
47. Ulmsten U, Johnson P, Rezapour M. A three year follow up of tension free vaginal tape for surgical treatment of female stress urinary incontinence. *Br J Obstet Gynaecol* 1999;**106**:345–50.
48. Kahn MA, Stanton SL. Posterior vaginal wall prolapse and its management. *Contemp Rev Obstet Gynaecol* 1997;**9**:303–310.
49. Milley PS, Nichols DH. A corrective investigation of the human rectovaginal septum. *Anat Rec* 1968;**163**:433–52.
50. Cundiff GW, Weidneer AC, Visco AG, *et al.* An anatomic and functional assessment of the discrete defect rectocoele repair. *Am J Obstet Gynaecol* 1998;**179**:1451–7.
51. Grody MHT. Posterior pelvis III: rectocele and perineal defects. In: Grody MHT. *Benign postreproductive gynecologic surgery.* New York: McGraw-Hill, 1995:247–76.

Chapter 19

Rectal prolapse

Alan P Meagher, David Z Lubowski, Michael L Kennedy

Rectal prolapse is not confined to humans, having been described in animals varying from emus to pythons.[1] In man the first description is said to be in the Ebers papyrus.[2] It is claimed that Hippocrates was the first to describe a treatment for this condition, hanging patients by the heels and shaking them.[3] In the 20th century our understanding of the etiology and treatment of rectal prolapse has advanced substantially, together with our knowledge of the symptoms of bowel dysfunction so often associated with it. A plethora of operative treatments for rectal prolapse have emerged during this time. While much has been learnt about the long-term results of some of these procedures, direct comparisons between different series of patients undergoing different procedures are of limited validity, and the next step in our understanding of this condition will come from the completion of prospective studies which compare long-term outcome following different operations.

RECTAL PROLAPSE IN CHILDREN

ETIOLOGY

Rectal prolapse in children is usually associated with a definite cause. Males and females are equally affected, most commonly children younger than 3 years.[4] The anatomy of young children, including vertical configuration of the sacrum and pelvis along with a mobile sigmoid colon is implicated as being of etiological importance.[5] Whereas in developed countries constipation and cystic fibrosis are common etiologies, in underdeveloped countries diarrhea is often causal. Malnutrition has been recognized as a predisposing factor,[6,7] possibly due to disappearance of the ischiorectal fat pad and loss of rectal support. In 1908 Lockhart-Mummery noted that 'rectal prolapse is a comparatively common affliction among children in that class which attends hospitals', and presumably the well nourished suffered this condition less frequently. In children with chronic respiratory disease, in particular cystic fibrosis when there is often associated diarrhea, rectal prolapse is common. In one study of 605 patients with cystic fibrosis 112 (19%) developed rectal prolapse; in one third of these the prolapse preceded diagnosis of cystic fibrosis.[8] Another study found that 23% of 386 children with cystic fibrosis developed rectal prolapse.[9] It has been suggested that a sweat test be carried out in all children with rectal prolapse in whom the cause is unknown. The condition has also been associated with meningomyelocele, spina bifida, Ehlers–Danlos syndrome, Hirschsprung's disease, and straining at urination due to phimosis.[4,10–12]

CLINICAL FINDINGS

Symptoms include straining at stool, perianal discomfort, passage of mucus and blood onto the nappy, abdominal pain, diarrhea, and symptoms of the cause of the prolapse. Often the sphincters are lax and there may be excoriation of the perianal skin. Malnutrition may be present.

TREATMENT

Conservative

Conservative management of the prolapse is initially attempted.[4,5,13] Although there are no large series outlining the long-term success rates of this treatment, it does appear that in the majority of patients this is successful. It is thought that normal development of the child's anatomy results in resolution of the condition. Stool softeners or anti-diarrheal medications may be used as indicated. Manual support of the perineum during defecation, and defecation in the recumbent position are said to be helpful.[4] Taping the buttocks together when the prolapse occurs between episodes of defecation may also be used. Children should not be allowed to sit for defecation longer than necessary. Malnourished children will require nutritional support.

Surgery

A number of surgical procedures have been described to treat childhood rectal prolapse, with control of the prolapse in over 95% of patients in almost all series. This suggests both that conservative treatment might be tried for longer periods in some patients and that the less invasive operative interventions should initially be used. Injection sclerotherapy has been described using various solutions including 30% saline,[14,15] 70% alcohol[16] and 50% dextrose in water.[17] Phenol has been used less often in children.[17,18] All have been associated with success rates of over 90%, although up to three injections may be required. Sclerotherapy may be used for both mucosal and full-thickness prolapse. Generally it is advised that sedation or general anesthesia is used. Via a transanal or perianal approach the sclerosant is injected circumferentially into the submucosal planes and perirectal tissues just above the dentate line and proximally for 6–8 cm. Complications, which include abscess formation and bleeding from injection sites, are uncommon. It has been suggested that because of its effectiveness and low morbidity injection therapy should be considered as the first treatment if conservative measures are not successful.[17]

Excellent results are also reported with anal encircling Thiersch procedures.[7,19–21] The suture, absorbable or non-absorbable, is placed around the anus under general anesthesia. Suture breakage or erosion through the skin may occur, as with adults. After three months the suture can be removed at a planned second procedure, by which time the prolapse will not recur. The Delorme's procedure has been applied successfully in children with no morbidity in one series of six patients.[22] Ekehorn's rectopexy employs a non-absorbable mattress suture placed trans-anally through the rectal ampulla, then through the lowermost part of the sacrum and overlying skin and tied over a dry gauze at the level of the sacrococcygeal ligament. The suture is removed after 10 days. Recent series report excellent results with minimal morbidity.[23]

Linear cauterization of the ano-rectum has also been reported in a large series of 73 patients, with successful control of the prolapse in all but two patients.[24] More complex operative procedures include posterior plication of the rectum via a perineal approach,[25] and the Lockhart-Mummery operation where, through a posterior perianal approach the presacral space is dissected and packed with mesh which is slowly removed over eight to ten days.[5,26] Alternatively Gelfoam has been used to pack the presacral space in one series of 100 patients, with complete cure reported in every case.[6] Perineal rectosigmoidectomy has also been used.[27] It appears that these procedures can be avoided in the majority of cases.

RECTAL PROLAPSE IN ADULTS

INCIDENCE

In most series of operations for rectal prolapse females outnumber males by about ten to one.[28–31] Amongst females the incidence rises steadily with age, whereas in males there does not appear to be such an increase.[32,33] The incidence of prolapse does not appear to be lower in nulliparous women, although these patients are less likely to suffer fecal incontinence.[34] Goligher found that in a series of 83 women 39 were nulliparous,[32] while in 183 women treated at St Mark's Hospital 72 were nulliparous[35] suggesting that the incidence of prolapse may be higher in women who have not borne children. This is a surprising observation since it does not seem to fit with the finding that about two thirds of women with rectal prolapse have neurogenic weakness of the pelvic floor,[36] which is usually a consequence of childbirth.

PREDISPOSING FACTORS

Senile dementia and mental illness are said to predispose to prolapse.[37] Goligher noted that in his series of 100 patients 64 were normal, 33 were 'rather odd' and three were psychotic.[38] Another series noted that 53% of patients had mental illness.[39] However, in a series of 187 patients from Birmingham only two had senile dementia.[13]

Many patients with rectal prolapse give a history of straining at stool. A subgroup of patients also has slow transit constipation.[40] One report describes patients whose prolapse is associated with a hypermotile sigmoid colon and fecal incontinence.[41] Both schistosomiasis and amoebiasis have been reported in Egypt.[42] Rectal prolapse is a recognized complication of systemic sclerosis, and is often associated with fecal incontinence in these patients.[43] Recently seven cases were reported of bulimia nervosa complicated by rectal prolapse. Laxative abuse, malnutrition, and increased intra-abdominal pressure associated with vomiting are proposed causes for this relationship.[44] There are also cases of acute rectal prolapse after ingestion of oral cathartics taken for medical investigations, which did not lead to recurrent prolapse.[45] One case of acute prolapse following blunt abdominal trauma eventually required surgical treatment.[46]

Rectal prolapse may be associated with an intra-abdominal mass such as ovarian tumor.[47] Although this may be coincidental, secondary constipation with consequent straining may be implicated. Increased joint mobility has been observed in patients with rectal prolapse compared with age- and sex-matched controls.[48] It is well recognized that occasionally a colonic polyp or carcinoma may cause intussusception and present as rectal prolapse. One study followed 70 consecutive patients treated for rectal prolapse for a mean time of 4.4 years, and compared their incidence of cancer with a control group of 350 patients.[49] The incidence of rectosigmoid cancer in the study group was statistically greater than the controls (5.7% v. 1.4%, $p < 0.02$) and the study concluded that patients with rectal prolapse should at least undergo flexible sigmoidoscopy.

PATHOLOGY

Using cineradiography with contrast material in the rectum, distal colon, small bowel (lying in the pouch of Douglas), vagina and bladder, Broden and Snellman studied patients during straining and demonstrated that the initial event in the production of a prolapse is a circumferential intussusception of the rectum, usually starting 6–8 cm from the anal verge. The apex passes down through the lower rectum and out of the anus. [50] In large prolapses the pouch of Douglas, which may contain loops of small bowel, also passes through the anus. Previously Moscowitz had proposed that rectal prolapse was due to a sliding hernia and that repair of this hernia, by obliteration of the deep peritoneal pouch of Douglas will treat the prolapse.[51]

CLINICAL FINDINGS

The majority of patients experience a rectal prolapse which reduces spontaneously after defecation. In some patients prolapse occurs spontaneously, which may be accompanied by discomfort and seepage of mucus. Not all patients are aware of the prolapse and fecal incontinence may be the presenting symptom.

Examination may reveal a typical prolapse appearance, with a lax sphincter which gapes on traction due to loss of internal sphincter tone. External sphincter squeeze may be reduced and the levators are flaccid and contract poorly. The skin at the anal verge appears thickened, with loss of corrugations, and prolapsing mucosa may be visible. When the patient strains down while lying in the left lateral position, the full thickness prolapse may appear. When this does not occur the prolapse may be demonstrated by straining while sitting on the toilet. An examination under anesthesia is then occasionally required to confirm that a full thickness prolapse is present. There may be an associated rectocele, enterocele or vaginal vault prolapse.

Not all patients with prolapse have weakness of the pelvic floor musculature, and in some cases there may be no abnormality on initial inspection. The sphincter then feels normal on digital examination and the prolapse often appears rather suddenly on straining down.

INVESTIGATIONS

In early studies of patients with rectal prolapse, Neill and colleagues showed that in two thirds of patients, sphincter function was similar to patients with fecal incontinence and that both groups had evidence of neurogenic sphincter weakness.[36] The remaining patients with prolapse had normal sphincter function and most were continent. An understanding of this distinction is important when predicting the likely outcome of surgery.

Anal manometry and electrophysiology quantify sphincter function and help in making this prediction. Manometry may identify weakness of the internal and external sphincters, with reduced resting and squeeze pressures as well as reduced sphincter length.[36,52] These features are indicative of both neurogenic sphincter weakness as well as mechanical dilatation of the internal sphincter. Pudendal nerve motor conduction studies will show prolonged latencies when a neuropathy is present.[53] Anal mucosal electrosensitivity will be reduced, reflecting a sensory deficit in the pudendal nerves,[54] but also possibly due to prolapse of relatively insensitive mucosa from the rectum or ano-rectal junction into the anal canal. Single fiber electromyography will confirm neurogenic change in the external sphincter. The internal sphincter may be thinner than normal, which may be demonstrated with endoanal ultrasound.[55]

Some patients with rectal prolapse are constipated, which may be associated with prolonged colonic transit time. This may be due to slow transit through the left colon or there may be a more diffuse abnormality affecting the left and right sides of the colon. This is demonstrated with radio-opaque markers or isotope colon transit studies.[56]

SURGICAL TREATMENT

Surgical treatment of rectal prolapse remains one of the most controversial and difficult areas in colorectal surgery. Given the widely differing views expressed in the literature and the large number of operations described, surgeons frequently base their preferences for various operations on anecdotal personal experience. For no particular scientific reason different operations have been in vogue in different continents, with the Ripstein rectopexy popular in North America and Australasia while the Wells-type procedures were practised in Europe. Perineal procedures lost popularity but recently there has been much renewed interest in both the Delorme's operation as well as perineal rectosigmoidectomy.

It is critical to define outcome measures after surgery:

- Incidence of recurrent prolapse.
- Restoration of continence.
- Incidence of postoperative constipation.
- Morbidity, particularly sexual dysfunction in males.

These factors often need to be balanced against one another and the choice of treatment must be tailored for the individual patient.

Most detailed texts on rectal prolapse devote considerable space to numerous operations that are rarely if ever performed such as the Gant–Miwa procedure, Lahaut's procedure, the Orr–Loygue rectopexy, the Moschowitz repair, the Hughes levator plication, and the Goligher–Graham levator repair. Although these operations may be of some interest, this chapter will concentrate on the procedures most commonly used. Although the authors do not practice or recommend the Thiersch procedures, these are still in use in some centers and will also be included. The following procedures will therefore be discussed:

1. **Perineal procedures**
   - Thiersch procedure
   - Delorme's procedure
   - Perineal rectosigmoidectomy
2. **Abdominal procedures**
   - Rectopexy
   - Resection rectopexy
   - Anterior resection.

PERINEAL PROCEDURES

Thiersch operation

Encirclement of the anal canal with silver wire was first described by Carl Thiersch in 1891.[57] Although never considered an ideal operation for prolapse in adults, it has been advocated by many for very debilitated patients as the procedure can be performed quickly with minimal dissection under regional or local anesthetic. The exact operative technique varies, but generally two incisions are made on opposite sides of the anal verge and curved clamps are used to create a tunnel around the anal canal and sphincters. Various materials have been used to encircle the anus, including knitted Dacron,[58] silastic rings,[59] stainless steel or silver wire, or nylon,[39] Dacron-reinforced silastic,[60] the Angelchik anti-reflux prosthesis,[61] Dacron-impregnated Silastic sheet,[62] a helical silastic encircler,[63] two separate silicone rubber perianal sutures,[64] a specially designed silicone elastomer surrounded by silicone-coated Dacron tape[65] and polypropylene mesh.[66]

Most series are small and there has been a notable decrease in published series over the last decade. This decline has been matched by increasing interest in the alternative perineal operations, Delorme's procedure and perineal rectosigmoidectomy. It does appear that recurrence rates with the Thiersch procedure are high, varying from 27% to 39% in three recent series of 15 to 41 patients.[39,58,59] In addition there are frequent reports of complications related to the placement of the foreign encircling material, such as sinus formation, infection including Clostridial myonecrosis,[67] cutting out, breakage, stretch, and fecal impaction, necessitating removal in up to 59% of cases.[39] For these reasons the present authors do not use the Thiersch operation.

Delorme's procedure

Edmond Delorme, a French military surgeon, was the first to describe transanal mucosal sleeve resection as a treatment of rectal prolapse. His initial report outlined the treatment of three patients, one of whom died postoperatively. Although this procedure did not initially achieve wide acceptance, recently there has been renewed interest.

Operative procedure (Fig. 19.1)

Full bowel preparation and antibiotics are given. The procedure may be carried out in the lithotomy or prone jack-knife position. The authors prefer the lithotomy position. The rectum is maximally prolapsed using a series of Babcock clamps placed circumferentially. Some surgeons infiltrate the submucosa with a 1:300 000 adrenaline solution and then use scissors or a cutting diathermy for dissection, but we prefer not to use any infiltration and rely on coagulation diathermy for the entire dissection. The mucosa is incised circumferentially at the dentate line, and a mucosal tube is dissected from the prolapsed bowel. Large submucosal vessels are either diathermized or ligated. The mucosa is usually easily dissected from the underlying muscle in this way and the coagulation diathermy technique allows the operation to proceed in a bloodless field. When there is an associated solitary rectal ulcer syndrome with edema and ulceration of the mucosa, then the mucosa may be adherent and the dissection may be more difficult. Once the dissection reaches the apex of the prolapse, the mucosal tube is dissected from within the prolapse for 1–2 cm, at which point it is excised. A series of 3/0 Vicryl sutures are then placed to plicate the prolapse. Each suture begins at the divided mucosa at the dentate line and then takes several bites of muscle, to end at the mucosa within the prolapse. The sutures are placed circumferentially and held, before being tied.

Results (Table 19.1)

It should be recognized that a comparison of studies is of limited value due to very variable patient selection for this operation. One study reports only performing the Delorme's procedure in patients who are 'poor candidates for a major abdominal approach'.[68] Another study found that the recurrence rate following Delorme's procedure was significantly lower in younger patients than in elderly or poor risk patients who were not suitable for an abdominal procedure (5% v. 22.5%).[69] When compared with large series of patients undergoing rectopexy the recurrence rate with Delorme's procedure appears to be higher.[70] This may be related to patient selection, although during a Delorme's procedure the decision regarding the length of mucosa to resect is difficult and some recurrences may be related to a learning curve with this procedure. In two studies largely with elderly or unfit patients, it was concluded that because of favourable results the Delorme procedure should be used more readily in all patients with rectal prolapse.[70,71]

Although morbidity reported in some publications is high this tends to relate to minor conditions such as

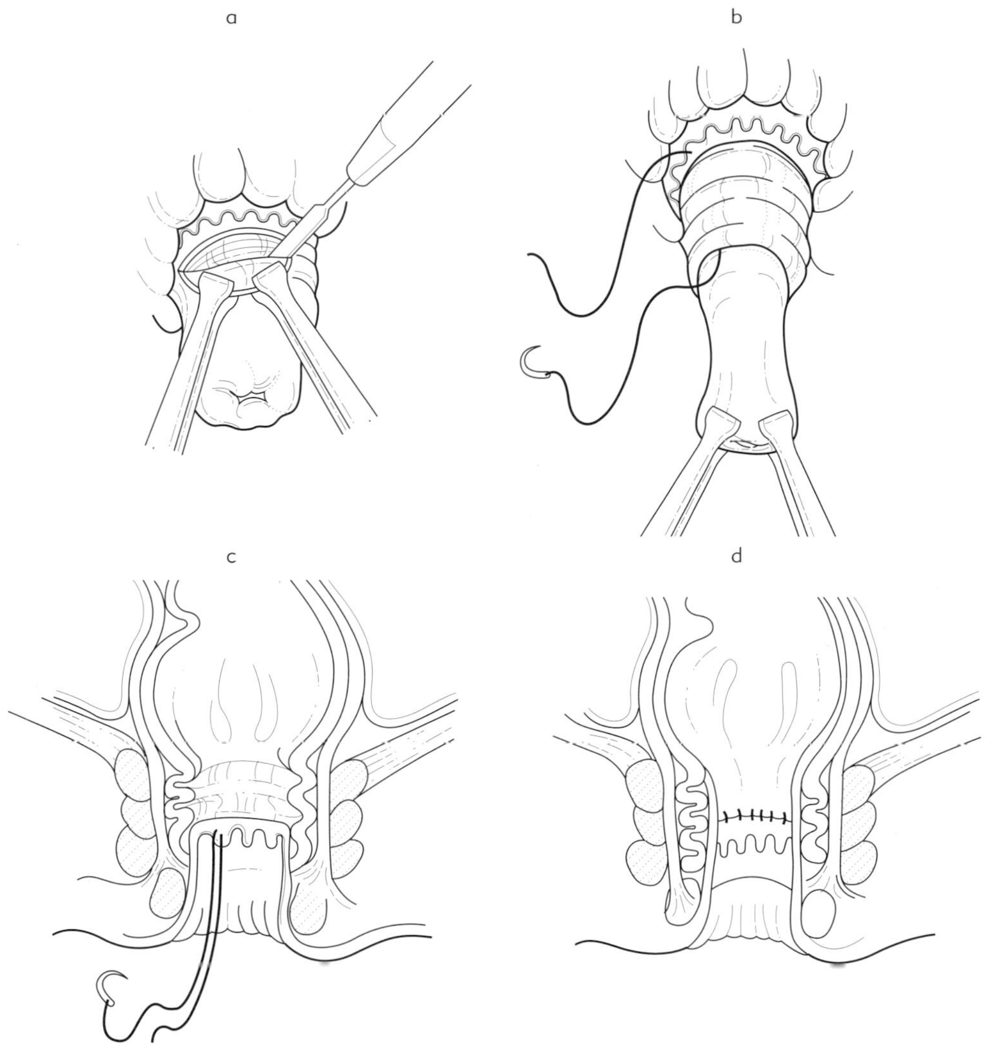

Figure 19.1 Delorme's procedure. (a) The mucosa is dissected for the prolapse. (b) A series of plicating sutures is placed, taking several bites of muscle. (c) Once all the sutures have been placed and held, they are tied to reduce the prolapse. (d) A corrugated muscular tube is created, theoretically creating a zone of pressure.

urinary tract infections or the patient's medical status such as cardiac failure. Operation-specific complications are rare and include hemorrhage from the suture line and late anastomotic stenosis.

Delorme's operation is often used to treat recurrent prolapse, being the indication for surgery in one third of the patients in one series.[70] This is usually following a previous abdominal procedure, although second or third Delorme's procedures have also been performed.

Constipation, which is relatively common after rectopexy, does not appear to be a complication of Delorme's procedure. In one study 50% of those who complained of constipation pre-operatively improved following operation,[70] and in another no patient developed constipation.[72] Measuring anal sphincter pressure, rectal compliance and sensation before and after surgery the volume of first rectal sensation decreased from a median of 140 ml preoperatively (which is abnormally high) to 65 ml after surgery ($p = 0.001$) and the maximal tolerable volume decreased from a median of 249 ml to 120 ml ($p = 0.001$).[72] Rectal compliance changed from a median of 143 mL/kPa to 12 mL/kPa ($p = 0.002$) and it was concluded that the improved rectal sensation and lower compliance were associated with a reduced incidence of defecation problems after Delorme's procedure. Although there was a 17% recurrence rate, the operation was proposed as the treatment of choice in patients with defecation disorders.

Table 19.1 Results of Delorme's procedure

	No. Pts	Mean follow-up (months)	Morbidity (%)	Mortality (%)	Recurrence (%)	Continence improved (%)
Uhlig, 1979[150]	44	NS	34	0	7	NS
Christiansen, 1981[151]	12	36	0	0	17	50
Houry, 1987[152]	18	18	NS	0	17	44
Gundersen, 1985[153]	18	42	17	0	6	NS
Monson, 1986[154]	27	35	0	0	8	83
Abulafi, 1990[155]	22	29	30	0	5	86
Graf, 1992[156]	14	18	7	0	21	55
Senapati, 1994[70]	32	24	6	0	12.5	46
Tobin, 1994[71]	49	20	8	0	22	80
Oliver, 1994[68]	40	47	25	2.5	20	68
Lechaux, 1995[69]	85	33	14	1	13.5	69
Plusa, 1995[72]	19	NS	0	0	NS	28
Kling, 1996[157]	6	11	0	0	17	67
Watts, 2000[79]	101	36[a]	5	4	30	89[b]

[a] Minimum 12 months.
[b] 35% completely continent; 89% unchanged or improved.

Perineal rectosigmoidectomy

This operation was first described by Mickulicz in 1889[73] in a patient with irreducible prolapse, and indeed remains the operation of choice for gangrenous or irreducible prolapse. Both Miles and Gabriel reported using this technique.[74,75] Following an early report from St Mark's Hospital in which the results were disappointing with a recurrence rate of 58% and a postoperative incontinence rate of 76%, the procedure fell out of favor.[76] However, Altemeier later popularized the technique of one-stage perineal rectosigmoidectomy and later added levatoroplasty to improve postoperative incontinence.[37] There is concern that poor postoperative bowel function after perineal rectosigmoidectomy may partly be related to replacing the compliant capacious rectum with narrowed sigmoid colon, and performing a stapled colonic J-pouch–anal reconstruction may be advantageous.[13]

Operative technique (Fig. 19.2)

The procedure is carried out in the prone jack-knife position to have appropriate access for the anastomosis. General anesthesia is preferred but spinal anesthesia can be used. Full bowel preparation and intravenous antibiotic cover are given. The rectum is prolapsed, and a circumferential incision is made through the mucosa about 1 cm beyond the dentate line. The level at which this incision and the subsequent dissection is made should take into account the length of the internal sphincter in the particular patient, so that the bowel will be divided at a point which allows complete preservation of the internal sphincter. The dissection is continued through the submucosa using the coagulation diathermy and large vessels are individually coagulated or ligated. Then the muscle layer of the rectum is divided in a similar way. The rectum is drawn down to expose the peritoneal reflection over the rectovaginal septum, which is incised to enter the peritoneal cavity. This is a key step in the procedure, which can at times be difficult if the sphincter is long and the levators are not neuropathic and weakened. Once the peritoneal cavity has been exposed, the rectum and sigmoid are drawn down as far as possible. If the sigmoid is tethered then only the distal sigmoid will be drawn down, but in other cases a greater length of sigmoid will be resectable. The sigmoid mesentery is ligated and divided. The levator muscles are then

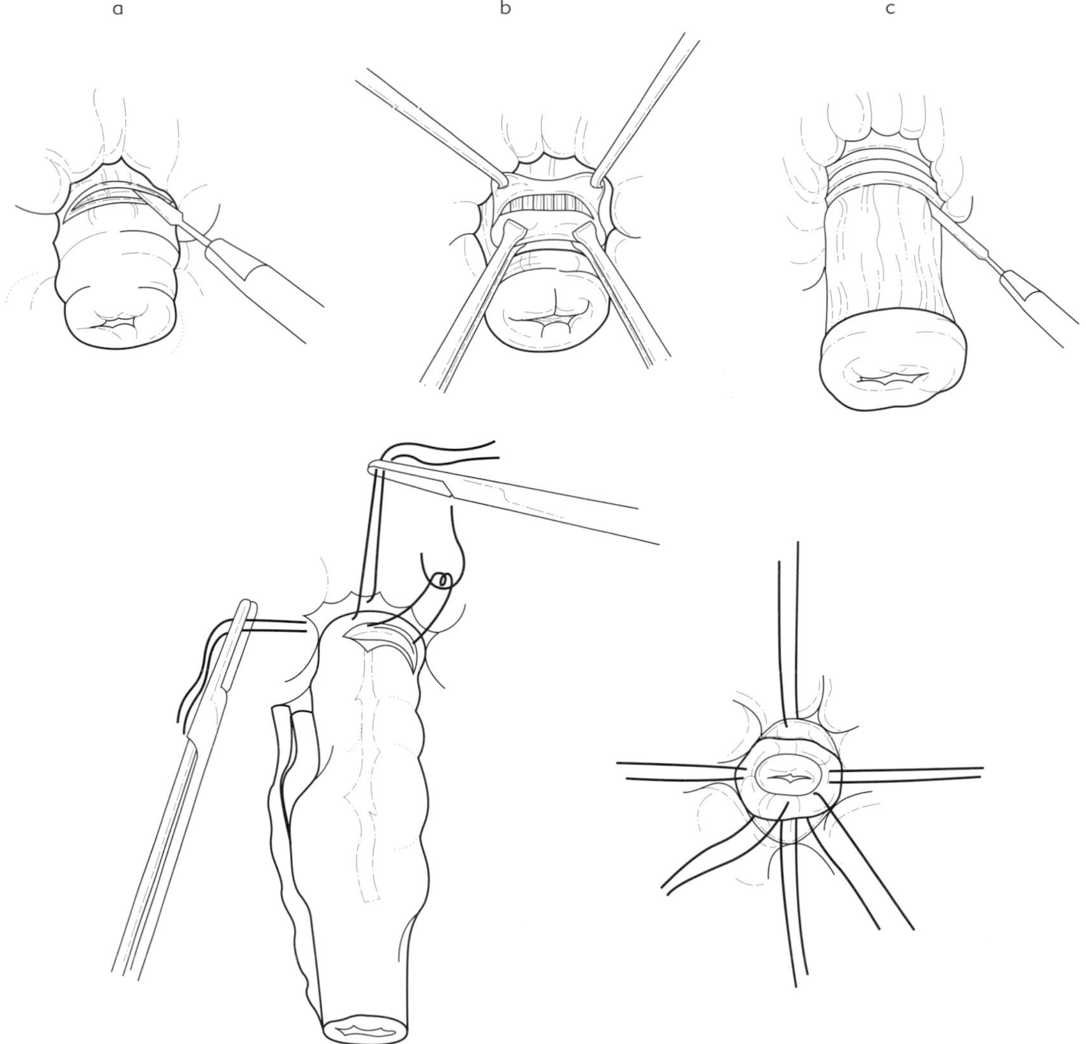

Figure 19.2 Perineal rectosigmoidectomy. (a) The outer tube is incised circumferentially. (b) The edge of the peritoneal reflection is opened. (c) The rectum and any mobile part of the sigmoid are drawn down and the segmental blood vessels are ligated. (d) The inner tube is incised and a series of interrupted sutures is placed. (e) The sutures are held until all have been placed around the circumference, before tying to complete the coloanal anastomosis.

plicated in front of the bowel using a series of 2/0 Vicryl sutures. The sigmoid colon is then divided and anastomosed to the anal canal using interrupted 3/0 Vicryl.

Results

Table 19.2 shows that the incidence of morbidity and mortality is low. Despite being a colo-anal anastomosis leak rates are very low. The duration of hospitalization was noted in five of the studies, varying from a median of 4 days[30] to a mean of 13.5 days.[77] Recurrence rates have improved since the initial disappointing results reported by Porter.[78] Several studies report low rates from 0% – 10%[30,37,77,79] but in others the incidence is higher.[80] The reason for this is unclear but it is our view that it is crucial to resect the entire length of sigmoid colon that can be drawn down, rather than only the length of rectum that prolapses readily.

Improvement in continence varies widely, ranging from 22% to 100%. The addition of levatorplasty appears to be important in restoring continence. One study found that of 11 patients who underwent levatorplasty 10 either improved or regained full continence postoperatively, compared with only 26 of 56 patients who underwent perineal rectosigmoidectomy alone.[30]

Table 19.2 Results of perineal rectosigmoidectomy

	No. Pts	Mean follow-up (months)	Morbidity	Mortality (%)	Recurrence (%)	Continence improved (%)
Porter, 1962[76]	110	NS	Anastomotic leaks: 2 Bleeding: 1	1	58	NS
Altemeier, 1971[37]	106	NS	26 Abscess: 4 Strictures: 2	0	3	NS
Friedman, 1983[158]	27	NS	Abscess: 1 Stricture: 1 Hematoma: 1	0	35	22
Gopal, 1984 + levatorplasty[77]	18	NS		6	6	NS
Watts, 1985[40]	33	22	NS	0	0	Worse in 16%
Prasad, 1986[159]	25	<36	0	0	0	100
Finlay, 1991[160]	17	24	Rectovaginal fistula: 1	6	6	NS
Thorne, 1992[80]	16	16	Bleeding: 1 Stricture: 1	0	13	44
Williams, 1992[30]	114	12	Bleeding: 3 Anastomotic leak: 1	0	10	54
Johansen, 1993 + levatorplasty[161]	20	26	Pelvic hematoma: 1	5	0	90
Ramanujam, 1994 + levatorplasty[162]	72 (9 acute)	48	Anastomotic leaks: 2	0	5.5	67

NS: not stated.

Postoperative constipation appears to be rare although it has not been carefully studied. Porter found that constipation was improved in 66% of cases.[78]

COMPARISON WITH OTHER PROCEDURES

A retrospective study compared the results of eight patients who underwent Delorme's procedure with 32 patients who underwent perineal rectosigmoidectomy and 21 patients who had perineal rectosigmoidectomy with levatoroplasty.[81] Recurrence rate was higher in the Delorme's group (38% v. 13% and 4% respectively) but complications related to the anastomosis were less common (0% v. 16% and 5%). The mean postoperative incontinence scores were worse in the Delorme's group (11.1 v. 6.7 and 4.9).

A prospective randomized trial compared 10 patients undergoing resection rectopexy with 10 patients having perineal rectosigmoidectomy, both with pelvic floor repair.[82] Following resection rectopexy continence to liquid and stool was achieved in nine patients with some soiling in two, compared with continence in eight patients with soiling in six following perineal rectosigmoidectomy. The median daily defecation frequency after resection rectopexy was 1 (range 1–3) compared with 3 (range 1–6) with rectosigmoidectomy. The mean resting anal canal pressure increased after resection rectopexy by 19.3 cm water compared with a decrease of 3.4 cm water after rectosigmoidectomy ($p = 0.003$). Rectal compliance was also higher after resection rectopexy. Despite the small numbers, the study does suggest that resection rectopexy offers superior functional results to perineal rectosigmoidectomy and should be used in patients who are fit for abdominal surgery.

ABDOMINAL PROCEDURES

Abdominal rectopexy

Rectopexy involves mobilization of the rectum to a varying degree followed by fixation to the sacrum.

Many surgeons believe that rectopexy is the 'gold standard' operation for prolapse, with the lowest recurrence rates and highest rates of improvement in continence. Postoperative constipation however has been found to be a significant problem in most series where close attention is paid to functional results. This is a central issue to the current debate about which operative method of fixation to the sacrum is optimal and whether rectopexy should be combined with colonic resection.

Ripstein's original procedure involved the wrapping of a material, usually polypropylene mesh or Teflon, around the anterior aspect of the rectum and fixing the material to the sacrum.[83,84] It has been suggested that this may cause constipation if the wrap is too tight or if the sigmoid colon folds over the upper edge of the wrap, complications possibly avoided by posterior rectopexy which leaves the anterior circumference of the rectum free.[85,86] Strictures at the wrap site have been reported in up to 17% of patients, requiring re-operation in some cases.[87–89] Rarely polypropylene mesh can become infected or erode into the rectum.[87,90] Ivalon (polyvinyl alcohol) rectopexy was popular for many years in Britain. The Ivalon sponge was wrapped posteriorly around the rectum, causing subsequent pelvic fibrosis and this was thought to decrease the risk of recurrence. However recurrence rates do not appear to be lower than with other methods, and since the Ivalon may occasionally become infected requiring removal, this method is now used much less frequently. One must question whether any foreign material is required as the results of simple suture rectopexy appear to be equally good in terms of recurrence (Table 19.3 and 19.4). Suture rectopexy is the preferred method used by the current authors.

Operative procedure

Bowel preparation and intravenous antibiotic cover are given. The Lloyd–Davies position with Trendelenburg tilt, and a lower midline incision are used. The peritoneum is incised on each side of the rectum and the posterior presacral plane is developed in front of the presacral nerves. The rectum is mobilized down to the tip of the coccyx using the diathermy point, and the levator muscles are clearly visualized. The anterior peritoneum is incised and the upper end of the rectovaginal space is exposed. The lateral ligaments are divided with the diathermy. The rectum is secured to the sacrum, either using a sheet of Marlex mesh placed posteriorly, or directly by suture. If mesh is to be used, four sutures of 3/0 Ethibond are placed in two rows just below the sacral promontory to fix the mesh, taking care to avoid the presacral nerves and venous structures. The rectum is drawn up firmly but should not be taught, and the lateral edges of the mesh are sutured to the lateral ligaments of the rectum using 3/0 Ethibond, encircling half or less of the rectal circumference (posterior rectopexy: Wells procedure, Fig. 19.3). Alternatively the mesh is wrapped anterior to the rectum and secured to the sacrum on each side of the rectum (anterior rectopexy: Ripstein procedure, Fig. 19.4). If mesh is not used, the sutures are placed in the sacrum and fixed directly to the tissues of the lateral ligaments (suture rectopexy, Fig. 19.5). A suction drain is placed in the pelvis, and the peritoneum is closed to prevent small bowel loops from entering the pelvis.

Results

Abdominal rectopexy is very effective in controlling the prolapse. Recurrence rates depend on the length of follow-up and range from 0% to 16%. The recurrence rates are not consistently better with any one method of rectopexy (Tables 19.3 and 19.4). Hence other factors, particularly restoration of continence and incidence of constipation, become important in determining an optimal procedure.

There are few studies which have accurately compared results of different methods of rectopexy. One prospective randomized study compared Ivalon sponge rectopexy in 31 patients to suture rectopexy in 32 patients.[91] There was no difference in postoperative morbidity and after a median follow-up of 47 months there was no difference in recurrence rates, with one patient in each group. Both incontinence and constipation were slightly more common in the Ivalon group (9 v. 5 patients, and 15 v. 10 patients respectively), and it was concluded that suture rectopexy is at least equivalent to the Ivalon sponge technique and is preferable.

There has been interest in the use of absorbable mesh for rectopexy. Galili *et al.* prospectively randomized 37 patients to standard polypropylene mesh or absorbable polyglycolic acid mesh.[92] No difference in outcome was found. Winde *et al.* compared two absorbable meshes, polyglycolic acid or polyglactin.[93] Again, no differences in outcome were noted. Although absorbable mesh may have some advantages over non-absorbable mesh, the avoidance of mesh altogether with simple suture rectopexy may be preferable. Recurrence rates are as low as 2% with sutures alone (Table 19.4).

Division of the lateral ligaments appears to reduce the recurrence rate. This probably reflects the extent of rectal mobilization and is accompanied by a higher incidence of postoperative constipation. In one study 26 patients undergoing posterior Marlex rectopexy were randomized to having the lateral ligaments divided (14 patients) or preserved (12 patients).[94] Incontinence improved in both groups, and with division of the lateral ligaments constipation increased from three patients before the operation to 10 after operation while there was no significant change in the other group ($p < 0.01$). Similarly the mean percentage time straining and number of patients using laxatives increased signifi-

Table 19.3 Results of abdominal rectopexy with mesh. Anterior or posterior rectopexy is noted.

		No. Pts	Mean follow-up (months)	Morbidity (%)	Mortality (%)	Recurrence (%)	Continence improved (%)	Constipation worsened (%)
Hilsabeck, 1981[163]	Posterior Marlex	14	22	NS	0	0 1 mucosal	NS	
Keighley, 1983[89]	Posterior Marlex	100	>24	NS	0	0 4 mucosal	64	NS
Hiltunen, 1991[164]	Posterior Marlex	54	36	22	0	2 6 mucosal	75	31
Yoshioka, 1989[90]	Posterior Marlex	165	36	19	0	1.5 7 mucosal	88	12
Cuthbertson, 1988[165]	Posterior Mersilene	104	60	23 Infected slings: 2	2	9.5	78	32
McMahan, 1987[86]	Posterior Gortex	23	16	NS	0	0 1 mucosal	0	NS
Holmstrom, 1986[130]	Anterior Marlex	108	81	3.7	2.8	4.1	59	13
Launer, 1982[88]	Anterior Teflon	57	63	28	0	12.2	41	18 obstructive symptoms
Tjandra, 1993[166]	Anterior Teflon	142	50	21	0.7	9	48	46 improved 28 worse
Roberts, 1988[167]	Anterior Teflon	135	41	52	0.7	9.6	78	69 improved; 31 same or worse
Leenen, 1989[168]	Anterior Teflon	64	30	28	0	0 2 mucosal	NS	NS
Jurgeleit, 1975[169]	Anterior Teflon	55	46	13	0	8	NS	NS
Morgan, 1980[170]	Anterior Teflon	64	72	1 reop to sling structure	2	2	NS	NS
Eisenstat, 1979[171]	Anterior Teflon	30	NS	2 obstructed sling	0	0	NS	NS
Winde, 1993[93]	Anterior PGA[a]	42	51	28	0	0 14 mucosal	55	Dec. const op. 47–17
Boulos, 1984[172]	Posterior Ivalon	32	120 median	NS	0	16	75	NS
McCue, 1991[173]	Posterior Ivalon	53	37	40% infected sponge	0	3.8	38	Overall improvement
Penfold, 1972[174]	Posterior Ivalon	101	72	6% 2 infections and removal	0	3	70: solid feces 33: liquid feces	29:def more difficult 24:def easier
Morgan, 1972[175]	Posterior Ivalon	150	±60	3% sepsis	2.6	4	53% improved	Constipation decreased from 65% to 27%
Mann, 1988[96]	Posterior Ivalon	66	58	39	0	9[b]	38% improved	46
Anderson, 1984[176]	Posterior Ivalon	42	50	9	2	2	75% improved	NS

[a] PGA Absorbable polyglycolic acid + polyglactin.
[b] Mucosal prolapse only in all six patients.

Table 19.4 Results of suture rectopexy							
	No. Pts	Mean follow-up (months)	Morbidity (%)	Mortality (%)	Recurrence (%)	Continence improved (%)	Constipation worsened (%)
Blatchford, 1989[177]	43	28	20	0	8	41	23
Carter, 1983[178]	32	NS	NS	0	3 9 mucosal	NS	NS
Graham, 1984[179]	28	18	11	4	0 11 mucosal	77	NS
Goligher, 1984[38]	52			0	2	NS	NS
Ejerblad, 1988[180]	46 (+ levator-plasty in 17)	80	0	0	4	69	'Substantial'

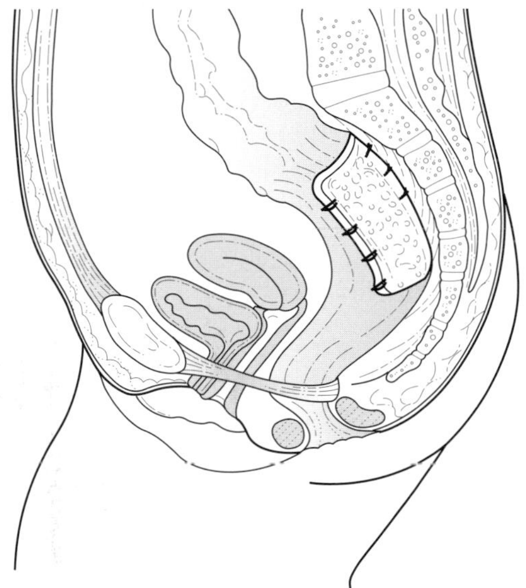

Figure 19.3 Posterior rectopexy. The mobilized rectum is fixed to the upper sacrum using a rectangle of mesh secured to the posterior half of the rectum.

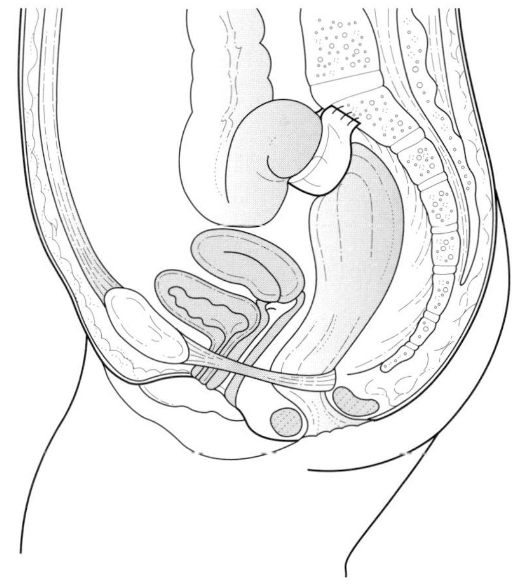

Figure 19.4 Anterior rectopexy. The rectum is fixed by placing an anterior mesh sling, which is sutured on each side to the sacrum.

cantly postoperatively when the lateral ligaments were divided, while there was no significant change in the other group. In addition, the rectal electrical sensory threshold increased in those in whom the ligaments were divided (preoperative 27.6 mA v. postoperative 56.7, $p < 0.01$), but not in those in whom they were preserved (39.0 mA v. 34.9 mA). However, six of the 12 patients with undivided ligaments suffered some degree of recurrent prolapse and four required a Delorme's procedure while two developed external mucosal prolapse only. None of those with divided ligaments developed recurrence.

In another study which was non-randomized the first group of 16 patients underwent posterior Marlex rectopexy with division of the lateral ligaments, then a consecutive group of 16 patients underwent the same procedure without lateral ligament division.[95] Clinical and physiological assessments were made before and 3, 6 and 12 months after surgery. Improvement in continence was similar in both groups. Bowel regulation problems significantly worsened postoperatively when the lateral ligaments were divided, whereas they were unchanged when the ligaments were preserved. At 12 months significantly more patients who had their

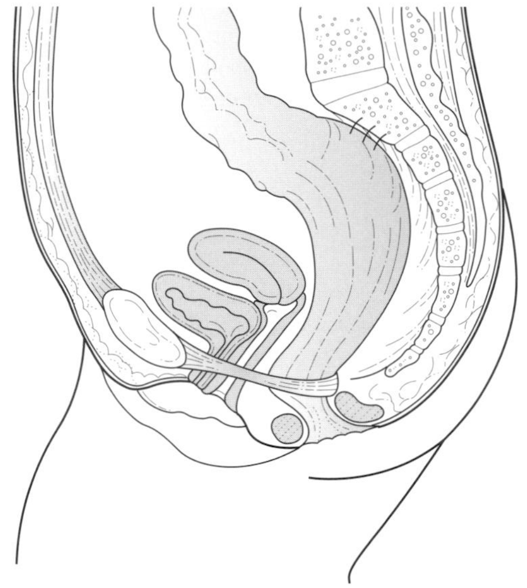

Figure 19.5 Suture rectopexy. The rectum is fixed directly to the sacrum without mesh.

ligaments divided complained of infrequent movements with use of laxatives or enemas (81% v. 47%, $p < 0.025$) while complaints of incomplete evacuation were also more common (88% v. 57%, $p < 0.025$), as was excessive straining at stool (80% v. 25%) and lack of urge to defecate (61% v. 19%, $p < 0.005$). Although follow-up was only one year, no recurrences occurred in either group.

There is considerable variation between different forms of rectopexy in restoration of continence and onset of constipation. The precise mechanism of constipation is unclear, but pre-existing constipation and the extent of rectal mobilization seem to be important. Hence with an extensive anterior and posterior mobilization almost half the patients developed constipation.[96] Other studies where the mobilization was less extensive report lower rates (Table 19.3). The constipation may in part be due to reactive thickening of the rectal wall. In a study of 57 patients before and three months after Ivalon sponge rectopexy it was found that there was a significant increase in the prevalence of constipation from 30% to 57% ($p < 0.01$).[97] Rectal wall thickness was assessed with CT scan before and after surgery, and was found to significantly increase. The authors felt that the increased thickness was due to rectal mobilization rather than the Ivalon sponge, and that constipation may be due to the thickened rectal wall impeding the passage of stool.

Dolk and colleagues studied 18 patients with constipation following rectopexy.[98] These patients were from a group of 108 patients of whom 35 developed severe postoperative constipation. The 18 patients underwent defecography, ano-rectal manometry, electromyography and colon transit studies. None showed a normal pattern in the parameters studied and in particular 13 had slow transit constipation. The authors suggested that patients should undergo careful preoperative investigations to try to identify those patients who would benefit from subtotal colectomy in association with rectopexy.

Another study examined 12 patients who suffered constipation after rectopexy.[99] Each underwent left colonic manometry, ano-rectal manometry, evacuation proctography and colonic transit studies. Results were compared with a group of ten healthy controls and another group of 12 patients with rectal prolapse. In the rectopexy group colonic transit times were significantly longer than the other groups. The left colonic manometric studies revealed significantly less basal motor activity in the rectopexy group. In addition the normal postprandial peristaltic rush was absent in rectopexy patients, whereas it was present in four of the seven rectal prolapse patients studied and seven of the ten healthy volunteers studied. Evacuation proctography and anal manometric studies were not different between the groups, and the authors concluded that constipation following rectopexy is related to acquired motility disturbances above the rectopexy rather than ano-rectal emptying abnormalities.

These studies have added weight to the argument for sigmoid resection in some patients and there has been much interest in this procedure.

Resection rectopexy

The combination of rectopexy and resection of the sigmoid colon was popularized by Frykman and Goldberg.[100] Originally the colonic resection was performed to decrease the risk of recurrence, but more recently interest has centered on the evidence that it is associated with a decreased incidence of debilitating constipation.

In the first large series with this procedure 138 patients were treated from 1953 to 1983, of whom nine had undergone subtotal colectomy.[40] There was no mortality and the recurrence rate was 1.9%. 43% of patients reported improved continence postoperatively. Constipation was not studied closely. A subsequent study from the same center examined in more detail the functional results of 47 patients undergoing suture rectopexy and colonic resection from 1979 to 1985. Thirty-seven patients underwent sigmoidectomy, eight had subtotal colectomy, and four underwent sigmoid colectomy followed by subtotal colectomy. Three (6.3%) developed full-thickness recurrence and four (8.5%) developed mucosal prolapse. Ten of 20 patients (50%) who had constipation preoperatively improved, including seven (70%) who underwent subtotal colectomy. Eight of 21 patients (38%) with preoperative incontinence improved. Continence worsened in six patients and four patients developed significant diarrhea, which did not correlate with the length of colon resected. Three patients, one with radiation proctitis, required a stoma for persisting incontinence.[101]

Husa *et al.* found that all but two patients with preoperative incontinence improved after resection-rectopexy, and of 16 patients who had constipation preoperatively only four remained constipated.[102] In a non-randomized study the results of posterior Marlex mesh rectopexy in 16 patients were compared with sigmoidectomy and suture rectopexy in 13 patients.[103] Hospital stay, morbidity, recurrence and improvement in continence were comparable. Postoperative constipation occurred in seven of 16 patients undergoing rectopexy alone, compared to one of 13 undergoing resection–rectopexy.

A prospective study of 42 patients undergoing resection–rectopexy[104] found that constipation improved from 44% to 26% ($p < 0.001$) and incontinence from 67% to 23% ($p < 0.001$), and this was associated with improved physiological parameters with maximum anal canal resting pressure and squeeze pressure each increased significantly, 37 mmHg to 46 mmHg, and 91 mmHg to 103 mmHg respectively. Total colonic transit time decreased from 48 hours to 39 hours, while the rectosigmoid transit time decreased from 21 to 13 hours ($p < 0.001$).

In a randomized study nine patients underwent suture rectopexy alone and nine underwent suture rectopexy and colectomy.[105] At 3 months, seven patients in the rectopexy group suffered severe constipation, compared with two in the resection–rectopexy group. Pre- and postoperative colonic transit studies confirmed significantly increased transit time in the rectopexy group, whereas there was no increase in the resection-rectopexy group. Another randomized study compared 15 patients undergoing resection–rectopexy with 15 patients undergoing polyglycolic acid posterior mesh rectopexy.[106] There were no cases of recurrent prolapse and continence improved similarly in each group. Constipation disappeared in three and seven patients after resection–rectopexy and rectopexy alone respectively. However, there were no new cases of constipation in the resection–rectopexy group while five of the rectopexy alone group developed severe constipation requiring colectomy in one, although interestingly, there was no significant change in the transit studies postoperatively. It was concluded that sigmoid colectomy was not associated with increased morbidity and reduced postoperative constipation.

Anterior resection

Treatment of rectal prolapse by anterior resection was first proposed by Muir in 1955, suggesting that fibrosis around the anastomosis would fix the rectum to the sacrum.[107] The operation has been popularized by the Mayo Clinic. In a review of 113 patients who underwent anterior resection between 1969 and 1990 the mean follow-up time was 7 years and the recurrence rate was 9%. Importantly, this large series demonstrated that recurrence continues to occur with prolonged follow-up after prolapse surgery, with 3%, 6% and 12% after 2, 5 and 10 years respectively. Operative mortality was 1%, while morbidity was 29%, including three anastomotic leaks.

In another study of 41 patients who underwent high anterior resection for rectal prolapse the mean follow-up was 6 years,[108] recurrence rate was 7%, there was no mortality and morbidity was 15%. In 90% incontinence improved. Seventeen patients had preoperative constipation which worsened in four cases and remained unchanged or improved in the rest. There were no anastomotic complications.

Anterior resection is therefore associated with a low recurrence rate, and functional outcome appears satisfactory. Selection of patients would be particularly important since incontinence would potentially be a problem in old or frail patients or if anal sphincter function was poor. The possibility of anastomotic complications also needs to be considered.

Laparoscopic operations

Most series have contained small patient numbers, and have outlined laparoscopic techniques for standard abdominal procedures such as sigmoid resection, suture rectopexy, or different methods of fixing mesh to the sacrum.[109–117] Laparoscopic-assisted perineal rectosigmoidectomy has also been described.[118]

Darzi *et al.* reported 29 patients undergoing laparoscopic posterior polypropylene mesh rectopexy.[119] The mean operating time was 95 minutes, only one open conversion was needed, and mean hospital stay was 5 days. There was no mortality and minimal morbidity, and after a mean follow-up of 8 months one patient developed mucosal prolapse.

Another study retrospectively compared the results of eight patients who underwent laparoscopic resection–rectopexy with ten age and sex matched patients who underwent laparotomy with resection–rectopexy.[120] There was no difference in morbidity or mortality. The mean operating time was longer for the laparoscopic group (177 v. 87 minutes), while the mean length of hospitalization, time to passage of flatus and introduction of oral intake were all less in the laparoscopic group.

Stevenson *et al.* reviewed 30 patients who underwent laparoscopic resection–rectopexy.[121] Median operating time was 185 minutes, median time to passage of flatus 2 days, and median hospital stay 5 days. Mortality rate was 3%, while the morbidity rate was 13%. After a median follow-up of 18 months 70% of those with preoperative incontinence had improved, and constipation was improved in 64%. There were no recurrent prolapses although two patients developed mucosal prolapse.

Solomon *et al.* have carried out a randomized trial in 40 patients.[122] Patients were told to expect discharge from hospital by day 5. Operating time was significantly longer with the laparoscopic than open technique, and 95% v. 47% of patients respectively were discharged by the fifth day. An independent assessment found that significantly more patients in the laparoscopic group tolerated food on day 2, and significantly lower amounts of analgesics were required up to day 5. Long-term follow-up is awaited.

It does appear that laparoscopic operations for rectal prolapse may well be associated with early recovery, but further follow-up is needed to evaluate recurrence rates and function.

FECAL INCONTINENCE AND PROLAPSE

Apart from the prolapse itself, fecal incontinence is the most important symptom in patients with rectal prolapse. The etiology of incontinence is often multifactorial: the prolapse acts as a direct conduit, the internal sphincter is weakened by repeated dilatation, and there may be a pudendal neuropathy which causes further weakness. Electromyographic changes of denervation have been demonstrated in the external sphincter and puborectalis in patients with prolapse,[53] perhaps due to the effect of chronic straining on pudendal nerve function.[123] In many cases incontinence improves substantially after surgical correction of the prolapse. The management of persistent postoperative incontinence is a particular problem.

Restoration of continence is an important endpoint in the management of prolapse. Overall, abdominal rectopexy is more likely to be successful than a perineal procedure. However some studies report a high rate of continence after both the Delorme's procedure as well as perineal rectosigmoidectomy. Addition of levatorplasty to perineal rectosigmoidectomy seems to be important. Undoubtedly the method of assessing continence varies considerably and studies are therefore not necessarily comparable. Improvement in continence is shown in Tables 19.1–19.4.

Not surprisingly, preoperative incontinence correlates with both low resting and squeeze anal pressures[52,124–126] and a short sphincter length.[52] Several studies have shown that restoration of continence is accompanied by significant improvement in resting pressure[127–131] indicating recovery of internal sphincter tone. Other studies have found that both resting and squeeze pressures improve postoperatively in patients who become continent.[124–126]

However not all studies have shown improvement in resting pressure after rectopexy[52,90] and other parameters may also be important in restoring continence. Rectal sensitivity to balloon distension and anal mucosal electrosensitivity have been found to improve[52] and improved sensation may therefore be an important factor. Preoperative parameters which have been found to predict return of continence are delayed leakage during saline infusion test, a narrow ano-rectal angle, minimal pelvic floor descent and a long anal canal.[90] Patients with prolonged pudendal nerve terminal motor latencies[132] and very low anal pressures are less likely to improve after rectopexy.[124,133]

There is however good evidence that internal sphincter function does improve after abdominal rectopexy. In an important study 22 patients underwent ambulatory electromyography of the internal and external sphincters and manometry before and after rectopexy.[129] There was significant improvement in the internal sphincter EMG frequency and resting anal pressure after operation, even though these variables remained significantly lower than those found in normal controls. Patients with fecal incontinence and rectal prolapse also have high pressure rectal waves associated with inhibition of the internal sphincter EMG and a fall in resting pressure,[134] and these changes are not seen in patients with neurogenic incontinence or in normal controls. These rectal pressure waves were abolished after surgery to correct the prolapse, suggesting that repair of the prolapse allows the internal sphincter to recover by removing the cause of persistent recto-anal inhibition.

POSTOPERATIVE FECAL INCONTINENCE

Persistent incontinence after repair of rectal prolapse has usually been treated by postanal repair. Most series have been small. One with careful follow-up studied 11 patients,[135] with clinical and ano-rectal physiology follow-up in nine. Seven had improved continence, with two continent to solid and liquid stool and five to solid stool only. Ano-rectal physiology tests showed that the anal canal became longer, the resting pressure was higher and there was less perineal descent. The best results were achieved in those without preoperative pudendal neuropathy.

Although some other series have found better results[96,136–138] this may be due to shorter follow-up and less detailed assessment. Most surgeons perform repair of the prolapse first, and then postanal repair if incontinence persists. This appears reasonable, as accurate prediction of improvement in continence is not possible.

We have used graciloplasty in a few patients with persisting incontinence, but there are no reports which have studied this in any detail. There has been some interest in biofeedback and studies are awaited.

INTERNAL RECTAL PROLAPSE

Increased use of defecating proctography has led to the recognition that incomplete rectal prolapse, intussusception that does not protrude through the anus, is relatively common. This can be associated with pain, a feeling of incomplete evacuation, bleeding and mucous discharge.[139] However internal intussusception is also a common finding in asymptomatic individuals, being observed on proctography in up to 23–50% of asymptomatic volunteers,[140,141] so that the importance of this radiological finding is difficult to establish.

Sun *et al.* hypothesized that full thickness rectal prolapse, anterior mucosal prolapse and solitary rectal ulcer syndrome have a common pathophysiology.[142] They studied 21 patients with full thickness prolapse, 24 with anterior mucosal prolapse, 11 with solitary rectal ulcer syndrome and 30 normal subjects. Similarities were found between the three patient groups, which all differed from the controls – basal and squeeze anal pressures were lower than the controls; pressures were lower during increases in intra-abdominal pressure; serial distention of the rectum caused rectal contractions far more commonly; the highest anal pressure was always higher than rectal pressure during rectal distention in normal subjects but not in the patients; and the threshold rectal volume causing the desire to defecate was significantly lower in each of the patient groups compared to the control group. It was suggested that the increased rectal sensitivity may encourage patients to strain when there is little stool in the rectum, initially causing anterior mucosal prolapse, ongoing straining and eventually full thickness prolapse.

Two clinical studies have not tended to support this theory. Allen-Mersch *et al.* studied 250 patients with anterior mucosal prolapse diagnosed in an out-patient department 10 years previously and only three were noted to develop full-thickness rectal prolapse.[143] The authors concluded that the development of some degree of anterior mucosal prolapse may be part of the normal aging process especially in women, and only uncommonly develops into full thickness prolapse. Mellgren *et al.* found that only two of 38 patients diagnosed with internal intussusception on proctography and not treated surgically developed full thickness rectal prolapse after a mean follow-up of 11.4 years.[144]

The place of surgical treatment of internal prolapse is still debated. We do not believe the literature supports the role of surgery.

Rubber band ligation has been reported to produce complete resolution of symptoms (bleeding, tenesmus, obstructed defecation) in 71% of patients and some improvement in a further 24%.[145] Other studies have also shown favorable results with rubber banding.[146,147]

Delorme's procedure has also been reported to produce relief of symptoms[148] but there are no studies which accurately correlate clinical improvement with control of the prolapse. Abdominal rectopexy was carried out in 37 patients with internal prolapse, 18 of whom also had solitary rectal ulcer syndrome.[149] On defecography 13 had anterior prolapse while 21 had circumferential prolapse. Twenty-six patients (70%) became asymptomatic, although 17 of these had solitary rectal ulcer syndrome and the procedure was not successful in the majority of patients with obstructed defecation without the solitary rectal ulcer syndrome.

SELECTION OF OPERATIVE PROCEDURE

There is no doubt that a perineal procedure is associated with less morbidity than abdominal rectopexy. In old or unfit patients our preference is for perineal rectosigmoidectomy and levatorplasty if the prolapse is large. With smaller prolapses a Delorme's procedure is preferred.

In younger female patients we carry out abdominal sutured rectopexy without mesh. If there is associated constipation or a history of constipation before the prolapse developed, then isotope colon transit studies are done and if slow colonic transit is present then resection rectopexy is carried out. The amount of colon resected depends on the severity of constipation and the pattern of colonic transit; in most cases sigmoid resection is adequate but if there is severe slow transit with total colonic inertia then total colectomy and ileorectal anastomosis with sutured rectopexy is carried out.

We are reluctant to advise abdominal rectopexy in young men, even though the actual risk of nerve damage is very small. Most men would therefore be treated with a perineal procedure. However if incontinence is severe or there is a recurrent prolapse then rectopexy may be needed. Nerve damage is more likely to affect the sympathetic nerves, causing retrograde ejaculation and infertility, and in young men we offer the option of preoperative collection of sperm for storage.

REFERENCES

1. Bodri MS, Sadanaga KK. Circumcostal cloacapexy in a python. *J Am Vet Med Assoc* 1991;**198**(2):297.
2. Buls JG. Rectal prolapse. In: Fazio VW (ed.) *Current therapy in colon and rectal surgery*. Toronto: B.C. Decker, 1990.
3. Eu KW, Seow-Choen F. Functional problems in adult rectal prolapse and controversies in surgical treatment. *Br J Surg* 1997;84(7):904–11.
4. Corman ML. Rectal prolapse in children. *Dis Colon Rectum* 1985;**28**(7):535–9.
5. Qvist N, Rasmussen L, Klaaborg KE, Hansen LP, Pedersen SA. Rectal prolapse in infancy: conservative versus operative treatment. *J Pediat Surg* 1986;**21**(10):887–8.
6. Nwako F. Rectal prolapse in Nigerian children. *Int Surg* 1975;**60**(5):284–5.
7. Narasanagi SS. Rectal prolapse in children. *J Indian Med Assoc* 1974;**62**(11):378–80.

8. Stern RC, *et al.* Treatment and prognosis of rectal prolapse in cystic fibrosis. *Gastroenterology* 1982;**82**(4):707–10.
9. Kulczcki LL, Shwachman H. Studies in cystic fibrosis of the pancreas: occurrence of rectal prolapse. *New Engl J Med* 1958;**259**:409–412.
10. Zempsky WT, Rosenstein BJ. The cause of rectal prolapse in children. *Am J Dis Child* 1988; **142**(3):338–9.
11. Douglas BS, Douglas HM. Rectal prolapse in the Ehlers-Danlos syndrome. *Aust Paediat J* 1973;**9**(2):109–10.
12. Traisman E, *et al.* Rectal prolapse in two neonates with Hirschsprung's disease. *Am J Dis Child* 1983;**137**(11):1126–7.
13. Keighley MRB, Williams NS. Rectal prolapse. In: Keighley MRB, Williams NS (eds). *Surgery of the anus, colon and rectum.* London: W.B. Saunders, 1999:794–842.
14. Kay NR, Zachary RB. The treatment of rectal prolapse in children with injections of 30 per cent saline solutions. *J Pediat Surg* 1970;**5**(3):334–7.
15. Dutta BN, Das AK. Treatment of prolapse rectum in children with injections of sclerosing agents. *J Indian Med Assoc* 1977;**69**(12):275–6.
16. Malyshev YI, Gulin VA. Our experience with the treatment of rectal prolapse in infants and children. *Am J Proctol* 1973;**24**(6):470–2.
17. Chan WK, *et al.* Injection sclerotherapy in the treatment of rectal prolapse in infants and children. *J Pediat Surg* 1998;**33**(2):255–8.
18. Wyllie GG. The injection treatment of rectal prolapse. *J Pediat Surg* 1979;**14**(1):62–4.
19. Thiersch C. Carl Thiersch 1822–1895. Concerning prolapse of the rectum with special emphasis on the operation by Thiersch [classical article]. *Dis Colon Rectum* 1988;**31**(2):154–5.
20. Groff DB, Nagaraj HS. Rectal prolapse in infants and children. *Am J Surg* 1990;**160**(5):531–2.
21. Oeconomopoulos CT, Swenson O. Thiersch's operation for rectal porlapse in infants and children. *Am J Surg* 1960;**100**:457–61.
22. Chwals WJ, *et al.* Transanal mucosal sleeve resection for the treatment of rectal prolapse in children. *J Pediat Surg* 1990;**25**(7):715–8.
23. Schepens MA, Verhelst AA. Reappraisal of Ekehorn's rectopexy in the management of rectal prolapse in children. *J Pediat Surg* 1993;**28**(11):1494–7.
24. Hight DW, *et al.* Linear cauterization for the treatment of rectal prolapse in infants and children. *Surg Gynecol Obstet* 1982;**154**(3):400–2.
25. Tsugawa C, *et al.* Posterior plication of the rectum for rectal prolapse in children. *J Pediatr Surg* 1995;**30**(5):692–3.
26. Lockhart-Mummery JP. Rectal prolapse. *BMJ* 1939;**18**:345–7.
27. Nash DF. Bowel management in spina bifida patients. *Proc R Soc Med* 1972;**65**(1):70–71.
28. Duthie GS, Bartolo DC. Abdominal rectopexy for rectal prolapse: a comparison of techniques. *Br J Surg* 1992;**79**(2):107–13.
29. Agachan F, *et al.* Results of perineal procedures for the treatment of rectal prolapse. *Am Surg* 1997;**63**(1):9–12.
30. Williams JG, *et al.* Treatment of rectal prolapse in the elderly by perineal rectosigmoidectomy. *Dis Colon Rectum* 1992;**35**(9):830–4.
31. Schlinkert RT, *et al.* Anterior resection for complete rectal prolapse. *Dis Colon Rectum* 1985; **28**(6):p.409–12.
32. Kupfer CA, Goligher JC. One hundred consecutive cases of complete prolapse of the rectum treated by operation. *Br J Surg* 1970;**57**(7):482–7.
33. Nicholls JR, Banarjee A. Rectal prolapse and solitary rectal ulcer syndrome. In: Nicholls RJ, Dozois RR (eds). *Surgery of the colon and rectum.* New York: Churchill Livingstones 1997:709–737.
34. Mortensen NJ, Vellacott KD, Wilson MG. Lahaut's operation for rectal prolapse. *Ann R Coll Surg Engl* 1984;**66**(1):17–8.
35. Hughes ESR. In discussion on rectal prolapse. *Proc Roy Soc Med* 1949;**42**:1007.
36. Neill ME, Parks AG, Swash M. Physiological studies of the anal sphincter musculature in faecal incontinence and rectal prolapse. *Br J Surg* 1981;**68**(8):531–6.
37. Altemeier WA, *et al.* Nineteen years' experience with the one-stage perineal repair of rectal prolapse. *Ann Surg* 1971;**173**(6):993–1006.
38. Goligher JC. *Surgery of the anus, colon and rectum.* 1984, London: Baillière Tindall, 1984:246–84.
39. Vongsangnak V, Varma JS, Smith AN. Reappraisal of Thiersch's operation for complete rectal prolapse. *J R Coll Surg Edinb* 1985;**30**(3):185–7.
40. Watts JD, *et al.* The management of procidentia. 30 years' experience. *Dis Colon Rectum* 1985; **28**(2):96–102.
41. Keighley MR, Shouler PJ. Abnormalities of colonic function in patients with rectal prolapse and faecal incontinence. *Br J Surg* 1984;**71**(11):892–5.
42. Aboul-Enein A. Prolapse of the rectum in young men: treatment with a modified Roscoe Graham operation. *Dis Colon Rectum* 1979;**22**(2):117–9.
43. Leighton JA, *et al.* Anorectal dysfunction and rectal prolapse in progressive systemic sclerosis. *Dis Colon Rectum* 1993;**36**(2):182–5.
44. Malik M, Stratton J, Sweeney WB. Rectal prolapse associated with bulimia nervosa: report of seven cases. *Dis Colon Rectum* 1997;**40**(11):1382–5.
45. Korkis AM, *et al.* Rectal prolapse after oral cathartics. *J Clin Gastroenterol* 1992; **14**(4):339–41.
46. Kram HB, *et al.* Rectal prolapse caused by blunt abdominal trauma. *Surgery* 1989;**105**(6):790–2.
47. Banerjee AK, Jackson BT, Nicholls RJ. Full thickness rectal prolapse associated with primary intraabdominal pathology. *Postgrad Med J* 1986;**62**(726):303–4.
48. Marshman D, *et al.* Rectal prolapse: relationship with joint mobility. *Aust NZJ Surg* 1987; **57**(11):827–9.
49. Rashid Z, Basson MD. Association of rectal prolapse with colorectal cancer. *Surgery* 1996; **119**(1):51–5.
50. Broden B, Snellman B. Procidentia of the rectum studied with cineradiography. A contribution to the discussion of causative mechanism. *Dis Colon Rectum* 1968;**11**(5):330–47.
51. Moschcowitz AV. The pathogenesis, anatomy and cure of prolapse of the rectum. *Surg Gynecol Obstet* 1912;**15**:7–10.
52. Bartolo DC, Duthie GS. The physiological evaluation of operative repair for incontinence and prolapse. *Ciba Found Symp* 1990;**151**:223–35; discussion 235–45.
53. Snooks SJ, Henry MM, Swash M. Anorectal incontinence and rectal prolapse: differential assessment of the innerva-

tion to puborectalis and external anal sphincter muscles. *Gut* 1985;**26**(5):470–6.
54. Miller R, *et al.* Differences in anal sensation in continent and incontinent patients with perineal descent. *Int J Colorectal Dis* 1989;**4**(1):45–9.
55. Tjandra JJ, *et al.* Endoluminal ultrasound is preferable to electromyography in mapping anal sphincteric defects. *Dis Colon Rectum* 1993;**36**(7):689–92.
56. McLean RG, *et al.* Colon transit scintigraphy in health and constipation using oral iodine-131-cellulose. *J Nucl Med* 1990;**31**(6):985–9.
57. Corman ML. Rectal prolapse. Surgical techniques. *Surg Clin North Am* 1988;**68**(6):1255–65.
58. Poole GV, Jr, *et al.* Modified Thiersch operation for rectal prolapse. Technique and results. *Am Surg* 1985;**51**(4):226–9.
59. Hunt TM, Fraser IA, Maybury NK. Treatment of rectal prolapse by sphincteric support using silastic rods. *Br J Surg* 1985;**72**(6):491–2.
60. Labow SB, *et al.* Modification of silastic sling repair for rectal procidentia and anal incontinence. *Dis Colon Rectum* 1985;**28**(9):684–5.
61. Ladha A, Lee P, Berger P. Use of Angelchik Anti-Reflux Prosthesis for repair of total rectal prolapse in elderly patients. *Dis Colon Rectum* 1985;**28**(1):5–7.
62. Horn HR, *et al.* Sphincter repair with a Silastic sling for anal incontinence and rectal procidentia. *Dis Colon Rectum* 1985;**28**(11):868–72.
63. Swerdlow H. The Encircler. A new instrument for the performance of the Thiersch procedure for rectal procidentia. *Dis Colon Rectum* 1986;**29**(2):145–7.
64. Earnshaw JJ, Hopkinson BR. Late results of silicone rubber perianal suture for rectal prolapse. *Dis Colon Rectum* 1987;**30**(2):86–8.
65. Khanduja KS, *et al.* A new silicone prosthesis in the modified Thiersch operation. *Dis Colon Rectum* 1988;**31**:380–83.
66. Sainio AP, Halme LE, Husa AI. Anal encirclement with polypropylene mesh for rectal prolapse and incontinence. *Dis Colon Rectum* 1991;**34**(10):905–8.
67. Rye BA, Seidelin C, Dueholm S. Perineal progressive myonecrosis following Thiersch's operation for rectal prolapse. *Ann Chir Gynaecol* 1987;**76**(2):136–7.
68. Oliver GC, *et al.* Delorme's procedure for complete rectal prolapse in severely debilitated patients. An analysis of 41 cases. *Dis Colon Rectum* 1994;**37**(5):461–7.
69. Lechaux JP, Lechaux D, Perez M. Results of Delorme's procedure for rectal prolapse. Advantages of a modified technique. *Dis Colon Rectum* 1995;**38**(3):301–7.
70. Senapati A, *et al.* Results of Delorme's procedure for rectal prolapse. *Dis Colon Rectum* 1994; **37**(5):456–60.
71. Tobin SA, Scott IH. Delorme operation for rectal prolapse. *Br J Surg* 1994;**81**(11):1681–4.
72. Plusa SM, *et al.* Physiological changes after Delorme's procedure for full-thickness rectal prolapse. *Br J Surg* 1995;**82**(11):1475–8.
73. Mickulicz J. Zur operativen behandlung dis prolapsus recti et coli invaginati. *Arch Klin Chir* 1889;**38**:74.
74. Miles WE. Rectosigmoidectomy as a method of treatment for procidentia recti. *J Roy Soc Med* 1933;**26**:1445–52.
75. Gabriel WB. The principles and practice of rectal surgery. London: HK Lewis, 1945.
76. Porter NH. Surgery for rectal prolapse. *BMJ* 1971; 3(766):113.
77. Gopal KA, *et al.* Rectal procidentia in elderly and debilitated patients. Experience with the Altemeier procedure. *Dis Colon Rectum* 1984;**27**(6):376–81.
78. Porter N. Collective results of operations for rectal prolapse. *Proc Roy Soc Med* 1962;**55**:1087–91.
79. Watts AM, Thompson MR. Evaluation of Delorme's procedure as a treatment for full-thickness rectal prolapse. *Br J Surg* 2000;**87**(2):218–22.
80. Thorne MC, Polglase AL. Perineal proctectomy for rectal prolapse in elderly and debilitated patients. *Aust NZJ Surg* 1992;**62**(10):791–4.
81. Agachan F, *et al.* Comparison of three perineal procedures for the treatment of rectal prolapse. *South Med J* 1997;**90**(9):925–32.
82. Deen KI, *et al.* Abdominal resection rectopexy with pelvic floor repair versus perineal rectosigmoidectomy and pelvic floor repair for full-thickness rectal prolapse. *Br J Surg* 1994;**81**(2):302–4.
83. Ripstein CB. A simple, effective operation for rectal prolapse. *Postgrad Med* 1969;**45**(3):201–4.
84. Ripstein CB. Procidentia: definitive corrective surgery. Dis Colon Rectum 1972;15(5):334–6.
85. Wells C. New operation for rectal prolapse. Proc Roy Soc Med 1959;52:602–603.
86. McMahan JD, Ripstein CB. Rectal prolapse. An update on the rectal sling procedure. Am Surg 1987;53(1):37–40.
87. Gordon PH, Hoexter B. Complications of the Ripstein procedure. *Dis Colon Rectum* 1978; **21**(4):277–80.
88. Launer DP, *et al.* The Ripstein procedure: a 16-year experience. *Dis Colon Rectum* 1982;**25**(1):41–5.
89. Keighley MR, Fielding JW, Alexander-Williams J. Results of Marlex mesh abdominal rectopexy for rectal prolapse in 100 consecutive patients. *Br J Surg* 1983;**70**(4):229–32.
90. Yoshioka K, Heyen F, Keighley MR. Functional results after posterior abdominal rectopexy for rectal prolapse. *Dis Colon Rectum* 1989;32(10):835–8.
91. Novell JR, *et al.* Prospective randomized trial of Ivalon sponge versus sutured rectopexy for full-thickness rectal prolapse. *Br J Surg* 1994;**81**(6):904–6.
92. Galili Y, Rabau M. Comparison of polyglycolic acid and polypropylene mesh for rectopexy in the treatment of rectal prolapse. *Eur J Surg* 1997;**163**(6):445–8.
93. Winde G, *et al.* Clinical and functional results of abdominal rectopexy with absorbable mesh-graft for treatment of complete rectal prolapse. *Eur J Surg* 1993;**159**(5):301–5.
94. Speakman CT, *et al.* Lateral ligament division during rectopexy causes constipation but prevents recurrence: results of a prospective randomized study. *Br J Surg* 1991;**78**(12):1431–3.
95. Scaglia M, *et al.* Abdominal rectopexy for rectal prolapse. Influence of surgical technique on functional outcome [see comments]. *Dis Colon Rectum* 1994;**37**(8):805–13.
96. Mann CV, Hoffman C. Complete rectal prolapse: the anatomical and functional results of treatment by an extended abdominal rectopexy. *Br J Surg* 1988;**75**(1):34–7.
97. Allen-Mersh TG, Turner MJ, Mann CV. Effect of abdominal Ivalon rectopexy on bowel habit and rectal wall. *Dis Colon Rectum* 1990;**33**(7):550–3.

98. Dolk A, *et al.* Slow transit of the colon associated with severe constipation after the Ripstein operation. A clinical and physiologic study. *Dis Colon Rectum* 1990;**33**(9):786–90.
99. Siproudhis L, *et al.* Constipation after rectopexy for rectal prolapse. Where is the obstruction? *Dig Dis Sci* 1993;**38**(10):1801–8.
100. Frykman HM, Goldberg SM. The surgical treatment of rectal procidentia. *Surg Gynecol Obstet* 1969; **129**(6):1225–30.
101. Madoff RD, *et al.* Long-term functional results of colon resection and rectopexy for overt rectal prolapse. *Am J Gastroenterol* 1992;**87**(1):101–4.
102. Husa A, Sainio P, von Smitten K. Abdominal rectopexy and sigmoid resection (Frykman–Goldberg operation) for rectal prolapse. *Acta Chir Scand* 1988;**154**(3):221–4.
103. Sayfan J, *et al.* Sutured posterior abdominal rectopexy with sigmoidectomy compared with Marlex rectopexy for rectal prolapse. *Br J Surg* 1990;**77**(2):143–5.
104. Huber FT, Stein H, Siewert JR. Functional results after treatment of rectal prolapse with rectopexy and sigmoid resection. *World J Surg* 1995;**19**(1):138–43; discussion 143.
105. McKee RF, et al. A prospective randomized study of abdominal rectopexy with and without sigmoidectomy in rectal prolapse. Surg Gynecol Obstet 1992;174(2):145–8.
106. Luukkonen P, Mikkonen U, Jarvinen H. Abdominal rectopexy with sigmoidectomy vs. rectopexy alone for rectal prolapse: a prospective, randomized study. Int J Colorectal Dis 1992; 7(4):219–22.
107. Muir EG. Rectal prolapse. *Proc Roy Soc Med* 1955; **48**:33–44.
108. Cirocco WC, Brown AC. Anterior resection for the treatment of rectal prolapse: a 20-year experience. *Am Surg* 1993;**59**(4):265–9.
109. Berman IR. Sutureless laparoscopic rectopexy for procidentia. Technique and implications. *Dis Colon Rectum* 1992;**35**(7):689–93.
110. Kusminsky RE, Tiley EH, Boland JP. Laparoscopic Ripstein procedure. *Surg Laparosc Endosc* 1992;2(4):346–7.
111. Ballantyne GH. Laparoscopically assisted anterior resection for rectal prolapse. *Surg Laparosc Endosc* 1992;2(3):230–6.
112. Cuesta MA, *et al.* Laparoscopic rectopexy. *Surg Laparosc Endosc* 1993;3(6):456–8.
113. Munro W, Avramovic J, Roney W. Laparoscopic rectopexy. *J Laparoendosc Surg* 1993; 3(1):55–8.
114. Cuschieri A, *et al.* Laparoscopic prosthesis fixation rectopexy for complete rectal prolapse. *Br J Surg* 1994;**81**(1):138–9.
115. Kwok SP, *et al.* Laparoscopic rectopexy. *Dis Colon Rectum* 1994;**37**(9):947–8.
116. Graf W, *et al.* Laparoscopic suture rectopexy. *Dis Colon Rectum* 1995;38(2):211–2.
117. Poen AC, *et al.* Laparoscopic rectopexy for complete rectal prolapse. Clinical outcome and anorectal function tests. *Surg Endosc* 1996;**10**(9):904–8.
118. Reissman P, *et al.* Laparoscopic-assisted perineal rectosigmoidectomy for rectal prolapse. *Surg Laparosc Endosc* 1995;5(3):217–8.
119. Darzi A, *et al.* Stapled laparoscopic rectopexy for rectal prolapse. *Surg Endosc* 1995;**9**(3):301–3.
120. Baker R, Senagore AJ, Luchtefeld MA. Laparoscopic-assisted vs. open resection. Rectopexy offers excellent results. *Dis Colon Rectum* 1995;**38**(2):199–201.
121. Stevenson AR, Stitz RW, Lumley JW. Laparoscopic-assisted resection-rectopexy for rectal prolapse: early and medium follow-up. *Dis Colon Rectum* 1998;**41**(1):46–54.
122. Solomon M, *et al.* Randomised controlled trial of laparoscopic vs open abdominal rectopexy. *Aust NZJ Surg* 2000;**70**:A60.
123. Lubowski DZ, *et al.* Increase in pudendal nerve terminal motor latency with defaecation straining. *Br J Surg* 1988;**75**(11):1095–7.
124. Williams JG, *et al.* Incontinence and rectal prolapse: a prospective manometric study. *Dis Colon Rectum* 1991;**34**(3):209–16.
125. Sainio AP, Voutilainen PE, Husa AI. Recovery of anal sphincter function following transabdominal repair of rectal prolapse: cause of improved continence? [published erratum appears in *Dis Colon Rectum* 1991 Dec;34(12):1108]. *Dis Colon Rectum* 1991;**34**(9):816–21.
126. Delemarre JB, *et al.* The effect of posterior rectopexy on fecal continence. A prospective study. *Dis Colon Rectum* 1991;**34**(4):311–6.
127. Schultz I, *et al.* Continence is improved after the Ripstein rectopexy. Different mechanisms in rectal prolapse and rectal intussusception? *Dis Colon Rectum* 1996;**39**(3):300–6.
128. Ihre T, Seligson U. Intussusception of the rectum-internal procidentia: treatment and results in 90 patients. *Dis Colon Rectum* 1975;**18**(5):391–6.
129. Farouk R, *et al.* Restoration of continence following rectopexy for rectal prolapse and recovery of the internal anal sphincter electromyogram. *Br J Surg* 1992;**79**(5):439–40.
130. Holmstrom B, Broden G, Dolk A. Results of the Ripstein operation in the treatment of rectal prolapse and internal rectal procidentia. *Dis Colon Rectum* 1986;**29**(12):845–8.
131. Hiltunen KM, Matikainen M. Improvement of continence after abdominal rectopexy for rectal prolapse. *Int J Colorectal Dis* 1992;**7**(1):8–10.
132. Birnbaum EH, *et al.* Pudendal nerve terminal motor latency influences surgical outcome in treatment of rectal prolapse [see comments]. *Dis Colon Rectum* 1996;**39**(11):1215–21.
133. Madden MV, *et al.* Abdominal rectopexy for complete prolapse: prospective study evaluating changes in symptoms and anorectal function. *Dis Colon Rectum* 1992;**35**(1):48–55.
134. Farouk R, *et al.* Rectoanal inhibition and incontinence in patients with rectal prolapse. *Br J Surg* 1994; **81**(5):743–6.
135. Setti Carraro P, Nicholls RJ. Postanal repair for faecal incontinence persisting after rectopexy. *Br J Surg* 1994;**81**(2):305–7.
136. Keighley MR, Matheson DM. Results of treatment for rectal prolapse and fecal incontinence. *Dis Colon Rectum* 1981;**24**(6):449–53.
137. Browning GG, Parks AG. Postanal repair for neuropathic faecal incontinence: correlation of clinical result and anal canal pressures. *Br J Surg* 1983;**70**(2):101–4.

138. Keighley MR, Fielding JW. Management of faecal incontinence and results of surgical treatment. *Br J Surg* 1983;**70**(8):463–8.
139. White CM, Findlay JM, Price JJ. The occult rectal prolapse syndrome. *Br J Surg* 1980; **67**(7):528–30.
140. Goei R, *et al.* Anorectal function: defographic measurement in asymptomatic subjects. *Radiology* 1989;**173**:137–41.
141. Shorvon PJ, *et al.* Defecography in normal volunteers: results and implications. *Gut* 1989; **30**(12):1737–49.
142. Sun WM, *et al.* A common pathophysiology for full thickness rectal prolapse, anterior mucosal prolapse and solitary rectal ulcer. *Br J Surg* 1989;**76**(3):290–5.
143. Allen-Mersh TG, Henry MM, Nicholls RJ. Natural history of anterior mucosal prolapse. *Br J Surg* 1987;**74**(8):679–82.
144. Mellgren A, *et al.* Internal rectal intussusception seldom develops into total rectal prolapse. *Dis Colon Rectum* 1997;**40**(7):817–20.
145. Mathai V, Seow-Choen F. Anterior rectal mucosal prolapse: an easily treated cause of anorectal symptoms. *Br J Surg* 1995;**82**(6):753–4.
146. Niv Y, Abu-Avid S, Oren M. Internal rectal prolapse: rubber-band ligation as treatment for a neglected disease. *Mt Sinai J Med* 1990;**57**(2):106–8.
147. Berman IR, Harris MS, Leggett IT. Rectal reservoir reduction procedures for internal rectal prolapse. *Dis Colon Rectum* 1987;**30**(10):765–71.
148. Berman IR. Different strokes for different folks in repair of rectal prolapse [letter: comment]. *Dis Colon Rectum* 1995;**38**(3):330.
149. van Tets WF, Kuijpers JH. Internal rectal intussusception – fact or fancy? *Dis Colon Rectum* 1995;**38**(10):1080–3.
150. Uhlig BE, Sullivan ES. The modified Delorme operation: its place in surgical treatment for massive rectal prolapse. *Dis Colon Rectum* 1979;**22**(8):513–21.
151. Christiansen J, Kirkegaard P. Delorme's operation for complete rectal prolapse. *Br J Surg* 1981;**68**(8):537–8.
152. Houry S, *et al.* Treatment of rectal prolapse by Delorme's operation. *Int J Colorectal Dis* 1987; **2**(3):149–52.
153. Gundersen AL, Cogbill TH, Landercasper J. Reappraisal of Delorme's procedure for rectal prolapse. *Dis Colon Rectum* 1985;**28**(10):721–4.
154. Monson JR, *et al.* Delorme's operation: the first choice in complete rectal prolapse? *Ann R Coll Surg Engl* 1986;**68**(3):143–6.
155. Abulafi AM, *et al.* Delorme's operation for rectal prolapse [see comments]. *Ann R Coll Surg Engl* 1990;**72**(6):382–5.
156. Graf W, *et al.* Delorme's operation for rectal prolapse in elderly or unfit patients. *Eur J Surg 1992;158*(10):555–7.
157. Kling KM, *et al.* The Delorme procedure: a useful operation for complicated rectal prolapse in the elderly [see comments]. *Am Surg* 1996;**62**(10):857–60.
158. Friedman R, Muggia-Sulam M, Freund HR. Experience with the one-stage perineal repair of rectal prolapse. *Dis Colon Rectum* 1983;**26**(12):789–91.
159. Prasad ML, *et al.* Perineal proctectomy, posterior rectopexy, and postanal levator repair for the treatment of rectal prolapse. *Dis Colon Rectum* 1986;**29**(9):547–52.
160. Finlay IG, Aitchison M. Perineal excision of the rectum for prolapse in the elderly. *Br J Surg* 1991;**78**(6):687–9.
161. Johansen OB, *et al.* Perineal rectosigmoidectomy in the elderly. *Dis Colon Rectum* 1993;**36**(8):767–72.
162. Ramanujam PS, Venkatesh KS, Fietz MJ. Perineal excision of rectal procidentia in elderly high-risk patients. A ten-year experience. *Dis Colon Rectum* 1994;**37**(10):1027–30.
163. Hilsabeck JR. Transabdominal posterior proctopexy using an inverted T of synthetic material. *Arch Surg* 1981;**116**(1):41–4.
164. Hiltunen KM, Matikainen M. Clinical results of abdominal rectopexy for rectal prolapse. *Ann Chir Gynaecol* 1991;**80**(3):263–6.
165. Cuthbertson AM, Smith JA. An abdominal repair for complete rectal prolapse. *Aust NZJ Surg* 1988;**58**(6):499–503.
166. Tjandra JJ, *et al.* Ripstein procedure is an effective treatment for rectal prolapse without constipation. *Dis Colon Rectum* 1993;**36**(5):501–7.
167. Roberts PL, *et al.* Ripstein procedure. Lahey Clinic experience: 1963–1985. *Arch Surg* 1988; **123**(5):554–7.
168. Leenen LP, Kuijpers JH. Treatment of complete rectal prolapse with foreign material. *Neth J Surg* 1989;**41**(6):129–31.
169. Jurgeleit HC, *et al.* Symposium: Procidentia of the rectum: teflon sling repair of rectal prolapse, Lahey Clinic experience. *Dis Colon Rectum* 1975;**18**(6):464–7.
170. Morgan B. The teflon sling operation for repair of complete rectal prolapse. *Aust NZJ Surg* 1980;**50**(2):121–3.
171. Eisenstat TE, Rubin RJ, Salvati EP. Surgical treatment of complete rectal prolapse. *Dis Colon Rectum* 1979;**22**(8):522–3.
172. Boulos PB, Stryker SJ, Nicholls RJ. The long-term results of polyvinyl alcohol (Ivalon) sponge for rectal prolapse in young patients. *Br J Surg* 1984;**71**(3):213–4.
173. McCue JL, Thomson JP. Clinical and functional results of abdominal rectopexy for complete rectal prolapse. *Br J Surg* 1991;**78**(8):921–3.
174. Penfold JC, Hawley PR. Experiences of Ivalon-sponge implant for complete rectal prolapse at St. Mark's Hospital, 1960–70. *Br J Surg* 1972;**59**(11):846–8.
175. Morgan CN, Porter NH, Klugman DJ. Ivalon (polyvinyl alcohol) sponge in the repair of complete rectal prolapse. *Br J Surg* 1972;**59**(11):841–6.
176. Anderson JR, Wilson BG, Parks TG. Complete rectal prolapse – the results of Ivalon sponge rectopexy. *Postgrad Med J* 1984;**60**(704):411–4.
177. Blatchford GJ, *et al.* Rectal prolapse: rational therapy without foreign material. *Neth J Surg* 1989;**41**(6):126–8.
178. Carter AE. Rectosacral suture fixation for complete rectal prolapse in the elderly, the frail and the demented. *Br J Surg* 1983;**70**(9):522–3.
179. Graham W, Clegg JF, Taylor V. Complete rectal prolapse: repair by a simple technique. *Ann R Coll Surg Engl* 1984;**66**(2):87–9.
180. Ejerblad S, Krause U. Repair of rectal prolapse by rectosacral suture fixation. *Acta Chir Scand* 1988;**154**(2):103–5.

Chapter 20

Dysfunctional voiding and urinary retention

J Quentin Clemens, Edward J McGuire

The term *dysfunctional voiding* refers to a lack of coordination between detrusor and urethra which cannot be explained by overt neurological causes. The clinical manifestations of dysfunctional voiding encompass a wide range of signs and symptoms which are often extremely bothersome to patients and their families, and in some cases, may be a risk to ureteral and renal function. Examples of such conditions include idiopathic detrusor instability, enuresis, vesicoureteral reflux, Hinman's syndrome, detrusor sphincter pseudodyssynergia, and urinary retention. These voiding disorders represent an intermediate level of dysfunction between the highly synchronized voiding seen in normal individuals, and overt discoordination seen after suprasacral spinal cord injury. An understanding of the mechanisms underlying these two functional extremes is helpful for understanding dysfunctional voiding.

GUARDING REFLEX

The guarding reflex is a phenomenon in which the external urethral sphincter activity (measured with an intraluminal transducer or with electromyography) increases progressively as the bladder fills. Urethral activity reaches a peak just before micturition, at which time the detrusor contraction is preceded by a complete relaxation of the external urethral sphincter. At low bladder volumes this reflex is *involuntary* and mediated by the autonomic nervous system. When the sensory threshold for bladder filling is reached, the guarding reflex may be *voluntarily* augmented through pudendal nerve-mediated contraction of the striated urethral sphincter. Afferent impulses from stretch receptors in the bladder wall travel in the pelvic nerve through the ascending spinal cord pathways to the brainstem.[1] Integrated supraspinal input to the thoracolumbar and sacral spinal cord produces detrusor relaxation via the sympathetic hypogastric nerves and increased urethral sphincter tone via the somatic (and possibly autonomic) pudendal nerve. In the presence of a complete spinal cord injury, the guarding reflex is lost.[2] Therefore, this reflex appears to be centrally mediated at a brainstem level.

While bladder distention results in increased urethral tone, it appears that afferent urethral signals via the pudendal nerve may also have a significant affect on the bladder. In non-human primates, stimulation of the external urethral sphincter results in profound detrusor inhibition. This is true even in the presence of suprasacral spinal cord transection, indicating that the effect is mediated through a sacral pathway.

Taken together, these observations provide a framework by which normal and abnormal bladder storage function can be understood. The lower urinary tract is a unique functional unit which requires input from both autonomic and somatic neurons in order to function appropriately. Communication between these two neural systems is accomplished by the external urethral sphincter, which may be considered the 'on/off' switch.[3] For instance, when an individual is asked to stop voiding, the initial event is a voluntary contraction of the external urethral sphincter (somatic efferent input to the external sphincter via the pudendal nerve, afferent output from the pudendal nerve to sacral cord) which is followed quickly by an involuntary cessation of the detrusor contraction (autonomic efferent input via the hypogastric and pelvic nerves). In contrast, the first event at the initiation of voiding is voluntary relaxation of the external urethral sphincter, which is followed by an autonomically-driven detrusor contraction. Altered coordination and sequencing of these autonomic and somatic systems has a profound effect on lower urinary tract function.

DETRUSOR SPHINCTER DYSSYNERGIA

Detrusor sphincter dyssynergia (DSD) refers to the presence of an involuntary, phasic detrusor contraction coupled with a simultaneous involuntary contraction of the external urethral sphincter. These opposing contractions result in urinary incontinence, large postvoid residual volumes, elevated intravesical pressures and pressure-driven upper urinary tract damage. DSD occurs in the presence of a suprasacral spinal cord injury in which descending supraspinal input to the lower urinary tract is lost. Afferent impulses from the bladder stretch receptors are not communicated above the level of the injury, but lower spinal reflex circuits are left intact. The lack of input from the pontine micturition centers results in a lack of sympathetic inhibition of the detrusor, and a lack of coordination of efferent neural impulses to the detrusor and urethral sphincter. With bladder filling, there is an inappropriate decrease in urethral pressure (lack of guarding reflex). When the bladder reaches a critical volume there is a sudden reflex detrusor contraction (spinal reflex). It is unclear what triggers the contraction, but increased afferent impulses from detrusor stretch receptors coupled with diminished urethral afferent signals probably play a role. The detrusor contraction is immediately followed by a contraction of the external urethral sphincter. The stimulus for the urethral contraction is also not known, but local urethral stretch receptors due to the urine bolus or an aberrant guarding reflex in response to the abrupt increase in detrusor wall tension during the detrusor contraction are likely factors. The urethral contraction has an inhibitory effect on the detrusor, but is poorly sustained. The result is a cyclic repetition of dyssynergic detrusor and urethral contraction, causing a sustained elevation of intravesical pressures and poor bladder emptying.

IDIOPATHIC DETRUSOR INSTABILITY

Idiopathic detrusor instability (DI) is a clinical diagnosis in which an unanticipated detrusor contraction occurs with little warning.[4] These contractions often occur without any discernible pattern, and may not be related to the amount of urine present in the bladder. If the patient is unable to inhibit the contraction, urge incontinence occurs. DI was initially felt to be a urodynamic diagnosis based on the findings of an involuntary rise in bladder pressure during a cystometrogram. However, as many as 50% of patients with complaints of urge incontinence may show no pressure rise on conventional urodynamics despite classic symptoms of urge incontinence. Furthermore, ambulatory urodynamic studies, where detrusor pressures are monitored during daily activities, demonstrate uninhibited detrusor contractions in a significant percentage of persons with complaints of DI but a 'normal' cystometrogram. Therefore, it appears that the sensitivity of conventional urodynamic testing is insufficient to diagnose many patients with DI.

The high false negative rate for conventional cystometrics may be explained by the phenomenon of urethral instability. During conventional urodynamic studies, many patients with DI do not demonstrate uninhibited bladder activity, but rather have a loss of the normal guarding reflex. Rather than a slow, progressive rise in urethral pressure with filling, these patients demonstrate poor sensation of bladder filling with intermittent decrease in urethral pressures.[5] Since the level of urethral activity is integrated with detrusor activity, the lower urethral pressures may trigger a detrusor contraction, or they may be the prodromal event in a contraction which is subsequently inhibited. The frequent false negative findings with conventional cystometrics may be explained by voluntary augmentation of the external urethral sphincter tone during the study when the subject's attention is focused on the bladder.

The initial treatment of detrusor instability includes timed voiding and anticholinergic therapy. Timed voiding, starting at frequent intervals and gradually lengthening the period between voids, is essential in order to prevent the sudden onset of urgency. By having the patient empty the bladder before the critical volume which triggers a detrusor contraction is reached, unanticipated detrusor contractility is avoided. This regimen alone has been reported to resolve symptoms in up to 80% of patients.[6] Anticholinergic therapy without behavioral modification is frequently ineffective because these agents do not alter the sudden unanticipated onset of urgency and incontinence which is the main complaint in patients with DI. Rather, anticholinergics allow the bladder to hold a higher volume before the abrupt sensation of fullness and urgency occurs. With a regimen of timed voiding and anticholinergics, a 60% reduction in urge incontinence episodes can be expected (Urinary Incontinence Guideline Panel, 1992).[7] However, patient compliance with chronic anticholinergic therapy tends to be poor due to anticholinergic side effects.

For patients who fail simple timed voiding exercises, further behavioral therapies utilizing pelvic floor exercises, biofeedback, and electrical stimulation may be used. The goal of these exercises is to inhibit detrusor contractions through central neural pathways (which mediate voluntary control of the bladder and striated sphincter) and through peripheral neural pathways (stimulation of the perineum which causes reflex detrusor inhibition).[8] Pelvic floor exercises involve repetitive, voluntary contractions of the pelvic muscles. As mentioned above, contraction of these muscles exerts a direct inhibitory effect on the detrusor. These exercises are designed to strengthen the pelvic floor muscles in order to maximize the amount of inhibition that occurs. Up to 50% of patients demonstrate a weak or absent voluntary pelvic floor contraction due to muscle atrophy or inability to isolate these muscles.[9] Such patients may benefit from adjunctive biofeedback. Biofeedback utilizes auditory or visual cues at the time of pelvic floor muscle contraction to teach the patient to properly isolate the pelvic floor muscles. Such cues may be obtained from cutaneous, needle, intravaginal or rectal sensors. In small series with limited numbers of patients, success rates as high as 80% have been reported.[10,11] The durability of these results is not known.

Electrical stimulation refers to the application of electric current to the peripheral autonomic or somatic nerves. For the treatment of detrusor instability, the stimulation is felt to activate local pelvic reflexes via autonomic afferent fibers from the rectum, vagina and genitals, and via somatic afferent fibers from the lower extremities and pelvic floor muscles.[12] These afferent impulses are inhibitory to the bladder parasympathetic efferent fibers carried in the pelvic nerve. Vaginal or anal probes, or surface patch electrodes are used to deliver the current. Two types of stimulation are used: chronic and maximal stimulation. Chronic stimulation is delivered at a current below the sensory threshold for 6 to 12 hours daily for several months. Maximal stimulation is delivered at a higher intensity in order to elicit a visible muscle contraction. This type of treatment is given 2–3 times per week, also for a period of months. All studies of electrostimulation for urge incontinence involve small numbers and limited follow-up intervals. In these studies approximately 20% of patients became dry with this therapy, and an additional 35% were significantly improved.[12]

Sacral nerve stimulation is another form of electrical stimulation in which an implanted electrode is used to apply current directly to the sacral nerve roots at the S3 level. The mechanism of action of this treatment has not been clearly elucidated, but the stimulation is postulated to activate afferent fibers of the pelvic nerve, pudendal nerve and muscle afferent fibers from the limbs, all of which have been shown to inhibit detrusor contractions via spinal reflexes.[13–16] While this type of stimulation is more precise than surface stimulation, a surgical procedure is required for electrode placement and not every patient responds to the therapy. Therefore a test stimulation is performed prior to implantation of the permanent stimulator. For the testing phase a temporary wire electrode is placed percutaneously under local anesthesia. Placement of the wire at the S3 nerve root is confirmed by a contraction of the levator muscles and ipsilateral big toe during stimulation at a voltage high enough to induce a somatic response. The test stimulation is performed at lower voltage (regulated by the patient) for 3 to 7 days, and daily voiding diaries are used to assess the response. Patients who demonstrate greater than 50% improvement in baseline voiding symptoms are offered surgical implantation of the permanent stimulator. Unfortunately, the response rate to the test stimulation has historically been low, ranging from 13 to 62%.[17–21] In addition, approximately 25% of patients who respond to the percutaneous trial fail to respond to the permanent implant.[17,20,22]

For implantation of the permanent stimulator, a small vertical incision is made over the sacrum, and the S3 foramen is identified. A single electrode is generally placed, although bilateral placement has also been described.[23] The electrode is fixed to the periosteum, and a lead extension is tunneled subcutaneously to the programmable stimulator, which is placed in a subcutaneous pocket over the abdomen. The stimulation parameters (voltage, timing) can be changed by the patient using a remote control device. Published results for the treatment of refractory urge incontinence due to idiopathic DI have been encouraging. Schmidt *et al.* treated 76 patients and found a significant decrease in incontinence episodes and pad use.[20] Complete continence was achieved in 47%, and at least a 50% reduction in leakage was demonstrated in an additional 28%. These results appeared to be durable to 18 months. Weil *et al.* performed a prospective randomized study and found a significant decrease in pad use, leakage episodes, and leakage severity in 20 treated patients compared with 22 controls.[21] Complete continence was achieved in 56%. At 36 months the actuarial failure rate was 32.4%. At a longer follow-up (mean 29 months), Bosch *et al.* reported a 90% or greater decrease in pad use and/or incontinent episodes in 11 of 18 patients (61%).[22] Infection rates have been quite low, but the reoperation rate is high (30–50%) due to lead migration or breakage, pain at the stimulator site, or lack of efficacy.[20–22]

ENURESIS

Enuresis indicates the presence of clinically significant wetting during childhood, as defined by the patient and family. Approximately 85% of children attain day-time and night-time dryness by the age of 5,[24] and therefore children who are referred at an earlier age are generally treated with watchful waiting. There is a 15% annual spontaneous resolution rate,[24] and virtually all patients will eventually become continent without treatment. However, if wetness becomes a social problem, intervention may be indicated. The wetting may occur during the day (diurnal enuresis) and/or at night (nocturnal enuresis), and may be associated with other voiding symptoms such as urgency and intermittent voiding (polysymptomatic enuresis) or no other symptoms (monosymptomatic enuresis).[25] Over 80% of enuretic children have isolated nocturnal enuresis.

During infancy, voiding occurs frequently (approximately 20 times per day) via reflex detrusor contractions when a critical intravesical volume, or some degree of detrusor muscular tension, is reached. Bladder wall mechanoreceptors sense an increase in wall tension and signal sensory neurons in the dorsal root ganglia of S2–4 which convey afferent information to the brainstem. The pontine micturition center returns a signal to parasympathetic neurons in the spinal cord which is transmitted to the bladder via the pelvic nerve and to the urethra via the pudendal nerve. Voiding is accomplished through coordinated relaxation of the urethral sphincter and contraction of the detrusor. For a child to attain continence, bladder capacity must increase, and volitional (cortical) control of the external urethral sphincter must be learned in order to inhibit and initiate voiding.[3,26] Day-time urinary control is generally attained before night-time continence.

As in adults, poor coordination between the bladder and urethra may result in voiding dysfunction, which is often manifested as enuresis in children. For instance, urodynamic studies of patients with diurnal and nocturnal enuresis frequently demonstrate a profound lack of appreciation of bladder filling. There is also a lack of awareness of a detrusor contraction or the prodromal events of a detrusor contraction (such as a decrease in urethral electromyographic activity and urethral closure pressure).[27] These findings are quite similar to those in adult patients with idiopathic detrusor instability. Patients experience a sudden, unanticipated detrusor contraction which they attempt to control with a volitional contraction of the external sphincter and pelvic floor. Despite these attempts, unwanted leakage (enuresis) occurs.

Patients with isolated nocturnal enuresis appear to have a loss of cortical appreciation of detrusor events which is less severe than those with daytime and night-time wetting. Contrary to previous thoughts, such patients are not abnormally deep sleepers.[28,29] On urodynamics, most will demonstrate uninhibited detrusor activity during provocative cystometry while asleep, but normal urodynamics when awake.[30] Koff has hypothesized that most enuretic children have a dual developmental delay, comprising afferent and efferent components.[31] The afferent component causes the cortex to fail to respond to bladder filling or detrusor contractions during sleep, while the efferent component results in failure of suppression of the micturition reflex. This hypothesis is supported by the fact that 30–40% of enuretic children have other subtle developmental delays, including speech defects, impaired motor skills, and decreased spatial or visual motor perception, which do not occur in nonenuretic controls.[32]

Numerous additional factors may be contributory to the development or persistence of enuresis in a given child. Genetics clearly play a role in many cases. If one parent has a history of enuresis the likelihood of his or her children having the condition is 40%. If both parents have a history of enuresis the likelihood rises to 70%.[33] Furthermore, the age at which wetting resolved in the parents is predictive of the age of continence for the children.[34] Genetic linkage analysis has identified loci for nocturnal enuresis on chromosomes 13q and 12q.[35,36]

Antidiuretic hormone (ADH) is produced by the posterior pituitary and has the effect of reducing urine output by increasing distal tubule water reabsorption in the nephron. Normally, ADH secretion is increased at night, causing a decrease in nocturnal urine production.[37] A deficiency in nocturnal ADH production has been observed in children with nocturnal enuresis and is hypothesized to contribute to the wetting by causing urine output to exceed functional bladder capacity.[38,39] This hypothesis is controversial, however, as these observations have not been confirmed by others.[40–43]

Psychological factors may contribute to wetting, especially in older children, but emotional disorders are not present in the vast majority of patients with enuresis.[44] Furthermore, successful treatment of the enuresis does not result in new somatic complaints,[45,46] and psychological treatment is ineffective in reducing wetting episodes.[47]

The mainstays of treatment for enuresis, as for idiopathic detrusor instability, are pharmacologic agents and behavioral therapy. Commonly used medications include anticholinergic agents (most commonly oxybutinin chloride), tricyclic antidepressants (imipramine), and DDAVP. Oxybutinin therapy is no better than placebo in patients with monosymptomatic nocturnal enuresis,[48] but in those with day-time voiding symptoms or urodynamic evidence of detrusor instability, success rates of 40–80% have been reported.[26,27,49] However, most enuretic children have isolated nocturnal wetting, and therefore anticholinergic therapy alone is not commonly indicated.

The exact mechanism of action of imipramine has not yet been determined, but it appears to be a weak anticholinergic and antispasmodic which also increases sympathetic input to the bladder and alters sleep patterns. Multiple placebo-controlled studies have demonstrated a cure rate of up to 30–40% for the treatment of monosymptomatic nocturnal enuresis,[50–52] but the recurrence rate following discontinuation of therapy is high.[51,53]

Despite the unclear relationship between ADH levels and the presence of nocturnal enuresis, DDAVP, a synthetic analog of vasopressin, has been widely used for the treatment of nocturnal enuresis. It may be administered as an intranasal spray or in oral tablet form. In a meta-analysis of 18 randomized controlled trials of intranasal DDAVP treatment, Moffatt *et al.* concluded that DDAVP is effective in reducing the number of wet nights, but only 25% of patients became completely dry.[54] The results with oral administration have been similar.[55,56] As with imipramine, discontinuation of the medication does not result in persistent cure. Long-term continence rates following cessation of therapy are no different than those seen for spontaneous resolution of the wetting.[51]

Behavioral therapy consists of timed voiding for diurnal enuresis and use of a night-time alarm for nocturnal enuresis. The purpose of timed voiding for diurnal enuresis is the same as for idiopathic detrusor instability – to promote bladder emptying before a volume is reached which triggers an uninhibited detrusor contraction. No formal studies of timed voiding alone for the treatment of diurnal enuresis have been performed, but timed voiding is almost universally used when pharmacologic agents are prescribed, and results with this combination have been good.[27] For refractory cases of nocturnal enuresis with idiopathic DI, intravesical biofeedback has also been used to inhibit unstable bladder contractions with a reported continence rate of 70%.[57]

For nocturnal enuresis, the best results have been obtained with the use of an enuretic alarm. This device consists of a sensor which is worn on the child's underclothes connected to a small alarm on the shirt or wrist. A tiny amount of moisture is sufficient to activate the alarm. When the alarm sounds the child (or parent) is awakened and voiding is completed into the toilet. Eventually the child gains the ability to awaken independently prior to an enuretic episode, or subconscious cortical inhibition of the detrusor contraction occurs and the child sleeps through the night. Average success rates of 60–80% have been reported.[51,58,59] In contrast to pharmacologic therapy, the relapse rate following discontinuation of alarm therapy is low, approximately 25%.[60,61] Furthermore, relapsers frequently respond to a repeat course of therapy.[58,62] Unfortunately, the enuretic alarm often must be used for 3 weeks or more before a decrease in wetting frequency is seen.[51,61] As a result, there is a high non-compliance rate. Improved compliance and short-term results have been reported with combination therapy using pharmacologic agents and the alarm.[63,64]

There have been few studies of nocturnal enuresis in adults over 18 years of age. The reported prevalence has varied between 1 and 4%.[65–67] The workup of these patients should exclude neurologic causes, infections, and anatomic bladder outlet obstruction as causes of the wetness. In the remainder of patients, detrusor instability is frequently found on urodynamics.[68] DDAVP treatment results in resolution of leakage in approximately 70% of patients, but wetness almost invariably recurs following discontinuation of treatment.[69] Night-time alarm use may result in durable continence, but the compliance rate with this therapy is generally low.[69] Patients with intermittent or random night-time leakage may be treated with single-dose DDAVP on evenings where leakage would be particularly distressing.

VESICOURETERAL REFLUX, URINARY TRACT INFECTIONS, AND DYSFUNCTIONAL VOIDING

A clear association between vesicoureteral reflux (VUR) and dysfunctional voiding exists.[70–72] In this context, dysfunctional voiding refers to neurologically normal children with symptoms of urinary urgency and frequency, diurnal and/or nocturnal incontinence, squatting maneuvers to prevent leakage, or an intermittent or interrupted urinary stream. Constipation and encopresis are also common.[73] These symptoms have been reported in 18% of children with VUR.[71] Conversely, 20–50% of children with dysfunctional voiding may be found to have VUR.[70,74,75] Abnormal urodynamic findings are present in 40–75% of patients with VUR, and include uninhibited detrusor contractions (most common) and/or external sphincter activity during voiding.[70,76–79]

The normal ureterovesical junction is extremely resistant to reflux, even in the presence of exceptionally high voiding pressures (>100 cmH_2O) which may occur in young boys. Therefore, the presence of reflux in a patient with dysfunctional voiding and a presumably normal ureterovesical junction cannot be explained by elevated voiding pressures alone. Rather, chronic functional obstruction due to discoordination of the bladder and outlet is felt to cause anatomic changes (bladder hypertrophy, saccule formation, etc.) which alter the dynamics of the ureterovesical junction and allow reflux to occur.[80] The functional obstruction is present whenever a detrusor contraction is opposed by an external sphincter which is incompletely relaxed. The incomplete sphincter relaxation is commonly a compensatory maneuver in response to an uninhibited detrusor contraction, but may be volitional as well. If the dysfunctional voiding pattern is allowed to continue, continued alterations in the ureterovesical junction anatomy allow reflux to occur at progressively lower pressures.

The presence of dysfunctional voiding in patients with vesicoureteral reflux is an adverse prognostic factor. Regardless of treatment for the reflux (medical or surgical), those with dysfunctional voiding symptoms experience significantly more urinary tract infections than those with normal voiding patterns.[71,73,81] In those with low grades of reflux who are managed medically, resolution of the reflux occurs more slowly in those with dysfunctional voiding.[72] After ureteral reimplantation, patients with dysfunctional voiding are more likely to exhibit persistent reflux.[73,82,83] Not surprisingly, treatment of dysfunctional voiding can improve these outcomes. Anticholinergic medications, which diminish uninhibited bladder activity and therefore prevent compensatory sphincter contractions from occurring, are the primary treatment. In most studies, treatment with these agents results in resolution of reflux in 50–90% of patients and a decrease in the rate of breakthrough urinary tract infections.[70,76,77]

HINMAN'S SYNDROME (NON-NEUROGENIC NEUROGENIC BLADDER)

The non-neurogenic neurogenic bladder originally described by Hinman[84] represents the most severe manifestation of dysfunctional voiding. This syndrome con-

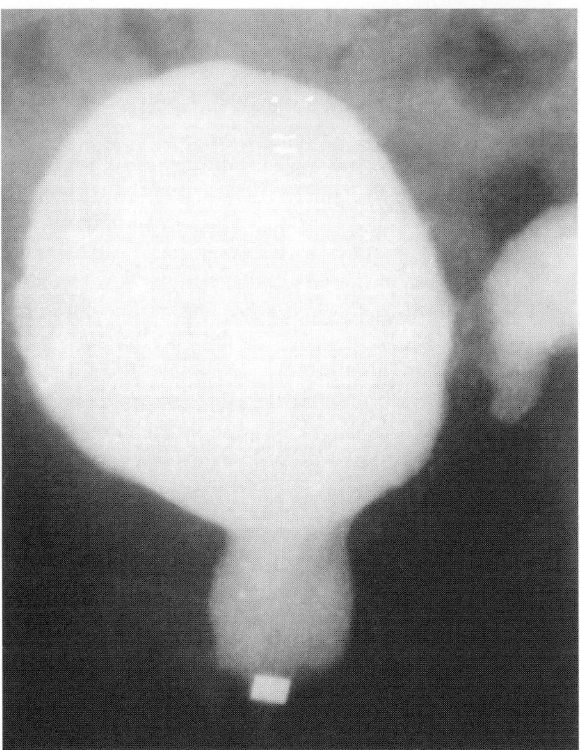

a

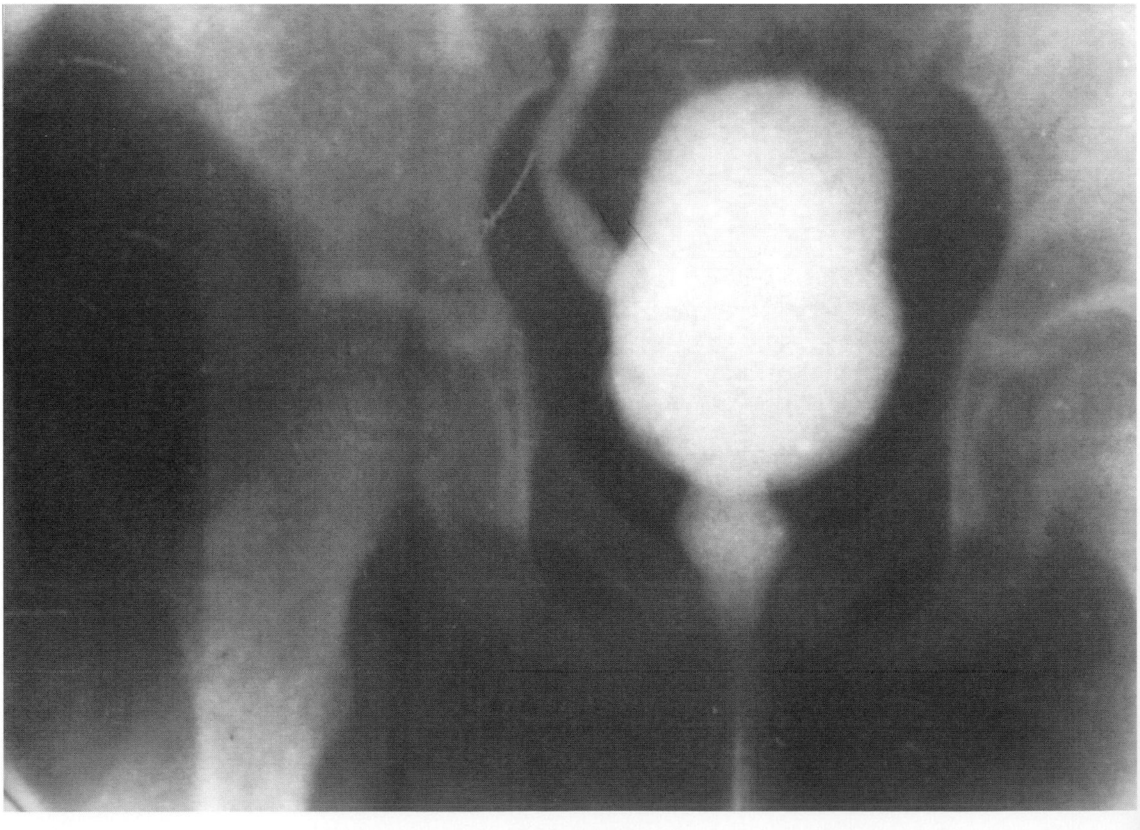

b

Figure 20.1 Fluoroscopic images during detrusor contractions in a neurologically normal patient with Hinman's syndrome (a) and a patient with a cervical spinal cord injury and detrusor sphincter dyssynergia (b). In each instance there is external urethral sphincter activity with voiding, a sustained elevation of intravesical pressure, and vesicoureteral reflux. The fluoroscopic images are indistinguishable.

sists of daytime and night-time incontinence, encopresis, bladder trabeculation, urinary tract infections, obstructive uropathy with vesicoureteral reflux, and a negative neurological examination. If untreated, end-stage bladder changes (fibrosis, decreased compliance, elevated intravesical storage pressures) may occur, and patients may progress to dialysis-dependent renal failure.[85,86] Most cases have been reported in children. Traditionally, these patients were thought to exhibit a volitional interruption of voiding brought on by psychological abnormalities, traumatic experiences or stress.[87] However, the presence of typical findings of this syndrome in newborn children argues against environmental factors as the cause in all cases.[56] Furthermore, careful urodynamic evaluation of children with Hinman's syndrome demonstrated that most patients have a sudden, unanticipated detrusor contraction which they attempt to inhibit by volitionally contracting the external sphincter.[27] The detrusor continues to contract against the closed sphincter, resulting in sustained elevations in intravesical pressure. The events are indistinguishable urodynamically or fluoroscopically from DSD (Fig. 20.1), and upper tract damage occurs via a similar mechanism, although in the case of Hinman's syndrome the external sphincter activity is volitional rather than reflex in nature. This pattern of voiding becomes habitual so that the patient has difficulty distinguishing voluntary from involuntary detrusor contractions; therefore, inappropriate sphincter activity occurs all of the time.[88]

Treatment is directed at protecting the upper tracts and achieving continence by lowering intravesical pressures and promoting effective bladder emptying. If end-stage bladder changes are absent, this may be effectively accomplished with timed voiding, anticholinergic medications, biofeedback, and/or intermittent self-catheterization.[27,89] When a significant psychological component is evident, psychotherapy is also indicated. Those who do not respond to conservative therapy may require surgical bladder enlargement to improve storage pressures.

PSEUDODYSSYNERGIA

The term 'pseudodyssynergia' has been used to refer to the presence of a contraction of the external urethral sphincter during voiding in young adult males.[90] The contraction may be observed as an increase in electromyographic activity or a narrowing of the urethra on fluoroscopy with concomitant increase in the intraluminal urethral pressure. The voiding pattern is frequently intermittent in nature, and may be associated with obstructive and irritative voiding symptoms. Frequently these patients are misdiagnosed as having 'chronic prostatitis'. Successful results with behavior modification and biofeedback have been reported.[91] It is important to distinguish this functional obstruction from an anatomic obstruction at the bladder neck which may be better treated with an ablative procedure.

URINARY RETENTION

Urinary retention results from anatomic bladder outlet obstruction, functional derangements of the bladder or urethra, or a combination of these factors. Common types of anatomic obstruction include benign prostatic hyperplasia or urethral strictures in males, and urethral occlusion following stress incontinence procedures in females. Treatment is directed at relief of the obstruction after which adequate voiding function is usually restored. A detailed discussion of the etiology and treatment of anatomic bladder outlet obstruction is beyond the scope of this chapter.

As discussed above, normal micturition is a centrally mediated event which requires afferent input to the brainstem and cortex. Voiding is accomplished by a coordinated relaxation of the external urethral sphincter followed by a sustained detrusor contraction. Neurologic disease or trauma which disrupts central pathways mediating afferent or efferent components of micturition may cause urinary retention. Suprasacral spinal cord injury commonly results in discoordinated bladder and urethral activity and impaired emptying (DSD, see above). Sacral spinal cord injury and lumbar myelomeningoceles cause damage to sensory and motor fibers to the bladder resulting in detrusor areflexia. Multiple sclerosis may affect any part of the central nervous system and can be associated with detrusor areflexia or DSD. Damage to the dorsal columns of the spinal cord from tabes dorsalis or pernicious anemia can result in loss of bladder sensation and consequent urinary retention.

Pathologic processes involving the peripheral nervous system have also been associated with urinary retention. Lumbar disc protrusion may impinge upon sacral nerve roots, causing detrusor areflexia, lower back pain, saddle anesthesia, and lower extremity weakness (cauda equina syndrome).

Neurotropic viruses such as herpes simplex or herpes zoster can cause transient urinary retention through involvement of the sensory dorsal root ganglia. Peripheral neuropathy from diabetes mellitus results in sensory and motor bladder dysfunction which may progress to urinary retention. Radical pelvic surgery (radical hysterectomy, abdominoperineal resection) may result in damage to the pelvic plexus, which contains preganglionic parasympathetic and postganglionic sympathetic nerve fibers. Unilateral injury results in urinary retention due to parasympathetic vesical denervation. Although partial sympathetic denervation also occurs with this type of injury, contralateral sympathetic fibers remain functional and the bladder neck remains closed. This type of injury usually recovers within 12–18 months. Bilateral pelvic plexus injury causes complete decentralization of the bladder and is permanent; associated findings include urinary retention, an open bladder neck, and decreased bladder compliance.[92]

Chronic urinary retention may occur in neurologically normal individuals as well. Most commonly this occurs after transient overdistention injuries to the bladder. Such injuries can be associated with anesthetic administration, pelvic prolapse, stress incontinence procedures, episodes of acute cystitis, excessive alcohol intake, and other conditions which acutely inhibit the bladder's ability to empty. Experimental evidence suggests that neuromuscular damage occurs after acute bladder overdistention. Animal studies have demonstrated degeneration of unmyelinated bladder wall nerve fibers, decreased detrusor contractility, and increased nuclear proliferation and bladder mass.[93–96] These changes can persist for weeks following a single overdistention episode.[95]

Fowler has described a syndrome of abnormal urethral sphincter electromyographic activity in women with idiopathic urinary retention.[97] This abnormal activity is hypothesized to cause incomplete sphincter relaxation during voiding. Subsequent ultrasonographic studies demonstrated increased external sphincter volume in these patients, suggesting that muscle hypertrophy may contribute to the voiding dysfunction.[98] The prevalence of these abnormal electromyographic patterns in the normal female population has not been studied.

Initial treatment of nonobstructive, non-neurogenic urinary retention includes intermittent catheterization at intervals sufficient to prevent vesical overdistention (usually less than 500–600 ml). Bethanechol chloride, a parasympathomimetic agent with relative in vitro selectivity for the bladder and gut, is frequently prescribed although objective evidence of its efficacy is lacking. Spontaneous recovery of voiding can occur, but it is currently not possible to predict when or if that will happen in a specific patient.

Patients with chronic idiopathic urinary retention have been successfully treated with sacral neuromodulation. The mechanism of action is not known. A pathologic voiding inhibition reflex has been postulated to exist, which is inhibited by afferent spinal cord input from the stimulator.[99] Other investigators have demonstrated a 'rebound' bladder contraction in animals when the electrical stimulation is interrupted.[100] In 20 treated patients, Shaker showed a decrease in postvoid residual volume from 78% to 10% of total bladder volume.[99] Elabbady treated eight patients and found a decrease in post-void residual volume from 85% to 29%, with a decrease in the catheterization frequency from 4.2 to 1.3 times per day.[101] Hohenfeller showed similar results (decrease in postvoid residual volume from 450 ml to 106 ml, decreased catheterization frequency from four times to once per day) in six patients.[23] Longer follow-up with larger numbers of patients is required, but these preliminary results clearly warrant further study.

VOLITIONAL/PSYCHOGENIC VOIDING DISORDERS

Traditionally, most types of dysfunctional voiding were felt to represent behavioral or psychological disorders. Terms such as 'lazy bladder syndrome' implied that poor habits were partly responsible for the symptoms. Uncontrolled studies were cited to demonstrate a high prevalence of psychosocial problems in families of dysfunctional voiders. Behavioral therapy and psychiatric counseling were recommended as initial therapy in order to identify and correct these factors. Today, although the precise etiology of dysfunctional voiding is still not well understood, it is recognized that the majority of patients with this problem demonstrate disordered coordination of the detrusor and urethra which is not under their control.[27] Behavioral therapy remains an integral part of treatment, but the goal of this therapy should be to help the patient regain control over a bladder which contracts abruptly and without warning, rather than to correct poor habits. Psychological factors are also important, as the stress and anxiety caused by the dysfunctional voiding symptoms may result in disadvantageous compensatory behavior. For instance, increased pelvic floor muscle tension due to constant fear of uncontrolled wetting may result in insufficient pelvic floor relaxation during normal voiding attempts.[88]

Although most cases of dysfunctional voiding may be attributed to involuntary factors, volitional or psychogenic voiding dysfunction does occur. The most frequent complaint is bladder pain, often accompanied by urinary retention. Other somatic complaints without clear diagnoses, and multiple emergency room and physician office visits are common. If intermittent catheterization has been prescribed, the patient may complain of pain or inability to catheterize. Despite this history, cystoscopy will often be normal indicating that catheterizations are not being performed. The neurologic examination is normal, and on urodynamics the guarding reflex is present as the bladder is filled. When asked to void, there may be a volitional lack of relaxation of the external urethral sphincter, which by itself is nondiagnostic. When multiple, severe complaints are present and are accompanied by a normal physical examination, a normal cystoscopy, and a normal urodynamic study except for lack of sphincter relaxation, volitional voiding dysfunction is likely. Such patients should be confronted and offered psychiatric counseling.

REFERENCES

1. De Groat WC. Anatomy and physiology of the lower urinary tract. *Urol Clin NA* 1993;**20**:383–401.
2. Siroky MB, Krane RJ. Neurologic aspects of detrusor sphincter dyssynergia with reference to the guarding reflex. *J Urol* 1982;**127**:953–7.
3. Park JM, Bloom DA, McGuire EJ. The guarding reflex revisited. *Br J Urol* 1997;**80**:940–45.
4. Griffiths D. Clinical aspects of detrusor instability and the value of urodynamics: a review of the evidence. *Eur Urol* 1999;**34** (Suppl):13–15.
5. Wise BG, Cardozo LD, Cutner A, Benness CJ, Burton G. Prevalence and significance of urethral instability in women with detrusor instability. *Br J Urol* 1993;**72**:26–9.
6. Frewen WK. A reassessment of bladder training in detrusor dysfunction in the female. *Br J Urol* 1982;**54**:372–3.
7. Urinary Incontinence Guideline Panel: Urinary incontinence in adults: clinical practice guideline. AHCPR Pub No 92-0038, Rockville, MD: Agency for Health Care Policy and Research, Public Health Service, US Department of Health and Human Services, March 1992.
8. Blaivas JG, Romanzi LJ, Heritz DM. Urinary incontinence: pathophysiology, evaluation, treatment overview, and nonsurgical management. In: Walsh PC, Retik AB, Vaughan ED Jr, Wein AJ (eds). *Campbell's Urology*. Philadelphia: WB Saunders, 1998;1007–1043.
9. Bump RC, Hurt WG, Fantl JA, Wyman JF. Assessment of Kegel pelvic muscle exercise performance after brief verbal instruction. *Am J Obstet Gynecol* 1991;**105**:322–9.
10. Cardozo LD, Abrams PD, Stanton SL, Feneley RC. Idiopathic bladder instability treated by biofeedback. *Br J Urol* 1978;**50**:521–3.
11. Kiolseth D, Madsen B, Knudsen LM, Norgaard JP, Djurhuus JC. Biofeedback treatment of children and adults with idiopathic detrusor instability. *Scand J Urol Nephrol* 1994;**28**:243–47.
12. Payne CK. Electrostimulation. In: O'Donnell PD. *Urinary incontinence*. St. Louis: Mosby, 1997;287.
13. Wyndaele JJ, Michielsen D, van Dromme S. Influence of sacral neuromodulation on electrosensation of the lower urinary tract. *J Urol* 2000;**163**:221–4.
14. Fall M, Lindstrom S. Electrical stimulation. A physiologic approach to the treatment of urinary incontinence. *Urol Clin NA* 1991;**18**:393–407.
15. Vodusek DB, Light JK, Libby JM. Detrusor inhibition induced by stimulation of pudendal nerve afferents. *Neurourol Urodynam* 1986;**5**:381.
16. Vodusek DB, Plevnik S, Vrtacnik P, Janez J. Detrusor inhibition on selective pudendal nerve stimulation in the perineum. *Neurourol Urodynam* 1988;**6**:389.
17. Schmidt RA. Applications of neurostimulation in urology. *Neurourol Urodynam* 1988;**7**:585–92.
18. Everaert K, Plancke H, Lefevere F, Oosterlinck W. The urodynamic evaluation of neuromodulation in patients with voiding dysfunction. *Br J Urol* 1997;**79**:702–707.
19. Janknegt RA, Weil EHJ, Eerdmans PHA. Improving neuromodulation technique for refractory voiding dysfunctions: two-stage implant. *Urology* 1997;**49**:358–62.
20. Schmidt RA, Jonas U, Oleson KA, *et al.* Sacral nerve stimulation for treatment of refractory urinary urge incontinence. *J Urol* 1999;**162**:352–7.
21. Weil EHJ, Ruiz-Cerda JL, Eerdmans PHA *et al.* Sacral root neuromodulation in the treatment of refractory urge incontinence: a prospective randomized clinical trial. *Eur Urol* 2000;**37**:161–171.
22. Bosch JLHR, Groen J. Sacral (S3) segmental nerve stimulation as a treatment for urge incontinence in patients with detrusor instability: results of chronic electrical stimulation using an implantable neural prosthesis. *J Urol* 1995;**154**:504–507.
23. Hohenfellner M, Schultz-Lampel D, Dahms S, Matzel K, Thuroff JW. Bilateral sacral neuromodulation for treatment for lower urinary tract dysfunction. *J Urol* 1998;**160**:821–4.
24. Forsythe WI, Redmond A. Enuresis and spontaneous cure rate: study of 1129 enuretics. *Arch Dis Child* 1974;**49**:259–63.
25. Tietjen DN, Husmann DA. Nocturnal enuresis: a guide to evaluation and treatment. *Mayo Clinic Proc* 1996;**71**:857–62.
26. Husmann DA. Enuresis. *Urology* 1996;**48**:184–93.
27. McGuire EJ, Savastano JA. Urodynamic studies in enuresis and the nonneurogenic neurogenic bladder. *J Urol* 1984;**132**:299–302.
28. Kales A, Kales JD, Jacobson A, Humphrey FJ 2nd, Soldatos CR. Effect of imipramine on enuretic frequency and sleep stage. *Pediatrics* 1977;**60**:431–6.
29. Mikkelsen EJ, Rapoport JL, Nee L, Gruenau C, Mandelson W, Gillin JC. Childhood enuresis: I. Sleep patterns and psychopathology. *Arch Gen Psychiat* 1980;**37**:1139–44.
30. Norgaard JP, Pedersen EB, Djurhuus JC. Diurnal antidiuretic hormone levels in enuretics. *J Urol* 1989;**134**:1029–31.
31. Koff SA. Cure of nocturnal enuresis: why isn't desmopressin very effective? *Peiat Nephrol* 1996;**10**:667–70.
32. Jarvelin MP. Developmental history and neurologic findings in enuretic children. *Dev Med Child Neurol* 1989;**31**:728–36.
33. Bakwin H. The genetics of enuresis. *Clin Dev Med* 1973;**48/49**:73–7.
34. Fergusson DM, Horwood LJ, Shannon FT. Factors related to the age of attainment of nocturnal bladder control: an 8-year longitudinal study. *Pediatrics* 1986;**78**:884–90.
35. Arnell H, Hjalmas K, Jagervall M, *et al.* The genetics of primary nocturnal enuresis: inheritance and suggestion of a second major gene on chromosome 12q. *J Med Genet* 1997;**34**:360–65.
36. Eiberg H, Berendt I, Mohr J. Assignment of dominant inherited nocturnal enuresis (ENUR1) to chromosome 13q. *Nat Genet* 1995;354–6.
37. George CPL, Messeril FH, Genest J, *et al.* Diurnal variation of plasma vasopressin in man. *J Endocrinol Metab* 1975;**41**:332–8.
38. Norgaard JP, Hansen JH, Wildschiot J. Sleep cystometries in children with nocturnal enuresis. *J Urol* 1989;**141**:1156–69.
39. Rittig S, Knudsen UB, Norgaard JP, Pedersen EB, Djurhuus JO. Abnormal diurnal rhythm of plasma vasopressin and urinary output in patients with enuresis. *Am J Physiol* 1989;**256**:F664–F671.

40. Eggert P, Kuhn B: Antidiuretic hormone regulation in patients with primary nocturnal enuresis. *Arch Dis Child* 1995;**73**:508–511.
41. Steffens J, Netzer M, Isenberg E, Alloussi S, Ziegler M. Vasopressin deficiency in primary nocturnal enuresis. Results of a controlled prospective study. *Eur Urol* 1993;**24**:366–70.
42. Kawauchi A, Watanabe H, Miyoshi K. Early morning urine osmolality in nonenuretic and enuretic children. *Pediat Nephrol* 1996;**10**:696–8.
43. Wille S, Aili M, Harris A, Aronson S. Plasma and urinary levels of vasopressin in enuretic and non-enuretic children. *Scand J Urol Nephrol* 1994;**28**:119–22.
44. Fergusson DM, Horwood LJ. Nocturnal enuresis and behavioral problems in adolescence: a 15-year longitudinal study. *Pediatrics* 1994;**94**:662–8.
45. Stromgen A, Thomsen PH. Personality traits in young adults with a history of conditioning-treated childhood enuresis. *Acta Psychiat Scand* 1990;**81**:538–41.
46. Moffatt MEK. Nocturnal enuresis: Psychological implications of treatment and nontreatment. *J Pediat* 1989;**114**:697–704.
47. Scharf MB, Pravda MF, Jennings SW, Kauffman R, Ringel J. Childhood enuresis: A comprehensive treatment program. *Psychiat Clin NA* 1987;**10**:655–66.
48. Lovering JS, Tallett SE, McKendry JB. Oxybutinin efficacy in the treatment of primary enuresis. *Pediatrics* 1988;**82**:104–106.
49. Kass EJ, Diokno AC, Montealegre A. Enuresis: principles of management and result of treatment. *J Urol* 1979;**121**:794–6.
50. Fritz GK, Rockney RM, Yeung A. Plasma levels and efficacy of imipramine treatment for enuresis. *J Am Acad Child Adolesc Psych* 1994;**33**:60–64.
51. Monda JM, Husmann DA. Primary nocturnal enuresis: a comparison among observation, impiramine, desmopressin acetate and bed-wetting alarm systems. *J Urol* 1995;**154**:745–8.
52. Kardash S, Hillman ES, Werry J. Efficacy of imipramine in childhood enuresis: a double-blind control study with placebo. *Can Med Assoc J* 1968;**99**:263–6.
53. Blackwell B, Currah J. The psychopharmacology of nocturnal enuresis. In: Kolvin I, MacKeith RC, Meadow SR (eds). *Bladder control and enuresis*. London: Heinemann Medical Books, 1973;231–57.
54. Moffatt MEK, Harlos S, Kirshen AJ, Burd L. Desmopressin acetate and nocturnal enuresis: how much do we know? *Pediatrics* 1993;**92**:420–25.
55. Skoog SK, Stokes A, Turner KI. Oral desmopressin: a randomized double-blind placebo controlled study of effectiveness in children with primary nocturnal enuresis. *J Urol* 1997;**158**:1035–1040.
56. Jayanthi VR, Khoury AE, McLorie GA, Agarwal SK. The nonneurogenic neurogenic bladder of early infancy. *J Urol* 1997;**158**:1281–5.
57. Hoekx L, Wyndaele JJ, Vermandel A. The role of bladder biofeedback in the treatment of children with refractory nocturnal enuresis associated with idiopathic detrusor instability and small bladder capacity. *J Urol* 1998;**160**:858–60.
58. Forsythe WI, Butler RJ. Fifty years of enuretic alarms. *Arch Dis Child* 1989;**64**:879–85.
59. Turner RK. Conditioning treatment of nocturnal enuresis: present status. In: Kolvin I, MacKeith RC, Meadow SR (eds). *Bladder control and enuresis*. London: Heinemann Medical Books, 1973;231–57.
60. Rushton HG. Nocturnal enuresis: epidemiology, evaluation, and currently available treatment options. *J Pediat* 1989;**114**:691–6.
61. Wille S. Comparison of desmopressin and enuresis alarm for nocturnal enuresis. *Arch Dis Child* 1986;**61**:30–33.
62. Scott MA, Barclay DR, Houts AC. Childhood enuresis: etiology, assessment, and current behavioral treatment. *Prog Behav Modif* 1992;**28**:83–117.
63. Sukhai RN, Mol J, Harris AS. Combined therapy of enuresis alarm and desmopressin in the treatment of nocturnal enuresis. *Eur J Pediat* 1989;465–67.
64. Maizels M, Ghandi K, Keating B, Rosenbaum D. How to diagnose and treatment for children who cannot control urination. *Curr Probl Pediat* 1993;**23**:402–450.
65. Cushing FC Jr, Baller WP. The problem of nocturnal enuresis in adults: special reference to managers and managerial aspirants. *J Psychol* 1975;**89**:203–213.
66. Wadsworth ML. Persistent enuresis in adults. *Am J Orthopsychiat* 1944;**14**:313.
67. Turner RK, Taylor PD. Conditioning treatment of nocturnal enuresis in adults: preliminary findings. *Behav Res Ther* 1974;**12**:41.
68. Karaman MI, Esen T, Kocak T, Akinci M, Tellaloglu S. Rationale of urodynamic assessment in adult enuresis. *Eur Urol* 1992;**21**:138–140.
69. Vandersteen DR, Husmann DA. Treatment of primary nocturnal enuresis persisting into adulthood. *J Urol* 1999;**161**:90–92.
70. Koff SA, Murtagh DS. The uninhibited bladder in children: effect of treatment on recurrence of urinary infection and on vesicoureteral reflux resolution. *J Urol* 1983;**130**:1138–41.
71. van Gool JD, Hjalmas K, Tamminen-Mobius T, Olbing H. Historical clues to the complex of dysfunctional voiding, urinary tract infection and vesicoureteral reflux. *J Urol* 1992;**148**:1699–1702.
72. Koff SA, Lapides J, Piazza DH. Association of urinary tract infection and reflux with uninhibited bladder contractions and voluntary sphincteric obstruction. *J Urol* 1979;**121**:373–5.
73. Koff SA, Wagner TT, Jayanthi VR. The relationship among dysfunctional elimination syndromes, primary vesicoureteral reflux and urinary tract infections in children. *J Urol* 1998;**160**:1019–22.
74. Schulman SL, Quinn CK, Plachter N, Kodman-Jones C. Comprehensive management of dysfunctional voiding. *Pediatrics* 1999;**103**:E31.
75. Allen TD. Vesicoureteral reflux as a manifestation of dysfunctional voiding. In: Hodson CJ, Kincaid-Smith P (eds). *Reflux nephropathy*. New York: Masson Publishing, 1979;171–80.
76. Homsy YL, Nsouli I, Hamburger B, Laberge I, Schick E. Effects of oxybutinin on vesicoureteral reflux in children. *J Urol* 1985;**134**:1168–71.
77. Seruca H. Vesicoureteral reflux and voiding dysfunction: a prospective study. *J Urol* 1989;**142**:494–8.
78. Taylor CM, Corkery JJ, White RHP. Micturition symptoms

and unstable bladder activity with primary vesicoureteral reflux. *Br J Urol* 1982;**54**:494–8.

79. Scholtmeijer RJ, Nijman RJM. Vesicoureteral reflux and videourodynamic studies: results of a prospective study after three years of follow-up. *Urology* 1994;**43**:714–18.
80. Koff SA. Relationship between dysfunctional voiding and reflux. *J Urol* 1992;**148**:1703–1705.
81. Snodgrass W. The impact of treated dysfunctional voiding on the nonsurgical management of vesicoureteral reflux. *J Urol* 1998;**160**:1823–5.
82. Noe HN. The role of dysfunctional voiding in failure or complication of ureteral reimplantation for primary reflux. *J Urol* 1985;**134**:1172–5.
83. Noe HN. The risk and risk factors of contralateral reflux following repair of simple unilateral primary reflux. *J Urol* 1998;**160**:849–50.
84. Hinman F Jr, Baumann FW. Vesical and ureteral damage from voiding dysfunction in boys without neurologic or obstructive disease. *J Urol* 1973;**109**:727–32.
85. Yang CC, Mayo ME. Morbidity of dysfunctional voiding syndrome. *Urology* 1997;**49**:445–8.
86. Kumar A, Banerjee GK, Goel MC, Mishra VK, Kapoor R, Bhandari M. Functional bladder neck obstruction: a rare cause of renal failure. *J Urol* 1995;**154**:186–89.
87. Hinman FJ. Non-neurogenic neurogenic bladder (the Hinman Syndrome) – 15 years later. *J Urol* 1986;**136**:769–77.
88. Bauer SB, Retik SB, Colodny AH, Hallett M, Khoshbin S, Dyro FM. The unstable bladder of childhood. *Urol Clin NA* 1980;**7**:321–36.
89. Hellstrom A-L, Hjalmas K, Jodal U. Rehabilitation of the dysfunctional bladder in children: method and 3-year follow-up. *J Urol* 1987;**138**:847–9.
90. Kaplan SA, Ikeguchi EF, Santarosa RP, *et al.* Etiology of voiding dysfunction in men less than 50 years of age. *Urology* 1996;**47**:836–9.
91. Kaplan SA, Santarosa RP, D'Alisera PM, *et al.* Pseudodyssynergia (contraction of the external sphincter during voiding) misdiagnosed as chronic nonbacterial prostatitis and the role of biofeedback as a therapeutic option. *J Urol* 1997;**157**:2234–7.
92. McGuire EJ. Neurovesical dysfunction after abdomino-perineal resection. *Surg Clin NA* 1980;**60**:1207–1213.
93. Sehn JT. Anatomic effect of distention therapy in unstable bladder: new approach. *Urology* 1978;**11**:581–7.
94. Ghoneim GM, Regnier CH, Biancani P, Johnson L, Susset JG. Effect of vesical outlet obstruction on detrusor contractility and passive properties in rabbits. *J Urol* 1986;**135**:1284–9.
95. Tammela TL, Levin RM, Monson FC, Wein AJ, Longhurst PA. The influence of acute overdistension on rat bladder function and DNA synthesis. *J Urol* 1993;**150**:1533–9.
96. Bross S, Schumacher S, Scheepe JR, *et al.* Effects of acute urinary bladder overdistention on bladder response during sacral neurostimulation. *Eur Urol* 1999;**36**:354–9.
97. Fowler CJ, Christmas TJ, Chapple CR, Fitzmaurice PH, Kirby RS, Jacobs HS. Abnormal electromyographic activity of the urethral sphincter, voiding dysfunction, and polycystic ovaries: a new syndrome? *Br J Med* 1988;**297**:1436–8.
98. Noble J, Dixon P, Rickards D, Fowler O. Urethral sphincter volumes in women with obstructed voiding and abnormal sphincter EMG activity. *Br J Urol* 1995;**76**:741–6.
99. Shaker HS, Hassouna M. Sacral rot neuromodulation in idiopathic nonobstructive chronic urinary retention. *J Urol* 1998;**159**:1476–8.
100. Schultz-Lampel D, Jiang C, Lindstrom S, Thuroff JW. Experimental results on mechanisms of action of electrical neuromodulation in chronic urinary retention. *World J Urol* 1998;**16**:301–304.
101. Elabbady AA, Hassouna MM, Elhilali MM. Neural stimulation for chronic voiding dysfunctions. *J Urol* 1994;**152**:2076–2180.

Chapter 21

Bladder dysfunction in neurological disorders

Michael J Swinn, Clare J Fowler

INTRODUCTION

The bladder performs only two functions – urine storage and emptying. The micturition frequency in a healthy adult with a bladder capacity of about 500 ml is likely to be about once every 3–4 hours. This means that for more than 98% of life, the bladder is in its storage mode. The current view is that the control of these two mutually exclusive activities is effected by neural programs which exist in the pons and that suprapontine influences act to 'switch' from one state to the other.

Normally, voiding is timed according to the perceived state of bladder fullness together with an assessment of the social appropriateness to do so. Connections between the pons and the sacral spinal cord must be intact, as well as the peripheral innervation arising from the most caudal segments of the sacral cord. The peripheral innervation passes through the cauda equina to the sacral plexus and via the pelvic and pudendal nerves to innervate the bladder and sphincter. Thus the innervation needed for physiological bladder control is extensive, requiring supra pontine inputs, intact spinal connections between the pons and the sacral cord, and intact peripheral nerves. A knowledge of the 'map' of the neurological control of the bladder allows the clinician to predict with some certainty what the likely effect a particular disorder of the nervous system will have on a patient's bladder function.

THE NEURAL CONTROL OF BLADDER FUNCTION

Barrington, working on the decerebrate cat in London in the 1920s, demonstrated that the 'middle pons was the level in the brain at which the motor tone of the bladder arises.'[1] Some 40 years later, Kuru carried out further studies in cats and suggested that the group of cells in the pons which when electrically stimulated resulted in a detrusor contraction be called 'Barrington's nucleus'.[2] Subsequent studies by de Groat's[3,4] and later Holstege's groups refined details of the localization of brainstem activity involved in bladder storage and voiding in animals.[5,6] Stimulation of a medial region in the dorsum of the pons results in an immediate decrease in urethral pressure and silence of pelvic floor EMG signal, followed by a rise in detrusor pressure. This region, which Holstege *et al.* called the 'M-region', is the same area as the pontine micturition centre (PMC) or Barrington's nucleus. Ultrastructural tracing studies demonstrated direct projections from the 'M-region' to the intermediolateral cell column of the sacral cord and the parasympathetic preganglionic bladder motor neurons in the cat.[7] Stimulation of a nucleus at the same level of the pons, but more laterally placed, the so-called 'L-region', results in a powerful contraction of the urethral sphincter.[5] Injection of radioactive leucine into the 'L-region' produced labeled fibers in Onuf 's nucleus,[5] the motor nucleus containing the anterior horn cells innervating the sphincters. It was therefore proposed that the 'L-region' be regarded as important for continence and the 'M-region' the site of activation for micturition.[6]

A brainstem mechanism whereby the bladder is 'switched' from voiding to storage, and vice versa, is now generally accepted as the model in experimental animals and now, as a result of PET scanning studies, in humans. There are, however, a number of other segmental reflexes controlling bladder and sphincter behavior which have been identified in experimental animals. The control of the bladder in newborn kittens, rat pups etc. is quite different from that in adult animals, and it seems likely that although various sacral segmental reflexes may be of functional significance in infancy, maturation allows pontine and supra-pontine mechanisms to develop a controlling influence. However, in pathological states these 'primitive' or infantile reflexes may re-emerge and in humans become clinically relevant. Most important in this respect is the C-fiber mediated reflex which emerges following disconnection from pontine regulatory influences as a consequence of spinal cord disease.

The descriptions of PET studies of male and female subjects during voiding have demonstrated that the neurological control of the bladder in man is essentially similar to that which had been demonstrated in experimental animals.[8,9] Right-handed volunteers were trained to void whilst lying in the scanner; in both studies a proportion of both the male and female subjects were unable to do this. The differences seen between the 'successful' and 'unsuccessful' voiders were of great interest. Focusing on the dorsomedial tegmentum of the pons it was shown that in successful voiders there was activity in a region of the medio-posterior pons. It was suggested that this is the human homolog of the so called 'M-region' in animals.[10] In the 'unsuccessful' voiders, a region in the ventrolateral pontine tegmentum was seen to be activated (Fig. 21.1). It was proposed that this is the region homologous to the 'L-region' of the cat.

BLADDER FUNCTION IN CENTRAL NERVOUS SYSTEM DISEASE

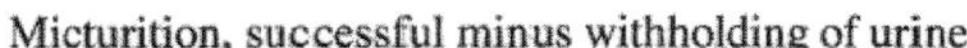

FRONTAL LOBE LESIONS

Prior to the findings of these functional brain imaging experiments in humans, all that was known about the cortical control of the bladder was based on clinical studies of patients with brain lesions. The most influential was that by Andrew and Nathan in 1964, who described 38 patients with disturbances of micturition resulting from lesions in the anterior frontal lobe.[11] In their series there were 10 patients with intracranial tumors, two with anterior frontal lobe damage following rupture of an aneurysm, four who had penetrating brain wounds and 22 patients who had undergone leucotomy. The authors explained that the leucotomy cases were the most useful in terms of localization of the important brain structures and they concluded that the area shown in Fig. 21.2 was critical for bladder control.

The typical clinical picture of frontal lobe incontinence they described was of a patient with severe urgency and frequency of micturition, and urge incontinence. Micturition was normally coordinated, indicating that the disturbance was in the higher control of these processes. The infrequency with which such patients are encountered was stressed by the authors explaining that they had each been collecting cases separately over a period of 24 years and only just prior to writing did they learn of each other's interest and combine to present a joint paper.[11]

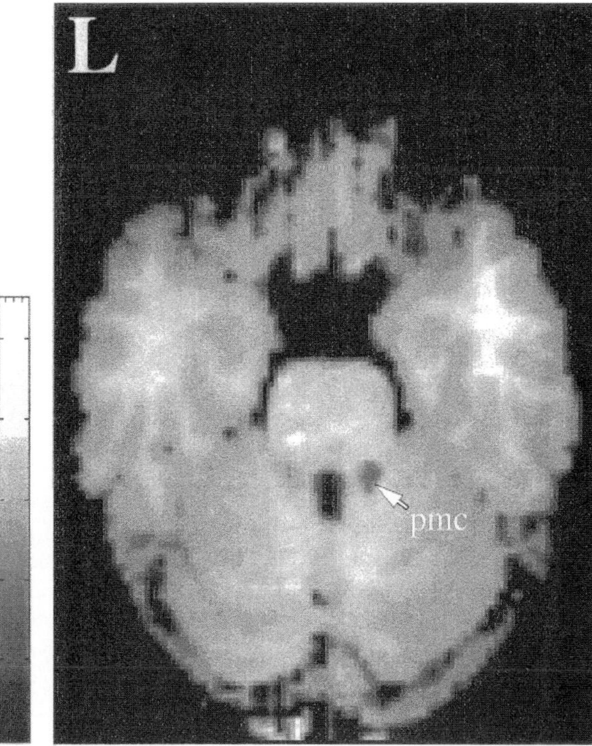

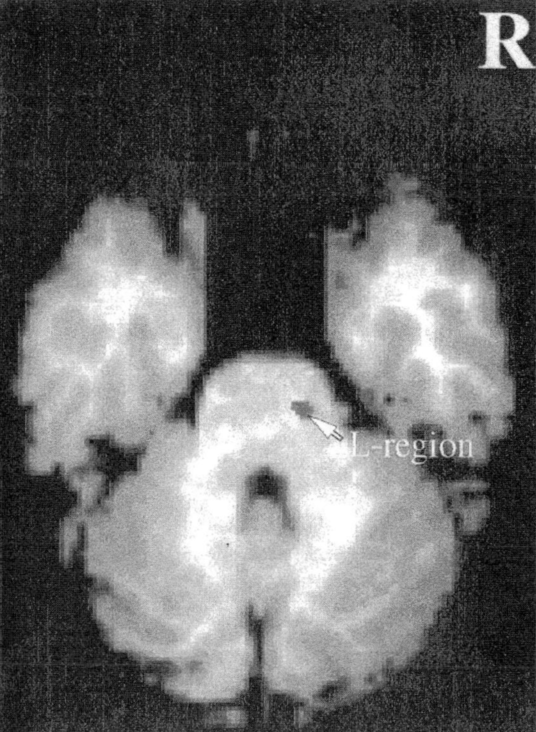

Figure 21.1 Brainstem activation in women who could (left) and could not void (right). The numbers on the color scale refer to the corresponding Z-scores (significance). From Ref. 9, with permission.

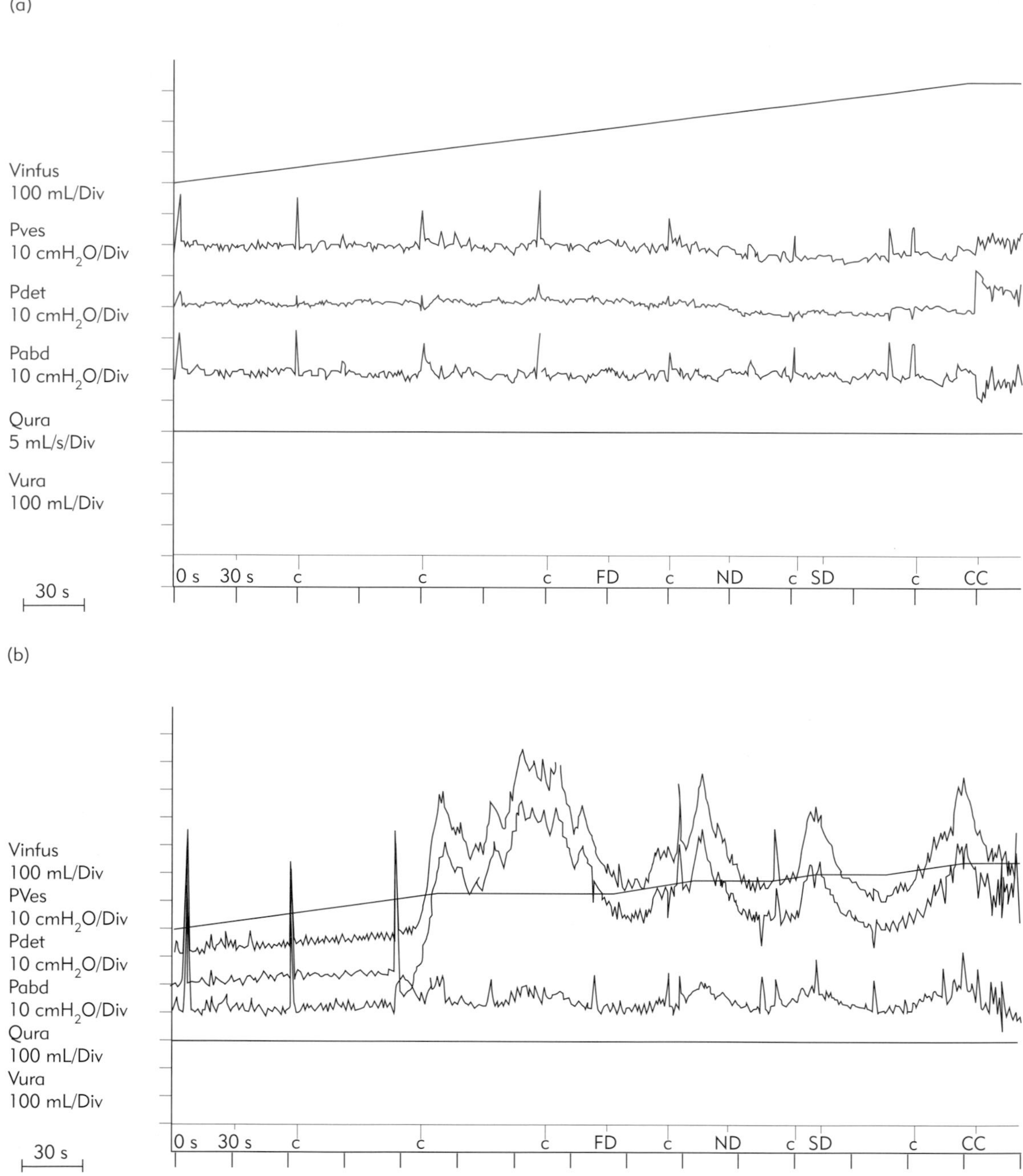

Figure 21.2 (a) Normal filling cystometry. Lines in the bladder and rectum continuously record the pressure as the bladder is slowly filled via a catheter. The rectal pressure is taken as being the same as abdominal pressure. Since the intravesical pressure is the sum of the detrusor pressure and the surrounding abdominal pressure, the detrusor pressure is calculated by subtraction. The patient is asked to cough regularly to ensure correct line positioning. This trace shows the detrusor pressure remaining low throughout filling. (b) Filling cystometry in a patient with a spinal cord injury. When about 100 ml of fluid has been infused into the bladder, a large hyperreflexic detrusor contraction is seen. Vinfus: volume infused; Pves: vesical pressure; Pdet: detrusor pressure; Pabd: abdominal pressure; Qura: flow of urine; Vura: volume of urine passed; c: cough; FD: first desire (to void); ND: normal desire (to void); SD: strong desire (to void); CC: cystometric capacity.

Although the 1964 paper by Andrew and Nathan has been the most influential in the study of frontal lobe control of the bladder, it was not in fact the first. In 1960 Ueki had published a paper of which Andrew and Nathan were unaware. Ueki, a Japanese neurosurgeon, had analysed the urinary symptoms of 462 patients who had surgery for brain tumors. He illustrated his conclusions with a diagram showing a strong positive influence on micturition of an area in the pons and an inhibitory input from the frontal lobe and bilateral paracentral lobules.[12]

Urinary retention has also been described in patients with brain lesions. Two of Andrew and Nathan's patients were in urinary retention at some stage.[11] More recently there have been three reports of elderly women with various forms of right frontal lobe pathology who had urinary retention. In two the underlying lesion was successfully treated and they recovered bladder function.[13,14]

CEREBROVASCULAR ACCIDENTS (CVAs)

There have been a number of studies of groups of patients who have had CVAs and subsequently developed urinary symptoms. The conclusions drawn from these groups of patients with disparate cortical lesions are that, in general, voiding is normally coordinated, no patients showing evidence of detrusor sphincter dyssynergia, and that the commonest finding on cystometry is detrusor hyperreflexia.[15–18]

Most recently Sakakibara *et al.*[19] reported on the bladder symptoms of 72 patients who had been admitted with an acute hemispheric stroke. When assessed at 3 months, 53% were found to have significant urinary complaints. The commonest problem was nocturnal frequency which affected 36%, while urge incontinence affected 29% and difficulty in voiding, 25%. Urinary retention was seen in the acute phase of illness in 6%. A significant positive correlation was found between the occurrence of a urinary disturbance and hemiparesis ($p < 0.05$) and a negative correlation with hemianopia ($p < 0.05$). Brain imaging techniques confirmed a more anterior location of brain lesions in the former group. Urodynamic studies of 22 symptomatic patients showed detrusor hyperreflexia in 68%, detrusor–sphincter dyssynergia in 14% and uninhibited sphincter relaxation in 36%. Patients with urinary retention had detrusor areflexia and a non-relaxing sphincter. No statistically significant correlation could be demonstrated between any particular lesion site and urodynamic findings. There was some indication that lesion size was related to the occurrence of urinary symptoms. The findings suggested that damage to the anteromedial frontal lobe and its descending pathway, and the basal ganglia, is mainly responsible for micturitional dysfunction in stroke patients.

Analysis of the symptoms of 532 patients seen within 7 days of their stroke found that the presence of urinary incontinence appeared to be a more powerful prognostic indicator for poor survival and eventual functional dependence than a depressed level of consciousness in this period.[20,21] It was suggested either that incontinence was the result of a severe general rather than a specific loss of function or that those who were incontinent were less motivated both to recover continence and more general neurological function. Outcome was so much better in those who remained or became dry that it seems possible that recovery of continence may promote morale and self-esteem which can actually hasten overall recovery.

PARKINSONISM

Although the basal ganglia have been shown to have an effect on micturition reflexes in experimental animals, there are several additional possible causes of urinary symptoms in a patient with parkinsonism. These include a number of possible neurogenic causes depending on the exact underlying neurological diagnosis as well as local urological problems. In Parkinson's disease (PD) bladder symptoms usually occur at an advanced stage of the disease and prostatic outflow obstruction should first be excluded in an elderly man. However, in a patient with severe urinary symptoms yet relatively mild parkinsonism a diagnosis of multiple system atrophy (MSA) should be considered.

The onset of urogenital symptoms in MSA may precede overt neurological involvement by some years and in a study of the duration of symptoms before the diagnosis of MSA was made erectile dysfunction and bladder symptoms began 4–5 years prior to the diagnosis and on average, 2 years before more specific neurological symptoms appeared. Almost half the male patients had had a transurethral prostatectomy but with lasting beneficial effect in very few.[22]

In MSA the central nervous system is affected at several different locations which are important for bladder control. It is thought that detrusor hyperreflexia is due to cell loss in the pontine region, whereas incomplete bladder emptying is due to loss of parasympathetic drive on the detrusor neurons following atrophy of cells in the intermediolateral cell columns of the sacral cord. In addition, anterior horn cell loss in Onuf's nucleus[23] results in denervation of the striated urethral sphincter so that the patient has a combination of bladder overactivity, together with incomplete emptying and a weak sphincter. There may be a marked change in bladder dysfunction during the progression of MSA. Although patients often present with detrusor hyperreflexia, over the course of ensuing months or years, a failure of bladder emptying may develop so that the post micturition residual volume increases.[24]

Table 21.1 Urogenital criteria which favor a diagnosis of MSA

- Urinary symptoms preceding or presenting with parkinsonism
- Urinary incontinence
- Post-micturition residual volume >100 ml
- Erectile dysfunction preceding or presenting with parkinsonism
- Worsening bladder control after urological surgery

Because of the motor neuron loss in Onuf 's nucleus, changes of chronic reinnervation in the motor units of both urinary and anal sphincters may be demonstrated and sphincter EMG may be contributory in making the diagnosis.[25,26] However if this test is not available there are clinical urological criteria which may assist in recognizing patients with MSA (Table 21.1) and should make a urological surgeon cautious about operating.[27]

In patients with Parkinson's disease (PD) there may be considerable difficulties in establishing the exact cause of any bladder symptoms, and treatment is often problematic. The bladder symptoms usually come on after many years of treatment for PD[27] and patients often show features of long-term side effects of levodopa. Typically they complain of urgency and frequency, and urge incontinence if poor mobility compounds with their bladder overactivity. Urodynamic studies in patients with PD have shown that the commonest urodynamic abnormality is detrusor hyperreflexia,[28–33] and there are several possible causes for this. The hypothesis which has been most widely proposed is that in health the basal ganglia have an inhibitory effect on the micturition reflex and with cell loss in the substantia nigra, detrusor hyperreflexia develops.

Studies that have looked at the effect of L-dopa or apomorphine on bladder behavior in patients with PD have produced conflicting results. In patients showing 'on–off ' phenomena cystometry in both states showed a lessening of hyperreflexia with L-dopa in some patients and a worsening in others.[30] A similar, unpredictable effect was found on detrusor hyperreflexia when subcutaneous apomorphine was given in one study[31] although in another all those with detrusor hyperreflexia improved.[33]

Although the hypothesis that bladder dysfunction is due primarily to basal ganglia disease is generally accepted, there are other factors which should be considered. A potentially correctable cause such as prostatic outflow obstruction should be considered in an older male patient. The poor reputation for outcome following prostatic surgery in patients with PD may well have been due to the inclusion of patients with MSA in studies of 'Parkinson's disease and the bladder'. However most publications in the last decade recognize the potential problem and give some statement about the certainty of neurological diagnosis. If there is convincing evidence of prostatic occlusion prostatectomy should be considered bearing in mind that some men with PD do benefit from a TURP.[27,34]

There may also be outflow obstruction in PD due to impaired relaxation or 'bradykinesia' of the urethral sphincter.[31,35] A study of subcutaneous apomorphine in patients with PD and urinary symptoms found that apomorphine reduced bladder outflow resistance and improved voiding in all 10 patients in the study.[31] It was proposed that this method of investigation be used to demonstrate the reversibility of outflow obstruction in men with PD before prostatic surgery be undertaken.

A final consideration is the possible effect of the dopaminergic medication on the detrusor muscle itself. Dopamine D1 and D2 receptors have been demonstrated in bladder biopsies using radioligand binding and autoradiographic techniques,[36] but the long-term effect on these receptors of exposure to L-dopa is not known.

BRAINSTEM LESIONS

In 1926 Holman noted that voiding difficulty could be a sign of posterior fossa tumors[37] and in a series of patients with brain tumors reported by Ueki, voiding difficulty occurred in 46 (30%) of 152 patients with posterior fossa tumors, while urinary incontinence occurred in only three (2%).[12] Renier *et al.* found urinary retention in 71% of 17 children with pontine glioma.[38] There are also reports of patients presenting with difficulty with micturition found to have various brainstem pathologies.[39,40,41]

In 1996 Sakakibara *et al.* reported the urinary symptoms of 39 patients with brainstem strokes.[42] Almost half had urinary symptoms, with nocturnal urinary frequency and voiding difficulty in 28%, urinary retention in 21% and urinary incontinence in 8%. These problems were more common following hemorrhage probably because the damage was usually bilateral. Urinary symptoms did not occur in those with lesions of the midbrain, but did occur in 35% of those with pontine lesions and 18% with medullary stroke. A correlation was found between urinary symptoms and sensory disturbance, abnormal eye movement and incoordination. Urodynamics in 11 symptomatic patients showed detrusor hyperreflexia in eight (73%), low compliance bladder in one (9%), detrusor areflexia in three (27%), non-relaxing sphincter on voiding in five (45%) and uninhibited sphincter relaxation in three (27%). The proximity of the medial longitudinal fasciculus to the presumed pontine micturition center in the dorsal pons means that a disorder of eye movement such as an internuclear ophthalmoplegia is highly likely in patients with pontine pathology causing a voiding disorder.

SPINAL CORD INJURY

Immediately following spinal cord transection and during the phase of spinal shock the bladder is acontractile but gradually, over the course of some weeks, reflex detrusor contractions develop in response to low filling volumes. This phenomenon is referred to as 'detrusor hyper-reflexia' when secondary to neurological disease and 'detrusor instability' when occurring in the neurologically intact. The resultant rises in intravesical pressure can be demonstrated using the technique of cystometry (Fig. 21.2). It has been proposed from studies in the cat that following spinal injury and damage to the pontine micturition center, C fibers emerge as the major afferents forming a spinal segmental reflex which results in automatic voiding.[43,44] It is assumed that the same pathophysiology occurs in man. The response to intravesical capsaicin (a C fiber neurotoxin) in patients with acute traumatic spinal cord injury[45] or chronic progressive spinal cord disease suggests this may be the case.[46]

A second type of abnormal bladder pressure rise can develop following spinal cord injury. This is the steady rise in pressure which occurs on filling and is due to the loss of active compliance of the normal bladder (Fig. 21.3). The precise mechanisms underlying this are not known.

The pathways that connect the pontine micturition centers to the sacral cord affect the reciprocal activity of the detrusor and sphincter needed to 'switch' between storage and voiding. Following disconnection from the pons this synergistic activity is lost so that the sphincter tends to contract during detrusor contraction, a condition known as 'detrusor–sphincter dyssynergia' (Fig. 21.4).

The combination of detrusor hyperreflexia, loss of compliance and detrusor–sphincter dyssynergia can be of such severity as to cause ureteric reflux, hydronephrosis and eventual upper renal tract damage. Prior to the introduction of modern treatments, renal failure was a common cause of death following spinal cord injury (SCI). The bladder problems of those with SCI must therefore be managed in such a way as to lessen the possibility of upper tract disease as well as provide the patient with adequate bladder control for a fully rehabilitated life. Those with SCI are often young and otherwise fit and it may be better for them to undergo surgery on their lower urinary tract with a view to fulfilling these two aims of management rather than be managed by the medical means which are more suitable for patients with progressive neurological disease.

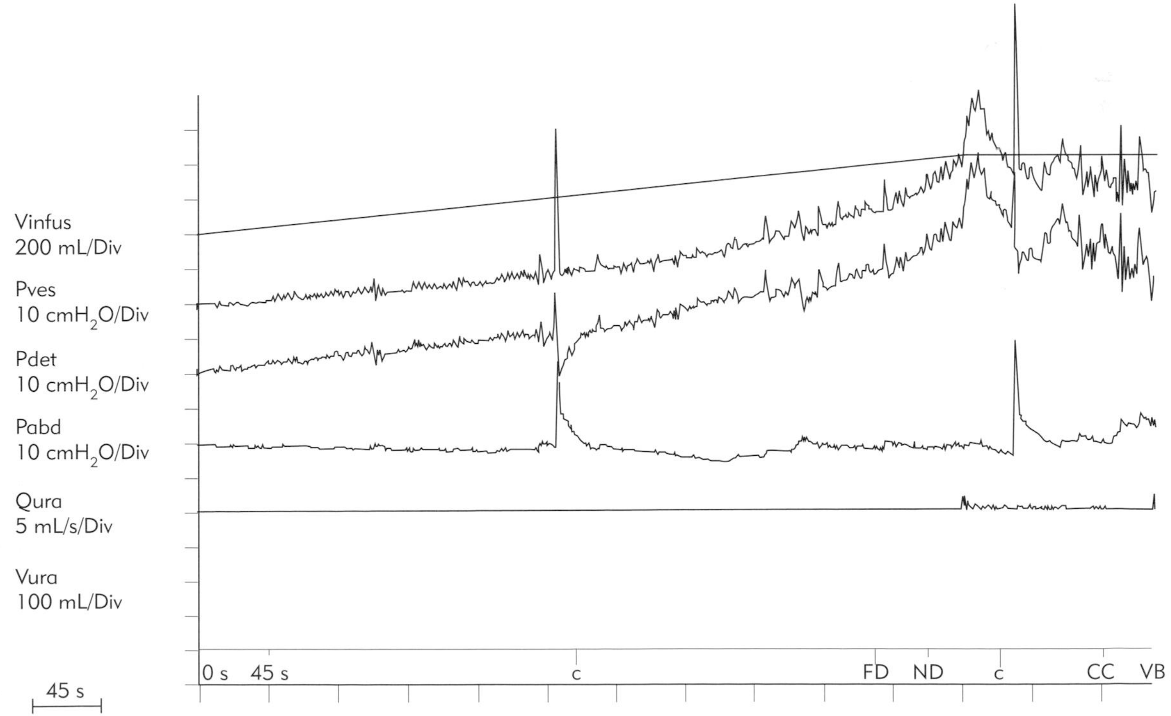

Figure 21.3 Filling cystometry showing loss of compliance. In this patient, as the bladder is slowly filled (50 mL/minute), there is a gradual increase in detrusor pressure. Abbreviations as in Fig 21.2.

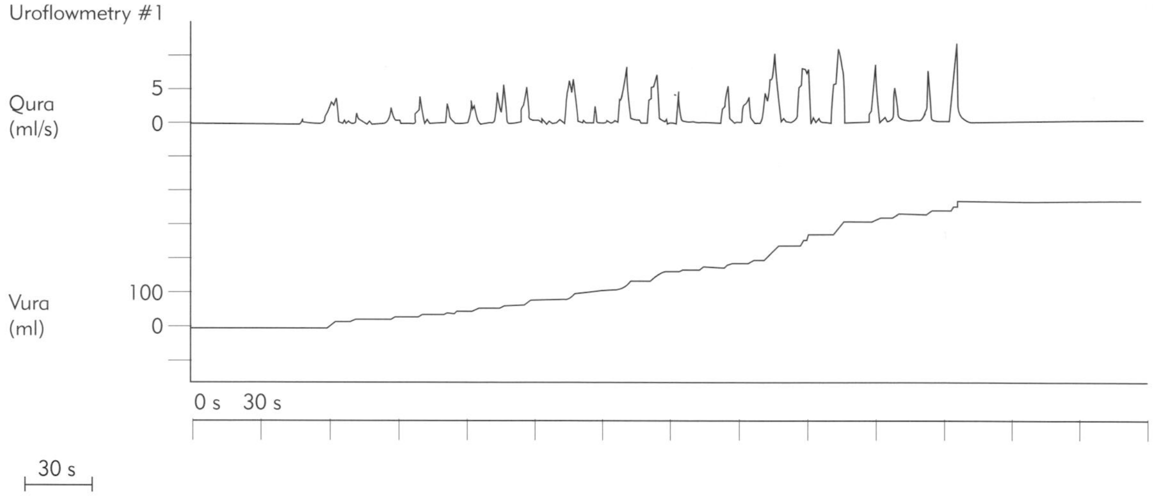

Figure 21.4 Simple flow test showing the interrupted stream of detrusor–sphincter dyssynergia.

SPINAL CORD DISEASE

The abnormally overactive small capacity bladder which characterizes spinal cord disease means that patients are troubled by urgency and frequency. If the detrusor hyperreflexia is severe and particularly if there is also a spastic paraparesis, urge incontinence is likely since impaired mobility may contribute to difficulty in reaching the toilet in time.

Poor neural drive on the detrusor muscle during attempts to void[47] together with an element of detrusor–sphincter dyssynergia means that there is likely to be incomplete bladder emptying and this may in turn exacerbate symptoms due to detrusor hyperreflexia. Although the process of voiding may have been equally severely disrupted by spinal cord disease as the process of storage, the symptoms of difficulty in emptying may be relatively minor compared to those of urge incontinence. It may be only on direct questioning that a patient admits to difficulty initiating micturition or an interrupted stream, or possibly to a sensation of incomplete emptying.[48]

A valuable clinical point is that because the innervation of the bladder arises more caudally than the innervation of the lower limbs, any form of spinal cord disease which causes bladder dysfunction is likely to produce clinical signs in the lower limbs unless the lesion is restricted to the conus. Indeed, this is a sufficiently reliable rule to be of great value when considering whether or not a patient has a neurogenic bladder due to spinal cord involvement.

Figure 21.5 shows the results of a study of the neurological cause of bladder symptoms in patients attending a Uro-Neurology department over a period of a few weeks. Given that the site of responsible pathology in MS is spinal[48] the diagram shows that spinal cord disease was responsible for bladder dysfunction in about half the patients. This conclusion is borne out by a study of the urinary complaints of 786 patients with neurological disorders consecutively admitted to hospitals in Catania, Sicily. Fifty-six percent had bladder symptoms and in 10% these were thought to be urological. Of the 438 patients with neurogenic bladder dysfunction, 74% had some form of spinal cord disease.[49] Specific disorders affecting the spinal cord are discussed below.

Multiple sclerosis

In patients with MS there is a strong association between bladder symptoms and the presence of clinical spinal cord involvement including paraparesis and upper motor neuron signs on examination of the lower limb.[48] Both clinical studies and more recently MRI studies have shown that approximately 75% of those with a diagnosis of MS have spinal cord involvement.[50] The estimated incidence of bladder dysfunction in MS is similar.[51]

The commonest urinary symptom that patients with MS complain of is urgency. All series of urodynamic studies of patients with MS have shown that this is due to underlying detrusor hyperreflexia.[52] Urge incontinence is likely to be a problem if the patient also has impaired mobility and this together with frequency means that many patients are reluctant to be far away from access to a toilet. The symptoms of impaired voiding are often less prominent and may only be elicited by direct questioning. Patients may volunteer or admit on direct questioning to hesitancy of micturition but the more disabled may find themselves unable to initiate micturition voluntarily, only emptying their bladders with an involuntary hyperreflexic contraction.

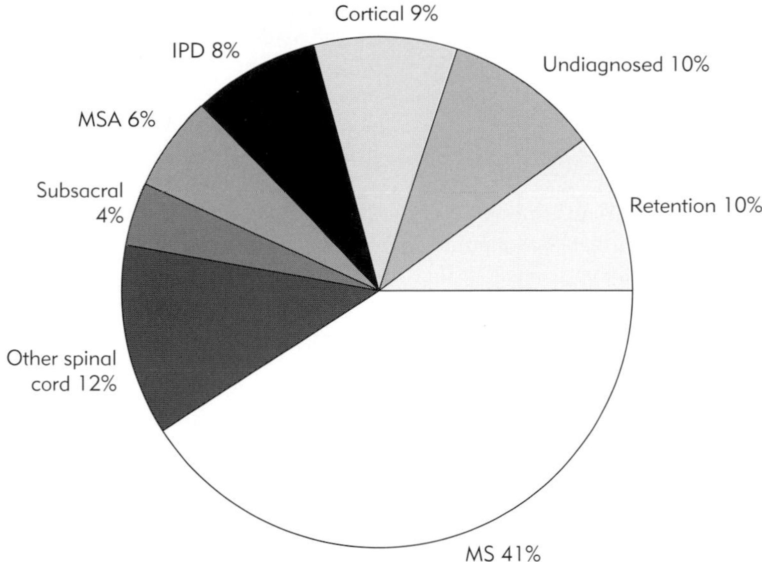

Figure 21.5 Pie diagram showing underlying neurological problem of 140 patients presenting over a 12-week period with bladder symptoms.

In addition to hesitancy, an interrupted urinary flow pattern may be reported. Evidence of incomplete emptying may not come from a reported sensation of continued fullness after voiding but rather the observation by the patient that having passed urine once they are able to do so again within just a few minutes.[48]

With progression of the neurological condition, bladder function deteriorates. This is because of worsening detrusor hyperreflexia together with decreasingly efficient bladder emptying in the context of worsening mobility and possibly also cognitive impairment. However, unlike the bladder dysfunction that follows spinal cord injury, MS very rarely causes upper urinery tract involvement.[53,54] The reason for this is not known but means that in patients with MS the emphasis in management needs to be on symptomatic relief.[55]

Cervical myelopathy

Early reviews stated that bladder disturbance was very rare in patients with cervical spondylosis although more recent studies have refuted this.[56,57] A variable combination of detrusor hyperreflexia and detrusor sphincter dyssynergia is the commonest urodynamic finding and the majority of patients with these abnormalities have long tract symptoms and signs. However, only recently was a relationship between bladder overactivity and pyramidal signs in patients with cervical cord pathologies demonstrated.[58] The neurogenic features of voiding disorder i.e. hesitancy, poor stream and incomplete emptying can be easily confused with those that occur due to obstruction of the bladder outlet.[57]

Syringomyelia

Although it is a benign pathology, syringomyelia can cause progressive spinal cord dysfunction due to expanding fluid within the central spinal canal. Bladder dysfunction usually occurs after other neurological deficits are established[59] although a case where retention was an early symptom has been described.[60]

Transverse myelitis

An unusual but consistent feature of transverse myelitis is that although there may be an excellent clinical recovery from a severe tetraparesis, bladder dysfunction may be the sole residual neurological sequel.[61] The explanation for this is not known but it may relate to the emergence of spinal segmental reflexes during the period of 'spinal shock', which then persist, unmodulated. This begs the question as to whether bladder function could ever be normalized if a treatment were found which enabled re-growth of axons through regions of damage in the spinal cord.

Tropical spastic paraparesis

Tropical spastic paraparesis (TSP), a progressive myelopathy due to infection by HTLV-1 virus, recognized especially in Japan and in patients of Caribbean origin. The myelopathy is slowly progressive over the course of a decade or more with an onset usually before the age of 40 and back pain is often prominent.[62] Proximal myopathy may be an associated feature. Detrusor hyperreflexia is the most common urodynamic abnormality;[63] urge incontinence due to detrusor hyperreflexia occurs as an early feature and may even be a presenting symptom.[64,65] Recently a characteristic thickening of lamina propria nerves seen on detrusor biopsy specimens from patients with TSP has been reported,[66] though the full significance of this remains to be determined.

Arteriovenous malformations (AVMs)

AVMs of the spinal cord may be difficult to recognize clinically but may cause bladder disturbance as a prominent, early feature. Although the majority occur in the thoracolumbar region, alterations to cord blood flow, and subsequent conus ischemia, mean that the patient may present with what appears to be a conus or cauda equina lesion.[67] Symptoms of voiding difficulty include hesitancy and urinary retention.[68]

Tethered cord

A mixture of upper and lower motor neuron signs in the legs is characteristic of a tethered cord, together with urinary symptoms. Typically asymmetric wasting of the calves and intrinsic muscles of the feet occurs but the prominent bladder symptoms and, possibly, extensor plantar responses suggests a diagnosis of a conus lesion rather than peripheral neuropathy or previous poliomyelitis. Although the majority of cases present in childhood, symptomatic onset in adulthood is probably not as rare as once thought.[69] Urodynamic studies show a mixed picture of detrusor hyperreflexia and incomplete bladder emptying and although an improvement in bladder function following a de-tethering procedure has been claimed, the operation is usually carried out to treat pain or prevent progression of neurological deficit.[70]

Cauda equina

Damage to the innervation of the bladder in the cauda equina is likely to affect both the anterior and posterior sacral roots containing somatic and parasympathetic fibres. The clinical picture is therefore typically of perineal sensory loss caused by damage to the S2–S4 roots together with loss of voluntary control of both anal and urethral sphincters, as well as sexual responsiveness. The second order parasympathetic innervation running to the detrusor from the spinal cord in the cauda equina terminates in the parasympathetic ganglia which often lie in the bladder wall. The detrusor is therefore not 'denervated' but is disconnected from central control following a cauda equina injury. The sympathetic innervation of the bladder neck may be preserved. A range of bladder dysfunctions has been described in patients with cauda equina lesions,[71,72,73] including detrusor hyperreflexia.[74]

The bladder dysfunction which occurs may not be a major complaint, the patient being more preoccupied by the profound genital sensory loss or inability to defecate normally. Although there are a number of papers reporting the bladder dysfunction that can occur with a cauda equina lesion there have been few reports on the devastating effect on the quality of life such a lesion can have. However the levels of compensation awarded in medicolegal cases reflect the fact that the loss of control of the pelvic organs and perineal sensation is catastrophic to quality of life.

BLADDER DYSFUNCTION DUE TO DISORDERS OF PERIPHERAL INNERVATION

Because of its extensive autonomic innervation, bladder dysfunction is most commonly seen in those generalised neuropathies that involve small nerve fibres (Table 21.2). Diabetic neuropathy is the commonest cause of a small fiber neuropathy. Small fiber involvement usually occurs as part of a distal, generalized sensory neuropathy but autonomic neuropathy can less commonly occur relatively independently.

Diabetes mellitus

Bladder involvement was once considered an uncommon complication of diabetes, but the greater use of techniques for studying bladder function have shown that the condition is often asymptomatic and discovered incidentally.[75] Bladder dysfunction in isolation does not occur and other symptoms and signs of generalized neuropathy can always be demonstrated in affected patients. The onset of the disorder is insidious over the course of several years with progressive loss of bladder sensation and impairment of bladder emptying eventually culminating in chronic low pressure urinary retention.[76,77] Urodynamic studies demonstrate impaired detrusor contractility, reduction in urinary flow rate and increased post-micturition residual volume with reduced bladder sensation.[78] It seems likely that there is involvement of the vesical sensory afferent fibers causing reduced awareness of bladder filling and of the parasympathetic efferent fibers to the detrusor, decreasing the ability of the bladder to contract. The density of acetyl cholinesterase positive staining nerves in the bladder wall has been shown to be reduced in diabetics.[79]

Table 21.2 Generalized neuropathies with small fiber involvement

- Diabetes
- Amyloidosis – inherited (FAP) and secondary
- Immune mediated neuropathy (AMSAN)
- Distal autonomic neuropathy (pan/cholinergic dysautonomia)
- Inherited neuropathies (HSAN)

Amyloidosis

Autonomic involvement occurs early in both inherited familial amyloid polyneuropathy (FAP) and when amyloidosis is secondary to myeloma or benign plasma cell dyscrasia. Typically there are features of somatic sensory involvement such as loss of pain and temperature sensation in the feet when the disease has advanced to produce autonomic involvement. A study of the urogenital complaints of 12 patients with FAP type I amyloidosis showed reduced bladder contractility and a reduced flow rate in most; two patients had a significant post-micturition residual volume.[80] All were generally very unwell with severe generalized neuropathy.

Immune mediated

About a quarter of patients with Guillain–Barré syndrome have bladder symptoms.[81,82] These are usually those with more severe neuropathy. The bladder symptoms appear after weakness is established. Both detrusor areflexia and bladder overactivity have been described.[82]

It is likely that acute distal autonomic neuropathy is a form of the Guillain–Barré syndrome. There have been a number of reports of distal autonomic neuropathy affecting both the sympathetic and parasympathetic systems. Painful urinary retention usually occurs in both cholinergic and pandysautonomia.[83]

Pelvic nerve injury

The peripheral innervation of the pelvic organs can be damaged by extirpative visceral surgery such as resection of rectal carcinoma, radical prostatectomy, or radical hysterectomy. The dissection necessary for rectal cancer is likely to damage the parasympathetic innervation to the bladder and genitalia, as the pelvic nerves take a medio-lateral course through the pelvis on either side of the rectum and across the apex of the prostate. The pelvic nerves may either be removed together with the fascia which covers the lower rectum, or may be damaged by a traction injury as the rectum is mobilized prior to excision.[84] A prospective study of patients undergoing sphincter sparing surgery for low rectal carcinomas in which each patient acted as their own control, showed that postoperatively there was a significant increase in post-micturition residual urine volume and in 15% there appeared to have been severe damage to the parasympathetic innervation of the detrusor resulting in long term painless retention, a poor stream, loss of normal bladder sensation during filling and near loss of detrusor contraction pressure.[85] The incidence of bladder dysfunction following an abdomino-perineal resection for rectal carcinoma is more than 15%.[86] Urinary incontinence following a radical prostatectomy or a radical hysterectomy which includes the upper part of the vagina is probably also due to damage to the parasympathetic innervation of the detrusor and, at least in the case of a radical prostatectomy, direct damage to the innervation of the striated urethral sphincter.[86,87]

URINARY RETENTION IN YOUNG WOMEN

Urinary retention or obstructed voiding in young women in the absence of overt neurological disease has long puzzled urologists and neurologists alike and in the absence of any convincing organic cause the condition has often been considered hysterical. Indeed the largest body of medical literature on the disorder refers to a condition of 'psychogenic urinary retention'.[88–96]

Typically the clinical history is of a young woman, aged between 20 and 30 years, who presents with retention and a bladder capacity in excess of 1 liter. The history is often that over the preceding 12 hours she has found herself unable to void and although by the time of presentation she may be highly uncomfortable, she does not have the sensations of extreme urgency that might be expected. There are no other clinical neurological features or laboratory investigations to support a diagnosis of MS and MRI of the brain, spinal cord and cauda equina is normal. The lack of sacral anesthesia makes the possibility of a cauda equina lesion improbable.

In 1988 Fowler *et al.* showed that a striking electromyographic (EMG) abnormality on concentric needle electrode examination of the striated muscle of the urethral sphincter was present in this syndrome.[97] The abnormal EMG activity is localized to the urethral sphincter and consists of a type of activity which would be expected to cause inappropriate contraction of the muscle.

Electromyographic analysis shows that the abnormal sphincter activity consists of two components, complex repetitive discharges (CRDs) and decelerating bursts.[98,99] It is known from other electromyographic studies that CRDs are due to direct spread of electrical activity from one muscle fiber to another. Single fiber EMG analysis of a CRD shows a very low 'jitter' indicating that the potentials forming a CRD are not the result of neuromuscular transmission.[100,99] Complex repetitive discharges have a characteristic sound over the audio output of the EMG machine resembling a motorcycle or helicopter. The other type of activity, the 'decelerating bursts' have been said to produce a sound reminiscent of recordings of whales singing in the ocean.[101] Indeed patients with urinary retention in the author's laboratory are referred to as being either 'whale noise' positive or negative. The hypothesis that this abnormal EMG activity causes impaired sphincter relaxation was recently confirmed in a study by Deindl *et al.*, who used special hooked-wire recording electrodes to record simultaneous EMG from the urethral sphincter, together with bladder pressure and urine flow measurements.[102]

Why this type of EMG activity should develop particularly in the urethral sphincter is not known. It is a type of activity which the striated urethral sphincter and to some extent the striated anal sphincter muscles are prone to develop but is rarely encountered in other striated muscles.[103] It is possible that it relates in some way to the size of the muscle fibers of the sphincters which are known to be of relatively small diameter,[104] but the observation by Fowler *et al.* that the women with urinary retention also often have polycystic ovaries raises the possibility that the activity is linked in some way to a hormonal abnormality which causes impaired muscle membrane stability, allowing direct spread of electrical impulses throughout the muscle.[97] The disorder may possibly be the manifestation of a focal, hormonal-dependent channelopathy.

Whatever the exact cause or nature of the EMG abnormality it is the commonest finding on concentric needle EMG of the striated muscle of the urethral sphincter in young women with retention. However, the clinical picture of a woman with this sphincter EMG abnormality, depends on the reaction of her detrusor muscle to the relative degree of outflow obstruction and the same EMG finding has been reported in women with obstructed voiding and detrusor instability.[105] Others have reported finding this activity in the urethral sphincter[98,101,106] with a variety of bladder disorders. In a survey of 477 patients referred for neuro-urological evaluation, the abnormality was found in 10% of women and often in association with an increased post-micturition residual volume or a history of recurrent infections.[103] Webb *et al.* found the same activity in eight out of 18 women in urinary retention,[107] but also found EMG abnormalities in the anal sphincter, whereas Jensen and Stien found the activity only rarely in the anal sphincter.

The natural history of this disorder was investigated recently by means of a questionnaire sent out to 155 women seen over the last 10 years. The peak age incidence was 26 years and retention was either of acute or chronic onset, chronic urinary retention being partial and somewhat more common in older women. The EMG abnormality is very rarely found in women over the age of 45 and almost never in postmenopausal women. Many of the women had experienced an interrupted urinary stream, but were unaware that this is abnormal. To the patients the difference between being in complete retention and able to pass some urine is tantamount and many, unaware of the extent of their incomplete emptying, frequently continue in partial retention with abnormal voiding for months or even years.[108] Unfortunately none of the women had themselves discovered an effective treatment and efforts to treat the condition by hormonal manipulation, injections of botulinum toxin,[109] or application of topical nitric oxide cream have been unsuccessful. However, the results of using the recently introduced sacral nerve stimulator are promising[110–112] and preliminary results indicate the urinary retention of women with this syndrome is highly responsive to neuromodulation:[108] a woman who has not passed urine *per urethram* for many months or even years may find that, within 24 hours of the insertion of a temporary stimulating lead though an S3 foramen and its connection to an external stimulator, she is able to void. The mechanism of action of this therapeutic intervention is uncertain.

URINARY RETENTION IN THE ELDERLY AND INSTITUTIONALIZED

Detrusor function appears to decline with age so that there is a relative impairment of bladder emptying leading to larger postvoid residual volumes with increasing age.[113] It has been proposed that these changes are due to degenerative changes in the detrusor muscle with characteristic electron microscopic abnormalities.[114] Although debate continues as to the specificity of the ultrastructural changes described, it now seems clear that there is primary detrusor pathology with aging and that not all bladder dysfunction is secondary to cortical disease, as was once thought. The commonest demonstrable abnormality of bladder function in the institutionalized elderly is detrusor overactivity.[115] The combination of involuntary detrusor contraction, i.e. detrusor hyperreflexia, leading to urge incontinence together with impaired contractile function causing incomplete bladder emptying has been termed DHIC,[116] but whether this is a single condition or due to detrusor malfunction occurring in combination with cortical dysfunction remains the subject of some discussion.[117]

The cause of urinary incontinence in dementia is probably multifactorial. Not all incontinent elderly persons are cognitively impaired, nor are all cognitively impaired elderly people incontinent. A study which looked at the association between cognitive impairment and bladder dysfunction concluded that urge incontinence and reduced bladder sensation were associated with reduced frontal lobe perfusion on SPECT brain imaging.[118] In a study of patients with cognitive decline, incontinence was associated with severe mental failure in pure Alzheimer's disease but preceded by severe cognitive impairment in diffuse Lewy body disease.[119] In a much less common cause of dementia, low-pressure hydrocephalus, urinary incontinence is a cardinal feature[120] and improvement in urodynamic function has been demonstrated within hours of lumbar puncture in patients with this rare disorder.[121]

Thus, in addition to the various possible neurogenic causes of impaired bladder control and the contribution of abnormal detrusor behavior in the elderly, the existence of concomitant urological disorders should be considered in each patient. Urinary incontinence in an elderly person is likely to be a complex problem and it is often the onset of incontinence which leads to institutionalization. The scale of the problem has significant socioeconomic consequences and the cost of containment of incontinence forms a significant proportion of the national budget for healthcare in countries with advanced healthcare systems.[122]

TREATMENT OF NEUROLOGICAL DISORDERS OF MICTURITION

DETRUSOR HYPERREFLEXIA

Oral anticholinergic medication is currently the most effective treatment for detrusor hyperreflexia. Until the recent introduction of tolterodine, oxybutynin was the most commonly used drug in the UK. This has a relatively selective effect on the parasympathetic innervation of the detrusor muscle but frequently causes a dry mouth. It is claimed that tolterodine has the same efficacy but causes less dry mouth. Oxybutinin can be given as a bladder instillation.[123] Where neither oxybutinin nor tolterodine are available, alternatives such as propantheline bromide or imipramine can be tried.

Desmopressin (DDAVP) spray, is a nasal spray preparation of a synthetic antidiuretic hormone, first introduced to treat diabetes insipidus. It is currently widely used by children with nocturnal enuresis but in the UK is also licensed for the treatment of patients with MS and night-time frequency.[124] One or two nasal puffs of DDAVP from a metered-dose spray administered on retiring reduces urine output for the following 6–8 hours and an oral preparation of DDAVP (Desmotabs) is now available with the same effect. Some patients with MS who were given Desmospray at night chose to use this during the day instead and a placebo controlled trial showed a significant reduction in voiding frequency in the 6 hours following treatment. An increase in night-time frequency does not seem to occur in those who use the medication during the day nor is there a significant change in serum sodium levels of the group.[125] If hyponatremia does occur, it usually happens within the first week or so of starting the medication, giving the chief symptoms of general malaise, headache and visible edema of the face and ankles. Rapid restitution of the sodium level occurs when the medication is stopped.

Although the prospect of using a nasal spray to control urinary frequency is often more appealing to a patient than performing self-catheterization, the prescription of DDAVP should be restricted to patients who understand that the medication is acting on the kidneys rather than the bladder, and that it must only be used once in 24 hours.

Intravesical capsaicin has been used to treat intractable detrusor hyperreflexia due to spinal cord disease on the basis that it has a neurotoxic effect on the C fiber afferents which drive volume-determined, reflex detrusor contractions. Capsaicin has a biphasic action; it is initially an irritant, but if applied in sufficiently high concentration its secondary effect is as a selective neurotoxin acting on unmyelinated afferent C fibers. Patients with detrusor hyperreflexia report an initial deterioration in their bladder symptoms lasting up to 10 days followed by a lessening of urgency and frequency which may last up to 6 months, when the instillation needs to be repeated.[46] A controlled study using capsaicin dissolved in alcohol versus the alcohol solution alone has shown capsaicin is the active ingredient.[45,126]

A study looking at the effectiveness of intravesical capsaicin in a group of patients with MS found it was most effective in those who were still ambulant.[127] An instillation of lignocaine prior to capsaicin does not appear to lessen the efficacy of the capsaicin and greatly improves patient tolerance of the procedure.[128] Resiniferatoxin, an ultrapotent capsaicinoid, is an extract from the plant *Euphorbia resinifera* and has been demonstrated to be 1000 times more neurotoxic than capsaicin for the same degree of pungency as capsaicin. Promising preliminary results have been reported using resiniferatoxin to deafferent the overactive bladder.[129,130] A recent review article concluded that on the basis of its fewer side effects, resiniferatoxin will prove to be clinically more useful than capsaicin.[131]

INCOMPLETE BLADDER EMPTYING OR URINARY RETENTION

Incomplete emptying can exacerbate detrusor hyperreflexia, and an overactive bladder constantly stimulated by a residual volume will respond by contracting and producing symptoms of urgency and frequency. Incomplete emptying is particularly likely to occur in patients with spinal cord disease due to a combination of detrusor sphincter dyssynergia occurring during attempts to void and poorly sustained detrusor contractions during the voiding phase.

The best way of managing incomplete emptying or retention has been to use intermittent catheterization. Sterile intermittent catheterization was first introduced in the 1960s,[132] but it was then found that a clean rather than sterile technique was adequate.[133] Performed for children with spina bifida and the elderly with disorders of complete bladder emptying,[134] it has proved highly effective in many patients with MS and various other bladder disorders characterized by incomplete emptying.

Patients are often unaware of the extent to which they empty incompletely and for this reason, measurement of this parameter is the single most important measurement to be made when planning bladder management.[135] The postvoid residual volume may be measured either with ultrasound or using 'in-out' catheterization. The advantage of the latter procedure is that it familiarizes the patient with catheterization and so makes teaching the technique of self-catheterization more readily acceptable. A generally accepted figure for significant residual volume is 100 ml.

Intermittent catheterization is best performed by the patient alone, who should be taught by someone experienced in the method. A main requirement for success with this technique is patient motivation; a degree of physical disability may usually be overcome provided the patient is sufficiently determined. As a general rule, if patients are able to write and feed themselves they are likely to be able to perform the technique. Sometimes tremor, impaired visual acuity, spasticity, adductor spasm, or rigidity may make it impossible for the patient to do self-catheterization and in such circumstances it may be performed by a partner or care assistant. Since the principle of this technique is to reduce the post-micturition residual, most patients are advised initially to perform the technique at least twice a day. There is, however, no fixed limit on how often it should be performed provided it is done regularly. Doing it only very occasionally provides the opportunity to introduce bacteria without the benefit of regular, complete bladder emptying. Although bacteriuria is noted in 50% of patients using clean intermittent self-catheterization (CISC), the incidence of symptomatic urinary tract infections is low. Hematuria in the early stages of learning the method is common.[136]

In spinal cord disease, a combination of intermittent self-catheterization and an oral anticholinergic, manages both aspects of bladder dysfunction, incomplete emptying and detrusor hyperreflexia. In a patient with a borderline significant residual volume, starting an anticholinergic may have the effect of further impairing bladder emptying. This should be suspected if the anticholinergic has some initial efficacy which then disappears. Also, it is advisable for a patient who has marked hesitancy and difficulty in initiating micturition to wait to start anticholinergic medication until CISC has been established, since there is otherwise a risk of developing complete urinary retention. This combined approach works well in all patients with neurogenic bladder dysfunction who have a combination of hyperreflexia and incomplete emptying.

Although a combination of anticholinergic medication with CISC is the optimal management for patients with detrusor hyperreflexia and incomplete bladder emptying, there comes a point when the patient is no longer able to perform self-catheterization, or when urge incontinence and frequency are unmanageable. In patients with spinal cord disease this point may be reached when the patient is no longer weight-bearing and is chair-bound and at this stage an indwelling catheter becomes necessary.

The most immediate simple solution is an indwelling Foley catheter, but the long-term ill effects of these are well-known. One of the major problems may be leakage of urine around the catheter which occurs when strong detrusor contractions produce a rapid urine flow that cannot drain fast enough. A common reaction to this is to insert a wider-caliber catheter, with the effect that the bladder closure mechanism becomes progressively stretched and destroyed. The detrusor contractions may be of sufficient intensity to extrude the 10- or 20-ml balloon from the bladder, further rupturing the bladder neck. The end result is then a totally incompetent bladder neck and urethra. Bladder stones and recurrent, resistant infections are also more likely in a bladder with an indwelling catheter.

A preferred alternative to an indwelling urethral catheter is a suprapubic catheter which can be inserted under local anesthetic. However, the procedure should only be undertaken by a trained urologist since there is a danger that bowel overlying the bladder may be punctured, especially in patients with small, contracted bladders. Once *in situ*, the catheter is left on constant drainage. Closing the urethra is a difficult urological procedure which is not usually attempted so that continence depends on the suprapubic drain remaining patent. Should the catheter become blocked or kinked, the patient leaks urethrally. Although by no means a perfect system, a suprapubic catheter is a better alternative to an indwelling urethral catheter and is often the method of choice in managing incontinence in patients for whom other means are no longer effective.[137]

If urge incontinence is the main problem and the bladder empties completely, some men are able to wear an external device attached around the penis. The simplest and least obtrusive is a self-sealing latex condom sheath, which can be put on each night or kept in place for up to 3 days. More elaborate body-worn appliances are also available. An effective external appliance for women has yet to be devised.

An extradural sacral nerve stimulator can be used to lessen detrusor instability when this proves resistant to anticholinergic medication. The principle by which it is effective is still far from clear but it seems likely that its action is through stimulation of pelvic afferents.[138] Implanting a stimulator is a two-stage procedure. The first stage, when the stimulating lead is inserted through an S3 foramen under local anesthetic, is performed as an outpatient. The lead is connected to an external stimulator for 3 days and if the patient's symptoms improve significantly during this time, as judged by measurement of residual volumes and recorded voided volumes, they are eligible for a permanent stimulator. This device is implanted in a subcutaneous pocket under general anesthesia; the stimulating lead tunneled subcutaneously back to the sacrum and the electrode implanted through the sacral foramen.[139,140]

In patients who have suffered a complete spinal cord transection but in whom the caudal section of the cord and its roots is intact, the implantation of a nerve root stimulator should be considered. This device was pioneered by Professor Giles Brindley and his collaborators, and more than 2000 have been implanted worldwide.[141,142] Stimulating electrodes are applied intrathecally to the lower sacral anterior roots (S2–S4) and the posterior roots are cut proximally. After the implant, adjustments are made to the stimulation parameters so that the patient obtains the maximum benefit from the stimulator, in terms of making the bladder contract for voiding, assisting defecation, or producing a penile erection. This is achieved by stimulating individual roots or combinations of roots. The major benefit from the stimulator is an improvement in urinary continence. This is usually achieved by a combination of increasing bladder capacity, due largely to the posterior rhizotomy that is performed, and improving bladder evacuation. Brindley has argued that women have greater potential gain from these stimulators than men since incontinence in women is more difficult to manage. Moreover, in men the dorsal rhizotomy that is a necessary part of the procedure will abolish any reflex erections that might otherwise be possible. These stimulators are only suitable for patients with complete spinal cord lesions rather than partial cord lesions or progressive neurological disease.

REFERENCES

1. Barrington F. The relation of the hind-brain to micturition. *Brain* 1921;**44**:23–53.
2. Kuru M, Yamamoto H. Fiber connections of the pontine detrusor nucleus (Barrington). *J Comp Neurol* 1964;**123**:161–85.
3. de Groat W. Nervous control of the urinary bladder of the cat. *Brain Res* 1975;**87**:201–211.
4. Noto H, Roppolo J, Steers W, de Groat W. Electrophysiological analysis of the ascending and descending components of the micturition reflex pathway in the rat. *Brain Res* 1991;**549**:95–105.
5. Holstege G, Griffiths D, de Wall H, Dalm E. Anatomical and physiological observations on supraspinal control of bladder and urethral sphincter muscles in the cat. *J Comp Neurol* 1986;**250**:449–61.
6. Griffiths D, Holstege G, de Wall H, Dalm E. Control and coordination of bladder and urethral function in the brain stem of the cat. *Neurourol Urodynam* 1990;**9**:63–82.
7. Blok B, Holstege G. Ultrastructural evidence for a direct pathway from the pontine micturition center to the parasympathetic preganglionic motorneurons of the bladder of the cat. *Neurosci Letts* 1997;**222**:195–8.
8. Blok B, Willemsen T, Holstege G. A PET study of brain control of micturition in humans. *Brain* 1997;**120**:111–21.
9. Blok B, Sturms L, Holstege G. Brain activation during micturition in women. *Brain* 1998;**121**:2033–42.
10. Blok B, Holstege G. Direct projections from the periaqueductal gray to the pontine micturition centre (M-region). An anterograde and retrograde tracing study in the cat. *Neurosci Letts* 1994;**166**:93–6.
11. Andrew J, Nathan PW. Lesions of the anterior frontal lobes and disturbances of micturition and defaecation. *Brain* 1964;**87**:233–62.
12. Ueki K. Disturbances of micturition observed in some patients with brain tumour. *Neurol Med Chir* 1960;**2**:25–33.
13. Yamamoto S, Soma T, Hatayama T, Mori H, Yoshimura N. Neurogenic bladder induced by brain abscess. *Br J Urol* 1995;**76**:272.
14. Lang E, Chesnut R, Hennerici M. Urinary retention and space-occupuing lesions of the frontal cortex. *Eur Neurol* 1996;**36**:43–7.
15. Khan Z, Hertanu J, Yang W, Melman A, Leiter E. Predictive correlation of urodynamic dysfunction and brain injury after cerebrovascular accident. *J Urol* 1981;**126**:86–8.
16. Tsuchida S, Noto H, Yamaguchi O, Itoh M. Urodynamic studies on hemiplegic patients after cerebrovascular accident. *Urology* 1983;**21**:315–18.
17. Kuroiwa Y, Tohgi H, Itoh M. Frequency and urgency of micturition in hemiplegic patients: relationship to hemisphere laterality of lesions. *J Neurol* 1987;**234**:100–102.
18. Khan Z, Starer P, Yang W, Bhola A. Analysis of voiding disorders in patients with cerebrovascular accidents. *Urology* 1990;**35**:263–70.
19. Sakakibara R, Hattori T, Yasuda K, Yamanishi T. Micturitional disturbance after acute hemispheric stroke: analysis of the lesion site by CT and MRI. *J Neurol Sci* 1996;**137**:47–56.
20. Wade D, Langton Hewer R. Outlook after an acute stroke: urinary incontinence and loss of consciousness compared in 532 patients. *Quart J Med* 1985;**56**:601–608.
21. Barer D, Mitchell J. Predicting the outcome of acute stroke: do multivariate models help? *Quart J Med* 1989;**70**:27–39.
22. Beck RO, Betts CD, Fowler CJ. Genito-urinary dysfunction in multiple system atrophy: clinical features and treatment in 62 cases. *J Urol* 1994;**151**:1336–41.
23. Sung JH, Mastri AR, Segal E. Pathology of the Shy–Drager syndrome. *J Neuropath Exp Neurol* 1978;**38**:253–68.
24. Sakakibara R, Hattori T, Tojo M, Yamanishi T, Yasuda K, Hirayama K. Micturitional disturbances in multiple system atrophy. *Jap J Psychiat Neurol* 1993;**47**:591–8.
25. Pramstaller P, Wenning G, Smith S, Beck R, Quinn N, Fowler C. Nerve conduction studies, skeletal muscle EMG, and sphincter EMG in multiple system atrophy. *J Neurol Neurosurg Psychiat* 1995;**58**:618–21.
26. Palace J, Chandiramani VA, Fowler CJ. Value of sphincter EMG in the diagnosis of multiple system atrophy. *Muscle Nerve* 1997;**20**:1396–403.
27. Chandiramani VA, Palace J, Fowler CJ. How to recognise patients with parkinsonism who should not have urological surgery. *Br J Urol* 1997;**80**:100–104.
28. Berger Y, Blaivas JG, De La Rocha ER, Salinas JM. Urodynamic findings in Parkinson's disease. *J Urol* 1987;**138**:836–8.
29. Pavlakis AJ, Siroky MB, Goldstein I, Krane RJ. Neurologic findings in Parkinson's disease. *J Urol* 1983;**129**:80–83.

30. Fitzmaurice H, Fowler CJ, Rickards D, *et al.* Micturition disturbance in Parkinson's disease. *Br J Urol* 1985;**57**:652–6.
31. Christmas TJ, Kempster PA, Chapple CR, Frankel JP, Lees AJ, Stern GM. Role of subcutaneous apomorphine in parkinsonian voiding dysfunction. *Lancet* 1988;**2**:1451–3.
32. Hattori T, Yasuda K, Kita K, Hirayama K. Voiding dysfunction in Parkinson's disease. *Jap J Psychiat Neurol* 1992;**46**:181–6.
33. Aranda B, Cramer P. Effect of apomorphine and L-dopa on parkinsonian bladder. *Neurourol Urodynam* 1993;12:203–209.
34. Staskin DS, Vardi Y, Siroky MA. Post-prostatectomy incontinence in the parkinsonian patient: the significance of poor voluntary sphincter control. *J Urol* 1988;**140**:117–18.
35. Galloway NTM. Urethral sphincter abnormalities in parkinsonism. *Br J Urol* 1983;**55**:691–3.
36. Escaf S, Cavallotti C, Ricci A, Vega J, Amentas F. Dopamine D1 and D2 receptors in the human ureter and urinary bladder: a radioligand binding and autographic study. *Br J Urol* 1994;**73**:473–9.
37. Holman E. Difficult urination associated with intracranial tumours of the posterior fossa. A physiologic and clinical study. *Arch Neurol Psychiat* 1926;**15**:371–80.
38. Renier WO, Gabreels FJM. Evaluation of diagnosis and non-surgical therapy in 24 children with a pontine tumour. *Neuropaediatrie* 1980;**11**:262–73.
39. Betts CD, Kapoor R, Fowler CJ. Pontine pathology and micturition dysfunction. *Br J Urol* 1992;**70**:100–102.
40. Manente G, Melchionda D, Uncini A. Urinary retention in bilateral pontine tumour: evidence for a pontine micturition centre in humans. *J Neurol Neurosurg Psychiat* 1996;**61**:528–36.
41. Sakakibara R, Hattori T, Fukutake T, Mori M, Yamanishi T, Yasuda K. Micturitional disturbance in herpetic brainstem encephalitis; contribution of the pontine micturition center (PMC). *J Neurol Neurosurg Psychiat* 1998;**64**:269–72.
42. Sakakibara R, Hattori T, Yasuda K, Yamanishi T. Micturitional disturbance and the pontine tegmental lesion: urodynamic and MRI analyses of vascular cases. *J Neurol Sci* 1996;**141**:105–110.
43. Thor K, Kawatani M, de Groat W. Plasticity in the reflex pathways of the lower urinary tract in the cat during postnatal development and following spinal cord injury. In: Goldberger M, Gorio A, Murray M. (eds). *Development and plasticity of the mammalian spinal cord.* 1986, Padova: Liviana Press.
44. de Groat W. Central neural control of the lower urinary tract. In: Bock G, Whelan J (eds). *Neurobiology of incontinence.* John Wiley, Chichester: 1990:27–56.
45. Wiart L, Joseph P, Petit H, Dosque J, de Seze M, Brochet B, *et al.* The effects of capsaicin on the neurogenic hyperreflexic detrusor. A double blind placebo controlled study in patients with spinal cord disease. Preliminary results. *Spinal Cord* 1998;**36**:95–9.
46. Fowler C, Beck R, Gerrard S, Betts C, Fowler C. Intravesical capsaicin for treatment of detrusor hyperreflexia. *J Neurol Neurosurg Psychiat* 1994;**57**:169–73.
47. Mayo M, Chetner M. Lower urinary tract dysfunction in multiple sclerosis. *Urology* 1992;**34**:67–70.
48. Betts CD, D'Mellow MT, Fowler CJ. Urinary symptoms and the neurological features of bladder dysfunction in multiple sclerosis. *J Neurol Neurosurg Psychiat* 1993;**56**:245–50.
49. Ventimiglia B, Patti F, Reggio E, Failla G, Morana C, Lopes M, *et al.* Disorders of micturition in neurological patients. *J Neurol* 1998;**245**:173–7.
50. Kidd D, Thorpe J, Thompson A, Kendall B, Moseley I, MacManus D, *et al.* Spinal cord MRI using multi-array coils and fast spin echo. *Neurology* 1993;**43**:2632–7.
51. Miller H, Simpson CA, Yeates WK. Bladder dysfunction in multiple sclerosis. *BMJ* 1965;**1**:1265–9.
52. Chancellor M, Blavias J. Multiple sclerosis. In: Chancellor M, Blaivas J (eds). *Practical neuro-urology*, Boston: Butterworth-Heinemann, 1995:119–37.
53. Sirls L, Zimmern P, Leach G. Role of limited evaluation and aggressive medical management in multiple sclerosis: a review of 113 patients. *J Urol* 1994;**151**:946–50.
54. Koldewijn E, Hommes O, Lemmens W, Debruyne F, van Kerrebroeck P. Relationship between lower urinary tract abnormalities and disease-related parameters in multiple sclerosis. *J Urol* 1995;**154**:169–73.
55. Litwiller S, Frohman E, Zimmern P. Multiple sclerosis and the urologist. *J Urol* 1999;**161**:743–57.
56. Katz P, Alberico A, Zampieri T, Fox L. Voiding dysfunction associated with cervical spondylotic myelopathy. *Neurourol Urodynam* 1988;**6**:419–24.
57. Hattori T, Sakakibara R, Yasuda K, Murayama N, Hirayama K. Micturitional disturbance in cervical spondylotic myelopathy. *J Spinal Disord* 1990;**3**:16–18.
58. Sakakibara R, Hattori T, Tojo M, Yamanishi T, Yasuda K, Hirayama K. The location of the paths subserving micturition: studies in patients with cervical myelopathy. *Auton Nerv Syst* 1995;**55**:165–8.
59. Sakakibara R, Hattori T, Yasuda K, Yamanishi T. Micturition disturbance in syringomyelia. *J Neurol Sci* 1996; **143**:100–106.
60. Amoiridis G, Meves S, Schols L, Przuntek H. Reversible urinary retention as the main symptom in the first manifestation of a syringomyelia. *J Neurol Neurosurg Psychiat* 1996;**61**:407–408.
61. Sakakibara R, Hattori T, Yasuda K, Yamanishi T. Micturition disturbance in acute transverse myelitis. *Spinal Cord* 1996;**34**:481–5.
62. Montgomery R, Cruickshank E, Robertson W, McMenemey W. Clinical and pathological observations on Jamaican neuropathy: a report on 206 cases. *Brain* 1964;**87**:425–62.
63. Saito M, Kondo K, Kato K, Gotoh M. Bladder dysfunction due to human T-lymphotropic virus type I associated myelopathy. *Br J Urol* 1991;**68**:365–8.
64. Cruickshank J, Rudge P, Dalgleish A, Newton M, Mclean B, Barnard R, *et al.* Tropical spastic paraparesis and human T cell lymphotrophic virus type I in the United Kingdom. *Brain* 1989;**112**:1057–90.
65. Imamura A, Kitagawa T, Ohi Y, Osame M. Clinical manifestations of human T-cell lymphotropic virus type-I-associated myelopathy and vesicopathy. *Urol Int* 1991;**46**:149–53.
66. Dasgupta P, Fowler C, Scaravilli F, Shah J. Bladder biopsies in tropical spastic paraparesis and the effect of intravesical capsaicin on nerve densities. *Euro Urol* 1996;**30(S2)**:237.

67. Aminoff M, Logue V, Clinical features of spinal vascular malformations. *Brain* 1974;**97**:197–210.
68. Murayama N, Yasuda K, Yamanishi T, Hattori T, Kitahara H, Shimazaki J. Disturbances of micturition in patients with spinal arteriovenous malformations. *Paraplegia* 1990;**27**:212–16.
69. Pang D, Wilberger J. Tethered cord syndrome in adults. *J Neurosurg* 1982;**57**:32–47.
70. Adamson A, Gelister J, Hayward R, Snell M. Tethered cord syndrome: an unusual cause of adult bladder dysfunction. *Br J Urol* 1993;**71**:417–21.
71. Nordling J, Meyhoff H, Olesen K. Cysto-urethrographic appearance of the bladder and posterior urethra in neuromuscular disorders of the lower urinary tract. *Scand J Urol Nephrol* 1982;**16**:115–24.
72. Pavlakis AJ, Siroky MB, Goldstein I, Krane RJ. Neurourologic findings in conus medullaris and cauda equina injury. *Arch Neurol* 1983;**4**:570–73.
73. Light J, Beric A, Petronic I. Detrusor function with lesions of the cauda equina, with special emphasis on the bladder neck. *J Urol* 1993;**149**:539–42.
74. O'Flynn KJ, Murphy R, Thomas DG. Neurogenic bladder dysfunction in lumbar intervertebral disc prolapse. *Br J Urol* 1992;**69**:38–40.
75. Ioanid C, Noica N, Pop T. Incidence and diagnostic aspects of the bladder disorders in diabetics. *Euro Urol* 1981; **7**:211–14.
76. Frimodt-Moller C. Diabetic cystopathy: A clinical study of the frequency of bladder dysfunction in diabetics. *Dan Med Bull* 1976;**23**:267–78.
77. Ellenberg M. Development of urinary bladder dysfunction in diabetes mellitus. *Ann Intern Med* 1980;**92**:321–3.
78. Buck A, Reed P, Siddiq Y, Chisholm G, Fraser T. Bladder dysfunction and neuropathy and diabetes. *Diabetologia* 1976;**12**:251–8.
79. Van Poppel H, Stessens R, Van Damme B, Carton H, Baert L. Diabetic cystopathy: neuropathological examination of urinary bladder biopsy. *Euro Urol* 1988;**15**:128–31.
80. Villaplana G, Rosino E, Cubillana P, Egea L, Pertusa P, Albacete M. Corino-Andrade disease (familial amyloidotic polineuropathy type 1) in Spain. *Neurourol Urodynam* 1997;**16**:55–61.
81. Zochodne D. Autonomic involvement in Guillain-Barré syndrome: a review. *Muscle Nerve* 1994;**17**:1145–55.
82. Sakakibara R, Hattori T, Kuwabara S, Yamanishi T, Yasuda K. Micturitional disturbance in patients with Guillain-Barré syndrome. *J Neurol Neurosurg Psychiat* 1997;**63**:649–53.
83. Kirby RS, Fowler CJ, Gosling J, Bannister R. Bladder dysfunction in distal autonomic neuropathy of acute onset. *J Neurol Neurosurg Psychiat* 1985;**48**:762–7.
84. Mundy A. An anatomical explanation for bladder dysfunction following rectal and uterine surgery. *Br J Urol* 1982;**54**:501–504.
85. Neal D, Williams N, Johnston D. A prospective study of bladder function before and after sphincter saving resections for low carcinoma. *Br J Urol* 1981;**53**:558–64.
86. Yalla S, Andriole G. Vesicourethral dysfunction following pelvic ablative surgery. *J Urol* 1984;**132**:503–509.
87. Leveckis J, Boucher N, Parys B, Reed M, Shorthouse A, Anderson J. Bladder and erectile dysfunction before and after rectal surgery for cancer. *Br J Urol* 1995;**76**:752–6.
88. Knox S. Psychogenic urinary retention after parturition resulting in hydronephrosis. *Br J Med* 1960;**2**:1422–4.
89. Larsen JW, Swenson WM, Utz DC, Steinhilber RM. Psychogenic urinary retention in women. *JAMA* 1963;**184**:697.
90. Margolis G. A review of the literature on psychogenic urinary retention. *J Urol* 1965;**94**:257–8.
91. Allen T. Psychogenic urinary retention. *South Med J* 1972;**65**:302–304.
92. Barrett D. Psychogenic urinary retention in women. *Mayo Clin Proc* 1976;**51**:351–6.
93. Montague DK, Jones LR. Psychogenic urinary retention. *Urol* 1979;**13**:30–35.
94. Bird JR. Psychogenic urinary retention. *Psychother Psychosom* 1980;**34**:45–51.
95. Bassi P, Zattoni F, Aragona F, Dal Bianco M, Calabro A, Artibani W. La retention psychogene d'urine chez la femme: aspects diagnostiques et therapeutiques. *J Urol* 1988;**94**:159–62.
96. Siroky M, Krane R. Functional voiding disorders in women. In: Krane R, Siroky M (eds). *Clinical neurourology*. Boston: Little Brown, 1991:445–57.
97. Fowler CJ, Christmas TJ, Chapple CR, Fitzmaurice PH, Kirby RS, Jacobs HS. Abnormal electromyographic activity of the urethral sphincter, voiding dysfunction, and polycystic ovaries: a new syndrome? *Br J Med* 1988;**297**:1436–8.
98. Dyro FM, Bauer SB, Hallett M, Khoshbin S. Complex repetitive discharges in the external urethral sphincter in a pediatric population. *Neurourol Urodynam* 1983;**2**:39–44.
99. Fowler CJ, Kirby RS, Harrison MJG. Decelerating bursts and complex reptitive discharges in the striated muscle of the urethral sphincter associated with urinary retention in women. *J Neurol Neurosurg Psychiat* 1985;**48**:1004–1009.
100. Trontelj J, Stolberg E. Bizarre repetitive discharges recorded with single fibre EMG. *J Neurol Neurosurg Psychiat* 1983;**46**:310–16.
101. Butler WJ. Pseudomyotonia of the periurethral sphincter in women with urinary incontinence. *J Urol* 1979;**122**:838–40.
102. Deindl F, Vodusek D, Bischoff C, Hartung R. Zwei verschieddene Formen von Miktionsstorungen bei jungen Frauen: Dyssynerges Verhalten im Beckenboden oder Pseudomyotonie im externen urethralen sphinkter? *Aktuelle Urol* 1997;**28**:88–94.
103. Jensen D, Stien R. The importance of complex repetitive discharges in the striated female urethral sphincter and male bulbocavernosus muscle. *Scand J Urol Nephrol* 1996;(Suppl.)**179**:69–73.
104. Gosling JA, Dixon JS, Critchley HOD. A comparative study of the human external sphincter and periurethral levator ani muscles. *Br J Urol* 1981;**53**:35–41.
105. Potenzoni D, Juvarra G, Bettoni L, Stagni G. Pseudomyotonia of the striated urethral sphincer. *J Urol* 1983;**130**:512–13.
106. Dibenedetto M, Yalla SV. Electrodiagnosis of striated urethral sphincter dysfunction. *J Urol* 1979;**122**:361–5.

107. Webb RJ, Fawcett PRW, Neal DE. Electromyographic abnormalities in the urethral and anal sphincters of women with idiopathic retention of urine. *Br J Urol* 1992;**70**:22–5.
108. Swinn M, Lowe E, Fowler C. The clinical features of non-psychogenic urinary retention (Fowler's syndrome) (Abstract). *Neurourol Urodynam* 1998;**17**:383–4.
109. Fowler CJ, Betts CD, Christmas TJ, Swash M, Fowler CG. Botulinum toxin in the treatment of chronic urinary retention in women. *Br J Urol* 1992;**70**:387–9.
110. Vapnek J, Schmidt R. Restoration of voiding in chronic urinary retention using the neuroprosthesis. *World J Urol* 1991;**9**:142–4.
111. Elabbady A, Hassouna M, Elhilali M. Neural stimulation for chronic voiding dysfunctions. *J Urol* 1994; **152**:2076–80.
112. Everaert K, Plancke H, Lefevere F, Oosterlinck W. The urodynamic evaluation of neuromodulation in patients with voiding dysfunction. *Br J Urol* 1997;**79**:702–707.
113. Malone-Lee J, Wahedna I. Characterisation of detrusor contractile function inrelation to old age. *Br J Urol* 1993;**72**:873–80.
114. Elbadawi A, Yall S, Resnick N. Structural basis of geriatric voiding function. IV Bladder outlet obstruction. *J Urol* 1993;**150**:1681–95.
115. Resnick N, Yalla S, Laurino E. The pathophysiology of urinary incontinence among institutionalized elderly persons. *New Engl J Med* 1989;**1989**:1–7.
116. Resnick N, Yalla S. Detrusor hyperactivity with impaired contractile function: an unrecognized but common cause of incontinence in elderly patients. *JAMA* 1987; **257**:3076–81.
117. Griffiths D, McCracken P, Harrison G, Gormley E, Moore K. Urge incontinence and impaired detrusor contractility in elderly people. *NeurourolUrodynam* 1997;**16**:251–6.
118. Griffiths D, McCracken P, Harrison G, Gormley E, Moore K, Hooper R, *et al.*Cerebral aetiology of urinary urge incontinence in elderly people. *Age Ageing* 1994;**23**:246–50.
119. Del-Ser T, Munoz D, Hachinski V. Temporal pattern of cognitive decline andincontinence is different in Alzheimer's disease and diffuse Lewy body disease. *Neurology* 1996;**46**:682–6.
120. Hakim S, Adams RD. The special clinical problem of symptomatic hydrocephalus with normal cerebrospinal fluid pressure. *J Neurol Sci* 1965;**2**:307–327.
121. Ahlberg J, Norlen L, Blomstrand C. Outcome of shunt operating on urinary incontinence in normal pressure hydrocephalus predicted by lumbar puncture. *J Neurol Neurosurg Psychiat* 1988;**51**:105–108.
122. Royal College of Physicians. *Incontinence. Causes, management and provision of Services.* London: RCP, 1995.
123. Vaidyananthan S, Soni B, Brown E, *et al.* Effect of intermittent urethral catheterisation and oxybutynin bladder instillation on urinary continence status and quality of life in a selected group of spinal cord injury patients with neuropathic bladder dysfunction. *Spinal Cord* 1998;**36**:409–414.
124. Hilton P, Hertogs K, Stanton S. The use of desmopressin (DDAVP) for nocturia in women with multiple sclerosis. *J Neurol Neurosurg Psychiat* 1983;**46**:854–5.
125. Hoverd P, Fowler C. Desmopressin in the treatment of daytime urinary frequency in patients with multiple sclerosis. *J Neurol Neurosurg Psychiat* 1998;**65**:778–80.
126. de Seze M, Wiart L, Joseph P, Dosque J, Mazaux J, Barat M. Capsaicin and neurogenic detrusor hyperreflexia. A double blind placebo-controlled study in 20 patients with spinal cord lesions. *Neurourol Urodynam* 1998;**17**:513–23.
127. De Ridder D, Chandiramani V, Dasgupta P, Van Poppel H, Baert L, Fowler CJ. Intravesical capsaicin as a treatment for refractory detrusor hyperreflexia: a dual centre study with long-term follow-up. *J Urol* 1997;**158**:2087–92.
128. Chandiramani VA, Petersen T, Duthie GS, Fowler CJ. Urodynamic changes during therapeutic intravesical instillations of capsaicin. *Br J Urol* 1996;**77**:792–7.
129. Cruz F, Guimaraes M, Silva C, Reis M. Suppression of bladder hyperreflexia by intravesical resiniferatoxin. *Lancet* 1997;**350**:640–41.
130. Lazzeri M, Beneforti P, Turini D. Urodynamic effects of intravesical resiniferatoxin in humans: preliminary results in stable and unstable detrusor. *J Urol* 1997;**158**:2093–6.
131. Chancellor M, de Groat W. Intravesical capsaicin and resiniferatoxin therapy: spicing up the ways to treat the overactive bladder. *J Urol* 1999;**162**:3–11.
132. Guttmann L, Frankel H. The value of intermittent catheterisation in the early management of traumatic paraplegia and tetraplegia. *Parap* 1966;**4**:63–84.
133. Lapides J, Diokno A, Gould F. Further observations on self catheterisation. *J Urol* 1976;**116**:169–71.
134. Webb R, Lawson A, Neal D. Clean intermittent self-catheterisation in 172 adults. *Br J Urol* 1990;**65**:20–23.
135. Fowler CJ. Investigation of the neurogenic bladder. *J Neurol Neurosurg Psychiat* 1996;**60**:6–13.
136. Bakke A. Physical and psychological complications in patients treated with clean intermittent catheterization. *Scand J Urol Nephro* 1993;**(Suppl.)150**.
137. Barnes DG, Shaw PJR, Timoney AG, Tsokos N. Management of the neuropathic bladder by suprapubic catheterization. *Br J Urol* 1993;**72**:169–72.
138. Lindstrom S, Fall M, Carlsson C-A, Erlandson B-E. The neurophysiological basis of bladder inhibition in response to intravaginal electrical stimulation. *J Urol* 1983;**129**:405–410.
139. Hassouna MM, Elhilali MM. Role of sacral stimulator in voiding dysfunction. *World J Urol* 1991;**9**:145–8.
140. Dijkema H, Weil E, Mijs P, Janknegt R. Neuromodulation of sacral nerves for incontinence and voiding dysfunctions. Clinical results and complications. *Euro Urol* 1993;**24**:72–6.
141. van Kerrebroeck P, Debruyne F. World wide experience with the Finetech-Brindley sacral anterior root stimulator. *Neurourol Urodynam* 1993;**12**:497–503.
142. Brindley G. Long term follow-up of patients with sacral anterior root stimulator implants. *Paraplegia* 1994;**32**:795–805.

Chapter 22

Constipation

Michael Camilleri, Lawrence A Szarka

INTRODUCTION AND DEFINITIONS

Constipation is a symptom that is poorly defined and may have multiple underlying causes. In the broadest sense, constipation refers to infrequent or qualitatively inadequate defecation. When patients complain of constipation, only a third of them describe infrequent bowel movements; the remaining patients complain of either straining or passage of hard stools.[1] An international working group has attempted to standardize the meaning of chronic constipation, in a consensus document which is now frequently referred to as the 'Rome definition'. The Rome definition requires two or more of the following complaints for at least 12 months when not taking laxatives:

1. Straining during >25% of bowel movements.
2. The sensation of incomplete evacuation on >25% of bowel movements.
3. Hard or pellety stools on >25% of bowel movements.
4. Less than three stools passed per week.[2]

The Rome definition also requires exclusion of irritable bowel syndrome (IBS). This is difficult because the symptoms of constipation-predominant IBS patients can overlap with Rome-consistent chronic constipation.[3] In addition, there is poor correlation between physiological measures of slow colonic transit and the Rome criteria for functional constipation.[3] Constipated people also frequently complain of many other symptoms, associated with their constipation, such as abdominal pain, bloating, distention, nausea, perineal pain, and the need for digital help to defecate.[4] Data from a large nationwide telephone-based survey suggest that failure to satisfactorily complete defecation is prevalent among participants who reported constipation.[5]

In this chapter current concepts of the different forms of constipation will be reviewed with regard to epidemiology, pathophysiology, evaluation and therapy. The focus of the second part of this chapter will be directed at the subgroup of patients with idiopathic slow transit constipation, because this group seems to be the most refractory to conventional treatment, requires greater utilization of medical resources than functional constipation, and includes some patients who need colectomy for the management of their constipation.

CLASSIFICATION

Simple constipation refers to a mild to moderate degree of infrequent or difficult passage of stool. Symptoms tend to be intermittent and minimally bothersome. Simple constipation responds readily to conservative measures such as increased fiber intake.[6,7]

There are also a number of local and systemic conditions that result in *secondary constipation*. Examples include mechanical obstruction, unwanted effects of medications[8] (Table 22.1), hypothyroidism, and hypercalcemia. Several neurological diseases may also cause constipation. These include Parkinson's disease, multiple sclerosis, autonomic neuropathy, and spinal cord injury. Additionally, constipation may be associated with primarily psychiatric disorders such as depression, anorexia nervosa, and a possible association of constipation with a history of previous or ongoing sexual abuse. In these disorders, treatment of the underlying disorder will help to resolve the symptom of constipation.

After simple and secondary constipation, there are three major clinical groups: constipation-predominant IBS, idiopathic slow transit constipation (ISTC), and rectosigmoid outlet delay.

Constipation predominant IBS occurs mostly in young women; abdominal pain is the most prominent symptom, and measurement of colonic transit time is not significantly different from that of healthy controls. It is essential to consider rectosigmoid outlet delay in these patients, because the two conditions often coexist.

Idiopathic slow transit constipation (ISTC) is found in a small group of patients, usually young or middle aged women, in whom there is no response to bulking agents or traditional laxatives. These patients feel the urge to defecate only rarely, if ever. The *sine qua non* of this group is slow colonic transit time on a scintigraphic or radio-opaque marker study. Colonic inertia is a term that has unfortunately been misused in the literature.

Table 22.1 Medications associated with a reported incidence of constipation of 3% or more

Analgesics	Cardiovascular drugs
Narcotics	**Calcium channel blockers**
Morphine	Nifedipine
Codeine	Verapamil
Fentanyl	**Antidysrhythmics**
Butorphanol	Disopyramide
Non-steroidal anti-inflammatories	Amiodarone
Diclofenac	Flecainide
Indomethacin	Mexiletine
Naproxen	Propafenone
Salicylates	**Lipid lowering agents**
Sulindac	Lovastatin
Nabumetone	Pravachol
Muscle relaxants and other analgesics	Cholestyramine
	Colestipol
Baclofen	**Antiplatelet**
Carisoprodol	Anagrelide
Tizanidine	**Antihypertensives**
Tramadol	Acebutolol
	Guanfacine
	Clonidine
Hematological/ oncological drugs	**Neurological drugs**
Filgrastim (G-CSF)	Bromocriptine
Erythropoietin	Pergolide
Carboplatin	Valproic acid
Vinblastine	Felbamate
Psychiatric drugs	**Gastrointestinal drugs**
Antidepressants	Mesalamine
Amoxapine	Pancreatin
Bupropion	Sandostatin
Clomipramine	
Fluoxetine	
Maprotiline	
Venlafaxine	
Sertraline	
Paroxetine	
Mirtazepine	
Tranquilizers	
Alprazolam	
Clozapine	
Olanzapine	
Risperidone	
Endocrine-drugs	**Miscellaneous agents**
Pamidronate	Leuprolide
Alendronate	Ondansetron
	Interferon alfa-2b
	Levofloxacin
	Nicotine

Many authors seem to have used this term interchangeably with ISTC. The term, inertia, should be reserved to describe a subgroup of patients with slow transit constipation in whom there is no colonic response to neuropharmacological stimulation, and physiologic reflexes are absent. Thus, the colon is truly inert.[9] Another term used more or less synonymously with colonic inertia in the literature is chronic intestinal (colonic) pseudo-obstruction.[10]

Outlet delay or *evacuation disorders* are terms that refer to conditions such as pelvic floor dysfunction, anismus and structural problems such as rectocele and mucosal prolapse or intussusception. Patients in this group may complain of difficult or prolonged defecation requiring manual disimpaction, or a feeling of anal blockage. These symptoms have reasonable specificity for this condition.[4] Many such patients give a history of antecedent vaginal childbirth or pelvic surgery that seems to be followed by constipation. The functional outlet delay may slow colonic transit, but this is usually secondary to the ineffective evacuation. A test of colonic transit alone cannot exclude such evacuation disorders, although selective 'hold-up' in the rectosigmoid is suggestive of outlet delay. The description and management of outlet delay and pelvic floor dysfunction is considered in detail elsewhere (Chapters 4, 5, 15, 16, 20, 28) in this book.

EPIDEMIOLOGY

The prevalence of constipation depends on what question is being asked, which population is asked and what the subjects mean when they are responding to the question. Further difficulty is caused by the heterogeneity of causation of constipation. Even idiopathic slow transit constipation is unlikely to be a single entity. In general, epidemiologic studies show that constipation in young and middle aged adults is approximately three times more prevalent in women than men and that the prevalence increases in both sexes with advancing age.[11]

In the broadest sense, it has been reported that 95% of the adult population in western countries have bowel movements between once every 2 days and twice daily.[12] Therefore, patients with a frequency of bowel movements less than this normal range can be considered to have abnormally infrequent defecation. Defecation frequency of less than three stools per week is reported by 4% of the population and 1% to 2% have less than two stools per week.[13] The prevalence of 'constipation' in the United States has been estimated to be anywhere from 2% to 34%.[14] This variability may be explained by the lack of concordance in the definition of constipation between studies, and by reliance on self-defined constipation in most epidemiologic studies. Failure to consider the role of constipating drugs in some epidemiological studies makes estimates of true prevalence of intrinsic bowel problems almost impossible. In the large United States Householders survey, Drossman *et al.* found the prevalence of functional constipation to be 3.6%, after people with IBS, functional bloating, or with any ano-rectal symptoms were excluded.[15] When chronic constipation was defined as the presence of straining and hard stools more than a quarter of the time or less than three stools per week, 16.8% of a random sample of a middle aged population (ages between 30 and 64 years) in Olmsted County, Minnesota reported constipation.[16]

The exact prevalence of rectosigmoid outlet delay or evacuation disorders is not known. In a survey of a healthy, middle aged, community population, the prevalence of any symptom compatible with outlet delay (feeling of anal blockage more than a quarter of the time, requiring greater than 10 minutes to accomplish defecation, and needing manual disimpaction with pressure in or around the anus to aid defecation) was found to be 11%.[14] Interestingly, only a small proportion (17%) of this group regarded themselves as being constipated. Outlet delay was found to be significantly more common in women, whereas chronic constipation without symptoms of outlet delay had an equal gender distribution. There is considerable overlap between the diagnostic groups of constipation, IBS, and outlet delay. In the same population cited above, 17% fulfilled the Rome criteria for IBS, and approximately one third of these or 5.2% of the total population met the definition for both chronic constipation and IBS.[17] Slightly less than half of the patients with both IBS and chronic constipation also had symptoms associated with outlet delay.

The epidemiology of constipation at tertiary referral centers is necessarily different from that in the community since it must be enriched with patients with more severe constipation. Among 70 patients referred to a tertiary gastroenterology motility clinic with non-diagnostic evaluations elsewhere and failure to respond to conventional approaches, Surrenti *et al.* reported that 37% had pelvic floor dysfunction, 27% had slow transit constipation, and 23% had IBS.[18] Half of these referred patients had some form of outlet delay: pelvic floor dysfunction, excessive perineal descent, anismus or some combination of these. These findings were confirmed by Koch *et al.* Among a group of 190 referred patients, they found outlet delay or disordered defecation in 59%, slow transit in 27%, a combination in 6%, and no demonstrable pathophysiological findings in 8%.[19] It remains unclear whether the outlet delays and abnormalities are a cause, or a result, of constipation and excessive straining, but at least in some patients the onset of outlet delay can be traced back to childbirth or pelvic surgery. In one prospective study of 200 women undergoing hysterectomy, 5% developed constipation.[20]

Finally, the burden of constipation seems greatest in the elderly. The prevalence of any form of constipation in the elderly community population is estimated at 40%, and it would be expected to be even higher among hospitalized or nursing home elderly patients.[21] Symptoms of outlet delay were reported by 24% in this community population.[21] In a systematically studied small cohort of elderly constipated patients, outlet delay was more frequent than slow transit.[22] Excessive perineal descent and failure of the rectoanal angle to open during defecation appears to be more prevalent among elderly women than men (Fig. 22.1).[23]

IMPACT OF CONSTIPATION: QUALITY OF LIFE AND HEALTHCARE UTILIZATION

The general well-being of patients with chronic constipation is lower than that of the general population. Glia and Lindberg used the psychological general well-being (PGWB) index and gastrointestinal symptom rating scale (GRS) to assess quality of life in 102 chronically constipated patients who were evaluated and classified into subgroups.[24] Overall, the mean PGWB index was substantially lower in the constipated group (score 85.5 compared with the healthy controls (score 102.9)). This decrease in quality of life score is in the same range as that for patients with dyspepsia. This study also suggested that patients with normal transit and more frequent stools had a paradoxically lower quality of life score compared with slow transit constipation patients with infrequent stools (PGWB scores: 82 v. 94, $p < 0.05$). Patients with outlet delay had a significant increase in the anxiety component of the PGWB index compared with constipated patients without outlet delay.

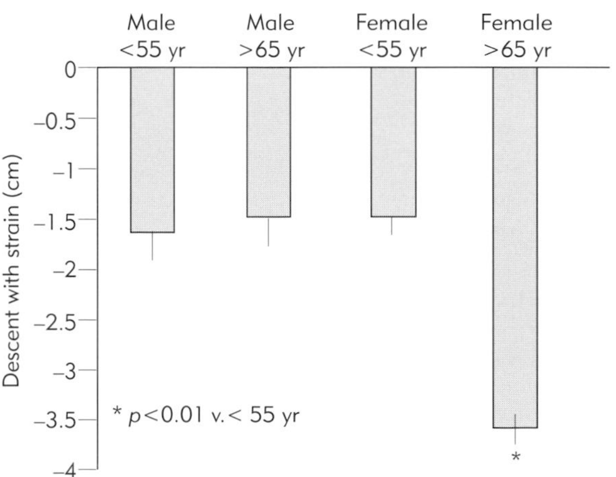

Figure 22.1 Extent of perineal descent during defecation in younger and older males and females. Excessive perineal descent in older females contributes to the failure of rectal evacuation and constipation. Data reproduced from Ref. 23.

It is estimated that only 10% of the population with functional bowel disorders present for medical care.[25] Even so, approximately 1.2% of the United States population seeks some form of medical consultation each year for constipation, with 5% of this population requiring subspeciality evaluation.[13] The exact economic burden of constipation in the community with regard to office visits, diagnostic tests, cost of prescription and non-prescription drugs, is not specifically known, but must be considerable. For the population that is referred for subspecialty evaluation, the mean cost of diagnostic tests alone was found to be $2752 (range $1150–$4792) in a publication in 1997.[26]

PHYSIOLOGY, PATHOPHYSIOLOGY AND ETIOLOGY

Constipation is a condition with high prevalence with some common causes (Table 22.2), but little is known about the true etiology of idiopathic constipation. In this section, we will review aspects of colonic physiology and pathophysiology in health and in constipation, as well as examine possible etiologies of idiopathic constipation.

INNERVATION

The motor and sensory functions of the colon are controlled by the nervous system of the gut, which comprises both intrinsic and extrinsic innervations.[27] The intrinsic nervous system consists of myenteric, submucosal and mucosal neuronal plexuses. The myenteric plexus regulates smooth muscle function (motility) and the submucosal plexus controls ion transport and absorptive processes. The extrinsic nervous system is composed of the parasympathetic and sympathetic autonomic innervation. Parasympathetic nerves reach the colon via the vagus nerves which supply the right colon; and the sacral parasympathetic nerves (S2–4), which enter in the distal colon and ascend intramurally for a variable distance to innervate the transverse colon, left colon and rectum. The chief parasympathetic excitatory neurotransmitters controlling motor function are acetylcholine, and the tachykinins, such as substance P.[28] Sympathetic nerves reach the gut along the arterial arcades of the superior and inferior mesenteric vessels. There is tonic sympathetic input into the gut, and this is generally excitatory to sphincters and inhibitory to non-sphincteric smooth muscle. The sympathetic effect is mediated primarily by the alpha-2 adrenergic system. Clonidine, an alpha-2 agonist, is known to decrease colonic tone and increase compliance, and the alpha-2 antagonist, yohimbine, has the opposite effect.[29] In contrast, alpha-1 and beta agonists do not appear to influence colonic tone, compliance or sensation.[30]

The functions of the enteric and extrinsic neurons are modulated by interneurons through a variety of neurotransmitters including acetylcholine, opioids, norepinephrine, serotonin, somatostatin, cholecystokinin, substance P, vasoactive intestinal peptide, neuropeptide Y and, doubtless, several others. Pharmacological studies have begun to elucidate the neurohumoral integration of colonic motility. The muscarinic anticholinergic agent atropine has been shown to reduce colonic tone in all its regions.[31] Cholecystokinin, in doses producing maximal pancreatic stimulation, does not stimulate colonic tone or phasic activity.[32] There are at least five types of serotonin receptors. Therefore; certain drugs have a potential role in modulation of sensory and motor activity of the colon. The most thoroughly studied are the 5HT-3 antagonists, such as ondansetron, which inhibit colonic tone and compliance,[33] and delay orocecal and colonic transit.[34] Agonists of the 5-HT_4 receptor stimulate acetylcholine release and seem to have a prokinetic effect.[35] The somatostatin analog, octreotide, also decreases postprandial colonic tone, but paradoxically increases phasic motility in the descending colon and rectum.[36] In resected colons from patients with constipation, abnormal distribution of several neuropeptides has been reported, but not consistently confirmed.[37]

Table 22.2 Common causes of constipation

Primary constipation
Idiopathic slow transit/colonic inertia
Irritable bowel syndrome
Functional outlet obstruction
Secondary constipation
Gastrointestinal:
Diverticulosis
Stricture
Polyps
Cancer
Ischemia
Endocrine/metabolic
Hypothyroidism
Hypercalcemia
Neurologic
Parkinson's disease
Multiple sclerosis
Autonomic neuropathy
Spinal cord injury
Sacral parasympathetic nerve damage
Psychiatric
Depression
Anorexia nervosa

EXTRINSIC NEUROPATHY

Damage to the autonomic nerves by trauma, infection, neuropathy and neurodegeneration may lead to motor, secretory, and sensory disturbances, most frequently resulting in constipation. Patients with spinal cord injury above the level of the sacral segments have delayed proximal and distal colonic transit attributable to loss of parasympathetic modulation.[38] In these patients, fasting colonic motility and tone are normal, but the response to feeding is generally reduced or absent.[39] Spinal cord lesions involving the sacral segments, or damage to the efferent nerves from these segments, disrupt the neural integration of rectosigmoid expulsion and anal sphincter control. In patients with these injuries, there is loss of contractile activity in the left colon,[40] and decreased rectal tone and sensitivity which may lead to colonic dilation and fecal impaction.[41]

Parkinson's disease and multiple sclerosis are two neurological diseases that are frequently associated with constipation. In Parkinson's disease, a reduction in the dopamine containing neurons and Lewy bodies in the myenteric plexus neurons has been described.[42] Additionally, failure to relax the striated muscles of the pelvic floor has been reported in Parkinson's disease, and this may be an extrapyramidal manifestation of the disease. Constipation is a common complication of multiple sclerosis, with a reported prevalence of 43% in one series.[43] Multiple sclerosis is associated with slow colonic transit and absence of the postprandial motor response in the colon,[44] probably due to spinal cord lesions disrupting parasympathetic control of the colon.

Constipation related to diabetes mellitus is thought to be secondary to autonomic dysfunction.[45] In a large group of diabetic patients screened for autonomic neuropathy, the prevalence of constipation was 22% among the diabetics with neuropathy, but only 9.2% in diabetics without neuropathy, which was not significantly different from the healthy control group.[46] Feldman *et al.* reported a questionnaire-based study of diabetics in a referral clinic; constipation was more prevalent in insulin dependent diabetes mellitus than in non-insulin dependent diabetes mellitus, and was associated with symptoms of dysautonomia and use of constipating drugs, e.g. calcium channel blockers.[47] It has been suggested that subclinical dysautonomia may have an important role in idiopathic STC as well. Altomare *et al.* studied a group of 23 patients who had documented slow transit without any features of outlet obstruction or IBS; 70% of constipated patients, but only 8% of healthy controls had an abnormal test of sympathetic postganglionic function (acetylcholine sweat spot test).[48] However, more extensive studies of autonomic function in a group of patients with severe constipation and symptoms suggestive of a possible dysautonomia revealed autonomic dysfunction uncommonly (four of 28 patients).[19]

The parasympathetic and sympathetic components of the extrinsic innervation also convey visceral sensory afferent inputs. The phenomenon of reduced rectal sensitivity has been reported in patients with ISTC compared with patients with normal transit constipation.[49] Careful studies by Bassotti *et al.* on constipated patients found that there were higher defecatory sensation thresholds and higher maximal rectal tolerable volumes, particularly in the group of patients with rectal outlet delay.[50] It is possible that this sensory dysfunction reflects the moderate rectal dilation or megarectum observed in patients with long standing symptoms.

ENTERIC NEUROPATHY

The most familiar condition involving a defect in the enteric nervous system is Hirschsprung's disease; this is usually present from birth and is identified in infancy or early childhood; onset of symptoms and diagnosis after the age of ten is rare.[51] Hirschsprung's disease is well characterized histologically by the absence of ganglion cells in the myenteric and submucosal plexuses and the presence of hypertrophied nerve trunks in the space normally occupied by the ganglion cells. The aganglionosis starts from the anal verge and extends proximally for varying distances. The normal development of the enteric nervous system is dependent on the presence of neurotrophic factors such as glial-derived nerve growth factor (GDNF) and endothelin-3.[52] Lack of nerve growth factor receptors in the muscle layers of the colon involved with Hirschsprung's disease has been demonstrated.[53] The enteric narrowing, and failure of relaxation in the aganglionic segment is thought to be due to the lack of neurons containing nitric oxide synthase.[54]

Idiopathic megarectum and megacolon can be either congenital or acquired, but the role of an enteric nervous system defect is less clear. In megacolon, the dilated segment shows normal phasic contractility, but decreased colonic tone.[55] Gattuso *et al.* studied a total of 30 patients with either megarectum or megacolon. Histological examination of megarectum specimens found significant thickening due to smooth muscle hypertrophy and fibrosis of the muscularis mucosa, circular muscle, and longitudinal muscle layers. There was also reduced density of neural tissue in the longitudinal muscle layer in the megarectum specimens, but no abnormality in specimens with idiopathic megacolon.[56] An acquired defect in the enteric nervous system, characteristically leading to constipation, occurs in Chagas' disease, which is caused by infection with *Trypanosoma cruzi* that causes destruction of myenteric neurons. Chagas' disease is common in South America, but does not occur indigenously in North America or Europe or in other parts of the world.

Acquired aganglionosis has also been reported due to circulating auto-antineuronal antibodies which may be associated with or without neoplasm.[57]

Earlier studies with routine light microscopy failed to identify consistent abnormalities in colons from patients with severe idiopathic constipation. Special stains and immunocytochemical methods have led to the re-exploration of the ultrastructure of the colon in idiopathic constipation. In resected colons of constipated patients, Krishnamurthy *et al.* have shown reduced numbers of argyrophilic neurons and structural abnormalities in argyrophilic neurons, such as decreased neuronal processes and variable sized nuclei in the ganglia.[58] Neurofilaments provide the basis for selective neuronal staining with silver. Variations in argyrophilicity (silver affinity) are due to the differing amounts of neurofilaments within neurons. Although the exact role of neurofilaments is undetermined, they are known to act as cytoskeletal elements and to have a role in axonal transport, which may be important for neurotransmitter delivery to the presynaptic area of the axon.[59] Further investigation of neuropathological changes in patients with ISTC by Schouten *et al.* confirmed that there was marked reduction or absence of neurofilament expression in the myenteric plexus along the entire length of colon in 17/29 specimens, and in segments of the colon in the remaining 12/29 specimens.[59]

The role of laxatives in damaging enteric neurons is unclear. The effect of known neurotoxins, such as vinca alkaloids, as well as conditions associated with axonal damage such as infantile neuroaxonal dystrophy and giant axonal neuropathy result in dense aggregation of neurofilament and increased density on silver staining or with immunohistological staining against neurofilament.[60] An early report of slight increase in argyrophilic staining after anthraquinone dosing in mice has not been confirmed;[60] Milner *et al.* showed no changes in colonic ultrastructure or of neuropeptide levels in rodents treated chronically with laxatives.[61] Increases in argyrophilic staining in the colon are not seen in humans with chronic laxative use; in contrast, argyrophilic neurons are reduced in number.[62] The etiologic significance of this reduction in argyrophilic staining and neurofilament expression in the enteric nervous system remains unresolved. More recent studies have focused on the interstitial cells of Cajal (ICC), which are thought to have an important role in the generation of intrinsic electrical activity and electromechanical coupling in the gut. Hagger *et al.* have studied the distribution of ICC in the different colonic regions,[63] and the 'volume' of ICC in the myenteric plexus of resected colon is diminished in idiopathic slow transit constipation.[64]

COLONIC MOTILITY

Understanding of motor physiology in the colon has advanced greatly with the application of manometry and other research techniques, more proximally in the colon and for longer durations. The normal colon displays short duration (phasic) contractions and a background contractility or tone. Myoelectrical studies have identified two phenomena: short spike bursts that may or may not be associated with phasic contractions, and long spike bursts associated with high amplitude propagated contractions (HAPCs).[29] Non-propagated phasic contractions have a role in segmenting the colon into haustra, which compartmentalize and facilitate mixing, retention of residue and formation of solid stool. HAPCs are characterized by an amplitude greater than 75 mmHg, propagation over a distance of at least 15 cm, and a propagation velocity of 0.15–2.2 cm/s.[65] HAPCs contribute to the mass movements in the colon. In health, HAPCs occur on average 5–6 times per day, most often postprandially and between 6 am and 2 pm.[65]

Patients with idiopathic slow transit constipation (ISTC) have reduced numbers of HAPCs. In one study, during a 24-hour period, the mean number of HAPCs in constipated patients was 2.6 compared with 6.1 in healthy subjects, and 30% of the constipated patients had no HAPCs at all.[66] The effect of meals on colonic motility is to increase phasic contractions and tone for about 2 hours.[67] The initial response seems to be vagus mediated since it can be stimulated by mechanical distention of the stomach alone. The subsequent response requires caloric ingestion and appears to be a hormonal effect.[68]

A study of colonic responsiveness to stimulation by ingestion of a 1000 kcal meal, found that there was a significantly reduced motor response in the idiopathic constipation patients, only 7% having any HAPCs compared with 45% in the control group.[69] The colon in ISTC is also less responsive to cholinergic stimulation. Challenge with edrophonium, a short-acting cholinesterase inhibitor, showed a complete absence of motor response in 12% of patients and significant attenuation of the motility index in ISTC compared with controls.[9]

Some patients with idiopathic constipation have other motility abnormalities in the gut, such as delayed gastric emptying and prolonged small bowel transit.[70,71] It is unclear whether these are reflex changes or part of a generalized gastrointestinal dysmotility.

COLONIC TRANSIT

Examinations of colonic ultrastructure, motility and myoelectrical events are relatively difficult; in contrast, the physiological endpoint of transit is readily quantifiable and has led to important descriptive differences between health and disease. In health, the ascending and transverse regions of the colon serve as reservoirs and the descending colon as a conduit.[72] The aboral movement of colonic contents is a discontinuous process, slow most of the time and very rapid at other times. Residue may be retained for prolonged periods in the right colon, and a mass movement may deliver the contents to the sigmoid colon in seconds.[73] In health, the average mouth to cecum transit time is about 6 hours and regional transit times by radiopaque marker methods through the right colon, left colon and sigmoid colon are about 12 hours each. Overall, the normal mean colonic transit time is 36 hours, but the range is wide.[74]

There are multiple factors that can affect gut transit rates. It was previously thought that the ileocolonic junction regulated transit; however, studies of transit in patients with right hemicolectomy, have not shown any significant differences in whole gut transit times despite loss of the ileocolonic sphincter.[75] Easily modifiable factors that can affect colonic transit include diet, caloric intake, liquid delivery to the colon, and presence of distal obstruction. As dietary fiber is increased, mean colonic transit time decreases, stool frequency increases and stool consistency becomes softer.[76] Decreased caloric intake slows colonic transit, but this is reversible when caloric intake is normalized.[77] The presence of outlet obstruction in patients with pelvic floor dysfunction is often associated with slow colonic transit and decreased postprandial colonic tone; these usually normalize once normal rectal propulsion is re-established by biofeedback training.[78] Failure to correct transit time after effective pelvic floor rehabilitation suggests that there is an associated colonic dysmotility. Voluntary suppression of defecation also markedly retards colonic transit.[79]

Fluid balance in the gut influences gastrointestinal transit. Approximately 9 liters of fluid enter the gut from oral intake and endogenous secretions. The small intestine delivers about 1.5 liters of fluid to the colon, where most is reabsorbed, leaving a maximum of 200 ml of water excreted in stool.[80] It has been postulated that, in constipation, an increased adrenergic tone results in increased absorption of water by the enterocytes and decreased secretion.[80] Osmotic laxatives, which increase fluid loading in the colon, accelerate ascending colonic transit.[81] However, the absorption reserve of the colon is large, and it is estimated that up to 3 liters of fluid can be reabsorbed by the colon in a 24-hour period, unless the rate of ileocolonic flow or colonic motility overwhelms the colon's capacitance and reabsorptive capacity.[82]

DEFECATION

Normal defecation requires a series of coordinated actions of the colon, rectum, pelvic floor and the anal sphincter muscles. The pelvic floor is composed of the striated puborectalis and levator ani muscles, which separate the pelvis from the perineum. The pelvic floor is in a state of tonic contraction.

The continence barrier (Fig. 22.2) is comprised of the normally contracted puborectalis muscle which is responsible for maintaining the acute recto-anal angle, and the internal and external anal sphincters which are contracted at rest and constitute the physiologic sphincter. The internal anal sphincter receives sympathetic innervation from the hypogastric nerves and parasympathetic innervation from the first, second, and third segments of the pelvic nerves.[83] The external anal sphincter is innervated by the pudendal nerves.[83]

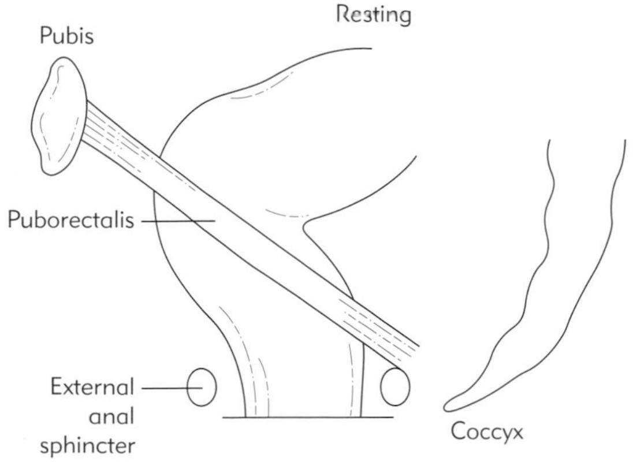

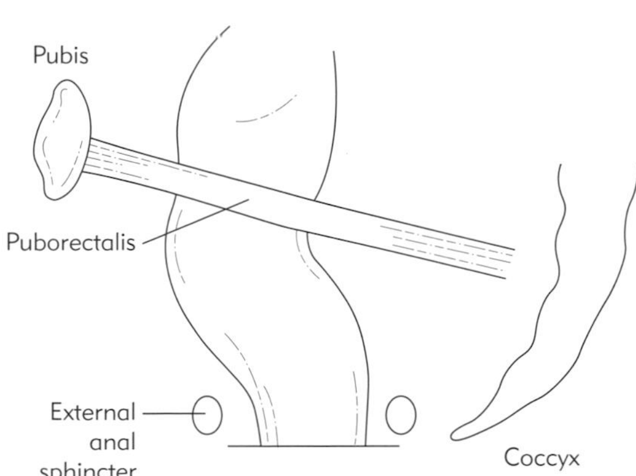

Figure 22.2 Pelvic floor and ano-rectal functions during continence and defecation. Cartoon shows sagittal view through the pelvis in the resting and straining postures. Coordinated functions of pelvic floor (puborectalis) and anal sphincter are essential for continence and defecation.

Normal defecatory function (Fig. 22.2) sometimes begins with a mass movement associated with a propagated peristaltic contraction originating in the proximal colon which moves a fecal bolus distally to the rectum. Filling of the rectum by a volume as small as 10 ml may be sensed, although the rectum can accommodate a volume of up to 300 ml before a sense of fullness and urge to defecate develops.[84] Distention of the rectum results in the relaxation of the internal anal sphincter (recto-anal inhibitory reflex) and simultaneous contraction of the external anal sphincter to maintain continence. The relaxation of the internal anal sphincter exposes the sensory receptor rich anal transition zone to the intraluminal contents and permits discrimination between solid or liquid stool, and gas (the 'sampling reflex').[85] When there is a socially convenient time and place to defecate, the person assumes the sitting position and flexion of the hips facilitates opening of the anorectal angle. Straining is associated with contraction of the diaphragm and rectus abdominus muscles, resulting in elevated intra-abdominal pressure. Coordinated relaxation of the pelvic floor muscles and external anal sphincter muscle results in further opening of the anorectal angle and a favorable pressure gradient between the rectum and the anus. Expulsion of stool is facilitated by the contraction of the rectum.

Constipation associated with impaired defecation may result from inappropriate contraction of the pelvic floor muscles.[86] This phenomenon, known as anal dyssynergia or anismus, may occur in symptomless individuals[87] but seems to be more common in patients with constipation.[13]

In some cases there is failure to raise intrarectal pressure sufficiently to expel stool despite relaxation of sphincters and pelvic floor.[88] Clinically, this can be observed by noting the lack of perineal descent with straining.[89]

Other causes of impaired defecation leading to constipation include rectocele, anatomical defects in the rectum, and the descending perineum syndrome. In women, the perineal body supports the anterior rectal wall at the anorectal junction but, above this, the unsupported rectovaginal septum can bulge anteriorly to form a rectocele. Imaging of defecation dynamics shows that rectoceles are common and that protrusions of at least 4 cm from the anterior rectal wall may be unassociated with symptoms.[90] Symptomatic rectoceles result in the appearance of a lump at the vaginal introitus with each straining effort. Digitation to support the posterior vaginal wall is then necessary to enable completion of defecation. Proctography during defecation may show preferential filling of a large rectocele with retained contrast material at the end of defecation.

In some patients, weakness of pelvic floor support results in the descending perineum syndrome which may cause obstruction to defecation by possibly two different mechanisms. First, pelvic floor weakness results in widening of the anorectal angle, weakening of the perineal body, and a more vertical orientation of the rectum. This arrangement favors intrarectal intussusception or rectal prolapse.[13] Second, it is possible that the lax pelvic floor does not provide the necessary rigidity for the extrusion of solid stool through the anal canal.[13] A weak pelvic floor may be identified on physical examination or scintigraphic or radiological tests as excessive perineal descent (> 4.0 cm) associated with straining.[91] This may also result in or be due to sacral nerve damage with secondary muscular atrophy. Electrophysiologic studies show partial denervation and prolonged latency on stimulation of the pudendal nerve which is characteristic of nerve damage. Histologically, there is frequently evidence of muscle fiber loss.[92] The underlying nerve injury has been associated with trauma during parturition and possibly repeated prolonged straining efforts.[92]

OTHER ETIOLOGIC FACTORS

The extensive biomass of colonic flora in the right hemicolon consists mainly of Gram-negative anaerobes. The bacterial flora and intraluminal pH are different in patients who have slow compared to normal transit.[93] Increased ability to digest fiber by the colonic flora may also lead to smaller stools in some patients. Another mechanism by which the bacterial flora may affect motility is by the production of secondary metabolites from the fermentation of unabsorbed polysaccharides, fatty acids, and bile acids. Some of these secondary metabolites (short chain fatty acids and metabolites of long chain fatty acids) seem to act as intraluminal mediators resulting in powerful peristaltic contractions and rapid movement of the intraluminal contents.[76] In two uncontrolled studies, manipulation of the bacterial flora with vancomycin, an antibiotic selective for Gram-positive anaerobes in the colon, has resulted in occasional long-term improvements in constipation.[94]

The role of female sex hormones in the etiology of ISTC also merits discussion. It is known that childhood constipation is equally prevalent by gender, yet ISTC is predominantly found in females of reproductive age, with onset most often around the time of puberty. As early as 1909, Arbuthnot Lane described a syndrome of 'intestinal stasis' in young women, who tended to have abdominal bloating, poor peripheral circulation, as well as conditions suggestive of hormonal abnormalities including amenorrhea, loss of female secondary sexual characteristics, infertility and an increased incidence of ovarian cysts.[95] Davies *et al.* reported changes in bowel function that varied with the phase of menstrual period; during the luteal phase, there was markedly decreased transit time, stool weight and increased hardness of stool.[96] However, other studies have not shown clinically significant differences in colonic transit attributable to gender or phase of menstrual cycle over and above intra-individual variation.[97,98] A report of improvement in constipation and other bowel symptoms in female patients by use of a gonadotropin-releasing hormone analog has not been replicated.[99]

DIAGNOSIS AND MANAGEMENT

Although patient reports of defecatory habits and symptoms are sometimes imprecise, an algorithmic, pragmatic approach based upon likely findings (Fig. 22.3) is helpful in diagnosis and treatment of these patients.

STEP 1

The first step in management is to diagnose or exclude the possibility of a stricture or a mass lesion in patients with new onset constipation above the age of 40. This can be done by colonoscopy or colon X-ray. Younger patients also require a colonic structural study to exclude rare conditions such as Hirschsprung's disease, megarectum or megacolon if there is a long history of constipation. Laboratory studies are useful to screen for such obvious underlying conditions as hypothyroidism and hypercalcemia. If these studies are normal, a therapeutic trial of fiber supplementation should be carried out. A large study by Voderholzer *et al.*[100] showed that in a heterogeneous group with constipation, dietary supplementation with 15–30 g fiber/day failed to achieve improvement in 80% of patients with slow transit constipation and in 63% of those with outlet delay. In contrast, 85% of the constipated patients without physiopathological findings (normal transit constipation without evacuation disorder) either improved or became symptom free.[100] Therefore, a trial of fiber is invaluable since it will most likely adequately treat the large proportion of patients with simple constipation as well as a small proportion of those with outlet delay and slow transit. The remainder, who do not respond to a trial of at least 12 g fiber/day, require more extensive investigation. These basic diagnostic and therapeutic steps can all be accomplished by the primary health care provider.

STEP 2

Symptoms of difficulty with defecation requiring manual disimpaction or a feeling of anal blockage with

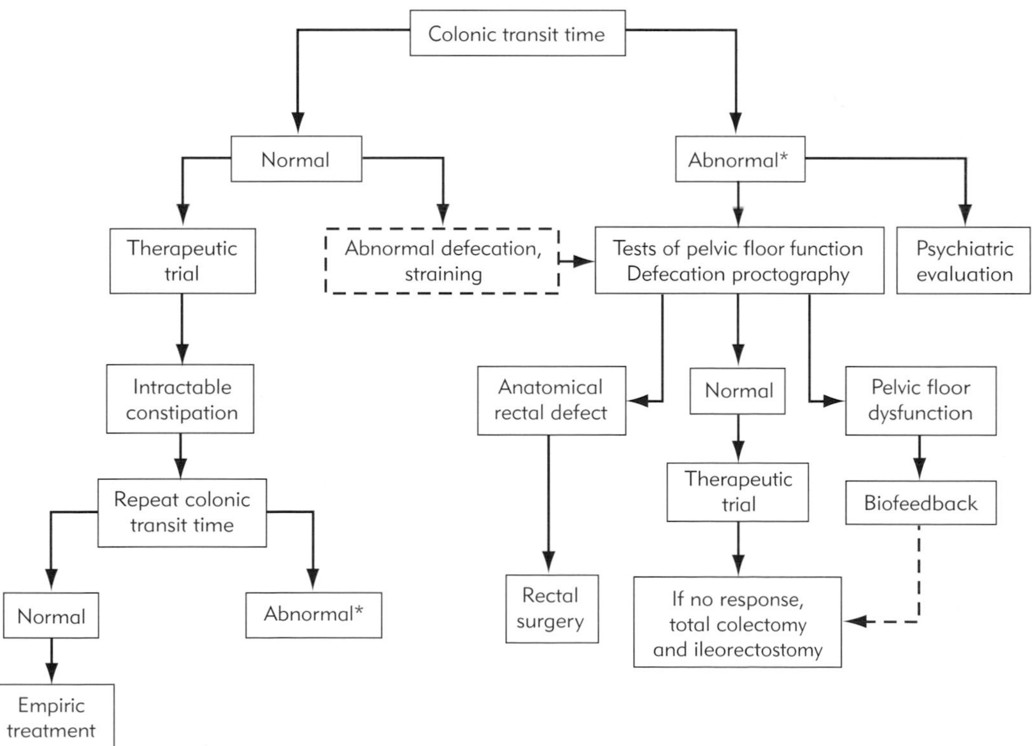

Figure 22.3 Algorithm for management of constipation in patients not responding to fiber supplementation and osmotic laxative. Adapted and reproduced with permission from Camilleri M, *et al.* Clinical management of intractable constipation. *Ann Intern Med* 1994;**121**:520–8.

prolonged defecation suggest rectal outlet delay (Fig. 22.3). Findings on examination of a lack of (< 1 cm) or excessive (>3.5 cm) perineal descent is also valuable, indicating puborectalis spasm or descending perineum syndrome. These factors should direct investigation by anorectal manometry with balloon expulsion. Anal manometry provides quantitative information on the anal sphincter tone at rest and pressures during squeeze. It is also helpful to assess rectal compliance (which is increased in megarectum or in patients with long history of outlet delay), threshold of urge perceptions and rectoanal inhibitory reflex.[101] The absence of internal anal sphincter relaxation in response to rectal distention suggests Hirschsprung's disease,[102] but a false positive result may occur with rectal volume enlargement due to prolonged fecal retention. A test of balloon expulsion (50 ml latex balloon) with the patient in the left lateral position should be performed routinely to screen for evacuation disorders. In healthy individuals, expulsion of the balloon occurs spontaneously or with the addition of a 200 g weight attached to the end of the balloon and hanging over a pulley at the level of the anal canal. A normal balloon expulsion test essentially excludes any important functional outlet delay.[103] In patients who have abnormalities of sphincter function or balloon expulsion, defecation scintigraphy or proctography should be performed. These tests are useful in determining the difference in recto-anal angle between rest and during straining and squeezing (normally at least 15 degrees). The extent of perineal descent can also be measured during straining.[19] Defecation proctography may give additional information when an anatomical defect (such as rectocele, enterocele or intussusception) is suspected. The combination of history, physical examination, and diagnostic tests will identify the subgroup of patients with outlet delay. After biofeedback retraining has established normal rectal expulsion, most patients become asymptomatic; however, a small number of patients will still be constipated. In these, repeat transit testing and, if necessary, treatment of associated ISTC, is indicated.

STEP 3

Patients who do not respond to fiber, and who do not have symptoms or physical findings suggestive of outlet delay, should have a colonic transit study. One of the most convenient methods to assess colonic transit uses radiopaque markers. In one of the popular methods, 24 markers are ingested at the same time of day on three successive days, and abdominal radiography is then performed on day 4 (and again on day 7 if all 72 markers are retained in the colon on day 4). The normal mean colonic transit time is 36 hours; thus, on average, 36 markers are expelled from the colon by day 4 of the transit study.[74] A whole gut transit time of 72 hours or more is considered abnormally prolonged. An alternative radioscintigraphic method (Fig. 22.4) gives a more detailed appraisal of regional colonic transit non-invasively.[104] Solid particles labeled with a relatively short half-life radioisotope (Indium-111) are formulated in a pH sensitive capsule coated with methacrylate polymer.[104] The methacrylate dissolves in the alkaline pH, that is characteristic of the distal small intestine. The terminal ileum then delivers its contents of isotopically labeled solid particles into the colon. Sequential gamma camera images quantify the amount of radioactivity in each region as the isotope traverses the colon, and the transit time is calculated, based upon the movement of the geometric center of the isotope mass.[72]

In patients who have constipation-predominant IBS, a colon transit study will usually reveal normal transit time, and the patient should be reassured of the significance of this and other normal study results. A minority of patients will have a structurally normal colon, no evidence of outlet delay, but slow colonic transit. Further evaluation in this group depends on which associated symptoms are present and what therapy is contemplated. Patients should be screened for evidence of dysautonomia, such as postural dizziness, palpitations, abnormal sweating patterns, difficulty emptying the urinary bladder, or problems with visual accommodation to bright lights.

Tests of autonomic function that are easily available and may be helpful include: measurement of blood pressure in the lying and standing positions, measurement of the interval between successive R waves on the EKG and its response to deep breathing, and the heart rate and blood pressure response to the Valsalva maneuver. In the presence of any upper gut symptoms, such as dysphagia, nausea, heartburn, early satiety and postprandial bloating, gastric emptying rates and small bowel transit should be measured and, if abnormal, esophageal and antroduodenal manometry may be necessary to determine whether there is a generalized dysmotility. It is important to identify these patients because the presence of generalized dysmotility is predictive of a poor outcome from colectomy.[105] Additionally, patients who have generalized dysmotility or autonomic dysfunction should undergo further investigation to evaluate the cause of the neuropathy such as diabetes, amyloidosis or a paraneoplastic syndrome.

Not infrequently, patients are thought to have ISTC, but have normal transit on objective testing. If symptoms do not suggest irritable bowel syndrome and a therapeutic trial of fiber and osmotic laxatives fails, a second transit study may demonstrate slow transit. If slow transit is not detected in subsequent testing, the patient should be treated medically and should not be offered colectomy.

Once the diagnosis of true idiopathic slow transit constipation is made, a therapeutic trial of laxatives is

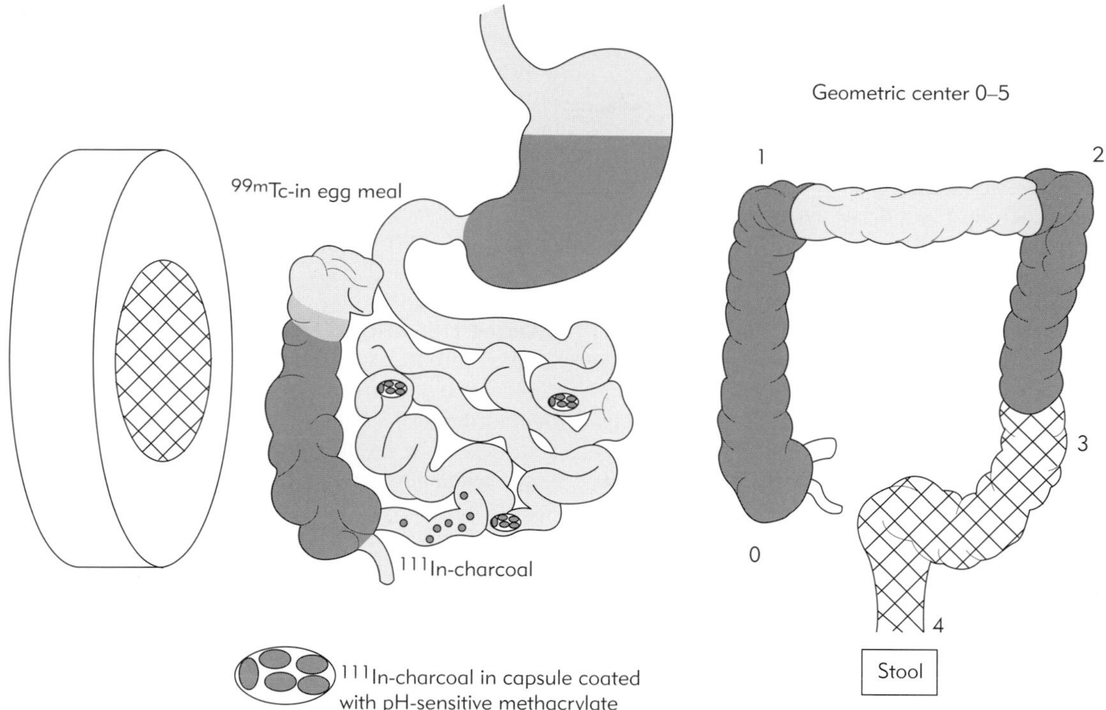

Figure 22.4 Scintigraphic method to evaluate gastric, small bowel and colonic transit. A delayed-release, pH-sensitive capsule delivers isotopically-labeled solid particles to the colon to estimate colonic transit. Geometric center refers to the weighted average of counts in four regions of colon and stool. Reproduced with permission from von der Ohe MR, Camilleri M. Measurement of small bowel and colonic transit: indications and methods. *Mayo Clin Proc* 1992;**67**:1169–79.

indicated. Only in non-responders is colonic manometry useful to further characterize the pathophysiology and stratify the patients to different types of treatment. Colonic manometry involves the use of several water-perfused, open-tipped manometry tubes or solid state transducers which can detect changes in intraluminal colonic pressure associated with strong contractions that occlude the lumen, but not with weak contractions. These devices can detect changes in contractile activity which occur normally following meals and also with pharmacological agents, such as with reversible inhibition of acetylcholinesterase activity caused by edrophonium or neostigmine.

As mentioned earlier, most patients with ISTC have not lost colonic responsiveness to such stimulation; it is only a small subset of ISTC patients that have true loss of colonic responsiveness and therefore may be categorized as colonic inertia. Patients with colonic inertia appear to have a worse prognosis and are likely to require subtotal colectomy with ileorectostomy.

THERAPY

After identifying and treating any underlying disorder, stepwise introduction of symptomatic treatment is required. We will review the available treatment options for idiopathic constipation with traditional laxatives, colonic prokinetics, experimental laxatives, biofeedback and surgical therapy.

BULK LAXATIVES

Bulk substances (bran, psyllium, ispaghula, methylcellulose) have considerable efficacy in most patients with simple constipation in a clinical trial setting where compliance and other favorable factors are maximized. Because fiber is efficacious, inexpensive and safe, it also forms the basic empirical tool since a therapeutic response identifies simple constipation. Conversely, patients who do not respond to an adequate trial of fiber (> 12 g/day) require evaluation with transit, ano-rectal motility, and pelvic floor studies. Bulk supplements increase stool weight by their water holding capacity, and by providing substrate for the colonic microflora to grow, thereby increasing the bacterial mass in stool.[106] It has been suggested that the bowel requires time, from weeks to months, in order to adapt to increased fiber intake, possibly because of the effect of fiber on the microflora. Occasionally, fiber supplementation may be poorly tolerated. It has been shown that all fiber supplements are associated with a similar degree of bloating sensation, gas formation and flatus, regardless of whether or not the fiber is fermentable by colonic bacteria.[107]

OSMOTIC LAXATIVES

Osmotic and saline laxatives include glycerine, lactulose, sorbitol or mannitol, magnesium salts (sulphate, citrate, and phosphate), and polyethylene glycol with electrolytes. Lactulose is a disaccharide that cannot be split by human intestinal enzymes and therefore it has an osmotic effect delivering more water to the colon. In the colon, lactulose is metabolized by the bacterial flora, increasing the concentration of short chain fatty acids and lowering the colonic pH, which may also result in an increase in colonic peristalsis.[108] The effectiveness of the osmotic laxatives appears to be equivalent. The magnesium compounds act not only by an osmotic effect, but also by increasing secretion and motility of the gut, possibly by enhancing cholecystokinin or some other hormonal mediator.[109] Since a significant amount of magnesium may be absorbed in the distal small bowel, toxicity may result if renal clearance is diminished. Polyethylene glycol is associated with less gas and bloating than other osmotic sugars/alcohols.

LUBRICANTS

Lubricants such as mineral oil and paraffin act by softening and lubricating the passage of stool. Because of predictable side effects such as fat-soluble vitamin malabsorption and less predictable events, such as lipoid pneumonitis due to aspiration in the elderly with swallowing problems, these agents are infrequently used.

STIMULANT LAXATIVES

The *polyphenolic compounds* and *anthranoid compounds* are both considered stimulant laxatives. The stimulant activity refers to the observed increase in colonic motor response including the presence of propagated high-pressure waves and augmentation of the normal colonic motor responses to the stimulus of meals.[110] Polyphenolic compounds include phenolphthalein and bisacodyl. Oxyphenacetin is no longer available due to its well described association with drug induced autoimmune hepatitis.[111] The polyphenolic drugs have multiple effects which include inducing a net fluid and electrolyte secretion into the lumen, stimulating mucosal prostaglandin E release, and increasing motor activity. Anthranoid derivatives are naturally occurring and include senna, cascara, nutmeg and aloes among others. These drugs induce a net secretion of fluid, but their mechanism of action may also include mediators such as prostaglandins.[112] The sennosides require hydrolysis by the colonic microflora and therefore have an action limited to the colon.[113] There is no evidence for small intestine mucosal damage with the sennosides. Likewise, long-term toxicity studies in experimental animals have not revealed changes in the smooth muscle layers or nervous plexuses in the colon.[114] While the overall safety of laxatives has been questioned, a meta-analysis of laxatives as a risk factor for colon cancer found a lower odds ratio for use of laxatives than for dietary factors such as fat, alcohol intake and low residue diet.[115] Since stimulant laxatives seem to have the effect of increasing colon motility without demonstrable toxic effects, it is not unreasonable to use these drugs for patients with ISTC in adequate doses and even for long-term maintenance therapy, if they are effective.

PROKINETICS AND NEWER DRUGS

More recently, a variety of novel medications have been employed in the treatment of refractory constipation. Pharmacological stimulation of gastrointestinal motility continues to be an area of active research. Of the currently available prokinetic medications, cisapride has been the most used in the treatment of constipation. Cisapride activated 5-HT_4 receptors on myenteric cholinergic nerves with consequent increased acetylcholine release.[36] The increased acetylcholine release results in smooth muscle contraction in the gut and is thought to be due to the partial agonist activity of cisapride at the 5-HT_4 receptor.[116] Placebo-controlled randomized clinical trials have shown that cisapride accelerates large intestinal transit time.[117] One study, involving the treatment of 126 idiopathic constipation patients with cisapride, 20 mg b.i.d., was associated with significant increase in spontaneous bowel movements and improvement in stool consistency compared to placebo.[118] Although cisapride appeared to have a useful prokinetic effect based upon initial trials, the drug has been disappointing in clinical practice. Furthermore, new safety concerns regarding the association of cisapride therapy with prolonged QT syndrome and fatal arrhythmias have dampened enthusiasm for the long-term use of this drug without evidence of unique benefit. Cisapride is only available by compassionate release protocol. Other prokinetic drugs, metoclopramide and domperidone do not have any apparent effects on colonic motility.[119] The remaining drug with prokinetic activity is erythromycin. Erythromycin has agonist activity at the motilin receptor and has known upper gut prokinetic effects. In a pilot study of 11 patients with ISTC, treatment with *per os* erythromycin, 1 g/day and 500 mg/day, resulted in significant shortening of colonic transit time and increase in stool frequency compared to baseline.[120]Unfortunately, the presence of the motilin receptor in the human colon has not been established, and the diarrheal effect of the antibiotic could account for the accelerated transit reported by Sharma *et al.* In any case, erythromycin is not an ideal agent because of its antibacterial activity and because of its poorly tolerated side effects of nausea and gastric upset. We await a non-antibiotic, motilin receptor agonist to study its effect in constipation.

Misoprostol, a prostaglandin E_1 analog, has been considered as treatment for refractory constipation. It is known that prostaglandins of the E series have a promotility effect on the gut. The laxative actions of the polyphenolic and anthranoid compounds may be partially related to increased mucosal prostaglandin production. In clinical use of misoprostol at 400–800 micrograms/day (for the prevention of drug induced peptic ulcers), cramping and diarrhea are common side effects. Roarty *et al.* studied the effects of misoprostol at doses between 600–2400 micrograms/day in an open-label study of 18 patients with refractory idiopathic constipation.[121] Six of the 18 patients did not tolerate the drug because of side effects, and the remaining patients all had a significant increase in bowel movement frequency. A previous study demonstrated that misoprostol decreases colonic transit time in patients with idiopathic constipation.[122]

There are also reports that colchicine stimulates intestinal motility in rats[123] and, in clinical practice, it can cause diarrhea at higher doses. A small pilot study using colchicine, 0.6 mg three times daily for 8 weeks, found significant acceleration of colonic transit time and increased stool frequency compared to baseline.[124]

While such reports are encouraging and point to future investigation, it is not appropriate at this time to treat patients with such drugs based on these few reports of small, open-label trials.

POLYETHYLENE GLYCOL

An iso-osmotic polyethylene glycol electrolyte solution (PEG) provides a non-absorbable moiety that increases intraluminal water by an osmotic effect. PEG is reported to be effective in acute fecal impaction and severe constipation.[125] Corazziari *et al.* reported a placebo controlled trial of small daily doses (250 ml twice daily) of PEG electrolyte solution in 48 constipated patients.[126] After 4 weeks, the PEG solution was found to accelerate colon transit time, increase frequency of bowel movements, and improve stool consistency.[126] In another study, 240 ml/day of PEG balanced electrolyte solution increased loose stools in opiate induced constipation.[127] Chronic use of low dose PEG solutions is a reasonable management strategy for patients refractory to other medical treatments.

EXPERIMENTAL THERAPIES

Recently, there has been increasing interest in exploiting the prokinetic effects of 5-HT_4 receptor agonists. In a one-week trial in constipation-predominant IBS patients, tegaserod, a 5-HT_4 partial agonist, significantly accelerated orocecal transit relative to placebo and accelerated colonic transit relative to pretreatment measurements.[128] In a study of healthy volunteers receiving prucalopride, a specific and selective 5-HT_4 agonist, significantly accelerated colonic transit was noted compared to placebo; gastric and small bowel transit were unaltered.[129] Large randomized, placebo-controlled trials of these drugs in patients with idiopathic constipation showed significant increases in spontaneous complete bowel movements.

The serendipitous observation that diarrhea developed in patients receiving experimental therapy for peripheral neuropathy with the nerve growth factor, neurotrophin-3 (NT-3), has led to interest in examining the effects of nerve growth factors on gastrointestinal motility. Studies of NT-3 in healthy volunteers and patients with idiopathic constipation found significant acceleration of orocecal and colonic transit in both groups.[130] Brain derived nerve growth factor (BDNF), had a similar effect in healthy volunteers.[131] While receptors for these nerve growth factors are present throughout the gut from early development through adulthood,[132] the mechanism of action of these novel compounds is unclear and merits further investigation.

CONSTIPATION-PREDOMINANT IBS

Rational treatment for constipation-predominant IBS patients is difficult. These patients have normal stool frequency, stool consistency, and colonic transit time; yet, they are unhappy and have a lower quality of life than the more physiologically perturbed patients with ISTC.[24] Prognosis may be most closely correlated with the presence or absence of major life stressors,[133] and it is difficult to justify the use of laxatives in this group. Fiber often exacerbates bowel symptoms such as pain and bloating.[134] Treatment of underlying visceral hypersensitivity may be currently accomplished by use of a non- or minimally constipating antidepressant such as trazodone or one of the selective serotonergic reuptake inhibitors (SSRIs). In the future, it is possible that novel treatments with agents as kappa opioid agonists, and 5HT_4 tagonists, or substance P antagonists might relieve the abnormal visceral sensations;[26] however, some may actually be deleterious for the symptom of constipation.

BIOFEEDBACK

Although there is a single report that biofeedback provides equal benefit to patients with severe constipation regardless of etiology,[135] the use of biofeedback and pelvic floor retraining is generally reserved for patients with documented rectal outlet delay. For this condition, the available studies show an impressive overall improvement rate of between 44% and 100% in symptoms or in objective parameters of ano-rectal function.[136]

SURGERY

Some patients fail all known laxatives and defecatory aids. When the diagnosis is ISTC or colonic inertia without generalized gut dysmotility or abnormal evacuation dynamics, the patient should be referred to an experienced surgeon for consideration of surgical management. Current surgical treatment of ISTC is a total colectomy with ileorectal anastomosis; in some patients, this has been performed as a laparoscopically assisted procedure.[137] In general, the results have not always been satisfactory, primarily due to inadequate selection of patients with undetected evacuation disorder, generalized dysmotility or significant psychological overlay. Colectomy and ileorectal anastomosis help the majority of ISTC patients. An outcome study of 59 patients[138] found that about 70% had satisfactory results, with four or less bowel movements per day; 10% had diarrhea or incontinence; and the remainder had persistent constipation. Overall, 90% reported that they were satisfied with the procedure.[138] Segmental colonic resections are rarely effective in relieving constipation and tend not to be considered.

For patients with megacolon, colectomy and ileorectal anastomosis are effective. When the rectum and sigmoid are dilated, a colo-anal anastomosis or a procto-colectomy with an ileal pouch anal anastomosis may be offered.[12] Generally, patients with occult rectoceles and descending perineal syndrome do not respond well to surgical management.[12] More significant rectoceles that selectively fill and do not empty on defecation proctography may be effectively resected. Patients with complete rectal prolapse are candidates for rectal mobilization and anterior resection.[12]

Patients who fail to have an adequate response to surgery may be managed by continued medical therapy, further biofeedback therapy for evacuation disorders, or, as a last resort, revisional surgery or lower descending colostomy, depending on the cause for the surgical failure.

REFERENCES

1. Sandler RS, Drossman DA, Nathan HP, *et al.* Symptoms, complaints and health care seeking behavior in subjects with bowel dysfunction. *Gastroenterology* 1984;**87**:314–8.
2. Drossman DA, Thompson WG, Talley NJ, *et al.* Identification of sub-groups of functional gastrointestinal disorders. *Gastroenterol Int* 1990;3:159–72.
3. Probert CS, Emmett PM, Cripps HA, *et al.* Evidence for the ambiguity of the term constipation: the role of irritable bowel syndrome. *Gut* 1994;**35**:1455–8.
4. Koch A, Voderholzer WA, Klauser AG, *et al.* Symptoms in chronic constipation. *Dis Colon Rectum* 1997;**40**:902–6.
5. Sandler RS, Galanko JC, Murray SC, *et al.* Symptom criteria for constipation subtypes in a U.S. national epidemiologic study of constipation. *Gastroenterology* 1998;**114**:A831.
6. Voderholzer WA, Schatke W, Muldorfer BF, *et al.* Clinical response to dietary fiber treatment of chronic constipation. *Am J Gastroenterol* 1997;**92**:95–8.
7. Turnbull GK, Lennard-Jones JE, Bartram CI. Failure of rectal expulsion as a cause of constipation: why fibre and laxatives sometimes fail. *Lancet* 1986;i(8484):767–9.
8. Mehta M. *PDR companion guide.* Montvale, NJ: Medical Economics Co, 1998:1316–8.
9. Bassotti G, Chiarioni G, Imbimbo BP, *et al.* Impaired colonic motor response to cholinergic stimulation in patients with severe chronic idiopathic (slow transit type) constipation. *Dig Dis Sci* 1993;**38**:1040–5.
10. Ghosh S, Papachrysostomou M, Batool M, *et al.* Long-term results of subtotal colectomy and evidence of idiopathic slow transit constipation. *Scand J Gastroenterol* 1996;**31**:1083–91.
11. Johnson JF, Sonnenberg A, Koch TR. Clinical epidemiology of chronic constipation. *J Clin Gastroenterol* 1989; **11**:525–36.
12. Bartolo DCC, Devroede G, Kamm MA, *et al.* Symposium on constipation. *Int J Colorectal Dis* 1992;**7**:47–67.
13. Lennard-Jones JE. Constipation. In: Feldman M, Scharschmidt BF, Sleisenger MH (eds). *Sleisenger and Fordtran's Gastrointestinal and Liver Disease*, 6th edn. Philadelphia: WB Saunders, 1998:174–97.
14. Talley NJ, Weaver AL, Zinsmeister AR, *et al.* Functional constipation and outlet delay: a population-based study. *Gastroenterology* 1993;**105**:781–90.
15. Drossman DA, Li Z, Andruzzi E, *et al.* U.S. householder survey of functional gastrointestinal disorders. Prevalence, sociodemography, and health impact. *Dig Dis Sci* 1993;**38**:1569–80.
16. Talley NJ. Who has functional disorders? In: *Gastrointestinal Motility: Proceedings of the Twelfth BSG-SB International Workshop*, 1991:45–7.
17. Locke GR. The epidemiology of functional gastrointestinal disorders in North America. In: Camilleri M (ed.) *Gastroenterology Clinics of North America: Gastrointestinal Motility in Clinical Practice*, Vol. 25. Philadelphia: WB Saunders, 1996:1–19.
18. Surrenti E, Rath DM, Pemberton JH, *et al.* Audit of constipation in a tertiary-referral gastroenterology practice. *Am J Gastroenterol* 1995;**90**:1471–5.
19. Koch A, Voderholzer WA, Klauser AG, *et al.* Symptoms in chronic constipation. *Dis Colon Rectum* 1997;**40**:902–6.
20. Read NW. Who is constipated? In: *Gastrointestinal Motility: Proceedings of the Twelfth BSG-SB International Workshop*, 1991:51–3.
21. Talley NJ, Fleming KC, Evans JM, *et al.* Constipation in an elderly community: a study of prevalence, and potential risk factors. *Am J Gastroenterol* 1996;**91**:19–25.
22. Merkel IS, Locher J, Burgio K, *et al.* Physiologic and psychologic characteristics of an elderly population with chronic constipation. *Am J Gastroenterol* 1993;**88**:1854–9.
23. Bannister JJ, Abouzekry L, Read NW. Effect of aging on anorectal function. *Gut* 1987;**28**:353–7.
24. Glia A, Lindberg G. Quality of life in patients with different types of functional constipation. *Scand J Gastroenterol* 1997;**32**:1083–9.
25. Camilleri M, Choi MG. Review article: Irritable bowel syndrome. *Aliment Pharmacol Ther* 1997;**11**:3–15.
26. Rantis PC, Vernava AM, Daniel GL, *et al.* Chronic constipation – is the work-up worth the cost? *Dis Colon Rectum* 1997;**40**:280–6.
27. Christensen J. Gross and microscopic anatomy of the large intestine. In: Phillips SF, Pemberton JH, Shorter RG (eds).

The large intestines: physiology, pathophysiology and disease. New York: Raven Press, 1996:13–35.

28. Camilleri M, Ford MJ. Review article: Colonic sensorimotor physiology in health and its alteration in constipation and diarrhoeal disorders. *Aliment Pharm Ther* 1998; 12:287–302.
29. Bharucha AE, Camilleri M, Zinsmeister AR, *et al.* Adrenergic modulation of human colonic motor and sensory function. *Am J Physiol* 1997;**273**:G997–1006.
30. Gillis RA, Dias Souza J, Hicks KA, *et al.* Inhibitory control of proximal colonic motility by the sympathetic nervous system. *Am J Physiol* 1987;**253**:G531–9.
31. Steadman CJ, Phillips SF, Camilleri M, *et al.* Control of muscle tone in the human colon. *Gut* 1992;**33**:541–6.
32. Snape WJ Jr, Carlson GM, Cohen S. Human colonic myoelectrical activity in response to prostigmin and the gastrointestinal hormones. *Am J Dig Dis* 1977;**22**:881–7.
33. von der Ohe MR, Hanson RB, Camilleri M. Serotonergic mediation of postprandial colonic tone and phasic responses in humans. *Gut* 1994;**35**:536–41.
34. Talley NJ, Phillips SF, Haddad A, *et al.* GR-38082F (ondansetron), a selective 5-HT3 antagonist, slows colonic transit in healthy man. *Dig Dis Sci* 1990;**35**:477–80.
35. Scarpignato C. Pharmacological stimulation of gastrointestinal motility: where we are and where we are going? *Dig Dis* 1997;**15**:112–36.
36. von der Ohe MR, Camilleri M, Thomforde G, *et al.* Differential regional effects of octreotide on human gastrointestinal motor function. *Gut* 1995;**36**:743–8.
37. Sjolund K, Fasth S, Ekman R, *et al.* Neuropeptides in idiopathic chronic constipation (slow transit constipation). *Neurogastroenterol Motil* 1997;**9**:143–50.
38. Keshavarzian A, Barnes WE, Bruninga K, *et al.* Delayed colonic transit in spinal cord-injured patients measured by Indium-111 Amberlite scintigraphy. *Am J Gastroenterol* 1995;**90**:1295–300.
39. Bruninga K, Camilleri M. Colonic motility and tone after spinal cord and cauda equina injury. *Am J Gastroenterol* 1997;**92**:891–4.
40. Devroede G, Lamarche J. Functional importance of extrinsic parasympathetic innervation to the distal colon and rectum in man. *Gastroenterology* 1974;**66**:273–80.
41. Devroede G, Arhan P, Duguay C, *et al.* Traumatic constipation. *Gastroenterology* 1979;**77**:1258–67.
42. Singaram C, Ashraf W, Gaumnitz EA, *et al.* Dopaminergic defect of enteric nervous system in Parkinson's disease patients with chronic constipation. *Lancet* 1995;**346**:861–4.
43. Hinds JP, Eidelman BH, Wald A. Prevalence of bowel dysfunction in multiple sclerosis. A population survey. *Gastroenterology* 1990;**98**:1538–42.
44. Glick ME, Meshkinpour H, Haldeman S, *et al.* Colonic dysfunction in multiple sclerosis. *Gastroenterology* 1982;**83**:1002–7.
45. Battle WM, Snape WJ Jr, Alavi A, *et al.* Colonic dysfunction in diabetes mellitus. *Gastroenterology* 1980;**79**:1217–21.
46. Maxton DG, Whorwell PJ. Functional bowel symptoms in diabetes – the role of autonomic neuropathy. *Postgrad Med J* 1991;**67**:991–3.
47. Feldman M, Schiller LR. Disorders of gastrointestinal motility associated with diabetes mellitus. *Ann Intern Med* 1983;**98**:378–84.
48. Altomare D, Pilot MA, Scott M, *et al.* Detection of subclinical autonomic neuropathy in constipated patients using a sweat test. *Gut* 1992;**33**:1539–43.
49. De Medici A, Badiali D, Corazziari E, *et al.* Rectal sensitivity in chronic constipation. *Dig Dis Sci* 1989;**34**:747–53.
50. Bassotti G, Chiarioni G, Vantini I, *et al.* Anorectal manometric abnormalities and colonic propulsive impairment in patients with severe chronic idiopathic constipation. *Dig Dis Sci* 1994;**39**:1558–64.
51. Barnes PRH, Lennard-Jones JE, Hawley PR, *et al.* Hirschsprung's disease and idiopathic megacolon in adults and adolescents. *Gut* 1986;**27**:534–41.
52. Milla PJ. Endothelins, pseudo-obstruction and Hirschsprung's disease. *Gut* 1998;**44**:148–52.
53. Kobayashi H, O'Brien DS, Puri P. Nerve growth factor receptor immunostaining suggests an extrinsic origin for hypertrophic nerves in Hirschsprung's disease. *Gut* 1994;**35**:1605–7.
54. Vanderwinden JM, De Laet MH, Schiffmann SN, *et al.* Nitric oxide synthase distribution in the enteric nervous system of Hirschsprung's disease. *Gastroenterology* 1993;**105**:969–73.
55. von der Ohe MR, Camilleri M, Carryer PW. A patient with megacolon and intractable constipation: evaluation for impairment of colonic muscle tone. *Am J Gastroenterol* 1994;**84**:1867–70.
56. Gattuso JM, Kamm MA, Talbot IC. Pathology of idiopathic megarectum and megacolon. *Gut* 1997;**41**:252–7.
57. Smith VV, Gregson N, Foggensteiner L, *et al.* Acquired intestinal aganglionosis and circulating autoantibodies without neoplasia or other neural involvement. *Gastroenterology* 1997;**112**:1366–71.
58. Krishnamurthy S, Schuffler MD, Rohrman CA, *et al.* Severe idiopathic constipation is associated with a distinctive abnormality of the colonic myenteric plexus. *Gastroenterology* 1985;**88**:26–34.
59. Schouten WR, ten Kate FJW, de Graaf EJR, *et al.* Visceral neuropathy in slow transit constipation: an immunohistochemical investigation with monoclonal antibodies against neurofilament. *Dis Colon Rectum* 1993;**36**:1112–7.
60. Smith B. The effect of irritant purgatives on the myenteric plexus in man and the mouse. *Gut* 1968;**9**:139–43.
61. Milner P, Belai A, Tomlinson A, *et al.* Effects of long-term laxative treatment on neuropeptides in rat mesenteric vessels and cecum. *J Pharm Pharmacol* 1992;**44**:777–9.
62. Smith B. Pathologic changes in the colon produced by anthraquinone purgatives. *Dis Colon Rectum* 1972;**16**:455–8.
63. Hagger R, Gharaie S, Finlayson C, *et al.* Regional and transmural density of interstitial cells of Cajal in human colon and rectum. *Am J Physiol* 1998;**275**:G1309–16.
64. He CL, Burgart L, Wang L, Pemberton J, Young-Fadok T, Szurszewski J, Farrugia G. Decreased interstitial cells of Cajal volume in patients with slow-transit constipation. *Gastroenterology* 2000;**118**:14–21.
65. Narducci F, Bassotti G, Gaburri M, *et al.* Twenty-four manometric recordings of colonic motor activity in healthy man. *Gut* 1987;**28**:17–25.
66. Bassotti G, Gaburri M, Imbimbo BP, *et al.* Colonic mass movements in idiopathic chronic constipation. *Gut* 1988;**29**:1173–9.

67. Snape WJ Jr, Wright SH, Battle WM, *et al.* The gastrocolic response: evidence for a neural mechanism. *Gastroenterology* 1979;**77**:1235–40.
68. Snape WJ Jr, Matarrazzo SA, Cohen S. Effect of eating and gastrointestinal hormones on human colonic myoelectrical and motor activity. *Gastroenterology* 1978;**75**:373–8.
69. Bassotti G, Chiarioni G, Imbimbo BP, *et al.* Impaired colonic motor response to eating in patients with slow transit constipation. *Am J Gastroenterol* 1992;**87**:504–8.
70. Stivland T, Camilleri M, Vassallo M, *et al.* Scintigraphic measurement of regional gut transit in idiopathic constipation. *Gastroenterology* 1991;**101**:107–15.
71. van der Sijp JRM, Kamm MA, Nightingale J, *et al.* Disturbed gastric and small bowel transit in severe idiopathic constipation. *Dig Dis Sci* 1993;**38**:837–44.
72. Proano M, Camilleri M, Phillips SF, *et al.* Transit of solids through the human colon: regional quantification in the unprepared bowel. *Am J Physiol* 1990;**258**:G856–62.
73. Ritchie JA. Colonic motor activity and bowel function. Part 1: Normal movements of the contents. *Gut* 1968;**9**:442–56.
74. Metcalf AM, Phillips SF, Zinsmeister AR, *et al.* Simplified assessment of segmental colonic transit. *Gastroenterology* 1987;**92**:40–7.
75. Phillips SF. The ileocolon. In: *Gastrointestinal Motility: Proceedings of the Twelfth BSG-SB International Workshop*, 1991:33–7.
76. Davies GJ, Crowder M, Reid B, *et al.* Bowel function measurements of individuals with different eating patterns. *Gut* 1986;**27**:164–9.
77. Chun AB, Sokol MS, Kaye WH, *et al.* Colonic and anorectal function in constipated patients with anorexia nervosa. *Am J Gastroenterol* 1997;**92**:1879–83.
78. Karlbom U, Pahlman L, Nilsson S, *et al.* Relationships between defecographic findings, rectal emptying, and colonic transit time in constipated patients. *Gut* 1995;**36**:907–12.
79. Klauser AG, Voderholzer WA, Heinrich CA, *et al.* Behavioral modification of colonic function. *Dig Dis Sci* 1990;**35**:1271–5.
80. Ewe K. Intestinal transport in constipation and diarrhea. *Pharmacology* 1988;**36**:73–84.
81. Barrow L, Steed KP, Spiller RC, *et al.* Scintigraphic demonstration of lactulose-induced accelerated proximal colon transit. *Gastroenterology* 1992;**25**:326–8.
82. Debongie JC, Phillips SF. Capacity of the human colon to absorb fluid. *Gastroenterology* 1978;**74**:698–703.
83. Rogers J. The anorectum. In: *Gastrointestinal Motility: Proceedings of the Twelfth BSG-SB International Workshop*, 1991:38–40.
84. Shelton AA, Welton ML. The pelvic floor in health and disease. *West J Med* 1997;**167**:90–8.
85. Miller R, Lewis GT, Bartolo DCC, *et al.* Sensory discrimination and dynamic activity in the anorectum: evidence using a new ambulatory technique. *Br J Surg* 1988;**75**:1003–7.
86. Schouten WR, Briel JW, Auwerda JJA, *et al.* Anismus: fact or fiction? *Dis Colon Rectum* 1997;**40**:1033–41.
87. Voderholzer WA, Neuhaus DA, Klauser AG, *et al.* Paradoxical sphincter contraction is rarely indicative of anismus. *Gut* 1997;**41**:258–62.
88. Roberts JP, Womack NR, Hallan RI, *et al.* Evidence from dynamic integrated proctography to redefine anismus. *Br J Surg* 1992;**79**:1213–8.
89. Halligan S, Thomas J, Bartram C. Intrarectal pressures and balloon expulsion related to evacuation proctography. *Gut* 1995;**37**:100–4.
90. Shrovon PJ, McHugh S, Diamant NE, *et al.* Defecography in normal volunteers: results and implications. *Gut* 1989;**30**:1737–42.
91. Harewood GC, Coulie B, Camilleri M, *et al.* Descending perineum syndrome: audit of clinical and laboratory features and outcome of pelvic floor retraining. *Am J Gastroenterol* 1999;**94**:126–30.
92. Snooks SJ, Barnes PRH, Swash M, *et al.* Damage to the innervation of the pelvic floor musculature in chronic constipation. *Gastroenterology* 1985;**89**:977–84.
93. Oufir LE, Flourie B, des Varannes SB, *et al.* Relations between transit time, fermentation products, and hydrogen consuming flora in healthy humans. *Gut* 1996; **38**:870–7.
94. Celik AF, Tomlin J, Read NW. The effect of oral vancomycin on chronic idiopathic constipation. *Aliment Pharmacol Ther* 1995;**9**:63–8.
95. Lane WA. Chronic intestinal stasis. *BMJ* 1909;**1**:1408–11.
96. Davies GJ, Crowder M, Reid B, *et al.* Bowel function measurements of individuals with different eating patterns. *Gut* 1986;**27**:164–9.
97. Turnbull GK, Thompson DG, Day S, *et al.* Relationships between symptoms, menstrual cycle and orocecal transit in normal and constipated women. *Gut* 1989;**30**:30–4.
98. Hinds JP, Stoney B, Wald A. Does gender or the menstrual cycle affect colonic transit? *Am J Gastroenterol* 1989; **84**:123–6.
99. Mathias JR, Clench MH. Relationship of reproductive hormones and neuromuscular disease of the gastrointestinal tract. *Dig Dis* 1998;**16**:3–13.
100. Voderholzer WA, Schatke W, Muldorfer BE, *et al.* Clinical response to dietary fiber treatment of chronic constipation. *Am J Gastroenterol* 1997;**92**:95–8.
101. Wald A. Colonic and anorectal motility testing in clinical practice. *Am J Gastroenterol* 1997;**89**:2109–15.
102. Tobon F, Reid NC, Talbert JL, *et al.* Nonsurgical test for the diagnosis of Hirschsprung's disease. *N Engl J Med* 1968;**278**:188–94.
103. Rao SS, Sun WM. Current techniques of assessing defecation dynamics. *Dig Dis* 1997;**15**:64–77.
104. Burton DD, Camilleri M, Mullan BP, *et al.* Colonic transit scintigraphy labeled activated charcoal compared with ion exchange pellets. *J Nucl Med* 1997;**38**:1807–10.
105. Redmond JM, Smith GW, Barofsky I, *et al.* Physiological tests to predict long-term outcome of total abdominal colectomy for intractable constipation. *Am J Gastroenterol* 1995;**90**:748–53.
106. Eastwood M. Faecal bulking agents. In: *Proceedings of the Twelfth BSG-SB International Workshop*, 1991:62–3.
107. Zumarraga L, Levitt MD, Suarez F. Absence of gaseous symptoms during ingestion of commercial fibre preparations. *Aliment Pharmacol Ther* 1997;**11**:1067–72.
108. Devroede G. Constipation. In: Sleisenger MH, Fordtran JS (eds). *Gastrointestinal disease: pathophysiology, diagnosis*

and management, 5th edn. Philadelphia: W.B. Saunders, 1993:837–64.
109. Godding EW. Laxatives and the special role of senna. *Pharmacology* 1988;**36**:230–6.
110. Staumont G, Frexinos J, Fioramonti J, *et al.* Sennasoids and human colonic motility. *Pharmacology* 1988;**36**:49–56.
111. Homberg JC, Abuaf N, Helmy-Khalil S, *et al.* Drug-induced hepatitis associated with anticytoplasmic organelle autoantibodies. *Hepatology* 1985;**5**:722–7.
112. Beubler E, Juan H. Effect of ricinoleic acid and other laxatives on net water flux and prostaglandin E release in the rat colon. *J Pharm Pharmacol* 1979;**31**:681–5.
113. Hietala P, Lainonen H, Marvola M. New aspects of metabolism of the sennosides. *Pharmacology* 1988;**36**:138–43.
114. Mengs U. Toxic effects of sennosides in laboratory animals and *in vitro*. *Pharmacology* 1988;**36**:180–7.
115. Sonnenberg A, Muller AD. Constipation and cathartics as risk factors for colorectal cancer: a meta-analysis. *Pharmacology* 1993;**43**:224–33.
116. Gardner VY, Beckwith JV, Heyneman CA, *et al.* Cisapride for the treatment of chronic idiopathic constipation. *Ann Pharmacother* 1995;**29**:1161–3.
117. Van Daele L, DeCuypere A, Van Kerckhove M. Routine radiological follow-through examination shows effect of cisapride on gastrointestinal transit: a controlled study. *Curr Ther Res* 1984;**36**:1038–44.
118. Muller-Lissner SA, the Bavarian Constipation Study Group. Treatment of chronic constipation with cisapride and placebo. *Gut* 1987;**28**:1033–8.
119. Brunton LL. Agents affecting gastrointestinal water flux and motility, digestants, and bile acids. In: Gilman AG, Rall TW, Neis AS, *et al.* (eds.). *Goodman and Gilman's The Pharmacological Basis of Therapeutics*, 8th edn. New York: Pergamon Press, 1990: 914–32.
120. Sharma SS, Bhargava N, Mathur S. Effect of oral erythromycin on colonic transit in patients with idiopathic constipation. *Dig Dis Sci* 1995;**40**:2446–9.
121. Roarty TP, Weber F, Soykan I, *et al.* Misoprostol in the treatment of chronic refractory constipation: results of a long-term, open-label trial. *Aliment Pharmacol Ther* 1997;**11**:1059–66.
122. Soffer EE, Metcalf A, Launspach J. Misoprostol is effective treatment for patients with severe chronic constipation. *Dig Dis Sci* 1988;**39**:929–33.
123. Sninsky CA, Lynch DF. Why should microtubular inhibitors induce frequent activity fronts (AF) of the migrating motor complex (MMC)? *Gastroenterology* 1986;**90**:1641–4.
124. Verne GN, Eaker EY, Davis RH, *et al.* Colchicine is an effective treatment for patients with chronic constipation: an open label trial. *Dig Dis Sci* 1997;**42**:1959–63.
125. Smith RG, Currie JJ. Whole gut irrigation: a new treatment for constipation. *BMJ* 1978;**8**:396–7.
126. Corazziari E, Badiali D, Habib FI, *et al.* Small volume iso-osmotic polyethylene glycol electrolyte balanced solution (PMF-100) in treatment of chronic nonorganic constipation. *Dig Dis Sci* 1996;**41**:1636–42.
127. Freedman MD, Schwartz HJ, Roby R, *et al.* Tolerance and efficacy of polyethylene glycol 3350/electrolyte solution versus lactulose in relieving opiate induced constipation: a double-blind, placebo-controlled trial. *J Clin Pharmacol* 1997;**37**:904–7.
128. Prather CM, Camilleri M, McKinzie S, *et al.* HTF919, a partial $5HT_4$ agonist, accelerates small bowel transit in patients with constipation-predominant irritable bowel syndrome. *Gastroenterology* (abstract, in press).
129. Bouras BP, Camilleri M, Burton D, *et al.* Selective stimulation of colonic transit by the benzofuran $5HT_4$ agonist, prucalopride, in healthy humans. *Gut* (in press).
130. Szarka LA, Camilleri M, Burton D, *et al.* Recombinant human neurotrophin-3 (NT-3) accelerates small bowel and colonic transit in healthy humans and patients with constipation. *Gastroenterology* (abstract, in press).
131. Coulie B, Camilleri M, Burton D, *et al.* Recombinant human brain derived neurotrophic factor accelerates colonic transit in humans. *Gastroenterology* (abstract, in press).
132. Hoehner JC, Wester T, Pahlman S, *et al.* Localization of neurotrophins and their high-affinity receptors during human enteric nervous system development. *Gastroenterology* 1996;**110**:756–65.
133. Bennett EJ, Tennant CC, Piesse C, *et al.* Level of chronic life stress predicts clinical outcome in irritable bowel syndrome. *Gut* 1998;**43**:256–61.
134. Lewis MJ, Whorwell PJ. Bran may irritate irritable bowel. *Nutrition* 1998;**14**:470–1.
135. Chiotakakou-Faliakou E, Kamm MA, Roy AJ, *et al.* Biofeedback provides long-term benefit for patients with intractable, slow and normal transit constipation. *Gut* 1998;**42**:517–21.
136. Rao SSC, Enck P, Loening-Baucke V. Biofeedback therapy for defecation disorders. *Dig Dis* 1997;**15**:78–92.
137. Young-Fadok TM, Pemberton JH, Camilleri M. A case-controlled study of laparoscopic total abdominal colectomy and ileorectal anastomosis (TAC-IRA) with open TAC-IRA for slow transit constipation (STC). Gastroenterology 2001;120:A476.
138. Lubowski DZ, Chen FC, Kennedy ML, *et al.* Results of colectomy for severe slow transit constipation. *Dis Colon Rectum* 1996;**39**:23-9.

Chapter 23

Irritable bowel syndrome

W Grant Thompson

Strictly speaking, the irritable bowel syndrome (IBS) is not a disease of the pelvic floor. It is a disorder of the intestines, although its exact nature is unknown. Nevertheless, the pelvic floor and anal sphincters are involved in an intimate way with the diarrhea and constipation that IBS patients suffer. Even if the pelvic floor's involvement is reactive, a discussion of the IBS is certainly appropriate in this book. Moreover many patients visiting gynecologists and perhaps urologists complain of 'pelvic' pain.[1] By this is usually meant lower abdominal pain, and the symptom often turns out to be part of the IBS. The pain may be severe and recurrent and IBS subjects are prone to abdominal surgery,[2-4] including hysterectomy.[5] Removal of a normal gall bladder, appendix or uterus cannot be expected to improve a patients' IBS symptoms.

A WORLD VIEW (FIG. 23.1)

The prevalence of IBS depends upon how the condition is defined (see below). Nevertheless, it appears that the one-year point prevalence of IBS in adults is between 10 and 20% worldwide. This was first reported in an unselected British population in 1980,[6] and has been duplicated in populations around the world,[7-9] even in China.[10] There are two studies of random population samples that indicate similar prevalences in the United States[11] and the UK.[12] In these studies it appears that female/male ratio is two to one, and that the prevalence is unaffected by age.

In sequential studies[13,14] it appears that while the point prevalence remains constant at 15 to 20%, the individuals in that IBS population change. There is thus a gain and loss into the IBS cohort such that the lifetime prevalence

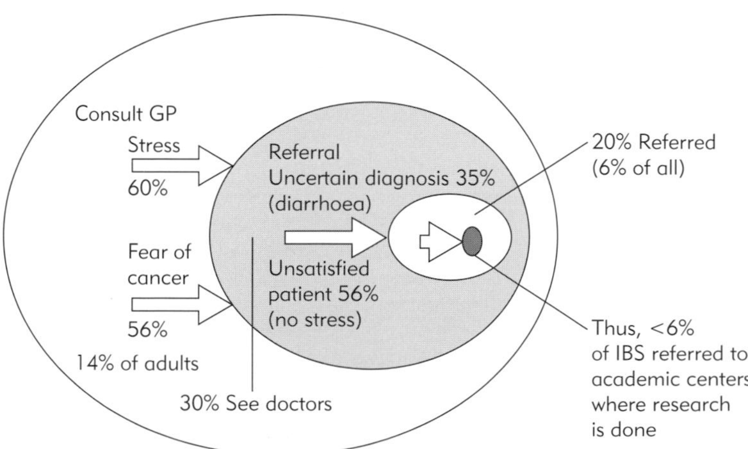

Figure 23.1 A world view of IBS: While 14% of adults have the IBS, only a minority (perhaps 35%) see general practitioners in England. Of those, only about 20% are referred to specialists; a still smaller percentage are referred to academic centers. Yet almost all the published literature on IBS originates in these centers. Much of the data presented in this literature are not necessarily applicable to non-patients, or patients in primary care. Moreover, specialists see only a fraction of IBS sufferers, but almost all patients with IBD. Therefore, comparisons of IBS and IBD in clinical studies carried out by specialists are not valid. Thus the IBS may seem different to different people: non-patients, patients, primary care physicians, gastroenterologists, surgeons, gynecologists and academicians (see text).

of IBS is much higher than 15 to 20%. Clinical studies in which patients who have a firm initial diagnosis are seen one to eight years later, find that most are symptomatic (Table 23.1).[13,15–18] This indicates that the IBS is a chronic or recurrent condition. It is also important to observe that in studies where the diagnosis of IBS was confidently made initially, few patients turn out later to have an organic gastrointestinal disease, and in no case could the original diagnosis have been said to be incorrect.[15–18]

Many epidemiological studies that have been done over the past 20 years show that most patients suffering from IBS symptoms do not seek medical care for them.[6–10] Therefore, it would seem that most of the population consider these symptoms to be part of life, like a muscle pain or headache, and don't seek medical attention. An important objective of current research is to discover why only a minority of people that see doctors do so.

Most individuals who become patients are cared for in primary care.[19,20] It appears that stress and the fear of serious disease such as cancer are important reasons for them to seek medical help.[20] At least in the UK, General Practitioners (GPs) do not find IBS to be a difficult problem,[19] nor are they prone to misdiagnose it. In contrast, those relatively few patients referred to gastroenterologists are often considered to be difficult to manage.

Individuals in the community who have IBS symptoms (non-patients) appear to have a psychosocial make-up that is similar to the remainder of the population.[21,22] However, those patients seen in academic centers have a high prevalence of depression,[23–28] anxiety,[27,28] panic,[27,29,30] and personality disorders. The commonest reasons given by the GPs for a referral to specialists are uncertain diagnosis, and an unsatisfied patient.[19] From the data, it seems that in primary care, diagnosis, reassurance and management of stress are important components of management. Gastroenterologists, on the other hand, should see that their mission includes firm confirmation of the diagnosis, and discovery and management of the reason for the patients' dissatisfaction. The latter may require psychological intervention.

IBS has been associated with many other conditions, such as fibromyalgia,[31,32] and chronic fatigue.[33] However, these data come from specialist centers, and may not hold true in a general practice setting.

COST

Based on a survey in Minnesota,[34] it has been estimated that in the United States IBS costs eight billion dollars annually. These costs embrace investigations, doctors' visits, prescription drugs and other treatments, but do not include non-prescription drugs, and time off work.

IBS is not a particularly disabling disorder for most patients, but it affects many people of all ages, and frequently engenders worries of other serious disease. Such worries generate many consultations and investigations. Indeed IBS appears to be the principal indication for conducting a barium enema examination.[35]

To be sure, a few IBS patients are severely troubled, even disabled by their symptoms and accompanying psychological circumstances. It is reasonable to suspect that most of the costs are generated by this subset of patients who not only contact their primary care physician, but also are referred on to specialists. These patients are vulnerable to over-investigation and inappropriate treatment.

The large amount of money directed towards the benign symptoms of IBS diverts resources from the management of more serious disease. The $8 billion annual cost would pay for over 10 000 liver transplants and their first year of postoperative care.

DEFINITIONS AND CRITERIA

To many, IBS is a diagnosis of exclusion. It consists of those gut symptoms that remain unexplained after extensive investigation of the intestinal tract. This costly approach is inappropriate and not only generates much cost, but also engenders much insecurity in the patient. Each new round of investigations increases the patient's anxiety, and lack of confidence in the physician and the diagnosis.

Table 23.1 Prognosis in irritable bowel syndrome[71]

Author	Patients	Years follow-up	Percent still symptomatic	Comment
Holmes, 1982[15]	77	6	57	New diagnosis in 4
Svendsen, 1985[16]	112	2	–	Organic disease in 3
Harvey, 1987[17]	97	5–8	74	No change in diagnosis
Owens, 1995[18]	112	32	–	Misdiagnosis in 3, observed Survival same as expected

In the last 20 years there has been an effort to enable physicians to arrive at a more positive diagnosis of IBS based on symptom criteria. The first step in that process was the development of the Manning Criteria (Table 23.2).[36] The table lists six symptoms which were found in a clinic to be more common in patients with a diagnosis of the irritable bowel syndrome, than in those with organic abdominal disease. These have been extensively used in divining the epidemiology of this disorder and as entry criteria for clinical trials.[12,37–39] Subsequently, Kruis published a similar study that confirmed some of the Manning criteria and listed features such as bleeding and weight loss that mitigate against a diagnosis of IBS (Table 23.3).[40]

The organizers of the 1988 International Congress of Gastroenterology in Rome commissioned a working team to develop guidelines for the management of IBS. A large component of this effort was the development of a consensus as to what constituted a diagnosis of IBS.[41] This was followed by a second working team that developed a classification system and criteria for all the functional gastrointestinal disorders (Table 23.4).[42] As a result of this activity the Rome criteria for the irritable bowel syndrome were published (Table 23.5).[43] These criteria identify pain as a cardinal feature of the IBS and emphasize the relationship of the pain to the disordered bowel habit. These criteria are now widely known and employed, and have become the accepted standard for entry of IBS patients into clinical trials of new IBS drugs.

In order to ensure that the criteria were in keeping with current information, a Rome II process was initiated. The results of that exercise were published in 1999,[44,45] and the new Rome II criteria are seen in Table 23.6. These criteria will need updating as validation studies and new information appear. Meanwhile, a questionnaire designed for Rome I can also be used for the Rome II criteria. The major differences between Rome I and Rome II are (i) that the requirement for the presence

Table 23.2 The Manning criteria: Symptoms more likely to be found in irritable bowel syndrome (IBS) than organic abdominal disease[a]

	Organic	IBS	Significance
Pain eased after bowel movement	9/30	25/31	$p < 0.01$
Looser stools at onset of pain	8/30	25/31	$p < 0.001$
More frequent bowel movements at onset of pain	9/30	23/31	$p < 0.01$
Abdominal distention	7/33	17/32	$p < 0.01$
Mucus per rectum	7/33	15/32	$0.05 < p < 0.1$
Feeling of incomplete emptying	11/33	19/32	$0.05 < p < 0.1$

[a]Manning *et al.*[36]

Table 23.2 Symptoms more likely to be found in irritable bowel syndrome (IBS) than organic abdominal disease[a]

	Organic	IBS	Significance
n (sample size)	299	108	
A. Abdominal pain	55%	96%	$p < 0.61$
B. Flatulence	50%	85%	$p < 0.4$
C. Iregularity	42%	85%	$p < 0.025$
A+B+C	0%	70%	$p < 0.0005$
Symptoms more than 2 years	39%	70%	$p < 0.0005$
Diarrhea and constipation	30%	65%	$p < 0.0005$
Pellety stools or mucus	38%	76%	$p < 0.0001$

[a]Kruis *et al.*[40]

Table 23.4 Functional gastrointestinal disorders[a]

(A) Functional esophageal disorders
A.1 Globus
A.2 Rumination syndrome
A.3 Functional chest pain of presumed esophageal origin
A.4 Functional heartburn
A.5 Unspecified functional esophageal disorder

(B) Functional gastroduodenal disorders
B.1 Functional (non-ulcer) dyspepsia
B.2 Aerophagia

(C) Functional bowel disorders
C.1 *Irritable bowel syndrome*
C.2 Functional abdominal bloating
C.3 Functional constipation
C.4 Functional diarrhea
C.5 Unspecified functional bowel disorder

(D) Functional abdominal pain
D.1 Functional abdominal pain syndrome
D.2 Unspecified functional abdominal pain

(E) Functional biliary pain

(F) Functional ano-rectal disorders
F.1 Functional incontinence
F.2 Functional ano-rectal pain
F.2A Levator syndrome
F.2B Proctalgia fugax
F.3 Pelvic floor dyssenergia
F.4 Unspecified functional ano-rectal disorder

[a]Thompson *et al.* (1999)[44,45]

Table 23.5 Rome I diagnostic criteria for the irritable bowel[a]

At least 3 months continuous or recurrent symptoms of:
1. *Abdominal pain or discomfort* which is:
   - relieved with defecation
   - and/or associated with a change in the frequency of stool
   - and/or associated with a change in the consistency of stool.

and

2. Two or more of the following, at least a quarter of occasions or days:
   - altered stool *frequency*
   - altered stool *form* (lumpy/hard or loose/watery stool)
   - altered stool *passage* (straining, urgency, or feeling of incomplete evacuation
   - passage of *mucus*
   - *bloating*, or feeling of abdominal distention.

[a]Thompson *et al.*[87]

of two of the associated symptoms (part 2) has been dropped and (ii) that in part 1, two of 'abdominal pain with defecation', 'abdominal pain associated with a change in consistency of stool', or 'abdominal pain associated with a change in the frequency of stool' are the required features, without which the diagnosis should not be made. This change was based on a factor analysis of a large group of patients and on other data;[46,47] (iii) In Rome I, it was required that the symptoms be present for at least 3 months. This is changed to: '12 weeks within the last 12 months'. Validation studies of the Rome II criteria are already underway.

Table 23.6 Rome II diagnostic criteria for the irritable bowel[a]

Twelve weeks within the last 12 months of:
Abdominal pain or discomfort which is:
- relieved with defecation
- and/or associated with a change in the frequency of stool
- and/or associated with a change in the consistency of stool.

[a]Thompson *et al.*[44,45]

The subdivision of IBS into diarrhea-dominant and constipation-dominant is a contentious issue. This terminology has largely come from industry personel testing pharmacological agents that, while aimed at the irritable bowel at large, do cause constipation or diarrhea. While designers of clinical trials for these drugs naturally wish to avoid patients that might be worsened by the drug to be tested, it is very uncertain that such a sub-division can be validated. Most IBS patients swing between constipation, diarrhea, and normal. In some instances patients have been known to switch from one to the other during a clinical trial run-in or baseline period.

THEORIES OF PATHOGENESIS

The etiology of IBS is unknown. Many individuals claim to have discovered the cause, but none of these have achieved universal approbation. It is very likely that none of the current popular explanations are the truth. Indeed these symptoms are so common that they might be considered to be part of the human condition. Nevertheless, these putative causes are worth exploring since they help provide an overall understanding of IBS. Moreover, each may be important in some individuals.

MOTILITY DISTURBANCE

One could make a *prima facie* case that IBS is a motility disorder. How else to explain the chaotic bowel habits of which these patients complain? Nevertheless, for a hundred years investigators using contrast techniques,[48] intracolonic pressure sensors,[49] colonic muscle electrical potential measurement[50] and so on have failed to find a distinctive motility pattern that is common to patients with IBS. Moreover, the abdominal pain and bloating which are such common features of IBS have not been

Box 23.1 Putative causes of IBS

- Motility disturbance
- Visceral hypersensitivity
- Psychopathology
- Diet
- Infection

temporally associated with changes in colon motility. It has been shown that balloon distention throughout the gut can usually find 'trigger points' that can reproduce the patients' abdominal pain both in quality and in location.[51,52] These facts do not distinguish between normal appreciation of abnormal motility or abnormal appreciation of normal motility.

VISCERAL HYPERSENSITIVITY

Thirty years ago it was shown that patients with IBS experienced pain with balloon distention at lower pressures and volumes than in those who did not.[53] In more recent years this observation has been put on a scientific footing,[54] but the phenomenon is insufficiently sensitive or specific to act as a diagnostic test for the syndrome. Nevertheless, because of this apparent altered sensitivity the notion of visceral hypersensitivity has arisen. In addition to balloon distention, the irritable gut appears to show a hyperactive response to eating, defecation, stress and other environmental phenomena. The hypersensitivity theory places the abnormality in the enteric nervous system and connections to the central nervous system. Since serotonin plays a major role in these central afferent pathways, a variety of agonists and antagonists to two serotonin (HT_3 and HT_4) receptors have been developed as possible IBS treatments.

There is evidence provided by positron emission tomography and other technology that the brain plays an important role in the perception of and modification of pain sensation.[55] It is of interest that, while IBS patients' gut may appear to be hypersensitive, their perception of somatic sensation is apparently normal.[56] IBS patients have a greater propensity to regard visceral sensations negatively,[57] and perception of gut sensations is greater with attention or anticipation, than when the subject is distracted.[58]

PSYCHOPATHOLOGY

Many studies show that depression, anxiety, and panic are more prevalent in IBS patients than in those with other gastrointestinal diseases (see above). However, almost without exception these studies have been done in tertiary care centers on subjects that are not typical of the population of people who have IBS. Indeed studies in the community find no difference in the psychosocial make-up of those individuals suffering from IBS from those who do not.[21,22] It may be that the very psychological problems noted in tertiary care centers are the factors that got them referred there in the first place.

Research is needed to determine the psychological makeup of IBS patients in primary care. In one study, seeking health care (not necessarily specialists) was not due to psychological factors.[59] Meanwhile, we cannot assume that IBS is caused by psychopathology, or that their concurrence in academic centers is more than a coincidence.

DIET

Many patients become convinced that food is the cause of their symptoms. To be sure, eating is a powerful stimulus to the colon and a hypersensitive gut may overreact. This is different from implying that a specific food causes an immediate gut reaction by its nature alone. Through a non-colonergic effect, fat exerts a strong gastrocolonic response.[60] It therefore makes sense to reduce the amount of fat in the diet. However, 'food allergy' must be an extremely rare cause of IBS symptoms.[61] In the first place food allergies generally cause symptoms in systems beyond the GI tracts such as urticaria or wheezing. Secondly, attempts to identify specific foods that cause IBS symptoms have been largely unsuccessful, and in one study a positive result may have been due to the fact that the patients had diarrhea, not IBS.[62] Lactose intolerance was once thought to explain IBS in many patients.[63,64] However it is rare amongst Caucasians, and recent studies suggest that even those with lactose intolerance can tolerate small amounts of milk.[65] Moreover, the symptoms of lactose intolerance are diarrhea and the passage of gas, so lactose intolerance cannot explain the constipation and the abdominal pain of IBS.

INFECTION

The discovery of *Helicobacter pylori* as the explanation for most chronic peptic ulcers has led researchers and gastroenterologists to ponder the possibility of a similar explanation for other gut disorders. Studies report the presence of inflammation in the colon and small bowel mucosa of individuals with IBS.[66,67] Indeed, many patients begin to experience IBS symptoms after an enteric infection.[68] However biopsies of a large series of individuals with and without IBS have shown no difference in the appearance of the colon mucosa.[38] This challenging theory needs much more research before it can be accepted or rejected.

OVERVIEW

The above hypotheses are not mutually exclusive. Several factors may appear to be at work in an individual with IBS. For now, it seems reasonable to consider these factors as irritants, contributing factors or epiphenomena, rather than causes. We will likely be surprised when the real cause(s) are known. The symptoms are so common, that it is tempting to consider them part of living, like menstrual cramps, headaches or myalgia. However, this point of view would be unacceptable to many sufferers.

DIAGNOSIS

IBS has no pathophysiological marker. It follows that we only know about the syndrome because of what patients tell us. Therefore IBS is a symptomatic diagnosis. Those who believe that IBS is a diagnosis of exclusion imply that every organic disease of the intestines must be excluded before a diagnosis of IBS can be made. This approach is not only incorrect but it is also very expensive, leads to much unnecessary testing and undermines the patient's confidence in the diagnosis. Thus IBS must be a positive diagnosis, one that is made on the basis of the patient's reported symptoms.

Although the Rome and Manning criteria were developed for research purposes they can also serve as a guide to clinicians (Tables 23.2 and 23.6). The more of the symptom items that are present the more likely is the individual to have IBS.[36,69]

Of course alarm symptoms such as bleeding, severe weight loss, fever or anemia cannot be explained by IBS. Any condition that affects 15% of the population is bound to sometimes coexist with organic disease. Nevertheless a strong IBS diagnosis made on the basis of symptoms in the absence of alarm features is a safe one and stands up over time (Table 23.1).[15–18]

Tests needed to support a diagnosis of IBS have been the subject of much debate. Since IBS has no known pathophysiology, no test will positively identify the phenomenon. Many gastroenterologists would recommend at least a sigmoidoscopy. If correctly done, the procedure can be a therapeutic tool. However, sigmoidoscopy seldom assists in the diagnosis, and biopsy of the colon is of no value if IBS symptoms are typical.[38] Only about 10% of GPs in England and family doctors in Canada[70] ever perform a sigmoidoscopy. Therefore, requiring this test for all IBS patients would make IBS a specialist's disease – an outcome that few would applaud.

No tests may be required in a young patient with a typical history of abdominal pain associated with defecation along with such features as bloating, mucus in the stool, chaotic bowel habit and a feeling of incomplete evacuation. If there is a family history of Crohn's disease, one might consider a small bowel enema or an ultrasound examination, but in most instances these are not necessary.

A patient over 45 years of age should have some type of colon examination, especially if there is a family history of colon cancer. In family practice the most practical test would normally be a barium enema. If the risk of cancer were high then a referral to a gastroenterologist for a colonoscopy would be wise. Remember though, the symptoms of IBS are not those of cancer of the colon. Nevertheless, the great prevalences of the two conditions suggests caution.

Special tests might be indicated under certain circumstances. In endemic areas one may wish to check for Giardia, and in non-Caucasians lactose intolerance is common. However these diseases cause diarrhea, not IBS and should be considered as aggravating factors rather than causes of the syndrome.

It is important that the physician feel confident with the diagnosis and to transmit that confidence to the patient. Once a patient has been investigated for IBS symptoms it is often counterproductive to re-investigate them at a later date. This practice can undermine the patients' confidence in the diagnosis and in the doctor. Such security is an important objective of therapy.

TREATMENT

It is a maxim that the more treatments there are for a condition, the less likely that any of them are effective. Such appears to be the case with IBS. This benign, fluctuating, chronic disorder affects vast numbers of people in different ways. For these reasons clinical trials are difficult to design and end-points are difficult to agree upon. Nonetheless, we can make use of what we do know about IBS to help most of our patients and protect them against over-investigation and over-treatment. The following are six principals upon which IBS management can be based.

1. A confident diagnosis

Only when a confident diagnosis is established can the physician confidently reassure the patient that no serious disease exists, and no bad prognosis awaits him or her.[71] Moreover, he or she is now in a position to explain to the patient what is known about IBS. The knowledge that many people suffer from these symptoms can be reassuring. The notion that the gut is hypersensitive is understandable and may help persuade the patient to eliminate irritating factors from their life such as stress, poor eating habits, drugs, caffeine, and alcohol.

Box 23.2 Management plan

- Confident diagnosis
- Consider patient's agenda
- Diet
- Critical use of drugs
- Psychosocial treatments
- Continuing care

A firm diagnosis followed by a reassuring discussion with the patient explaining the symptoms may lead to a better outcome.[72] Patients who receive sufficient attention early on are more likely to feel better, and are less likely to complain about their symptoms, or use the health care system.[18]

2. Consideration of the patient's agenda

Most patients with IBS do not seek medical help.[6–12] Those that do often have an agenda that may not be directly related to IBS itself. In primary care, patients appear to be worried about the possibility of cancer, or other serious disease and require some management of stress.[19] In secondary care, the issues are often uncertainty about the diagnosis and dissatisfaction with the management. Also in secondary care there is much comorbidity: depression, anxiety, panic attacks, personality disorders, and other somatic syndromes such as fibromyalgia. A few see their symptoms as means to such secondary gain as the compliance of a spouse or the acquisition of disability insurance benefits.

Whatever the patient's IBS complaints, these other agenda items must be dealt with or at least recognized. A depressed patient with IBS is unlikely to improve until the depression has been adequately treated.

3. Diet

There is much controversy about the role of diet in IBS. Because eating stimulates the gastrocolonic response, an episode of diarrhea is often falsely attributed to a specific food. A salad for instance is unlikely to stimulate immediate diarrhea. Hypervigilant patients may remove many important nutrients from the diet and this needs correction and monitoring. Our attitudes towards foods are modified by our experiencees. Despite many beliefs and attitudes, few, if any, foods have been established as a cause of IBS. While some foods may cause diarrhea, they are unlikely to account for the full syndrome. Nonetheless it is worth looking for dietary substances that might irritate the hypersensitive bowel such as caffeine, sorbitol or alcohol. Fat stimulates the gastrocolonic response,[73] so a low lipid intake can be recommended.

Several studies have examined the effect of bran and psyllium on the IBS.[74] None of them have shown convincing success. Nonetheless it does appear that dietary fiber can improve the constipation part of IBS. If the patient reports periods of hard or pebbly stools one might consider giving bran or psyllium supplements (a sufficiently high fiber diet is too difficult to achieve). A patient might be started on a tablespoon of bran or psyllium with breakfast increasing the doses at weekly intervals until they are is taking three or four tablespoons a day. It should be emphasized that this is aimed at eliminating the constipated stools, but that its overall effect on the syndrome may not be great. One hospital center reports that IBS symptoms often worsen after bran,[75] but experience at such a center must differ from that in primary care.[76]

Perhaps most importantly, sensible eating habits should be encouraged. Individuals who rush through their meals, eat one large meal a day exclusively, or persistently eat junk food can expect some improvement if they are persuaded to eat regular meals in an atmosphere insulated from their stressful surroundings. Also, some diets that are proposed in the lay press or the internet are dangerous, and may cause weight loss or nutritional defects. These have no rational basis for benefit, and should be discouraged.

4. Critical use of drugs

No drug has been proven effective for the whole syndrome.[77,78] Even the drugs under clinical trial have constipating or diarrheogenic effects that may limit their indications to subtypes of IBS. While one may wish to use a drug for its placebo effect it is at best a diversion (Table 23.7). Moreover, one needs to consider the implications of putting a young person on a drug of unproven benefit and unknown long-term effects for long periods. Table 23.8 shows the drugs approved by licensing authorities in several different Western countries. The lack of agreement between licensing authorities on the effectiveness of drugs for IBS speaks volumes about the confidence with which one can recommend the use of these 'approved' drugs.

Nevertheless, if a patient has a predominant, troublesome symptom within the IBS syndrome certain drugs may be of value (Table 23.9). The use of bulking agents in constipation is discussed above. Some patients are so concerned about having an episode of diarrhea perhaps with soiling, that they fear to go to work or to social engagements. The strategic use of an anti-diarrheal agent such as Loperamide (Imodium™) might be helpful in this instance. This drug may help a patient function, but care should be taken not to precipitate an episode of constipation. Analgesics are usually unhelpful for the

Table 23.7 The placebo response: Percent of subjects responding to placebo in clinical trials of IBS

Author	Trial substance	% Placebo response
Lichstein, 1967	Belladonna	30
Wayne, 1969	Librax	38
Soltoft, 1975	Bran	69
Fielding, 1982	Domperidone	57
Lucey, 1987	Bran	71

Table 23.8 Drugs officially approved for IBS in five countries

Country Generic name of drug	Trade name	Action
Australia		
Dicyclomine	Merbentyl	Anticholinergic
Alverine	Alvercol	Papaverine-like
Hyoscine	Donnatab	Anticholinergic
Atropine		
Scopolamine		
Mebeverine	Colofac	Antispasmodic
Peppermint oil	Mintec	Carminative
Canada		
Bentylol	Dicyclomine	Anticholinergic
Propantheline	Probanthine	Anticholinergic
Hyocyamine	Levsin	Anticholinergic
Hyocyamine, atropine, scopolamine + phenobarbital	Donnatal	Anticholinergic
Pinovarium	Dicetel	Calcium channel blocker
Trimebutane	Modulon	Kappa opiate antagonist
Peppermint oil	Colpermin	Carminative
France		
Prifinium	Riabal	Anticholinergic
Alverine	Spasmaverine	Papaverine-like
Mebeverine	Colopriv	Antispasmodic
Pinaverium	Dicetel	Calcium channel blocker
Trimebutane	Debridat	Kappa opiate antagonist
United Kingdom		
Propantheline	Pro-banthine	Anticholinergic
Alverine	Spasmonal	Antispasmodic from papaverine
Mebeverine	Colofac	Antispasmodic
Peppermint oil	Colpermin	Carminative
USA		
Dicyclomine	Bentyl	Anticholinergic
Hyoscyamine	Levsin	Anticholinergic
Hyoscyamine, atropine, scopolamine + phenobarbitol	Donnatol	Anticholinergic

Note: no drug is supported by a randomized controlled trial that satisfies the criteria of Klein. References: Australia Prescription Practices Guide 1995; CPS 1997 (Canada); Vidal 1995 (France); MIMS 1996 (UK); Physicians' Desk Reference 1997 (USA).

abdominal pain. However if the pain is chronic and troublesome such that it is interfering with an individual's life, low-dose antidepressant therapy may be useful.[79,80]

5. Psychosocial treatments

Clinical trials of psychological treatments are even more difficult to perform than drug trials. Not surprisingly, such trials are open to much criticism[81] and none have satisfactorily proven efficacy. This has not prevented many psychological treatments from being introduced. These are often available regionally such as hypnotherapy in England,[82] and biofeedback[83] and cognitive behavioral therapy[84] in certain cities in North America. If such a treatment is available in the community many patients may benefit from the experience, but we are not yet in a position to prove efficacy. The physician should retain overall control of the patient's care, and complete cure should not be promised. Rather, the emphasis should be on improved occupational and social functioning. Those patients whose pain is chronic, severe and disabling may benefit from referral to a pain clinic.

6. Continuing care

The troubled, chronically affected IBS patient needs continuing care. This is best offered by the family physician who can ensure that the patient's diet is a safe one and that if some form of alternative medicine is used by the patient[85,86] that it is not harmful. The advantage of

Table 23.9 Drugs for a dominant symptom in irritable bowel syndrome

Symptom	Drug	Dose
Diarrhea	Loperamide	1–2 tablets when necessary, maximum 6 tablets daily
	Cholestyramine	1 scoop or packet with meals
Constipation	Psyllium	1 tbsp bid with meals, then adjust
	Methylcellulose	1 tbsp bid with meals, then adjust
	Calcium polycarbophil	1 g qd to qid
	Lactulose	1–2 tbsp bid (may cause bloating)
	70% Sorbitol	1 tbsp bid (may cause bloating)
Abdominal pain	Anticholinergic/ antispasmodic	Take AC, if pain is PC
	Tricyclic antidepressants	For intractable pain

AC: before meals; PC: after meals.

continuing care by a single family doctor is a coherent medical record and protection against repeated investigations and harmful treatments.

SUMMARY

IBS is a dysfunction of the intestine that meets the outside world at the pelvic floor. It affects a great many adults worldwide. Only a minority of IBS subjects consult physicians, and even fewer subjects are referred to specialists. While we know much about the psychosocial profiles of subjects seen at academic centers, we know little about those seen in primary care, and those who consult gynecologists and urologists. Despite many theories we do not know the cause(s) of IBS, but many environmental irritating factors can be identified. The diagnosis can only be made by careful attention to symptoms. In the absence of alarm symptoms or family history of disease, few investigations are needed, especially in the young. Since there is no cure, or even proven effective palliation, management rests on a confident diagnosis, consideration of the patient's reasons for consulting, sensible employment of diet, drugs and psychotherapy, and continuing care. Currently, IBS diverts a large amount of health care resources from other, sometimes very serious diseases, so an economical approach to the syndrome is of great public importance.

REFERENCES

1. Longstreth GF, Preskill DB, Youkeles L. Irritable bowel syndrome in women having diagnostic laparoscopy or hysterectomy. *Dig Dis Sci* 1990;**35**:1285–90.
2. Burns DG. The risk of abdominal surgery in irritable bowel syndrome. *South Afr Med J* 1986;**70**:91.
3. Fielding JF. Surgery and the irritable bowel syndrome: the singer as well as the song. *J Ir Med* 1988;**76**:33–4.
4. Doshi M, Heaton KW. Irritable bowel syndrome in patients discharged from surgical wards with non-specific abdominal pain. *Br J Surg* 1994;**81**:1216–8.
5. Prior A, Stanley KM, Smith ARB, Read NW. Relationship between hysterectomy and the irritable bowel: a prospective study. *Gut* 1992;**33**:814–7.
6. Thompson WG, Heaton KW. Functional bowel disorders in apparently healthy people. *Gastroenterology* 1980;**79**: 283–8.
7. Drossman DA, Sandler RS, McKee DC, Lovitz AJ. Bowel patterns amongst subjects not seeking health care. *Gastroenterology* 1982;**83**:529–34.
8. Bommelaer G, Rouch M, Dapoigny M, *et al.* Epidemiologie des troubles fonctionnels dans une population apparement saine. *Gastroenterol Clin Biol* 1986;**10**:7–12.
9. Dent OF, Goulston KJ, Zubrzycki J, Chapuis PH. Bowel symptoms in an apparently well population. *Dis Colon Rectum* 1986;**29**:243–7.
10. Bi-zhen W, Qi-Ying P. Functional bowel disorders in apparently healthy chinese people. *Chinese J Epid* 1988;**9**:345–9.
11. Drossman DA, Li Z, Andruzzi E, *et al.* U.S. householder survey of functional gastrointestinal disorders: prevalence, sociodemography and health impact. *Dig Dis Sci* 1993;**38**:1569–80.
12. Heaton KW, O'Donnell LJD, Braddon FEM, Mountford RA, Hughes AO, Cripps PJ. Symptoms of irritable bowel syndrome in a British urban community: consulters and non-consulters. *Gastroenterology* 1992;**102**:1962–7.
13. Talley NJ, Weaver AL, Zinsmeister AR, Melton LJ. Onset and disappearance of gastrointestinal symptoms and functional gastrointestinal disorders. *Am J Epidemiol* 1992;**136**:165–77.
14. Kay L, Jorgensen T. Abdominal symptom associations in a longitudinal study. *Internat J Epidemiol* 1993;**22**:1093–1100.
15. Holmes KM, Salter RH. Irritable bowel syndrome – a safe diagnosis. *Br Med J* 1982;**285**:1533–4.
16. Svendsen JH, Munck LK, Andersen JR. Irritable bowel syndrome: prognosis and diagnostic safety. A 5-year follow up study. *Scand J Gastroenterol* 1985;**20**:415–8.
17. Harvey RF, Mauad EC, Brown AM. Prognosis in the irritable bowel syndrome: a five-year prospective study. *Lancet* 1987;**2**:963–5.
18. Owens DM, Nelson DK, Talley NJ. The irritable bowel syndrome: long term prognosis and the patient–physician interaction. *Ann Intern Med* 1995;**122**:107–12.
19. Thompson WG, Heaton KW, Smyth GT, Smyth C. Irritable bowel syndrome: the view from general practice. *Eur J Gastroenterol Hepatol* 1997;**9**:689–92.
20. Thompson WG, Heaton KW, Smyth GT, Smyth C. Irritable bowel syndrome in general practice. *Gastroenterology* 1997;**112**: A837.
21. Drossman DA, McKee DC, Sandler RS, *et al.* Psychosocial factors in the irritable bowel syndrome. A multivariate study of patients and nonpatients with irritable bowel syndrome. *Gastroenterology* 1988;**95**:701–8.
22. Whitehead WE, Bosmajian L, Zonderman A, *et al.* Psychological distress associated with irritable bowel syndrome: comparison of community and medical clinic factors. *Gastroenterology* 1988;**95**:709–14.
23. Young SJ, Alpers DH, Norland CC, Woodruff RA. Psychiatric illness and the irritable bowel syndrome. Practical implications for the primary physician. *Gastroenterology* 1976;**70**:162–6.
24. Drossman DA. Depression and the gastrointestinal disorders. *Clini Adv Treat Depression* 1987;**1**:8–11.
25. Toner BB, Garfinkel PE, Jeejeebhoy KN, Scher H, Shulhan D, Gasbarro ID. Self-schema in irritable bowel syndrome and depression. *Psychosom Med* 1990;**52**:149–55.
26. Walker EA, Roy-Byrne PP, Katon WJ. Irritable bowel syndrome and psychiatric illness. *Am J Psych* 1990;**147**:567–72.
27. Walker EA, Katon WJ, Jemelka RP, Roy-Byrne PP. Comorbidity of gastrointestinal complaints, depression, and anxiety in the epidemiological catchment area (ECA) study. *Am J Med* 1993;**92**: (Suppl.)1A:26–30.
28. Tollefson GD, Tollefson SL, Pederson M, Luxenberg M, Dunsmore G. Comorbid irritable bowel syndrome in patients with generalized anxiety and major depression. *Ann Clin Psychiat* 1991;**3**:215–22.
29. Lydiard RB, Laraia MT, Howell EF, Ballenger JC. Can panic disorder present as irritable bowel syndrome. *J Clin Psychiat* 1986;**47**:470–3.

30. Marshall JR. Are some irritable bowel syndromes actually panic disorders? *Postgrad Med* 1988;**83(6)**:206–9.
31. Triadafilopoulos G, Simms RW, Goldenberg DL. Bowel dysfunction in fibromyalgia syndrome. *Dig Dis Sci* 1991;**36**:59–64.
32. Veale D, Kavanagh G, Fielding JF, Fitzgerald O. Primary Fibromyalgia and the irritable bowel syndrome: different expressions of a common pathogenic process. *Br J Rheum* 1991;**30**:220–2.
33. Gamberone JE, Gorard DA, Dewsnap PA, Libby GW, Farthing MJ. Prevalence of irritable bowel syndrome in chronic fatigue. *J R Coll Phy Lond* 1997;**30**:512–3.
34. Talley NJ, Gabriel SE, Harmsen WS, Zinsmeister AR, Evans RW. Medical costs in community subjects with irritable bowel syndrome. *Gastroenterology* 1995;**109**:1736–41.
35. Thompson WG, Patel DG, Tao H, Nair RC. Does uncomplicated diverticular disease produce symptoms? *Dig Dis Sci* 1982;**27**:605–8.
36. Manning AP, Thompson WG, Heaton KW, Morris AF. Towards positive diagnosis of the irritable bowel. *BMJ* 1978;**2**:653–4.
37. Olibuyide IO, Olawuyi F, Fassanmade AA. A study of irritable bowel syndrome diagnosed by Manning criteria in an African population. *Dig Dis Sci* 1995;**40**:983–5.
38. McIntosh D, Thompson WG, Patel D, Barr JR, Guindi M. Is rectal biopsy necessary in irritable bowel syndrome? *Am J Gastroenterol* 1992;**87**:1407–9.
39. Crowell MD, Dubin NH, Robinson JC, *et al.* Functional bowel disorders in women with dysmenorrhoea. *Am J Gastroenterol* 1994;**89**:1973–7.
40. Kruis W, Thieme CH, Weinzierl M, Schussler P, Hall J, Paulus W. A diagnostic score for the irritable bowel syndrome. Its value in the exclusion of organic disease. *Gastroenterology* 1984;**87**:1–7.
41. Thompson WG, Dotevall G, Drossman DA, Heaton KW, Kruis W. Irritable bowel syndrome: guidelines for the diagnosis. *Gastroent Int* 1989;**2**:92–5.
42. Drossman DA, Funch-Jensen P, Janssens J, Talley NJ, Thompson WG, Whitehead WE. Identification of subgroups of functional bowel disorders. *Gastroent Int* 1990;**3**:159–72.
43. Thompson WG, Creed FH, Drossman DA, Heaton KW, Mazzacca G. Functional bowel disorders and functional abdominal pain. *Gastroent International* 1992;**5**:75–91.
44. Thompson WG, Longstreth GF, Drossman DA, Heaton KW, Irvine EJ, Muller-Lissner SA. Functional bowel disorders and functional abdominal pain. *Gut* 1999;**45(Suppl)**:II43–7.
45. Thompson WG, Longstreth GF, Drossman DA, *et al.* 4. Functional bowel disorders and D. Functional abdominal pain In: Drossman DA, Corazziari E, Talley NJ, Thompson WG, Whitehead WE (ed). *The functional gastrointestinal disorders,* 2nd edn. Washington: Degnon 1999.
46. Taub E, Cuevas JL, Cook EW, Crowell MD, Whitehead WE. Irritable bowel syndrome defined by factor analysis. *Dig Dis Sci* 1995;**40**:2647–55.
47. Whitehead WE, Crowell MD, Bosmajian L, *et al.* Existence of irritable bowel syndrome supported by factor analysis of symptoms in two community samples. *Gastroenterology* 1990;**98**:336–40.
48. Cannon WB. The movements of the intestine studied by means of roentgen rays. *Am J Physiol* 1902;**6**:251.
49. Connell AM. The motility of the pelvic colon. Part II Paradoxical motility in diarrhoea and constipation. *Gut* 1962;**3**:342–8.
50. Snape WJ, Carlson GM, Cohen S. Colonic myoelectric activity in the irritable bowel syndrome. *Gastroenterology* 1976;**70**:326–30.
51. Swarbrick ET, Hegarty JE, Bat L, Williams CB, Dawson AM. Site of pain from the irritable bowel syndrome. *Lancet* 1980;**2**:443–6.
52. Moriarty KJ, Dawson AM. Functional abdominal pain: further evidence that whole gut is affected. *BMJ* 1982;**284**:1670–2.
53. Ritchie JA. Pain from distension of the pelvic colon by inflating a balloon in the irritable bowel syndrome. *Gut* 1973;**14**:125–32.
54. Whitehead WE, Holtkotter B, Enck P, *et al.* Tolerance for rectosigmoid distention in irritable bowel syndrome. *Gastroenterology* 1990;**98**:1187–92.
55. Aziz Q, Thompson DG. Brain-gut axis in health and disease. *Gastroenterology* 1998;**114**:559–78.
56. Cook IJ, van Eeden A, Collins SM. Patients with irritable bowel syndrome have greater pain tolerance than normal subjects. *Gastroenterology* 1987;**93**:727–33.
57. Tzavella K, Riepl R, Klauser AG, Voderholzer WA, Shindlbeck NE, Muller-Lissner SA. Decreased substance P levels in rectal biopsies from patients with slow transit constipation. *Eur J Gastroenterol Hepatol* 1996;**8**(1207):1211.
58. Accarino AM, Azpiroz F, Malagalada JR. Attention and distraction. *Gastroenterology* 1999;**113**:415–22.
59. Talley NJ, Boyce PM, Jones M. Predictors of health care seeking for irritable bowel syndrome: a population study. *Gut* 1999;**41**:394–8.
60. Sullivan MA, Cohen S, Snape WJ. Colonic myoelectrical activity in irritable bowel syndrome. Effect of eating and anticholinergics. *New Engl J Med* 1978;**298**:878–83.
61. Zwetchkenbaum JF, Burakoff R. Food allergy and the irritable bowel syndrome. *Am J Gastroentrol* 1988;**83**:901–4.
62. Jones A, Shorthouse M, McLaughlan P, *et al.* Food intolerance: a major factor in the pathogenesis of the irritable bowel syndrome. *Lancet* 1982;**2**:1115–7.
63. Weser E, Rubin W, Ross L, Sleisenger MH. Lactase deficiency in patients with irritable bowel syndrome. *N Engl J Med* 1965;**273**:1070–5.
64. Newcomer AD, McGill DB. Irritable bowel syndrome: role of lactase deficiency. *Mayo Clin Proc* 1983;**59**:339–41.
65. Suarez FL, Savaiano DA, Levitt MD. A comparison of symptoms after the consumption of milk or lactose-hydrolyzed milk by people with self-reported severe lactose intolerance. *New Engl J Med* 1995;**333**:1–4.
66. Collins SM. The immunoregulation of enteric neuromuscular function: implications for motility and inflammatory disorders. *Gastroenterology* 1996;**111**:1683–99.
67. Weston AP, Biddle WL, Bhatia PS, Miner PB. Terminal ileal mucosal mast cells in irritable bowel syndrome. *Dig Dis Sci* 1993;**38**:1590–5.
68. Gwee KA, Graham JC, McKendrick NW, *et al.* Psychometric scores and persistence of irritable bowel after infectious diarrhoea. *Lancet* 1996;**347**:150–3.
69. Thompson WG. Gastrointestinal symptoms in the irritable bowel compared with peptic ulcer and inflammatory bowel disease. *Gut* 1984;**25**:1089–92.

70. Glaser SR. Utilization of sigmoidoscopy by family physicians in Canada. *Can Med Assoc J* 1994;**150**:367–71.
71. Thompson WG. *Gut reactions.* New York: Plenum, 1989.
72. Swedlund J, Sjoden L, Ottosson JO, Doteval G. Controlled study of psychotherapy in irritable bowel syndrome. *Lancet* 1983;**2**:589–91.
73. Wright SH, Snape WJ, Battle W, *et al.* Effect of dietary components on gastrocolonic response. *Am J Physiol* 1980;**238**:228–32.
74. Heaton KW, *et al.* Dietary fibre. *Eur J Gastroenterol Hepatol* 1993;**5**:569–91.
75. Francis CY, Whorwell PJ. Bran and irritable bowel syndromes: time for reappraisal. *Lancet* 1994;**344**:39–40.
76. Thompson WG. Doubts about bran. *Lancet* 1994;**344**:3.
77. Klein KB. Controlled treatment trials in the irritable bowel syndrome: a critique. *Gastroenterology* 1988; **95**:232–41.
78. Talley NJ, Nyren O, Drossman DA, *et al.* The irritable bowel syndrome: toward optimal design of controlled treatment trials. *Gastroenterol International* 1994;**6**:189–211.
79. Clouse RE, *et al.* Antidepressant therapy in 138 patients with irritable bowel syndrome: a five-year clinical experience. *Aliment Pharmacol Therap* 1994;8409–16.
80. Myren J, Lovland B, Larssen SE, Larsen S. Psychopharmacologic drugs in the treatment of the irritable bowel syndrome a double blind study of effect of trimipramine. *Ann Gastroenterol Hepatol* 1984;**20**:117–23.
81. Talley NJ, Owen BK, Boyce P, Paterson K. Psychological treatments for irritable bowel syndrome: a critique of controlled clinical trials. *Am J Gastroenterol* 1996;**91**:277–86.
82. Whorwell PJ. Hypnotherapy in the irritable bowel syndrome. *Stress Med* 1987;**3**:5–7.
83. Whitehead WE. Biofeedback treatment of gastrointestinal disorders. *Biofeedback Self Regul* 1992;**17**:59–76.
84. van Dulman AM, Fennis JF, Bleijenberg G. Cognitive-behavioural group therapy for irritable bowel syndrome: effects and long-term follow-up. *Psychosomat Med* 1996;**58**:508–514.
85. Smart HL, Mayberry JF, Atkinson M. Alternative medicine consultations and remedies in patients with the irritable bowel syndrome. *Gut* 1986;**27**:826–8.
86. Verhoef MJ, Sutherland LR, Brkich L. Use of alternative medicine by patients attending a gastroenterology clinic. *Can Med Assoc J* 1990;**142**:121–5.
87. Drossman DA; Richter J; Talley NJ, *et al. Functional gastrointestinal disorders.* Boston: Little, Brown 1994.

Chapter 24

Fecal incontinence – pathophysiology and management

A James Eccersley, Norman S Williams

DEFINITION AND EPIDEMIOLOGY

In Coloproctology and the Pelvic Floor, the authors defined major fecal incontinence as the 'frequent and inadvertent voiding per anum of formed stool'.[1] They discussed separately minor fecal soiling, incontinence of flatus and incontinence associated with diarrhea. Conversely, other authors have defined anal incontinence as the 'loss of anal sphincter control ... resulting in unwanted release of gas, liquid or solid stool'.[2] Whilst all modalities of incontinence can affect lifestyle, this chapter reflects the fact that physicians and surgeons dealing with incontinence tend to concentrate on the management of gross incontinence of solid and liquid stool.

As a result of this imprecise definition and the reluctance of patients and physicians to report the problem,[3] the prevalence of fecal incontinence is poorly defined. In a telephone survey in Wisconsin, 2.2% of the population reported anal incontinence, half of whom were incontinent to solid or liquid stool.[4] This survey identified that women were 50% more likely to report incontinence, and that poor general health rather than age was strongly associated with incontinence. Studies using anonymous questionnaires have identified higher rates of incontinence with 4.8% of a population without known bowel disease reporting a disturbance in control of solid stool, and 6.7% encountering difficulty with liquid stool.[5] In many studies females appear to be more commonly affected and increased age decreased the length of time that defecation could safely be deferred. However a recent Australian postal study revealed that men were apparently more affected by anal incontinence (including incontinence of flatus) than women.[6] Unsurprisingly chronic digestive disorders are associated with a higher incidence of fecal incontinence, with a questionnaire study in Germany[7] reporting that 1.4% of healthy controls and 12% of those with inflammatory bowel disease encountered involuntary loss of stool.

The symptoms of fecal incontinence are also poorly defined; most authors have assessed the severity of the disorder by the frequency of incontinence to each modality of stool (i.e. solid, liquid and flatus). A linear unweighted scoring system such as that developed at the Cleveland Clinic, Florida[8] (Table 24.1) is easy to use, but may over-report scores in those with frequent yet mild symptoms (i.e. incontinence to flatus) and underscore those with more distressing yet rarer episodes of incontinence to solid stool. Non-linear scoring systems that

Table 24.1 Cleveland Clinic Incontinence Scoring System[2]

Type of incontinence	Never	Rarely	Sometimes	Usually	Always
Solid	0	1	2	3	4
Liquid	0	1	2	3	4
Gas (flatus)	0	1	2	3	4
Wears pad	0	1	2	3	4
Lifestyle alteration	0	1	2	3	4

Score of 0: perfect continence; score of 20: complete incontinence. Never: 0; Rarely: <1/month; Sometimes: <1/week, but >1/month; Usually: <1/day, but >1/week; Always: daily or worse. The incontinence score is determined by adding points from the above table, which takes into account the type and frequency of incontinence and the extent to which it alters the patient's life.

weight incontinence of solids higher than other symptoms[9] have been developed or extended to include domains on lifestyle disturbance and urgency.[10] A recent study of existing systems showed a high degree of agreement between observers and scoring systems,[11] but the varied systems used by surgeons worldwide confounds the comparison of treatment outcomes between centers.[12]

The social impact of fecal incontinence has been best studied in those with congenital ano-rectal anomalies, in whom incontinence has been shown to be associated with significant social educational and psychological morbidity.[13,14] In adults generic quality of life indices are also significantly impaired in those with incontinence,[15] but there is no validated disease specific quality of life index. The financial impact of fecal incontinence is unknown, although a recent study[9] estimated the costs of appliances at between $200 and $500 per annum. The costs of surgical treatment are also substantial, with the same study reporting an average (insurance based) cost of sphincter repair at $17 000.

PATHOPHYSIOLOGY

Continence appears to involve the physiological interaction of rectal motility and sensation with the activity of smooth and striated muscle. Since this interaction is complex and incompletely understood, the pathophysiology underlying an individual's incontinence is often difficult to elucidate. Some authors attempt to differentiate passive incontinence from urge incontinence, arguing that each reflects a different pathophysiological process. Indeed there is some evidence that passive incontinence may be related to internal sphincter defects whilst urge incontinence is associated with external sphincter defects.[16] However many patients present with mixed symptoms of both passive leakage and urgency, and in many cases incontinence can be caused by disturbed rectal storage or sensation. A binary classification of symptoms into urge or passive incontinence tends to be an oversimplification. In our clinical practice we find it better to integrate findings from the clinical history, examination and investigations[17] to deduce the etiology of incontinence and then formulate a management plan. Hence we discuss the pathophysiology of incontinence by reference to the anatomical structure or physiological function which appears to be impaired, accepting that in many cases the etiology is multifactorial.

EXTERNAL SPHINCTER INJURY

The commonest cause of fecal incontinence is sphincter injuries related to birth trauma. In the western world, the availability of specialist midwifery services appears to have reduced the incidence of obstetric sphincter injury. Although overt external sphincter injuries present after fewer than 1% of all deliveries, endosonographic studies suggest that occult sphincter injuries occur in 6–30% of women after their first childbirth.[18] Instrumental delivery, particularly with forceps, appears to increase the risk of both sphincter injury and pelvic floor denervation, although the prolonged second stage of labor which necessitated obstetric intervention is probably the underlying cause of the obstetric injury.[19] External sphincter injuries occur by a direct mechanical tear (or a surgical episiotomy) traversing the fibers of the transverseii perineii and entering the external sphincter.

In some obstetric injuries the damage to the external anal sphincter is limited to the outermost fibers. This situation leads to partial interruption of the external anal sphincter with a segment of non-contractile scar tissue bridging the gap in the perimeter of the sphincter ring. Anal resting pressure, 85% of which is attributed to the internal sphincter, is likely to be normal. The coordinated tightening of the external sphincter as part of the anal sampling reflex response to rectal distention is preserved, but the anal pressure during sampling is likely to be lowered and less well maintained. Such a defect may be asymptomatic or may lead to seepage of a little soft or liquid stool during sampling or episodes of raised intra-abdominal pressure alone. The patient may report soiling, but often learns that defecation as soon as the rectum begins to fill can reduce the frequency of soiling. This need for prompt defecation may be misinterpreted as rectal urgency. In these incomplete sphincteric injuries, biofeedback may be successful because the sensory retraining increases discrimination of rectal filling, whilst squeeze exercises improve the strength and stamina of the remaining sphincter ring.

In a more severe tear, fibers of a radial segment of the external anal sphincter may be torn through to the intersphincteric plane, and the muscle ends may become separated by scar tissue. In these circumstances, the squeeze pressure is usually significantly reduced. In addition the anal canal may develop a keyhole or gutter deformity which may be seen or felt during clinical examination, through which soft stool can seep despite sphincter contraction. A complete external sphincter defect is likely to lead to more frequent incontinence of liquid and even solid stool. In addition the closing reflex may be weakened resulting in post-defecatory soiling.

Endoanal ultrasonography can be used to differentiate between complete and incomplete external sphincter disruption. This differentiation is important because incomplete defects may respond to non-operative therapies such as biofeedback,[20] whilst complete defects which cause more severe incontinence may require more interventional treatment.[21] The large variability of results from the reported series of biofeedback may be at least partially explained by the fact that most authors have failed to discriminate between the degree to which the external anal sphincter is disrupted.

INTERNAL SPHINCTER INJURY

The advent of endoanal ultrasonographic imaging has increased our knowledge of internal sphincter injury as a cause of incontinence. Several studies have shown that internal sphincter injuries occur in up to 35% of women during childbirth. Such injuries may occur in the absence of any structural damage to the external anal sphincter where it is thought that the smooth muscle is injured by a shearing force placed on the ano-rectum during the second stage of labor. In an isolated internal sphincter injury, the resting anal pressure may be low but if the external sphincter is intact the squeeze function should be preserved. In cases of internal sphincter disruption, physiotherapy to decrease the fatigability of the intact external sphincter may be beneficial.

The most caudal fibers of the internal sphincter may be divided as a therapeutic maneuver for chronic anal fissure. Lateral rather than posterior sphincterotomy is to be preferred because the divided internal sphincter is better supported by the external sphincter laterally than in the midline, so gutter formation and soiling is less likely. Digital anal stretch procedures should be avoided since they have been shown to cause widespread sphincter defects[22] and may result in a higher incidence of incontinence. Iatrogenic incontinence due to a gutter deformity or sphincter disruption may also occur after hemorrhoidectomy and surgery for fistula-in ano; advancement flap anoplasty may be a therapeutic option in such cases.

NEUROPATHIC INCONTINENCE

The reduced pudendal nerve conduction velocity frequently induced by childbirth adversely affects the coordinated control of the posterior pelvic floor. This traction neuropraxia leads to the histological and physiological changes of denervation/reinnervation with the pelvic floor muscles which are discussed elsewhere within this book. Whilst pudendal nerve function and continence returns to near normal within 6 months in the majority of women, a degree of (sub-clinical) denervation may well persist in some women.[23] After further childbirth or the menopause (when changes in the hormonal milieu may further weaken the pelvic floor) the patient may develop clinical symptoms of incontinence.

Changes in pudendal nerve conduction can also be induced by repetitive straining and any sensory denervation of the ano-rectum induced by an obstructed delivery may lead to disturbed evacuation. The consequent need to strain at stool may further exacerbate the traction neuropathy, and recent studies have identified that around one third of incontinent women have a coexisting rectal evacuation disorder.

Pudendal neuropathy alone does not necessarily result in incontinence; there are a number of reports of advanced pudendal neuropathy identified in patients with normal continence.[24]

AUTONOMIC NEUROPATHY

Even an uncomplicated vaginal delivery may lead to a reduction in both anal resting and squeeze pressure,[25] and there is mounting evidence that traction on the pelvic floor during labor may injure the autonomic nerves as well as the pudendal nerve. The consequent autonomic neuropathy may lead to internal sphincter denervation. As a result the internal sphincter appears normal during endosonography, but is hypotonic and exhibits poor reflex control. The evidence that autonomic neuropathy rather than anatomical disruption alone causes postnatal sphincter dysfunction arises from a number of studies. These suggest that affected women have a global (circumferential) reduction in sphincter tone rather than a segmental sphincter weakness[26] following childbirth. Therapeutic internal sphincterotomy also causes a global reduction in resting sphincter tone as shown by vector volume studies[27] perhaps by interference with the autonomic regulation of sphincter tone.

The reduction in anal defense mechanisms after anterior resection has also been attributed to colonic and pelvic floor denervation, with post-denervation hypersensitivity of the smooth muscle in the rectal remnant and internal anal sphincter.[28] Diseases such as diabetes mellitus which are known to cause both somatic and autonomic neuropathy may also lead to denervation and dysfunction of both the internal and external sphincters.[29]

SENSORY IMPAIRMENT AND RECTAL EVACUATORY DISORDERS

The role of disturbed sensation in the etiology and pathophysiology is becoming increasingly apparent. In such cases sphincter function may be normal, but blunted anorectal sensation with impaired reflex external sphincter contraction during the sampling reflex leads to soiling and incontinence.[30] A common manifestation of this condition is fecal impaction with overflow incontinence, which typically occurs in institutionalized elderly people who have both reduced sensation and poor rectal motility. Disimpaction by mechanical or pharmacological means may eliminate incontinence, but sensation may remain disturbed and regular toileting as well as the treatment of any correctable underlying metabolic or endocrine disease are important.

The process of defecation is complex and poorly understood, and many cases of incontinence in the presence of normal sphincter structure may be related to impaired evacuation. This may be due to an intrinsic neuropathy of the colon and rectum, as is increasingly recognized in ano-rectal anomalies.[31] Alternatively there may be an anatomic distortion of the rectum such as a rectocele which prevents emptying but leads to post-defecatory soiling. This rectal dysfunction is similar to the overflow incontinence identified in fecal impaction, where sphincter function is often found to be normal.

There is also a group of patients who either for unknown reasons or as a result of undergoing rectal surgery for a variety of conditions are left with a small capacity hypersensitive rectum. In such cases we have been able to identify high pressure rectal contractions during ambulatory rectal motility studies which appear to coincide with epidodes of urgency and frank incontinence. Surgical methods of rectal augmentation, which appear to improve capacity and normalize rectal motility, may be appropriate in some instances in this group and are discussed later.

CONGENITAL CAUSES OF FECAL INCONTINENCE

Although relatively uncommon, an important cause of incontinence in childhood and younger adults are the congenital pelvic floor anomalies. In the UK, 2.8 per 10 000 infants have ano-rectal malformations,[32] half of which are associated with other congenital malformations. Low malformations, in which pelvic floor and sphincter musculature are essentially normal but the anus is closed by a membrane, are relatively easy to treat by a 'cutback' procedure in the neonatal period. However up to 50% of these infants have abnormal bowel function in later life.[33]

Higher malformations where the formation of the levator plate as well as both external and internal sphincters are abnormal cause a more profound disturbance of the continence mechanism. In high ano-rectal atresia, rudimentary fibers of the internal anal sphincter complex have been identified within the recto-urogenital fistula.[34] Attempts to incorporate these smooth muscle fibers within the reconstructed anal canal have not yet been shown to restore continence. More than half the infants with high ano-rectal malformations will have disturbed continence in later life, with effects on education and social function.[35] Traditionally high anomalies were repaired by synchronous abdomino-perineal pullthrough, although the more recent posterior sagittal approach in which the puborectalis and external sphincter is split in the midline and repaired under direct vision appears to improve outcome.

Even with satisfactory pullthrough surgery, bowel function in ano-rectal anomalies is likely to be compromised by disturbed ano-rectal sensation and colonic dysmotility. Recent studies have revealed that the propagation of colonic peristaltic activity in those with high ano-rectal anomalies is deficient,[36] a finding which may be associated with abnormalities of enteric nerves.[37] Biofeedback retraining of the pelvic floor is frequently ineffective in this group of patients,[38] although bowel management programs,[39] regular enemata and colonic irrigation may improve function.

Children may also develop encopresis, a disorder of bowel control often related to psychological stress. In this condition, soiling is usually related to disturbed patterns of evacuation. Bowel management and biofeedback programs, which reinforce the child's development of a regular and effective bowel habit, have been shown to have a high success rate in this condition.[40] In view of the partially psychogenic nature of this condition, surgical intervention should be avoided unless megacolon has developed.

MEDICAL TREATMENT

Inevitably the majority of patients presenting to physicians with fecal incontinence will not need or want surgical intervention. Medical treatment can successfully reduce the frequency and severity of incontinence symptoms. In almost all patients, dietary interventions are the first step in controlling incontinence. Patients with incontinence exacerbated by chronic diarrhea justify investigation to exclude conditions such as gluten intolerance or pancreatic exocrine insufficiency. A low fat diet and the use of bile salt binding agents such as cholestyramine may also reduce the frequency of bowel action, for example in post-cholecystectomy diarrhea.

Fiber supplementation has sometimes been promoted as a ubiquitous 'cure-all' for bowel disorders, but increased insoluble fiber intake may be unhelpful because it both decreases transit time and increases stool bulk creating a larger volume of softer stool for the incompetent sphincter to deal with. Soluble fiber supplements undergo colonic fermentation with the production of more flatus and a more acidic stool, both of which may exacerbate rather than relieve symptoms.

Anti-diarrhea medications containing Loperamide,[41] Codeine or Diphenoxylate[42] can greatly reduce symptoms, particularly in cases of incontinence exacerbated by chronic diarrhea. Loperamide may have to be used in larger doses than those prescribed for sporadic diarrhea, and some patients find that Loperamide syrup is more effective than capsule preparations. Topical skin protecting creams such as Orobase® also have a role in relieving the perianal pain and pruritis associated with chronic soiling.

Anal plugs similar in construction to vaginal tampons may also have a role in the medical management of incontinence, but unpublished studies in the UK suggest that only around half of the users can tolerate their regular use; those with blunted anal canal sensation after surgery or neurological disorders appear to be the most likely to succeed with these devices.

Simple pelvic floor exercises described elsewhere in this volume may also benefit those with milder incontinence. The role of biofeedback in improving pelvic floor function is discussed in a later chapter; the reported results of biofeedback are difficult to interpret because the casemix varies between series. Biofeedback is most likely to be successful in those with only partial rather than complete sphincter defects in whom sphincter symmetry and rectal capacity is preserved.[43,44] Studies which have included full sphincter manometry and endoanal ultrasound in all participants suggest that less than 50% of patients with confirmed sphincter defects respond successfully to biofeedback.[45,21] Biofeedback may be augmented with electrical stimulation of the pelvic floor,[46] and in a recent randomized study only the addition of electrical stimulation to a standard biofeedback regimen improved sphincter tone.[47]

EXTERNAL SPHINCTER REPAIR FOR OBSTETRIC TRAUMA

Sphincter repair performed at the time of a third or fourth degree obstetric sphincter injury can have a high success rate, but in those whom the degree of sphincteric injury is overlooked or in whom the primary repair dehisces, delayed repair is necessary. Up to 85% of women with third degree tears have endosonographic evidence of a persistent external anal sphincter defect after primary repair, and incontinence to solid or liquid stool is found in 8% of women after a primary repair of a third degree injury.[48]

The timing of delayed repair of obstetric sphincter injuries has been widely debated, but most authors advocate delaying surgery for at least 2 months after the original injury to allow the separated sphincter ends to undergo fibrosis and for any infection or edema to subside. After childbirth patients may need to be encouraged to report symptoms of incontinence since sphincter repair surgery is more successful if undertaken at a younger age.[49]

TECHNIQUE OF DIRECT SPHINCTER REPAIR

Originally direct sphincter repair was performed by end-to-end sutured apposition of the separated edges of the external sphincter, but results were disappointing. Numerous studies since suggest that superior results are achieved with an overlapping repair, as first described by Sir Alan Parks.[50] In our practice patients suitable for anterior sphincter repair are selected on the basis of intractable symptoms unresponsive to conservative treatment. Prior to consideration of surgery all patients are investigated with endoanal ultrasound to confirm the presence and site of an external sphincter defect and to detect coexisting defects elsewhere in the sphincteric complex. In this context, endoanal ultrasound has been shown to have a high correlation with the findings at surgery[51] and histology.[52] Whilst patients with two separate defects within the external sphincter or a coexisting internal sphincter defect can be treated by overlapping repair, results are less good and transposition myoplasty may be a better option. Pudendal nerve conduction studies, manometry and ano-rectal sensory testing are also important components of planning the optimal treatment strategy. Neither pudendal neuropathy nor sensory dysfunction are contraindications to surgery, but some surgeons consider that bilateral pudendal neuropathy renders a successful outcome less likely, a consideration which is discussed below.

Surgery is performed under general anesthetic after full bowel preparation with stimulant or osmotic laxatives. We favor the lithotomy position although others, particularly in North America, routinely use the prone jack-knife position. An elliptical circumanal incision is made at the edge of the pigmented anal skin and sharp dissection is used to free the external sphincter remnants. The lateral part of the external sphincter on each side is mobilized from surrounding fat and from the underlying internal sphincter up to the level of the pelvic floor. This should permit a tension free overlap of healthy sphincter muscle by at least half an inch (15 mm). The fibrotic tissue within the sphincter defect is excised and the healthy sphincter tissue on either side is overlapped and secured using interrupted non-absorbable sutures, typically Ethibond® (PTFE) or Prolene® (Polypropylene), placed in a mattress configuration (Figs 24.1 to 24.3).

In some cases the perineal body and the anterior pelvic floor is deficient, and in such cases we favor anterior levatorplasty to tighten the anterior pelvic floor. This is performed prior to construction of the overlapping sphincter repair by suturing the two limbs of the puborectalis together in the midline using non-absorbable sutures. This and other additional procedures are discussed below.

Usually the wound is closed using interrupted absorbable sutures, although in cases where the perineal body is deficient or there is a traumatic cloaca, a V-Y plasty or the rotation of flaps from the inner thigh to cover the wound may be necessary. Some surgeons leave a suction drain in the subcutaneous tissues, whilst others do not close the skin wound but leave it to heal by secondary intention.

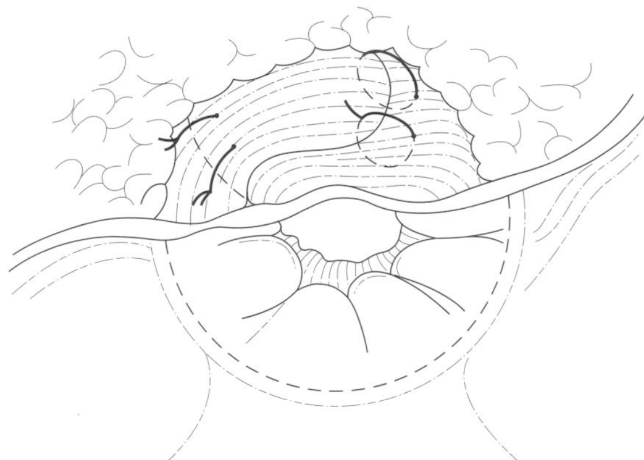

Figure 24.1 Drawing of a completed overlapping anterior sphincter repair.

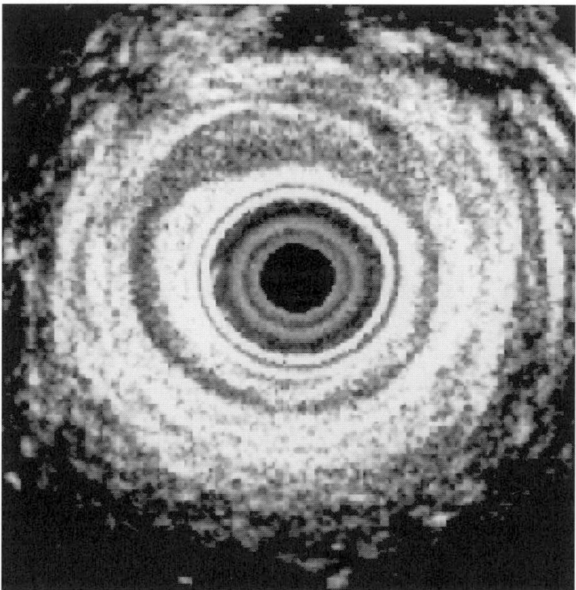

Figure 24.2 Endoanal ultrasound of a successful overlapping anterior sphincter repair.

The optimal timing for reintroduction of diet postoperatively and the use of a covering loop stoma are both controversial. We do not routinely use a stoma except in repeat sphincter repair or in cases with a traumatic cloaca. However the patient is kept on a liquid diet for several days after surgery and daily wound irrigation is encouraged. The use of antidiarrheal drugs to 'confine the bowels' may cause fecal impaction in up to 10%; we favor the routine use of stool softeners to prevent this painful complication. In an audit of the various peri-

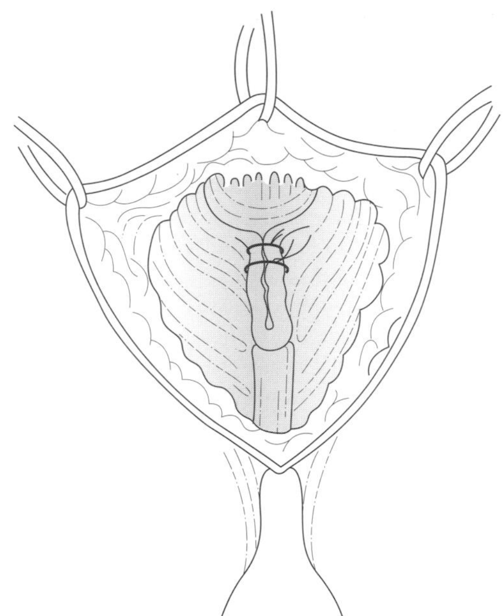

Figure 24.3 Completed postanal repair.

operative management regimes used at St Marks Hospital, similar outcomes and complication rates were obtained whether a stoma, laxatives or antidiarrheal drugs were used.[53] A randomized American study showed that bowel confinement strategies were associated with more episodes of impaction and increased in-hospital expenditure when compared with the early reintroduction of a full diet.[54]

In obstetric trauma, success rates as high as 80% have been reported, with success related to significant increases in voluntary squeeze pressure[58] and an increase in anal canal length.[59] In the few studies reporting longer term follow-up there is a decline in continence,[61] so it is unlikely that the benefits of surgery are permanent. Some authors argue that the results of overlapping sphincter repair are poorer in patients with a pudendal neuropathy[55,62] although a succession of more recent studies dispute this.[58,59,63] Most authors agree that functional and physiological results are probably poorer in older patients and in those with coexistent evacuatory disorders. Nevertheless, an overlapping sphincter repair remains the primary treatment of any intractably incontinent patient in whom a definite external sphincter defect can be detected at endosonography.

SPHINCTER REPAIR FOLLOWING NON-OBSTETRIC TRAUMA

Delayed sphincter repair is also a good therapeutic option in patients with a single sphincter defect after external trauma. In a series of patients undergoing

Table 24.2 The results of overlapping sphincter repair

Series	Etiology	Number	% Continent to solid and liquid	Poorer outcome in neuropathy?	Notes
Browning[55]	Obstetric	13	84%	Yes	65% had stoma
Browning[55]	Mixed	84	64%		
Engel[56]	Post fistula	20	65%		
Engel[57]	External trauma	52	69%		95% had stoma
Engel[58]	Obstetric	53	79%	No	25% had stoma
Hool[59]	Mixed	51	80%	No	
Laurberg[60]	Obstetric	19	47%	Yes	
Londono-Schimmer[61]	Mixed	128	50%	Yes	Long-term follow-up
Wexner[62]	Obstetric	17	76%	Yes	Incorporated internal sphincter reefing
Young[63]	Obstetric	56	87%	No	Age and stoma did not affect outcome

Note: Success rates are calculated from the percentage of patients usually continent to solid and liquid stool or improved after surgery; the definition of success may differ from that in the original papers since there is no standard outcome measure.

sphincter repair for a single defect following external trauma, who were selected to exclude those with severe concomitant rectal injuries or sepsis, 69% regained good continence.[57] A defunctioning stoma was used in almost all cases, and a successful outcome was associated with significant increases in both resting and squeeze pressure rather than with the nature of the original trauma. Delayed overlapping sphincter repair can also restore acceptable continence in 65% of patients who were previously rendered incontinent by surgical procedures for complex fistula in ano.[56]

INTERNAL SPHINCTER REPAIR

In an effort to improve the outcome of sphincteroplasty a trial of simultaneous sutured imbrication of the internal sphincter[64] has been attempted. This procedure did not appear to offer any benefit since continence was restored in around two-thirds of patients whether or not imbrication was added to the external sphincter repair. This negative finding was confirmed in another non-randomized series of overlapping sphincter repairs.[62] Similarly internal sphincter plication does not appear to improve the outcome of pelvic floor repairs performed for neuropathic incontinence.[65] Only one study of overlap repair of the internal anal sphincter after iatrogenic injuries has demonstrated a useful improvement in continence, but even in this report endosonography revealed persistent internal sphincter defects in all patients.[66]

REPEAT SPHINCTER REPAIR

Inevitably there are cases in which the first attempt at sphincter repair fails to achieve satisfactory improvement in continence. In such circumstances repeated investigation by endosonography and manometry is appropriate before deciding on subsequent therapeutic options. If the repair is intact on endosonography, biofeedback retraining may yield useful improvements in the symptoms of incontinence and avoid the need for further surgery even in patients with pudendal neuropathy.[67] If a persistent sphincter defect is felt to be responsible for the ongoing symptoms of incontinence, further surgery may be offered. In a recent small series, both continence score and ability to defer defecation was improved in 65% of patients undergoing a second or third overlapping sphincter repair.[68] In this series, failure was associated with a persisting sphincter defect on endosonography. Conversely, the later addition of a post anal repair after failed anterior sphincter repair appears to be less successful.[69] Transposition of muscle from the gluteus[70] or the use of a simultaneous unstimulated gracilis wrap[90] has also been described in conjunction with a sphincter repair in such circumstances. Others would advocate that a failed sphincter repair despite endosonographic evidence of an intact overlap is an indication for a stimulated graciloplasty,[71] antegrade colonic irrigation or perhaps an artificial bowel sphincter; options which are discussed later in this chapter.

POSTANAL REPAIR

The operation of postanal repair, originally developed by Parks, is performed under general anesthetic with the patient placed in either the Lloyd-Davies or more commonly in the prone jack-knife position. A posterior circumanal incision is made and extended into the intersphincteric space to the level of the pelvic floor. The decussating fibers of the puborectalis posterior to the ano-rectal junction are plicated or reefed together, usually with interrupted non-absorbable sutures. The posterior component of the external sphincter is tightened by a further series of interrupted sutures, before the skin is closed primarily.

Originally the procedure was believed to work by tightening the posterior pelvic floor and accentuating the ano-rectal angle, and was advocated in neurogenic or idiopathic fecal incontinence. Early studies identified changes in functional anal canal length,[72] resting tone[73] or ano-rectal angle postoperatively, but no consistent effect of the procedure on commonly measured ano-rectal parameters has ever been demonstrated.

Follow-up studies of the results of postanal repair have been disappointing, with reports that less than half the patients have improved continence a median of 2 years later, despite improvements in anal manometric indices.[74] Perhaps as a result, it appears that postanal repair has become less frequently performed within Britain during recent years.[75]

No-one has been able to replicate the successful outcome described in the original reports of the procedure, but it may still have a role in treating neuropathic incontinence. Since we know that neuropathic incontinence frequently involves sensory as well as motor abnormalities, the high rates of failure and postoperative evacuatory difficulties are not altogether unexpected but can lead to patient dissatisfaction.

ANTERIOR LEVATORPLASTY AND PELVIC FLOOR REPAIR

Anterior levatorplasty is performed via a transverse perineal incision. After dissection in the rectovaginal septum, muscle fibers of levator ani within the pelvic floor are exposed and tightened by a series of interupted sutures passed from side-to-side. This has the effect of reforming the perineal body and appears to improve anal tone, although a non-randomized trial failed to show any difference in outcome when compared with postanal repair.[76] Reports suggest that anterior levatorplasty is more likely to benefit those with obstetric rather than neuropathic incontinence, but only around 50% benefit in the longer term.[77] As a result the procedure is not usually performed alone, but may be a useful adjunct to overlapping sphincter repair in the presence of a traumatic cloaca.

The combination of a postanal repair with an anterior levatorplasty has been termed a total pelvic floor repair. In one randomized trial comparing the combined procedure to postanal repair or anterior levatorplasty alone,[78] only the patients having a total pelvic floor repair gained a significant improvement in anal canal length. As a result, two thirds of the total pelvic floor repair patients enjoyed restored continence, compared to only one third of those treated by other techniques. In another report 65% of women with neuropathic fecal incontinence treated by this method gained improved continence, but only 14% were fully continent.[79] Conversely in a randomized Dutch study comparing total pelvic floor repair with postanal repair,[80] less than half of the patients in either group benefited from surgery, and there was no consistent change in ano-rectal physiological indices.

TRANSPOSITION MYOPLASTY

In the absence of sufficient sphincteric tissues to achieve a direct sphincter repair surgeons have transposed healthy skeletal muscle from the buttock or thigh to the anal region in order to replace or augment the original sphincters. Both the gracilis and the gluteus maximus muscles have been used for this purpose because their vascular supplies are sufficiently plastic to permit transposition to the pelvic floor.

THE TECHNIQUE OF GRACILOPLASTY (THE GRACILIS NEOSPHINCTER) (FIG. 24.4)

The procedure is performed under general anaesthetic in the Lloyd-Davies position. We prefer to prepare the bowel preoperatively and favor the use of a defunctioning stoma, especially in those patients who have previously had extensive perianal surgery. The gracilis muscle is mobilized via a medial thigh incision, and the distal tendon is divided just above its insertion at the *pes anserinus*. The neurovascular pedicle is located on the inner aspect of the muscle at about one-quarter of the way from the groin to the knee; this neurovascular pedicle forms the fulcrum about which the distal three-quarters of the gracilis is rotated in order to reach the perineum. Although there are minor blood vessels within the lower thigh which contribute to the muscles' vascular supply the previously described premobilization and division of distal vessels is probably not of benefit, and no longer forms part of our routine practice.

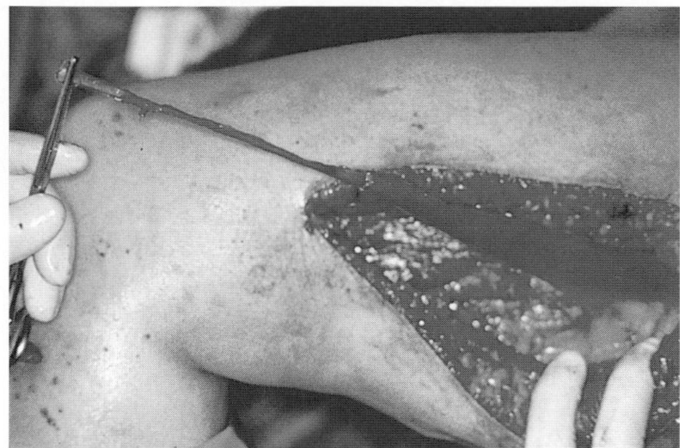

Figure 24.4 The gracilis muscle is mobilized from the thigh. (Courtesy Medtronic Interstim, Maastrict, Netherlands.)

Through two lateral circumanal incisions and an additional upper thigh incision, a tunnel is created for the body of the gracilis to be passed from the thigh to encircle the anal canal. Various configurations of gracilis wrap around the anus have been described, but most authors use the gamma configuration where the initial part of the wrap passes anteriorly to the anus, and after making a 360° loop, the distal muscle is fixed with a non-absorbable suture (e.g. Ethibond®) to the contralateral ischial tuberosity. Adduction of the thigh into a neutral position is necessary before securing the distal muscle. Since the contractile function of striated muscle is partially dependent on muscle tension, some authors have attempted to perform anal manometry intraoperatively although this may be unreliable in an anesthetized patient. We believe that adequate tension of the transposed muscle can be judged by creating a neosphincter which is snug rather than tight around a 1.5 cm dilator or an experienced surgical digit.

THE ELECTRICALLY STIMULATED (DYNAMIC) GRACILOPLASTY

Unlike the external anal sphincter, which is a fatigue resistant muscle containing predominantly slow-twitch fibers, both gracilis and gluteus are composed of a high percentage of type II fast-twitch fibers which are unable to maintain a sustained contraction. After unstimulated myoplasty the improvement in continence is reliant on either passive tightening of the anal canal by the encircling muscle, or on active but poorly sustained squeeze. When biofeedback or exercise has been used to enhance muscle contraction, several authors from the 1950s to the present day have reported reasonable improvements in bowel control.

There had been anecdotal reports for many years that electrical stimulation of the transposed muscle could improve continence, but it was not until the 1970s that chronic low-frequency skeletal muscle was shown to be able to transform muscle fiber-type to a predominantly slow-twitch morphology. During the 1980s, the advances in implanted pacemaker technology permitted surgeons working in both the UK[81] and The Netherlands[82] to simultaneously demonstrate that chronic electrostimulation could induce controllable yet fatigue-resistant contractile activity within the transposed human gracilis. This phenomenon of phenotypic transformation of muscle fiber-type has since been demonstrated by manometry, histology and electromyography. Electrical stimulation has also been used with a similar therapeutic aim after gluteal myoplasty.

Electrical stimulation to create a dynamic graciloplasty can be delivered either to the nerve to gracilis itself by fixing a neural electrode directly over the nerve, or by the use of an intramuscular electrode. Theoretically direct neural stimulation offers more complete recruitment of the muscle fibers, leading to a greater degree of fiber-type transformation and fatigue resistance.[83] Since lower voltage requirements appear to be necessary to induce muscle contraction, direct neural stimulation may also prolong the life of the stimulator battery. Unfortunately some neural electrodes, particularly those used in early series, can become dislodged and require surgical revision. For this reason some authors argue that intramuscular electrostimulation can reduce the morbidity of the procedure,[84] but no direct comparative study has ever been performed.

Whichever type of electrode is used, it is connected by a tunnelled lead to a pulse generator or stimulator which is implanted subcutaneously in the abdominal wall. The stimulator delivers low frequency (10 or 12 Hz) pulsatile output which is capable of producing a tetanic contraction in the transformed muscle. Initial voltages of 0.5–1 V are required to induce contraction but a degree of peri-electrode fibrosis necessitates slow increases in the voltage to between 1 and 3 volts after 3 years. The attending surgeon can adjust all stimulation parameters using a lap-top style computer which communicates with the implanted pulse generator by a radiofrequency coil held adjacent to the abdominal wall. The patient uses a hand-held radiotelemetry controller to turn off the stimulator and relax the graciloplasty prior to defecation; patients using the latest generation of controllers can also alter the strength of gracilis contraction by increasing or decreasing the stimulating voltage within preset limits (Fig. 24.5).

If electrical stimulation is to be used it seems logical to be in a position to initiate stimulation as soon as possible after surgery in order to prevent disuse atrophy of the transposed gracilis. Therefore we usually fix an electrode plate over the nerve to gracilis at the time of initial surgery and commence stimulation within 2

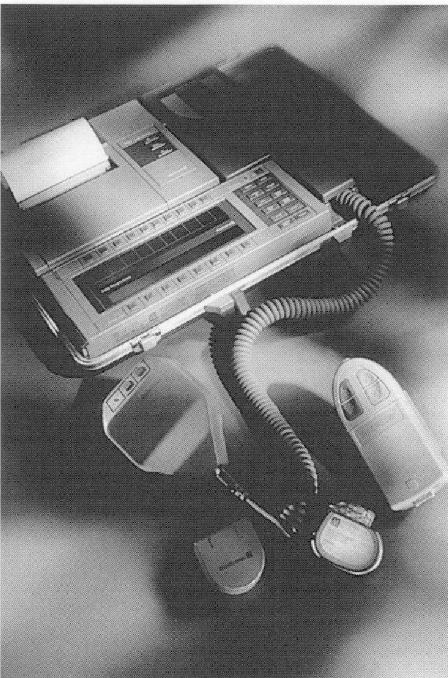

Figure 24.5 The programmer, stimulator and hand-held controller used in dynamic graciloplasty. (Courtesy of Medtronic A/A.)

weeks of transposition. Later implantation of either a neural or an intramuscular electrode can be performed, but the unstimulated gracilis is known to lose up to one-third of its bulk within 6 weeks.

As a result of the rapid fatigue of the untransformed (predominantly fast-twitch) muscle, initial stimulation is started intermittently, with cyclical activation and contraction of the muscle every few seconds. The length of activation time is increased over 6 to 8 weeks until the graciloplasty develops fatigue resistance, at which time continuous activation of the gracilis may be commenced, and any defunctioning stoma can be reversed. It is also possible to commence very low frequency stimulation continuously at 2 Hz; there is evidence from animal studies that this may result in faster fiber-type conversion.[85]

THE OUTCOME OF UNSTIMULATED GRACILOPLASTY (TABLE 24.3)

The analysis of results for unstimulated graciloplasty is difficult since many series consist of cases of mixed etiology and the method of outcome assessment is often poorly explained. Although most reports describe a significant improvement in anal squeeze function, our experience is that a considerable proportion of the patients also encounter evacuatory difficulty. If graciloplasty alone is unsuccessful at restoring continence, the addition of electrostimulation may improve sphincter pressures, but it will only restore continence if evacuatory function is normal.

Bilateral graciloplasty where both gracili are utilized in a number of configurations has also been described. In one technique each muscle is wrapped around the contralateral anal canal and joined in the posterior midline. In a small series, eight out of ten patients gained increases in anal canal length and tone associated with apparent reduction in the frequency of their incontinence.[91] Evacuatory dysfunction was not reported in this series, but in other series of bilateral dynamic graciloplasty evacuatory problems have been reported.

THE OUTCOME OF ELECTRICALLY STIMULATED (DYNAMIC) GRACILOPLASTY (TABLE 24.4)

Patients coming forward to graciloplasty have usually failed to respond to conventional sphincter or pelvic floor repair procedures. Yet almost all authors have reported that resting anal pressures with stimulation are unchanged by surgery, whilst electrical stimulation can increase squeeze pressure significantly to values comparable to normal control populations.[99] A number of quality of life indices can be improved by surgery[95,100] although a large number of complications including electrode migration, stenosis, infection, anal erosion and electronic failure have been reported,[101] particularly with early stimulation devices.[84] More

Table 24.3 The results of unstimulated graciloplasty for fecal incontinence

Author	Number	Etiology	Number (%) improved	Comments
Yoshika[86]	6	Mixed	0 (0%)	High sepsis rate
Christiansen[87]	12	Trauma	6 (50%)	
Faucheron[88]	22	Mixed	15 (68%)	Reports evacuatory difficulty
Sielezneff[89]	8	Mixed	8 (100%)	Included biofeedback exercises
Eccersley[90]	12	Trauma	8 (67%)	Two were later stimulated; high rate of sepsis and evacuatory difficulty

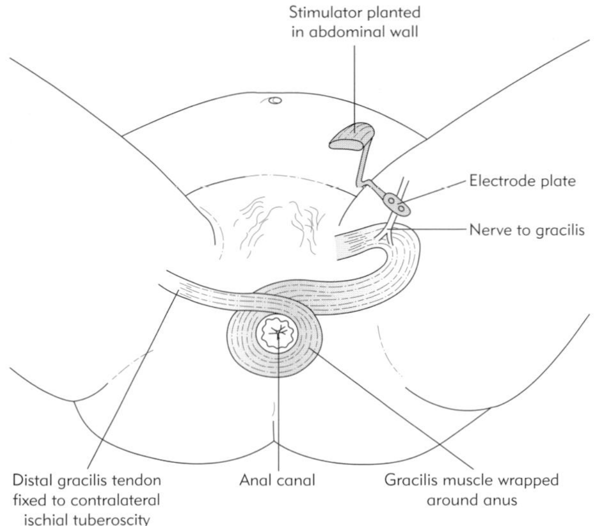

Figure 24.6 The gracilis wrap around the anal canal. A stimulator is implanted in the anterior abdominal wall and tunnelled subcutaneously to the nerve to gracilis.

recently a multicenter[98] trial of intramuscular stimulation has reported that '85 of 128 graciloplasty patients (66%) achieved and maintained a successful outcome.' Only half of the patients with congenital anomalies achieved success, whereas 70% of those with traumatic incontinence responded to the therapy. The surgery was associated with a major wound complication rate of over 30%.

The fact that rectal evacuation may be disturbed after graciloplasty has been increasingly reported in recent published series. The majority of the patients coming forward for the procedure have failed to respond to conventional medical and surgical treatments. Most have little residual sphincter function, and many have pelvic floor denervation and evacuatory disturbances. This problem appears to be especially prevalent in those who previously had ano-rectal anomalies. These patients probably have a rectal evacuatory disorder which is exacerbated by further attempts at sphincter augmentation, and we believe that antegrade colonic irrigation (discussed below) may be a useful adjunctive or alternative treatment strategy.

GLUTEOPLASTY

This procedure involves the transposition of the medial fibers of gluteus maximus on their intact neurovascular bundle to encircle the anal canal. One, or more commonly, both glutei have been used to perform this repair. The glutei are predominantly fast twitch muscles, but with postoperative retraining approximately half of the patients with conditions refractory to conventional repair procedures have regained good or excellent continence.[102] Although gluteal myoplasty has recently been favorably compared with total pelvic floor repair as a treatment for neuropathic fecal incontinence,[103] the gluteal procedure appears to have a higher rate of wound infection, a risk of anal stenosis, and evacuatory

Table 24.4 The results of dynamic (electrically stimulated) graciloplasty

Series	Number	Mode of stimulation	Number (%) improved	Comments
Korsgen[92]	4	Neural	1 (25%)	Rectal evacuatory problems in three
Sielezneff[93]	16	Neural (13/16)	12 (75%)	High revision rate, but only two had impaired evacuation
Christiansen[94]	13	Intramuscular	6 (50%)	Three had impaired evacuation
Baeten[95]	52	Intramuscular	38 (73%)	Rectal sensation important to success
Royal London[96]	60	Neural	36 (60%)	Colonic irrigation in 75% of congenitals
Rosen[97]	10	Intramuscular	9 (90%)	20% Needed rectal irrigation
Wexner[84]	27	Mixed	13 (43%)	Most complications in neural group
Multicenter[98]	128	Intramuscular	85 (66%)	30% Major wound complication rate

difficulty. Of the eleven patients treated with an electrostimulated gluteoplasty in a recent report, only five (45%) achieved a successful outcome.[98]

THE ARTIFICIAL ANAL SPHINCTER (FIG. 24.7)

There are inevitably patients in whom no sphincter or pelvic floor reconstructive procedures have succeeded. In such cases a totally implanted artificial anal sphincter may be utilized. The technology of an artificial sphincter was originally developed for use in urology, but has subsequently been modified for anal incontinence.

Prior to implantation of the device, the patient must be carefully assessed as digital dexterity is required to operate the device. The ABS (Artificial Bowel Sphincter®, American Medical Systems, Minnesota, USA) which is currently the most widely used system, involves the implantation of a hydraulic cuff around the anal canal. This cuff is connected by totally implanted siliconized tubing to a saline reservoir implanted above the inguinal ligament and to a valved inflation device placed within the scrotum or labia majora. On activation, the hydraulic pressure within the reservoir fills the cuff and occludes the previously incompetent anal canal. When the patient wishes to defecate, the scrotal or labial valve is squeezed and the cuff deflates for several minutes. After evacuation, the cuff re-expands to maintain anal closure.

Early series reported high failure rates due to anal canal erosion, sepsis or mechanical failure.[104] Subsequent reports where the ABS has been specifically designed for use in anal incontinence appear to have more promising short-term results, with the majority of patients enjoying improved continence. The cuff can exacerbate evacuatory difficulties and one series identified that almost half the patients needed regular enemata.[105] The devastating complication of sepsis in an implanted foreign body may possibly be reduced by careful aseptic technique and bowel preparation, although there is little evidence to support this. Recent reports from Scotland describe a novel implantable sphincter which appears less likely to become infected since it is placed around the closed rectum at laparotomy, and has a pressure profile that is unlikely to cause mucosal erosions.[106]

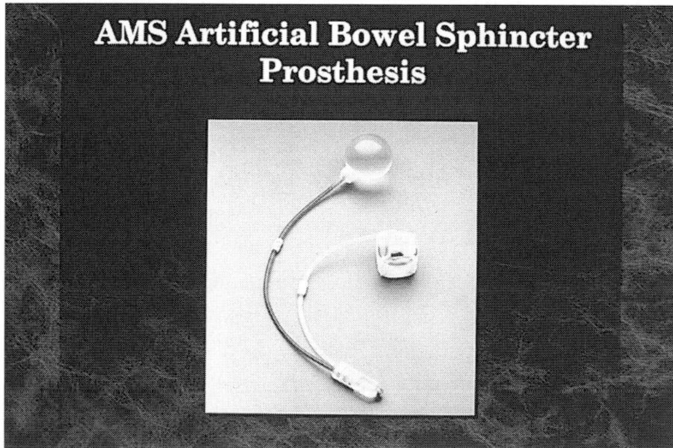

Figure 24.7 The Artificial Bowel Sphincter before implantation, showing cuff, reservoir and valve. (Courtesy of American Medical Systems Inc, Minneapolis, Minn, USA.)

ANTEGRADE COLONIC IRRIGATION

It will be apparent from the above review that many cases of incontinence resistant to biofeedback or conventional surgery have an underlying rectal evacuatory disorder as a result of both sensory and motor disturbances within the ano-rectal complex. The use of rectal enemas is one method of improving symptoms of disturbed evacuation, and irrigation with a customized rectal catheter has been found to be beneficial in between 40 and 60% of these complex cases.[107]

Antegrade colonic irrigation, where water and/or a pro-kinetic agent is instilled via a catheter introduced into the proximal colon, can also improve evacuation and promote fecal continence by ensuring regular colonic emptying. The most popular route for antegrade irrigation in children has been via an appendicostomy created at open surgery or sometimes laparoscopic surgery,[108] where around 75% of children with incontinence following previously treated high ano-rectal anomalies can regain continence.[109] Complications of stenosis at the appendiceal orifice and reflux of colonic contents[110] together with the fact that the appendix may be absent or of too narrow a caliber to permit successful antegrade irrigation in adults, led us to develop the valved colonic conduit in adult patients.

THE COLONIC CONDUIT (FIG. 24.8)

The colonic conduit provides a catheterizable channel leading from the skin to the colonic lumen that incorporates a full thickness intussuscepted valve to prevent reflux.[111] To accomplish this, the transverse colon is mobilized and divided at the hepatic flexure. The proximal transverse colon is intussuscepted to form an anti-reflux valve. The afferent limb is then narrowed using a linear stapling device and tunneled through the anterior abdominal wall to form a small continent orifice. Colonic continuity is restored by an end to side anastomosis between the ascending and distal transverse colon. Following surgery the patient is taught to catheterize the conduit daily with a urethral catheter and irrigate using 2 pints (1 litre) of tap water warmed to body temperature (Fig. 24.9). This method of antegrade colonic irrigation has also been particularly

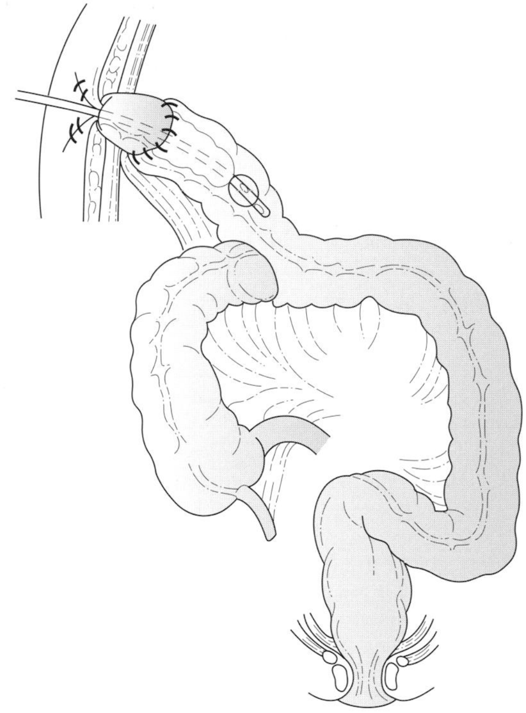

Figure 24.8 The colonic conduit sited in the transverse colon and tunneled through the anterior abdominal wall. A catheter is passed into the conduit through the abdominal wall, and the balloon has been inflated. (Reproduced with permission of Blackwell Science Ltd., from *Br J Surg*, 1995;**82:**1319; original artwork by Gillian Lee.)

utilized in adults with incontinence related to disordered rectal evacuation, where high rates of success have been reported.[112] A high level of nursing support and patient motivation is required for successful use of these techniques, but it is applicable for patients in whom major structural defects or impaired evacuation prohibit successful reconstruction.[113]

RECTAL AUGMENTATION

There is a group of previously overlooked patients who, as the result of previous surgery or disease, have greatly reduced rectal capacity. These patients experience severe urgency of defecation and urge incontinence even when sphincter function is normal or has been restored by surgery. The underlying pathophysiology appears to be a reduced rectal capacity and consequent volume hypersensitivity. The situation is in some ways analogous to the 'anterior resection syndrome' encountered after straight colo-anal anastomoses, and part of the pathophysiology may be related to the autonomic denervation described in this condition.

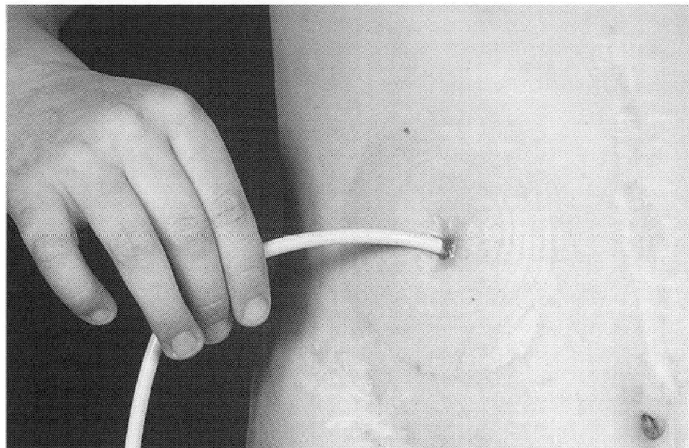

Figure 24.9 Intubation of the continent orifice of the colonic conduit with a latex catheter prior to antegrade colonic irrigation.

Whilst biofeedback and even forcible rectal dilatation[114] may help some such patients, surgical construction of an enlarged rectal pouch may also offer some benefit. Routes to increase rectal capacity include the construction of a J-pouch. Although this technique is easily applicable at the time of a primary colo-anal anastomosis, it is impractical in a patient with an intact yet shrunken rectum. For this reason we have begun to develop the technique of a ileo-rectoplasty, where a patch of ileum is incorporated into the rectum to increase its storage capacity in a fashion similar to the clam ileo-cystoplasty. A segment of vascularized ileum, 12–15 cm in length, is isolated from the small bowel by cross-stapling. Small bowel continuity is restored with a standard anastomosis. The isolated ileal segment is stapled over the anterior rectal wall using a linear stapling device, with the result that the ileal patch increases rectal capacity. In our early experience in three patients, rectal capacity (as demonstrated by increases in the rectal sensory volumes) is considerably improved, with a concomitant reduction in the symptoms of urge incontinence. Ambulatory rectal motility studies have shown the ablation of the high pressure waves formerly associated with considerable urgency and incontinence.

CONCLUSION

Scientific understanding of and treatment for fecal incontinence has advanced greatly in the last decade. However there remains a great deal more yet to be discovered; in particular the autonomic innervation of the ano-rectum is poorly understood. Clearly many patients debilitated by mild or moderate incontinence may benefit from medical therapy and the increased use of biofeedback technologies to retrain the pelvic floor. Patients with external sphincter defects unresponsive to conservative therapy should be offered sphincter repair surgery even if they have evidence of concomitant internal sphincter defects or pelvic floor denervation.

Patients with structurally intact sphincters but profound incontinence due to neuropathy may benefit from postanal or pelvic floor repair; but graciloplasty may be just as effective as these procedures. In recent years it has become apparent that rectal evacuation is frequently disturbed in pelvic floor disorders; both biofeedback and antegrade colonic irrigation may help patients whose poor sphincter function is compounded by evacuatory difficulty. Complex reconstructive procedures such as the electrically stimulated graciloplasty or even artificial sphincters may offer the hope of restored continence to those who would previously have been condemned to a lifetime of disability.

REFERENCES

1. Henry MM, Swash M, Phillips RKS, *et al.* Faecal incontinence. In: Henry MM, Swash M (eds). *Coloproctology and the pelvic floor*, 2nd edn. Oxford: Butterworth Heinemann, 1992:257–304.
2. Oliveira L, Wexner SD. Anal incontinence. In: Beck DE, Wexner SD (eds). *Fundamentals of anorectal surgery*, 2nd edn. London: WB Saunders, 1998:115–52.
3. Leigh RJ, Turnberg LA. Faecal incontinence: the unvoiced symptom. *Lancet* 1982;**1**:1349–51.
4. Nelson R, Norton N, Cautley E, Furner S. Community based prevalence of anal incontinence. *JAMA* 1995;**274**:559–61.
5. Giebel GD, Lefering R, Troidl H, Blochl H. Prevalence of fecal incontinence: what can be expected? *Int J Colorect Dis* 1998;**13**:73–77.
6. Lam TC, Kennedy ML, Chen FC, Lubowski DZ, Talley NJ. Prevalence of fecal incontinence: obstetric and constipation related risk factors; a population-based study. *Colorectal Dis* 1999;**1**:197–203.
7. Enck P, Bielefeldt K, Rathmann W, *et al.* Epidemiology of faecal incontinence in selected patient groups. *Int J Colorect Dis* 1991;**6**:143–6.
8. Jorge JMN, Wexner SD. Etiology and management of fecal incontinence. *Dis Colon Rectum* 1992;**36**:77–97.
9. Mellgren A, Jensen L, *et al.* The long-term cost of fecal incontinence. *Dis Colon Rectum* 1999;**42**:857–63.
10. Lunniss P, Kamm MA, Phillips RKS. Factors affecting continence after surgery for anal fistula. *Br J Surg* 1994;**81**:1382–5.
11. Vaizey CJ, Carapeti E. Cahill JA. Kamm MA. Prospective comparison of faecal incontinence grading systems. *Gut* 1999;**44**:77–80.
12. Pescatori M, Anastasio G, Bottini C, Mentasti A. New grading and scoring for anal incontinence. *Dis Colon Rectum* 1992;**35**:482–7.
13. Diseth TH, Emblem R. Somatic function, mental health and psychosocial adjustment of adolescents with anorectal anomalies. *J Pediat Surg* 1996;**31**:638–43.
14. Rintala R, Mildh L, Lindahl H. Fecal continence and quality of life for adult patients with an operated high or intermediate anorectal malformation. *J Pediat Surg* 1994;**29**:777–80.
15. Sailer M, Bussen D, Debus ES, *et al.* Quality of life in patients with benign anorectal disorders. *Br J Surg* 1998;**85**:1716–9.
16. Engel AF, Kamm MA, Bartram CI, Nicholls RJ. Relationship of symptoms in faecal incontinence to specific sphincter abnormalities. *Int J Colorectal Dis* 1995;**10**:152–5.
17. Keating JP, Stewart PJ, *et al.* Are special investigations of value in the management of patients with fecal incontinence? *Dis Colon Rectum* 1997;**40**:896–901.
18. Sultan AH, Kamm MA, *et al.* Anal sphincter disruption during vaginal delivery. *N Engl J Med* 1993;**329**:1905–11.
19. Groutz A, Fait G, *et al.* Incidence and obstetric risk factors of postpartum anal incontinence. *Scand J Gastroenterol* 1999;**34**:315–8.
20. Norton C, Kamm MA. Biofeedback for faecal incontinence. *Br J Surg* 1999;**86**:1159–63.
21. Leroi A-M, Dorival M-P, *et al.* Pudendal neuropathy and severity of incontinence but not presence of an anal sphincter defect may determine the response to biofeedback therapy in fecal incontinence. *Dis Colon Rectum* 1999;**42**:762–9.
22. Nielsen MB, Rasmussen OO, Pedersen JF, Christiansen J. Risk of sphincter damage and anal incontinence after anal dilatation for fistula in ano. *Dis Colon Rectum* 1993;**36**:677–80.
23. Ryhammer AM, Laurberg S, Hermann AP. No correlation between perineal position and pudendal nerve terminal motor latency in healthy perimenopausal women. *Dis Colon Rectum* 1998;**41**:350–3.
24. Wakeman R, Allen-Mersh T. Puborectalis and external anal sphincter paralysis with preservation of fecal continence. *Dis Colon Rectum* 1989;**32**:980–1.
25. Wynne J, Myles J, Jones I, *et al.* Disturbed anal sphincter function following vaginal delivery. *Gut* 1996;**39**:120–4.
26. Roberts P, Coller J, *et al.* Manometric assessment of patients with obstetric injuries and faecal incontinence. *Dis Colon Rectum* 1990;**33**:16–20.
27. Williams N, Scott NA, Irving MH. Effect of lateral sphincterotomy on internal anal sphincter function. A vector manometry study. *Dis Colon Rectum* 1995;**38**: 700–4.
28. Rao GN, Drew PJ, Lee PWR, *et al.* Anterior resection syndrome is secondary to sympathetic denervation. *Int J Colorectal Dis* 1996;**11**:250–8.
29. Jameson JS, Scott AD. Medical causes of faecal incontinence. *Eur J Gastro Hepatol* 1997;**9**:428–30.
30. Sun WM, Read NW, Miner PB. Relationship between rectal sensation and anal function in normal subjects and patients with faecal incontinence. *Gut* 1990;**31**:1056–61.
31. Nagashima M, Iwai N, *et al.* Motility and sensation of the rectosigmoid and the rectum in patients with anorectal malformations. *J Pediat Surg* 1992;**27**:1273–7.
32. Office for National Statistics. Congenital anomaly statistics 1995–6. London: The Stationary Office, 1998:2–4.
33. Rintala R, Lindahl H, Rasanen M. Do children with repaired low anorectal malformations have normal bowel function? *J Pediat Surg* 1997;**32**:823–6.
34. Rintala R, Lindahl H, Sariola H, *et al.* The rectourogenital connection in anorectal malformations is really an ectopic anal canal. *J Pediat Surg* 1990;**25**:665–8.

35. Rintala R, Mildh L, Lindahl H. Faecal continence and quality of life for adult patients with an operated high or intermediate anorectal malformation *J Pediat Surg* 1994;**29**:777–80.
36. Rintala RJ, Marttinen E, *et al.* Segmental colonic motility in patients with anorectal malformations. *J Pediat Surg* 1997;**32**:453–6.
37. Kenny SE, Connell MG, Rintala RJ, *et al.* Abnormal colonic interstitial cells of Cajal in children with anorectal malformations. *J Pediat Surg* 1998;**33**:130–2.
38. Iwai N, Iwata G, Kimura O, Yanagihara J. Is a new biofeedback therapy effective for fecal incontinence in patients who have anorectal malformations? *J Pediat Surg* 1997;**32**:1626–9.
39. Pena A, Guardino K, *et al.* Bowel management for fecal incontinence in patients with anorectal malformations. *J Pediat Surg* 1998;**33**:133–7.
40. Arhan P, Faverdin C, *et al.* Biofeedback re-education of faecal continence in children. *Int J Colorectal Dis* 1994;**9**:128–33.
41. Arnbjornsson E, Breland U, *et al.* Effect of Loperamide on faecal control after rectoplasty for high imperforate anus. *Acta Chir Scand* 1986;**152**:215–6.
42. Harford W, Krejs G, *et al.* Acute effect of diphenoxylate with atropine in patients with chronic diarrhea and fecal incontinence. *Gastroenterology* 1990;**78**:440–3.
43. Ko CY, Tong J, *et al.* Biofeedback is effective therapy for fecal incontinence and constipation. *Arch Surg* 1997;**132**:829–34.
44. Glia A, Gylin M, *et al.* Biofeedback training in patients with fecal incontinence. *Dis Colon Rectum* 1998;**41**:359–64.
45. Rieger N, Wattchow D, *et al.* Prospective trial of pelvic floor retraining in patients with fecal incontinence. *Dis Colon Rectum* 1997;**40**:821–6.
46. Osterberg A, Graf W, *et al.* Is electrostimulation of the pelvic floor an effective treatment for neurogenic faecal incontinence? *Scand J Gastroenterol* 1999; **34**:319–24.
47. Fynes M, Marshall K, *et al.* A prospective randomized study comparing the effect of augmented biofeedback with sensory biofeedback alone on fecal incontinence after obstetric trauma. *Dis Colon Rectum* 1999;**42**:753–61.
48. Poen AC, Felt-Bersma RJF, Strijers RLM, *et al.* Third degree obstetric perineal rupture (Abstract). *Gastroenterology* 1998;**118**:A822.
49. Rasmussen OO, Puggaard L, Christiansen J. Anal sphincter repair in patients with obstetric trauma – age affects outcome. *Dis Colon Rectum* 1999;**42**:193–5.
50. Parks AG, McPartlin JF. Late repair of injuries of the anal sphincter. *J Roy Soc Med* 1971;**64**:1187–9.
51. Romano G, Rotondano G, *et al.* External anal sphincter defects: correlation between pre-operative anal endosonography and intra-operative findings. *Br J Radiol* 1996;**69**:6–9
52. Sultan AH, Kamm MA, *et al.* Anal endosonography for identifying external sphincter defects confirmed histologically. *Br J Surg* 1994;**81**:463–5.
53. Ingham-Clark C, Rihani H, Nicholls RJ, *et al.* Peri-operative management of patients undergoing anal sphincter repair. (Abstract). *Br J Surg* 1997;**84**:38–9.
54. Nessim A, Wexner SD, *et al.* Is bowel confinement necessary after anorectal surgery? *Dis Colon Rectum* 1999;**42**:16–23.
55. Browning GGP, Motson RW. Anal sphincter injury. *Ann Surg* 1984;**199**:352–7.
56. Engel A, Lunniss PJ, *et al.* Sphincteroplasty for incontinence after surgery for idiopathic fistula in ano. *Int J Colorectal Dis* 1997;**12**:323–5.
57. Engel A, Kamm MA, *et al.* Civilian and war injuries of the perineum and anal sphincters. *Br J Surg* 1994;**81**:1069.
58. Engel A, Kamm MA, Sultan AH, *et al.* Anterior anal sphincter repair in patients with obstetric trauma. *Br J Surg* 1994;**81**:1231–4.
59. Hool GR, Lieber ML, Church JM. Postoperative anal canal length predicts outcome in patients having sphincter repair for fecal incontinence. *Dis Colon Rectum* 1999;**42**:313–8.
60. Laurberg S, Swash M, Henry MM. Delayed external sphincter repair for obstetric tear. *Br J Surg* 1988;**75**:786–8.
61. Londono-Schimmer E, Garcia-Duperly R, *et al.* Overlapping anal sphincter repair for faecal incontinence due to sphincter trauma: five year follow-up functional results. *Int J Colorectal Dis* 1994;**9**:110–3.
62. Wexner SD, Marchetti F, Jagelman DG. The role of sphincteroplasty for fecal incontinence reevaluated: a prospective physiological and functional review. *Dis Colon Rectum* 1991;**34**:22–30.
63. Young CJ, Mathur MN, Eyers AE, Solomon MJ. Successful overlapping anal sphincter repair. *Dis Colon Rectum* 1998;**41**:344–9.
64. Briel J, de Boer L, Hop WCJ, Schouten WR. Clinical outcome of anterior overlapping external anal sphincter repair with internal anal sphincter imbrication. *Dis Colon Rectum* 1998;**41**:209–14.
65. Deen KI, Kumar D, Williams JG, *et al.* Randomized trial of internal anal sphincter plication with pelvic floor repair for neuropathic fecal incontinence. *Dis Colon Rectum* 1995;**38**:14–8.
66. Leroi AM, Kamm MA, Weber J, *et al.* Internal anal sphincter repair. *Int J Colorectal Dis* 1997;**12**:243–5.
67. Jensen LL, Lowry AC. Biofeedback improves functional outcome after sphincteroplasty. *Dis Colon Rectum* 1997;**40**:197–200.
68. Pinedo G, Vaizey CJ, Nicholls RJ, *et al.* Results of repeat anal sphincter repair. *Br J Surg* 1999;**86**:66–9.
69. Engel A, Brummelkamp W. Secondary surgery after failed postanal or anterior sphincter repair. *Int J Colorectal Dis* 1994;**9**:187–90.
70. Enriquez-Navascues JM, Devesa-Mugica JM. Traumatic anal incontinence role of unilateral gluteus maximus transposition supplementing and supporting direct anal sphincteroplasty. *Dis Colon Rectum* 1994;**37**:766–9.
71. Romano G, Rotondano G, *et al.* External anal sphincter defects: correlation between pre-operative anal endosonography and intra-operative findings. *Br J Radiol* 1996;**69**:6–9.
72. Womack N, Morrison J, Williams NS. Prospective study of the effects of post anal repair in neurogenic faecal incontinence. *Br J Surg* 1988;**75**:48–52.
73. Keighley MRB, Fielding JWL. Management of faecal incontinence and results of surgical treatment. *Br J Surg* 1983;**70**:463–8.

74. Jameson JS, Speakman CTM, Darzi A, Chia YW, Henry MM. Audit of postanal repair in the treatment of fecal incontinence. *Dis Colon Rectum* 1994;**37**:369–72.
75. Varma JS, Binnie NR, Kawimbe B, *et al.* A regional audit of the investigation and treatment of pelvic floor disorders. *Int J Colorectal Dis* 1993;**8**:66–70.
76. Orrom WJ, Miller R, *et al.* Comparison of anterior levatorplasty and postanal repair in the treatment of idiopathic incontinence. *Dis Colon Rectum* 1991;**34**:-305–10.
77. Osterberg A, Graf W, *et al.* Long-term results of anterior levatorplasty for fecal incontinence. *Dis Colon Rectum* 1996;**39**:671–5.
78. Deen KI, Oya M, Ortiz J, Keighley MRB. Randomized trial comparing three methods of pelvic floor repair for neuropathic faecal incontinence. *Br J Surg* 1993;**80**:794–8.
79. Korsgen S, Deen KI, Keighley MRB. Long-term results of total pelvic floor repair for postobstetric fecal incontinence. *Dis Colon Rectum* 1997;**40**:835–9.
80. van Tets WF, Kuijpers JHC. Pelvic floor procedures produce no consistent changes in anatomy or physiology. *Dis Colon Rectum* 1998;**41**:365–9.
81. Williams NS, Patel J, George BD, *et al.* Development of an electrically stimulated neoanal sphincter. *Lancet* 1991;**338**:1166–9.
82. Konsten J, Baeten CG, Havemith MG, Soeters PB. Morphology of dynamic graciloplasty compared with the anal sphincter. *Dis Colon Rectum* 1993;**36**:559–63.
83. Konsten J, Baeten CG, *et al.* Follow-up of anal dynamic graciloplasty for fecal continence. *World J Surg* 1993;**17**:404–9.
84. Mavrantonis C, Wexner SD. Stimulated graciloplasty for treatment of intractable fecal incontinence. *Dis Colon Rectum* 1999;**42**:497–504.
85. Altomare DF, Boffoli D, *et al.* Fast-to-slow muscle conversion by chronic electrostimulation: effects on mitochondrial respiratory chain function with possible implications for the gracilis neosphincter procedure. *Br J Surg* 1996;**83**:1569–73.
86. Yoshioka K, Keighley MRB. Clinical and manometric assessment of gracilis muscle transplant for fecal incontinence. *Dis Colon Rectum* 1998;**31**:767–9.
87. Christiansen J, Sorensen M, Rasmussen O. Gracilis muscle transposition for faecal incontinence. *Br J Surg* 1990;**77**:1039–40.
88. Faucheron J-L, Hannoun L, Thorne C, Parc R. Is fecal continence improved by nonstimulated gracilis muscle transposition. *Dis Colon Rectum* 1994;**37**:979–83.
89. Sielezneff I, Bauer S, Bulgare JC, Sarles JC. Gracilis muscle transposition in the treatment of faecal incontinence. *Int J Colorectal Dis* 1996;**11**:15–8.
90. Eccersley AJP, Lunniss PJ, Williams NS. Unstimulated graciloplasty in traumatic faecal incontinence. *Br J Surg* 1999;**86**:1071–2.
91. Kumar D, Hutchinson R, Grant E. Bilateral gracilis neosphincter construction for treatment of faecal incontinence. *Br J Surg* 1995;**82**:1645–7.
92. Korsgen S, Keighley MRB. Stimulated gracilis neosphincter – not as good as previously thought. *Dis Colon Rectum* 1995;**38**:1331–3.
93. Sielezneff I, Malouf AJ, Bartolo DC, *et al.* Dynamic graciloplasty in the treatment of patients with faecal incontinence. *Br J Surg* 1999;**86**:61–5.
94. Christiansen J, Rasmussen O, Lindorff-Larsen K. Dynamic graciloplasty for severe anal incontinence. *Br J Surg* 1998;**85**:88–91.
95. Baeten C, Geerdes B, Adang E, *et al.* Anal dynamic graciloplasty in the treatment of intractable fecal incontinence. *N Engl J Med* 1995;**332**:1600–5.
96. Stuchfield B, Eccersley AJP. The modern management of faecal incontinence. In: Porrett T & Daniel N (eds). *Essential coloproctology*, 1st edn. London: Whurr Publishers, 1999:292–317.
97. Rosen HR, Novi GN, Zoech G, *et al.* Restoration of anal sphincter function by single-stage dynamic graciloplasty with a modified (Split sling) technique. *Am J Surg* 1998;**175**:187–93.
98. Madoff RD, Rosen HR, Baeten CG, *et al.* Safety and efficacy of dynamic muscle plasty for anal incontinence: lessons from a prospective, multicenter trial. *Gastroenterology* 1999;**116**:549–56.
99. Mander BJ, Williams NS. The electrically stimulated gracilis neosphincter. *Eur J Gastro Hepatol* 1997;**9**:435–41.
100. Eccersley AJP, Maw A, Williams NS. Quality of life can be improved by anorectal reconstruction (Abstract). *Int J Colorectal Dis* 1997;**12**:130.
101. Altomare DF, Rinaldi M, Pannarale OC, Memeo V. Electrostimulated gracilis neosphincter for faecal incontinence. *Int J Colorectal Dis* 1997;**12**:308–12.
102. Devesa JM, Madrid JM, Gallego BR, *et al.* Bilateral gluteoplasty for fecal incontinence. *Dis Colon Rectum* 1997;**40**:883–8.
103. Yoshioka K, Ogunbiyi OA, Keighley MRB. A pilot study of total pelvic floor repair or gluteus maximus transposition for postobstetric neuropathic fecal incontinence. *Dis Colon Rectum* 1999;**42**:252–7.
104. Wong WD, Jensen LJ, Bartolo DC, Rothenberger DA. Artificial anal sphincter. *Dis Colon Rectum* 1996;**39**:1345–51.
105. Lehur P-A, Michot F, *et al.* Results of artificial bowel sphincter in severe anal incontinence. *Dis Colon Rectum* 1996;**39**:1352–5.
106. Hajivassiliou CA, Finlay IG. Effect of a novel prosthetic anal neosphincter on human colonic blood flow. *Br J Surg* 1998;**85**:1703–7.
107. Briel JW, Schouten WR, Vlot EA, *et al.* Clinical value of colonic irrigation in patients with continence disturbances. *Dis Colon Rectum* 1997;**40**:802–5.
108. Webb HW, Barraza MA, Crump JM. Laparoscopic appendicostomy for management of fecal incontinence. *J Pediat Surg* 1997;**32**:457–8.
109. Wilcox DT, Kiely EM. The Malone antegrade colonic enema procedure: Early experience. *J Pediat Surg* 1998;**33**:204–6.
110. Koyle MA, Kaji DM, Duque M, *et al.* The Malone antegrade continence enema for neurogenic and structural fecal incontinence and constipation. *J Urol* 1995;**154**:759–61.
111. Maw A, Williams NS. The colonic conduit for disorders of colorectal evacuation. *Persp Colon Rectal Surg* 1998;**11**:43–65.

112. Hughes SF, Williams NS. Continent colonic conduit for the treatment of faecal incontinence associated with disordered evacuation. *Br J Surg* 1995;**82**:1318–20.
113. Dick A, McCallion W, *et al.* Antegrade colonic enemas. *Br J Surg* 1996;**83**:642–3.
114. Alstrup NI, Rasmussen O, Christiansen J. Effect of rectal dilatation in fecal incontinence with low rectal compliance. *Dis Colon Rectum* 1995;**38**:988–9.

Chapter 25

Solitary rectal ulcer, rectocele, hemorrhoids and pelvic pain

Leo P Lawler, James W Fleshman

SOLITARY RECTAL ULCER

INTRODUCTION

Crueilhier is credited with the first report of this entity in 1829.[1] The term we now commonly use was introduced by a St Mark's surgeon, Lloyd-Davies, in the 1930s.[2] The first full clinical descriptions of solitary rectal ulcer syndrome (SRUS) came from Madigan and Morson.[3,4] Over time, the usual clinical problems associated with SRUS became manifest as bleeding, altered bowel habit, mucus discharge and proctalgia fugax (intermittent pain and rectal spasm).

PATHOPHYSIOLOGY

Pathological findings

Gross

Macroscopically, the ulcer in SRUS is usually an erythematous, friable, thickened patch of mucosa. However, it may be more advanced forming a circumferential, deep, ulcer exposing rectal muscle with surrounding heaped mucosa (Fig. 25.1).

Although classically described on the anterior wall, the ulceration has been found at other sites.[5,6] It has been polypoid in some cases.[6–8] A SRUS can be found anywhere from 5 to 12 cm from the anal verge. This may be due to ischemia caused by internal intussusception of the rectum or pressure of the rectal wall against the anal canal during ineffectual straining to evacuate. This area is frequently mistaken for a flat cancer and has often resulted in rectal resection.

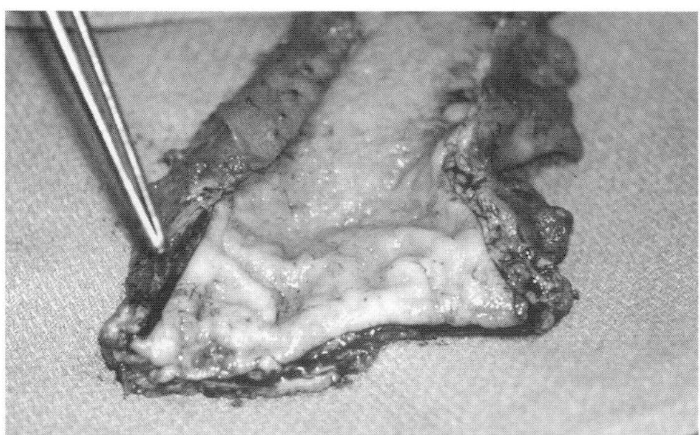

Figure 25.1 Rectal specimen showing heaped ridges of mucosa in a thickened rectal wall.

Histology

Histologically, the ulcer shows a lamina propria replaced by fibroblasts and smooth muscle fibers extending from a thickened muscularis mucosa, and shortening of the crypts.[9–11] The histological features in SRUS and complete rectal prolapse are similar. However, in SRUS there is greater rectal wall thickening and collagen deposition, possibly representing a response to repeated trauma.

Architectural derangement of the muscle fibers may be unique to SRUS.[10] It has been suggested that the continued urge to defecate stimulates the muscularis enough over time to cause its hypertrophy. However, the defecatory urge may, in fact, be secondary to the muscular hypertrophy itself caused by an unknown local process. In some patients, the region of the ulcer takes on an appearance similar to sphincter muscle and thus may represent an area of abnormal increased pressure.[10]

Over time, the histological features resemble chronic ischemia, and transitional epithelium develops. Glands may be trapped in the submucosa during the repeated injury and healing process, and result in the entity of colitis cystica profunda. Colitis cystica profunda has been reported in 6% of cases.[12] It has also been postulated that abnormal muscle contractions may force the glands into the submucosa. Biopsies of colitis cystica profunda may sometimes be mis-interpreted as cancer because of the deep aberrant position of the glands below the muscularis mucosa. However, the pathologist should be able to determine that the glands are otherwise histologically normal. Heavy deposition of collagen fibers by fibroblasts has been observed by electron microscopy, probably representing attempts at healing in response to trauma. This should not be misinterpreted as a desmoplastic response to an invasive cancer.

Etiological agents

The following have been suggested as possible etiological agents for the solitary rectal ulcer:

- Hyperactive anal sphincters
- Weak anal sphincters
- Raised electrosensory threshold of the rectal mucosa
- Raised intrarectal pressures
- Internal rectal intussusception
- Rectal prolapse
- Systemic disease
- Paradoxical puborectalis action
- Digital trauma to the distal rectum.

The pathophysiologic findings in the setting of a solitary rectal ulcer include altered electrosensitivity of the rectal wall, microvascular abnormalities in the submucosa, and thickening of the muscularis propria. The cause and effect relationships remain unclear. Defecation disorders noted to have an association with SRUS are failure of the puborectalis to relax, rectal prolapse, internal rectal intussusception, increased anorectal angle, abnormal perineal descent and decreased anorectal sensitivity to ballon inflation.[13]

Defecation disorder

Constipation and fecal impaction may play a role in the etiology of SRUS. Stercoral ulceration has a similar appearance but can usually be related to an adherent piece of stool. Personality disorder, manual disimpaction, autoeroticism and ergotamine suppositories (ischemia) have all been implicated in the etiology. Self-manipulation probably has a limited role in the development of this condition,[14] although, in the past, many people were accused of such behavior because of our lack of understanding of this problem. However, digital rectal evacuation may indeed account for some ulcers.[14-16] Digitalizing to evacuate is reported in varying percentages of patients ranging from 8 to 90%.

Systemic disease

SRUS has also been associated with systemic disease relating it to recurrent oral ulcerations, erythema nodosum, sacroileitis and HLA B-27 histocompatibility antigen.[17] Systemic lupus erythematosus has been suggested as a source of vasculitis which may cause the typical ulcer of SRUS.

Pelvic floor abnormality

Abnormal perineal descent has been observed in patients with SRUS.[18] However, since perineal descent is felt to be a sign of pelvic floor dysfunction or outlet obstruction, it should not be misconstrued as a primary source of SRUS.

Sphincter dysfunction

Both hyperactive and weak sphincters have been noted in patients with SRUS. Inappropriate Puborectalis Muscle contraction is not universal however. Van Outyrve confirmed on ultrasound the failure of the puborectalis to relax in a series of patients with SRUS.[19] He implicated the inappropriate PRM relaxation as the direct cause of the increased load on the rectal wall and consequent muscularis propria enlargement.

Abnormal pudendal nerve terminal motor latencies (PNTML), and single fiber electromyography (EMG) have been reported suggesting sphincter function compromise due to pudendal nerve injury.[20] It is difficult to determine whether patients with SRUS develop pudendal nerve damage due to the excessive straining associated with the syndrome, or whether a weak external sphincter from pudendal neuropathy may be a result of obstetric trauma. A compromised sphincter may allow the rectal mucosa to prolapse and ulcerate.

Straining at stool is common in this patient population and paradoxical overactivity of the anal sphincter has been reported.[20] The resulting high intrarectal pressures may have a role in mucosal trauma, especially if the intussuscepting rectum is pushed down to the closed anal canal. High intrarectal pressures may also expose the rectal wall to high transmural gradients.[21] Womack suggested that raised intrarectal pressures, aggravated by the inappropriate sphincter contraction, caused venous engorgement and ulceration. He noted increased EMG activity in the external anal sphincter and high voiding pressures in the SRUS group. Excessive straining to overcome the inappropriate sphincter contraction was suggested as a cause for the rectal prolapse in SRUS in that study.

Electrosensory threshold

An impaired electrosensory threshold has been seen in patients with SRUS.[22] Conversely, Sun *et al.*[23] suggest that the combination of rectal hypersensitivity and anal sphincter weakness leads to prolapse and SRUS. Rectal hypersensitivity causes abnormal straining and a continued urge to evacuate. This eventually results in mucosal prolapse and high intrarectal pressures. The evolution of rectal prolapse from mucosal prolapse is not guaranteed. One could speculate that impaired sensitivity is a late finding and hypersensitivity is an early finding in prolapse and SRUS.

Intussusceptions defecating proctography

Defecatory proctography has revealed an association between rectal intussusception and SRUS.[7,24] However, internal intussusception is seen in normal subjects. It has been suggested that the configuration of the intussusception with its apex directed toward the rectal lumen, rather than the anal canal and the associated thickened folds, separates the SRUS form of intussusception from normal individuals.[25] The association of internal intussusception and SRUS makes a very attractive hypothesis that local ischemia at the lead point of the intussusceptum is a cause of SRUS.

Rectal prolapses

It has been suggested that solitary rectal ulcer and complete rectal prolapse share a common pathophysiology,[21,23,26] mainly because they are often found together and therefore there is guilt by association.[6,21] Many authors continue to believe SRUS to be the consequence of rectal prolapse which causes an inflammation in the wall of the prolapsed rectum.[24,26–29]

Madigan *et al.* showed that only 30% of patients with SRUS had prolapse, but Womack *et al.* found a higher incidence.[4,21] The histologic features of SRUS and prolapse are similar.[4,26] The physiologic findings of low anal pressure, sensitive and reactive rectum, abnormal perineal descent, prolonged pudendal nerve terminal motor latencies and increased fibre density of the external anal sphincter are also seen in both conditions.[20,21,23,30] However, these are two distinct conditions in terms of the symptom complex and histologic features. Both may be part of a spectrum of the same disease. Whatever the subtle differences in pathophysiology, the findings of straining and the symptom of incomplete evacuation are more prominent in the solitary rectal ulcer group. Rutter *et al.* have suggested that the trauma and ischemia suffered by the prolapsing rectum due to excessive straining leads to the ulcer.[5] Kang *et al.*[31] showed that patients with SRUS, who had differing degrees of prolapse, also had different physiologic features depending on the degree of prolapse. They suggested that this was evidence for different disease entities causing SRUS, SRUS with prolapse, and SRUS with intussusception.

Management

Evaluation

The initial step in dealing with patients with SRUS is to clearly document the predominant symptom complex, which may include any combination of straining, digitalization, pain, laxative use, etc. This provides a baseline so that the response after treatment can be clearly documented. Physical examination may reveal an ulcerated lesion 6–8 cm above the dentate line with a surrounding raised edematous edge or, indeed, a polypoid excrescence. However, Thomson *et al.* described lesions thought to represent part of the spectrum of this disorder that were neither ulcerated nor solitary.[32]

Investigations such as manometry, defecography, barium enema and endorectal ultrasound may show some of the associated features or exclude other conditions. There is no consensus on the best investigation algorithm, though all of these tools have been used to varying extent.[7,19,24,25] Some would argue that just visualizing the lesion with rigid sigmoidoscopy and performing biopsy is adequate.[2] If the lesion is proximal to the rectum, inflammatory bowel disease must be excluded.

Barium enema may reveal ulceration, polypoid mass, stricture, granularity and rectal fold thickening but will seldom be adequate and usually requires direct visualization and biopsy for confirmation.[33] It has been suggested that defecating proctography is more appropriate than barium enema as the contrast study of choice, due to its inherent ability to evaluate associated conditions (Fig. 25.2). Defecating proctography may reveal the exaggerated impression of an overactive puborectalis.[25] The configuration of the intussusception and the thickness of the rectal folds may give evidence that this is associated pathology and not incidental.[25] A defecatory disorder may be documented by incomplete or delayed emptying. Prolapse and pelvic floor descent may be observed.

Anal manometry is intiated if the patient describes local incontinence. The possibility that incontinence is associated with rectal prolapse warrants performing pudendal nerve terminal motor latencies. Pudendal neuropathy is partially reversible and has been shown to influence outcome if a sphincter repair is contemplated.[34,35]

Defecographic evidence of non-relaxation of the puborectalis muscle should be confirmed with balloon expulsion[36] or anal electromyography[24] before assuming this is a true component of the symptom complex. Defecography is a non-physiologic test usually performed in an embarrassing 'public' setting and causes false positives for puborectalis problems, such as paradoxical puborectalis contraction during defecation.

Our preference for workup is:

- digital examination with the patient straining to expel the finger in order to evaluate the puborectalis sling (the puborectalis sling felt posteriorly at the level of the ano-rectal ring should move posteriorly to relax as the patient strains to expel rectal contents);
- proctosigmoidoscopy (biopsy if indicated);
- defecography (confirmed with balloon expulsion);
- colonoscopy to clear the rest of the colon of pathology.

It is sometimes difficult to distinguish colitis cystica profunda from adenocarcinoma. A biopsy reveals aberrantly placed *normal* glands with mucin lakes and a minimal desmoplastic reaction. A high index of suspicion is needed to make the diagnosis and communication of the suspicion of SRUS/colitis cystica profunda to the pathologist is sometimes essential to make the diagnosis of this benign condition. Colitis cystica profunda

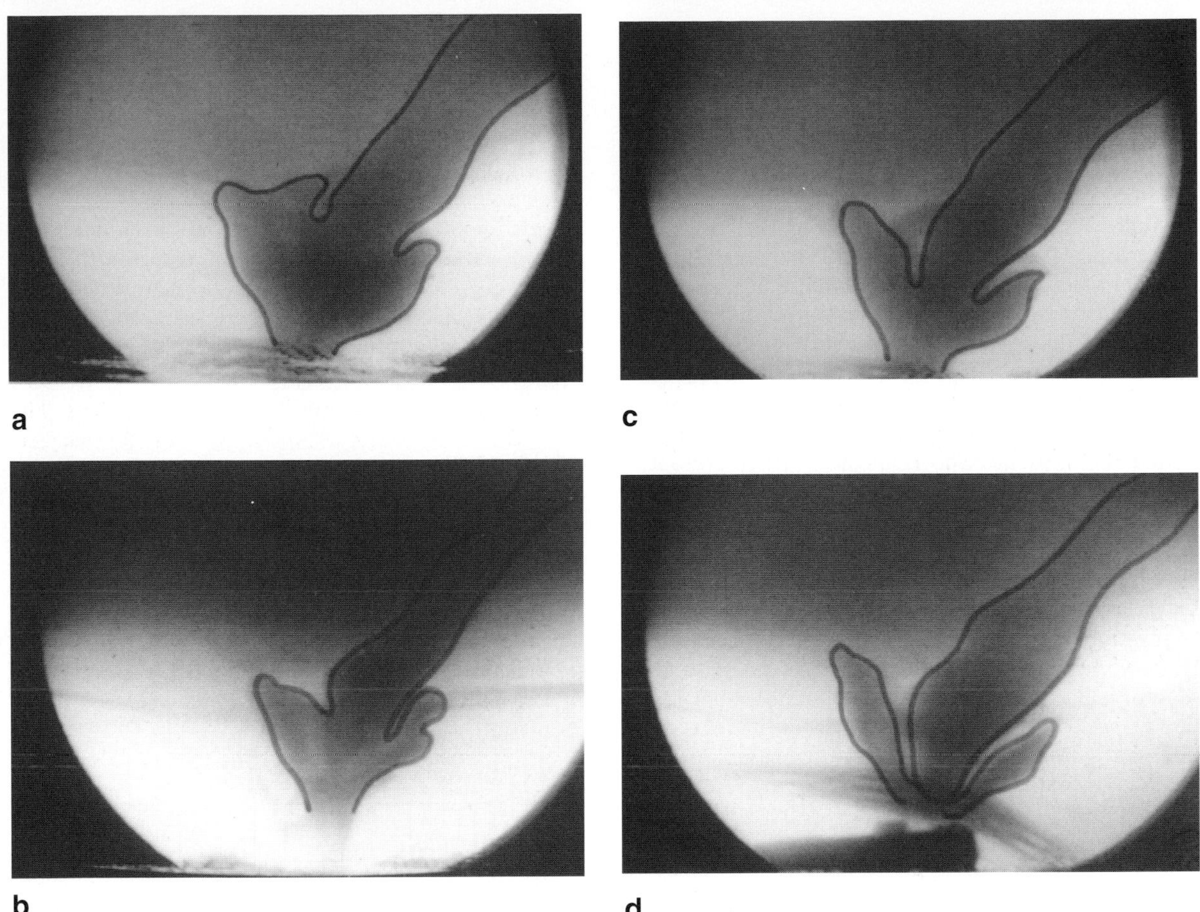

Figure 25.2 Defecography shows anterior rectocele. (a) Formation of lead point in mid rectum. (b) Early funneling of rectum. (c) Advanced funneling of rectum. (d) Full intussusception of mid rectum to anus.

as an entity is not an indication for resection. Awareness of its existence can prevent an unnecessary procedure in most patients.

Treatment

Conservative

The first line of treatment for any pelvic floor abnormality, especially SRUS, is high fiber diet and bowel management.[37] Enough fiber (insoluble) should be taken to expand the stool in the rectal vault, restore the normal sensation of a need to evacuate, and consolidate the stool in such a way that one large movement empties the rectum and the patient feels empty. This has taken as much as 18 g of psyllium husk daily in patients in our clinic. The patient is encouraged not to strain to defecate. Hydrocortisone enemas, local anesthetic and sucralfate retention enemas have all been suggested.[38]

Biofeedback for non-relaxing puborectalis involving pelvic floor coordination, posture, toilet schedule, and use of accessory muscles has shown some success.[8,12,39] This can be accomplished as an outpatient.[40] Biofeedback addresses a toileting behavior disorder with excessive straining. It may also be used as an adjunct to surgery. Vaizey *et al.* prospectively treated 13 patients with EMG biofeedback, and noted resolution of symptoms in four and improvement in four at 9-month follow-up.[39] However, the ulcer did not heal completely in any of this group.

Surgery

Surgical approaches in patients with SRUS involve the following:

- Rectopexy
- Coloanal anastomosis
- Anterior resection
- Local therapy
- Delorme's procedure.

Approaches that involve local excision, rectopexy and fecal diversion have all been employed and there is no consensus on the ideal operation. Operative management should be selected on a case by case approach. Most local therapies involve transanal local excision, cauterization of the ulcer base, injection of sclerosant, Nd-YAG laser of the ulcer or coverage of the area with human fibrin sealant.[8,12] Local treatments are more successful if there is no full thickness prolapse[8] and if they are limited to ulcers within reach of the anoscope.

Rectopexy, anterior resection of the rectosigmoid colon or colostomy is indicated for those failing conservative therapy or minor transanal surgery.[8,9,12,41] Haray found that those patients ultimately requiring surgery had long-standing symptoms or full thickness prolapse.[2] A retrospective review of patients with SRUS, treated with Ivalon sponge rectopexy at St Mark's Hospital, suggested that patients who responded well to rectopexy had evacuation times less than 15 seconds.[42] Patients who required prolonged evacuation did not respond as well to this surgery. In an earlier publication, this same group had suggested that anteroposterior rectopexy provided better resolution of SRUS compared with posterior rectopexy and anterior excision of the rectum. They correlated the finding of intussusception on defecating proctography with good response to abdominal rectopexy.[43] However, rectopexy alone for patients with intussusception results in continued constipation postoperatively and may produce less satisfying results from that point of view.[44]

Results with rectal excision and coloanal anastomosis have been disappointing.[45,46] In the setting of massive bleeding, a colostomy may be the best procedure. A low anterior resection becomes very difficult when the ulcer is at 6–8 cm and the rectum is very thick and inflamed. As a result, often a coloanal anastomosis is necessary to be able to avoid a permanent colostomy. The rectum in these circumstances becomes too thick to accept a transverse stapler across the rectum above the anal canal. The bowel fractures with closure of the stapler and an anastomosis is not possible. It is better to perform a rectopexy and re-evaluate in a month if possible. Only if bleeding is life threatening should a low anterior resection be contemplated.

If there is a causative relationship between prolapse or intussusception in this condition, treatment of these may yield benefit. In those with depressive illness, appropriate antidepressive therapy is indicated prior to biofeedback therapy.

RESULTS

Operative treatment of SRUS in its advanced stages is usually successful. Medical treatment has a variable outcome and depends on the underlying etiology of the SRUS. Surgical treatment should probably not be recommended until medical treatment has been tried.

It has been suggested that the finding of obstructed defecation is a predictor of poor surgical outcome.[42] Constipation often becomes worse after a rectopexy for SRUS. Each method of treatment must be evaluated on the basis of resolution of symptoms as well as objective healing of the solitary rectal ulcer. Table 25.1 provides a summary of results from a number of series. There are no good randomized trials to compare conservative and operative therapies. Not all series reported outcome based on symptoms. However, conservative measures aimed at eliminating straining or paradoxical contraction of the puborectalis muscle seem to be equally as successful as an operative approach.

CONCLUSION

Solitary rectal ulcer syndrome is not a psychological disease. Medical treatment with high doses of fiber together with pelvic floor retraining may be successful and should be attempted before surgical repair. Surgical repair of SRUS should be tailored to the associated problems: low anterior resection in patients with constipation, and rectopexy in patients with severe internal intussusception and fecal incontinence.

RECTOCELE

INTRODUCTION

Rectocele is defined as a hernial protrusion of the anterior rectal wall and the posterior vaginal wall into the vagina and through the vaginal introitus (Fig. 25.3). Rectoceles are classified by their position relative to the vagina: low, middle and high. It is part of a 'pelvic laxity syndrome' and may be associated with cystocele and cystoeurethrocele. Also, middle and high rectoceles are more commonly associated with enterocele and cystocele because their etiology is related to the lax pelvic floor (Fig. 25.4). However, low rectoceles are usually associated with scarring and shortening of the anterior anal sphincter mechanism.

It was Redding who first recognized rectocele as a source of symptoms such as constipation, anal pain and bleeding.[47] Murthy *et al.*[48] and Klevin *et al.*[49] both showed correlation between the size of the anterior bulge and intensity of symptoms. It must be remembered that rectocele is found in the normal population,[50,51] and there is a spectrum of symptoms not always correlating with size. Improved imaging, such as defecography and dynamic MRI, detect more abnormalities which may not be clinically relevant. A rectocele which is 2 cm in depth is generally big enough to cause symptoms. This is not always the case, however. Obviously, the size of the rectocele is less important than the symptoms it produces. The impact of the recto-

Table 25.1 Summary of results of treatment for solitary rectal ulcer comparing a number of series.

Author	Patients	Approach	Outcome
van den Brandt-Gradel	21	High fiber No straining	15 no symptoms healing 10.5 m 6 no change
Vaizey CJ		Biofeedback Abdominal rectopexy	Symptoms improved in majority 50% symptoms improved Rectal ulcer may persist with symptom improvement
Sitzler PJ	66	49 rectopexy 9 Delorme 2 anterior resection 4 stoma	Failed 22 of 49 4 Failed 4 Failed Overall stoma rate 30% Surgery satisfactory in 55–60%
Vaizey CJ	13	Biofeedback	4 asymptomatic 4 improved No complete healing of ulcer
Costalat G	22	Intersphincteric rectopexy or abdominal rectopexy 3 Proltapsectomy	2 failed 80% symptoms improved
Tjandra JJ	69	Bulk laxative Bowel retraining	29% no change in symptoms 19% improved 29% surgery
Zargar SA	6	Topical sucralfate	4 complete relief 2 improved 1 recurrence
Nicholls RJ	14	Anterior posterior rectopexy	Symptoms improved in 12 Defecation attempts decreased Lavatory time decreased 2 constipation 1 tenesmus
Martin CJ	51	Roughage Sponge rectopexy	Benefit in 66% 50% satisfactory
Binnie NR	14 17	Conserv. or surgery Biofeedback with surgery	High recurrence rate: 15 episodes 4 episodes recurrence

cele may depend on the presence of associated abnormalities, such as nonrelaxing puborectalis or anal incontinence.

PATHOPHYSIOLOGY

Uhlenhuth provided one of the early descriptions of the female equivalent of Denonvillier's fascia.[52] Situated deep in the pelvic cavity at the pelvic outlet, the rectovaginal septum separates the dorsal (rectal) compartment from the ventral urogenital compartment. Richardson demonstrated tears in this septum in individuals with rectocele. Most commonly, this manifests as a transverse separation immediately above the attachment to the perineal body.[53] Trauma, such as obstetrical injury, seems to have a role in weakening the rectovaginal septum. The sphincter is shortened and the perineal body is thinned. It has been postulated that thinning of the rectovaginal septum and/or pelvic denervation, secondary to hysterectomy, may contribute to formation of a rectocele.[54] The possibility exists that a vaginal hysterectomy puts a woman at more risk of rectocele than a total abdominal hysterectomy, due to the increased rectovaginal trauma and pelvic floor denervation induced by the transvaginal approach. It has also been noted that some patients have associated paradoxical sphincter contraction and raised mean resting rectal pressures.[55,56] The postmenopausal state with supporting tissue laxity cannot be discounted in the pathogenesis.

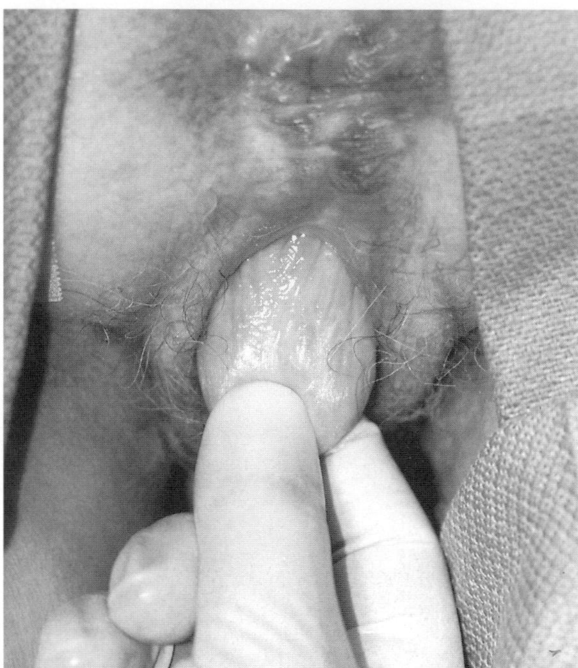

Figure 25.3 Full vaginal prolapse of anterior rectocele. Patient in prone jackknife position.

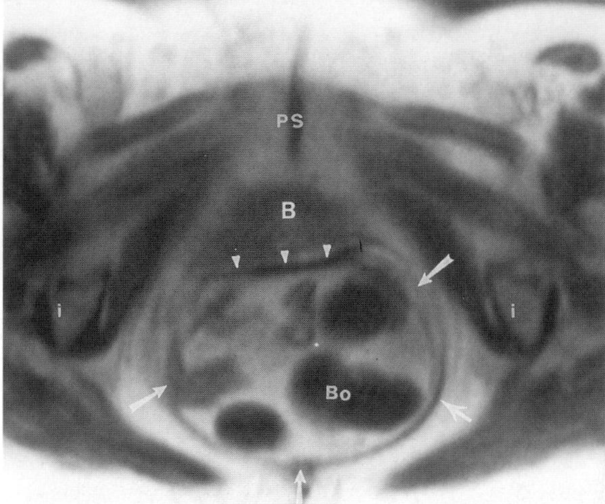

Figure 25.4 Axial MRI image during straining. Contained within a distortion of the pouch of Douglas (white arrows) can be seen bowel loops (Bo) comprised of enterocele and sigmoidocele and rectocele. The abnormality is clearly seen posterior to the low signal vaginal cuff (white arrowheads) and low signal bladder neck (B). The ischial tuberosities (I) and symphysis pubis (PS) give anatomic orientation. (Courtesy of Dr Vamsi Narra, Mallinckrodt Institute of Radiology, St Louis.)

It is unclear where rectocele fits in the pathogenesis of constipation and the role constipation has in the etiology of a rectocele.[57,58] A rectocele is usually found in the setting of other pelvic problems and thus may share a common etiology. However, it is clear at this point that the etiology of rectocele may be different in each individual, with different implications for evaluation and therapy.[59]

MANAGEMENT

Indications for treatment

Indications for treatment of a rectocele include disturbance of evacuation, rectal pain, a need to aid evacuation by stenting the posterior vaginal wall digitally, stool pocketing, protrusion through the introitus, and a symptomatic lump in the perineal body or posterior vagina. Repair may also be indicated if repair of an associated cystocele or enterocele is required.[60] Occasionally, a rectocele will produce enough vaginal wall prolapse to cause significant bleeding, which responds only to rectocele repair.

Clinical evaluation

This includes:

- History
- Physical exam including digital rectal exam
- Proctosigmoidoscopy
- Manometry
- Defecography
- Dynamic MRI
- Transrectal ultrasound
- Pudendal nerve terminal motor latency
- Balloon expulsion.

Thorough evaluation including assessment of the need for surgery and factors affecting the surgical approach, requires a history and physical examination as well as defecography for the majority of patients.[61]

In some cases, anorectal manometry may be of value. The exact role of dynamic MRI is still under review. Eventually, dynamic MRI may replace defecography and TRUS to evaluate pelvic floor anatomy. The use of an intra-rectal coil provides exquisite detail of pelvic structures but may impair mobility since the coil is stiff. Dynamic MRI can elucidate pelvic floor hernias, enteroceles, cystoceles, rectoceles, internal intussusception, sigmoidoceles and anal sphincter defects[62] (Fig. 25.5). Our current standard approach involves performing a fast dynamic sequence using a half Fourier transform turbo-spin echo producing live images during rest and straining. Our standard measurements involve either pubococcygeal or pubosacral reference lines, and lines perpendicular to bladder neck, cervix and pelvic floor

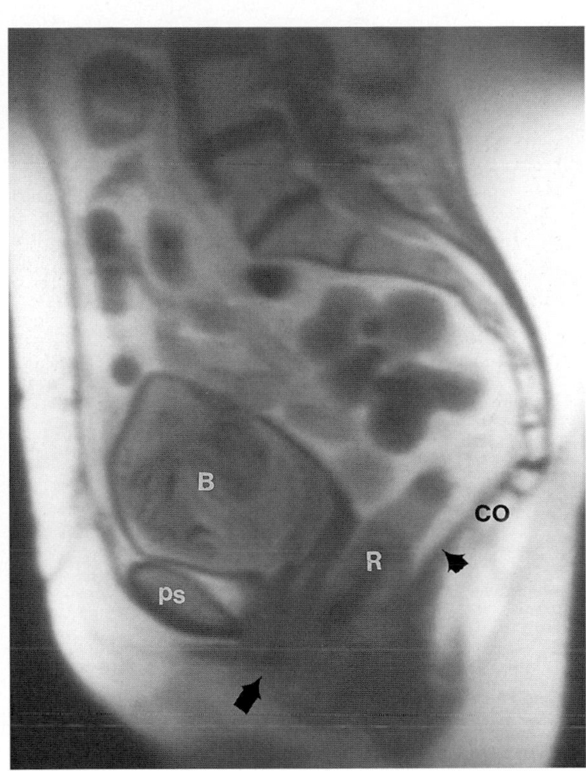

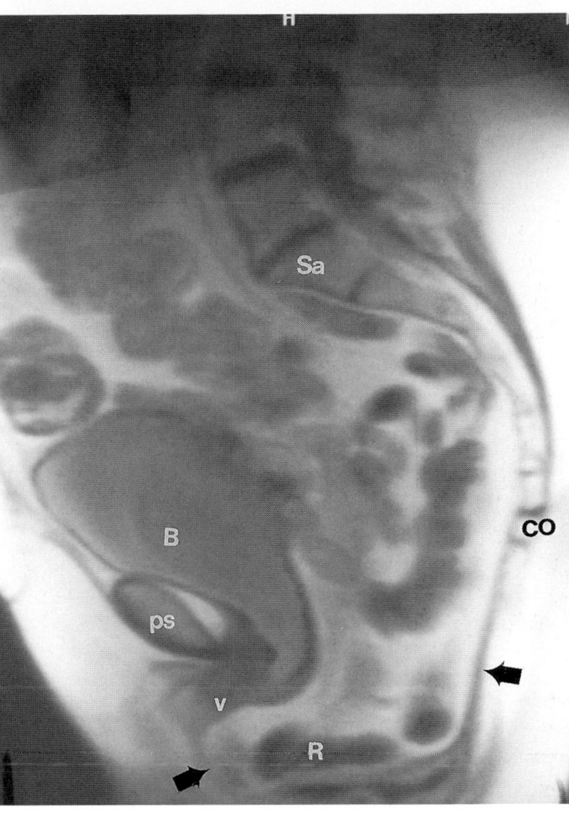

a b

Figure 25.5 Sagittal MRI images at rest (a) and straining (b). Compared with rest (b), a well-demarcated low signal levator muscle is noted (a, arrows), descending with Valsalva in this patient with marked pelvic floor weakness. Note also the rectum [R] enters the capacious pouch thus formed and is posterior to the vagina (v) and introitus. The anatomical landmarks of sacrum (Sa), coccyx (CO) and pubic symphysis (ps) are also seen. (Courtesy Dr Vamsi Narra, Mallinckrodt Institute of Radiology, St. Louis.)

(Fig. 25.6). More experience is needed to define the role of dynamic MRI in the evaluation of these problems. Other tests, such as axial imaging contrast studies and ultrasound, are recommended on an individual basis but are not part of the routine work-up of an uncomplicated rectocele. There is little doubt that the correct choice of tests based on clinical history optimizes the chances of a good outcome.[49]

The history may reveal the need to digitally aid evacuation, thought by some to be a good indication for surgery and a predictor of good response to surgery.[49] Factors such as difficult evacuation, as well as the sensation of a mass in the vagina, may become apparent. The obstetric history and gynecological history, particularly of hysterectomy, must be sought as they are often implicated in the pathogenesis. It is also important to look for, and to note, associated conditions commonly found in this setting such as incomplete urinary voiding, suggesting bladder herniation or urinary bladder outlet obstruction. Once one has defined the rectocele, the next step is to be cognizant of those other conditions that may influence the final decision regarding the likely success of any intervention. A leading condition among those to be considered is that of obstructed defecation which is evidenced by excessive and prolonged straining at defecation on a regular basis. The causes of obstructed defecation include anal stenosis, non-relaxing puborectalis, internal intussusception, megarectum and sigmoidocele.

Digital rectal examination may reveal the weak anterior rectal wall. It is difficult to differentiate an enterocele, sigmoidocele and rectocele by vaginal examination. It is also difficult to evaluate the size of the rectocele and impossible to measure its ability to empty. Due to these limitations, one is obliged to proceed to other investigations in the evaluation of a symptomatic rectocele.

The role of defecography (evacuation proctography) is to document the presence of a rectocele (Fig. 25.7), its

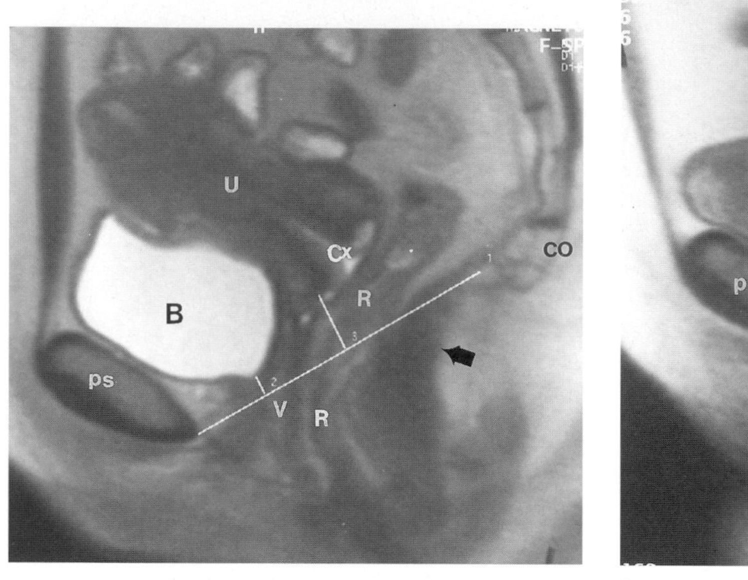

a

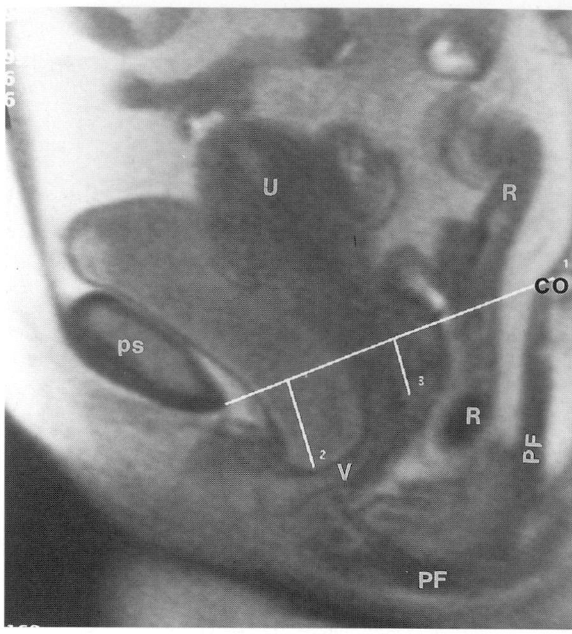

b

Figure 25.6 Sagittal MRI images at rest (a) and straining (b). The pubococcygeal line (1), base of bladder (2) and external cervical os (3) are illustrated. Also seen are the anatomical landmarks of uterus (U), cervix (Cx), coccygeus (CO) and symphysis pubis (ps). Note: with straining, the descent of the pelvic floor (a, arrow; b, PF) as well as bladder neck, vagina (V) and rectum (R). All MRI images were obtained using a half Fourier transform turbo-spin echo with cine imaging. Each image was obtained in less than half a second. (Courtesy Dr Vamsi Narra, Mallinckrodt Institute of Radiology, St Louis.)

size and whether any associated conditions exist such as intussusception, enterocele and cystocele. Upper gastrointestinal and bladder contrast material must be employed during the test to achieve this goal. Vaginal contrast is also essential to identify disruption of the normal vaginal contour by the anterior rectal wall. The rectum is evacuated at the end of defecography and the ability to evacuate the rectocele is assessed. Note is made of the retention of any contrast within the rectocele. This alone has been used as an indication for surgery. However, for most surgeons it is an important, but not essential, factor in deciding whether an operation is indicated. Mellgren *et al.* have suggested hesitation in advising surgical intervention if the cavity empties completely.[63] Others have seen improvement in symptoms even if a rectocele is repaired which empties completely. The retention of contrast is thought to be due to the anterior wall inverting over the anal canal as it emptied to close off the anterior portion of the rectocele. Van Dam *et al.* evaluated the role of defecography and showed that the parameters of rectocele size, internal intussusception, rectal evacuation, perineal descent or radiological signs of anismus had no effect on correction of symptoms after operative repair.[64] They saw the role of defecography as documenting the rectocele and any associated abnormalities such as enterocele. Defecography is also useful as an objective means of assessing the surgical outcome. Physiological studies, such as manometry, pudendal nerve terminal motor latency and balloon compliance did not contribute to surgical decision making in this study. However, if incontinence or diarrhea are present, anal physiology testing may have a role.

Ano-rectal manometry is useful to evaluate the anal sphincter mechanism preoperatively to determine whether combined sphincter reconstruction and endorectal repair of the rectocele might be beneficial. The best method for evaluating the anatomy of the anal sphincter is transrectal ultrasound, using a 10 MHz transducer on a rotating probe. The anal cap attachment for the Bruel and Kjaer instrument enables clear evaluation of the internal and external anal sphincter (Fig. 25.8). Typically, in the patient with associated sphincter dysfunction, there is some scarring in the rectovaginal septum and there may be varying amounts of separation of the ends of one or both of the internal or external sphincter. Anal manometry is best used to document reduced rest and squeeze pressures before any planned repair and then after repair to compare pressures and document any residual deficit. However, it is not essen-

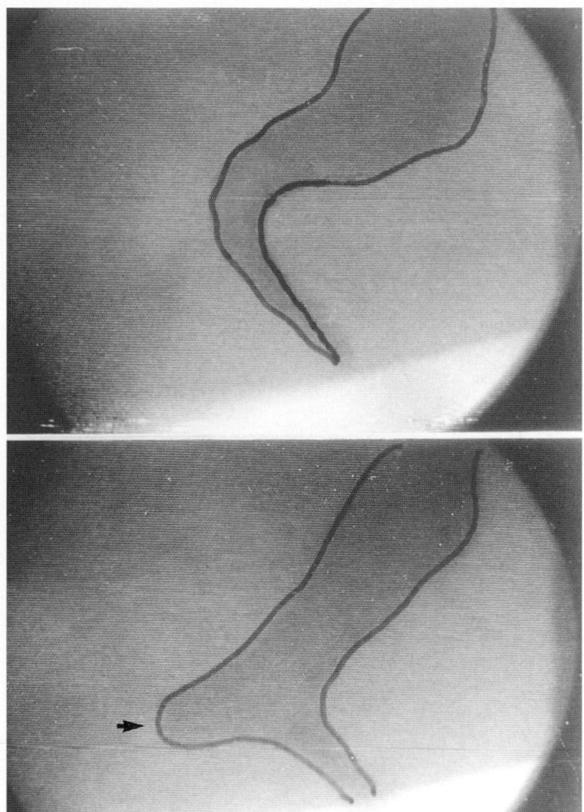

Figure 25.7 Defecography allows measurement of anterior bulge into posterior vagina and documents retention of material within the rectocele.

tial in the planning process. The data provided by manometry makes comparison with studies in the literature much easier and is essential in patients being studied to evaluate a procedure. Vectorography of the anal canal is not as useful as the combination of TRUS and anal manometry.

Proctosigmoidoscopy may be employed to rule out associated pathology that may complicate the surgical outcome.

Intervention

Each individual with a symptomatic rectocele deserves an initial trial of non-operative treatment. Conservative measures, such as dietary manipulation with high fiber intake, bulk laxative (psyllium 18 g/day), topical vaginal estrogens (for the postmenopausal woman) and a pessary (in the posthysterectomy patient), result in variable responses in terms of reducing the bulge of the rectocele and its symptoms. They may occasionally obviate the need for surgery, especially if the patient is unwilling or unable to have surgery.

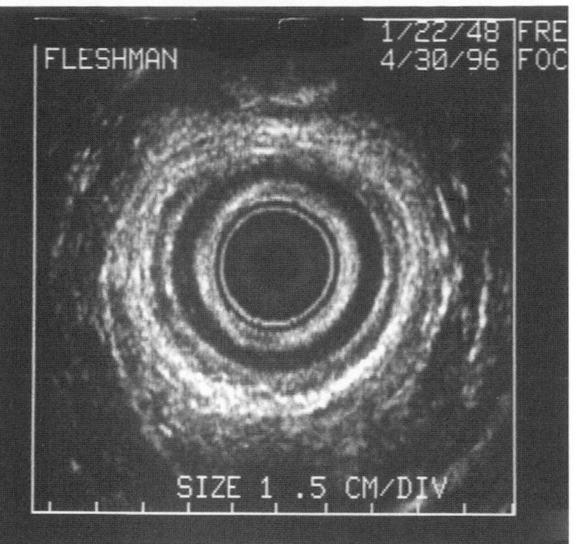

Figure 25.8 Endosonographic image of normal mid-level anal sphincter. Thick dark line is internal sphincter. White multiechogenic lines outside internal sphincter represents external anal sphincter.

Once the condition becomes refractory to medical management, surgery is considered. Surgical approaches are divided into transvaginal, transrectal and transabdominal, or combinations thereof; each has their own proponents distributed among the field of gynecology and colorectal surgery. In some cases a combined approach that embraces disciplines, as well as techniques, may be warranted. Repair of the vaginal wall alone in patients with a rectocele may be succesful; if not sufficient the anterior rectal wall must also be repaired.

Arnold found transvaginal and transrectal approaches equally effective in terms of symptomatic relief.[60] The surgeon's familiarity with the chosen approach seems to be the most important factor influencing the procedure of choice, as well as outcome.

Transrectal repair of rectocele was first advocated in 1968 by Sullivan *et al.*[65] The transrectal approach offers the opportunity to treat associated ano-rectal pathology.[66] Sehapayak showed decreased infection rates with the endorectal approach.[67] The most popular transrectal approach entails raising an anterior quadrant mucosal flap to a level above the suprasphincteric portion of the rectovaginal septum through a transverse incision above the dentate line (Fig. 25.9). Subsequently, the internal sphincter and rectal wall are plicated to reduce the redundant tissue in the anterior rectum. This vertical suture line is then folded horizontally to pull the upper anterior rectal wall down to the anal canal and sutured across the width of the rectum. The redundant portion of the mucosal flap created by this downfolding

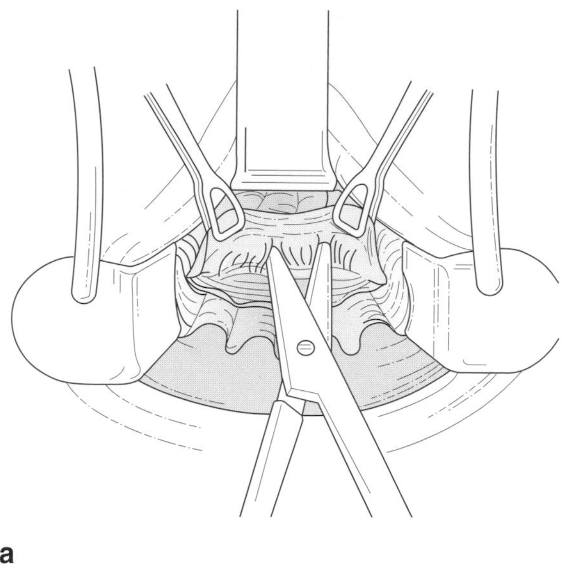

a

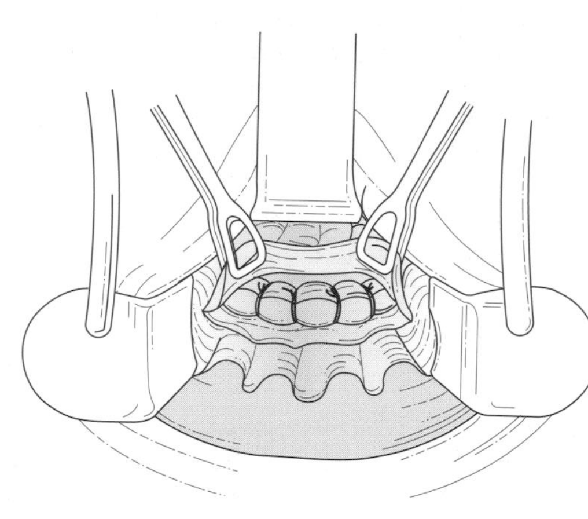

b

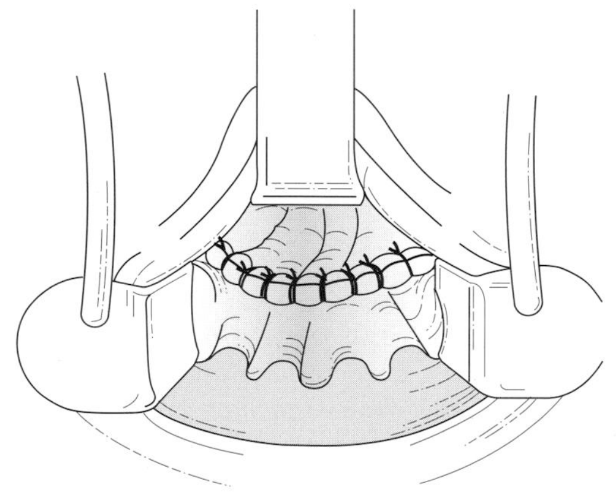

c

Figure 25.9 (a) A mucosal flap is raised around the anterior half of the anal canal for approximately 5–8 cm. (b) The anterior rectal wall muscle is folded down to the distal anal canal and reefed horizontally. (c) The redundant mucosa is excised and the new mucocutaneous junction restored across the anterior anal canal.

is then resected and the edges are approximated at the dentate line.

The obliterative suture technique is a more expedient approach.[68] Several parallel lines of absorbable suture are placed in a vertical direction extending upwards in the rectum across the anterior rectum to plicate the rectocele through an endoanal approach without raising a flap. Mucosal necrosis and scarring occur during the healing process and the redundant anterior rectal wall shrinks to obliterate most of the anterior bulge.

In the setting of a previous severe obstetric injury and associated anal sphincter disruption, some authors advocate a transperineal approach. The rectocele can be separated from the vagina before performing a levatorplasty, at the level of the pubococcygeus muscle, and plicating the rectocele from the perineal body approach. The external muscular component of the rectum is plicated longitudinally across the midline. The redundant mucosa is not removed. As part of this procedure, an anterior overlapping anal sphincter muscle repair can be performed. This results in restoration of the perineal body, reduction of the rectocele, and wide separating of the anterior rectal wall from posterior vagina, as well as improved anal sphincter function.

In the setting of a high rectocele, enterocele or cystocele, the transanal approach is relatively contraindicated. Some authors have indicated that the transanal approach carries increased risk of damage to the anal sphincter and should be avoided in those with an already lax sphincter.[69] If a sphincter repair is not contemplated as part of the procedure, the continued retraction during surgery may cause further harm to the sphincter mechanism. Ho *et al.*[69] found significant impairment in the resting and squeeze pressures although the rate of fecal incontinence was not increased.

Reported incontinence rates after rectocele repair vary, ranging up to 30%. Unfortunately, anal manometry data is not available in these reports to document the state of the sphincter before and after the repair so as to record the real effect of the procedure itself on the sphincter mechanism. In such cases a different approach, such as a transvaginal one, may be entertained or, as suggested, a repair combined with a sphincter reconstruction. In these circumstances, it is best to evaluate the sphincter with manometry and transrectal ultrasound.

The combined transanal and transvaginal repair involves a posterior colporrhaphy, then excision of redundant mucosa from the anterior rectal wall through the transanal approach with attendant transverse plication of the muscular layer.

The transvaginal repair may not give adequate symptomatic relief.[70,71] It has been suggested that the transvaginal repair be reserved for those without evidence of obstructed defecation as the latter, if present, may have a more complex pathogenesis than the prolapse of the anterior low rectal wall alone. A transvaginal approach, which does not address other factors, may lead to early recurrence of the rectocele or failure to resolve the symptoms because of its limited ability to address all aspects of the symptom complex.

The transabdominal approach is more suited for those with attendant cystocele, enterocele or sigmoidocele. Watson *et al.* have described a procedure which addresses the 'fallen pelvic floor' (Fig. 25.10) by suspending the rectovaginal septum and perineal body with a nylon mesh sling fixed to the sacrum.[72] This repositioning of the pelvic diaphragm seems to eliminate all the associated 'collapse' problems seen in an increasingly large group of patients (Fig. 25.11). However, it is not recommended for the patient with an isolated rectocele, most likely due to previous anal sphincter injury or hysterectomy. A non-absorbable suture attached to a 'y' shaped nylon mesh is tied over the perineal body to bring the vertical portion of the mesh down into the rectovaginal septum. The two limbs of the 'y' are then pulled up to the sacrum on either side of the rectum to hoist the pelvic floor cephalad. This technique is similar to one described by Sullivan for suspending all of the structures of the pelvic floor using mesh.[73] The rectovaginal septum is dissected all the way down to the anal sphincter from the transabdominal approach before using a special 'forked suture passer' to place the nylon suture through the perineal body skin.

RESULTS

When addressing the question of results, one must be aware of the problem or problems for which the therapy was employed. Surgical intervention may be employed for multiple symptoms assumed due to the presence of a rectocele. Only by careful follow-up will the true success of a particular repair be known. Most, if not all techniques result in a change in the rectovaginal septum that eliminates the rectocele bulge.

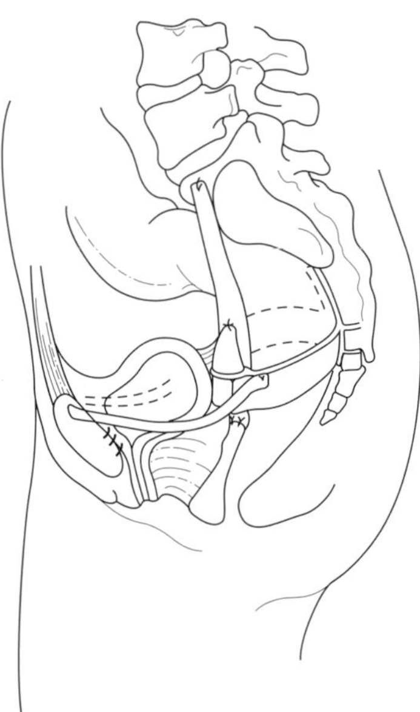

Figure 25.10 The pelvic floor and perineal body behind the vagina are suspended using slivers of mesh material or proline suture and ultimately attached to the anterior sacrum.

Arnold reported that in his 4 year experience, 50% patients were still symptomatic.[60] Watson *et al.* noted they had removed the need to digitally aid evacuation in most of their patients.[72] Murthy *et al.* showed excellent results and ascribed this in part to strict selection criteria.[49]

There have been numerous reports attesting to the success of the transanal approach.[74,75] Sullivan *et al.*[65] showed 97.5% success with 151 patients treated. Shapayak, using a transanal approach, demonstrated 98% success in 355 patients.[67] Jansen's *et al.*[76] series revealed 92% success with 72 patients using a transrectal approach. Mellgren *et al.*[63] reported an improvement in the symptom of constipation in 88% of patients and complete resolution in 52% of patients. Murthy *et al.* had excellent results which were attributed, in part, to strict selection criteria.[49] In their series, all patients who were offered a rectocele repair reported the sensation of a vaginal mass or bulge that required digital support, a confirmed rectocele on defecography, digitalization via the vagina to achieve evacuation, a very large rectocele with anterior wall prolapse through the vaginal introitus, and retention of barium in the rectocele on defecography. They reported 33 patients who underwent rectocele repair, 31 transanally and two

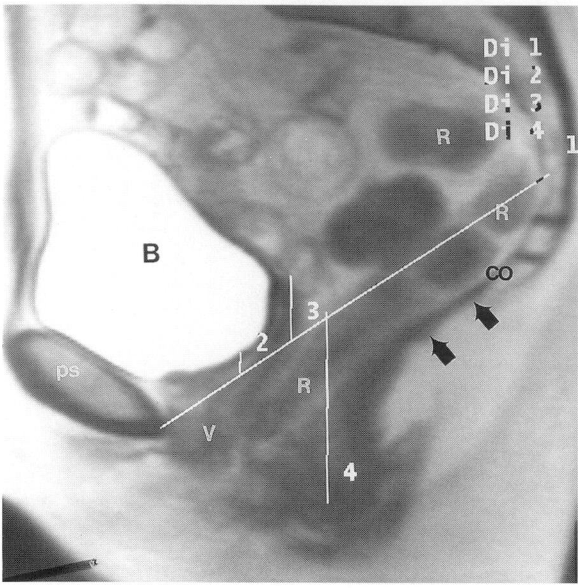

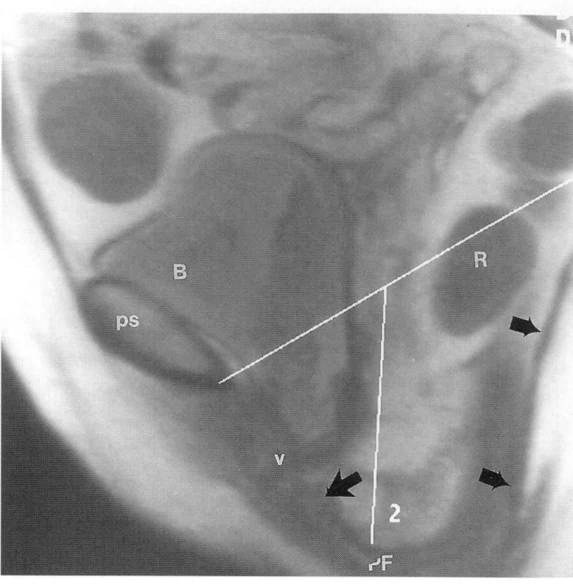

a b

Figure 25.11 Sagittal MRI images at rest (a) and straining (b). Lines are drawn from the pubosacral line (1) to mark the bladder neck (2), vaginal cuff (3), and pelvic floor (4). The pubosacral line as opposed to the pubococcygeal line is favored by some authors. These lines were not drawn perpendicular to the pubosacral line which we currently use as a standard. Marked pelvic floor weakness and descent (black arrows and PF) are noted. (Courtesy Dr Vamsi Narra, Mallinckrodt Institute of Radiology, St Louis.)

transabdominally. Overall, 92% of patients reported improvement of preoperative symptoms and were satisfied with the operation. The symptom of anterior rectal bulge had improved or resolved in 80% of patients. By restoring the rectovaginal septum, Sarles had excellent results in 11 of 16 patients.[77]

In patients with non-relaxation of the puborectalis muscle, or pelvic floor outlet obstruction, correction of the rectocele may not improve the symptoms of constipation. No serious study has evaluated the outcome after correction of rectocele in this group of patients with pelvic floor dysfunction. Continued straining to evacuate places the repair at risk of failure and in addition, the repair may add to the outlet obstruction. It is our policy to correct the symptoms of outlet obstruction before attempting repair. Table 25.2 summarizes the results of most larger series of rectocele repair. Unfortunately, once again all reports do not mention symptom improvement in the outcomes. No randomized trial comparing the different approaches is available.

The anatomical result of surgical correction should be a decrease in the size of the rectocele and raising of the pelvic floor. Karlbom *et al.* noted that rectocele repair does, indeed, improve rectal emptying and this is accompanied by improvement of symptoms.[78]

Complications

Complications of rectocele repair include non-specific postoperative problems such as infection as well as the specific impact of rectovaginal fistula. This latter complication occurred in very few patients (1/355) undergoing transanal repair in the studies reviewed,[67] but may be more likely to occur in those patients who develop abscess or infection after repair. Any injury to the rectal mucosa may result in direct communication with the vagina and a fistula is the result.

Dyspareunia is a recognized part of the symptom complex that is the rectocele. It is seen both before and after surgery. It has been postulated to be related to using the levators to repair the posterior vaginal wall. Urinary retention is probably the most common complication reported but is usually self-limiting and related to pain and spasm induced in the pelvic floor muscles when sutures are placed to tighten the pelvic floor outlet.[49]

CONCLUSION

A rectocele found on physical examination or defecography is not in itself an indication for an operation. Only if the rectocele can be shown to be directly responsible for associated symptoms should a repair be attempted. Adequate preoperative evaluation to docu-

Table 25.2 Summary of results of rectocele repair comparing a number of larger series

Author	No. patients	Approach	Success	Preconstip Defecation	Postconstip Defecation	Incontinence	Anal physiology	Complication
Ho H-Y	21	Transanal	All satisfied	Yes	Better	No	Resting and squeeze impaired	
Capps WF	51	Transrectal	76% excellent			No		41% urine retention; 8% infection
Janssen LW	76	Endorectal ant wall	38 Excellent	Yes 72% Post 5%		No		2 bleeds 1 free fluid
Karlbom U	34		79%	All				79% better
Khubchandani IT	59	Sullivan Endorectal	37 excellent					
Mellgren A	25	Posterior colporrhaphy; Perineorrhaphy; Transvaginal	88% better Paradoxical PRS not improved	6	Vaginal digitalization improved		Normal resting pressure post Sx	
Murthy VK	35	Transanal 31 Transabdominal 2	92% better	11%	58% Vaginal digitalization better			1 Impaction
Sehapayak S	355	Sullivan Transrectal	98% better; 49% excellent; 35% good					5.6% infection; 1 fistula 44% urine retention
Van Dam JH	74	Combined Transrectal and vaginal	37 excellent; 13 good	59%				
Arnold MW	64	35 Transanal 29 Transvaginal			50% of preop constipation still had it; less pain in transanal			
Watson WJ					8 of 9 pre constipation relieved			

ment stool trapping, pelvic floor or sphincter dysfunction, obstructed defecation or other associated problems should allow the surgeon to select those patients who will respond well to a rectocele repair. Correction of pelvic floor outlet obstruction should be achieved before attempting a repair. This data-driven process of selecting patients also allows the surgeon to select the appropriate operative approach if medical treatment has failed to help the patient.

HEMORRHOIDS

INTRODUCTION

The management of symptomatic hemorrhoids remains a vexing problem. Patients present with a spectrum of complaints ranging from minor inconvenience to severe debility and ill health.

PATHOLOGY AND PATHOPHYSIOLOGY

Hemorrhoids are submucosal vascular and connective tissue cushions which are arranged around the anal canal and are most commonly located in the right anterolateral, right posterolateral and left lateral positions.[79] The normal physiological role of hemorrhoidal tissue is proposed to be engorgement at the time of defecation to protect the underlying muscle, allowing the anus to dilate during defecation and then allowing complete closure of the anal canal at rest. The protective or physiologic effect of the non pathologic hemorrhoidal cushions has not been critically defined. The pathologic enlargement or prolapse of these structures is, however, well documented.[80] Hemorrhoid disease can be subdivided into the following types, as shown in Table 25.3.

Internal hemorrhoids are located above the dentate line and *external hemorrhoids* are below the dentate line. Each has a slightly distinctive natural history. Internal hemorrhoids are covered by rectal and transitional mucosa and may bleed, prolapse, or discharge mucus. The deposition of mucus or small amounts of stool on the anoderm causes symptoms of pruritus. If incarcerated at the outer ring of the anal canal, hemorrhoid tissue may thrombose or necrose. As internal hemorrhoid are not somatically innervated they must become incarcerated to produce pain. Thus anal pain is not caused by internal hemorrhoidal thrombosis in constipation. External hemorrhoids may thrombose and this causes a lot of pain and should an external thrombosis erode through the skin, bleeding will ensue. The richly innervated skin overlying an external thrombosis is a source of both pain and itching. Skin tags results from resolution of chronic hemorrhoids. Hemorrhoids are often associated with constipation and straining.

Table 25.3 Types of hemorrhoid

Type	Degree	Definition
Internal	First	Bleed
	Second	Bleed, prolapse and reduce spontaneously
	Third	Bleed, prolapse, require manual reduction Minor – with bowel motion Major – without bowel motion
	Fourth	Minor – can't reduce Major – internal and external
External		Below the dentate line
Mixed		Communication between internal and external

The pathophysiology of the hemorrhoid disease appears to be one end of the spectrum of normal function. It is thought that increased vascular pressure generated during straining leads to excessive engorgement and dilatation of the vascular pedicles[81–83] (Fig. 25.12).

The pathophysiology of the various presentations of hemorrhoidal disease include:

- Bleeding
- Pain
- Pruritus ani
- Mucus discharge
- Squamous change
- Incarceration
- Thrombosis
- Skin tags
- Disordered defecation.

Bleeding

Trauma to the fragile vessels beneath the stretched mucosa of the internal hemorrhoid during the passage of stool at defecation leads to bleeding. Alternatively, external hemorrhoid may cause bleeding by a clot eroding through skin. Bleeding from both internal and external hemorroids is bright red. Arterial blood that has stagnated in the rectum or that arising from venous vessels, of course, is darker.

Pain

The stretched, sensitive skin overlying a thrombosed and engorged external hemorrhoid induces pain. Internal hemorroids which are not ulcerated do not cause pain. Pain is most often caused by an anal fissure, or by cryptoglandular abscess disease.

Pruritus ani

Perianal itching is thought to arise from the compromised anal hygiene that results from skin tags, large external hemorrhoids and prolapsed mixed hemorrhoids. This is also aggravated by mucus discharge from internal hemorrhoids.

Mucus discharges

Irritation of the columnar epithelium overlying the internal hemorrhoids results in pathologic mucus discharge. Chronic moisture bathing the perianal area results in excoriation, deep rogation, thickening of the dermal layer, pseudocolumnar epithelium, and epidermal barrier breakdown.

Squamous changes

The columnar epithelium of exposed, chronically prolapsed hemorrhoids undergoes squamous adaptive change. The pseudoepithelialization of the mucosa may

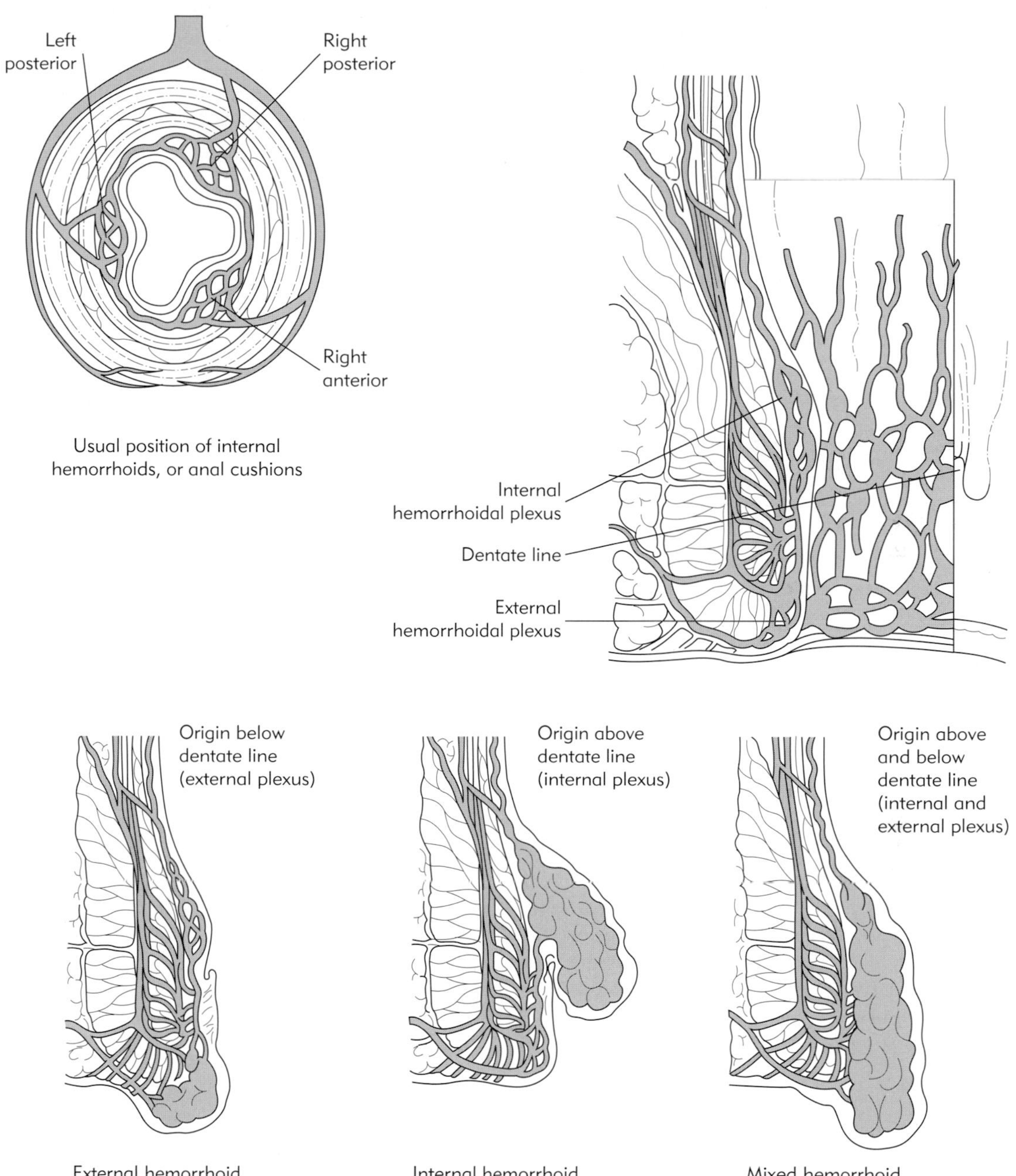

Figure 25.12 Anatomy and types of hemorrhoids. (Copyright 1985. Novartis. Reprinted with permission from Novartis Medical Education, illustrated by John A. Craig, MD. All rights reserved.)

result in bleeding, incarceration, or even polyp formation on the hemorrhoidal column.

Incarcerations

An internal hemorrhoid may become trapped outside the anal verge and induce spasm of the internal sphincter. This leads to a vicious cycle that culminates in massive local edema, thrombosis and severe pain. If swelling progresses to the point of occluding arterial inflow, strangulation and eventually necrosis occur.

Thrombosis

Obstructed venous outflow causes thrombosis. The external plexus of the entire anal canal circumference may be involved or it may be a localized site. This may lead to necrosis of the overlying skin and 'gangrene' or ulceration and extrusion of clot. The risk of portal pyelophlebits is very low but occurs after incarceration, strangulation and gangrene of the internal hemorrhoids.

Skin tags

Skin tags in the three quadrants at the anal verge result from the involution of an external hemorrhoid over time. After the thrombosis and edema resolve, any remaining skin tags are usually soft, pliant skin folds. This is in contrast to the thickened, atypically located, weeping skin tags of Crohn's disease.

Disordered defecation

There is a cause and effect relationship between disordered defecation and hemorrhoidal disease. Endless ineffective straining at defecation against a tight sphixter leads to engorgement of the vascular pedicles. Thereon, an increase in internal sphincter activity and ultra slow anal waves has been found in patients with hemorrhoids.[84,85] Increased resting anal pressure has also been documented. However, the finding that the resting anal pressure returns to normal after passage of a proctoscope or after a hemorrhoidectomy, even without anal dilatation, has led some to believe that the increased resting anal pressure is due to the presence of hemorrhoids and is not a cause of hemorrhoids primarily.[86]

Hypertrophy of the external anal sphincter muscle has also been observed in hemorrhoids.[87,88] When hypertrophied, the external anal sphincter contraction may lead to increased anal canal resting pressure since 20% of resting anal pressure is due to external anal sphincter activity, further aggravating the tendency to strain. J.P. Thompson[89] suggested that a lax anal canal epithelium that slides inferiorly to displace the anal cushions may cause prolonged bleeding and anal discharge.

MANAGEMENT

Evaluation

The evaluation of the patient with hemorrhoidal disease includes assessment of the peculiar risk factors, such as stool, habit and diet. Physical evaluation must include the observation of patient performing a Valsalva maneuver to measure the degree of hemorrhoidal prolapse, or extraction of the hemorrhoids during anoscopy. Anoscopy is the minimum endoscopic procedure required to evaluate the hemorrhoids. In the setting of rectal bleeding, especially in patients over 40 years of age or those in a high risk group for neoplasia, it is important to exclude more sinister disease, and colonoscopy has become the preferred endoscopic procedure in most institutions to accomplish this goal.

The pressure generated by the anal canal may or may not, however, show a relationship to hemorrhoidal disease measurement but is of predictive value in planning the treatment regimen except when there is concomitant anal incontinence.

Treatment

The presence of enlarged hemorrhoids in itself is not an indication for surgery. Treatment must be based on symptoms. The least invasive method is obviously the best. Constipation, aberrant behavior and disordered defection must be treated or altered before treating the hemorrhoids themselves.

Non-surgical treatment

An initial conservative approach involves stool modification with bulk forming agents and fiber, and avoidance of prolonged straining. Attempts to reach the daily recommended insoluble fiber requirement of 25 g without fiber supplements are difficult. Several formulations of psyllium husk provide an inert, non-laxative means of regulating bowel habits. Symptoms may be alleviated by topical analgesics and warm soaks. Soaking in a warm tub has been shown to reduce rest pressure and eliminate spasm. Skin tags may just require attention to hygiene.[90] Such a conservative regimen will alleviate symptoms of bleeding and discharge in nearly all first and 2nd degree hemorrhoids.

Surgery

The treatment of complicated and uncomplicated hemorrhoids differs. Incisional and non-incisional approaches are available and include:

- Maximal anal dilatation
- Internal sphincterotomy
- Elastic ligation
- Photocoagulation
- Electrocoagulation
- Sclerosis
- Laser therapy
- Cryosurgery
- Excisional hemorrhoidectomy.

These approaches should be selected based on the type of hemorrhoid and the presumed underlying pathophysiology.

Addressing the sphincters

The fact that anal pressures are raised in patients with hemorrhoids has been used to justify stretching or cutting the internal anal sphincter. The reduction of resistance to rectal evacuation may reduce the engorgement or bleeding from internal hemorrhoids. However, the underlying tissue abnormality is unaffected. The Lord procedure (maximal four finger dilatation) is mentioned here only for completeness.[91] It does not improve symptoms, does decrease resting anal canal pressures and does decrease ultra-slow waves. However, with its attendant risk of incontinence and the superior success of other approaches, it is now rarely used. The insertion of four fingers into the anal canal and application of lateral traction has been shown to result in multiple fractures of the internal anal sphincter as seen on endoanal ultrasound. The associated leakage of gas and mucus makes it an unacceptable approach to hemorrhoidal disease.[92,93]

Incisional sphincterotomy is indicated only if the hemorrhoidal disease is associated with an anal fissure. It is safer than the Lord's procedure as there is more control over the intentional sphincter disruption. Closed lateral anal sphincterotomy is very safe and results in a very low rate of incontinence.[94,95]

Addressing the hemorrhoid feeding vessels

Elastic ligations

This approach should be employed for second, and third degree hemorrhoids.[96-99] The principle is, firstly, interval placement of elastic rings at the vascular pedicle well above the dentate line causing necrosis and sloughing and leaving a scar.[97] One should avoid placement near the sensitive anoderm or anal transitional zone and limit the amount of internal sphincter included in the ligation[100] (Fig. 25.13). Capture of sphincter or ligation of innervated epithelium results in severe pain and anal spasm. This is usually readily apparent when the procedure is being performed without anesthesia in the outpatient clinic. Urinary retention may result from the injudicious placement of the bands or multiple ligations at a single visit. Full thickness rectal ligation may also lead to sepsis. However, sepsis as a complication is very rare. It has been associated with immune compromise (leukemia, AIDS, diabetes) and should be treated aggressively with hospital admission, removal of the rubber bands, intravenous antibiotics, and debridement of any necrotic tissue. Failure to do so may result in death of the patient. If the bands fall off prematurely, hemorrhage may occur but is usually not significant. In theory, patients should avoid non-steroidal anti-inflammatory drugs for 7 to 10 days after ligation. Suture ligation of the exposed vessels at the base of the scar is rarely necessary but very effective in controlling the bleeding.

Photocoagulation

Heat is applied to three or four sites 5 mm deep at the pedicle, 3 mm above the dentate line, inducing thrombosis and fibrosis. This is utilized in first and second degree hemorrhoids and has results comparable to elastic ligation.[101]

Sclerosis

Sclerotherapy was one of the first local outpatient methods of treating early stage bleeding hemorrhoids. In this approach, one injects 5% phenol in almond oil, or some other sclerosing agent, into the submucosa at the base of first and second degree hemorrhoids. This results in an acute inflammatory response and sclerosis of the vessels. The particular complications of this approach are ulceration, oleogranuloma, allergic reaction and prostate infection (if deep injection occurs). Its effectiveness is equal to elastic ligation though large hemorrhoids do not respond well.[102,103] Sclerotherapy is usually reserved for the treatment of bleeding first degree hemorrhoids if ligation is not possible. Obviously, surgeon preference is a major influence in the choice of this technique.

Address hemorrhoidal tissue

Harmonic scalpels

The harmonic scalpel is also being considered as another modern tool for performing excisional hemorrhoidectomy. Better control of bleeding and less collateral tissue injury are the proposed advantages of the harmonic scalpel in hemorrhoid surgery.[104]

Excisional hemorrhoidectomy

This still remains the gold standard for treatment and the modality by which all others are judged. The following surgical approaches are considered:

- Excise with open wounds – Milligan Morgan.[105]
- Excise with closed wounds – Ferguson.[106]
- Circumferential – Whitehead.[107]

This is the treatment of choice for patients with large, third and fourth degree hemorrhoids with the following:

- A large external component or mixed hemorrhoid
- Thrombosis
- Incarceration and severe pain
- Impending gangrene
- Bleeding in a patient requiring anticoagulation
- Difficult hygiene due to the presence of mixed hemorrhoids.

Excisional hemorrhoidectomy may be performed in several different ways using different techniques, tools and methods of wound closure. The basic principles for any technique are ligation and control of the vascular pedicle well above the dentate line, excision of the redundant prolapsing internal hemorrhoid tissue in such a way to avoid incising the underlying internal

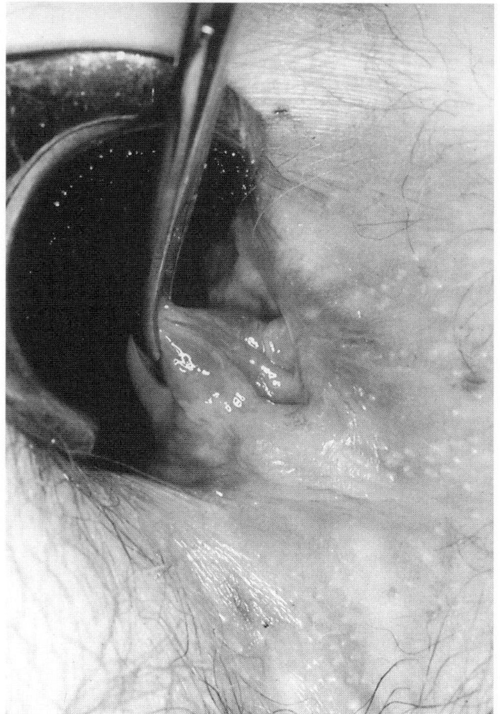

a

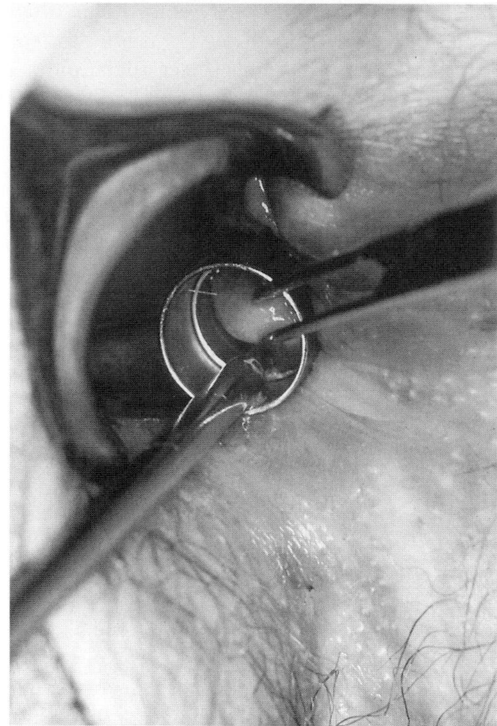

b

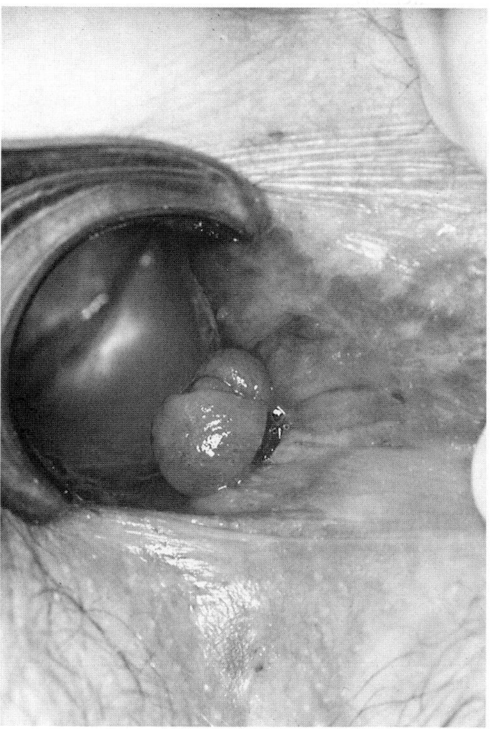

c

Figure 25.13 (a) The internal hemorrhoid (right anterior lateral position in this patient) is grasped on the mucosal surface 2 cm above the dentate line. Patient is in prone jackknife position. (b) The ligator is directed toward the wall of the rectum to pull the tissue up into the anal canal as the mucosal pedicle is pulled through the central opening of the ligator. (c) The rubber band is in place at the base of the ligated right anterior internal hemorrhoid.

sphincter, removal of the extra skin overlying external hemorrhoids and preservation of adequate anoderm to prevent cicatricial scarring and compromise of anal canal opening. The rates of incontinence, stenosis, recurrence and sepsis should all be low.[108]

The most popular technique in the US is the closed (Ferguson) hemorrhoidectomy.[106] This technique removes an ellipse of mucosa and anoderm, as well as underlying hemorrhoidal vessels and connective tissue, and ligates the vessels 3–4 cm above the dentate line to fix the pedicle to the internal sphincter. The elliptical defect is then closed from the vascular pedicle out to the tip of the skin defect in a linear suture line usually aimed radially out from the anal canal. This approach results in low recurrence and complication rates and probably reduces healing time and discomfort because of the closed wounds. Unfortunately, the suture lines open during the healing period in a significant group of patients, thus offsetting the presumed advantages of closure.

The Milligan–Morgan technique was popularized at St Mark's Hospital in the late 19th century and continues to be used extensively in Great Britain.[105] Ligation of the vascular pedicle, elliptical excision of the mucosa, anoderm, vessels and connective tissue are similar to the closed approach. With this technique, however, only the mucosal defect is reapproximated to the level of the dentate line and the skin defect is left open to close secondarily. Excellent recurrence and complication rates have been achieved, and high levels of patient satisfaction have been reported in the stoic British population.

A combination of internal elastic ligation and excision of internal and external components, respectively, is possible with excellent results. This technique can be tailored to meet the needs of the individual patient and the surgeon should be familiar with all of them.

The circumferential 'Whitehead' hemorrhoidectomy can be utilized to manage acute gangrene of incarcerated, strangulated mixed hemorrhoids.[107] This technique requires particular attention to preserving anoderm and maintaining the mucocutaneous junction within the anal canal after excision of the necrotic hemorrhoidal plexus. The best description of this technique, and comparison of this technique with standard three or four quadrant excisional hemorrhoidectomy, is from the Mayo Clinic.[109] The injection of hyaluronidase into the intersphincteric groove and thrombosed tissues usually allows reduction of the incarcerated pedicles and subsequent three quadrant excision. The complications of Whitehead hemorrhoidectomy are fairly severe and include anal stenosis and mucosal ectropion. Indeed, several operative procedures have been described to correct long-term complications of ectropion and stenosis which utilize advancement of skin into the anal canal to replace the excised anoderm.[110,111]

Laser

Carbon dioxide and Nd–Yag lasers have been used to vaporize overlying tissue and cause an ulcer and fixation.[112,113] These tools have also been employed to perform an excisional hemorrhoidectomy. Superficial CO_2 lasers have resulted in late hemorrhage, and the Nd–Yag lasers carry the potential risk of burning too deep and causing an intersphincteric abscess. Even so, randomized, prospective trials have shown laser assisted hemorrhoidectomy to be as safe as conventional, excisional hemorrhoidectomy.[114–116] The use of laser has never been convincingly shown to reduce pain and complications as originally touted. Expensive equipment, a definite learning curve and the need for safety measures during the procedure have limited the use of this technique to a few centers which tend to specialize in, and advertise the use of, lasers.

SUMMARY

The selection of the appropriate method for treating hemorrhoids is currently based on two factors: (i) surgeon training and experience; and (ii) availability of technology. Table 25.4 summarizes the results of treatment of hemorrhoids in a number of series reports. The reader must understand that each approach has advantages and disadvantages. There are no data that direct us to one correct method of treating the different degrees of hemorrhoid. However, a general principle should be to use a conservative non-operative approach initially if possible. Only after persistent disease indicates medical failure should an operative approach be selected. The least invasive method, which results in the least amount of morbidity in the hands of the surgeon, is then selected. This may vary according to surgeon and technology availability.

Treatment of acute thrombosis or incarceration of internal hemorrhoids

Incarceration and thrombosis of the entire hemorrhoidal tissue complex is a rare occurrence. This is a painful condition and frightening to observe. The most common setting for this condition is the postpartum patient after prolonged labor. Initially, bed rest and stool softeners should be offered to the patient in conjunction with analgesia. Epinephrine and hyaluronidase can be injected to reduce the incarcerated hemorrhoids. Subsequently, an excisional hemorrhoidectomy is performed if the naturally occurring sclerosis of the thrombosed vessels does not maintain the hemorrhoids in their anatomic position, or if necrosis occurs necessitating debridement (Fig. 25.14). Internal sphincterotomy is sometimes used if sphincter spasm is a consideration. Care must be taken to avoid causing incontinence if a sphincterotomy is performed and is generally to be avoided in the female patient.

Table 25.4 Summary of results of treatments of hemorrhoids from a number of series

Author	No. patients	Grade	Approach	Success	Complication
A. Results of excisional hemorrhoidectomy					
Hosch SB	34	2, 3	Parks v. Milligan Morgan	All satisfactory	Milligan Morgan – more pain; Parks – less hospital stay
Andrews BT	20	2, 3, Thrombosed	Diathermy v. Milligan Morgan	No difference in pain; No significant difference	
Bleday R	2100	Bleeding, prolapse; Thrombosis 80% Gr 3, 4 15% Gr 2	45% conservative 9.3% Surgery – sphincterotomy, hemorrhoidectomy 44% band		Urine retention 20%; Hemorrhage 2.4%
Khubchandani M	84		Whitehead		6 urine retention; 3 bleed; 3 stenosis; No ectropion
Wolff BG	484		Whitehead		1% fistula; 6.9% flap loss; stenosis 0.2%
Ganchrow MI	2038		Ferguson hemorrhoidectomy	95% symptom relief	4% complications; 2% bleeding 0.1% mortality
McConnell JC	441		Closed Hemorrhoidectomy	1 reoperation; 7% residual symptoms	
Cheng FC	120	Gr 2	Hemorroidectomy Injection Rubber band MAD	24 of 30 cured 18 of 30 cured 25 of 30 cured 24 of 30 cured	Pain in all; 2 stenosis; 2 hemorrhage 26 of 30 painless; no complications 25 of 30 painless; no complications
Lewis AA	112	Failed injection	Hemorrhoidectomy MAD Rubber band Cryosurgery	Most effective Recurrence, surgery Recurrence, surgery Recurrence, surgery	
Hosch SB	34	Gr 3 or 4	Parks v. Milligan Morgan	Both satisfactory results; More pain	No serious complications; No serious complication
Harvrylenko SP	121 101		Milligan Morgan Staple device		32% pain, 21% urine retention, 3% hemorrhage; No complications
B. Conservative approach					
Ibrahim S	91		Diathermy vs scissors	No difference in pain	1 urine retention; 2 bleeds
Ambrose NS	135	1,2	Photocoagulation Sclerotherapy	59% excellent; 7 repeat therapy 50% excellent; results comparable; 1 repeat therapy	None None
Ambrose NS	268		Photocoagulation vs sclerotherapy	Results comparable	
Asfar SK	123 125		Anal stretch Sphinecterotomy		Severe pain 96%; urine retention 39%; soiling 57% Severe pain 6%; urine retention 4%; soiling 6%

Author	No. patients	Grade	Approach	Success	Complication
Bat L	512	Internal	Banding	82% success; 58% excellent; 24% improved; 11% failed	6 bleed; 3 urine retention; 3 thrombotic hemorrhoids; 1 abscess; 24 minor complications
Santos G	189		Phenol	63 cured 26 better	
Wroblowski	266	31% Gr 1 28% Gr 2 34% Gr 3 7% Gr 4	Banding	80% better 69% symptom free 7% hemorrhoidectomy required	
Dencker			Sclerotherapy	Poor v. Milligan Morgan; 21% well; short-term benefit only	
Alexander-Williams J			Sclerotherapy	Short-term benefit	
Baritzal and Slosberg	670		Banding		4% pain 3% slight bleed
Steinberg	125		Banding	89% cured or improved; 44% symptom free	
Gehamy RA				76% symptom free	
Wilson MC	100		Cryosurgery	94% satisfactory	
Savin S	444		Cryosurgery	431 symptom free	
Walls ADF		15 Gr 1 48 Gr 2 37 Gr 3	Lord's maximal; anal dilatation	75 symptom free; 22 unsuccessful; all failed at 3 months; 19 subsequent surg	
McCaffrey J	50			36 symptom free; 4 subsequent surgery	40% incontinence
Schouten WR			Internal sphincterotomy	75% cured	
MacRae HM	Meta-analysis			Gr 1–3, banding best; Hemorrhoidectomy has better response; Hemorrhoidectomy has more complications; Banding better than sclerotherapy	
Keighley MR	216	Symptomatic	Anal dilatation Rubber band	MAD better than sphincterotomy or diet; MAD alone reduced anal pressure Better than cryosurgery or diet	
Oh C	1000		Cryosurgery	90% satisfied	33% mild to moderate pain

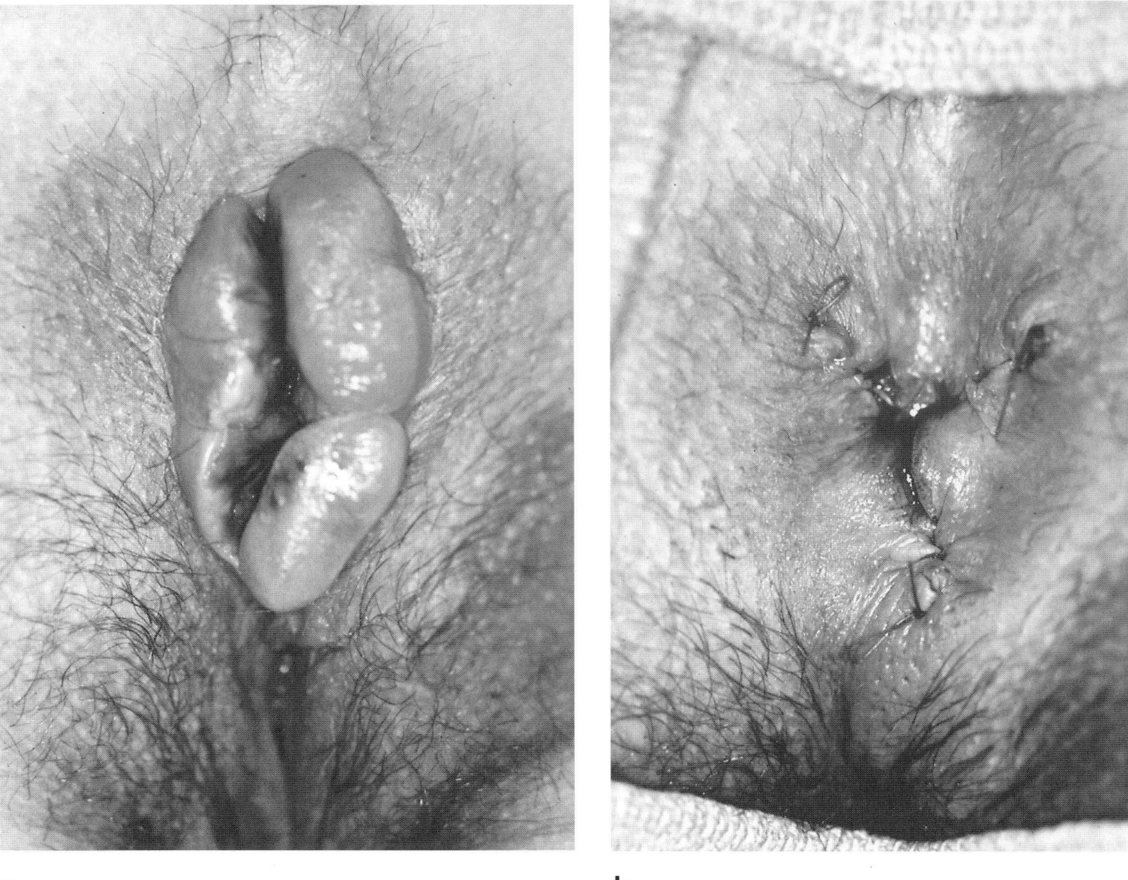

Figure 25.14 (a) Circumferential thrombosed gangrenous mixed incarcerated hemorrhoids. (Patient is in prone jackknife position). (b) Following three quadrant closed excisional hemorrhoidectomy, adequate tissue is present to prevent anal

Acute thrombosis of external hemorrhoids

Local anesthesia and incision of the thrombosed hemorrhoid with clot enucleation is employed in this situation. Subsequent definitive treatment is required to prevent recurrence.

Preventive treatment

Based on the edict that prevention is better than cure, patients and clinicians alike have sought preventive therapies for hemorrhoidal disease. Prevention has a number of goals which include preventing development of hemorrhoids *de-novo* in an at-risk population, prevention of progression of disease to higher grades, and finally preventing a recrudescence of disease in a patient who has already received definitive therapy. It is the propensity of the disease to recur that has driven this search.

Bowel habit and the disorders of function are intimately related. To this end, diet content, particularly fiber, has been implicated in the pathogenesis of hemorrhoids. Various diseases of the colon and rectum have been linked to the Western low fiber diet.[117,118] Studies have shown benefit regarding symptoms with the institution of a diet that increases fecal bulk.[119] Moesgaard showed statistically significant decreased bleeding and pain with this diet, though pruritus, secretion and prolapse were not affected.[120] If the disease also includes high anal sphincter pressures, one is less likely to meet success with diet management alone.[121] Keighley[121] found no change in anal pressure in those hemorrhoid patients with pressures measured at 74 mmHg or more; 73% were no better or required further treatment. Dietary management may also complement the surgical procedure such as in the study by Jensen[122] where the results with rubber band ligation were better in those patients on bran than those who were not. This study showed a significant improvement in long-term outcome for 4th degree hemorrhoid treatment, with 45% symptom recurrence in band ligation alone versus 15% in those also on the roughage diet.

Faulty bowel habit with prolonged straining is thought to generate a high shearing force causing the engorged hemorrhoidal tissue to prolapse and bleed.[123] Therefore, attempts have been made to correct faulty bowel habits that exacerbate this process. Even those who do not believe constipation *per se* is the problem have noted abnormal sphincter pressures and defecation dynamics[124] that could lend themselves to approaches such as biofeedback. More simplistically, it has been suggested that people adopt a process of 'controlled defecation' which entails passing the stool bolus, using their rectal squeeze to reduce the hemorrhoidal engorgement and then sitting relaxed until the next urge arrives. This is as opposed to continued straining at the stool. Suggestions go as far as to consciously reduce the time spent on the toilet and avoidance of habits such as reading during defecation which are thought to lead to unnecessary, ineffective and damaging straining.[125]

CONCLUSION

In conclusion, this chapter details current thinking, diagnosis and management techniques for solitary rectal ulcer, rectocele and hemorrhoids. As always, these diseases have continued to constitute a large part of any colorectal practice and a significant portion of pelvic floor disease. There remains a need for more detailed understanding of normal defecation, and of defecatory disorders, especially straining at stool and constipation. We now have a greater understanding of the dynamic interrelationships of the pelvic floor, its sphincters and supporting structures. The biggest lesson that can be learned is that we have moved far beyond a simple surgical repair of the problem. Each of these conditions requires a thorough evaluation of the patient and a customized therapy that addresses bowel physiology, sphincter control and the anatomic sequelae that result from their derangement.

Our armamentarium includes preventive, conservative and major surgical procedures. Nonetheless, there still remain unanswered questions regarding the physiology and pathophysiology of these diseases.

REFERENCES

1. Crueilhier J. Ulcere chronique du rectum. In: *Anatomie pathologique du corps humain*. Paris: JB Baillière, 1829.
2. Haray PN, Morriss-Stiff GJ, Foster ME. Solitary rectal ulcer syndrome – an underdiagnosed condition. *Int J Colorectal Dis* 1997;**12**:313–5.
3. Madigan MR. Solitary rectal ulcer of the rectum. *Proc R Soc Med* 1964;**57**:403.
4. Madigan MR, Morson BC. Solitary rectal ulcer of the rectum. *Gut* 1969;**10**:871.
5. Rutter KRP, Riddell RH. The solitary ulcer syndrome of the rectum. *Clin Gastroenterol* 1975;**4**:505.
6. Martin CJ, Parks TG, Biggart JD. Solitary rectal ulcer syndrome in Northern Ireland 1971–80. *Br J Surg* 1981;**68**:744–7.
7. Mahieu PHG. Barium enema and defecography in the diagnosis and evaluation of the solitary rectal ulcer syndrome. *Int J Colorectal Dis* 1986;**1**:85–90.
8. Tjandra JJ, Fazio VW, Church JM, *et al.* Clinical conundrum of solitary rectal ulcer. *Dis Colon Rectum* **35**:227–34.
9. Saul SH. Solitary rectal ulcer syndrome; its clinical and pathological underdiagnosis. *Am J Surg Pathol* 1985;**9**:411.
10. Kang YS, Kamm MA, Engel AF, Talbot IC. Pathology of the rectal wall in solitary rectal ulcer syndrome and complete rectal Prolapse. *Gut* 1996;**38**:587–90.
11. Franzin G, Dina R, Scarpa A, Frattan A. The evolution of the solitary ulcer of the rectum: an endoscopic and histopathological study. *Endoscopy* 1982;**14**:131.
12. Binnie NR, Papachrysotomou M, Clare N, Smith AN. Solitary rectal ulcer: the place of biofeedback and surgery in the treatment of the syndrome. *World J Surg* 1992;**16**:836–40.
13. Keighley MRB, Shoulder P. Clinical and manometric features of the solitary rectal ulcer syndrome. *Dis Colon Rectum* 1984;**27**:507.
14. Thomson H, Hill D. Solitary rectal ulcer: always a self induced condition? *Br J Surg* 1908;**67**:784.
15. Contractor TQ, Contractor QQ. Traumatic solitary rectal ulcer in Saudi Arabia – a distinct entity? *J Clin Gastroenterol* 1995;**221**(4):298–300.
16. Antia FP. Solitary rectal ulcer (digital bowel evacuation: mucous colitis). *Indian J Gastroenterol* 1987;**6**:45.
17. Tandon RK, Atmakuri SP, Mehra NK, Malaviya AN, Tandon HD, Chopra P. Is solitary rectal ulcer syndrome a manifestation of systemic disease? *J Clin Gastroenterol* 1990;12:286–90.
18. Ho YH, Ho JMS, Parry BR, Goh HS. Solitary rectal ulcer syndrome: the clinical entity and anorectal physiological findings in Singapore. *Aust NZ J Surg* 1995;**65**:93–7.
19. van Outryve MJ, Pelckmans PA, Fierens H, van Maercke YM. Transrectal ultrasound study of the pathogenesis of solitary rectal ulcer syndrome. *Gut* 1993;**34**:1422–6.
20. Snooks SJ, Nicholls RJ, Henry MM, Swash M. Electrophysiological and manometric assessment of the pelvic floor in solitary rectal ulcer syndrome. *Br J Surg* 1985;**72**:313–33.
21. Womack NR, Williams NS, Holmfield JH, Morrison JF. Pressure and prolapse – the cause of solitary rectal ulceration. *Gut* 1987;**28**:1228.
22. Yo YH, Ho JM, Parry BR, Goh HS. Solitary rectal ulcer syndrome: the clinical entity and anorectal physiological findings in Singapore. *Aust NZ J Surg* 1995;**65**(2):93–97.
23. Sun WM, Read NW, Bonelly TC, Bannister JJ, Shorthouse AJ. A common pathophysiology for full thickness rectal prolapse, anterior mucosal prolapse and solitary rectal ulcer. *Br J Surg* 1989;**76**:290–5.
24. Kuijpers HC, Scheve RH, Hoedmakers HTC. Diagnosis of functional disorders of defecation causing the solitary rectal ulcer syndrome. *Dis Colon Rectum* 1986;**29**:126–9.
25. Halligan S, Nicholls RJ, Bartram CI. Evacuation proctography in patients with solitary rectal ulcer syndrome:

anatomic abnormalities and frequency of impaired emptying and prolapse. *Am J Roengenol* **164**:91–5.
26. Mackle EJ, Parks TG. The pathogenesis and pathophysiology of rectal prolapse and solitary rectal ulcer syndrome. *Clin Gastroenterol* 1986;**15**:985–1002.
27. Duff TH, Wright FF. Acute and chronic ulcers of the rectum. *Surg Gynecol Obstet* 1981;**153**:398–400.
28. Levine DS. 'Solitary' rectal ulcer syndrome. Are 'solitary' rectal ulcer syndrome and 'localized' colitis cystica profunda analogous syndromes caused by rectal prolapse? *Gastroenterology* 1987;**92**:243–53.
29. Pescatori M, Maria G, Mattana C, *et al.* Clinical picture and pelvic floor physiology in the solitary rectal ulcer syndrome. *Dis Colon Rectum* 1985;**28**:862–7.
30. Lubowski DZ. Solitary rectal ulcer syndrome: pathophysiology and treatment. In: Henry MM, Swash M (eds). *Coloproctology and the pelvic floor.* London: Butterworth–Heinemann, 1985:305–15.
31. Kang YS, Kamm MA, Nicholls RJ. Solitary rectal ulcer and complete rectal prolapse: one condition or two? *Int J Colorect Dis* 1995;**10**:87–90.
32. Thomson G, Clark A, Handyside J, Gillespie G. Solitary ulcer of the rectum – or is it? A report of six cases. *Br J Surg* 1981;**68**:21–4.
33. Frezko P, O'Connell D, Riddell R, Frank P. Solitary rectal ulcer syndrome radiologic manifestations. *AJR* 1980; **135**:499–506.
34. Chen AS, Luchtefeld RG, Senagore AJ, MacKeigan JM, *et al.* Pudendal nerve latency: does it predict outcome of anal sphincter repair? *Dis Colon Rectum* 1998;**41**:1005–1009.
35. Simmang C, Birnbaum EH, Kodner IJ, *et al.* Anal sphincter reconstruction in the elderly: does advancing age affect outcome? *Dis Colon Rectum* 1994;**37**:1065.
36. Fleshman JW, Dreznik Z, Cohen E, Fry RD, *et al.* Balloon expulsion test facilitates diagnosis of pelvic floor outlet obstruction due to nonrelaxing puborectalis muscle. *Dis Colon Rectum* 1992;**35**:1019–29.
37. van den Brandt-Gradel V, Huibregtse K, Tygat GNJ. Treatment of solitary rectal ulcer syndrome with high fiber diet and abstention of straining at defecation. *Dig Dis Sci* 1984;**29**:1005–8.
38. Zargar SA, Khuroo MS, Mahajan R. Sucralfate retention enemas in solitary rectal ulcer. *Dis Colon Rectum* 1991;**34**:455–7.
39. Vaizey CJ, Roy AJ, Kamm MA. Prospective evaluation of the treatment of solitary rectal ulcer syndrome with biofeedback. *Gut* 1997;**41**:817–20.
40. Fleshman JW, Dreznik Z, Meyer K, Fry RD, *et al.* Outpatient protocol for biofeedback therapy of pelvic floor outlet obstruction. *Dis Colon Rectum* 1992;**35**:1–7.
41. Tjandra JJ, Fazio VW, Petras RE, *et al.* Clinical and pathological factors associated with delayed diagnosis in solitary rectal ulcer syndrome. *Dis Colon Rectum* 1993;**36**:146–53.
42. Halligan S, Nicholls RJ, Bartram CI. Proctographic changes after rectopexy for solitary rectal ulcer syndrome and preoperative factors for successful outcome. *Br J Surg* 1995;**82**:314–7.
43. Nicholls RJ, Simpson JNL. Anteroposterior rectopexy in the treatment of the solitary rectal ulcer syndrome without overt rectal prolapse. *Br J Surg* 1986;**73**:222–4.
44. Fleshman JW, Kodner IJ, Fry RD. Internal intussusception of the rectum: a changing perspective. *Netherland J Surg* 1989;**41**:145–48.
45. Panis Y, Perrin H, Poupard B, *et al.* Coloanal anastomosis for benign lesions: long-term functional results in 11 patients. *Eur J Surg* 1996;**162**:555–9.
46. Sitzler PJ, Kamm MA, Nicholls RJ, McKee RF. Long-term outcome of surgery for solitary rectal ulcer syndrome. *Br J Surg* 1998;**85**:1246–50.
47. Redding MD. The relaxed perineum and anorectal disease. *Dis Colon Rectum* 1965;**8**:279–82.
48. Klevin FM, Maglinte DD, Horback JA, Benson JT. Pelvic prolapse: assessment with evacuation proctography (defecography). *Radiology* 1992;**184**:547–51.
49. Murthy VK, Orkin BA, Smith LE, Glassman LM. Excellent outcome using selective criteria for rectocele repair. *Dis Colon Rectum* 1996;**39**:374–8.
50. Bartram CJ, Turnbull GK, Lennard-Jones JE. Evacuation proctography, an investigation of rectal expulsion in twenty subjects without defecatory disturbance. *Gastrointest Radiol* 1988;**13**:72–80.
51. Shorovan PJ, McHugh S, Diamant NE, Somers S, Stevenson GW. Defecography in normal volunteers, results and implications. *Gut* 1989;**30**:1737–49.
52. Uhlenhuth E, Wolfe WM, Smith EM, Middleton EB. The rectovaginal septum. *Surg Gynecol Obstet* 1948;**86**:148–63.
53. Richardson AC. The rectovaginal septum revisited: its relationship to rectocele and its importance in rectocele repair. *Clin Obstet Gynecol* 1993;**36**:976–83.
54. Beson JT. Female pelvic floor disorders: investigation and management. New York: WW Norton, 1992:380–89.
55. Mellgren A, Lupez A, Schultz I, *et al.* Rectocele is associated with paradoxical anal sphincter reaction. *Int J Colorectal Dis* 1998;**13**:13–16.
56. Joahannson C, Nilsson BY, Holmstrom B, *et al.* Association between rectocele and paradoxical sphincter response. *Dis Colon Rectum* 1992;**35**:503.
57. Siproudhus L, Dautrremes S, Ropert A, *et al.* Dyschezia and rectocele – a marriage of convenience? *Dis Colon Rectum* 1993;**36**:1030.
58. Yoshioka K, Matsui Y, Yamada O, *et al.* Physiologic and anatomic assessment of patients with rectoceles. *Dis Colon Rectum* 1991;**34**:704.
59. Macks MM. The rectal side of rectocele. *Dis Colon Rectum* 1967;**10**:387–8.
60. Arnold MW, Stewart WRC, Aguilar PS. Rectocele repair, four years experience. *Dis Colon Rectum* 1990;**33**:684–7.
61. Halverson AL, Orkin BA. Which physiologic tests are useful in patients with constipation? *Dis Colon Rectum* 1998;**41**:735–9.
62. Healy JC, Halligan S, Reznek RH, *et al.* Patterns of prolapse in women with symptoms of pelvic floor weakness: assessment with MR imaging. *Radiology* 1997;**203**:77–81.
63. Mellgren A, Anzen B, Nilsson B-Y, *et al.* Results of rectocele repair: a prospective study. *Dis Colon Rectum* 1995;**38**:7–13.
64. Van Dam JH, Ginai AZ, Gosselink MJ, *et al.* Role of defecography in the predicting of clinical outcome in rectocele repair. *Dis Colon Rectum* 1997;**40**:201–7.

65. Sullivan ES, Leaverton GH, Hardwick CE. Transrectal perineal repair: an adjunct to improved function after anorectal surgery. *Dis Colon Rectum* 1968;**1**:106–14.
66. Capps WF Jr. Rectoplasty and perineoplasty for symptomatic rectocele: a report of fifty cases. *Dis Colon Rectum* 1975;**18**:237–43.
67. Sehapayak S. Transrectal repair of rectocele: an extended armamentarium of colorectal surgeons: a report of 355 cases. *Dis Colon Rectum* 1985;**8**:22–33.
68. Block IR. Transrectal repair of rectocele using obliterative suture. *Dis Colon Rectum* 1986;**29**:707–11.
69. Ho Y-H, Ang M, Nyam D, Tan M, Seow-Choen F. Transanal approach to rectocele repair may compromise anal sphincter pressures. *Dis Colon Rectum* 1998;**41**:354–58.
70. Nichols DH, Randall CL. *Vaginal surgery*, 3rd edn. Baltimore: Williams and Wilkins, 1989.
71. Oster S, Astrup A. A new vaginal operation for recurrent and large rectocele using dermis transplant. *Acta Obstet Gynecol Scand* 1981;**60**:493–5.
72. Watson SJ, Loder PB, Halligan S, *et al.* Transperineal repair of symptomatic rectocele using Marlex mesh: a clinical, physiologic and radiologic assessment of treatment. *Am Coll Surg* 1996;**183**:257–61.
73. Sullivan ES, Stranburg CO, Sandoz IL, *et al.* Repair of total pelvic prolapse: an overview. *Perspect Colon Rectal Surg* 1990;**3**:119–31.
74. Khubchandani IT, Clancy JP, Rosen L. Endorectal repair of rectocele revisited. *Br J Surg* 1997;**84**:89–91.
75. Khubchandani IT, Sheets JA, Stasik JJ, Hakki AR. Endorectal repair of rectocele. *Dis Colon Rectum* 1983;**26**:792–6.
76. Jansen LW, Van Dijke CF. Selection criteria for anterior rectal wall repair in symptomatic rectocele and anterior wall rectal prolapse. *Dis Colon Rectum* 1994;**37**:1100–7.
77. Sarles JC, Arnaud A, Selezneff I, Olivier S. Endorectal repair of rectocele. *Int J Colorectal Dis* 1989;**4**:167–71.
78. Karlbaum K, Graf W, Nilsson S, Pahlman L. Does surgical repair of rectocele improve rectal emptying? *Dis Colon Rectum* 1996;**39**:1296–1302.
79. Fry RD, Kodner IJ. Anorectal disorders. *CIBA Clin Symp* 1985;**37**(6).
80. Haas PA, Fox TA Jr, Haas GP. The pathogenesis of hemorrhoids. *Dis Colon Rectum* 1984;**27**:442–50.
81. Sun WM, Peck RJ, Shorthouse AJ, Read NW. Hemorrhoids are associated, not with hypertrophy of the internal anal sphincter, but with hypertension of anal cushions. *Br J Surg* 1992;**79**:592–4.
82. Gibbons CP, Bannister JJ, Read NW. Role of constipation and anal hypertonia in the pathogenesis of hemorrhoids. *Br J Surg* 1988;**75**:656–60.
83. Saint-Pierre A, Treffot MJ, Martin PM. Anal pressure in haemorrhoids and anal fissure. *Br J Surg* 1982;**134**:608–10.
84. Arabi Y, Alexander-Williams J, Keighley M. Anal pressures in hemorrhoids and anal fissures. *Am J Surg* 1977;**134**:608–10.
85. Sun WM, Read NW, Shorthouse AJ. Hypertensive anal cushions as the cause of high anal pressures in patients with hemorrhoids. *Br J Surg* 1990;**77**:458–62.
86. Read MG, Read NW, Haynes WG. A prospective study of the effect of hemorrhoidectomy on sphincter function and fecal incontinence. *Br J Surg* 1982;**69**:396–8.
87. Teramoto JL, Parks AG, Swash M. Hypertrophy of the external and internal sphincter in hemorrhoids: a histometric study. *Gut* 1981;**22**:45–8.
88. Hancock BD. Internal sphincter and the nature of hemorrhoids. *Gut* 1977;**18**:651–5.
89. Thompson JP, Leicester RJ. Hemorrhoids: pathophysiology and clinical features. In: Henry MM, Swash M (eds). *Coloproctology and the pelvic floor*. London: Butterworths, 1985:195–216.
90. Burkitt DP, Graham-Stewart CW. Haemorrhoids: postulated pathogenesis and proposed prevention. *Postgraduate Med J* 1975;**51**:631.
91. Lord PH. Diverse methods for managing hemorrhoids, dilatation. *Dis Colon Rectum* 1973;**16**:180.
92. Snooks S, Henry MM, Swash M. Faecal incontinence after anal dilatation. *Br J Surg* 1984;**711**:617–8.
93. Eisenhammer S. Anal sphincterotomy and dilatation: a criticism. *Dis Colon Rectum* 1974;**17**:493–52.
94. Asfar SK, Juma TH, Ala-Edeen T. Hemorrhoidectomy and sphincterotomy: a prospective study comparing the effectiveness of anal stretch and sphincterotomy in reducing pain after hemorrhoidectomy. *Dis Colon Rectum* 1988;**31**:181–5.
95. Schouten WR, van Vroonhooven TJ. Lateral internal sphincterotomy in the treatment of hemorrhoids. *Dis Colon Rectum* 1986;**29**:869–872.
96. Barron J. Office ligation of hemorrhoids. *Am J Surg* 1963;**105**:563–70.
97. Rothberg R, Rubin RJ, Eisenstadt T, Salvati EP. Rubber band ligation hemorrhoidectomy: long-term results. *Dis Colon Rectum* 1985;**28**:291–3.
98. Steinberg DM, Liegois H, Alexander-Williams J. Long-term review of rubber band ligation of hemorrhoids. *Br J Surg* 1975;**62**:144–6.
99. Wrobleski DE, Gorman ML, Veidenheimer MC, Coller JA. Long-term evaluation of rubber ring ligation in hemorroidal disease. *Dis Colon Rectum* 1980;**23**:478–482.
100. Shemesh EI, Kodner IJ, Fry RD, Neufeld DM. Severe complication of rubber band ligation of internal hemorrhoids. *Dis Colon Rectum* 1987;**30**:199–200.
101. Templeton JL, Spence RA, Kennedy TL, *et al.* Comparison of infrared coagulation and rubber band ligation for first and second degree hemorrhoids: a randomized prospective clinical trial. *BMJ* 1983;**286**:1387–9.
102. Dencker H, Hjorth N, Norryd C, *et al.* Comparison of results of different methods of treating hemorrhoids. *Acta Chir Scand* 1973;**139**:742–5.
103. Alexander-Williams J, Crapp AR. Conservative management of hemorrhoids. Part 1: injection, freezing, and ligation. *Clin Gastroenterol* 1975;**4**:595.
104. Lacock WS, Trus TL, Hunter JG. New technology for the division of short gastric vessels during laparoscopic Nissen Fundoplication: a prospective, randomized trial. *Surg Endosc* 1996;**10**:71.
105. Milligan ETC, Morgan CN, Jones LE, *et al.* Surgical anatomy of the anal canal and operative treatment of hemorrhoids. *Lancet* 1937;**2**:1119–24.
106. Ferguson JA, Heaton JR. Closed hemorrhoidectomy. *Dis Colon Rectum* 1959;**2**:176.
107. Whitehead W. The surgical management of hemorrhoids. *BMJ* 1882;**1**:148.

108. Bleday R, Pena JP, Rothenberger DA, *et al.* Symptomatic hemorrhoids: current incidence and complications of operative therapy. *Dis Colon Rectum* 1992;**35**:477.
109. Wolff BG, Culp CE. The Whitehead hemorrhoidectomy: an unjustly maligned procedure. *Dis Colon Rectum* 1988;**31**:587–90.
110. Caplin DA, Kodner IJ. Repair of anal stricture and mucosal ectropion by simple flap procedure. *Dis Colon Rectum* 1986;**29**:92–4.
111. Ferguson JA. Repair of the Whitehead deformity of the anus. *Surg Gynecol Obstet* 1959;**108**:115.
112. Yu JC, Eddy HJ Jr. Laser: a new modality for hemorrhoidectomy. *Am J Proctol Gastroenterol Colon Rectal Surg* 1985;**36**:9.
113. Iwagaki H, Higuchi Y, Fuchimoto S, Orita K. The laser treatment of hemorrhoids: results of a study on 1816 patients. *Japan J Surg* 1989;**19**:658–61.
114. Wang JY, Chang-Chien CR, Chen J-S, *et al.* The role of lasers in hemorrhoidectomy. *Dis Colon Rectum* 1991;**34**:78–82.
115. Chia YW, Darzi A, Speakman CTM, *et al.* Carbon dioxide laser hemorrhoidectomy: does it alter anorectal function or decrease pain compared to conventional hemorrhoidectomy? *J Colorectal Dis* 1995;**10**:22–4.
116. Hodgson WJB, Morgan J. Ambulatory hemorrhoidectomy with CO_2 laser. *Dis Colon Rectum* 1995;**38**:1265–9.
117. Burkitt DP, Walker AR, Painter NS. Dietary fiber and disease. *JAMA* 1974;**229**:1068–74.
118. Burkitt DP. Hemorrhoids, varicose veins and deep venous thrombosis: epidemiologic features and suggestive causative factors. *Can J Surg* 1975;**18**:483–8.
119. Burkitt DP. Fiber as protective against gastrointestinal diseases. *Am J Gastroenterol* 1984;**79**:249–52.
120. Moesgaard F, *et al.* High-fiber diet reduces bleeding and pain in patients with hemorrhoids: a double-blind trial of Vi-Siblin. *Dis Colon Rectum* 1982;**25**:454–6.
121. Keighley MR, *et al.* Prospective trials of minor surgical procedures and high-fibre diet for haemorrhoids. *BMJ* 1979;**2**:967–9.
122. Jensen SL, *et al.* Maintenance bran therapy for prevention of sympytoms after rubber band ligation of third-degree haemorrhoids. *Acta Chir Scand* 1988;**154**:395–8.
123. MacLeod JH. Rational approach to treatment of hemorrhoids based on a theory of etiology. *Arch Surg* 1983;**118**:29032.
124. Gibbons CP, *et al.* Role of constipation and anal hypertonia in the pathogenesis of haemorrhoids. *Br J Surg* 1988;**75**:656–60.
125. Marx FA. Prevention of hemorrhoids by controlled defecation. *Dis Colon Rectum* 1993;**36**:1084.

Chapter 26

Neurological disorders and the pelvic floor

Michael Swash, Michael M Henry

Although much of this book is concerned with understanding of idiopathic urinary and fecal incontinence, and of incontinence associated with childbirth, much incontinence is due to disease of the central or peripheral nervous system, including disorders of the cauda equina and of the lumbo-sacral plexus. Idiopathic stress urinary and fecal incontinence, a disorder of complex and multifactorial etiology, has a major neurogenic causative component due to damage to the distal parts of the innervation of the pelvic floor striated sphincter muscles.[1,2] This seems to be due to recurrent stretch induced injury to this innervation.[3] When the connective tissues of the pelvic floor are damaged during childbirth there is additional susceptibility to nerve damage of this type, as well as disruption of the normal anatomical and pressure relationships of structures in the lower urinary and anal tracts. In addition, direct injury to the external anal sphincter plays a role in fecal incontinence. These complex relationships underly modern concepts of the role of suspensory procedures in the surgical repair of these functional incontinence syndromes.

A classification of the neurological causes of incontinence is given in Table 26.1. Other pelvic floor disorders occur in patients with neurological disease, but the relationship between these disorders and the neurological disease is usually indirect. For example, senile dementia is often accompanied by fecal impaction with overflow incontinence of feces and urinary incontinence. In addition, rectal prolapse is very common in this group of patients perhaps because of the abnormal stresses caused in the expulsion processes by the overfilling, and by the resultant damage to the smooth musculature of the anorectum and to its locally-mediated reflexes. It is likely these functional disorders result from inadequate personal care, as well as from the failure of central nervous system pathways. Similar secondary abnormalities occur in bladder function; chronic overfilling reduces bladder sensitivity to filling and overflow incontinence occurs. Thus incontinence in central nervous system disorders may have several inter-related underlying causes. Modification of one of these, however, for example, fecal impaction or bladder infection, may improve continence even though the primary abnormality of function, e.g., the central nervous system disorder has not been addressed.

Certain pre-existing conditions, e.g. irritable bowel syndrome, long suspected to be associated with a particular personality type, may be important in modifying

Table 26.1 Neurological causes of incontinence

Upper motor neuron lesions
Cerebral lesions
Dementia
Cerebrovascular disease
Hydrocephalus
Multiple sclerosis
Tumors (especially frontal tumors)
Traumatic encephalopathy
Cerebral infections
Spinal cord lesions
Trauma
Cord compression
Multiple sclerosis
Ischemia
Lower motor neuron lesions
Conus medullaris
Multiple sclerosis
Ischemia
Spinal dysraphism
Degenerative disease; especially primary autonomic failure
Multiple system atrophy (MSA)
Cauda equina lesions
Lumbosacral trauma
Lumbosacral disc prolapse
Lumbar canal stenosis and spondylosis
Ankylosing spondylitis
Peripheral nerve lesions
Pudendal/perineal stretch injury and neuropathy
Childbirth-associated injuries to innervation of pelvic floor
Intra-pelvic lesions; e.g. tumors, sepsis and endometriosis
Proximal diabetic neuropathy
Autonomic neuropathy?

the expression of bowel disorder in the presence of acquired CNS lesions. However, urgency of micturition occurring as a pre-existing trait is not important in the development of acquired bladder functional disorders due to CNS lesions.

The neural basis of normal bowel and bladder control has been dealt with elsewhere in this book. Disorders of continence and of colo-anal function that have a neurogenic basis can be classified using this approach, and this is useful in planning investigation and management in clinical practice. The elderly are particularly likely to be affected by disorders of multifactorial causation (Table 26.2). The central nervous system is able to modulate the activity of peripheral structures within a wide range of functional states. Thus, when there is damage to the peripheral structure, including nerves, muscles, the viscera themselves, elastic tissue and suspensory ligaments, the central nervous system has the capacity to compensate by overaction and modulation of the pattern of control activity. During aging, and with disease, this central control system is gradually brought to a point where full functional compensation is no longer possible and a disorder of continence develops. When the control system itself is disordered, this compensatory system is further threatened.

CENTRAL NERVOUS SYSTEM LESIONS

Lesions in the central nervous system may cause incontinence by interruption of the descending and ascending pathways concerned with modulation of the sphincter control system, or by interfering with the functioning of the central processes in the brain that constitute the higher level synthesis of sphincter control (storage) and of micturition and defecation (voiding). Lesions in the central control system in the brain, brainstem, and spinal cord rostral to the sacral nucleus of Onuf are upper motor neuron lesions with respect to the effector organs.

Voluntary control of the bladder and rectum is represented in the cerebral cortex, just as are other functions of the body that are consciously perceived. Kleist[4] indicated from studies of head-injured German soldiers in the First World War that the bladder and rectum are both represented on the medial surfaces of the cerebral hemispheres, with the motor and sensory representations situated adjacent to each other across the Rolandic fissure of the brain, a view confirmed by Förster and later by Penfield and Rasmussen.[5] However, lesions situated discretely at this site have not been reported to cause disorders of continence of urine or feces. Contemporary PET and functional MRI studies have shown that the cortical representation of micturition more or less conforms to these older ideas, but that there are other parts of the cerebral cortex that are concerned with the integration of afferent innervation, and with the generation of decisions to withhold micturition and in the sensation of the urge to micturate.[6,7] There is less understanding of defecation, but it is assumed that similar central neural processes are involved.[8]

Table 26.2 Multifactorial causes of incontinence and pelvic floor dysfunction

- Incontinence in the elderly
- Incontinence in confusional states
- Fecal impaction
- Immobility
- Rectal prolapse
- Ano-rectal, vaginal and perineal discomfort and pain
- Constipation

FRONTAL LOBE LESIONS

Frontal lobe lesions, particularly lesions of the inferior and medial surfaces of the frontal lobes, are well-known to be associated with incontinence. Thus meningiomas arising from the falx cerebri, or from the olfactory groove, that impinge on the medial and inferior surfaces of the frontal cortex bilaterally, may present with incontinence.[9] In these patients incontinence consists of inappropriate defecation or micturition. Rather than the involuntary emptying of the contents of the bladder or bowel to the embarrassment of the patient, a normal excretory act occurs, without understanding on the part of the patient that this is carried out in an inappropriate context. This is not urge or stress incontinence. This type of incontinence, consisting of loss of the critical functions of the brain, with reversion to an infantile pattern of non-toilet trained habits is particularly characteristic of frontal lobe lesions. It is therefore frequent in dementia, multiple strokes, post-traumatic encephalopathy, and in some patients with multiple sclerosis, in addition to focal lesions of the frontal lobes, such as extrinsic or intrinsic tumors. Patients with multifocal disorders such as multiple sclerosis or multi-infarct states will have lesions in different parts of the central nervous system, including deep central white matter, and the pattern of incontinence will be complex, with features of urgency and inappropriate behavior occurring together.

Single large hemispheric strokes are often associated with both incontinence and dysphagia in the acute phase of the illness. As the patient begins to recover function these two functional disorders resolve. It is presumed that these functional deficits result from a combination of the single large lesions in the hemisphere interrupting frontally dependent pathways for voiding and storage of urine and feces.[10] Despite the bilateral representation of continence-related functions in the brain there is a tendency for these functions to be predominantly functionally lateralized to one hemisphere, usually the right side. Conditioning studies, using magnetic cortical stimulation as the conditioning stimulus, have suggested that there is an inbuilt asymmetry of the cortical response in the esophageal swallowing response[11] and it may be that for defecation and micturition there is a similar asymmetry in the cortical arrangements. This has been linked to the asymmetry of brain function that is a feature of handedness, especially in right handed subjects, and may be important in the development of fecal incontinence following unilateral pudendal lesions in some subjects.[1,12,13] Similar asymmetry to the pudendal innervation of the pelvic sphincters has been found in animal studies in both the anal sphincter,[14] and in the urinary sphincter.[15] Thus, asymmetry of the organization of the neural control system extends from the cortex to the muscles of continence themselves, and has both anatomical and physiological significance.

MULTIPLE SCLEROSIS

The cause of incontinence in multiple sclerosis is not necessarily always of this type, however. Many such patients have fecal impaction as a consequence of their immobility with overflow of feces through a patulous anus, itself the result of reflex relaxation of the anal sphincter stimulated by the rectal distention. In addition multiple sclerosis also leads to incontinence from conus medullaris lesions, causing weakness and denervation of the pelvic floor striated sphincter muscles.[16] Multiple sclerosis is a common disease, especially in people of Scandinavian origin, and therefore there are relatively large numbers of affected people in Western Europe and the USA. The prevalence is about 160/100 000 in the UK, with a higher incidence and prevalence in Northern Scotland. As many as 70% of people with MS experience fecal incontinence,[17] and the incidence of urinary disorder, with incontinence, poor bladder emptying or uncontrollable urgency is even higher.[18] Bladder and bowel dysfunction is the third most important discomfort in MS after spasticity and incoordination.[19] No detailed data on the pattern of bowel functional abnormality in patients with MS, based on physiological and anatomical lesion analysis are available, perhaps because of the complexity of the problem in the context of the varied location and extent of lesions in MS, and the difficulty, even with modern MR imaging, in accurately delineating lesions, especially in the spinal cord. However, Mathers *et al.*[20] showed that it was possible to localize certain dysfunctional physiological disturbances using a combination of peripheral and central electrophysiological techniques, including cortical stimulation to evaluate cortical pathways to the external anal sphincter in MS patients, and Jameson *et al.*[21] have evaluated the clinical syndromes of pelvic floor dysfunction in MS. These include pelvic floor incoordination, constipation, incontinence, impaction, reduced anal sphincter squeeze pressure, and impaired ano-rectal sensation. In MS the principal bladder abnormalities are detrusor sphincter dyssynergia, retention of urine, and urgency with incontinence.[22] Rarely MS may present with urinary incontinence, probably due to demyelination in the region of the conus medullaris of the spinal cord.

HYDROCEPHALUS

Urinary incontinence is a distinctive presenting feature of patients with decompensated hydrocephalus. In these patients there is no evidence of functional disturbance of cortical neuronal function, and the urinary incontinence is thought to result from damage to the descending pathways between the cortex and the brainstem, caused by direct pressure effects on them as they project through the corticospinal pathway around the lateral side of the distended lateral ventricles, or from axonal stretch injury in the brain at this site. The corticomotor pathway from the medial surface of the hemisphere is more likely to be deformed by expansion of the lateral ventricle, affecting the motor fibers that take origin from the lateral surface of the hemisphere. The latter project to motor neurons innervating upper limb and bulbar muscles and there is therefore also an association between the development of incontinence and the finding of features of a slowly progressive spastic paraplegia, without involvement of the upper limbs, as the hydrocephalus advances. The typical clinical features of 'occult hydrocephalus' therefore consist of incontinence, spastic paraparesis with a shuffling, apractic gait pattern, and extensor plantar responses.[23] Differential diagnosis from degenerative disease causing dementia is not always easy, since there may be ventricular dilatation in both disorders. In degenerative brain diseases, however, such as Alzheimer's disease, there is also cortical atrophy. In occult or frank hydrocephalus the temporal horns are usually dilated. This is not a feature of the early stages of degenerative brain disease, although it may develop in the later phase when there is generalized cortical and central atrophy of the brain.

BRAINSTEM DISEASE

In brainstem vascular disease there is loss of supranuclear control of the sacral centers for defecation and micturition, so that in the absence of obstruction to normal micturition or defecation, or of infection, an automatic pattern of evacuation may be established. If the lesion disrupts the pontine centers for defecation and micturition, or for storage, however, retention may result, with overflow incontinence. It is presumed that the centers for fecal and urinary storage and voiding are located close to each other in the brainstem, although evidence on this point in humans, based on functional imaging data is so far available only for the urinary system.

Most lesions in the brainstem, for example, tumors, infarcts or hemorrhage, and demyelination, produce relatively extensive and complex functional disturbances, often with sensory impairment. There is then usually impairment of the normal appreciation of filling of the ano-rectum and bladder, resulting in overfilling, distention, and loss of locally-mediated reflexes in the bladder and bowel wall. Thus, there is loss of normal visco-elasticity of the wall of the ano-rectum and bladder, loss of the normal smooth muscle tone in these organs, and loss of the normal storage function of these organs. Retention of urine, in particular, is followed by recurrent urinary tract infection and stiffening of the bladder wall causing abnormal filling and sensory characteristics. These secondary factors can assume importance beyond the functional abnormality in the neural control system itself.

Sakakibara *et al.*[24] described a patient with Herpes simplex encephalitis involving the brainstem who presented with hiccup and coma with breathing disturbance, and developed nocturnal frequency of micturition, urinary incontinence, voiding difficulty and residual urine during the recovery phase. This was probably due to involvement of the pontine urinary storage and voiding centres, demonstrated by MR imaging in this patient, lesions that were predominantly right sided. Brainstem stroke has also been associated with micturitional disturbance, especially when the lesion is pontine,[25] and Ueki[26] in reporting that voiding difficulty is common in pontine tumors pointed out that Holman[27] had described this in 1926. Betts *et al.*[28] and Manente *et al.*[29] have also provided clinical evidence, from observations of patients with pontine tegmental tumors, for the existence of a pontine micturition center in humans.

PARKINSON'S DISEASE AND RELATED DISORDERS

Constipation is very common in Parkinson's disease, occuring in up to 80% of patients.[30] This intractable constipation is probably due, at least in part, to involvement of gut neurons by the disease process, as shown by the presence of Lewy bodies in myenteric plexus neurons. This is associated with slowed gut transit times.[31] Mathers *et al.*[32] reported outlet obstruction at the anal sphincter in some patients with Parkinson's disease, due to spontaneous and paradoxical contraction of the pelvic floor muscles, that they likened to anismus, but they felt that this was a form of focal dystonia of these muscles in this disease. They showed that this abnormality was responsive to treatment with dopaminergic agents, and was thus pharmacologically mediated.[33] Impairment of the defecation reflex in untreated 'off phase' Parkinson's disease shown by Mathers *et al.*[32,33] was confirmed by Ashraf *et al.*[34]

In progressive autonomic failure incontinence and impotence are major clinical features due to degeneration of autonomic pathways in the spinal cord, and of the Onuf nucleus neuroes in the sacral segments that innervate the urinary and anal sphincter muscles.

SPINAL CORD LESIONS

Glickman and Kamm[35] found that bowel disorders were a common source of disability and distress after spinal cord injury. In their questionnaire-based study of 115 consecutive patients with spinal cord injury 95% required at least one therapeutic method to induce defecation. Half were dependent on others for toileting, and 49% required longer than 30 minutes to complete their toilet procedure. Major fecal incontinence was often sudden and unpredictable. Problems related to bowel management were rated as nearly as troublesome as problems with mobility. Glickman and Kamm noted that after spinal cord injury the bowel loses part of its extrinsic autonomic innervation, leading to slow transit.[36] This causes loss of the normal postprandial intestinal hurry. Normal function of the sacral parasympathetic outflow to the left colon and rectum is essential for the initiation of normal defecation. There may also be loss of the somatic innervation of the external anal sphincter and pelvic floor. Diarrhea, for example, caused by laxatives can therefore lead to incontinence in the spinally-injured person. Colostomy may produce an improvement in quality of life. Low spinal injuries, e.g. at the thoraco-lumbar segmental junction will leave the sympathetic innervation but disconnect the sacral parasympathetic innervation from central control, although this latter innervation will be still connected autonomously to the bowel.

Nathan and Smith[37,38] demonstrated the location of the afferent and efferent pathways in the spinal cord subserving micturition and, presumably, also defecation. In spinal cord lesions, these pathways may be disrupted, resulting in separation of the pontine detrusor and storage mechanisms from the effector organs. This usually results in absence of evacuation responses, although 'mass' reflex evacuation may occur with certain cutaneous stimuli. Patients with complete spinal transection show lower resting pressures derived from the internal anal sphincter, diminished or absent anal and rectal sensation, but normal or exaggerated recto-anal reflexes following rectal distention. In addition they may show spontaneous high-amplitude rectal contraction at low distention volumes, without the ability to control this response.[39] Some afferent information from the gut can reach the brain though vagal afferents, even when there is a high spinal transection, leading to complexities in the interpretation of data, and to the patient stating that they have a sense of dull, painful rectal filling at high filling pressures.

CAUDA EQUINA LESIONS

Cauda equina lesions, for example due to sudden major disk prolapse unrelieved for several hours, may produce a devastating and permanent clinical deficit, with weakness of muscles innervated by the lower lumbar and sacral segments. Recognition of cauda equina or intra-pelvic lesions in the innervation of the pelvic floor muscles depends on a careful history and examination. The patient will usually describe low back or intra-pelvic pain or discomfort, often induced by movement or by certain postures. Sometimes, in patients with lumbosacral spondylosis, with narrow spinal canal (spinal stenosis), micturition is only possible with the spine held in a certain posture (usually in an exaggerated or maximally extended posture). Men usually develop ejaculatory impotence or even failure of erection as the cauda equina lesion or intra-pelvic lesion progresses.

Cauda equina compression is an acute emergency, that may develop as a sudden syndrome with major central disk prolapse, or may develop in the context of a long history of sciatica, almost always bilateral, when there is a sudden extension of pre-existing disk prolapse in the central part of the lumbo-sacral canal, causing compression of the cauda equina. The clinical disorder is often asymmetrical, and pain is felt not only in the back, but in the buttocks and perinuem, as well as in a more complete bilateral sciatic distribution. There may be a history of sciatica or of previous lumbosacral laminectomy. Sciatica is often bilateral, indicating the central location of the diskal prolapse. Sometimes cauda equina compression arises postoperatively, following laminectomy and disk excision, when there has been hemorrhage at the operative site with compression of the cauda equina nerve roots by hematoma.

The patient may be aware of loss of sensation in the perineum, or of loss of the normal sensations of bladder or bowel filling, and of loss of the sensation of urination and passage of feces during attempted micturition and defecation respectively. There is weakness of hip abduction and extension with relative sparing of hip flexion. Ankle and toe movements may be affected, especially lateral movement and abduction. Knee flexion is weak but the quadriceps are often unaffected. The knee and ankle reflexes are normal. The plantar responses are flexor, if obtainable. There is sensory loss in the same segments extending up the back of the calves to the posterior thighs and buttocks, thus having a characteristic 'saddle' distribution that extends forwards into the genitalia.

There is retention of urine with overflow and retention of feces with intractable difficulty in initiating micturition or defecation, and with loss of the normal sensation of bladder and rectal filling. There is no sense of the desire to void or defecate. The anal reflex and the cremasteric reflex are absent. The anal canal is patulous and loaded with feces. There is no anal response to coughing, and there is no anal squeeze response to volitional activity. The anal reflex is absent. There is marked perineal descent or straining, and the whole perineum is weak and feels 'ballooned' on examination of the rectum or vagina. The bladder is usually full and painless. The external anal sphincter is atrophic and denervated. The bladder requires an indwelling catheter for drainage, and destrusor activity is greatly reduced. Sexual function is absent or severely compromised after cauda equina lesion. Cystometry and ano-rectal manometry reveal essentially toneless organs, and EMG evaluation shows a few remaining abnormal polyphasic potentials in the perianal muscles.

It is important to recognize the development of signs of this syndrome at a much earlier stage than that described here, and MR imaging is the urgent diagnostic method of choice for definitive diagnosis. The prognosis of cauda equina lesions, almost always due to compression by disk, or to infiltration by metastatic tumor, is poor, regardless of surgical or medical therapy. Only with rapid surgical intervention in the case of compressive lesions is there any prospect of useful recovery of function. Gleave and Macfarlane[40] suggested that operation within 48 hours was necessary for a good outcome, but they felt that 'the die was cast' as soon as cauda equina compression had occurred and factors related to the severity of the compressive lesion determined the prognosis. Shapiro[41] came to a similar conclusion when the syndrome was of acute onset but pointed out that the outcome was better when the syndrome had developed over a few weeks.

CONUS MEDULLARIS LESIONS

The conus medullaris is sometimes the site of initial involvement in multiple sclerosis, causing presentation with urinary retention and overflow incontinence, difficulty initiating defecation and sensory impairment. In conus lesions the sensory loss is more extensive than in cauda equina disorders, extending onto the lower abdominal wall, and involving the anterior thighs as well as the lower lumbosacral segments. This results from involvement of the posterior columns and spinothalamic pathways in the conus. Since the lesion is often intrinsic, for example in conus tumors or penetrating trauma to the conus, this sensory disorder may be dissociated in type, involving pain and temperature more strikingly than touch and position sense. The conus is not a common site for cord infarction. Penetrating trauma is a relatively uncommon cause of conus lesion; this sometimes results from injury during attempted lumbar puncture or regional anesthesia, attempted at an unusually rostral level. Extrinsic lesions such as disk compression and extrinsic tumors, including metastases, usually present with pain before neurological deficit develops.

Conus lesions cause weakness that is partly the result of interruption of the sacral lower motor neuron outflow from the conus region, and partly due to damage to the corticospinal tracts in this terminal part of the spinal cord, causing weakness also of hip flexion and dorsiflexion of the feet. The plantar responses are extensor, and the ankle jerks are increased, although the knee jerks, representing the L4 segments, rostral to the lesion, are normal. Sensory loss extends beyond the distribution of that found in the cauda equina lesion described above, onto the anterior aspects of the legs and thighs and sometimes onto the lower abdominal wall. There may be more marked involvement of large fiber sensation; i.e. of position sense and light touch and vibration, than of pin-prick sensibility, a finding different from that found in cauda equina lesions. The prognosis in conus lesions, as in cauda lesions is generally poor, but depends on the etiology. There may be considerable recovery after penetrating trauma by an iatrogenic needle injury. Compressive lesions have a poor prognosis. In multiple sclerosis recovery may occur.

Following recovery, there may be residual burning, dysesthetic pain in the sacral dermatomes from spinothalamic damage, in addition to bladder and bowel dysfunction. The latter is due to interruption of the spinal connections to the Onuf nucleus system, and to the parasympathetic outflow. Weakness is also a problem, with features of both upper and lower motor neuron syndrome. There is weakness of hip flexion, representing corticospinal involvement in the conus medullaris white matter, with extensor plantar responses and brisk knee reflexes. The ankle jerks may be reduced or increased dependent on whether or not there is predominant lower or upper motor involvement. The anal canal is patulous and the anal reflex absent. Sexual function is severely affected, but it may be possible to obtain a partial erection, and sometimes ejaculation is also partially preserved. Orgasmic responses are diminished.

PERIPHERAL NERVOUS SYSTEM LESIONS

Damage to the somatic afferent and efferent nervous pathways to the ano-rectum results from lesions in the lumbosacral spine, for example cauda equina disease[42] due to lumbosacral spondylosis, tumors, sacral meningomyelocele, or trauma. It may also occur with intra-pelvic disease involving the sacral plexus, especially intra-pelvic metastases or traumatic fracture to the bony pelvis. Peripheral neuropathy may only rarely produce a similar functional disturbance, for example in some patients with diabetic proximal neuropathy, or with mononeuropathies involving the pudendal or perineal nerves as in traumatic injuries or even polyarteritis nodosa. Diabetes mellitus may also be associated with incontinence of both feces and urine, due to autonomic and sensorimotor neuropathy. The commonest neurogenic lesion of these nerves is that resulting from injury sustained in childbirth with vaginal delivery, as discussed elsewhere in this book.[43,44] Except in familial amyloidotic polyneuropathy, a disorder that selectively involves the autonomic nervous system, incontinence is a rare feature of polyneuropathy.

CLUES TO RECOGNITION OF A NEUROLOGICAL CAUSE FOR INCONTINENCE

It is important to recognize neurological disease causing urinary or fecal incontinence since investigation and management will be different, at least until the neurological disorder has been dealt with, so far as this is possible. Certain features are particularly important in suggesting a neurological cause.

PAIN AND SENSORY AND MOTOR SYMPTOMS IN CAUDA EQUINA COMPRESSION

Pain is common in any neurological disease involving sensory nerve roots. Pain is the principal early feature of cauda equina compression, by disk protrusion, tumor or infection. The pain is typically sharp and burning in character, with a shooting component induced by movement that radiates in a sciatic or lumbo-sacral dermatomal distribution, that is into the buttocks and perineum, and down the backs of the thighs toward the lateral foot. There is a sensory disturbance, in addition to pain, consisting of altered sensitivity in the affected sacral and lumbar segments.

BLADDER AND BOWEL

Inability to defecate, often misinterpreted as constipation, is a common initial manifestation of cauda equina and conus lesions. This is accompanied by retention of urine with overflow, and by the other features noted above involving pain, sensory symptoms, and weakness. The onset of urinary retention and bowel disorder should always be considered carefully after spinal surgery, and in people with a history of sciatica, especially when the latter has been bilateral. Always examine the anal reflex. A patulous anus and absence of the anal reflex are strongly suggestive of cauda equina lesion in the appropriate clinical context.

SENSORY LOSS

Sensory loss or sensory impairment extending into the buttocks suggest cauda equina or conus medullaris syndrome.

TENDON REFLEXES

The knee jerks are normal, but may be increased in conus lesions if the lesion extends rostrally into the lumbar cord level. The ankle jerks may be reduced, absent or normal. Therefore, preserved ankle jerks do not exclude cauda equina compression.

WEAKNESS

This involves hip extensors, thigh flexors and evertors of the ankle, but not knee extensors or extensors of the large toe. Ankle dorsiflexion may be scarcely affected. There is more difficulty standing and walking than expected from examination in the supine position. Always try to get your patient to stand and be suspicious if this is difficult.

REFERENCES

1. Laurberg S, Swash M, Snooks SJ, Henry MM. Neurologic cause of idiopathic incontinence. *Arch Neurol* 1988; **45**:1250–53.
2. Kiff ES, Swash M. Slowed conduction in the pudendal nerves in idiopathic (neurogenic) faecal incontinence. *Br J Surg* 1984;**71**:614–16.
3. Snooks SJ, Henry MM, Swash M. Abnormalities in peripheral and central nerve conduction in anorectal incontinence. 1985;**78**:294–300.
4. Kleist K. Kriegsverletzungen des Gehirnes. In: Bonhoeffer K (ed.) *Handbuch der Arztlichen Erfahrungen im Weltkriege 1914/1918. Band IV; Geistes- und Nervenkrankheiten.* Leipzig-Verlag, 1922;1343–69.
5. Penfield W, Rasmussen T. *The cerebral cortex of man.* Macmillan: New York, 1950.
6. Blok BF, Willemsen A-T, Holstege G. A PET study on brain control of micturition in humans. *Brain* 1997;**120**:111–21.
7. Blok BFM, Sturms LM, Holstege G. Brain activation during micturition in women. *Brain* 1998;**121**:2033–42.
8. Hobday DI, Aziz Q, Thacker N, *et al.* A study of the cortical processing of ano-rectal sensation using functional MRI. *Brain* 2001;**124**:361–8.
9. Andrew J, Nathan PW. Lesions of the anterior frontal lobes and disturbances of micturition and defaecation. *Brain* 1964;**87**:233–62.
10. Gelber DA, Good DC, Laven LJ, *et al.* Causes of urinary incontinence after acute hemispheric stroke. *Stroke* 1993;**24**:378–82.
11. Hamdy S, Enck P, Aziz Q, *et al.* Laterality effects of human pudendal nerve stimulation on corticoanal pathways: evidence for functional asymmetry. *Gut* 1999;**45**:58–63.
12. Sangwan YP, Coller JA, Barrett RC, *et al.* Unilateral pudendal neuropathy; significance and implications. *Dis Colon Rectum* 1996;**39**:249–51.
13. Sangwan YP, Coller JA, Barrett RC, *et al.* Unilateral pudendal neuropathy; impact on outcome of anal sphincter repair. *Dis Colon Rectum* 1996;**39**:686–9.
14. Wunderlich M, Swash M. The overlapping innervation of the two sides of the external anal sphincter by the pudendal nerves. *J Neurol Sci* 1983;**59**:97–101.
15. Morita T, Kizu N, Kondo S, *et al.* Ipsilaterality of motor innervation of the canine urethral sphincter. *Urol Int* 1988;**43**:149–56.
16. Swash M, Snooks SJ, Chalmers DHK. Parity as a factor in incontinence in multiple sclerosis. *Arch Neurol* 1987; **44**:405–508.
17. Hinds JP, Eidelman BH, Wald A. Prevalence of bowel dysfunction in multiple sclerosis. *Gastroenterology* 1990; **98**:1538–42.
18. Chia YW, Gill KP, Jameson JS, *et al.* Paradoxical puborectalis contraction is a feature of constipation in patients with multiple sclerosis. *J Neurol Neurosurg Psychiat* 1996;**60**:31–5.
19. Bauer HJ, Firnhaber W, Winkler W. Prognostic criteria in multiple sclerosis. *Ann NY Acad Sci* 1965;**122**:551.
20. Mathers SE, Ingram DA, Swash M. Electrophysiology of motor pathways for sphincter control in multiple sclerosis. *J Neurol Neurosurg Psychiat* 1990;**53**:955–60.
21. Jameson JS, Rogers J, Chia YW, *et al.* Pelvic floor function in multiple sclerosis. *Gut* 1994; **35**:388–90.
22. Betts CD, d'Mellow MT, Fowler CJ, *et al.* Urinary symptoms and the neurological features of bladder dysfunction in multiple sclerosis. *Gut* 1993;**56**:245–50.
23. Hakim S, Adams RD. The special clinical problem of symptomatic hydrocephalus with normal cerebrospinal fluid pressure. *J Neurol Sci* 1965;**2**:307–315.
24. Sakakibara R, Hattori T, Fukutake T, *et al.* Micturitional disturbances in herpetic brainstem encephalitis: contribution of the pontine micturition centre. *J Neurol Neurosurg Psychiat* 1998; **64**:269–72.
25. Sakakibara R, Hattori T, Yasuda K, *et al.* Micturitional disturbance and the pontine segmental lesion; urodynamic and MRI analyses of vascular cases. *J Neurol Sci* 1996;**141**:105–110.
26. Ueki K. Disturbances of micturition observed in some patients with brain tumour. *Neurol Med Chir (Tokyo)* 1960;**2**:25–33.
27. Holman E. Difficult urination associated with intracranial tumours of the posterior fossa. *Arch Neurol* 1926;**15**:371–80.
28. Betts CD, Kapoor R, Fowler CJ. Pontine pathology and voiding dysfunction. *Br J Urol* 1992; **67**:100–102.
29. Manente G, Melchionda D, Uncini A. Urinary retention in bilateral pontine tumour; evidence for a pontine micturition centre in humans. *J Neurol Neurosurg Psychiat* 1996;**61**:528–9.
30. Edwards L, Quigley EMM, Hofman R, Pfeiffer RF. Gastrointestinal symptoms in Parkinson's disease. *Mov Disord* 1993;**8**:83–6.
31. Jost WH, Schrimgk K. Constipation in Parkinson's disease. *Klin Wochenschr* 1991;**69**:906–909.
32. Mathers SE, Kempster PA, Law PJ, *et al.* Anal sphincter dysfunction in Parkinson's disease. *Arch Neurol* 1989;**46**:1061–4.
33. Mathers SE, Kempster PA, Swash M, Lees AJ. Constipation and paradoxical puborectalis contraction in anismus and Parkinson's disease. *J Neurol Neurosurg Psychiat* 1988;**51**:1503–1507.
34. Ashraf W, Pfeiffer RF, Quigley EMM. Anorectal manometry in the assessment of anorectal dysfunction in Parkinson's disease; a comparison with chronic idiopathic constipation. *Moy Disord* 1994;**9**:655–63.
35. Glickman S, Kamm MA. Bowel dysfunction in spinal cord injured patients. *Lancet* 1996;**347**:1651–3.

36. Menardo G, Bausano G, Corazziari E, *et al.* Large bowel transit in paraplegic patients. *Dis Colon Rectum* 1987; **30**:924–8.
37. Nathan PW, Smith MC. The centropetal pathway from the bladder and urethra within the spinal cord. *J Neurol Neurosurg Psychiat* 1951;**14**:262–89.
38. Nathan PW, Smith MC. The centrifugal pathway for micturition within the spinal cord. *J Neurol Neurosurg Psychiat* 1958;**21**:177–89.
39. Greving I, Tegenthoff M, Nedjat S, *et al.* Anorectal functions in patients with spinal cord injury. *Neurogastroenterol Mot* 1998;**10**:509–515.
40. Gleave JRW, MacFarlane R. Prognosis for recovery of bladder function following lumbar central disc prolapse. *Br J Neurosurg* 1990;**4**:205–210.
41. Shapiro S. Cauda equina syndrome secondary to lumbar disc herniation. *Neurosurgery* 1993; **32**:743–7.
42. Swash M, Snooks SJ. Slowed motor conduction in lumbosacral nerve roots in cauda equina lesions. *J Neurol Neurosurg Psychiat* 1986;**49**:808–816.
43. Snooks SJ, Swash M, Setchell M, Henry M. Injury to innervation of the pelvic floor sphincter musculature in childbirth. *Lancet* 1984;**2**:546–50.
44. Laurberg S, Swash M. Effects of aging on the anorectal sphincters and their innervation. *Dis Colon Rectum* 1989;**32**:737–42.

Chapter 27

Biofeedback in Pelvic Floor Disorders

Paul Enck, Frauke Musial

HISTORY OF BIOFEEDBACK IN PELVIC FLOOR DISORDERS

The term 'biofeedback' describes a therapeutic technique. The basis of biofeedback is 'learning through reinforcement' in the tradition of I.P. Pavlow and B.F. Skinner: if a behavior is followed by reward or punishment as 'feedback', this increases or decreases, respectively, the chances that it will be repeated. This type of learning is also called *instrumental learning*, or operant conditioning.

While Skinner and others restricted operant conditioning to observable behavior, it was subsequently shown that even functions of the autonomic nervous system can be influenced by operant conditioning. A body function, which cannot be perceived by the subject under normal conditions can be measured by a device and in turn demonstrated to the subject. The reinforcer in adult humans is usually the 'knowledge of results', but additional verbal or other positive 'signals' may also be helpful.

The beginning of biofeedback training in pelvic floor disorders is marked by a case report by Kohlenberg[33] in 1973. The author treated a 13-year-old boy with fecal incontinence (encopresis and soiling) after colorectal surgery for (questionable) Hirschsprung's disease 2 years before. At the time of the study the boy was supposed to undergo colectomy. Using a 3-cm balloon across the anal canal, the subject was taught to increase the anal pressure, but it remains unclear from the publication whether the authors provided feedback from the anal sphincter (resting pressure) only or from the external anal sphincter and rectum as well. The treatment resulted in a resting pressure increase from 35 mmHg baseline to about 50 mmHg. Consequent clinical improvement was poorly documented and reported.

The first report of EMG biofeedback in adult-type fecal incontinence, in contrast, is not biofeedback-theory generated, but a rather accidental observation by neurophysiologists. In 1967, Haskell and Rovner[24] showed that patients could utilize the auditory display of needle EMG activity of the external anal sphincter during clinical investigation to improve control over external anal sphincter function. Patients were instructed to synchronize voluntary contractions with electrically applied stimuli to the muscle and to perform home exercises. Patients with only partial denervation showed good improvement of incontinence symptoms. Due to the discomfort of this procedure, this technique did not gain a following until it was replaced by transcutaneous EMG recording, first reported by MacLeod in 1979.[43]

At this time, the historical roots of biofeedback training had already been forgotten by investigators using this technique. Consequently, its specific application in the treatment of constipation – from 1980 onwards[11] – was predominantly proposed and performed by pediatric and adult surgeons. Another case report in 1979 may also be a landmark for the conversion of a psychology-generated and theory-driven therapeutic strategy into clinical medical routine. Schiller *et al.*[53] successfully used the rectal infusion of saline as a training mode to improve sphincter function in a patient with incontinence and chronic diarrhea.

LITERATURE ON BIOFEEDBACK THERAPY IN PELVIC FLOOR DISORDERS

To date there have been 27 papers published concerning biofeedback for fecal incontinence, and a total of 25 papers reporting treatment of chronic constipation. They will be reviewed here. This review extends and updates a previous survey on the same subject.[12]

Excluded from this analysis are various case reports in the literature and all studies dealing with biofeedback treatment of constipation in children. Biofeedback in children is the subject of a recent excellent review paper.[40] Furthermore, applications of biofeedback other than in patients with incontinence, constipation and ano-rectal pain are also excluded from this report. The literature on biofeedback in fecal incontinence is much more comprehensive than in urinary incontinence.

BIOFEEDBACK TREATMENT OF FECAL INCONTINENCE

The 27 data-based studies reported in peer-reviewed international journals (see Tables 27.1 and 27.4) derive from almost as many centers around the world, these being either gastroenterological or surgical clinics or institutions closely associated with them. None of the studies has been undertaken in a psychological setting. This indicates that although biofeedback training is of psychological origin its application in (lower) intestinal dysfunction is restricted to medical settings in which invasive diagnostic and therapeutic approaches are available.

A total of almost 650 patients of all ages (predominantly women) have been treated. A single study[63] used geriatric patients only. Except for the five studies reported later, the patients entered into these studies had heterogeneous causes of fecal incontinence, depending on whether the setting was surgical or medical. While the initial studies had rather small sample sizes, the patient population has increased over the years, as has the duration of patients' follow-up after treatment. A recent multicenter trial across three different laboratories in the USA[44] included 72 patients followed for at least 2 years[9,13] (see Table 27.3).

While the initial studies from the Baltimore group focused on internal and external sphincter muscle *coordination* as the major goal of biofeedback training, subsequently sensory components as well as voluntary muscle control were included in the treatment program (see Table 27.2). This occurred because some of the investigators involved had shown that sensory perception from the rectum is necessary for treatment[62] and

Table 27.1 Biofeedback studies in fecal incontinence (1)

First author	Year	Ref.	*n*	Age	Range	Sex (F:M)	Origin[a]
Engel	1974	14	7	40.7	6–54	5:2	5:2
Cerulli	1979	7	50	46.0	5–97	36:12	35:14
Goldenberg	1980	20	12	n.r.	12–78	6:6	6:6
Wald	1981	57	17	46.9	10–79	11:6	4:13
Latimer	1984	36	8	30.1	8–72	4:4	5:3
Whitehead	1985	63	18	72.7	65–92	15:3	3:15
Buser	1986	5	13	53.6	13–66	7:6	9:4
McLeod	1987	41	113	56.0	25–88	67:46	79:34
Berti Riboli	1988	2	21	61.0	14–84	15:6	15:6
Loening-Baucke	1990	40	8	63.0	35–78	8:0	n.r.
Miner	1990	42	25	54.6	17–76	17:8	16:9
Chiarioni	1993	8	14	48.1	24–76	10:4	3:11
Keck	1994	31	15	39.0	29–65	13:2	6:9
Guillemot	1995	22	24	60.7	39–78	19:5	3:19
Sangwan	1995	51	28	52.9	30–74	22:6	13:25
Rao	1996	47	19	50.0	17–78	20:2	14:5
Ko	1997	32	25	63.0	31–82	21:4	25:3
Rieger	1997	49	30	68.0	29–85	28:2	27:3
Patankar	1997	45	25	66.0	34–85	13:12	8:17
Patankar[b]	1997	44	72	70.0	34–87	43:29	30:42
Glia	1998	19	26	61	32–82	22:4	19:7
All			570		5–97	401:169	

[a]Surgical/obstgetrical v. medical patients; [b]multicenter trial; n.r.: not reported.

Table 27.2 Biofeedback studies in fecal incontinence (2)

First author	Year	Ref.	Init[a]	End.[b]	C[c]	S[d]	V[e]	No of sessions	Add.[f]
Engel	1974	14	yes	yes	yes	no	no	1–4	no
Cerulli	1979	7	yes	yes	yes	yes	no	1	no
Goldenberg	1980	20	yes	no	no	yes	no	>1	no
Wald	1981	57	yes	no	yes	yes	yes	1 + 1	home
Latimer	1984	36	yes	yes	yes	yes	yes	8 (2/wk)	home
Whitehead	1985	63	yes	yes	no	no	yes	8 (2/wk)	home
Buser	1986	5	yes	yes	no	yes	yes	1–3	home
McLeod	1987	41	no	yes	no	no	yes	3.3	no
Berti Riboli	1988	2	yes	yes	yes	yes	yes	12 (2/wk)	no
Loening-Baucke	1990	40	yes	yes	yes	yes	yes	3	home
Miner	1990	42	yes	yes	yes	yes	yes	3	no
Chiarioni	1993	8	yes	yes	no	no	yes	2 + 1	home
Keck	1994	31	yes	yes	no	yes	yes	3 (1–7)	home
Guillemot	1995	22	yes	yes	no	no	yes	4 wk	home
Sangwan	1995	51	no	yes	no	yes	yes	33.75 (1–7)	home
Rao	1996	47	yes	yes	yes	yes	yes	7 (4–13)	home
Ko	1997	32	yes	no	no	no	yes	5 (2–13)	home
Rieger	1997	49	(yes)	no	no	no	yes	6	home
Patankar	1997	45	no	no	no	no	yes	7 (5–11)	home
Patankar[g]	1997	44	no	no	no	no	yes	7 (2–11)	home
Glia	1998	19	yes	yes	no	yes	yes	max. 10	no

[a]Initial evaluation (manometry, EMG).
[b]End evaluation (manometry, EMG).
[c,d,e]Treatment goals: coordination, sensitivity, voluntary contraction.
[f]Additional treatment (home training).
[g]Multicenter study.
()Indicate that only some of the patients were evaluated.

determines the outcome.[58] Two studies[36,42] have shown that sensory retraining is probably the most important factor in biofeedback training in incontinence.

The availability of non-invasive transcutaneous EMG biofeedback devices for clinical and for home training has fostered the training of voluntary anal sphincter muscle contraction as the major goal in biofeedback, while other goals have tended to diminish (see Table 27.2). Also, while most earlier studies have incorporated initial as well as terminal evaluation of physiological functions of the pelvic floor by means of manometry, EMG and other diagnostic tools, this comparison has not been made in more recent papers as biofeedback has been incorporated into routine clinical management.[44,45]

Despite broad agreement that biofeedback is the treatment of choice in patients with fecal incontinence, the treatment modalities vary in consistency; neither the total number of training sessions, nor their frequency, the duration of treatment, or the supplementation of therapy by home training with or without devices have been agreed upon (Table 27.3). Most recent studies do claim to

Table 27.3 Biofeedback studies in fecal incontinence[3]

Author	Year	Ref.	Criteria[a]	Type[b]	Follow-up[c]	Effi.[d]	Control[e]
Engel	1974	14	n.r.	interv	6–16 mo	57	no
Cerulli	1979	7	>90%	n.r.	4–108 wk	72	no
Goldenberg	1980	20	n.r.	n.r.	10–96 wk	83	no
Wald	1981	57	>75%	interv	2–38 mo	71	no
Latimer	1984	36	n.r.	diary	6 mo	88	within subjects
Whitehead	1985	63	>75%	diary	6 mo	77	waiting list
Buser	1986	5	n.r.	n.r.	16–30 mo	92	no
McLeod	1987	41	>90%	subj	6–60 mo	63	no
Berti Riboli	1988	2	>90%	n.r.	3 mo	86	no
Loening-Baucke	1990	40	>75%	diary	12 mo	50	convent treatment
Miner	1990	42	subj.	diary	<2 years	76	3-arm crossover
Chiarioni	1993	8	>75%	interv	14.5 mo	85	no
Keck	1994	31	subj.	interv	8 mo (1–23)	73	no
Guillemot	1995	22	subj.	diary	30 mo (24–36)	56	no treatment
Sangwan	1995	51	subj.	interv	20 mo (4–47)	75	no
Rao	1996	47	>67%	diary	1 year	53	no
Ko	1997	32	n.r.	diary	not done	87.5	no
Rieger	1997	49	>80%	interv	6–12 mo	67	no
Patankar	1997	45	>75%	subj.	not done	70	no
Patankar[f]	1997	44	>75%	subj.	not done	83.3	no
Glia	1998	19	>50%	interv	21 mo (12–46)	53.7	no

[a]Efficacy criteria: % decrease in incontinence symptoms.
[b]Evaluation by: interview, diary; subjective rating.
[c]Follow-up in weeks, months or years.
[d]% patients improved.
[e]Control group employed.
[f]Multicenter study. n.r.: not reported.
() Indicate that follow-up was not performed on all patients.

incorporate home exercises, but these are usually not controlled for compliance and efficacy (Fig. 27.1).

Symptom evaluation was mostly done with the help of diary cards which monitor progress in the course of treatment; however, others have used interview techniques and questionnaires. Estimating the efficacy of incontinence therapy by means of diary cards is reasonable because events are frequent and the recording period long (a week or longer). This is much more difficult with infrequent events, as is the case of patients with chronic constipation (see below).

Of the 21 studies published, all but one report a success rate greater than 50%, with efficacy criteria ranging between 75 to 90% reduction in the frequency of incontinence events. The overall success (% improved patients) is approximately 70%.

Only five out of 21 studies attempted to control the effect of treatment prospectively by including control

Table 27.4 Biofeedback studies in fecal incontinence in homogeneous patient groups

Author	Year	Ref.	*n*	Pathology	Age	Sex	Eval[a]	Duration	Control	Eff[b]
Wald	1984	59	11	diabetes	52.2	8:3	M	n.r.	no	73
van Tets	1996	56	12	neurogenic	48.0	n.r.	M,E	12 wk home	no	0
Ho	1996	27	13	LAR, Col	62.1	3:10	M	4 wks, 1/wk	no	76
Hämäläinen	1996	23	11	prolapse	61.2	9:2	M	4–6 wk presurg	no treat	90
Jensen	1997	28	28	sphinc surg	34.0	n.r.	diary	3–4 sess/wk	no	89

[a]Manometry, EMG.
[b]Efficacy: % patients improved.

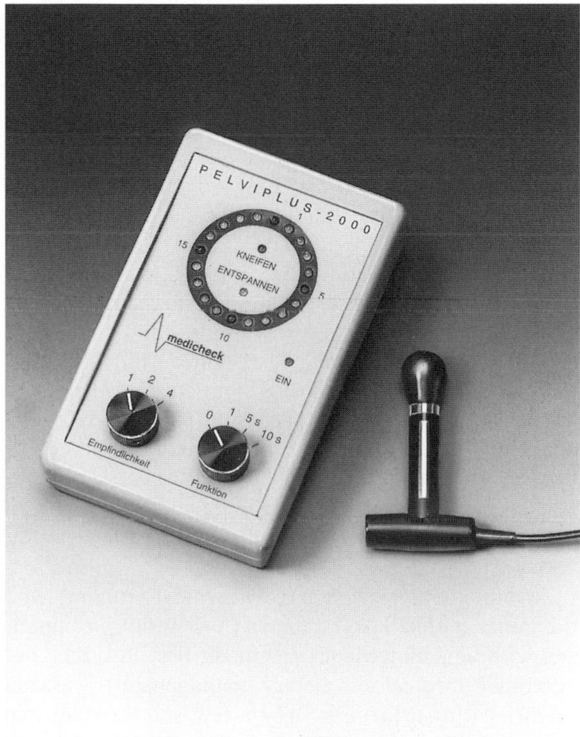

Figure 27.1 One out of many available biofeedback devices for clinical as well as home training. The external anal sphincter EMG amplitude is recorded by an anal plug electrode (front) and displayed as number of lights of the circle (courtesy Medicheck, Essen, Germany).

groups; in a few others post-hoc comparison of good and poor responders was used. Further studies used healthy control samples only for comparison with patients' manometric data before and after treatment.

In these five controlled studies, the strategies used were quite different. One used a conventional treatment group for comparison,[40] another provided no treatment for the control group;[22] in both cases no random group assignment was done. A third study used a behavioral modification strategy as a second treatment, and had patients who received no treatment on a waiting list, this time with random assignment.[63] The two studies which used a more sophisticated control strategy were Latimer's A-B-A-C-A-D-A design study[36] and Miner's comparison of different training components in a three-arm design: sensory training, voluntary contraction training, and sphincter coordination.[42] Both authors concluded that the most effective component is rectal filling sensation retraining.

BIOFEEDBACK TRAINING IN FECAL INCONTINENCE IN HOMOGENEOUS PATIENT GROUPS (Table 27.4)

In addition, five studies have been published in which homogeneous patient groups were tested, including patients with diabetes mellitus,[59] patients with various surgical conditions (prolapse, sphincter surgery, low anterior resection and colectomy),[23,27,28] and patients with 'idiopathic (neurogenic) fecal incontinence'.[56] It is surprising and noteworthy to find that only the latter group had a poor outcome. Unfortunately, documentation is poor in this study: neither EMG data prior to treatment nor incontinence symptoms before, during and after treatment are reported; the data does not differentiate between individuals; and while in the men increase in squeeze pressure was small, at least some patients showed marked improvement of the anal sphincter performance. Biofeedback training consisted of home training with four outpatient visits, but again, compliance of their patient to the program is not reported.

The only controlled study is the one by Hämäläinen[23] who used a 'no treatment by biofeedback' control group in patients undergoing surgery for rectal prolapse. Biofeedback was performed before surgery for 4 to 6 weeks to reduce postsurgery incontinence. It is questionable whether such a prospective study would still show significant improvement after operation in comparison with controls if a non-specific treatment option – to control for attention and other psychological effects, and/or of a specific treatment option, e.g. pelvic floor exercises without biofeedback support had been used.

BIOFEEDBACK TREATMENT OF CHRONIC CONSTIPATION

The application of biofeedback training in chronically constipated patients has a much shorter tradition, but obviously is gaining more attention today since a total of 25 papers have been published in the last 12 years. More than 700 patients have been treated in many different centers, and all but one[48] were surgical departments. This presumably indicates that surgeons more often than internists are confronted by patients with therapy-refractory chronic constipation[6] (Table 27.5). Interestingly, although surgery and surgery-associated physiological laboratory testing which revealed two types of constipation, slow colonic transit and 'outlet obstruction'-type ('spastic pelvic floor syndrome', anismus, pelvic floor dyssynergia); only the latter is subject to biofeedback treatment in most studies (see below).

Patients with chronic constipation are on the average younger in age than their incontinent counterparts, but female predominance persists. A history of constipation may date back into childhood in some, or a few months only in other patients. The mechanism by which functional outlet obstruction occurs is still unknown, and it is questionable whether all patients represent one clinical entity only. At least one study[46] claims to have identified different types of 'anismus', and another has suggested at least one cause of anismus to be sexual abuse in childhood or adulthood.[37]

Because the diagnosis of functional outlet obstruction is based only in part on clinical symptoms (laxative use, necessity for excessive straining, digital assistance with defecation), all studies have used elaborate laboratory testing to confirm the diagnosis: this usually includes manometry, defecography or related imaging techniques, anal sphincter EMG, and balloon expulsion tests. Most centers have also used large bowel transit studies to *exclude* slow transit constipation, but others[3] have ignored this or have challenged its necessity by consecutive inclusion of patients with constipation of both types.[34,35] While one can assume that colonic transit measurement may be comparable across centers, neither manometry nor defecography are standardized clinical procedures so far, and the same holds true for balloon expulsion. No agreement is currently available for how many and which tests need to be abnormal to confirm the diagnosis.

Probably the most surprising finding is that most centers have *not* included psychological evaluation of the patients included (Table 27.6), although it has been known for many years that many patients with chronic constipation suffer from overt psychopathology. In some studies, treatment failure has been attributed to psychopathology,[3,37,55] and psychological counseling was offered.

While two groups[3,10] suggested the necessity for hospital admission and inpatient treatment of 4 weeks and longer, subsequent experience has shown that outpatient management is feasible without loss of efficacy. From an economic standpoint, this modification was necessary to allow biofeedback treatment to become more widely accepted.[1] Whether or not single treatment sessions[38] will become the preferred and most effective mode in most patients is, however, questionable.

Treatment efficacy is usually assessed by comparing clinical symptoms prior to and after treatment, but some studies,[15,38,43] have evaluated sphincter performance during the physiological tests instead. Outcome is sometimes assessed by diary card, but often by reviews, interviews and questionnaires. It has to be borne in mind that these evaluation techniques are even more unreliable when the event to be recorded – e.g. defecation – is infrequent in nature. However, stool diaries would need to be used for longer periods of time than in patients with fecal incontinence to achieve the same sensitivity.

Different from incontinence training, re-education of paradoxical pelvic floor behavior is achieved in a shorter period of time – within a few sessions – and maintained for longer after the training has finished. Only one study found the results disappointing,[31] but did find efficacy in selected patients. This indicates that patient selection – and the appropriate diagnostic tools to differentiate between slow transit and outlet obstruction – may still be a matter of controversy. Sensitivity and specificity of these diagnostic tests (manometry, EMG, defecography, transit studies) may vary significantly.

While all studies compared treatment outcome with the initial complaints of patients (A–B design), comparison with non-biofeedback treatment (e.g. through conventional medical or dietary management) was not performed (or achieved). Only a few studies state that failure of standardized conventional treatment (dietary management) was a prerequisite for entering the study. It is, however, tempting to speculate whether a similar response may also be gained by other strategies, and may be due to non-specific placebo effects.

Two studies[4,18] compared different types of biofeedback signal on outcomes of therapy: EMG recording from the anal sphincter muscle – recorded transcutaneously through anal plug devices – versus a feedback signal from a pressure signal (balloon, manometry catheter). It was found that neither was superior over the other. However, pressure sensor in the anal canal carries a risk: the signal may be distorted through confounding pressure events (increases) in the rectum. A further study[46] compared the efficacy of biofeedback therapy

Table 27.5 Biofeedback studies in chronic constipation (1)

First author	Year	Ref.	*n*	Age	Range	Sex (F:M)	Duration (yrs)
Bleijenberg	1987	3	10	32.0	10–48	n.r.	> 6 yrs
Weber	1987	60	22	n.r.	18–35	22:0	n.r.
Lestar	1991	38	16	42.5	n.r.	10:6	n.r.
Kawimbe	1991	30	15	45.0	22–76	12:3	8.8
Dahl	1991	10	9	41.0	20–60	15:0	18 (4–40)
Wexner	1992	61	18	67.7	10–84	13:5	26.9
Fleshman	1992	15	9	49.4	35–62	8:1	n.r.
Turnbull	1992	55	7	35.7	29–42	7:0	12 (1–30)
Keck	1994	31	12	62.0	17–82	10:2	n.r.
Papachrysostymou	1994	43	22	42.0	32–50	17:5	3–25
Bleijenberg	1994	4	20	37.0	20–50	15.5	7 (2–15)
Koutsomanis	1994	34	20	34.0	18–53	18:2	n.r.
Koutsomanis	1995	35	60	40.5	20–64	53:7	13
Siproudhis	1995	54	27	46.0	21–77	20:7	35 mo (6–192)
Leroi[a]	1996	37	15	41.2	n.r.	15:0	n.r.
Ho	1996	26	62	48.0	n.r.	28:24	4.8
Park	1996	46	68	65.9	15–90	44:24	20
Ko	1997	32	17	50.0	22–82	12:5	8.1
Rao	1997	48	25	50.0	21–87	16:10	n.r.
Glia	1997	18	26	55.0	28–78	23:3	11
Karlbohm	1997	29	28	46.0	22–72	23:5	9 (1–30)
Rieger	1997	50	19	63.0	16–78	18:1	n.r.
Patankar	1997	45	30	65.3	33–86	24:6	n.r.
Patankar[b]	1997	44	116	73.0	33–85	88:28	n.r.
Chiotakakou[c]	1998	9	100	40.0	10–79	87:13	n.r.
Total			773		10–90	601:162	

[a]Sexually abused women; [b]multicenter study; [c]long-term follow-up. n.r.: not reported.

between two groups of patients with different types of anismus and showed that only those patients with 'classical' anismus, i.e. with a shortening of the ano-rectal angle with attempts to strain, profit from therapy.

In a more recently published study,[35] the investigators compared a group which received verbal feedback by an instructor with a group receiving feedback by visual display of pelvic floor EMG during straining. It was shown that the response rate was similar in both groups and resulted in symptom improvement of approximately 50%. The authors conclude that 'training in abdominal muscle contraction with pelvic floor

Table 27.6 Biofeedback studies in chronic constipation[2]

First author	Year	Ref.	Man[a]	Def[b]	Trans[c]	EMG[d]	Expul[e]	Psychol[f]
Bleijenberg	1987	3	no	yes	yes	yes	no	(yes)
Weber	1987	60	yes	no	no	no	no	no
Lestar	1991	38	yes	no	no	no	yes	no
Kawimbe	1991	30	yes	yes	no	yes	yes	no
Dahl	1991	10	yes	yes	yes	yes	yes	yes
Wexner	1992	61	yes	yes	yes	yes	no	no
Fleshman	1992	15	yes	yes	yes	yes	yes	yes
Turnbull	1992	55	yes	yes	yes	yes	no	yes
Keck	1994	31	yes	(yes)	(yes)	(yes)	yes	(yes)
Papachrysostymou	1994	43	yes	yes	yes	yes	yes	no
Bleijenberg	1994	4	yes	no	no	yes	yes	yes
Koutsomanis	1994	34	yes	yes	yes	no	yes	no
Koutsomanis	1995	35	no	no	yes	yes	yes	no
Siproudhis	1995	54	yes	yes	no	no	yes	no
Leroi	1996	37	(yes)	no	no	yes	no	yes
Ho	1996	26	yes	yes	yes	yes	no	??
Park	1996	46	yes	yes	yes	yes	no	yes
Ko	1997	32	yes	(yes)	yes	yes	(yes)	no
Rao	1997	48	yes	yes	yes	no	yes	no
Glia	1997	18	yes	yes	yes	yes	yes	no
Karlbohm	1997	29	yes	yes	yes	yes	no	no
Rieger	1997	50	yes	yes	(yes)	yes	yes	no
Patankar	1997	45	no	no	no	no	no	no
Patankar[f]	1997	44	no	no	no	no	no	no
Chiotakakou	1998	9	no	no	(yes)	(yes)	no	(yes)

[a,b,c,d,e]Diagnostic evaluations by manometry, defecography, EMG, colonic transit, balloon expulsion, and psychology; [f]multicenter trial; () indicates that the test was not performed in all patients.

relaxation is equally effective with or without a measuring device'; but admit that constant encouragement and praise by an instructor is necessary, as is a 'good rapport between patient and instructor'.

From a psychological standpoint, it is not surprising to learn that verbal instruction and reinforcement can be as effective a feedback mode as a visual or auditory mediated technical feedback display – it may only be surprising for physicians not used to being with their patients for longer that a few minutes. The more important question is whether constant verbal instruction is the more practical (and affordable) way of providing biofeedback than through simply designed technical measurement devices. These may be taken home, which would allow more training, in more privacy, and with lower total costs.[1] Interestingly, about half of the

Table 27.7 Biofeedback training in chronic constipation[3]

First author	Year	Ref.	Follow-up[a]	Sessions	Add[b]	Con[c]	Eval[d]	Eff[e]
Bleijenberg	1987	3	7 (1–18)	daily	yes	no	n.r.	70.0
Weber	1987	60	no	2–4		no	n.r.	18.2
Lestar	1991	38	no	1	yes	no	test	68.7
Kawimbe	1991	30	6.2	2/day	yes	no	diary	86.7
Dahl	1991	10	6	5	yes	no	diary	77.8
Wexner	1992	61	9 (1–17)	9	no	no	diary	88.9
Fleshman	1992	15	>6	2×6	no	no	test	100
Turnbull	1992	55	2–4 yrs	15	yes	no	diary	85.7
Keck	1994	31	1–8	3	yes	no	tel interv	58.0
Papachrysostymou	1994	43	no	>3	yes	no	test	86.0
Bleijenberg	1994	4	no	8	yes	yes	diary	50.0
Koutsomanis	1994	34	6–12	2–6	yes	no	diary	50.00
Koutsomanis	1995	35	2–3	1–7	no	yes	diary	50.0
Siproudhis	1995	54	1–36	1–7	no	no	n.r.	51.8
Leroi	1996	37	6–10	16	no	no	n.r.	66.7
Ho	1996	26	no	4	yes	no	diary	90.3
Park	1996	46	no	11	no	yes	diary	25/86[f]
Ko	1997	32	no	4	yes	no	quest	76.0
Rao	1997	48	<2	2/wk,2–4 wks	yes	no	diary	92.0
Glia	1997	18	no	1–2/wk <10 wk	yes	yes	diary	57.6
Karlbohm	1997	29	>1 yr	8	no	no	quest	43.0
Rieger	1997	50	>6	6 (1/wk)	yes	no	quest	12.5
Patankar	1997	45	no	7 (5–11), 1/wk	no	no	diary	84.0
Patankar	1997	44	no	8 (2–14), 1/wk	no	no	diary	84.0
Chiotakakou	1998	9	12–44	4 sess (1–4)	no	no	tel interv	57.0

[a]follow-up in months; [b]additional home training; [c]control group employed? [d]type of evaluation; [e]efficacy in % of patients reporting improvement.
[f]depending on the type of anismus.
n.r.: not reported.

studies – and not those claiming biofeedback to be helpful in *all* cases of chronic constipation – have incorporated home training procedures into the treatment program but, as with fecal incontinence, patient compliance to such training advice has never been studied in controlled trials.

BIOFEEDBACK THERAPY IN CHRONIC ANAL OR RECTAL PAIN

Another recent application of biofeedback training has been reported for treatment for chronic anal[16] or rectal pain[17,21] and levator ani syndrome.[25] It remained obscure and not shown by physiological data how re-training of

Table 27.8 Biofeedback studies in pain syndromes

First author	Year	Ref.	*n*	Diagnosis	Age	Sex (F:M)	Eval	Sessions	Cont[a]	Eff[b]
Grimaud	1991	21	12	anal pain	54.0	8:4	interv	8	no	100
Ger	1993	16	14	rectal pain	71.0	8:6	quest	>6	yes[c]	43
Gilliland	1997	17	86	rectal pain	68.0	55:31	interv	2–7	no	35
Heah	1997	25	16	levator ani syndrome	50.1	7:9	interv	n.r.	no	87

[a]Control group employed?
[b]Efficacy in % improved patients.
[c]Change into other therapy arm but not randomized.
n.r.: not reported.

striated pelvic floor muscle contractions and relaxations would allow the pain to subside if it originated from contraction of smooth muscle, as in proctalgia fugax, or from the rectum, as in IBS, or the external anal sphincter or levator ani muscle. The description of patients is poor in these studies. As long as the inclusion criteria and the physiological characteristics of these patients are not comparable, we will continue to see small sized studies with rather heterogeneous results.

SUMMARY

Biofeedback therapy of pelvic floor disorders has gained wide acceptance and has become the major conservative approach for the patient with fecal incontinence and constipation. Despite broad agreement about its efficacy, the modes of treatment have not been standardized, and the major components of their success not identified. New applications, such as in patients with ano-rectal pain syndromes have been tested adequately. It is tempting to speculate whether in another few years behavioral medicine approaches such as biofeedback training will become a legitimate and recognized part of clinical management.

REFERENCES

1. (Anonymous). Anismus and biofeedback. *Lancet* 1992;**339**:217–8.
2. Berti Riboli F, Frascio M, Pitto G, Reboa G, Zanolla R. Biofeedback conditioning for fecal incontinence. *Arch Phys Med Rehabil* 1988;**69**:29–31.
3. Bleijenberg G, Kuijpers HC. Treatment of the spastic pelvic floor syndrome with biofeedback. *Dis Colon Rectum* 1987;**30**:108–11.
4. Bleijenberg G, Kuijpers HC. Biofeedback treatment of constipation: Comparison of two methods. *Am J Gastroenterol* 1995;**89**:1021–6.
5. Buser WD, Miner PB. Delayed rectal sensation with fecal incontinence. Successful treatment using anorectal manometry. *Gastroenterology* 1986;**91**:1186–91.
6. Camilleri M, Phillips SF, Loening-Baucke V, Anuras S, Schuffler MD, Krishnamurthy S. Colectomy for severe constipation. *Dig Dis Sci* 1988;**33**:1196–8.
7. Cerulli MA, Nikoomanesh P, Schuster MM. Progress in biofeedback conditioning for fecal incontinence. *Gastroenterology* 1979;**76**:742–6.
8. Chiarioni G, Scattolini C, Bonfante F, Vantini I. Liquid stool incontinence with severe urgency: anorectal function and effective biofeedback treatment. *Gut* 1993;**34**:-1576–80.
9. Chiotakakou-Faliakou E, Kamm MA, Roy AJ, Storrie JB, Turner IC. Biofeedback provides long term benefit for patients with intractable, slow and normal transit constipation. *Gut* 1998;**42**:517–21.
10. Dahl J, Lindquist BL, Tysk C, Leissner P, Philipson L, Järnerot G. Behavioral medicine treatment in chronic constipation with paradoxical anal sphincter contraction. *Dis Colon Rectum* 1991;**34**:769–76.
11. Denis P, Crayon G, Galmiche JP. Biofeedback: The light at the end of the tunnel? Maybe for constipation. *Gastroenterology* 1980;**80**:23–4.
12. Enck P. Biofeedback training in disordered defecation. A critical review. *Dig Dis Sci* 1993; **38**:1953–60.
13. Enck P, Däublin G, Lübke HJ, Strohmeyer G. Long-term efficacy of biofeedback training for fecal incontinence. *Dis Colon Rectum* 1994;**37**:997–1001.
14. Engel BT, Nikoomanesh P, Schuster MM. Operant conditioning of rectosphincteric responses in the treatment of fecal incontinence. *N Engl J Med* 1974;**290**:646–9.
15. Fleshman JW, Dreznik Z, Meyer K, Fry RD, Carney R, Kodner IJ. Outpatient protocol for biofeedback therapy of pelvic floor outlet obstruction. *Dis Colon Rectum* 1992;**35**:1–7.
16. Ger GC, Wexner SD, Jorge JMN, *et al.* Evaluation and treatment of chronic intractable rectal pain – a frustrating endeavor. *Dis Colon Rectum* 1993;**36**:139–45.
17. Gilliland R, Heymen JS, Altomare DF, Vickers D, Wexner SD. Biofeedback for intractable rectal pain. *Dis Colon Rectum* 1997;**40**:190–6.
18. Glia A, Gylin M, Gullberg K, Lindberg G. Biofeedback retraining in patients with functional constipation and paradoxical puborectalis contraction. *Dis Colon Rectum* 1997; **40**:889–95.

19. Glia A, Gylin M, Akerlund JE, Lindfors U, Lindberg G. Biofeedback training in patients with fecal incontinence. *Dis Colon Rectum* 1998;**41**:359–64.
20. Goldenberg DA, Hodges K, Hersh T, Jinich H. Biofeedback therapy for fecal incontinence. *Am J Gastroenterol* 1980;**74**:342–5.
21. Grimaud JC, Bouvier M, Naudy B, Guien C, Salducci J. Manometric and radiologic investigations and biofeedback treatment of chronic idiopathic anal pain. *Dis Colon Rectum* 1991;**34**:690–5.
22. Guillemot F, Bouche B, Gower-Rousseau C, *et al.* Biofeedback for the treatment of fecal incontinence. *Dis Colon Rectum* 1995;**38**:393–7.
23. Hämäläinen KPJ, Raivio P, Natila S, Palmu A, Mecklin JP. Biofeedback therapy in rectal prolapse patients. *Dis Colon Rectum* 1996;**39**:262–5.
24. Haskell B, Rovner H. Electromyography in the management of the incompetent anal sphincter. *Dis Colon Rectum* 1976;**10**:81–4.
25. Heah SM, Ho YH, Tan M, Leong AFP. Biofeedback is effective treatment for levator ani syndrome. *Dis Colon Rectum* 1997;**40**:187–9.
26. Ho YH, Tan M, Goh HS. Clinical and physiologic effects of biofeedback in outlet obstruction defecation. *Dis Colon Rectum* 1996;**39**:520–4.
27. Ho YH, Chiang JM, Tan M, Low JY. Biofeedback therapy for excessive stool frequency and incontinence following anterior resection or total colectomy. *Dis Colon Rectum* 1996;**39**:1289–92.
28. Jensen LL, Lowry AC. Biofeedback improves functional outcome after sphincteroplasty. *Dis Colon Rectum* 1997;**40**:197–200.
29. Karlbohm U, Hallden M, Eeg-Olofsson, Pahlman L, Graf W. Result of biofeedback in constipated patients. A prospective study. *Dis Colon Rectum* 1997;**40**:1149–55.
30. Kawimbe BM, Papachrysostomou M, Clare N, Smith AN. Outlet obstruction constipation (anismus) managed by biofeedback. *Gut* 1991;**32**:1175–9.
31. Keck JO, Staniunas RJ, Coller YES, *et al.* Biofeedback training is useful in fecal incontinence but disappointing in constipation. *Dis Colon Rectum* 1995;**37**:1271–6.
32. Ko CY, Tong J, Lehman RE, Shelton AA, Schrock TR, Welton ML. Biofeedback is effective therapy for fecal incontinence and constipation. *Arch Surg* 1997;**132**:829–34.
33. Kohlenberg RJ. Operant conditioning of human anal sphincter pressure. *J Appl Behav Anal* 1973;**6**:201–8.
34. Koutsomanis D, Lennard-Jones JE, Kamm MA. Prospective study of biofeedback treatment for patients with slow and normal transit constipation. *Eur J Gastroenterol Hepatol* 1994;**6**:131–7.
35. Koutsomanis D, Lennard-Jones JE, Roy AJ, Kamm MA. Controlled randomised trial of visual biofeedback versus muscle training without a visual display for intractable constipation. *Gut* 1995;**37**:95–9.
36. Latimer PR, Campbell D, Kasperski J. A component analysis of biofeedback in the management of fecal incontinence. *Biofeedback Self-Regulat* 1984;**9**:311–24.
37. Leroi AM, Duval V, Roussignol C, Berkelmans I, Reninque P, Denis P. Biofeedback for anismus in 15 sexually abused women. *Int J Colorect Dis* 1996;**11**:187–90.
38. Lestar B, Penninckx F, Kerremans R. Biofeedback defaecation training for anismus. *Int J Colorect Dis* 1991;**6**:202–7.
39. Loening-Baucke V. Efficacy of biofeedback training in improving faecal incontinence and anorectal physiologic function. *Gut* 1990;**31**:1395–1402.
40. Loening-Baucke V. Biofeedback training in children with functional constipation. A critical review. *Dig Dis Sci* 1996;**41**:65–71.
41. MacLeod JH. Management of anal continence by biofeedback. *Gastroenterology* 1987;**93**:291–4.
42. Miner PB, Donelly TC, Read NW. Investigation of the mode of action of biofeedback in treatment of fecal incontinence. *Dig Dis Sci* 1990;**35**:1291–8.
43. Papachrysostomou M, Smith AN. Effects of biofeedback on obstructed defecation – reconditioning of the defecation reflex. *Gut* 1994;**35**:252–6.
44. Patankar SK, Ferrera A, Levy JR, Larach SW, Williamson PR, Perozo SE. Biofeedback in colorectal practice. A multicenter, statewide, three-year experience. *Dis Colon Rectum* 1997;**40**:827–31.
45. Patankar SK, Ferera A, Larach SW, *et al.* Electromyographic assessment of biofeedback training for fecal incontinence and chronic constipation. *Dis Colon Rectum* 1997;**40**:907–911.
46. Park UC, Choi SK, Piccirillo MF, Verzaro R, Wexner SD. Patterns of anismus and the relation to biofeedback therapy. *Dis Colon Rectum* 1996;**39**:768–73.
47. Rao SSC, Welcher KD, Happel J. Can biofeedback therapy improve anorectal function in fecal incontinence? *Am J Gastroenterol* 1996;**91**:2360–66.
48. Rao SSC, Welcher KD, Pelsang RE. Effects of biofeedback therapy on anorectal function in obstructed defecation. *Dis Dis Sci* 1997;**42**:2197–2205.
49. Rieger NA, Wattchow DA, Sarre RG, *et al.* Prospective trial of pelvic floor retraining in patients with fecal incontinence. *Dis Colon Rectum* 1997;**40**:821–6.
50. Rieger NA, Wattchow DA, Sarre RG, *et al.* Prospective study of biofeedback for treatment of constipation. *Dis Colon Rectum* 1997;**40**:1143–1148.
51. Sangwan YP, Coller JA, Barrett RC, Roberts PL, Murray JJ, Schoetz DJ. Can manometric parameters predict response to biofeedback therapy in fecal incontinence. *Dis Colon Rectum* 1995;**38**:1021–25.
52. Scheuer M, Kuijpers HC, Bleijenberg G. Effect of electrostimulation on sphincter function in neurogenic fecal incontinence. *Dis Colon Rectum* 1994;**37**:590–4.
53. Schiller LR, Santa Ana C, Davis GR, Fordtran JS. Fecal incontinence in chronic diarrhea. Report of a case with improvement after training with rectally infused saline. *Gastroenterology* 1979;**77**:751–3.
54. Siproudhis L, Dautreme S, Ropert A, *et al.* Anismus and biofeedback: who benefits? *Eur J Gastroenterol Hepatol* 1995;**7**:547–52.
55. Turnbull GK, Ritvo PG. Anal sphincter biofeedback relaxation treatment for women with intractable constipation symptoms. *Dis Colon Rectum* 1992;**35**:530–6.
56. van Tets WF, Kuipers JHC, Bleijenberg G. Biofeedback treatment is ineffective in neurogenic fecal incontinence. *Dis Colon Rectum* 1996;**39**:992–4.
57. Wald A. Biofeedback therapy for fecal incontinence. *Ann Int Med* 1981;**95**:146–9.

58. Wald A. Biofeedback for neurogenic fecal incontinence: rectal sensation is a determinant of outcome. *J Ped Gastroenterol Nutr* 1983;**2**:302–6.
59. Wald A, Tunuguntla AK. Anorectal sensorimotor dysfunction in fecal incontinence and diabetes mellitus. *N Engl J Med* 1984;**310**:1282–7.
60. Weber J, Ducrotte P, Touchais JY, Roussignol C, Denis P. Biofeedback training for constipation in adults and children. *Dis Colon Rectum* 1987;**30**:844–6.
61. Wexner SD, Cheape JD, Jorge JMN, Heyman SR, Yesgelman DG. Prospective assessment of biofeedback for the treatment of paradoxical puborectalis contraction. *Dis Colon Rectum* 1992;**35**:145–50.
62. Whitehead WE, Engel BT, Schuster MM. Perception of rectal distension is necessary to prevent fecal incontinence. In: Adam G, Meszaros I, Banyai EI (eds). *Advances in physiological sciences. Vol. 17, Brain and behavior.* Budapest, 1981:203–9.
63. Whitehead WE, Burgio KL, Engel BT. Biofeedback treatment of fecal incontinence in geriatric patients. *J Am Geriat Soc* 1985;**33**:320–4.

SECTION 5

Consequences of pelvic floor dysfunction and its treatment

Chapter 28

Prevention and management in pelvic floor disorders

Christine Norton

PREVENTION OF PELVIC FLOOR PROBLEMS

A considerable folklore has arisen around the subject of preventing pelvic floor dysfunction, in particular preventing urinary incontinence. To read some authors it might be concluded that if all childbirth were well managed and if women practised regular pelvic floor exercise (PFE) throughout their adult years, then incontinence would not occur. However, there is minimal research to substantiate these assumptions, and it simply is not known what proportion of problems could be prevented, and how practical prevention is in the real world.

Research on prevention of any health problem is notoriously expensive and difficult to conduct, usually requiring very large-scale and lengthy longitudinal studies. Even with major killer diseases little has as yet been proven about prevention. It is difficult to envisage funding for prevention studies in pelvic floor disorders becoming more readily available as there has been none to date. Therefore, when discussing preventing pelvic floor dysfunction, good studies do not exist, and most suggestions are speculative, and are based on known risk factors and associations. Although fully understanding risk factors is the essential first step in preventing incontinence, the subject has been poorly documented.[1]

Prevention can be considered in several stages. *Primary* prevention aims to prevent disease from developing by removing its causes or predisposing risk factors (e.g. preventing pregnancy or avoiding vaginal delivery). *Secondary* prevention aims to detect asymptomatic disease early and prevent symptoms developing once risk factors are present (e.g. practising postnatal exercises for women who have some evidence of pelvic floor impairment but who are as yet asymptomatic). *Tertiary* prevention aims to stop symptoms from getting worse, reduce complications and prevent chronic disabilities.

Both urinary and fecal incontinence are multifactorial, and although the sphincter muscles and pelvic floor are fundamentally important, they are by no means the only causative factor in fecal incontinence, urinary incontinence or pelvic organ prolapse. For example, fecal continence also depends upon gut motility and stool consistency, amongst other factors. Urinary continence also involves detrusor function. Both are influenced by neurological integrity, psychosocial and emotional factors and the physical environment. Bump and Norton[1] have suggested a model for prevention of pelvic floor problems (Fig. 28.1), with factors which may predispose, incite or promote pelvic floor dysfunction or lead to decompensating and symptom development.[1] For each individual presenting with symptoms of pelvic floor dysfunction there will be an interplay of factors which has led to symptoms and the relative weight of influences will vary considerably.

Urinary and fecal incontinence and prolapse often coexist, but when they do it would be simplistic to assume that the common mechanism is always pelvic floor damage or dysfunction. For example, Khullar[2] has found a prevalence rate for fecal incontinence of 15% on direct questioning among women attending a urodynamic clinic (this rose to 26% among the same women on a more impersonal postal questionnaire). However, the women with coexisting urinary and fecal incontinence were more likely to have a urodynamic diagnosis of detrusor instability than genuine stress incontinence, suggesting possible neurological, motility or anxiety disorders may be the common link rather than the pelvic floor.[2] There is an association between idiopathic detrusor instability and the irritable bowel syndrome.[3] Stress and urge urinary incontinence have different associated risk factors.[4] It is also common in clinical practice to encounter a woman with a clear history of obstetric trauma, and evidence of anal sphincter disruption on endoanal ultrasound, who has never the less been asymptomatic for some years and has developed fecal incontinence at a later date, presumably when some additional factor has altered bowel function or muscle integrity.

There is a small but growing movement to create multidisciplinary 'pelvic floor clinics', where the

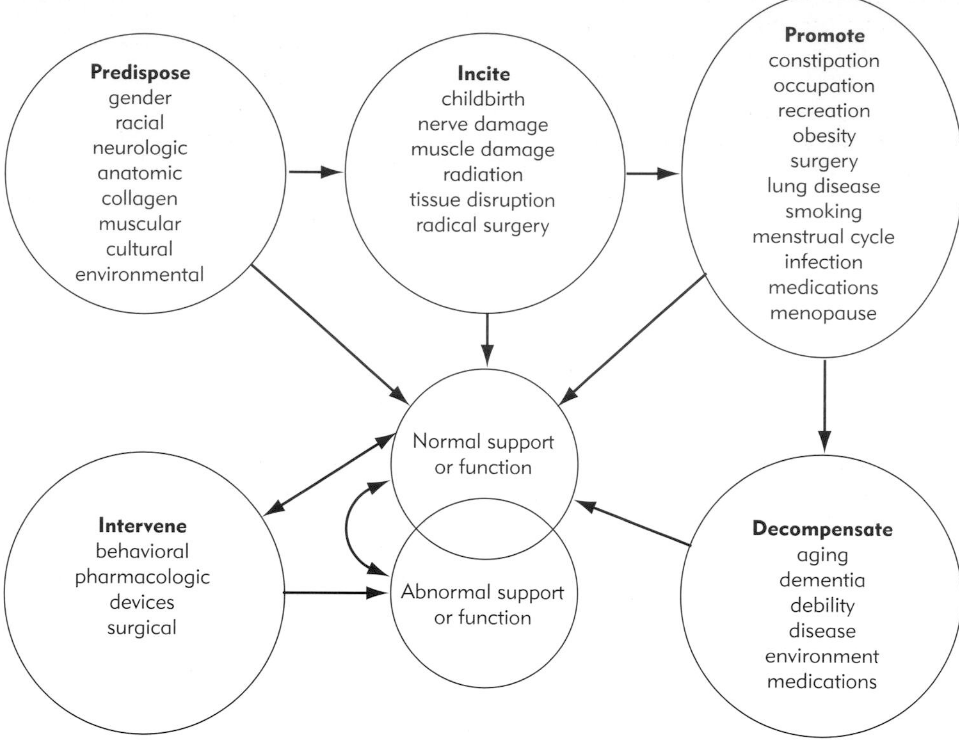

Figure 28.1 Model for the development of pelvic floor dysfunction in women.

urogynecologist, colorectal surgeon, specialist nurse and physiotherapist work together to increase mutual understanding of the interconnections between problems and attempt to dispense with the compartmentalization of pelvic floor problems.[5] To date there has been remarkably little cross-fertilization and sharing of expertise between these disciplines. There needs to be more awareness that treatments for one problem may cause new symptoms to appear in another organ system, leading to severe quality of life restrictions.

CHILDBIRTH

A survey of female obstetricians has found that nearly one third would opt for a cesarean delivery for herself in a first uncomplicated pregnancy to avoid the risk of perineal trauma.[6] The preference for cesarean delivery was even more striking in the presence of perceived risk factors – for example 68% would personally want a section if the anticipated birth weight were over 4.5 kg. In such a climate, it is surely time to put greater resources into research on preventing birth-related trauma to the pelvis. The solution is not to offer routine cesarean delivery, but to investigate ways of preventing maternal birth trauma.[7] If those most at risk of perineal trauma can be identified it should be possible to provide a rational basis for selective use of operative delivery.

In several large-scale epidemiological studies of fecal incontinence, more men than women are reported to have fecal incontinence.[8–10] However, in clinical practice, many more women than men present for help. Are women less tolerant of the symptom?

Childbirth is undoubtedly the major factor cited in causation of pelvic floor dysfunction. However, some epidemiological studies have suggested that most urinary problems start in pregnancy, not *de novo* after delivery.[11]

It is known that childbirth, in particular vaginal delivery, instrumental delivery, abnormal presentations, a prolonged active second stage of labor, birth weight over 4 kg, higher maternal age and first baby are all independent risk factors for subsequent anal incontinence.[12,13] If instrumental delivery is required, forceps seem to be more likely to cause damage than vacuum extraction,[12,13] although other studies have found equivalent rates with both forceps and vacuum delivery.[14] More than three or four births and more than three cesarean deliveries also seem to pose an increased risk. Elective, but not emergency cesarean delivery has been found to be protective.[14] Flatus incontinence is a permanent feature after 1.2% of first births, 1.5% second births and 8.3% third deliveries.[15] Others have found much higher rates of flatus incontinence (25%), which can be troublesome, but that it improves with time.[13] Women with pre-existing irritable bowel syndrome are prone to increased urgency of defecation and flatus incontinence after delivery.[16]

Urinary incontinence is likewise associated with forceps delivery, episiotomy, prolonged second stage and a large baby and an occiput posterior position.[17] Some women may be predisposed to damage by a weaker type of collagen, with poorer initial connective tissue. Isolated breaks in the fascial attachment of the pelvic floor may be as important as direct neuromuscular damage.[16]

Midline episiotomy is commonly practised in the USA. It has been found to increase the risk of subsequent risk of fecal incontinence threefold and to double the risk of flatus incontinence, compared to a spontaneous tear. Women with a midline episiotomy are five times more likely to have fecal incontinence than those with an intact perineum at 3 months postpartum.[18] Mediolateral episiotomy has not been shown to be so clearly related to subsequent fecal incontinence, but neither has it been shown to be protective and may even weaken the pelvic floor.[12] There is a conflict of opinion as to whether routine liberal use of episiotomy is protective (especially if combined with PFE[19]) or whether it should be abandoned altogether.[20]

The active pushing phase of the second stage of labour may be important, with pushing for more than one hour associated with increased risk of neuromuscular injury.[17] Cesarean delivery does seem to be protective against both urinary[21] and fecal incontinence,[22] although rates tend to equalize after two cesarean births.

A third degree obstetric tear leads to subsequent bowel symptoms in over 80% of women[23] and it has been suggested that the common obstetric practice of end-to-end repair should be replaced with a colorectal-style overlap sphincter repair, preferably under anesthetic in an operating theater.[12] Early studies have suggested that the technique of overlap repair is feasible in the immediate post-delivery period and may produce better results.[24]

There is debate about how to manage subsequent deliveries in women known to have sustained some anal sphincter damage already. Some would advocate allowing another vaginal delivery, on the basis that the damage has already been done, while others would repair the sphincter and plan for future cesarean births.[12]

It is commonly assumed that pelvic floor exercises during pregnancy or after delivery are protective against urinary incontinence. The evidence for this is equivocal. It has been found that women who actively exercise may recover continence earlier and have stronger muscles and less incontinence in the short term than those who do not[25] but there are no significant differences in pelvic muscle strength or in symptoms at 12 months after delivery.[26] Other workers have found some evidence that antenatal exercises are protective, but not completely so,[21] but this was a retrospective study. There may be an independent variable (such as general health awareness or level of fitness) that leads some women to do pelvic floor exercises and to subsequently experience less postnatal incontinence. Pre-pregnancy body mass was inversely correlated with incontinence. It may be that women who exercise the pelvic floor increase their awareness and so are able to better use these muscles under conditions of stress that threaten to cause leakage of urine.[27] Women with a pre-existing weakness in these muscles should maybe be targeted as those most likely to benefit from exercise. There are no data on the role of PFE in preventing fecal incontinence, although PFE have been shown to be of benefit in treating postnatal fecal incontinence, with anal biofeedback and electrical stimulation showing better results than vaginal biofeedback without stimulation in symptomatic women.[28]

It is notoriously difficult to motivate even symptomatic women to practice regular pelvic floor exercises, with dropout rates of over 50% in some studies.[29] Logically, it would be even more difficult to motivate symptom-free women to exercise. These exercises are very tedious and many women find it difficult to know if anything useful is being achieved. It has been found that pelvic floor exercises do not increase squeeze strength or EMG activity compared with controls in symptom-free nulliparous women.[30]

There is some evidence that women with urinary incontinence do not seek professional help because of a sense of guilt at having not done PFE postnatally. When incontinent women were interviewed and asked why they had not sought help, a sense of guilt was often expressed, a feeling that incontinence is their own fault because advice was ignored, or at least not complied with. Women felt that health professionals would not be sympathetic and so they did not present, even if the incontinence was bothersome.[31] It is possible that blanket advice to women to do these exercises either antenatally or postnatally, without any support or monitoring is not helpful in prevention of later problems and is actually counterproductive in that it discourages symptomatic women from seeking appropriate help.

SURGERY

There is some evidence that surgical solutions for one pelvic floor problem may unmask another and cause it to become symptomatic, or even possibly create new problems by distorting the anatomy or disrupting the nerve supply. For example, repairing a vaginal prolapse may unmask a tendency to urinary or fecal incontinence as the prolapse was actually supporting a cystocele or rectocele. Colposuspension is known to create new symptoms of prolapse in a proportion of patients.[32] Repair of a rectocele corrects the anatomical defect for three quarters of women undergoing posterior colporrhaphy, but there is not a clear relationship between anatomical defect and dysfunction. Repair of a rectocele has been found to create *de novo* fecal incontinence in 7% in one series, with some patients also reporting new sexual dysfunction (9%), rectal evacuation difficulties (11%) and poor control of flatus.[33]

Hysterectomy has been found in retrospective studies to change bowel function,[34] with over one third of women reporting newly decreased bowel frequency or difficulty with evacuation. It is postulated that the associated factors might include damage to the hypogastric nerve plexus during surgery, hormonal changes, or a common thread of chronic abdominal discomfort and anxiety in polysymptomatic women. Only 59% reported normal bowel function prior to hysterectomy.[35] Hysterectomy may be associated with later urinary incontinence, but the evidence is equivocal and the direction of causality is uncertain.[1] It may be that the surgery disrupts the pelvic nerve plexus and structural support to the bladder. However, often the primary reason for hysterectomy is pelvic floor dysfunction and so it may be a symptom rather than a cause of the problem.[1]

Several common ano-rectal procedures are associated with an increased risk of fecal incontinence. Lateral sphincterotomy to relieve a chronic painful anal fissure has been reported to result in minor symptoms of passive soiling (22%) and flatus incontinence (35%) and in major fecal incontinence in 5% of cases.[36] It is known that in women, who have a naturally shorter anal canal than men and a normal anterior ring of sphincter which is incomplete proximally, that it is not uncommon for a sphincterotomy to extend for the full length of the internal anal sphincter.[37] Surgical hemorrhoidectomy is reported to result in varying rates of fecal incontinence. Given that the reported rates do vary widely, it may be that variations in surgical technique or surgeon's skill are important. There does seem to be an increased willingness to take these 'minor' procedures more seriously and not leave them to the most inexperienced surgical trainees. Increased use of 'chemical sphincterotomy' (e.g. GTN or diltiazem), and injection or banding of hemorrhoids, with surgery reserved for the most severe or resistant cases, may lead to fewer future problems. In most countries, the practice of anal stretch seems to have fallen into disrepute because of subsequent problems with fecal incontinence,[38] except in pediatric practice, where presumably the internal sphincter is more elastic and less prone to fragment.

Men may benefit from PFE after radical prostatectomy, with men who exercise having a lesser degree and duration of urinary incontinence.[39]

LIFESTYLE

A body mass index (BMI) of 30 or over is an independent risk factor for urinary incontinence,[4] but it is not proven that weight loss is protective nor that it alleviates established urinary incontinence except in the morbidly obese requiring surgery for weight loss. Extra weight may impair the blood flow or nerves to the pelvic floor and this may be reversible.[1] There is no evidence about the effect of BMI on fecal incontinence.

Race also seems to be important, with Asian and white races more prone to pelvic floor problems,[4,17] and black women less so. While this does not give scope for primary prevention, it may enable secondary prevention programs to be targeted to those most at risk.

Smoking is a known risk factor for urinary incontinence and prolapse (OR 2.9),[1] presumably via chronic coughing, but there may be also less general health awareness in smokers than in non-smokers. It is also known that nicotine stimulates distal colonic motility and may therefore exacerbate a tendency to fecal urgency.[40] Caffeine stimulates both bladder and bowel as well as acting as a diuretic.[41]

Athletes who undertake a lot of high-impact exercise are more prone to stress urinary incontinence.[1] Excessive exercise may also be a factor in rectal prolapse. People whose jobs involve a lot of heavy lifting are more likely to need vaginal prolapse surgery than the general population (OR 1.6).[42]

A common factor in the genesis of pelvic floor problems may be chronic straining with perineal descent from constipation, with subsequent pelvic floor damage (direct or neurological)[43,44] resulting in prolapse, or urinary or fecal incontinence. Straining at stool in young women has been found to be associated with later prolapse and stress urinary incontinence.[45]

Many drugs are known to affect bladder and bowel function. It is beyond the scope of this chapter to review these, but prescribers should be aware of unintended side effects on urinary or fecal incontinence.

It may be that a number of lifestyle modifications, such as regulating bowel habit and avoiding straining, not smoking, regular physical exercise, estrogen replacement if indicated and weight loss may help to prevent the development of incontinence in at risk women.[1]

POST-SURGICAL

Patients with an ileoanal anastomosis have been found to develop a larger volume neorectum and less frequent stools at 3 and 6 months postoperatively with progressive balloon dilatations of the neorectum before ileostomy closure.[46] Average stool frequency was 6 per day in the group who underwent dilations, as opposed to 9 per day in a non-dilated group 6 months after surgery, but no information on fecal incontinence was given.

Formation of an ileoanal pouch reservoir is associated with fecal incontinence in some patients. Fecal soiling at night can be particularly troublesome. Surgical techniques that may overcome this are discussed elsewhere, but two studies have attempted to optimize function by additional conservative measures. Pelvic floor exercises, with or without additional balloon dilatation of the reservoir prior to ileostomy closure have not been found to be of benefit in improved continence of feces when compared with controls who did not have these treatments.[47,48]

OLDER PEOPLE

While it is impossible to halt aging *per se* there may be some factors commonly associated with aging which increase the risk of urinary incontinence and are amenable to modification (Table 28.1). Resnick has coined the mnemonic DIAPPERS to summarize these (Delirium/confusional state; Infection (symptomatic UTI); Pharmaceuticals; Psychological; Excessive urinary output; Restricted mobility; Stool impaction).[49] It is suggested that reversing these factors may be protective.[50] Maintaining functional mobility, cognitive function and good control of blood glucose levels (and hence secondary neuropathy) in diabetes may each have a role.[51] Many older people may tread a fine dividing line between continence and incontinence and for many it is necessary to plan coping to avoid development of frank symptoms because they cannot cope with the bladder or bowel.[52]

It has been suggested by an expert consensus meeting that 'healthy bladder habits' might be beneficial in preventing later problems. These included an adequate fluid intake, avoiding straining and constipation, and recognition of signs which should lead to seeking help.[53]

The incidence of fecal incontinence increases with advancing age. In frail nursing home patients, it is associated with male sex, dementia, immobility, stroke, diarrhea and possibly excessive fibre or laxative use.[54,55] New cases are also associated with acute diarrhea or impaction, severe cognitive decline and with much higher mortality that in patients who are continent.[56] The use of enemas and suppositories are negatively correlated with fecal incontinence. A striking feature of fecal incontinence in long-term and nursing home care is the huge variation in prevalence between different institutions with seemingly similar patient profiles. One study has found rates from 27% to 95%, suggesting that different bowel management regimes may be the most important factor. It would seem that laxatives are largely unsuccessful in preventing faecal incontinence in frail older people and should possibly be used less.[54]

Table 28.1 Risk factors associated with urinary incontinence in older people

- Advancing age, female sex
- Cognitive impairment
- Impaired mobility
- Functional disability
- Constipation
- Chronic cough
- Diabetes mellitus
- Cerebrovascular disease
- Hypnosedatives
- Diuretics
- Previous gastrointestinal surgery
- Urinary tract infections
- Lower urinary tract symptoms

Source: Ref. 50.

MENOPAUSE AND HORMONE REPLACEMENT

Prevalence studies often suggest a lower prevalence of urinary incontinence in women in the immediate postmenopausal years than in younger women.[57] This casts some doubt on the common assertion of patients that symptoms started at menopause, and on the role of hormone deficiency in causation of pelvic floor symptoms.

Hormone replacement therapy (HRT) is commonly used in clinical practice to treat urinary incontinence in postmenopausal women. However, objective evidence for efficacy is lacking, although subjective rating of symptoms by patients may improve.[58] The preventive value of hormone replacement is unknown, although estrogen receptors throughout the female genitourinary tract and in the pelvic floor musculature make this a possibility.

One study has suggested some benefit from HRT in postmenopausal women with fecal incontinence.[59] Resting and squeeze anal pressures were increased, as was the maximum volume tolerated in the rectum. The presence of an anal sphincter defect did not preclude symptomatic benefit. 90% of women reported some improvement and 25% became symptom-free. These results must be viewed with caution as it was a small (20 patient) uncontrolled study, and it has been suggested with urinary incontinence that subjective wellbeing rather than objective improvement may be the mode of action.[58] However, it does raise the question of the role of prophylactic HRT in preventing fecal incontinence in older women. It is known that hormone replacement can increase collagen and elastic tissue in the pelvic floor, that there are estrogen receptors in the external anal sphincter,[60] and that anal pressures have a tendency to decrease with advancing age.[61] It is theoretically possible that HRT could decrease or even reverse this trend. It would need a very large longitudinal study to investigate this. Meanwhile, clinically any postmenopausal woman in whom HRT is not contraindicated may be considered for a trial of therapy, particularly if there are also signs of atrophic changes vaginally.

PEOPLE WITH DISABILITIES

The prevalence of urinary and fecal incontinence is high in those with major neurological disabilities. Many people with physical disabilities have multiple predisposing factors for urinary and fecal incontinence, including neurogenic bladder or bowel syndromes and difficulties with accessing a toilet quickly and independently. Many cannot take continence for granted and will need to actively manage elimination (for example using intermittent self-catheterization) to prevent incontinence from developing. It is recognized that repeated use of valsalva to empty the bladder or bowel may lead to prolapse (rectal or vaginal). The ideal approach will often be multidisciplinary, with consideration not only of the organic dysfunction, but of the toileting facilities and the lifestyle of the individual and any involved carers.[62,63] Sometimes very simple solutions, such as the use of suppositories to give control over the timing of bowel evacuation, will be effective. A step-wise approach has been found to be successful in bowel management in spina bifida[64] and this approach is often useful in other conditions (Table 28.2). At other times a complex package of care which may include surgery may be appropriate. Many new options such as antegrade colonic irrigation, sacral nerve stimulation and implantation of prostheses are becoming available which may prevent incontinence in this group.

CHILDREN

It is known that constipation is the major factor in many children with soiling. The genesis of such constipation often seems to involve a complex interplay of family dynamics, toilet training practices, diet and minor painful ano-rectal conditions which lead to voluntary holding of stool and subsequent hard stool which is uncomfortable to evacuate, thus encouraging further holding of stool.[65] Systematic advice and a structured toileting program has been found to be effective in some children, and biofeedback to teach correct defecation dynamics has been found to augment the effectiveness of conservative measures in children with fecal incontinence in one study.[66] However, biofeedback has been found not to be any better than conservative measures alone in a larger study (non-randomized) by the same group[67] and in a randomized study by another group.[68]

It may be that teaching parents that the aim of toilet training should not be to reward retention of stool, but to reward correct placement of stool in the toilet, combined with greater attention to healthy eating and general exercise, as well as the possibly harmful effects of toilet training too early or aggressively, might go a long way to preventing the misery of childhood soiling. Early bowel management for children with neurological disorders such as spina bifida might prevent the chronic over-distention that is so often found when bowel training is eventually attempted. It is not certain what role chronic constipation plays in the eventual development of megarectum and megacolon, and it has been suggested that active management of childhood constipation could prevent many such problems from arising.[66] It is recommended that children developing encopresis secondary to chronic constipation should have intensive laxative treatment as a first choice to treat the problems and prevent long-term sequelae.[68]

Table 28.2 Protocol for progressive steps in bowel program

1. Bowel clean-out if hard stool is present in the rectal vault or palpable above the descending colon.
2. Appropriately soft stool consistency with diet and bulking agents.
3. Glycerine suppositories 20 minutes after meal. Ten minutes later on toilet, limited to less than 40 minutes, relieving skin pressure every 10 minutes.
4. Dulcolax suppository in place of glycerine.
5. Digital stimulation – 20 minutes post-suppository every 5 minutes × 3.
6. Timed oral medication, timed so that bowel movement would otherwise occur half to 1 hour after anticipated triggered bowel timing.

MANAGING PELVIC FLOOR PROBLEMS

MINIMIZING THE IMPACT OF INCONTINENCE

There is no doubt that urinary and fecal incontinence have a major negative impact on quality of life for many people. Individualized assessment and appropriate treatment of the underlying cause should lead to cure or adequate bladder or bowel control in the majority of cases.[52,69] However, there remains a significant minority of patients who fail to respond to treatment and who are left with urine or stool leakage sufficient to significantly restrict quality of life.

It is important not to assume that all those with symptoms find them bothersome or would want help. Indeed, several studies have suggested that up to half of patients with urinary incontinence do not want professional intervention.[70]

Those patients with residual bothersome symptoms which have failed to resolve need information and advice in order to minimize the impact of their symptoms. The patient who understands the nature of the problem can start to plan practical coping strategies, and there are many sources of information, such as books,[71–73] not for profit organizations and, increasingly, electronic media. Modification of diet and fluid intake, and simple measures for skin care and odor control will minimize the impact of symptoms for some people.

Some patients with a rectocele need simple reassurance that the symptoms are not sinister and can often be taught how to evacuate the bowel more effectively. Public awareness about bowel cancer is rightly increasing with active publicity drives. Many presenting with any bowel dysfunction are afraid that cancer may be the underlying cause. Prompt investigation and appropriate reassurance may allay anxiety and lead to decreased symptoms.

INCONTINENCE PRODUCTS

There is a huge variety of products designed to cope with incontinence.[52] Many different styles of absorbent pad will cope with most urinary incontinence. However, pads are much less acceptable for fecal incontinence.

An anal plug has been developed to help people with fecal incontinence. It is designed to be worn inside the rectum to plug the entrance to the anus from the inside. It comes wrapped in a water-soluble film, for ease of insertion. This film dissolves once inside the rectum, and the plug opens into the cup shape, with a string for removal from the anus.

Some people find an anal plug uncomfortable, or that it gives a constant feeling of needing to open the bowels. It has to be taken out before a bowel action, and so is not suitable for someone who needs to open the bowels very frequently. An evaluation of the plug found that 11 of 14 patients (71%), withdrew because of discomfort.[74] This will obviously be less of a problem when ano-rectal sensation is impaired.

ODOR CONTROL AND SKIN CARE

Meticulous personal hygiene and prompt disposal of soiled materials do not always ensure good odor control, and this can be the most embarrassing aspect of incontinence. Proprietary deodorants may be helpful. There are numerous other tips which can be tried.[71] Skin care can be problematic, particularly in the presence of diarrhea, double incontinence or a fistula. There is little research on or evaluation of the different products available and it is often a case of trial and error to find a skin care regime that eases soreness.

EDUCATION AND PUBLIC AWARENESS

Taboos on talking about bowel and bladder problems are slowly lifting, but there remain considerable barriers to public awareness of symptoms of pelvic floor dysfunction and they still cannot be discussed with the same openness as other medical problems. The World Health Organization has recognized the importance of promoting positive attitudes and educating the public so that those with a clinically significant problem can be empowered to seek help without shame or embarrassment.[5] The media have a part to play in this and are slowly coming to cover these topics.

An expert consensus meeting on prevention of incontinence agreed the following target groups for education about prevention:

- The general public on healthy habits and when to seek help.
- Teachers and schools on healthy habits, drinking and toilet facilities.
- People with neurological disease, with information that management is possible.
- Government bodies, health insurers, organizations of health professionals and national organizations whose members are in high risk groups for incontinence.[53]

PROFESSIONAL EDUCATION

Education of the various professionals who may be called on to help patients with pelvic floor problems is sadly lacking. Family practitioners, general nurses and specialist doctors, nurses and physiotherapists lack structured training in most instances, although accredited specialist training is becoming available in some countries.[5] Two thirds of newly qualified family doctors in the UK have been found to have between one and four hours training about incontinence; one third had received no training at all. About 92% of family doctors in practice for 5 years or more had received no training on incontinence and 80% of all doctors felt that their training was inadequate. Knowledge was found to be poor, with 76% having 'no idea' of the prevalence of incontinence.[76]

It has been found that the knowledge of doctors and nurses involved with childbirth may be inadequate. Many are unable to say which muscles are being repaired during perineal repairs and the majority feel that their training is inadequate.[77]

CONTINENCE SERVICES

There is no country in the world that has developed comprehensive continence services which are seen to be adequately meeting the needs of the population.[5] Most services are fragmented between urologists, gynecologists, colorectal surgeons, specialist nurses and physiotherapists, in varying combinations. There is no research on the best model for service delivery, although in the UK patients living in an area with access to a nurse specialist have been found to be more likely to have had appropriate referral, investigation and treatment of incontinence, and are more satisfied with the service, than those who live in areas with no specialist nurse access.[78]

There can be little doubt that the treatment offered for some pelvic floor conditions will depend largely upon what type of practitioner is consulted. For example, a woman presenting with a rectocele might be offered vaginal posterior repair by a gynecologist, transrectal or transperineal repair by a colorectal surgeon and evacuation training and biofeedback by a nurse or physiotherapist. There is little cross-boundary research to define the most effective approach. Much more of this collaborative research is needed to define the future contributions to a combined pelvic floor clinical service. The future should see much greater collaboration, multidisciplinary research and education to minimize the incidence and impact of pelvic floor problems.

REFERENCES

1. Bump RC, Norton PA. Epidemiology and natural history of pelvic floor dysfunction. *Obstet Gynecol Clin North Am* 1998;**25**(4):723–46.
2. Khullar V, Damiano R, Toozs-Hobson P, Cardozo L. Prevalence of faecal incontinence among women with urinary incontinence. *Br J Obstet Gynaecol* 1998; **105**:1211–3.
3. Monga AK, Marrero JM, Stanton SL, Lemieux M-C, Maxwell JD. Is there an irritable bladder in the irritable bowel syndrome? *Br J Obstet Gynaecol* 1997;**104**:1409–12.
4. Brown JS, Grady D, Ouslander JG, Herzog AR, Varner RE, Posner SF. Heart and Estrogen/Progestin Replacement Study (HERS) Research Group. Prevalence of urinary incontinence and associated risk factors in postmenopausal women. *Obstet Gynecol* 1999;**94**(1):66–70.
5. Norton C, Baracat F, Gartley CB, *et al.* Promotion, organisation and education in continence care. In: Abrams P, Khoury S, Wein A (eds). *Incontinence – First International Consultation on Incontinence* (World Health Organization). Monaco: Health Publications Ltd.; 1999;**21**:837–68.
6. Al-Mufti R, McCarthy A, Fisk NM. Obstetricians' personal choice and mode of delivery. *Lancet* 1996;**347**:544.
7. Sultan AH, Stanton SL. Preserving the pelvic floor and perineum during childbirth – elective caesarean section? *Br J Obstet Gynaecol* 1996;**103**:731–4.
8. Drossman DA, Li Z, Andruzzi E, Temple RD, Talley NJ, Thompson WG. U.S. householder survey of functional gastrointestinal disorders. *Dig Dis Sci* 1993;**38**(9):1569–80.
9. Johanson JF, Lafferty J. Epidemiology of fecal incontinence: the silent affliction. *Am J Gastroenterol* 1996;**91**(1):33–6.
10. Nakanishi N, Tatara K, Naramura H, Fujiwara H, Takashima Y, Fukunda H. Urinary and faecal incontinence in a community-residing older population in Japan. *J Am Geriat Soc* 1997;**45**:215–9.
11. Cook VAM, Osborn JL, Malone-Lee J. Pregnancy and not delivery associated with postpartum incontinence in primigravid women. *Neurourol Urodynam* 1999;**18**(4):292–3.
12. Sultan AH, Kamm MA. Faecal incontinence after childbirth. *Br J Obstet Gynaecol* 1997;**104**:979–82.
13. Zetterstrom JP, Lopez A, Anzen B, Dolk A, Norman M, Mellgren A. Anal incontinence after vaginal delivery: a prospective study in primiparous women. *Br J Obstet Gynaecol* 1999;**106**(4):324–30.
14. MacArthur C, Bick DE, Keighley MRB. Faecal incontinence after childbirth. *Br J Obstet Gynaecol* 1997;**104**:46–50.
15. Ryhammer AM, Bek KM, Laurberg S. Multiple vaginal deliveries increase the risk of permanent incontinence of flatus and urine in normal premenopausal women. *Dis Colon Rectum* 1995;**38**:1206–9.
16. Donnelly VS, O'Herlihy C, Campbell DM, O'Connell PR. Postpartum fecal incontinence is more common in women with irritable bowel syndrome. *Dis Colon Rectum* 1998;**41**(5):586–9.
17. Handa VL, Harris TA, Ostergard DR. Protecting the pelvic floor: obstetric management to prevent incontinence and pelvic organ prolapse. *Obstet Gynecol* 1996;**88**(3):470–8.
18. Signorello LB, Harlow BL, Chekos AK, Repke JT. Midline episiotomy and anal incontinence: retrospective cohort study. *Br Med J* 2000;**320**:86–90.
19. Taskin O, Wheeler JM, Yalcinoglu AI. The effects of episiotomy and Kegel exercises on postpartum pelvic relaxation: a prospective controlled study. *J Gynecol Surg* 1996;**12**:123–7.
20. Klein MC, Gauthier RJ, Robbins JM. Relationship of episiotomy to perineal trauma and morbidity, sexual dysfunction, and pelvic floor relaxation. *Am J Obstet Gynecol* 1994;**171**:591–8.
21. Wilson PD, Herbison RM, Herbison GP. Obstetric practice and the prevalence of urinary incontinence three months after delivery. *Br J Obstet Gynaecol* 1996;**103**(2):154–61.
22. Sultan AH, Kamm MA, Hudson CN, Thomas JM, Bartram CI. Anal sphincter disruption during vaginal delivery. *New Engl J Med* 1993;**329**:1905–11.
23. Sultan AH, Kamm MA, Hudson CN, Bartram CI. Third degree obstetric and sphincter tears: risk factors and outcome of primary repair. *Br Med J* 1994;**308**:887–91.
24. Sultan AH, Monga AK, Kumar D, Stanton SL. Primary repair of obstetric anal sphincter rupture using the overlap technique. *Br J Obstet Gynaecol* 1999;**106**(4):318–23.
25. Morkved S, Bo K. The effect of postpartum pelvic floor muscle exercise in the prevention and treatment of urinary incontinence. *Internat Urogynecol J Pelvic Floor Dysfunct* 1997;**8**(4):217–22.
26. Sampselle CM, Miller JM, Mims BL, DeLancy JOL, Ashton-Miller JA, Antonakos CL. Effect of pelvic muscle exercise on transient incontinence during pregnancy and after birth. *Obstet Gynecol* 1998;**91**:406–12.
27. Miller JM, Ashton-Miller JA, DeLancy JOL. The knack: a precisely timed pelvic muscle contraction can be used within a week to reduce leakage in urinary stress incontinence. *Gerontologist* 1996;**36**:328.
28. Fynes MM, Marshall K, Cassidy M, *et al.* A prospective, randomized study comparing the effect of augmented biofeedback with sensory biofeedback alone on fecal incontinence after obstetric trauma. *Dis Colon Rectum* 1999;**42**(6):753–8.
29. Wilson PD, Herbison GP. A randomized controlled trial of pelvic floor muscle exercises to treat postnatal urinary incontinence. *Internat Urogynecol J Pelvic Floor Dysfunct* 1998;**9**(5):257–64.
30. Thorp JM, Stephenson H, Jones LH, Cooper G. Pelvic floor (Kegel) exercises – a pilot study in nulliparous women. *Internat Urogynecol J* 1994;**5**:86–9.

31. Ashworth PD, Hagan MT. Some social consequences of non-compliance with pelvic floor exercises. *Physiotherapy* 1993;**79**(7):465–71.
32. Wiskind AK, Creighton SM, Stanton SL. The incidence of genital prolapse after the Burch colposuspension. *Am J Obstet Gynecol* 1992;**167**:399–404.
33. Kahn MA, Stanton SL. Posterior colporrhaphy: its effects on bowel and sexual function [see comments]. *Br J Obstet Gynaecol* 1997;**104**(1):82–6.
34. Taylor T, Smith AN, Fulton PM. Effect of hysterectomy on bowel function. *Br Med J* 1989;**299**:300–1.
35. van Dam JH, Gosselink MJ, Drogendijk AC, Hop WC, Schouten WR. Changes in bowel function after hysterectomy. *Dis Colon Rectum* 1997;**40**(11):1342–7.
36. Khubchandani I, Reed JF. sequelae of internal sphincterotomy for chronic fissure in ano. *Br J Surg* 1989;**76**:431–4.
37. Sultan AH, Kamm MA, Nicholls RJ, Bartram CI. Prospective study of the extent of internal sphincter division during lateral sphincterotomy. *Dis Colon Rectum* 1994;**37**:1031–3.
38. Snooks SJ, Henry MM, Swash M. Faecal incontinence after anal dilatation. *Br J Surg* 1984;**71**:617–8.
39. Van Kampden M, De Weerdt W, Van Poppel H, De Ridder D, Feys H, Baert L. Effect of pelvic-floor re-education on duration and degree of incontinence after radical prostatectomy: a randomised controlled trial. *Lancet* 2000;**355**:98–102.
40. Rausch T, Beglinger C, Alam N, Meier R. Effect of transdermal application of nicotine on colonic transit in healthy nonsmoking volunteers. *Neurogastroenterol Mot* 1998;**10**:263–70.
41. Brown SR, Cann PA, Read NW. Effect of coffee on distal colon function. *Gut* 1990;**31**:450–3.
42. Jorgensen S, Hein HO, Gyntelberg F. Heavy lifting at work and risk of genital prolapse and herniated lumbar disc in assistant nurses. *Occupa Med* 1994;**44**:47–9.
43. Snooks SJ, Barnes PRH, Swash M, Henry MM. Damage to the innervation of the pelvic floor musculature in chronic constipation. *Gastroenterology* 1985;**89**:977–81.
44. Lubowski DZ, Swash M, Nicholls RJ. Increases in pudendal nerve terminal motor latency with defecation straining. *Br J Surg* 1988;**75**:1095–7.
45. Spence-Jones C, Kamm MA, Henry MM. Bowel dysfunction: a pathogenic factor in uterovaginal prolapse and urinary stress incontinence. *Br J Obstet Gynaecol* 1994;**101**:147–52.
46. Telander RL, Perrault J, Hoffman AD. Early development of the neorectum by balloon dilatations after ileoanal anastomosis. *J Pediat Surg* 1981;**16**(6):911–6.
47. Jorge JM, Wexner SD, Morgado PJ, James K, Nogueras JJ, Jagelman DG. Optimization of sphincter function after the ileoanal reservoir procedure. *Dis Colon Rectum* 1994;**37**:419–23.
48. Oresland T, Fasth S, Nordgren S, Swenson L, Akervall S. Does balloon dilatation and anal sphincter training improve ileo-anal pouch function? *Internat J Colorectal Dis* 1988;**3**:153–7.
49. Resnick NM. Urinary incontinence. *Lancet* 1995;**346**:94–9.
50. Fonda D, Resnick NM, Kirschner-Hermanns R. Prevention of urinary incontinence in older people. *Br J Urol* 1998;**82**(Suppl.)1:5–10.
51. Luft J, Vriheas-Nichols AA. Identifying the risk factors for developing incontinence: can we modify individual risk? *Geriat Nurs* 1998;**19**(2):66–71.
52. Norton C (ed.) *Nursing for continence*, 2nd edn. Beaconsfield: Beaconsfield Publishers 1996.
53. Cottenden A, Gartley CB, Norton C, *et al. Consensus statement of the first international conference for the prevention of incontinence (Danesfield House)*. Wilmette, Illinois: Simon Foundation for Continence, 1997.
54. Brocklehurst JC, Dickinson E, Windsor J. Laxatives and faecal incontinence in long-term care. *Nurs Stand* 1999; **13**(52):32–6.
55. Johanson JF, Irizarry F, Doughty A. Risk factors for fecal incontinence in a nursing home population. *J Clin Gastroenterol* 1997;**24**(3):156–60.
56. Chassagne P, Landrin I, Neveu C, *et al.* Fecal incontinence in the institutionalized elderly: incidence, risk factors, and prognosis. *Am J Med* 1999;**106**(2):185–90.
57. Jolleys JV. Reported prevalence of urinary incontinence in women in a general practice. *Br Med J* 1988;**296**:1300–2.
58. Fantl JA, Cardozo L, McClish D. Estrogen therapy in the management of urinary incontinence in postmenopausal women: a meta-analysis. First report of the hormones and urogenital therapy committee. *Obstet Gynecol* 1994;**83**:12–8.
59. Donnelly V, O'Connell PR, O'Herlihy C. The influence of oestrogen replacement on faecal incontinence in postmenopausal women. *Br J Obstet Gynaecol* 1997;**104**:311–5.
60. Haadem K, Ling L, Ferno M, Graffner H. Oestrogen receptors in the external anal sphincter. *Am J Obstet Gynecol* 1991;**164**:609–10.
61. Laurberg S, Swash M. Effects of aging on the anorectal sphincters and their innervation. *Dis Colon Rectum* 1989;**32**:737–42.
62. White H, Norton C. Aids to continence for people with physical disabilities. In: *Nursing for continence*, 2nd edn. Beaconsfield: Beaconsfield Publishers 1996; Chapter 13, 299–316.
63. Norton C, Henry M Investigation and treatment of bowel problems. In: Fowler C (ed) *Neurology of bladder, bowel, and sexual dysfunction*. Boston: Butterworth Heinemann, 1999;**12**:185–207.
64. King JC, Currie DM, Wright E. Bowel training in spina bifida: importance of education, patient compliance, age, and anal reflexes. *Arch Phys Med Rehab* 1994;**75**(3):243–7.
65. Clayden GS, Agnarsson U. *Constipation in childhood*. Oxford: Oxford University Press, 1991.
66. Loening-Baucke V. Modulation of abnormal defaecation dynamics by biofeedback treatment in chronically constipated children with encopresis. *J Pediat* 1990;**116**(2):214–22.
67. Loening-Baucke V. Biofeedback treatment for chronic constipation and encopresis in childhood: long-term outcome. *Pediatrics* 1995;**96**(1 Pt 1):105–10.
68. van der Plas RN, Benninga MA, Buller HA, *et al.* Biofeedback training in treatment of childhood constipation: a randomised controlled study. *Lancet* 1996;**348**(9030):776–80.
69. Kamm MA. Faecal incontinence: clinical review. *Br Med J* 1998;**316**:528–32.
70. Lagro-Janssen ALM, Smits AJA, Van Weel C. Women with urinary incontinence – self-perceived worries and general

practitioner's knowledge of the problems. *Br J Gen Pract* 1991;**40**:331–4.

71. Norton C, Kamm MA. *Bowel control – information and practical advice.* Beaconsfield: Beaconsfield Publishers, 1999.
72. Toozs-Hobson P, Cardozo L. *Urinary incontinence in women.* London: British Medical Association/Dorling Kindersley, 1999.
73. Schuster MM, Wehmueller J. *Keeping control: understanding and overcoming faecal incontinence.* London: John Hopkins Press 1994.
74. Christiansen J, Roed-Petersen K. Clinical assessment of the anal continence plug. *Dis Colon Rectum* 1993;**36**(8):740–2.
76. Jolleys JV, Wilson J. GPs lack confidence (letter). *Br Med J* 1993;**306**:1344.
77. Sultan AH, Kamm MA, Hudson CN. Obstetric perineal trauma: an audit of training. *J Obstet Gynaecol* 1995;**15**:19–23.
78. Roe B, Doll H, Wilson K. Help seeking behaviour and health and social services utilisation by people suffering from urinary incontinence. *Internat J Nurs Stud* 1999;**36**(3):245–53.

Chapter 29

Application of theory to surgical management of female pelvic floor disorders

Peter E P Petros

SUMMARY

The International Continence Society (ICS) guideline offers surgical treatment only for stress incontinence in the absence of detrusor instability. The ICS paradigm is analysed and re-interpreted in terms of an anatomical classification specifying dysfunction in three compartments of the vagina based on the Integral Theory of female urinary incontinence. According to this theory, an external mechanism driven by the pelvic floor muscles assists opening and closure by stretching the connective tissue of urethra and anus. Connective tissue (CT) laxity invalidates this mechanism, causing dysfunction of opening and closure. The site of CT laxity is diagnosed using a pictorial algorithm which also acts as a guide for a series of new minimally invasive surgical methods characterized by reduced postoperative pain and catheterization. This anatomical approach is not inconsistent with ICS concepts. It also potentially addresses several other pelvic floor dysfunctions besides stress incontinence. These include bladder instability, fecal dysfunction, uterovaginal prolapse, and pelvic pain of otherwise unknown origin.

WHY THEORIES ARE IMPORTANT

All medical management is based on hypothesis. Scientific theories are universal statements. Popper [1] noted that by using such universal laws, it is possible to give causal explanations, and predict singular events. Ideally a theory should be simply expressed, consistent and falsifiable.

In order to accommodate practical necessity (daily usage of a theory), and progress (new theories, paradigm shifts etc.), Popper proposes two rules of methodology:

1. Scientific statements can never reach a point where they can be regarded as finally verified, i.e. no matter how powerful, they must always be open to replacement by another concept. Popper had a Darwinian attitude to hypotheses: they must struggle to maintain their primacy.
2. Once a hypothesis has been proven to some degree of validity it should not be allowed to drop out without good reason; i.e. unless it can be replaced by another hypothesis which is 'better testable', or following falsification of one of the consequences of the hypothesis. Popper recognized that hypotheses, even imperfect ones, can be usefully employed to direct research and activity. In pelvic floor disorders, therefore, it follows that before any competing management system can be introduced, the existing ICS system must not only be modified, its competitor must 'better explain' existing observations treatment success and failure.

AIMS OF THIS CHAPTER

Though Popper's guidelines create an imperative for refutation of existing hypotheses, and in particular, the ICS definitions, the aim of this chapter is to reinterpret the various ICS definitions and descriptions in terms of anatomical dysfunction; to incorporate these into a diagnostic classification specifying laxity in three compartments of the vagina; to explain in terms of the Integral Theory[2,3] why minimally invasive surgical repair in these compartments may improve not only stress incontinence, but also symptoms of bladder instability and abnormal emptying;[4] and to introduce a new test, 'simulated operations' which may help predict success or otherwise of these operations.

A CRITICAL ANALYSIS OF THE PRESSURE TRANSMISSION THEORY

The two theories which rely on raised intra-abdominal pressure to close the urethra[5,6] logically predict that a bladder neck elevation operation would not only cure stress incontinence, but also improve the 'cough pressure transmission ratio' (Faysal et al.[7]). The demonstration of both appeared to confirm the pressure transmission theory. However, these theories also predict that, during micturition, straining should close the urethra, causing urine flow to cease. However, straining generally causes flow to increase. Furthermore, these theories predict that during coughing, the pressure outside the urethra must always be higher than inside the urethra. Direct measurement in equivalent positions inside and outside the urethra while coughing during the intravaginal slingplasty operation[8] demonstrated that the pressure generated inside the urethra was far higher than outside the urethra. These observations seriously question the validity of pressure transmission theories.

A CRITICAL ANALYSIS OF 'DETRUSOR INSTABILITY'

The incontinence literature of the past 20 years has been dominated by the concept of detrusor instability. Yet nowhere has detrusor instability (DI) been defined as a theory or hypothesis. It was introduced into clinical thinking by an expert committee.[9] The term 'detrusor instability' (DI) as defined by the International Continence Society (ICS)[9,10] relates only to symptoms of frequency, urgency and nocturia if they are associated with a raised phasic detrusor pattern on testing. Without confirmation of DI, such symptoms are not attributed to an unstable bladder, as the previous generic term 'bladder instability' is not defined by the ICS. The concepts surrounding DI appear to have been inspired by observations of a high incidence of DI in patients with failed surgical operations for incontinence plus the not infrequent discovery of an effort-induced detrusor contraction (clearly not stress incontinence) as a cause of urine loss.[11] The ICS does not recommend[9,10] surgery in patients with urodynamically diagnosed detrusor instability (DI). Urodynamics are advised preoperatively, as symptoms are said to be unreliable. It is also stated[10] that DI should correlate with symptoms and signs, as asymptomatic continent patients may have DI.[10] Put another way, one must use urodynamics because symptoms are unreliable, and symptoms because urodynamics are unreliable.

Such recommendations by the ICS[9,10] are a major source of confusion. Furthermore, such statements cannot be challenged (are not 'falsifiable').[1] Popper[1] states that all 'meaningful statements' must be capable of being finally decided with respect to their truth and falsity; i.e. if there is no possible way to determine whether a statement is true, then that statement has no meaning. 'It is always possible to find some way of evading falsification, for example by introducing *ad hoc* an auxiliary hypothesis, or by changing *ad hoc* a definition'.[1] The original ICS definition of 'detrusor instability' specified a detrusor pressure rise to 15 cm water.[9] Subsequently, the ICS definition was modified,[10] so that it is now defined as a phasic pressure rise only, with no pressure limits specified. The objective standard used to validate subjective symptoms was itself now a subjective parameter.

Even the core practices of the ICS recommendations are being challenged. A large multicenter trial demonstrated that urodynamics were not predictive of surgical failure, neither was surgery contraindicated in the presence of an unstable bladder.[12] DI was not found to be a predictor of surgical failure with the intravaginal slingplasty (IVS) operation,[4] and was found postoperatively in many entirely asymptomatic patients cured of both stress and instability symptoms.[4] DI was found in 70% of asymptomatic women.[13] According to Popper's criteria, DI cannot now be considered either as an index of pathogenesis or a predictor of surgical failure.

The etiological basis of DI is unknown, but is generally attributed either to a neurological defect, or to some abnormality within the bladder itself. Urine loss may occur with handwashing provocation, possibly because of interruption of a central inhibitory pathway.[14] It is difficult to explain handwashing urine loss by a detrusor muscle abnormality or by neurologically based theories. A local lesion cannot be influenced by handwashing. A neurological lesion causes bladder instability precisely because it is not subject to the body's neurological control systems.

Examination according to Popper's criteria reveals several flaws in the ICS process of definition. First and foremost, a scientific term cannot be defined in a way which prevents it being challenged (falsified). Secondly, it is not valid to extrapolate from the particular to the general ('induction'). Association of failed surgery with DI in some patients cannot be extrapolated to a general rule that surgery is contraindicated in the presence of DI. Thirdly, one has to be certain that replacing an old term ('bladder instability') with a new term ('detrusor instability') does not cause confusion. Popper warns against introducing new words ('linguistics') which may not be as precise as previous descriptions. The term DI has been a major source of confusion for practitioners, especially if frequency, urgency and nocturia are present without associated 'DI'. And yet nearly all contradictions associated with the term DI disappear at once if, as proposed below, DI is regarded as a urodynamic expression of a prematurely activated micturition reflex.

THE 'INTEGRAL THEORY' – AN ALTERNATIVE TO THE ICS PARADIGM

The Integral Theory is a universal theory of female urinary function and dysfunction.[2,3] It is also a method of management.[3,4] According to this theory, a normal bladder has only two stable modes, open (voiding) or closed (storage). Inability to adequately achieve either state is defined as dysfunction. Central to this theory is the external musculoelastic mechanism assisting urethral opening and closure (Fig. 29.1). Connective tissue transmits the muscle forces. Thus connective tissue degeneration (laxity) may cause inadequate closure and opening. Clearly a damaged muscle[15] may modify the contractile strength of the muscles (Fig. 29.1). However, high cure rates for a range of pelvic floor symptoms following connective tissue repair,[4] indicate that muscle damage[15] may be more a modifying rather than a principal factor in causation of urinary dysfunction.

1. **During normal urethral closure**, three opposite directional forces, one forward, one backward, and one downward (Fig. 29.2 and 29.3), all generated by pelvic floor contraction, stretch the lower and upper parts of the vagina in opposite directions against the suspensory ligaments to effect urethral closure during stress.[2,3]

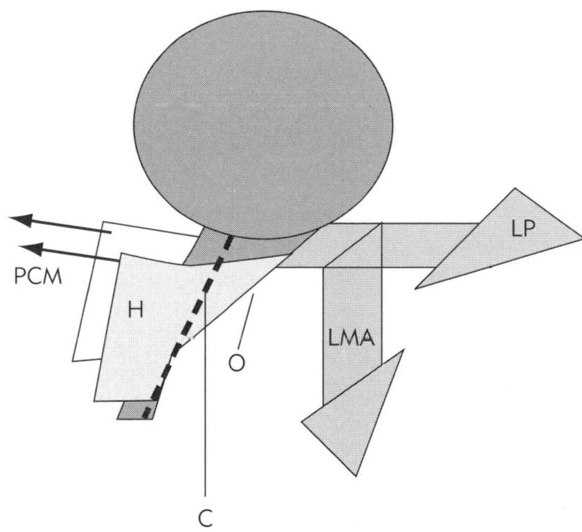

Figure 29.1 External connective tissue mechanism for opening and closure of the urethra. This represents a schematic sagittal representation of the bladder, urethra, and vaginal hammock. During closure, the anterior portion of pubococcygeus muscle (PCM) stretches the vaginal hammock (H) forwards to close the urethra from behind. At the same time, the levator plate (LP) and longitudinal muscle of the anus (LMA) stretch the upper vagina and bladder base backwards and downwards to close the bladder neck. The broken line 'C' demarcates the 'closed' position of the hammock. During micturition PCM relaxes. The vector forces LP and LMA stretch the hammock backwards to open out the urethra. Line 'O' represents the 'open' position of the hammock. Connective tissue laxity in 'H' or the upper vagina may cause inadequate transmission of the muscles forces required to close or open the urethra.

2. **During micturition,**[3] the forward force relaxes; the backward and downward forces combine to stretch the vagina, and therefore, urethra, during micturition (funneling, Fig. 29.4).
3. **A peripheral musculoelastic feedback control mechanism.**[2,3] 'N', Fig. 29.5, represents the volume and pressure receptors at the bladder base.[16] The nerve endings 'N' fire off at a critical pressure.[16] During bladder filling, the urethral pressure rises because of striated muscle contraction, (Fig. 29.3).[17] Contraction of Cm stretches the vaginal membrane below 'N'. This supports the urine column, preventing the afferent signal Oa to the brain CTX. The forward muscle forces (Fig. 29.3), and (Om) the backward/downward muscle forces (Fig. 29.4).
4. **Modulation of the afferent signal by central control.**[2,3] The afferent mechanism (Oa) is processed at facilitatory ('O') and inhibitory ('C') centers in the brain (Fig. 29.5). If convenient to micturate, the cortical centre 'CTX' inhibits 'C' and instructs 'O' to acclerate Oa. The efferent signals (Oe), in turn, proceed to relax the striated urethral sphincter (SM), relax the forward contractile muscle force, stimulate detrusor contraction (Od), and contract the backward and downward opening muscles (Om). In this way, the outflow tract is opened out as in Fig. 29.4, and the bladder contracts to empty. If inconvenient to empty, CTX suppresses all opening channels ('O'), and stimulates all closure channels ('C').

AN ALTERNATIVE CONCEPT FOR DETRUSOR INSTABILITY – PREMATURE ACTIVATION OF THE MICTURITION REFLEX

Because of the way it has been defined, it has been difficult in the past to challenge 'detrusor instability' as the gold standard in all aspects of the ICS paradigm. It cannot be argued, however, that uncontrolled urine loss is the end-point of 'detrusor instability'. It was found on direct observation during a handwashing test that symptoms of urgency, in fact, had a 97% correlation with actual urine loss.[18] Furthermore, the events associated with urine loss in 115 patients with a history of bladder instability undergoing a provocative handwashing test,[19] Table 29.1, were similar to what could be expected during normal micturition, each manifestation separated by a time delay of a few seconds. An anatomical rationale for DI is presented to explain ICS definitions or descriptions, which are indicated with italics.

Damage may occur in all three compartments (zones), causing laxity (Fig. 29.6). Laxity in any of the three zones may prevent the three muscle forces from stretching the vagina sufficiently to support the column of urine above 'N', so that symptoms of instability,

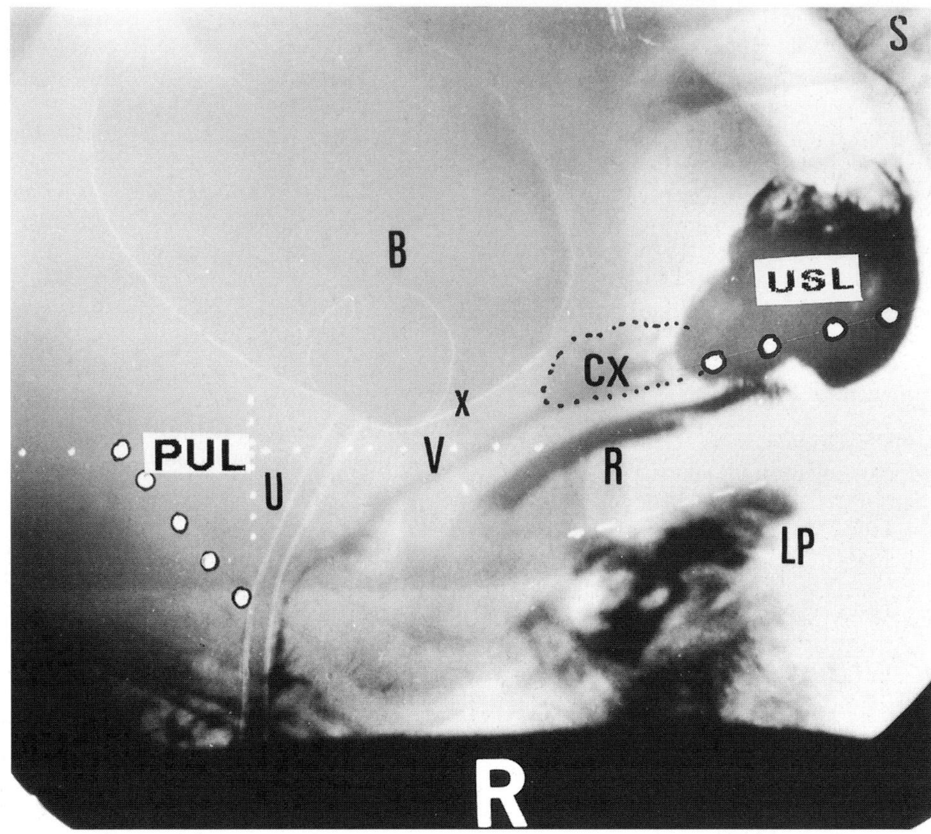

Figure 29.2 Resting position of pelvic organs. Continent patient. This is a sitting lateral X-ray in the resting position with a full bladder (B) incorporating a Foley catheter; the Foley balloon, opacified with radio-opaque dye outlines vagina (V), rectum (R) and levator plate (LP); superior border of LP: broken lines; the diagonal line composed of small solid circles represents pubourethral ligaments (PUL) anteriorly, and uterosacral ligaments (USL) posteriorly. CX: cervix; X: attachment of bladder base to vagina). U: urethra. The intersecting white dotted horizontal and vertical lines are drawn from fixed bony points.

frequency, urgency and nocturia may occur in any compartment (Fig. 29.7). According to[2,3] the bladder has two states only, open (micturition) and closed (storage). The 'open' circuit '0' (Fig. 29.5) is depicted by unbroken lines, and the 'closed' circuit 'C' by broken lines. Vaginal laxity may predispose to increased afferent impulses from 'N' ('0_a', Fig. 29.5), (*sensory urgency*). The cortex, (CTX, Fig. 29.5), may respond by activating the neurological closure circuit 'C'. This centrally blocks the afferent impulses (0a), the efferent impulses (0e), and causes the stricted muscle to contract, supporting the urine column, reducing stimulation of 'N'. The suppression circuit 'C' struggles for supremacy with the micturition circuit '0'. Because of the time lag associated with feedback circuits, this struggle is depicted graphically during urodynamic testing as a phasic (bell-shaped) pattern: seen simplistically, as the micturition reflex '0' predominates, the detrusor contracts, and detrusor pressure rises ('*detrusor instability*'). As 'C' gradually wrests control of the neural pathways, the detrusor pressure falls back to the baseline. Bladder training, pelvic floor exercises, electrotherapy, neurological lesions, mechanical causes such as cystocele are consistent with this scheme. Bladder training improves the central mechanism, pelvic floor exercises and electrotherapy improve muscle function. Bladder inflammation or tumor may stimulate 'N',

Table 29.1 Manifestations of the micturition reflex on handwashing provocation in 115 patients with a history of urge incontinence[19]

Manifestation	% of total (n=115)
Sensory urgency	93
Urethral relaxation	79
Detrusor contraction	49
Urine loss	45

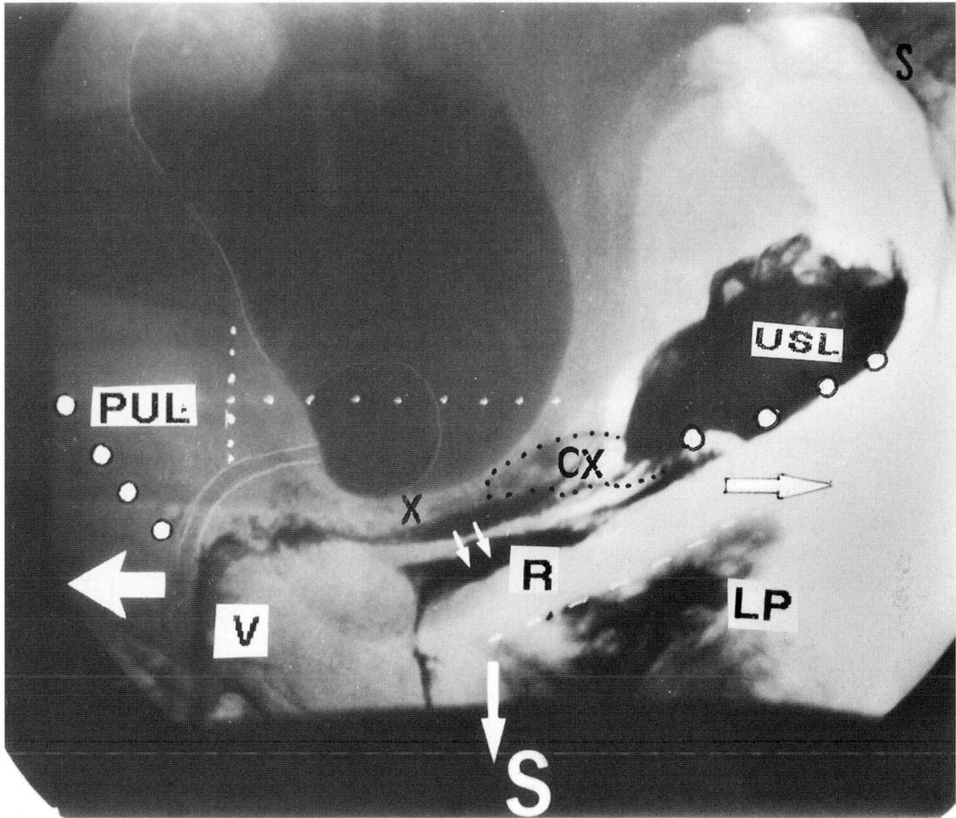

Figure 29.3 Active closure (coughing or straining). Same patient and labeling as in Fig. 29.2. Compared to Fig. 29.2, bladder neck, upper vagina and rectum appear to have been pulled backwards and downwards (arrows) by downward angulation of the superior border of levator plate (LP). With reference to the dotted white lines, the ascending vagina and urethra appear to have been pulled forwards (arrow), creating a right-angled bend of the Foley catheter tube.

causing excess afferent (0a) impulses (urgency symptoms). Multiple sclerous or other neurological lesions may interfere with 'C' at all levels in the brain and spinal cord causing uninhibited passage of impulses through the brain, and urine loss. Spinal cord transection may block both afferent (0a) and efferent 0e impulses causing neurogenic urinary retention.

Midcompartment laxity in the form of a cystocele may prevent the directional muscle forces (Fig. 29.7) from stretching the vaginal membrane to support 'N'. This may invalidate the peripheral neurological control mechanism, and result in urgency.

Finally, it is important to note that cystometry gives only a 'snapshot' of a particular set of circumstances which exist in the bladder control system over the time of measurement. Interpretation of data[20] from a handwashing test using a simple feedback equation ($X_{NEXT} = cX\ (1-X)$, where $X<1$) allows a more global perspective of how the processes underlying the formation of detrusor pressure may influence actual recorded results.

CONVERGENCE OF THE PATHOGENESIS OF UTEROVAGINAL PROLAPSE, AND FECAL AND URINARY INCONTINENCE

Figure 29.6 demonstrates how the fetal head may damage the various pelvic ligaments, and vaginal and rectal tissue, causing laxity of these tissues. Congenital connective tissue laxity may cause similar problems. In this context, symptoms and urodynamic findings are considered to be mainly secondary to anatomical defects.

AN ANATOMICAL CLASSIFICATION – A GUIDE TO SURGICAL CORRECTION OF DYSFUNCTION

It is evident on examining the radiographs (Fig. 29.2–4), that the forward and backward forces act against the anterior ligamentous supports of the vagina (PUL), and the downward force against the posterior ligaments ('USL'). Thus the anterior and posterior ligaments create

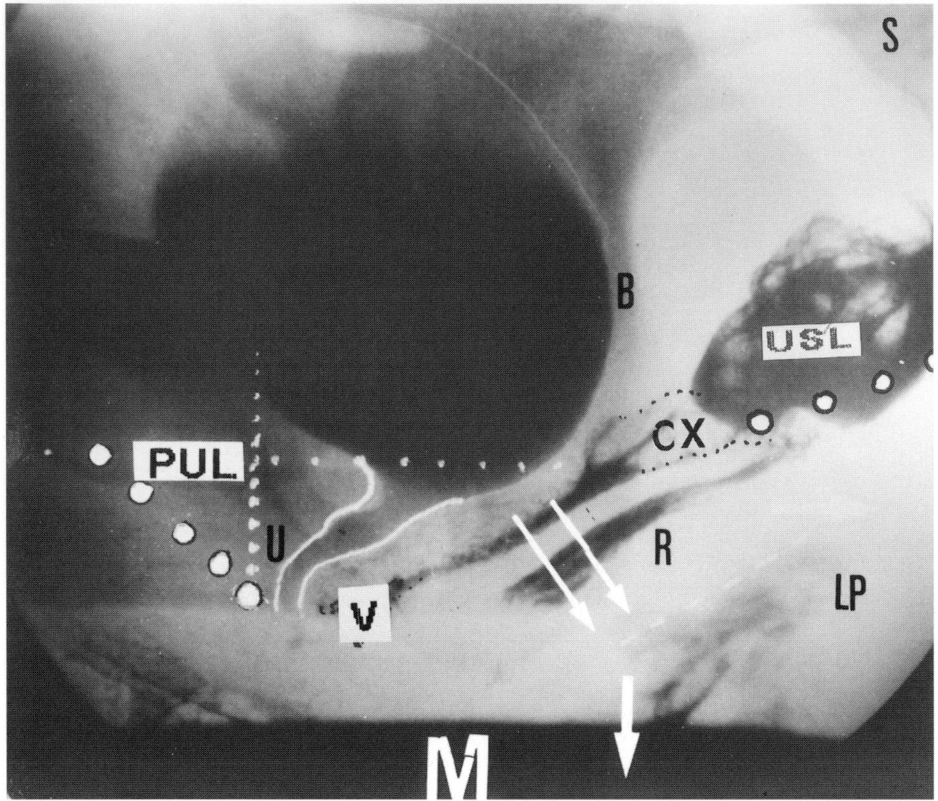

Figure 29.4 Micturition. Same patient and labeling as in Fig. 29.2. With reference to Figs 29.2 and 29.3, relaxation of the forward force permits urethra and bladder neck to be opened out by the downward and backward forces (arrows). Movements of upper vagina, bladder, rectum, and levator plate appear identical to those seen during closure.

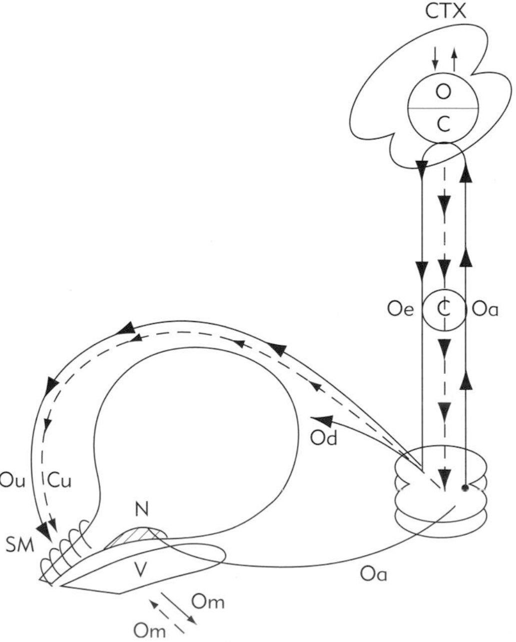

Figure 29.5 Schematic outline of central and peripheral control of the micturition reflex. This is a sagittal schematic representation of bladder, urethra, vagina, spinal cord and brain. 'N': nerve endings at bladder base; SM: intraurethral striated muscle sphincter. 'C' and 'O' are equivalent to the inhibitory and facilitatory micturition centers in the brain. They also represent the paths for the closure circuit 'C' (broken lines) and for the open (micturition) circuit 'O' (unbroken lines) – afferent outflow (Oa) from 'N' to spinal cord and brain, and efferent flow (Oe) to detrusor (Od), urethra (Ou) and pelvic muscles (Om, Cm). CTX: cortex. The two directional arrows below vagina (V) represent the muscle forces acting during the micturition (Om) and closure (Cm) reflexes.

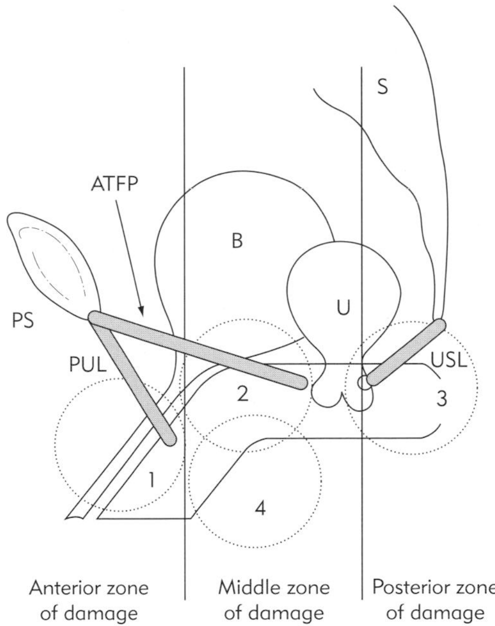

Figure 29.6 Damage to vagina at childbirth. The circles represent the fetal head overstretching the connective tissue of vagina and its supporting ligaments as it descends through the birth canal. 1: Hammock and pubourethral ligament (PUL) laxity; 2: cystocele and arcus tendineus fasciae pelvis (ATFP) laxity; 3: uterosacral/cardinal (USL) ligament laxity (uterine prolapse and enterocele); 4: rectocele, endoanal mucosa, external anal sphincter

a demarcation of the vagina into three compartments (Fig. 29.7). If the ligaments are lax, then the muscle forces acting during opening (Fig. 29.4), and closure (Fig. 29.3) may be compromised. A good analogy is a trampoline. If the membrane (vagina) or springs (ligaments) are loose, the membrane cannot be tensioned. The pictorial algorithma (Fig. 29.7) collates parameters associated with each compartment.

CORRELATION OF FUNCTIONAL ANATOMY WITH THE CLASSIFICATION

With reference to Fig. 29.3, it can be seen that the vaginal hammock is pulled forwards against PUL during effort. Therefore laxity in either the vaginal hammock or PUL (anterior compartment; Fig. 29.7) may cause stress incontinence. With reference to Fig. 29.4, it is clear that the forward force has relaxed. The backward and downward forces (arrows) open out the outflow tract during micturition. Therefore inability to empty the bladder adequately may be caused by laxity in the middle and posterior compartments. It has been found serendipitously that fecal incontinence was cured with the IVS operation[21] and pelvic pain with reconstruction of the posterior ligaments.[22] Therefore these symptoms are associated with the anterior and posterior compartments. Although substantially accurate in its predictions, the algorithm is no more than a guide. No specific parameter is always present in terms of a particular compartmental defect, and almost any symptom may be caused by any compartmental defect. For example, stress and fecal incontinence may, in some instances, be improved by repairing the posterior compartments only, especially in post-hysterectomy incontinence.

SIMULATED OPERATION – A NEW METHOD FOR PREDICTING SURGICAL CURE OF STRESS INCONTINENCE AND BLADDER INSTABILITY

These methods directly test the Integral Theory's predictions in a deductive way.[1] Selectively supporting specific connective tissue structures in the three zones (compartments) of vagina as in the algorithm (Fig. 29.7), may relieve urgency, prevent urine loss with stress, and change urodynamic parameters such as closure pressure and detrusor instability.

ANTERIOR COMPARTMENT

The support of an artery forcep on one side exactly at midurethra reinforces PUL (Fig. 29.2). This decreases or eliminates supine urine loss with coughing, and performed under ultrasound control, reverses bladder neck descent and funneling. This process is shown in a real observation on the website http://www.cs.curtin.edu.au/~bvk/petros/results.html. This maneuver frequently reduces urgency,[20] and also increases the 'cough transmission ratio' (CTR). Tightening the hammock may also control urine loss and increase CTR.[2] Neither of these maneuvers elevates the bladder neck. The raised CTR can be explained by reference to the formula P=F/A (Pressure = Force/Area). A firm anchoring point increases the force applied (F), and this stretches and narrows the urethral cavity (A) so that pressure (P) increases.

MIDDLE COMPARTMENT

Gentle digital support of the bladder base in patients with instability symptoms (DI) alleviated urge symptoms[20] and even urodynamic detrusor instability in some cases. This maneuver works by restoring the integrity of the peripheral neurological control mechanism (Fig. 29.5). Middle zone laxity may prevent the posterior force stretching the vagina to full extension during micturition as seen in Fig. 29.4. Opening out of

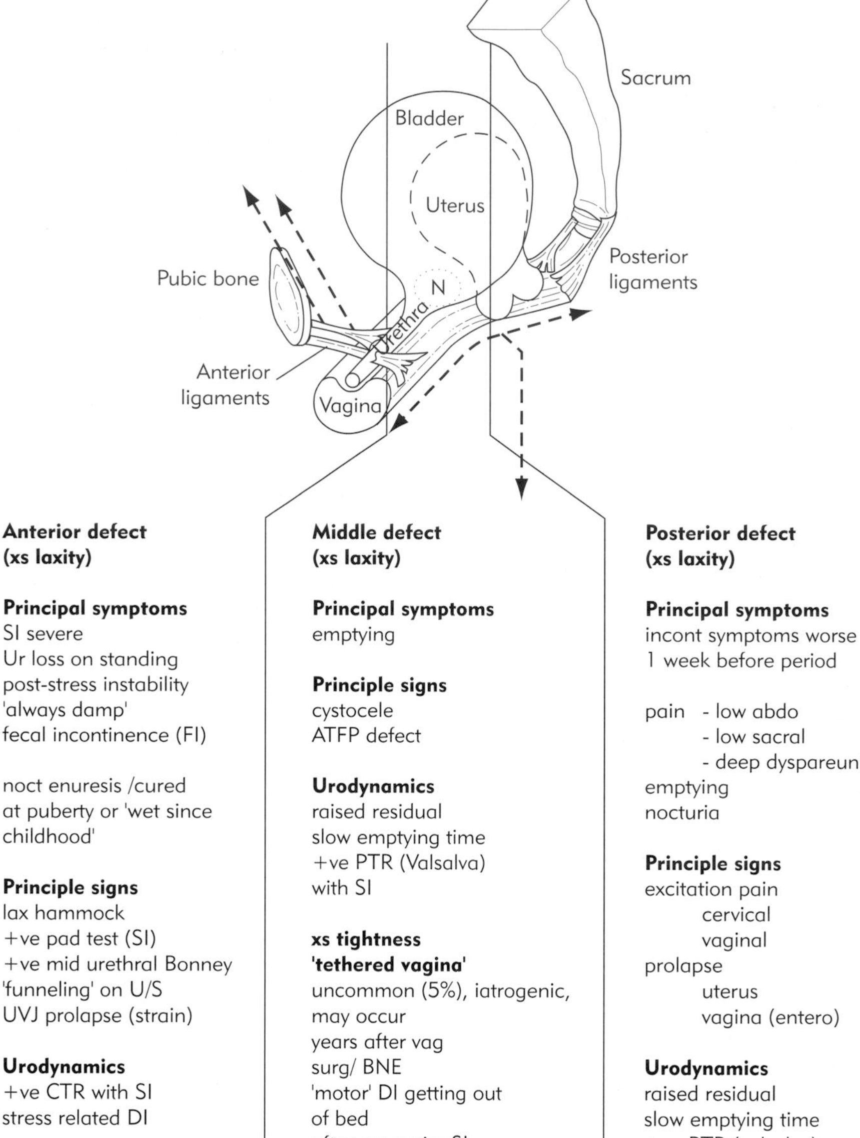

Figure 29.7 **Diagnostic pictorial algorithm. This is a schematic 3-dimensional view of bladder supported by vagina. The arrows represent directional striated muscle forces. 'N' indicates stretch receptors at bladder base.**

the urethra is suboptimal, and this, in turn, increases the resistance of the urethra, resulting in symptomatic inadequate emptying. Urethral resistance is extremely sensitive to outflow diameter (in proportion to the 4th power). Thus, halving of outflow diameter increases the urethral resistance by a factor of 16. Significant decrease in urine leakage on insertion of the Continence Guard in patients with urge incontinence[23] supports the concept that vaginal laxity may be an important cause of urinary dysfunction. The

Continence Guard stretches the middle zone of the vagina, supporting 'N' (Fig. 29.5).

POSTERIOR COMPARTMENT

Palpation of the prolapsed cervix or vaginal vault in patients with low abdominal pelvic pain of otherwise unknown origin generally reproduces that pain.[21] It is frequently possible to control urge symptoms by gently stretching the posterior fornix of the vagina with the bottom part of a bivalve speculum. Repair of the posterior ligaments significantly improves bladder emptying.[4]

SURGICAL TESTING OF THE ANATOMICAL CLASSIFICATION

Site-specific connective tissue repair according to the pictorial algorithm (Fig. 29.7) directly tests the Integral Theory's predictions in a deductive way[1] by relieving urgency, stress, emptying difficulty, and by changing urodynamic parameters such as closure pressure and detrusor instability.[3,4]

URINARY INCONTINENCE

The anatomical classification was directly tested by prospectively repairing ligamentous laxity in the three zones of the vagina according to the algorithm (Fig. 29.7).[4] There was no selection of patients, i.e. no patient was excluded from surgery. Repair of the anterior zone defect gave a high cure rate for stress incontinence, and repair of the other zones improved symptoms of urge, frequency, nocturia, and abnormal emptying.[4] Urodynamically diagnosed 'detrusor instability' was not a negative prognostic factor.[4] At 21 months follow-up, cure rates for symptoms were: stress incontinence 88% (n = 85) and 6% improvement; frequency 85% (n = 42), nocturia 80% (n = 30), urge incontinence, 86% (n = 74), emptying symptoms, 50% (n = 65). Surgical tightening of the posterior ligaments cured pelvic pain of otherwise unknown origin in 85% of patients.[22] Similar results for stress incontinence were reported with the tension-free vaginal tape (TVT) operation.[24] Like the Intravaginal Slingplasty (IVS) procedure, TVT repairs the anterior compartment, and works by creation of an artificial pubourethral ligament.

FECAL INCONTINENCE

Twenty-five patients presenting with both urinary and fecal incontinence reported 90% cure of their fecal incontinence for a minimum of 6 months (mean 26 months, range 6–48 months) after IVS surgery.[21] The external anal sphincter was normal in all 25 patients (100%). The internal anal sphincter (IAS) was normal in 18 patients (72%). There was no change in the morphology of the (damaged) IAS in the three patients who underwent postoperative ultrasound assessment. In three patients, fecal incontinence recurred simultaneously with occurrence of vaginal herniations in the posterior and middle parts of the vagina. Surgical repair of the uterosacral and arcus tendineus fasciae pelvis ligaments, plus endoanal suturing of prolapsed anal mucosa in one instance restored fecal continence. It was deduced from this experience that the anatomical classification (Fig. 29.7) may also apply for fecal dysfunction. This hypothesis is summarized in Figs. 29.8–29.10.

In essence, the same three directional forces which close the lower urinary tract, stretch, angulate, and close the rectum against the same pelvic ligaments (PUL and USL). This is evident on comparing Fig. 29.2 with Fig. 29.3. During anorectal closure, contraction of puborectalis (PRM) (Fig. 29.10), anchors the anus. The backward (LP) and downward (LMA) forces stretch and close the rectum against the now-anchored anus. This action creates the ano-rectal angle. The forward muscle force (PCM) anchors the anus. During defecation, relaxation of PRM allows LP and LMA to open out the ano-

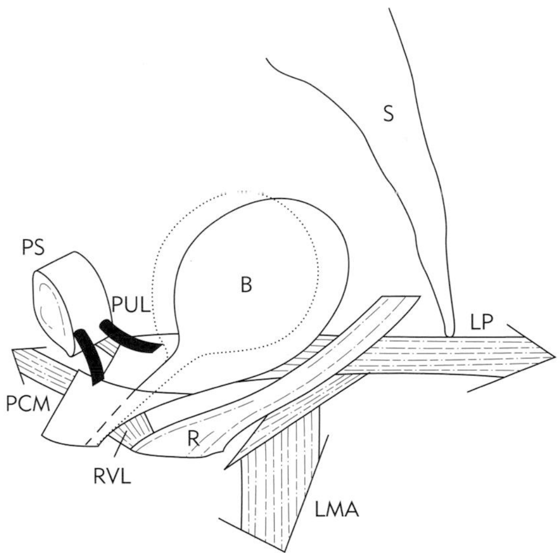

Figure 29.8 How vaginal and anterior ligamentous laxity may inactivate ano-rectal opening and closure. Three striated muscle forces, levator plate (LP) anterior portion of pubococcygeus (PCM) and longitudinal muscle of the anus (LMA) stretch the vagina and rectum against the pubourethral ligament (PUL). It is hypothesized that this action closes off both bladder neck and anorectal angle, and that PUL laxity may inactivate all three forces, so that leakage occurs. The normal closed position of bladder (B), is indicated by dotted lines. RVL: rectovaginal fascia.

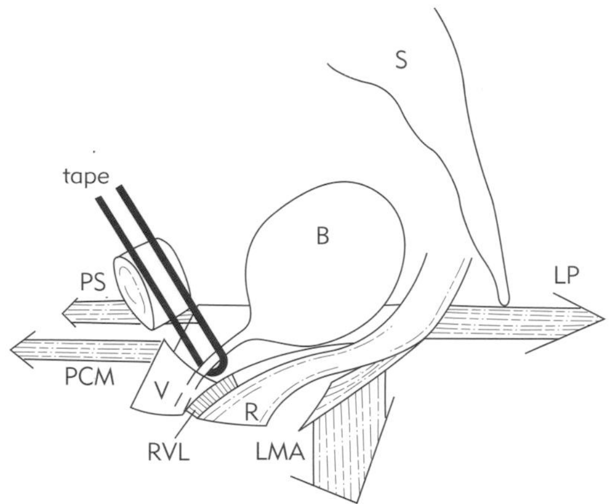

Figure 29.9 How restoration of the anterior ligamentous supports of vagina may restore ano-rectal closure. With reference to Fig. 29.8, it is hypothesized that the tape restores the insertion point of levator plate (LP) and anchors the anus via RVL; contraction of LP and LMA stretch the rectum (R) against a now rigid anchoring point, creating a rotational force around the tape; this action closes off the rectum at the ano-rectal junction. Labeling as in Fig. 29.8.

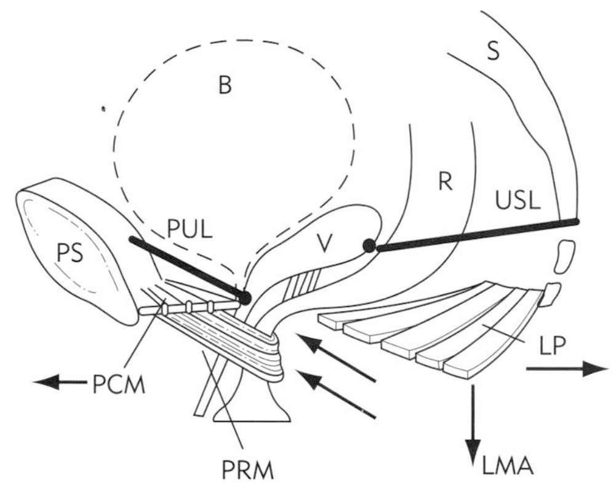

Figure 29.10 The muscle forces which create ano-rectal closure in the female. Schematic representation of the pelvic floor structures, with ano-rectal angle in the closed position. The middle part of pubococcygeus muscle (PCM) has been cut away to reveal the underlying puborectalis muscle (PRM). The bladder is represented by dotted lines. PCM: anterior portion of pubococcygeus muscle; V: vagina; R: rectum; LP: levator plate; LMA: force generated by the longitudinal muscle of the anus; PUL: pubourethral ligament; PS: pubic symphysis; S: sacrum; USL: uterosacral ligament. Arrows represent the directional forces created by the pelvic muscles. LMA is a striated muscle which surrounds the rectum, but is not attached to it.[26] LMA originates from LP, PCM and PRM, and inserts into the superficial and deep external anal sphincters and their related fascia.[26] It is to be distinguished from the longitudinal muscle of the rectum, a smooth muscle which forms part of the rectal wall.

rectal angle. PCM continues to contract, and this prevents the anterior wall of the anus collapsing inwards during defecation. Ligamentous laxity would weaken application of the muscle forces, and so cause dysfunction in both opening and closure of the anus, much as occurs in the urethra. With reference to Fig. 29.6, anal mucosa which has been dislocated from the wall of anus and rectum (i.e. prolapsed) may act as an irritant to cause incontinence.

AN ANATOMICAL CONNECTIVE TISSUE EXPLANATION FOR ICS DEFINITIONS AND DESCRIPTIONS

The remaining part of this chapter groups the ICS definitions and descriptions into dysfunctions of opening and closure. An anatomical explanation has been more completely presented elsewhere.[25]

DYSFUNCTIONS OF CLOSURE

With reference to Fig. 29.1 (Table 29.2), connective tissue (CT) laxity may prevent urethral closure (forward arrows explaining the ICS descriptions. If the three directional forces cannot stretch the vagina sufficiently to support the urine column, stress incontinence will develop. If there is high sensitivity in the stretch receptors, 'N' may fire off prematurely ('detrusor instability'), and if sufficiently severe, 'motor urgency'. All the other descriptions in the section 'CT plus peripheral neurological' follow naturally from this process.

Table 29.2 ICS definitions or descriptions: anatomical correlations[25]

Dysfunctions of closure	Dysfunctions of opening
Connective tissue (CT) only	**Connective tissue (CT) only**
Genuine stress incontinence	Slow flow
Unconscious incontinence	Feeling of not having emptied
Continuous leakage	Postmicturition dribble
Dribble incontinence	Dyssynergia
Interrupted flow	
CT plus peripheral neurological	**CT plus peripheral neurological**
Detrusor instability	Detrusor acontractility
Low bladder capacity	Under activity
Sensory urgency	Overflow incontinence
Frequency	Difficulty in initiation of flow
Nocturia	
Motor urgency	
Neurological only	**Neurological only**
Site specific multiple sclerosis	Spinal cord transection
Site specific brain tumor	Site specific multiple sclerosis
	Site specific brain tumor

DYSFUNCTIONS OF OPENING

With reference to Fig. 29.1 and 29.4, vaginal laxity may prevent opening out of the outflow tract by the backward and downward forces (arrows). Inability to stretch open the urethra greatly increases its resistance to flow (to the 4th power). Increased resistance to flow may explain all the symptoms grouped under "Dysfunctions of opening CT only" Table 29.2. If there is a combination of low sensitivity stretch receptors and lax tissues, further activation of 'N' either by urine in the proximal urethra or by muscle stretching may not occur. The patient may experience symptoms as in the section 'CT plus peripheral neurological'.

NEUROLOGICAL PROBLEMS

The site of the lesion is critical here. Multiple sclerosis may interfere with any tract, afferent, efferent, or central inhibitory. Spinal cord transection or damage to efferent fibers may prevent relaxation of 'Cm' (Fig. 29.5) a prerequisite for micturition, or activation of the backward/downward forces which open the outflow tract, (Fig. 29.4).

CONCLUSION

It is possible to re-interpret most of the ICS classifications and descriptions as dysfunctions of opening and closure only, consistent with the Integral Theory's anatomical classification. The same anatomical classification used to diagnose and manage urinary dysfunction in the female may also apply to ano-rectal opening and closure dysfunctions, and to selected cases of pelvic pain of otherwise unknown origin.

REFERENCES

1. Popper KR. A survey of some fundamental problems. On the problem of a theory of scientific method. Theories. Falsifiability. The problem of the empirical basis. Degrees of testibility. Simplicity. The logic of scientific discovery. London: Unwin, Hyman, 1980;27–146.
2. Petros PE, Ulmsten U. An integral theory of female urinary incontinence. *Acta Scand O&G* 1990;(Suppl. 153)**69**:1–79.
3. Petros P, Ulmsten U. An integral theory and its method for the diagnosis and management of female urinary incontinence. *Scand J Urol Nephrol* 1993;(Suppl.)**27** (153) Part 1:1–93.
4. Petros PE. New ambulatory surgical methods based on an anatomical classification of urinary dysfunction improve stress, urge, and abnormal emptying, *Int J Urogynecol* 1997;**8**:270–78.
5. Enhorning G. Simultaneous recording of intravesical and intraurethral pressure. *Acta Chir Scand* 1961;(Suppl.)**27**:61–8.
6. De Lancey JOL. 'Structural support of the urethra as it relates to stress incontinence: the hammock hypothesis. *Am J Obst Gynecol* 1994;**170**(6):1713–23.
7. Faysal MH, Constaninou CE, Rother LF, Govan DE. The impact of bladder neck suspension on the resting and stress urethral pressure profile: a prospective study comparing controls with incontinent patients preoperatively and postoperatively. *J Urol Neurol Urodyn J Urol* 1981;**125**:55–60.
8. Petros PE, Ulmsten U. Urethral pressure increase on effort originates from within the urethra, and continence from musculovaginal closure: *Neurourol Urodyn* 1995;**14**:337–50.
9. Bates P, Bradley WE, Glen E, *et al.* First report on the standardisation of terminology of lower urinary tract function. *Br J Urol* 1976;**48**:39–42.
10. Abrams P, Blaivas J, Stanton S, Andersen J. Standardisation of terminology of lower urinary tract function. *Scand J Urol Nephrol* 1988;(Suppl.)**114**.
11. Bates CP. The unstable bladder. *Clin Obst Gynaecol* 1978;**5**(1):109–122.
12. Black N, Griffiths J, Pope C, Bowling A, Abel P. Impact of surgery for stress incontinence on morbidity: cohort study. *Br Med J* 1997;**315**:1493–8.
13. van Doorn van Waalwijk ESC, Remmers A, Jaknegt RA. Conventional and extramural ambulatory urodynamic testing of the lower urinary tract in the female. *J Urol* 1992;**147**(5):1319–25.
14. Mayer R, Wells T, Brink C, Diokno A, Cockett A, Handwashing in the cystometric evaluation of detrusor instability. *Neurourol Urodyn* 1991;**10**:563–9.
15. Swash M, Henry MM, Snooks SJ. Unifying concept of pelvic floor disorders and incontinence. *J Roy Soc Med* 1985;**78**:906–911.
16. Morrison JB. The physiological mechanism involved in bladder emptying. *Scand J Urol Nephrol* 1997; **29**(Suppl. 184):15–18.
17. Chantraine A, de Laval J, Depireux P. Adult female intra and peri-urethral electromyographic study. *Neurourol Urodyn* 1990;**9**:139–44.
18. Petros PE, Ulmsten U. Urge incontinence history is an accurate predictor of urge incontinence. *Acta Obstet Gynecol Scand* 1992;**71**:537–9.
19. Petros PE, Ulmsten U. Bladder instability in women: A premature activation of the micturition reflex. *Neurourol Urodyn* 1993;**12**:235–9.
20. Petros PE. Detrusor instability and low compliance may represent different levels of disturbance in peripheral feedback control of the micturition reflex. *Neurourol Urod* 1998 (in press).
21. Petros PE. Cure of urinary and fecal incontinence by pelvic ligament reconstruction suggests a connective tissue aetiology for both. *Int J Urogyne* 1999;**10**:356–360.
22. Petros PE. Severe chronic pelvic pain in women may be caused by ligamentous laxity in the posterior fornix of the vagina. *Aust NZ Obstet Gyanaecol* 1996;**36**(3):349–53.
23. Thyssen HH, Sander P, Lose G. Vaginal device (Continence Guard) in the treatment of urge incontinence in women. *Neurourol Urodyn* 1997;**16**(5):484–6.
24. Ulmsten U, Falconer C, Jomaa M, Lanner L, Nilsson CG, Olsson I. A multicentre study of tension-free vaginal tape for surgical treatment of stress incontinence. *Int Urogynecol J* 1988;**9**: 212–213.

25. Petros PE, Ulmsten U. An anatomical classification – a new paradigm for management of lower female urinary dysfunction. *Euro J Obstet Gynecol Reprod Biol* 1998; 80:87–94.

26. Courtney H. Anatomy of the pelvic diaphragm and anorectal musculature as related to sphincter preservation in ano-rectal surgery. *Am J Surg* 1950;**79**:155–173.

Chapter 30

Effects of pelvic floor surgery

Steven D Wexner, Rong H Zhao

INTRODUCTION

All surgical procedures performed near the pelvic floor, whether for the treatment of urologic, gynecologic or colorectal diseases may alter fecal continence. Normal continence depends upon multiple components of the pelvic floor and their appropriate interaction. These factors include the internal and external sphincters, puborectalis muscle, ano-rectal angle, rectal sensation, anorectal reflexes, rectal capacity, and compliance. This chapter will summarize the current literature about the functional outcome of pelvic surgery relative to the above-listed parameters and therefore ultimately their impact upon fecal continence.

EFFECTS OF PELVIC FLOOR SURGERY: FECAL INCONTINENCE

ANAL PROCEDURES

Anal fissures

Anal dilatation

Manual dilatation of the anus was first described by Recamier in 1829 and subsequently reintroduced by Goligher and Lord in 1969.[1,2] Although the rationale, efficacy and complication rates have been questioned by some authors, it became transiently accepted as a therapy for anal fissures, hemorrhoids, and anal stenosis. However, after more widespread adoption, it was noted that some patients developed anal incontinence after anal dilatation. MacDonald and coworkers reported a group of 100 consecutive patients who underwent manual dilatation of the anus.[3] During a 76–100 month follow-up period, three patients died from unrelated causes: 27 of the remaining 97 patients (21 females and six males) developed incontinence (major incontinence in seven, minor incontinence in 20). Similarly, Nielsen *et al.* found incontinence in 12.5% of their patients.[4]

It is widely believed that incontinence following anal dilatation is attributable to anal sphincter injury. Speakman and co-authors reported anal manometry and ultrasonography in 12 men who presented with incontinence following anal dilatation.[5] All patients had a low resting pressure and 11 had a disrupted internal anal sphincter, 10 of whom had extensively fragmented sphincters. This finding indicated that the injury to the internal sphincter plays a significant role in impairing continence following anal dilatation. Moreover, in the same study, an external sphincter defect was identified in three cases further impairing continence.

Other subsequent studies have confirmed that the ultrasonographic demonstration of the sphincter defects after anal dilatation are not always related to incontinence. Nielsen and colleagues found that ultrasonographic sphincter defects were identified in 13 of 20 patients who complained of incontinence; they were also noted in the other 11 patients none of whom complained of incontinence.[4] Although sphincter defects do not always result in incontinence after anal dilatation, they may become more significant with advancing age or after additional anal surgery or vaginal delivery. Other studies exist on hemorrhoidectomy with anal dilatation, which confirm an increased risk of incontinence. For all of these reasons, anal dilatation has never gained widespread popularity.

Fissure

Partial lateral internal anal sphincterotomy has been accepted by most surgeons as the surgical treatment of choice for anal fissure. It effectively overcomes the spasm of the internal anal sphincter that prevents the fissure from healing and treats mild anal stenosis when present. A laterally placed sphincterotomy incision heals much faster than does a posterior sphincterotomy, and the relief of pain from anal fissure is usually dramatic. Posterior sphincterotomy is associated with an increased frequency of 'keyhole' deformity and a reported incidence of fecal incontinence of 43%.[6]

Studies that have compared lateral internal sphincterotomy with sphincter stretching[7,8] or with fissurectomy and posterior midline sphincterotomy[9] revealed that the results with internal sphincterotomy were superior to those with either of the other two operations. For all the above mentioned operations there is a wide variation of results, with recurrence rates ranging from 10–30% after manual dilatation of the anus[8,10,11] and from 0–15% after lateral internal sphincterotomy. Similarly incontinence has been reported from 0–34% after manual dilatation of the anus[8,11,12] compared with 0–15% after lateral internal sphincterotomy. Early complications of lateral internal sphincterotomy include euchymosis (2.4%), hemorrhage (0.5%), perianal abscess (1%), fistula in ano (2.6%) and hemorrhoidal prolapse (0.3%).[7,9,13–18] In addition to the surgical trauma, Van Tets *et al.*[19] suggested that the use of anal retractors might cause postoperative incontinence.

In a recent published report by Hananel and Gordon[20] impaired control was found in 1.7% and fecal soiling in 0.69% of all patients who were operated upon (n = 291) and in 0.75% and 0.38% in patients after lateral internal sphincterotomy; in more than 50% of the patients the incontinence was temporary. These findings mirrored those reported by Abcarian[21] who noted that problems related to control of flatus were temporary. Walker *et al.*[22] reported a high rate of complications (3% major and 36% minor) and Khubchandani and Reed[23] reported alterations in control of flatus in 35.1%, soiling of underclothing in 22%, and accidental bowel movements in 53% of patients. One of the factors related to this wide variation may be the lack of proper definition of incontinence and different durations of follow-up in these series. Keighley *et al.*[24] reported that the incontinence usually occurs within 4 months after inadequate sphincterotomy. Similarly Hananel and Gordon[20] noted that all of the complications in their series occurred early during the postoperative period.

Lateral internal sphincterotomy permanently decreases the elevated resting pressure in most patients with anal fissure; fortunately, this reduction only correlates with healing of the fissure and not with the development of incontinence. Similarly, Melange *et al.*[25] noted that incontinence after lateral internal sphincterotomy does not correlate with either resting or maximum squeeze pressures, a finding also confirmed by Garcia-Aguilar.[26] The authors suggested that incontinence after lateral internal sphincterotomy is due to the shorter functional length of the anal canal and to the length of the sphincterotomy. However, the high pressure zone length was not significantly different between incontinent patients and continent controls. Ultrasonography has enabled assessment of the extent of sphincter division following sphincterotomy. Sultan *et al.*[27] revealed that in contrast to lateral internal sphincterotomy in males, division of the internal sphincter in females tends to be more extensive than intended. Accordingly, they hypothesized that this difference could be related to the short anal canal in females.

Fistula surgery

The aim of treatment of anal fistula is to eradicate it without disturbing anal continence;[28] this goal can be achieved by multiple methods. One of the most common techniques is laying open of an intersphincteric or trans-sphincteric fistula,[29,30] provided all the primary and secondary tracts are addressed. However, this procedure can result in incontinence both by damage to the external anal sphincter and by creation of a 'gutter' deformity. However, laying open high trans-sphincteric, suprasphincteric, or extra-sphincteric fistulas involves division of most or all of the sphincter which can also compromise continence. Other operations aimed to preserve continence include rerouting the fistula tract,[31] closing the internal opening,[32] endorectal advancement flaps,[33–36] fistulotomy with primary repair of the sphincter, and seton placement.

The incidence of incontinence after fistulotomy varies from 18–52%, with soiling in up to 35–45% of patients.[37–40] According to Van Tets' study of complicated fistulas,[41] the location and level of internal openings appeared to be independent factors, related to the occurrence of continence disorders after fistulotomy. Intuitively, the more cephalad the internal opening, the more muscle will be divided and thus the greater the anticipated decrease in pressures. Scar tissue and deformities in symmetry may also contribute to imperfections in continence after fistulotomy; posterior fistulotomy may add the problem of a keyhole deformity. Lunniss *et al.*[42] studied anal physiology before and 3 months after fistula surgery in 55 consecutive patients who underwent fistula surgery. Incontinence was related to both low postoperative resting pressures in the distal anal canal and to blunted epithelial electrosensitivity. Interestingly, there was no association with squeeze pressure; thus attempts to preserve the external while sacrificing the internal anal sphincter may be misguided. The relative importance of the internal sphincter has been confirmed in a study of 25 patients successfully treated with a loose seton. This method sacrificed the internal while preserving the external sphincter. Sixteen of the 25 patients reported some deterioration of continence.[43] Even when the external sphincter was not divided and the seton was removed, after several weeks continence disorders occurred in 62% of patients; thus incontinence was not caused exclusively by an impaired external sphincter but by other abnormalities such as endoanal fibrotic scar and impaired internal sphincter function. The fear of incontinence from sphincter division has led to staged fistulotomy, which has recurrence rates ranging between 0–3%.[44–46] Functional outcome is moderate however after procedures with two or more stages. Fecal incontinence occurs in 0–8%[44] and minor incontinence in approximately 60%[43,44,46] of patients. Although other treatments including core excision and advancement flaps may cause less functional disturbance, the healing is less certain. In a recent retrospective study by Miller and Finan[47] advancement flap with core fistula tract excision resulted in healing of 20 of 26 complex fistulas with 'minimal' disturbance of continence and few complications. In general, every attempt should be made to preserve the sphincters, especially anteriorly in women.

Hemorrhoidectomy

Hemorrhoidectomy is a recognized treatment of prolapsing hemorrhoids. Ho *et al.*[48] evaluated 24 patients who underwent anal physiology testing 6 weeks and 3 months postoperatively. The changes which occurred 3 weeks after hemorrhoidectomy included a significant drop in maximum squeeze pressure, an increase in the electrosensory threshold in the upper and middle thirds of anal canal, and a decrease in the frequency of ultra slow waves. The physiology studies were repeated after 3 months, at which time the wounds were completely healed without complications. The findings included a significant decrease in maximum resting and squeeze pressure, absence of ultra-slow waves, increase in rectal compliance, and normalized electrosensory threshold. Raised anal pressure and ultra-slow wave activity were found in patients with prolapsed hemorrhoids, possibly due to vascular hypertension in the anal cushions. Normal resting anal canal pressures and the disappearance of ultra-slow waves may be related to reduction in postoperative anal pressure, but the patients who had ultra slow waves before surgery did not have significantly higher anal pressures than did their ultra-slow wave-free counterparts. The external sphincters were hypertrophied, probably from hyperactivity in response to the irritating anal mass, as well as the constant fear of soiling from the discharge associated with hemorrhoids.

One study has suggested that rectal compliance impairment may be related to a higher rectal pressure required to expel stool past obstructing hemorrhoids.[49,50] The improved rectal compliance after surgery may be related to re-establishment of normal bowel habits with diminished straining. Another hypothesis is that patients with chronic hemorrhoids may have impaired anal sphincter pressures secondary to either increased perineal descent, pudendal neuropathy, or both.[51] However, this finding was not substantiated in the study by Ho *et al.*

The lack of concordance is not surprising. In an analysis of over 200 patients[52] there was no relationship between perineal descent and pudendal nerve terminal motor latencies. Specifically, even latencies greater than 2.4 ms or perineal descent greater than 7.0 cm failed to relate to each other. In addition, the anal electrosensory threshold has been noted as raised in the upper and middle thirds of the anal canal, probably related to insensitive rectal mucosa prolapsing into the anus.[50] After surgery there was impairment of the upper anal canal sensation at 6 weeks possibly due to the granulating surgical wound; after complete healing the sensation was again normalized. The same study noted that although maximum voluntary contraction pressures were preoperatively elevated, there was a significant postoperative decrease.

These deteriorations in function indicate that these changes are secondary to and not the cause of hemorrhoids: they also mitigate against a routine concomitant sphincterotomy.

Partial puborectalis muscle resection

Partial puborectalis muscle resection has been recommended for the treatment of puborectalis syndrome.[53,54] Although a good postoperative anorectal function has been noted in an initial series of 46 patients, few further results were presented. Although the ideal treatment of paradoxical puborectalis contraction should aim to restore normal muscle function rather than to remove or divert normal tissue, the very few patients who have a definite diagnosis of puborectalis hypertrophy but do not respond to conservative therapy, may be candidates for partial resection of the puborectalis muscle.[55] In 1964, Wasserman[56] proposed spasmodic hypertrophy of the puborectalis muscle and in his report of four cases, three patients underwent partial resection of the puborectalis muscle with excellent results. Partial puborectalis resection was also advocated by Wallace,[53] based on his series of 44 cases that included 33 adults and 11 children; the surgery was successful in 33 cases (75%). More recently (1989), Yu *et al.*[54] reported partial resection of the puborectalis muscle in 18 selected patients with puborectalis hypertrophy with successful results in 15 of these patients (83%). Barnes *et al.*[57] however, reported a series of nine patients who underwent complete division of the puborectalis muscle. Only two patients (24%) obtained relief while seven patients had symptomatic improvement, suggesting that the complete division of the puborectalis muscle is not as effective as partial resection. Moreover, the rate of fecal incontinence (five cases, 56%) is much higher after complete puborectalis division.

These data indicate several factors might affect the surgical outcome. Firstly, thorough preoperative evaluation of anal physiology and colonic transit study are very important to help exclude coexisting anatomic outlet obstruction or colonic inertia. They also allow the differential diagnosis between puborectalis hypertrophy and paradoxical puborectalis contraction. Only very few of the patients with paradoxical puborectalis contraction have muscle hypertrophy and even fewer may respond well to partial puborectalis excision without incontinence. This procedure should therefore be restricted to those few patients who have definite evidence of outlet obstruction caused by hypertrophy of puborectalis muscle, and who fail to respond to conservative therapy. However, it may be safer to restrict its use due to the potential for incontinence. If surgery is undertaken, the width of the puborectalis muscle to be resected should be approximately 1.5 cm so as to prevent the occurrence of postoperative adhesions which may in turn cause recurrence of the symptoms. Yu has suggested that postoperative balloon dilation of the rectum may prevent adhesion occurrence.[54]

ABDOMINAL PROCEDURES

Sphincter sparing operations

Anal sphincter-saving operations are obviously preferred to permanent stomas after resections for both rectal cancer and mucosal ulcerative colitis.

Ileoproctostomy

This operation removes all of the diseased large intestine but preserves the rectum, the anal canal, and the anal sphincter. Early data from the Mayo Clinic verified the safety of the procedure and revealed a satisfactory outcome.[58] Half of the patients reported less than eight stools per day, with good continence and without medication. However, the other half of patients had more diarrhea, poorer continence, and required treatment for proctitis. The disadvantage of this operation is that the diseased mucosa remains in place and can cause symptoms of proctitis. Accordingly, these patients require regular surveillance for proctitis, dysplasia, and cancer. For these reasons, about one fourth of patients require proctectomy by 8 years after surgery.[58–62] The postoperative incidence of cancer has been reported to range from 4–6%[59–61] to 35% at a 25 year follow-up.[63]

Ileal pouch-anal anastomosis

Restorative proctocolectomy or ileal pouch anal anastomosis aims to excise all of the diseased mucosa, create a neorectal reservoir, and preserve sphincteric function. In this manner, respectively, the risks of carcinoma, dysplasia, and proctitis are obviated, a storage chamber is fashioned, and continence can be preserved. The pouch is fashioned utilizing the terminal 30–50 cm of the ileum, as regardless of design the pouch should be easy to construct and of satisfactory capacity and distensibility to efficiently evacuate. Nasmyth[64] *et al.* noted that daily stool frequency was inversely related to capacity and compliance. Harms *et al.*[65] noted a statistically significant improvement regardless of whether S or W pouch configuration was utilized. Specifically, daily stool frequency at 2 and 12 months was 8.7 and 5.6, respectively, for the S pouch ($p < 0.05$) and 7.5 and 4.4, respectively, for the W pouch ($p < 0.01$). Similarly, compliance was noted to improve during this same time interval from 6.9 cc/mmHg to 8.9 cc/mmHg in the S pouch ($p < 0.05$) and from 7.8 cc/mmHg to 10.6 cc/mmHg in the W pouch group ($p < 0.05$). W and K pouches have the advantages of being more spherical and therefore of larger capacity.[66,67] Although the larger size may decrease the frequency of evacuation, the alternate reservoir designs are more difficult to construct.[66–68] Regardless of pouch design, evacuation has been noted to be less than in control (normal) rectums. Specifically, Heppell[69] noted that 72% of the J pouch emptied versus 67% of the S pouch volume. However, in normal controls, rectal emptying was noted to be 90%. Thus overall, regardless of pouch design, emptying is similar. In a prospective randomized design comparing two 15 cm J pouch limbs, two 20 cm J pouch limbs, four 7.5 cm W pouch limbs, and four 10 cm W pouch limbs, Miller *et al.* noted fairly similar results in all groups[70] However, in no circumstance is emptying as good as noted in a normal rectum.

The advantages of the H and the S pouches are that they have efferent limbs which theoretically allow the pouch to reach the distal anal canal with less tension on the ileal mesentery as may happen with J or W design.[68] However, an added disadvantage of these configurations is incomplete emptying due to a long efferent limb. The efferent limb should be no more than 1–2 cm long. Therefore, some of the theoretical advantages to tension-free anastomosis are obviated by a structural outlet obstruction.

Although mucosectomy theoretically decreases the risk of carcinoma it does not obviate it.[71,72] Moreover a significant problem with mucosectomy has been incontinence due to a variety of factors including injury to the internal anal sphincter and its enervation, anal dilatation, and ablation of the rectoanal inhibitory reflex. Wexner *et al.*[73] noted that after mucosectomy, 60% of patients reported the use of a protective pad at night. In a similar fashion, Kelly *et al.*[74] presented a 5 year mean follow-up of 1193 patients with nocturnal continence imperfections found in 55% of patients. These two series thus achieved almost identical results confirming their validity. More recently, Becker[75] reported a 13-year follow-up of his 418 patients. He noted that the decreased resting tone gradually recovered 'toward' normal but that seepage rates were, similar to studies by Wexner *et al.*[73] and Kelly *et al.*,[74] 50% in the postoperative period declining to 20% in one year.

In an effort to improve continence. Holdsworth *et al.* suggested[76] that non-mucosectomy would avoid decreased sensation of the abnormal canal, preserve the rectoanal reflex, and maintain better discrimination of the flatus. During the following year, Keighley *et al.*[77] reported the results of 12 patients who had undergone transanal mucosectomy as compared to 10 patients who underwent an intraabominal mucosectomy. The hypothesis of Holdsworth *et al.*[76] was confirmed in that the rates of incontinence and soiling decreased from 30%

and 50% to 20% and 10%, respectively, comparing the mucosectomy and non-mucosectomy groups. During that same year, Johnston *et al.*[78] analyzed the results of 24 patients after mucosectomy as compared with 12 patients without mucosectomy. While only 10 of 24 patients in the former group were completely continent, 11 of 12 patients in the latter group reported complete continence to liquids ($p < 0.001$). Not surprisingly, comparing the preoperative to postoperative resting pressures, the former group decreased from 85 cmH_2O preoperatively to the postoperative value of 40 cmH_2O which was significantly different than was the preoperative to postoperative change in the non-mucosectomy group of 116 cmH_2O to 7 cmH_2O ($p < 0.001$). Moreover, while no change in the resting or high pressure zone was noted in the mucosectomy group, the high pressure zone was significantly shorter in the postoperative than in the preoperative period in the non-mucosectomy group, suggesting a sacrifice of the cephalad portion of the internal anal sphincter during the stapling procedure. Shortly thereafter, Liljeqvist[79] compared 38 patients in whom mucosectomy was eliminated to 34 patients in whom it was performed. While 92% of the former group was completely continent, this finding was noted in only 65% of patients in the latter group, confirming the initial results. Harms *et al.*[65] attributed these significant differences to a change in resting pressure from 69 ± 5 mmHg preoperatively to 47 ± 3 mmHg postoperatively in their series ($p < 0.0005$).[65]

It may be worth the significant sacrifice in normal continence by mucosectomy if the risk of carcinoma was truly eliminated. However, as noted by Tsunoda *et al.*,[80] the risk of dysplasia is indeed minimal. Specifically, when retrospectively analysed, the mucosal strippings in 110 patients who had undergone restorative proctocolectomy contained no carcinoma. There was only a single case of low-grade dysplasia and no high-grade dysplasia in this group for a 0.9% dysplasia incidence. More recently, Thompson-Fawcett[81] assessed 20 anal canals which had been removed by proctectomy utilizing a computer mapping of median length. They noted that the median lowest point of columnar epithelium was actually 1.1 cm cephalad to the lower border of the internal anal sphincter. The median length of the anal transitional zone was variable at 0.62 mm in inflammatory conditions and 0.43 mm in non-inflammatory ones. The median lowest extent of the columnar epithelium was 0.18 cm cephalad to the dentate line whereas the median highest point of squamous epithelium was 1.85 cm above the dentate line. Moreover, of the three tissue types, transitional, squamous, and columnar, the relative prevalence of these tissue types decreased from 1.8 cm^2 in the first group to 0.2 cm^2 in the second group to 0.08 cm^2 in the columnar group. Thus the risk of dysplasia or cancer is indeed very small given the small surface area and variable length of this type of mucosa. Lastly, O'Connell *et al.*[82] analysed the muscular cuffs and ileoanal anastomoses after proctectomy for failed ileal pouch-anal anastomosis. Known viable mucosal islands were noted in 21% of patients in one or both of these locations.

One could aggressively try to extirpate all mucosa. However, Corry *et al.*[83] reported upon direct vision *ex vivo* mucosectomy of a 5 cm piece of rectum striving for macroscopic clearance of mucosa. In the five patients without mucosal ulcerative colitis, one had no mucosal cells left on the mucosal layer, one had some mucosal remnants, three actually had full-thickness remnants despite attempted mucosectomy under optimal conditions. Even in the five non-inflamed rectums in which the maneuver was attempted, in one, some mucosal remnants were noted. The authors concluded that 'even when rectal mucosectomy was carried out under direct vision, there is a risk of retaining diseased mucosa'. Overly aggressive mucosectomy, however, may further damage the sphincter muscle. Becker *et al.*[84] reported that in 66 of 79 patients who underwent mucosectomy in his expert hands, smooth muscle was identified after mucosectomy. This extirpation of portions of the internal anal sphincter was associated with decreased anal sphincter pressures, increased stool frequency, and increased nocturnal leakage for up to 12 months after surgery. Conversely, utilizing the double stapled technique, the change in pressures and therefore the poor function after rectal mucosectomies seems to be reduced. It would not be worth this price or the risk if recurrence of dysplasia or carcinoma was significant. However, Haray *et al.*[85] analysed 109 patients at a mean follow-up of 2.6 years after non-mucosectomy with ileal pouch-anal anastomosis. No dysplasia was noted in either the distal tissue 'donuts' or any of the biopsy specimens during the annual follow-up. Ziv *et al.*[86] noted very similar findings. Thus in the overall balance, avoidance of mucosectomy does not increase the risk of carcinoma, dysplasia, or proctitis to any meaningful degree but may indeed serve to optimize postoperative function. Only a large multicentered patient-blinded prospective randomized trial will answer the question. To date three small series have failed to do so.[87–89]

Coloanal anastomosis

A better understanding of tumor biology has led to universal adoption of Heald's technique of total mesorectal excision.[90–92] While an increasing number of surgeons have now reported local recurrence rates without adjuvant therapy of 10% or less, a functional price has been paid by removing the rectal reservoir.[93–98] Specifically, Otto *et al.*[99] evaluated incontinence after lower anastomosis. They noted that the rectoanal inhibitory reflex, which had been present prior to surgery in 94% of patients, was present in only 17% after low anterior resection and only increased to a 25% prevalence at last follow-up.

Similarly, anal sensation decreased from a minimum threshold volume of 43 ml preoperatively to 29 ml during the postoperative interval increasing to 43 ml at the time of last follow-up. Using a five point continence grading system, Otto *et al.* noted that all 17 patients had grade 1 incontinence before surgery whereas in the immediate postoperative period only three remained in that category with seven patients in group 2, five in groups 3 and 2 in group 4. At the time of last follow-up, an additional six patients had reverted to continence grade 1 category and none remained in grade 4, but five patients remained in grade 2 and two in grade 3. Furthermore, the mean stool frequency of 1.1 per day noted before surgery increased to 4.5 in the postoperative period and then decreased again to 1.8 per day at the time of last follow-up.

The aberrations in continence are clearly related to the level of the anastomosis. Matzel *et al.*[100] analysed these changes, stratifying groups of patients by anastomotic levels: 3 or less centimeters from the anal verge, 4–6 cm, 7–9 cm, or 10 or more centimeters above the anal verge. The groups included 3, 12, 20, and 13 patients each without any significant differences in the median range of ages or in the gender distribution. Similarly, the mean follow-up was not different among the groups. The most significant finding was obviously the amount of residual rectum which was 0.5 cm in the ≤3 cm group, 2.3 cm in the 4–6 cm group, 5.1 cm in the 7–9 cm group, and 8.9 cm in the ≥10 cm group. As the level of anastomosis decreased, daily stool frequency increased, the incidence of incontinence increased, the ability to discriminate flatus from stool decreased, the incidence of anal soreness decreased, and the incidence of incomplete evacuation increased. Furthermore, many physiologic derangements were also noted to be dependent upon the level of anastomosis, including the presence of rectoanal inhibitory reflex, sensory thresholds to urgency and maximum tolerable, and threshold volume, and compliance. All of these are detrimental effects if the anastomoses are exacerbated by both pre and postoperative adjuvant therapy.[101–103] In an effort to improve the function after low anastomosis, simultaneously Parc and Tiret[104] and Lazorthes[105] introduced the colonic J pouch. Both of these initial publications suggested that the addition of a J shaped neorectal reservoir fashioned of the left colon would significantly decrease stool frequency. Subsequently, an initial small prospective randomized series by Seow-Choen *et al.*[106] confirmed these earlier suspicions. A more recent large prospective randomized study[107] confirmed that the addition of a reservoir as compared to a straight coloanal anastomosis is associated with significant improvements lasting for at least one year including bowel frequency per 24 hours, the incidence of urgency, and incontinence. A third prospective randomized study[108] confirmed the same findings. The reasons for these improvements were subsequently noted by Hallbook *et al.*[109] Specifically the J pouch compliance was significantly better for at least one year after surgery as compared to the straight coloanal anastomosis. Joo *et al.*[110] and more recently Lazorthes[111] noted that these improvements persisted for at least 2 years after surgery.

As with the ileal J pouch, some debate centers around the optimal configuration and size. Because of technical limitations, only J shaped reservoirs have been attempted. However, in a prospective randomized trial, Hida *et al.*[112] compared 20 age- and tumor location-matched patients who underwent construction of 5 cm × 5 cm J pouches with an equal cohort of patients who underwent 10 cm × 10 cm J pouches. Significant functional improvements were noted in the 10 cm × 10 cm group including increases in maximal tolerable volume, threshold volume, and compliance. However, from a functional view, this pouch was actually too large as balloon expulsion, maximum neorectal pressure, and five minute saline evacuation were all better in the 5 cm × 5 cm group. Thus an excessively large pouch may inhibit its appropriate and complete emptying. Banerjee *et al.*[113] utilized a mathematical model to establish the optimal dimensions of a colonic J pouch and arrived upon a 6–7 cm length of each limb. Most recently, Dehni *et al.*[114] compared the colonic J pouch to a low anterior resection. The 47 patients in the J pouch group were compared to 34 patients in the low anastomosis group for a minimum 3-year follow-up (mean, 5 years). The groups were matched for gender, age, stage, and use of adjuvant therapy. Daily stool frequency was 1.6 per day in the former and 2.8 per day in the latter group ($p < 0.001$). Furthermore, stool clustering was noted in 30% of the J and 71% of the low anastomosis group ($p = 0.003$). Antidiarrheal medications and restricted diets were also needed more often in the low anastomosis than in the J pouch group. Other authors have confirmed some of the findings, including Wang *et al.*[115] However, if a high anterior resection can be undertaken the outcome will be superior to that offered by a colonic J pouch. Ramirez *et al.*[116] compared 10 patients who underwent colonic J pouch with anastomosis created at a mean of 3.5 (range 2–4.5) cm as compared with ten patients who underwent a high anterior resection with anastomosis situated at a mean 12.7 (range 9.5–60.0) cm. Bowel frequency per 24 hours was 2.2 in the J pouch and 1.9 in the anterior resection group.

Continence was normal in 80% of the J pouch and 100% of the high anterior resection group. There were no differences between the incidences of urgency or incomplete evacuation between the two groups. The authors found that as compared to high anterior resection, there were no significant differences in maximum resting pressure, maximum squeeze pressure, maximum tolerable volume, threshold volume, or mucosal electrosensitivity. Thus despite the functional superiority of the colonic J pouch as compared with a low anastomosis, the remaining rectum, if it can be retained with a high anastomosis, is even more superior. This finding was echoed by Hida *et al.*[117] when they compared anastomoses from 1 to 4 cm cephalad to the anal verge, 5 to 8 cm cephalad to the anal verge and 9 to 12 cm cephalad to the anal verge. Five centimeter by 5 cm colonic J pouches were constructed in the first two groups and were compared to patients who underwent straight anastomoses in these two groups. Patients with anastomoses situated 9 to 12 cm at the anal verge did not undergo colonic J pouch but instead underwent a straight coloanal anastomosis. The J pouch offered significantly better results for the number of bowel movements per day and at night, the incidences of urgency, soiling, incontinence, use of a pad, and superior patient satisfaction as compared to the straight coloanal anastomosis.

In addition to problems in continence created by extirpation of the rectum, even with construction of the neorectal reservoir, additional imperfections in continence may result from a sphincter injury. Horgan *et al.*[118] assessed anal sphincter resting pressures at various stages during an anterior resection. They noted that the introduction of the circular stapling device, even when properly used, was associated with a significant level of transient decreased resting pressures. More recently Farouk *et al.*[119]utilized anal ultrasound 3, 6, 9, 12, and 24 months after anterior resection. Seven of 39 (18%) patients had persistent clinically significant anterior anal sphincter defects, including six of eight patients in whom a 31 mm stapler had been utilized, one of 27 in whom the 29 mm stapler was used, and none of the four patients in whom the 28 mm stapler had been chosen to effect the anastomosis. These ultrasonographic defects correlated well with significant changes noted in the resting pressure lasting up to 6–9 months after surgery.

EFFECT OF ADJUVANT RADIOTHERAPY ON THE ANORECTAL FUNCTION OF PATIENTS WITH RECTAL CARCINOMA

Birnbaum and co-workers[120] studied both early and chronic effects of preoperative pelvic radiation on anorectal function. Firstly, they evaluated the anorectal function of 20 patients with rectal carcinoma by anal manometry at 4 weeks after the patients received 4500 cGy external beam radiation. The mean minimal sensory threshold was significantly higher after radiation than before. They subsequently reported the manometric and clinical results 14 to 42 months after radiotherapy in 10 of the same 20 cases. The increased minimum sensory threshold noted at 4 weeks after radiation had decreased to initial baseline at later follow-up. There were no significant differences in mean maximum squeeze or resting pressures, sphincter profile, or rectoanal inhibitory reflex as compared to before radiation. Clinically, all patients reported normal anal function except one who was incontinent before treatment who remained incontinent. After treatment the authors concluded that preoperative radiotherapy had only minimal effects on anal sphincter function either immediately or after 1–4 years.

In contrast to sphincter function, the rectal reservoir function is clearly impaired by postoperative radiotherapy. Lewis and colleagues[121] reported the results of nine patients who received a curative anterior resection for rectal carcinoma followed by postoperative radiotherapy as compared with 50 patients treated by surgery alone. The study revealed that maximum resting and squeezing pressures were similar in the two groups, but the high pressure zone length and pressure profile were markedly abnormal. The difference between the pressures of rectum and anal canal was decreased and the length of the high pressure zone was also shorter. The capacity, compliance of the neorectum, and the amount of distention of the neorectum required to produce maximum inhibition of the anal sphincter during the rectoanal inhibitory reflex were all significantly reduced. Clinically, major fecal leakage necessitating the daily use of a pad occurred more frequently in patients who received surgery and radiotherapy than in those treated by surgery alone (33% v. 10%). Other studies confirmed decreased rectal capacity and compliance in the patients after pelvic irradiation for prostate carcinoma,[122,123] uterine cervical cancer,[124] and anal carcinoma.[125] Some patients had disturbed gas-stool discrimination, urgency, a sense of residual stool, and soiling after radiotherapy.

Although the use of adjuvant radiotherapy may decrease local recurrence for increased survival it is not administered without a potential price in terms of adverse functional sequelae. Lundby *et al.*[126] reported a prospective randomization of 93 patients, 44 of whom had no preoperative radiotherapy and 49 of whom had preoperative radiotherapy. There were no significant differences between the cohorts relative to mean age, gender distribution, or tumor stage or location. However, there were statistically significant differences favoring the non-radiotherapy group in terms of stool frequency (more than five bowel movements per day, 2 vs 18, respectively, $p < 0.01$), the incidence of loose or liquid stool (2% vs 25%, $p < 0.02$), fecal urgency (12% vs 41%, $p < 0.003$), fecal incontinence (5% vs 49%, $p < 0.001$), the use of pads (0 vs 26%, $p < 0.001$), or the ability to differentiate between stool and gas (95% vs 77%, $p < 0.014$). In this manner, evaluating postoperative radiotherapy, Arnaud *et al.*[127] analysed 172 patients, 84 of whom were randomized to receive 46 Gy (5 days per week over 30–80 days) versus 88 patients in whom no radiotherapy was utilized. There were no differences between the two groups relative to gender, Karnofsky index, tumor stage or extension, tumor differentiation, or the presence of venous invasion. At a median follow up of 85 months, the radiotherapy group had a significantly higher incidence of functional problems relative to the rectum. Kollmorgen *et al.*[103] compared 41 patients who had postoperative chemoradiotherapy versus 49 patients who did not. The groups were well matched for the length of follow-up as well as anastomotic height and gender. There were once again significant differences favoring the non-radiotherapy group relative to the median number of bowel movements per day (7 vs 2) the incidence of 'clustered' bowel movements (42% vs 3%), the incidence of nocturnal bowel movements (46% vs 14%), the incidence of liquid stools on a 'sometimes' or 'always' basis (29% vs 5%), the incidence of regular use of antidiarrheal agents (58% vs 5%), the incidence of perianal skin irritation (41% vs 12%), or the patient noting significantly poorer function than had been preoperatively present (93% vs 61%). Furthermore, there were differences in favor of the non-radiotherapy group relative to the incidence of 'frequent' incontinence (17% vs 0%), the incidence of 'occasional' incontinence (39% vs 7%), the incidence of wearing a pad (41% vs 10%), or the inability to defer bowel evacuation for more than 15 minutes (78% vs 19%).

The specific damages of radiotherapy are undoubtedly related to impairment in rectal capacity and compliance. Iwamoto *et al.*[124] analysed patients who had undergone between 4.2 and 5.0 Gy external beam radiotherapy for cervical carcinoma. They noted significant decreases even in the normal rectum and maximum tolerable volume, rectal compliance, and maximum tolerable pressure. These physiologic changes were noted even in asymptomatic patients and were progressive over time. Therefore, it is not surprising that when the rectum is excised and replaced by a neorectum, radiotherapeutic changes are even more profound. These changes can have a significant detrimental effect on quality of life as noted by Dahlberg *et al.*[128] These authors analysed 171 recurrence-free patients, 84 of whom had been randomized to preoperative low-dose radiotherapy (25 Gy) as compared with 87 patients who had surgery alone. The patients were analysed 80 months after prospective randomization for radiotherapy and after anterior resection. Between the two groups, patients had been well matched for gender, age, stage, and anastomotic height. The patients who had undergone radiotherapy a mean of 80 months earlier, as compared to their non-radiotherapy colleagues, were more likely to have incontinence for loose stool, require the use of a pad, experience perianal excoriation, note fragmented evacuation, and complain of urgency ($p < 0.003$ for all). In fact 30% of patients after radiotherapy noted impairment of social life, a difficulty stated by only 10% of patients who did not receive radiotherapy ($p < 0.003$).

Based on the above observations, preoperative radiotherapy may provide patients with better anorectal functional results than does postoperative radiotherapy. Injury of the myenteric plexus and smooth muscle manifested as vasodilatation, epithelial swelling and meganucleosis, lack of mitotic activity, and patchy fibroblastic proliferation in the lamina propria, can all be found in the rectum after irradiation.[129–131] These reduced the sensory functions, anal capacity and compliance. In the anal canal, radiotherapy may damage the epithelium and anal cushions.[125] It may cause the mild changes of sphincter pressure without the clinically significant disturbance of anal canal function. Therefore one must be very cognizant of the functional hazards of pelvic radiation.

REFERENCES

1. Goligher JC, Graham NG, De Dombal FT, Giles GR, Clark CG. The value of stretching of anal sphincters in the relief of pain after haemorrhoidectomy. *Br J Surg* 1969;**56**(5):390.
2. Lord PH. A day-case procedure for the cure of third-degree haemorrhoids. *Br J Surg* 1969;**56**(10):747–9.
3. MacDonald A, Smith A, McNeill AD, Finlay IG. Manual dilatation of the anus. *Br J Surg* 1992; **79**(12):1381–2.
4. Nielsen MB, Rasmussen OO, Pedersen JF, Christiansen J. Risk of sphincter damage and anal incontinence after anal dilatation for fissure-in-ano. An endosonographic study. *Dis Colon Rectum* 1993;**36**(7):677–80.
5. Speakman CT, Burnett SJ, Kamm MA, Bartram CI. Sphincter injury after anal dilatation demonstrated by anal endosonography. *Br J Surg* 1991;**78**(12):1429–30.
6. Magee HR, Thompson HR. Internal anal sphincterotomy as an out-patient operation. *Gut* 1966; **7**(2):190–3.
7. Hoffmann DC, Goligher JC. Lateral subcutaneous internal sphincterotomy in treatment of anal fissure. *Br Med J* 1970;3(724):673–5.
8. Jensen SL, Lund F, Nielsen OV, Tange G. Lateral subcutaneous sphincterotomy versus anal dilatation in the treatment of fissure in ano in outpatients: a prospective randomised study. *BMJ (Clin Res Ed)* 1984;**289**(6444): 528–30.
9. Abcarian H. Surgical correction of chronic anal fissure: results of lateral internal sphincterotomy vs. fissurectomy–midline sphincterotomy. *Dis Colon Rectum* 1980;23(1):31–6.
10. Collopy B, Ryan P. Comparison of lateral subcutaneous sphincterotomy with anal dilatation in the treatment of fissure in ano. *Med J Aust* 1979;2(9):461–2, 487.
11. Marby M, Alexander-Williams J, Buchmann P, *et al.* A randomized controlled trial to compare anal dilatation

with lateral subcutaneous sphincterotomy for anal fissure. *Dis Colon Rectum* 1979;22(5):308–11.

12. Millar DM. Subcutaneous lateral internal anal sphincterotomy for anal fissure. *Br J Surg* 1971; **58**(10):737–9.
13. Gingold BS. Simple in-office sphincterotomy with partial fissurectomy for chronic anal fissure. *Surg Gynecol Obstet* 1987;**165**(1):46–8.
14. Gordon PH, Vasilevsky CA. Symposium on outpatient anorectal procedures. Lateral internal sphincterotomy: rationale, technique and anesthesia. *Can J Surg* 1985;**28**(3):228–30.
15. Hsu TC, MacKeigan JM. Surgical treatment of chronic anal fissure. A retrospective study of 1753 cases. *Dis Colon Rectum* 1984;**27**(7):475–8.
16. Lewis TH, Corman ML, Prager ED, Robertson WG. Long-term results of open and closed sphincterotomy for anal fissure. *Dis Colon Rectum* 1988;**31**(5):368–71.
17. Notaras MJ. The treatment of anal fissure by lateral subcutaneous internal sphincterotomy – a technique and results. *Br J Surg* 1971;**58**(2):96–100.
18. Ravikumar TS, Sridhar S, Rao RN. Subcutaneous lateral internal sphincterotomy for chronic fissure-in-ano. *Dis Colon Rectum* 1982;**25**(8):798–801.
19. van Tets WF, Kuijpers JH, Tran K, Mollen R, van Goor H. Influence of Parks' anal retractor on anal sphincter pressures. *Dis Colon Rectum* 1997;**40**(9):1042–5.
20. Hananel N, Gordon PH. Lateral internal sphincterotomy for fissure-in-ano – revisited. *Dis Colon Rectum* 1997; **40**(5):597–602.
21. Abcarian H. Surgical correction of chronic anal fissure: results of lateral internal sphincterotomy vs. fissurectomy – midline sphincterotomy. *Dis Colon Rectum* 1980;23(1):31–6.
22. Walker WA, Rothenberger DA, Goldberg SM. Morbidity of internal sphincterotomy for anal fissure and stenosis. *Dis Colon Rectum* 1985;**28**(11):832–5.
23. Khubchandani IT, Reed JF. Sequelae of internal sphincterotomy for chronic fissure in ano. *Br J Surg* 1989;**76**(5):431–4.
24. Keighley MR, Greca F, Nevah E, Hares M, Alexander-Williams J. Treatment of anal fissure by lateral subcutaneous sphincterotomy should be under general anaesthesia. *Br J Surg* 1981; **68**(6):400–1.
25. Melange M, Colin JF, Van Wymersch T, Vanheuverzwyn R. Anal fissure: correlation between symptoms and manometry before and after surgery. *Int J Colorectal Dis* 1992;**7**(2):108–11.
26. Garcia-Aguilar J, Belmonte Montes C, Perez JJ, Jensen L, Madoff RD, Wong WD. Incontinence after lateral internal sphincterotomy: anatomic and functional evaluation. *Dis Colon Rectum* 1998; **41**(4):423–7.
27. Sultan AH, Kamm MA, Nicholls RJ, Bartram CI. Prospective study of the extent of internal anal sphincter division during lateral sphincterotomy. *Dis Colon Rectum* 1994;**37**(10):1031–3.
28. Williams JG, Rothenberger DA, Nemer FD, Goldberg SM. Fistula-in-ano in Crohn's disease. Results of aggressive surgical treatment. *Dis Colon Rectum* 1991;**34**(5):378–84.
29. Shouler PJ, Grimley RP, Keighley MR, Alexander-Williams J. Fistula-in-ano is usually simple to manage surgically. *Int J Colorectal Dis* 1986;**1**(2):113–5.
30. Vasilevsky CA, Gordon PH. The incidence of recurrent abscesses or fistula-in-ano following anorectal suppuration. *Dis Colon Rectum* 1984;**27**(2):126–30.
31. Mann CV, Clifton MA. Re-routing of the track for the treatment of high anal and anorectal fistulae. *Br J Surg* 1985;**72**(2):134–7.
32. Reznick RK, Bailey HR. Closure of the internal opening for treatment of complex fistula-in-ano. *Dis Colon Rectum* 1988;**31**(2):116–8.
33. Aguilar PS, Plasencia G, Hardy TG Jr, Hartmann RF, Stewart WR. Mucosal advancement in the treatment of anal fistula. *Dis Colon Rectum* 1985;**28**(7):496–8.
34. Wedell J, Meier zu Eissen P, Banzhaf G, Kleine L. Sliding flap advancement for the treatment of high level fistulae. *Br J Surg* 1987;**74**(5):390–1.
35. Jones IT, Fazio VW, Jagelman DG. The use of transanal rectal advancement flaps in the management of fistulas involving the anorectum. *Dis Colon Rectum* 1987;**30**(12):919–23.
36. Shemesh EI, Kodner IJ, Fry RD, Neufeld DM. Endorectal sliding flap repair of complicated anterior anoperineal fistulas. *Dis Colon Rectum* 1988;**31**(1):22–4.
37. Seow-Choen F, Nicholls RJ. Anal fistula. *Br J Surg* 1992;**79**(3):197–205.
38. Marks CG, Ritchie JK. Anal fistulas at St Mark's Hospital. *Br J Surg* 1977;**64**(2):84–91.
39. Lilius HG. Fistula-in-ano, an investigation of human foetal anal ducts and intramuscular glands and a clinical study of 150 patients. *Acta Chir Scand* (Suppl.) 1968;**383**:7–88.
40. Parks AG, Gordon PH, Hardcastle JD. A classification of fistula-in-ano. *Br J Surg* 1976; **63**(1):1–12.
41. Van Tets WF, Kuijpers HC. Continence disorders after anal fistulotomy. *Dis Colon Rectum* 1994; **37**(12):1194–7.
42. Lunniss PJ, Kamm MA, Phillips RK. Factors affecting continence after surgery for anal fistula. *Br J Surg* 1994;**81**(9):1382–5.
43. Kennedy HL, Zegarra JP. Fistulotomy without external sphincter division for high anal fistulae. *Br J Surg* 1990;**77**(8):898–901.
44. Pearl RK, Andrews JR, Orsay CP, *et al.* Role of the seton in the management of anorectal fistulas. *Dis Colon Rectum* 1993 J;**36**(6):573–7; discussion 577–9.
45. Ramanujam PS, Prasad ML, Abcarian H. The role of seton in fistulotomy of the anus. *Surg Gynecol Obstet* 1983;**157**(5):419–22.
46. Williams JG, MacLeod CA, Rothenberger DA, Goldberg SM. Seton treatment of high anal fistulae. *Br J Surg* 1991;**78**(10):1159–61.
47. Miller GV, Finan PJ. Flap advancement and core fistulectomy for complex rectal fistula. *Br J Surg* 1998;**85**(1):108–10.
48. Ho YH, Seow-Choen F, Goh HS. Haemorrhoidectomy and disordered rectal and anal physiology in patients with prolapsed haemorrhoids. *Br J Surg* 1995;**82**(5):596–8.
49. Hancock BD. Measurement of anal pressure and motility. *Gut* 1976;**17**(8):645–51.
50. Roe AM, Bartolo DC, Vellacott KD, Locke-Edmunds J, Mortensen NJ. Submucosal versus ligation excision haemorrhoidectomy: a comparison of anal sensation, anal sphincter manometry and postoperative pain and function. *Br J Surg* 1987;**74**(10):948–51.

51. Bruck CE, Lubowski DZ, King DW. Do patients with haemorrhoids have pelvic floor denervation? *Int J Colorectal Dis* 1988;3(4):210–4.
52. Jorge JM, Wexner SD, Ehrenpreis ED, Nogueras JJ, Jagelman DG. Does perineal descent correlate with pudendal neuropathy? *Dis Colon Rectum* 1993;**36**(5):475–83.
53. Wallace WC, Madden WM. Experience with partial resection of the puborectalis muscle. *Dis Colon Rectum* 1969;**12**(3):196–200.
54. Yu DH. Puborectalis syndrome: a cause of obstinate constipation. *Chung Hua Wai Ko Tsa Chih* 1989;**27**(5):267–8, 316.
55. Yu D-H. Surgical treatment for puborectalis hypertrophy. In: Wexner SD, Bartolo DCC and (eds.) *Constipation – aetiology, evaluation and management*. London, Butterworth Heinemann 1995
56. Wasserman JF. Puborectalis syndrome, rectal stenosis due to anorectal spasm. *Dis Colon Rectum* 1964;**7**:87–98.
57. Barnes PRH, Hawley PR, Presto DM, *et al.* Experience of posterior division of the puborectalis muscle in the management of chronic constipation. *Br J Surg* 1985;**72**:475–7.
58. Farnell MB, Van Heerden JA, Beart RW Jr, Weiland LH. Rectal preservation in nonspecific inflammatory disease of the colon. *Ann Surg* 1980;**192**(2):249–53.
59. Baker WN, Glass RE, Ritchie JK, Aylett SO. Cancer of the rectum following colectomy and ileorectal anastomosis for ulcerative colitis. *Br J Surg* 1978;**65**(12):862–8.
60. Johnson WR, McDermott FT, Hughes ES, Pihl EA, Milne BJ, Price AB. Carcinoma of the colon and rectum in inflammatory disease of the intestine. *Surg Gynecol Obstet* 1983;**156**(2):193–7.
61. Hawley PR. Ileorectal anastomosis. *Br J Surg* 1985;**72**(Suppl):S75–6.
62. Leijonmarck CE, Lofberg R, Ost A, Hellers G. Long-term results of ileorectal anastomosis in ulcerative colitis in Stockholm County. *Dis Colon Rectum* 1990;**33**(3):195–200.
63. Grundfest SF, Fazio V, Weiss RA, Jagelman D, Lavery I, Weakley FL, Turnbull RB Jr. The risk of cancer following colectomy and ileorectal anastomosis for extensive mucosal ulcerative colitis. *Ann Surg* 1981;**193**(1):9–14.
64. Nasmyth DG, Johnston D, Godwin PG, Dixon MF, Smith A, Williams NS. Factors influencing bowel function after ileal pouch-anal anastomosis. *Br J Surg* 1986;**73**(6):469–73.
65. Harms BA, Pahl AC, Starling JR. Comparison of clinical and compliance characteristics between S and W ileal reservoirs. *Am J Surg* 1990 Jan;**159**(1):34–9; discussion 39–40.
66. Nicholls RJ, Lubowski DZ. Restorative proctocolectomy: the four loop (W) reservoir. *Br J Surg* 1987;**74**(7):564–6.
67. Oresland T, Fasth S, Nordgren S, Hallgren T, Hulten L. A prospective randomized comparison of two different pelvic pouch designs. *Scand J Gastroenterol* 1990;**25**(10):986–96.
68. Fonkalsrud EW. Total colectomy and endorectal ileal pull-through with internal ileal reservoir for ulcerative colitis. *Surg Gynecol Obstet* 1980;**150**(1):1–8.
69. Heppell J, Belliveau P, Taillefer R, Dube S, Derbekyan V. Quantitative assessment of pelvic ileal reservoir emptying with a semisolid radionuclide enema. A correlation with clinical outcome. *Dis Colon Rectum* 1987;**30(2)**:81–5.
70. Miller AS, Williamson MER, Lewis WG, Sagar PM, Holdsworth PJ, Johnston D. Prospective controlled trial of duplicated (J) versus quadruplicated (W) ileal reservoirs for ulcerative colitis. *Br J Surg* (Suppl.) 1996;**83**:1.
71. Puthu D, Rajan N, Rao R, Rao L, Venugopal P. Carcinoma of the rectal pouch following restorative proctocolectomy. Report of a case. *Dis Colon Rectum* 1992;**35**(3):257–60.
72. Stern H, Walfisch S, Mullen B, McLeod R, Cohen Z. Cancer in an ileoanal reservoir: a new late complication? *Gut* 1990;**31**(4):473–5.
73. Wexner SD, Jensen L, Rothenberger DA, Wong WD, Goldberg SM. Long-term functional analysis of the ileoanal reservoir. *Dis Colon Rectum* 1989;**32**(4):275–81.
74. Kelly KA. Anal sphincter-saving operations for chronic ulcerative colitis. *Am J Surg* 1992; **163**(1):5–11.
75. Becker JM. What is the better surgical technique in ileal pouch-anal anastomosis? Mucosectomy. *Inflamm Bowel Dis* 1996;**2**:151–4.
76. Holdsworth PJ, Sagar PM, Lewis WG, Williamson M, Johnston D. Internal anal sphincter activity after restorative proctocolectomy for ulcerative colitis: a study using continuous ambulatory manometry. *Dis Colon Rectum* 1994;**37**(1):32–6.
77. Keighley MR. Abdominal mucosectomy reduces the incidence of soiling and sphincter damage after restorative proctocolectomy and J-pouch. *Dis Colon Rectum* 1987;**30**(5):386–90.
78. Johnston D, Holdsworth PJ, Nasmyth DG, *et al.* Preservation of the entire anal canal in conservative proctocolectomy for ulcerative colitis: a pilot study comparing end-to-end ileo-anal anastomosis without mucosal resection with mucosal proctectomy and endo-anal anastomosis. *Br J Surg* 1987;**74**(10):940–4.
79. Liljeqvist L, Lindquist K, Ljungdahl I. Alterations in ileoanal pouch technique, 1980 to 1987. Complications and functional outcome. *Dis Colon Rectum* 1988;**31(12)**:929–38.
80. Tsunoda A, Talbot IC, Nicholls RJ. Incidence of dysplasia in the anorectal mucosa in patients having restorative proctocolectomy. *Br J Surg* 1990;**77(5)**:506–8.
81. Thompson-Fawcett MW, Warren BF, Mortensen NJ. A new look at the anal transitional zone with reference to restorative protocolectomy and the columnar cuff. *Br J Surg* 1998;**85**(11):1517–21.
82. O'Connell PR, Pemberton JH, Weiland LH, *et al.* Does rectal mucosa regenerate after ileoanal anastomosis? *Dis Colon Rectum* 1987;**30**(1):1–5.
83. Corry DG, Feakins R, Williams NS. The effectiveness of experimental mucosectomy. (abstract) *Br J Surg* 1997;**84(Suppl.)**:57–58.
84. Becker JM, LaMorte W, St. Marie G, Ferzoco S. Extent of smooth muscle resection during mucosectomy and ileal pouch-anal anastomosis affects anorectal physiology and functional outcome. *Dis Colon Rectum* 1997;**40**(6):653–60.
85. Haray PN, Amarnath B, Weiss EG, Nogueras JJ, Wexner SD. Low malignant potential of the double-stapled ileal pouch-anal anastomosis. *Br J Surg* 1996;**83**(10):1406.
86. Ziv Y, Fazio VW, Sirimarco MT, Lavery IC, Goldblum JR, Petras RE. Incidence, risk factors, and treatment of dysplasia in the anal transitional zone after ileal pouch-anal anastomosis. *Dis Colon Rectum* 1994;**37**(12):1281–5.
87. Seow-Choen F, Tsunoda A, Nicholls RJ. Prospective randomized trial comparing anal function after hand sewn

ileoanal anastomosis with mucosectomy versus stapled ileoanal anastomosis without mucosectomy in restorative proctocolectomy. *Br J Surg* 1991;**78**(4):430–4.
88. Reilly WT, Pemberton JH, Wolff BG, *et al.* Randomized prospective trial comparing ileal pouch-anal anastomosis performed by excising the anal mucosa to ileal pouch-anal anastomosis performed by preserving the anal mucosa. *Ann Surg* 1997;**225**(6):666–76.
89. Luukkonen P, Jarvinen H. Stapled vs hand-sutured ileoanal anastomosis in restorative proctocolectomy. A prospective, randomized study. *Arch Surg* 1993;**128**(4):437–40.
90. Carlsen E, Schlichting E, Guldvog I, Johnson E, Heald RJ. Effect of the introduction of total mesorectal excision for the treatment of rectal cancer. *Br J Surg* 1998;**85**(4): 526–9.
91. Heald RJ, Moran BJ, Ryall RD, Sexton R, MacFarlane JK. Rectal cancer: the Basingstoke experience of total mesorectal excision, 1978–1997. *Arch Surg* 1998;**133**(8):894–9.
92. MacFarlane JK, Ryall RD, Heald RJ. Mesorectal excision for rectal cancer. *Lancet* 1993; **341**(8843):457–60.
93. Aitken RJ. Mesorectal excision for rectal cancer. *Br J Surg* 1996;**83**(2):214–6.
94. Arbman G, Nilsson E, Hallbook O, Sjodahl R. Local recurrence following total mesorectal excision for rectal cancer. *Br J Surg* 1996;**83**(3):375–9.
95. Bernstein MA, Amarnath B, Weiss EG, Nogueras JJ, Wexner SD. Total mesorectal excision without adjuvant therapy for local control of rectal cancer: a North American experience. *Technique Coloproctol* 1998;**2**:11–15.
96. Carter P. Evaluation of a policy of total mesorectal excision for rectal and rectosigmoid cancers. *Br J Surg* 1997;**84**(12):1749–50.
97. Enker WE, Thaler HT, Cranor ML, Polyak T. Total mesorectal excision in the operative treatment of carcinoma of the rectum. *J Am Coll Surg* 1995;**181**(4):335–46.
98. Karanjia ND, Schache DJ, North WR, Heald RJ. 'Close shave' in anterior resection. *Br J Surg* 1990;**77**(5):510–2.
99. Otto IC, Ito K, Ye C, *et al.* Causes of rectal incontinence after sphincter-preserving operations for rectal cancer. *Dis Colon Rectum* 1996;**39**(12):1423–7.
100. Matzel KE, Stadelmaier U, Muehldorfer S, Hohenberger W. Continence after colorectal reconstruction following resection: impact of level of anastomosis. *Int J Colorectal Dis* 1997;**12**(2):82–7.
101. Dahlberg M, Glimelius B, Graf W, Pahlman L. Preoperative irradiation affects functional results after surgery for rectal cancer: results from a randomized study. *Dis Colon Rectum* 1998;**41**(5):543–9; discussion 549–51.
102. Graf W, Ekstrom K, Glimelius B, Pahlman L. A pilot study of factors influencing bowel function after colorectal anastomosis. *Dis Colon Rectum* 1996;**39**(7):744–9.
103. Kollmorgen CF, Meagher AP, Wolff BG, Pemberton JH, Martenson JA, Illstrup DM. The long-term effect of adjuvant postoperative chemoradiotherapy for rectal carcinoma on bowel function. *Ann Surg* 1994;**220**(5):676–82.
104. Parc R, Tiret E, Frileux P, Moszkowski E, Loygue J. Resection and colo-anal anastomosis with colonic reservoir for rectal carcinoma. *Br J Surg* 1986;**73**(2):139–41.
105. Lazorthes F, Fages P, Chiotasso P, Lemozy J, Bloom E. Resection of the rectum with construction of a colonic reservoir and colo-anal anastomosis for carcinoma of the rectum. *Br J Surg* 1986; **73**(2):136–8.
106. Seow-Choen F, Goh HS. Prospective randomized trial comparing J colonic pouch-anal anastomosis and straight coloanal reconstruction. *Br J Surg* 1995;**82**(5):608–10.
107. Hallbook O, Pahlman L, Krog M, Wexner SD, Sjodahl R. Randomized comparison of straight and colonic J pouch anastomosis after low anterior resection. *Ann Surg* 1996;**224**(1):58–65.
108. Ho YH, Tan M, Seow-Choen F. Prospective randomized controlled study of clinical function and anorectal physiology after low anterior resection: comparison of straight and colonic J pouch anastomoses. *Br J Surg* 1996;**83**(7):978–80.
109. Hallbook O, Nystrom PO, Sjodahl R. Physiologic characteristics of straight and colonic J-pouch anastomoses after rectal excision for cancer. *Dis Colon Rectum* 1997;**40**(3):332–8.
110. Joo JS, Latulippe JF, Alabaz O, Weiss EG, Nogueras JJ, Wexner SD. Long-term functional evaluation of straight coloanal anastomosis and colonic J-pouch: is the functional superiority of colonic J-pouch sustained? *Dis Colon Rectum* 1998;**41**(6):740–6.
111. Lazorthes F, Gamagami R, Chiotasso P, Istvan G, Muhammad S. Prospective, randomized study comparing clinical results between small and large colonic J-pouch following coloanal anastomosis. *Dis Colon Rectum* 1997;**40**(2):1409–13.
112. Hida J, Yasutomi M, Fujimoto K, *et al.* Functional outcome after low anterior resection with low anastomosis for rectal cancer using the colonic J-pouch. Prospective randomized study for determination of optimum pouch size. *Dis Colon Rectum* 1996;**39**(9):986–91.
113. Banerjee AK, Parc R. Prediction of optimum dimensions of colonic pouch reservoir. *Dis Colon Rectum* 1996; **39**(11):1293–5.
114. Dehni N, Tiret E, Singland JD, *et al.* Long-term functional outcome after low anterior resection: comparison of low colorectal anastomosis and colonic J-pouch-anal anastomosis. *Dis Colon Rectum* 1998;**41**(7):817–22; discussion 822–3.
115. Wang JY, You YT, Chen HH, Chiang JM, Yeh CY, Tang R. Stapled colonic J-pouch-anal anastomosis without a diverting colostomy for rectal carcinoma. *Dis Colon Rectum* 1997; **40**(1):30–4.
116. Ramirez JM, Mortensen NJ, Takeuchi N, Smilgin Humphreys MM. Colonic J-pouch rectal reconstruction – is it really a neorectum? *Dis Colon Rectum* 1996;**39**(11):1286–8.
117. Hida J, Yasutomi M, Maruyama T, *et al.* Indications for colonic J-pouch reconstruction after anterior resection for rectal cancer: determining the optimum level of anastomosis. *Dis Colon Rectum* 1998;**41**(5):558–63.
118. Horgan PG, O'Connell PR. Shinkwin CA. Kirwan WO. Effect of anterior resection on anal sphincter function. *Br J Surg* 1989;**76**(8):783–6.
119. Farouk R, Duthie GS, Lee PW, Monson JR. Endosonographic evidence of injury to the internal anal sphincter after low anterior resection: long-term follow-up. *Dis Colon Rectum* 1998; **41**(7):888–91.
120. Birnbaum EH, Myerson RJ, Fry RD, Kodner IJ, Fleshman

JW. Chronic effects of pelvic radiation therapy on anorectal function. *Dis Colon Rectum* 1994;**37**(9):909–15.

121. Lewis WG, Williamson ME, Kuzu A, *et al.* Potential disadvantages of post-operative adjuvant radiotherapy after anterior resection for rectal cancer: a pilot study of sphincter function, rectal capacity and clinical outcome. *Int J Colorectal Dis* 1995;**10**(3):133–7.
122. Varma JS, Smith AN, Busuttil A. Correlation of clinical and manometric abnormalities of rectal function following chronic radiation injury. *Br J Surg* 1985;**72**(11):875–8.
123. Varma JS, Smith AN, Busuttil A. Function of the anal sphincters after chronic radiation injury. *Gut* 1986;**27**(5): 528–33.
124. Iwamoto T, Nakahara S, Mibu R, Hotokezaka M, Nakano H, Tanaka M. Effect of radiotherapy on anorectal function in patients with cervical cancer. *Dis Colon Rectum* 1997;**40**(6):693–7.
125. Broens P, Van Limbergen E, Penninckx F, Kerremans R. Clinical and manometric effects of combined external beam irradiation and brachytherapy for anal cancer. *Int J Colorectal Dis* 1998;**13**(2):68–72.
126. Lundby L, Juhl Jensen V, Overgaard J, Laurberg S. Deleterious colorectal function after adjuvant postoperative radiotherapy for colorectal cancer: A randomized study. (abstract) *Dis Colon Rectum* 1997;**40**:A34.
127. Arnaud JP, Nordlinger B, Bosset JF, *et al.* Radical surgery and postoperative radiotherapy as combined treatment in rectal cancer. Final results of a phase III study of the European Organization for Research and Treatment of Cancer. *Br J Surg* 1997; **84**(3):352–7.
128. Dahlberg M, Glimelius B, Graf W, Pahlman L. Preoperative irradiation affects functional results after surgery for rectal cancer: results from a randomized study. *Dis Colon Rectum* 1998; **41**(5):543–9; discussion 549–51.
129. Anseline PF, Lavery IC, Fazio VW, Jagelman DG, Weakley FL. Radiation injury of the rectum: evaluation of surgical treatment. *Ann Surg* 1981;**194**(6):716–24.
130. Sandeman TF. Radiation injury of the anorectal region. *Aust NZ J Surg* 1980;**50**(2):169–72.
131. Haboubi NY, Schofield PF, Rowland PL. The light and electron microscopic features of early and late phase radiation-induced proctitis. *Am J Gastroenterol* 1988;**83**(10):1140–4.

Chapter 31

Psychological aspects of pelvic floor disorders

Barbara K Bruce, Christopher D Sletten

INTRODUCTION

Pelvic floor disorders may result in chronic constipation, chronic pelvic pain or sexual dysfunction. Psychological variables are considered to be important in the development and maintenance of these disorders, as well as in their successful treatment. This chapter reviews the psychological distress and comorbid psychiatric diagnoses frequently observed in these populations. It also describes how psychological approaches may enhance treatment effectiveness and improve clinical outcomes.

CONSTIPATION

Psychological factors have been implicated in the etiology, maintenance, and management of constipation. Lifestyle can significantly impact constipation. Physicians routinely address behavioral changes associated with constipation at every level of severity. Psychological distress is frequently observed in this population, and is beginning to be understood as an important variable in the etiology and maintenance of some types of constipation. As we will discuss below, there is a high prevalence of comorbid psychiatric disorders in patients with intractable constipation that merit attention in their own right. The success of behavioral interventions such as biofeedback in treating some forms of constipation does not require that psychological variables be causal. However, the identification of psychological factors and their appropriate management or treatment will improve outcomes in this population whether other indicators suggest medical management, surgery or biofeedback as primary treatment options.

The very definition of constipation is subjective and is significantly influenced by a number of psychological variables. Childhood experiences such as physical or sexual abuse, toilet training, and parental models of so-called 'normal' defecation help to shape the subjective complaint of constipation. Also of importance, these factors and other personality variables likely determine which patients will seek medical attention for constipation complaints.

There is a widely held belief among patients with constipation that one must have a bowel movement daily or else be considered constipated. Studies of the normal population suggest significant variability exists in what defines a 'normal' bowel habit with 'normal' ranging from three bowel movements a week to three bowel movements a day.[1] Similar findings are noted for individuals over the age of 60.[2] Despite the fact that the majority of the elderly population have bowel movements within this normal range, as many as 50% of the elderly use laxatives.[3]

The definition of constipation always includes complaints of infrequent defecation, as well as difficulties with defecation. The duration of complaints is generally not included in the definition. Associated symptoms often include abdominal pain, feelings of bloating or distention, and loss of appetite.

TYPES OF CONSTIPATION

In the absence of anatomic or organic causes, constipation is considered to be a functional bowel disorder. As such, it has been divided into four types: slow transit constipation, normal transit constipation or constipation predominant irritable bowel syndrome (IBS), pelvic floor dysfunction, and combined disorder which includes patients with slow transit plus pelvic floor dysfunction.

Slow transit constipation

Patients with slow transit constipation complain of reduced frequency of defecation and associated symptoms of abdominal pain and bloating. Often patients present with a many-year history of such complaints. Patients are most often women. Investigations reveal a normal colon, yet transit studies reveal a marked delay in the movement of radio-opaque markers or a radioisotope-labeled meal along the colon. The cause of the delay in slow transit constipation is unknown.

Normal transit constipation or constipation predominant irritable bowel syndrome

Patients diagnosed with constipation predominant IBS and normal transit constipation both have normal pelvic floor functioning and normal anal sphincter tone in the presence of normal transit. Patients with normal transit constipation also typically fulfill sufficient criteria to be classified as IBS.[4] The presence of pain that is relieved with defecation further confirms the diagnosis of IBS. Patients exhibit normal transit time, yet present with significant abdominal pain, bloating, and periods of diarrhea alternating with constipation. Patients report loose stools often with the onset of pain. Table 31.1 contains the Rome criteria for the definition of IBS. These criteria have become a widely acceptable set of criteria that define IBS.[5]

Pelvic floor dysfunction

Constipation or obstructed defecation resulting from pelvic floor dysfunction has also been referred to as nonrelaxing puborectalis syndrome,[6] pelvic floor dyssynergia-type constipation,[7] and anismus.[8] Although the physical exam is normal in these patients, the pelvic floor is observed to fail to relax when the patient attempts defecation. Patients report difficulty in the initiation of defecation and a feeling of incomplete evacuation. A common finding is the need to utilize digital evacuation to assist defecation. Patients report pelvic pain or perianal pain associated with the complaints noted above. Patients report spending long periods of time on the toilet in an attempt to have a bowel movement.

The cause of pelvic floor dysfunction is unknown and no neurological basis for this disorder has been identified.[6,9] Pelvic floor dysfunction is thought to be an abnormal learned response that has been hypothesized to result in some patients from sexual assault[6] or sexual abuse.[10] In children, the presence of large, painful bowel movements is thought to contribute to the development of pelvic floor dysfunction.[11]

IMPACT

Constipation is considered to be a common complaint in the general population. Prevalence rates show that 1.2% to 4% of adults have subjective complaints of constipation.[12,13] Other studies suggest that the prevalence may be as high as 34% in women over the age of 65 and 30% in men over the age of 65.[3,14,15] Studies have established that the patients who seek treatment for bowel complaints with a diagnosis of IBS are different than the patients who cope with bowel complaints on their own.[16,17] Similar studies have yet to be done on patients with primary constipation complaints. The data reviewed below target patients presenting to GI specialists or tertiary referral centers only.

Table 31.1 Diagnostic criteria for definition of irritable bowel syndrome[5]

At least 3 months continuous or recurrent symptoms of:

1. Abdominal pain or discomfort which is:
   - relieved with defecation;
   - and/or associated with a change in frequency of stool;
   - and/or associated with a change in consistency of stool; and
2. Two or more of the following, at least a quarter of occasions or days:
   - altered stool frequency (either more than three bowel movements per day or fewer than three bowel movements per week);
   - altered stool form (lumpy/hard or loose/watery stool);
   - Altered stool passage (straining, urgency, or feeling of incomplete evacuation);
   - Passage of mucus;
   - Bloating or feeling of abdominal distention.

Because the diagnosis of these disorders requires radiological studies or manometry the constipation disorders population prevalence is unknown. The prevalence of these types of constipation has been studied in patients presenting to tertiary referral centers. In this setting, the prevalence of pelvic floor or combined disorder ranges from 8% to 74% of the patients seen, but are most typically found in the 30% to 50% range.[4,9,18–20]

A recent study found that 10% of patients seen by gastroenterologists meet criteria for a diagnosis of IBS.[21] Other similar studies place the number of new patients seen in this setting with diagnosis of IBS at 13%[22] to 50%.[23] A total of 23% of a tertiary sample were diagnosed with IBS and 27% were diagnosed with slow transit constipation.[4]

QUALITY OF LIFE

Chronic constipation can severely disrupt functioning and impair quality of life. Recent studies examined patients with chronic constipation of a variety of causes and found a negative impact on general well-being and quality of life,[24] as well as functional status and quality of life in the elderly.[25] Normal transit patients with chronic constipation were found to have poorer quality of life than slow transit constipation patients suggesting the presence of increased suffering in this group.[24]

Researchers compared patients with IBS to patients with inflammatory bowel disease on a number of psychological variables including self-perceived functional disability.[26] Results indicated that IBS patients view themselves as disabled across domains of physical, social, family, occupational, and emotional role functioning. Further, they rated themselves as equal to or more disabled than a sample of patients with serious organic GI disease.

PSYCHOLOGICAL DISTRESS

Psychological distress is commonly observed in patients with chronic constipation. Psychological functioning has been investigated with regard to its etiological significance in the development of chronic constipation, as well as its role in determining treatment-seeking behavior in this population.

The most consistent finding across the literature is the high frequency of psychological distress found in normal transit constipation and IBS. The potential overlap between these two types of constipation is significant as discussed previously, because normal transit patients typically fulfill sufficient criteria to be classified as IBS.[4]

Psychosocial concerns have been observed in normal transit patients and include a high degree of antidepressant use and involvement in psychiatric counseling.[27] Subsequent research has specifically assessed psychological distress in these patients utilizing the Hopkins Symptom Checklist.[28,29] These data showed that normal transit patients had greater levels of psychological distress when compared with slow transit constipation patients and GI control patients. Similar findings were reported in response to the MMPI with normal transit patients showing more psychopathology than slow transit patients.[30] Other researchers found normal transit patients to be more depressed than slow transit constipation or pelvic floor dysfunction patients, but did not find differences between the groups on an overall measure of psychological distress.[31]

One group of researchers examined differences between normal transit and slow transit constipation patients with regard to the psychological variables of psychological distress, depression, and illness behavior.[32] Results showed that both constipated groups were more distressed and depressed than a healthy non-GI control group. However, the variable that did separate the two constipated groups was type of response to the Illness Behavior Questionnaire.[33] Significant differences were observed with normal transit patients exhibiting abnormal illness behavior in the areas of hypochondriasis and disease affirmation. This study suggests that normal transit patients may misperceive, misinterpret or overestimate bodily sensations or bodily functions or have misconceptions regarding what normal bowel habits should be. These factors have been hypothesized to lead to psychological distress that results in seeking medical care in a manner out of proportion to the bowel complaints.[34]

Similarly, IBS patients who present for care have been found to have high levels of psychological distress, as well as a high frequency of co-morbid psychiatric disorders across a large number of studies.[26,35–41] Further, these studies reveal that 50% to 100% of irritable bowel patients assessed have co-morbid psychiatric diagnoses, primarily depressive and anxiety disorders. It is important to note that the irritable bowel patients who present for medical care appear to be more distressed than patients with IBS identified in the community.[17]

When IBS patients are compared to an organic GI disease sample, a depressed sample, and healthy volunteers, irritable bowel patients looked more depressed than the depressed sample. They also showed elevations across six of the eight sub-scales of the Illness Attitude Scale that assesses abnormal illness-related fears, beliefs, and attitudes.[42] Similar to the normal transit patients, IBS patients reported bodily sensations that were worrisome and difficult to ignore. The patients endorsed beliefs and fears regarding having serious illness that doctors may not have correctly diagnosed. These researchers proposed that such illness attitudes may prompt an individual to focus anxiously on physical sensations resulting in the high rate of health care seeking behavior observed in this patient group.

Patients with chronic constipation resulting from pelvic floor dysfunction and combined disorder are also observed to have a high frequency of current and lifelong psychiatric disorders.[43,44] In particular, the presence of an eating disorder or history of an eating disorder appears disproportionately high in pelvic floor patients. Further, pelvic floor patients were observed to have more anxiety suggesting a link with increased muscle tension.[24]

Inconsistent reports of psychological distress in slow transit constipation are found in the literature. Generally, these patients have been observed to have normal psychological profiles interpreted as evidence of their adaptation to longstanding bowel dysfunction.[28] But other researchers have observed psychosocial disturbance in slow transit constipation as well.[45] In one study, elderly patients with slow transit constipation were found to have high scores across dimensions of depression, anxiety, obsessive–compulsive symptoms, and increased focus on somatic symptoms.[46] Further research is needed to better understand the role of psychological distress in this group of constipation patients.

LIFESTYLE FACTORS

A number of lifestyle factors are associated with constipation including reduced food and fiber intake. Both of these alterations are thought to prolong the time residue remains in the small bowel. Inadequate hydration and physical inactivity are also linked to constipation. Physical inactivity prolongs transit time while increased exercise increases colonic propulsive activity.[47]

In a study of elderly ambulatory outpatients, constipated subjects reported eating fewer meals as well as fewer calories per day. In this study, caloric intake appeared more important than fiber consumption or other dietary guidelines in contributing to constipation.[46]

Clinically, patients with chronic constipation are frequently observed to dramatically alter their food intake and composition of diet in an effort to manage their bowel complaints. Further, the literature fails to address the use, overuse, abuse, and dependence upon laxatives that is observed in the population of patients with chronic constipation. Together dietary factors and laxative overuse can become very complex and difficult to manage in these patients.

Behavioral strategies that target lifestyle factors are fundamental to the management of chronic constipation. Normalizing food intake, addressing a diet lacking in fiber, addressing a need for ample liquids, lack of exercise, prudent use of laxatives, and basic stress management principles are important components in the treatment of constipation regardless of severity. Habit training or instructing patients in the establishment of a routine time to defecate can be an extremely effective behavioral strategy.

CLINICAL CASE: LIFESTYLE FACTORS

A 44-year-old divorced mother of two teenage daughters presented to a tertiary gastroenterology practice with complaints of severe and chronic constipation. She was diagnosed with a combined disorder involving both anismus and delayed colonic transit. Patient described a 2-hour commute to a fast-paced job as a receptionist in a large law firm. She reported waking at 4 am early morning to start her working day. She ate lunch, if she ate at all, at her desk. Her job required her to get a replacement if she left her desk for any reason including going to the bathroom. Rather than impose on co-workers or focus attention on her bowel complaints, the patient ate as little as possible during the day to avoid needing a bathroom break. The patient was home by 7 pm where she prepared the evening meal and managed family and household tasks until 11 pm at which time she fell into bed depleted. Upon psychological evaluation, the patient had no formal psychiatric disorder, and no current depressive symptoms, and little psychological distress. She had no time in the day for defecation and no set defecating schedule. Food intake was significantly restricted. Upon evaluation, she was exhausted due to chronic sleep deprivation, yet determined to financially provide for her children as sole breadwinner. Her food intake, defecation, and sleep patterns were chronically impaired. Constipation would likely not be successfully resolved until significant changes in lifestyle took place in addition to the pelvic floor biofeedback program recommended to her.

CO-MORBID PSYCHIATRIC DISORDERS

A high prevalence of co-morbid psychiatric disorders is found in patients with chronic constipation. Direct attention to the evaluation and treatment of these psychiatric disorders may be required to successfully impact constipation complaints.

Depression

Complaints of constipation are frequently observed in patients who are clinically depressed. Researchers found that 27% of patients with major depression reported the onset of constipation or significant worsening of constipation after the onset of depression.[48] Other studies placed the rate of constipation in depressed patients to fall at 28% to 60%.[49–51]

Effective treatment of depression will likely resolve constipation complaints in these patients, but caution is warranted in that antidepressants with anticholinergic properties can slow transit time and exacerbate existing constipation. The selective serotonin reuptake inhibitors have no anticholinergic properties and are viewed as an effective alternative for the treatment of depression in patients with constipation or in patients with concomitant depression and the presence of an eating disorder.[47]

CLINICAL CASES: DEPRESSION

A 36-year-old female nurse, married mother of two young children presented with a 20 plus year history of constipation managed on her own until the death of her father 2 years ago. Since that time, the constipation had become severe, intractable and not responsive to laxatives or enemas. The patient was diagnosed with major depression several months after her father's death. She had a significant weight loss, suicide attempt, sleep disturbance, loss of concentration, feelings of guilt, and hopelessness. She had been under psychiatric care for a year and a half and was taking a number of antidepressants at the time of evaluation. Patient continued to experience severe constipation and was diagnosed with delayed colonic transit and pelvic floor dysfunction. Psychological evaluation at the time of her medical work-up revealed only partially treated depression with the continued presence of suicidal thoughts and many symptoms of depression. Recommendations included more aggressive treatment of her depression in addition to the pelvic floor biofeedback program initially recommended.

A 45-year-old attorney with chronic history of constipation-predominant IBS presented to a tertiary medical center with symptoms of worsening constipation and significant disability. Patient had not been able to work and had applied for long-term disability. She reported significant concern that she may have an 'accident' at work and was unable to eat on work-days to prevent this from happening. She had experienced a significant weight loss. She reported severe abdominal pain, bloating, gas following the ingestion of any food so she restricted all of her food intake to the evening. Psychological evaluation revealed chronic sleep disturbance, because she spent much of the night on the toilet due to her abdominal complaints. Additionally, she described severe exhaustion and hopelessness, as well as suicidal ideation. She had no psychiatric history and forcefully rejected the idea that depression was an important component of her struggle. Psychiatric evaluation was recommended that she refused. Feedback was provided to her gastroenterologist regarding her depressive symptoms and debilitation, as well as recommendations that she receive treatment for depression.

Anxiety disorders

In addition to the high levels of general psychological distress found in chronic constipation patients, a number of anxiety disorders are also observed in patients with constipation. These include bowel obsessions, defecation rituals, obsessive–compulsive disorder, panic disorder, and generalized anxiety disorder.

Bowel obsessions and defecation rituals have been reported in patients with chronic constipation. The essential focus of bowel obsessions is the irrational fear of losing control of one's bowels in public. Any number of rituals or ritualistic behaviors are devised to supposedly prevent such an event from occurring. Examples include severe restriction of food, spending excessive time on the toilet, attempting to time bowel movements or even becoming house-bound to avoid leaving home thus avoiding the social activities in which such an accident could conceivably occur. Clinically, patients often present with dramatic preoccupation with bowel functioning and an alteration of lifestyle around bowel concerns with a need to complete defecation rituals. One researcher in the field notes that bowel obsessions are best conceptualized as a variant of obsessive–compulsive disorder.[52] Such symptoms have also been diagnosed as an atypical presentation of panic disorder,[53] agoraphobia without panic attacks,[54,55] social phobia,[54,56] and a specific phobia such as 'bowel movement phobia'.[57] Other researchers found an association between constipation and obsessive–compulsive disorder in women but not in men in a large randomly sampled population data set from the Epidemiologic Catchment Area Project.[58]

Effective pharmacologic and behavioral treatment has been demonstrated with nearly complete resolution of bowel complaints with effective treatment of the anxiety disorder. Tricyclic antidepressants including clomipramine, imipramine, and trazodone used in conjunction with behavior therapy have been extremely effective in the treatment of bowel obsessions.[59–63] Behavioral treatment has included exposure and response prevention, self-control treatment and cognitive–behavioral treatment with success.[52,55,57,64]

North and colleagues[58] suggest the use of newer agents of the selective serotonin reuptake inhibitor variety such as sertraline and fluoxetine in the treatment of obsessive–compulsive symptoms in constipated patients, because these drugs are not associated with the constipating effects observed in anticholinergic antidepressants such as clomipramine. Further, they recommend screening chronically constipated patients for obsessive–compulsive disorder, because obsessive–compulsive disorder is viewed as a very treatable psychiatric disorder.

CLINICAL CASE: BOWEL OBSESSION

A 54-year-old surgeon presented to a tertiary care center with complaints of severe constipation. He was diagnosed with disordered defecation and non-relaxing puborectal muscles following medical work-up that showed normal colon transit and abnormal pelvic floor studies. Psychological evaluation revealed significant preoccupation with bowel functioning and elaborate and bizarre rituals to stool. Patient was particularly fearful that he would need to have a bowel movement during surgery. His entire life revolved around actions that would prevent this from happening. These included total restriction of food the day before surgery, and hours of time attempting to have a bowel movement on the days before surgery. The time in the bathroom consisted of many ritualistic steps to try and achieve a bowel movement that included daily enemas, laxatives, suppositories, cigarettes, coffee, and so on. The patient could not travel for fear he would need to spend an inordinate amount of time in the bathroom and other passengers such as on an airplane would note this. The same factor prevented him from visiting others' homes or having guests in his own home. The patient had a significant history of social anxiety describing considerable difficulty having bowel movements in college, because of the large, open dormitory bathrooms and his concerns regarding scrutiny from others. The patient was referred for behavioral treatment of the obsessive–compulsive and social anxiety components of his bowel difficulties in addition to the pelvic floor biofeedback recommended.

CLINICAL CASE: SOCIAL ANXIETY

A 45-year-old professional musician presented to a tertiary medical center with multiple year history of intractable constipation and associated symptoms of severe abdominal pain, cramping back pain, and bloating. Patient described laxative dependence with high number of laxatives taken each day to have daily bowel movements. Patient experienced an 'accident' on stage many years before after taking a strong laxative.

Table 31.2 DSM-IV Criteria for Panic Attack[66]

A discrete period of intense fear or discomfort, in which four (or more) of the following symptoms developed abruptly and reached a peak within 10 minutes:

1. Palpitations, pounding heart or accelerated heart rate
2. Sweating
3. Trembling or shaking
4. Sensations of shortness of breath or smothering
5. Feeling of choking
6. Chest pain or discomfort
7. Nausea or abdominal distress
8. Feeling dizzy, unsteady, lightheaded, or faint
9. Derealization (feelings of unreality) or depersonalization
10. Fear of losing control or going crazy
11. Fear of dying
12. Paresthesias (numbness or tingling sensations)
13. Chills or hot flushes

Patient then became extremely preoccupied with preventing such an accident in the future. He spent 3 to 4 hours a day on the toilet. He reported significant anxiety if unable to have a bowel movement before a performance. Patient was diagnosed with pelvic floor dyssynergia with normal colon transit. Patient had seen a psychiatrist and several antidepressants had been prescribed in the past which were of little benefit. Patient was referred to cognitive–behavioral treatment in addition to his pelvic floor biofeedback retraining program to address the significant performance anxiety that had become chronic.

Panic disorder

Panic disorder has been linked to IBS in multiple studies.[38,39,65] Panic disorder is an anxiety disorder characterized by abrupt development of four or more of the symptoms listed in Table 31.2 which shows the DSM-IV criteria for diagnosis of panic attack.[66] The criteria for panic attack include gastrointestinal symptoms of nausea and abdominal distress. It has been suggested that a diagnostic overlap may exist between IBS and panic disorder.[67] In one series of patients with panic disorder and IBS, a substantial improvement was observed in GI symptoms after treatment of panic disorder with Alprazolam.[68] Other studies have shown tricyclic antidepressants and cognitive–behavior therapy to be effective in the treatment of panic disorder and IBS.[69–72]

Blanchard,[40] in his extensive work with irritable bowel patients notes that generalized anxiety disorder is the most common anxiety disorder observed in these patients. Table 31.3 contains the diagnostic criteria for generalized anxiety disorder.[73] The essential feature of generalized anxiety disorder is worry in the presence of at least three of six psychophysiological symptoms.

Table 31.3 DSM-IV Criteria for Generalized Anxiety Disorder[73]

A. Excessive anxiety and worry (apprehensive expectation) occurring more Days than not for at least 6 months, about a number of events or activities (such as work or school performance).
B. The person finds it difficult to control the worry.
C. The anxiety and worry are associated with three (or more) of the following six symptoms (with at least some symptoms present for more days than not for the past 6 months). Note: Only one item is required in children.
   1. Restlessness or feeling keyed up or on edge
   2. Being easily fatigued
   3. Difficulty concentrating or mind going blank
   4. Irritability
   5. Muscle tension
   6. Sleep disturbance (difficulty falling or staying asleep, or restless unsatisfying sleep).
D. The focus of the anxiety and worry is not confined to features of an Axis I disorder, e.g. the anxiety or worry is not about having a panic attack (as in panic disorder), being contaminated (as in obsessive–compulsive disorder), being away from home or close relatives (as in separation anxiety disorder), gaining weight (as in anorexia nervosa), or having a serious illness (as in hypochondriasis), and the anxiety and worry do not occur exclusively during post-traumatic stress disorder.
E. The anxiety, worry, or physical symptoms cause clinically significant distress or impairment in social, occupational, or other areas of functioning.
F. The disturbance is not due to the direct physiological effects of a substance (e.g. a drug of abuse, a medication) or a general medical condition (e.g. hyperthyroidism) and does not occur exclusively during a mood disorder, a psychotic disorder, or a pervasive developmental disorder.

Eating disorders

The presence of a formal eating disorder is a critical factor in the evaluation of constipation. Tables 31.4–31.6 contain the DSM-IV diagnostic criteria for anorexia nervosa, bulimia nervosa, and eating disorder not otherwise specified.[74] The hallmark of these disorders is a severe disturbance in eating behavior.

It is not surprising to find that constipation is a frequent complaint in patients with eating disorders and is considered by the majority of eating disordered patients to be among their most debilitating symptoms.[47,75,76] Researchers found that despite complaints of severe constipation in a sample of anorexic patients, colonic transit is normal or returns to normal once they are successfully treated in a refeeding program.[77] These researchers caution attempts at evaluation or treatment of constipation in the presence of an eating disorder and recommend, instead, a program of refeeding.

Table 31.4 Diagnostic Criteria for Anorexia Nervosa[74]

A. Refusal to maintain body weight at or above a minimally normal weight for age and height (e.g. weight loss leading to maintenance of body weight less than 85% of what expected; or failure to make expected weight gain during periods of growth, leading to body weight less than 85% of that expected).
B. Intense fear of gaining weight or becoming fat, even though under-weight.
C. Disturbance in the way in which one's body weight or shape is experienced, undue influence of body weight or shape on self-evaluation, or denial of the seriousness of the current low body weight.
D. In postmenarchal females, amenorrhea, i.e. the absence of at least three consecutive menstrual cycles. (A woman is considered to have amenorrhea if her periods occur only following hormone, e.g. estrogen administration.)

Specify type:
Restricting type: during the current episode of anorexia nervosa, the person has not regularly engaged in binge-eating or purging behavior (i.e. self-induced vomiting or the misuse of laxatives, diuretics, or enemas).

Binge-eating/purging type: during the current episode of anorexia nervosa, the person has regularly engaged in binge-eating or purging behavior (i.e. self-induced vomiting or the misuse of laxatives, diuretics, or enemas).

As seen in the DSM-IV criteria defining the eating disorders, the purging behavior that often accompanies the restriction of food or binge eating includes the chronic use of laxatives or more rarely enemas. The majority of patients with anorexia nervosa and bulimia nervosa abuse laxatives, often after binge eating, but many use laxatives on a daily basis and in quantities much larger than the recommended dosage.[78,79] One researcher notes that bulimics may take up to 50 to 100 laxative pills per day.[79]

The overuse/abuse/dependence upon laxatives and chronic use of enemas observed in patients with chronic constipation is striking. Whether self-initiated or physician prescribed, patients frequently present to a tertiary gastroenterology practice with a long history of laxative dependence and the absence of spontaneous bowel movements. A large percentage of such patients have a current eating disorder diagnosis and/or a history of a formal eating disorder with a previous inpatient psychiatric treatment and very low body weights.[44,43]

A laxative abuse syndrome has been described as a variant of Munchausen syndrome in that patients surreptitiously abuse laxatives while simultaneously presenting for medical care for complaints of chronic constipation.[80,81] Patients with laxative abuse syndrome often have a concurrent formal eating disorder with

Table 31.5 Diagnostic Criteria for Bulimia Nervosa[74]

A. Recurrent episodes of binge eating. An episode of binge eating is characterized by both of the following:
   1. Eating, in a discrete period of time (e.g. within any 2-hour period), an amount of food that is definitely larger than most people would eat during a similar period of time and under similar circumstances.
   2. A sense of lack of control over eating during the episode (e.g. a feeling that one cannot stop eating or control what or how much one is eating).
B. Recurrent inappropriate compensatory behavior in order to prevent weight gain, such as self-induced vomiting; misuse of laxatives, diuretics, enemas, or other medications; fasting or excessive exercise.
C. The binge eating and inappropriate compensatory behaviors both occur, on average, at least twice a week for 3 months.
D. Self-evaluation is unduly influenced by body shape and weight.
E. The disturbance does not occur exclusively during episodes of anorexia nervosa.

Specify type:
Purging type: during the current episode of bulimia nervosa, the person has regularly engaged in self-induced vomiting or the misuse of laxatives, diuretics, or enemas.

Non-purging type: during the current episode of bulimia nervosa, the person has used other inappropriate compensatory behaviors, such as fasting or excessive exercise, but has not regularly engaged in self-induced vomiting or the misuse of laxatives, diuretics, or enemas.

Table 31.6 Diagnostic Criteria for Eating Disorder not Otherwise Specified[74]

The eating disorders not otherwise specified category is for disorders of eating that do not meet the criteria for any specific eating disorder. Examples include:
1. For females, all of the criteria for anorexia nervosa are met except that the individual has regular menses.
2. All of the criteria for anorexia nervosa are met except that, despite significant weight loss, the individual's current weight is in the normal range.
3. All of the criteria for bulimia nervosa are met except that the binge eating and inappropriate compensatory mechanisms occur at a frequency of less than twice a week or for a duration of less than 3 months.
4. The regular use of inappropriate compensatory behavior by an individual of normal body weight after eating small amounts of food (e.g. self-induced vomiting after the consumption of two cookies).
5. Repeatedly chewing and spitting out, but not swallowing, large amounts of food.
6. Binge-eating disorder; recurrent episodes of binge eating in the absence of the regular use of inappropriate compensatory behaviors characteristic of bulimia nervosa.

strong desire for weight loss. Baker and Sandle review the many complications associated with laxative abuse.[82]

CLINICAL CASES: EATING DISORDER

A 42-year-old male teacher presented with complaints of severe postprandial abdominal pain and bloating, constipation, and significant weight loss. He had lost 50 pounds over the preceding year. He was diagnosed with pelvic floor dysfunction and malnutrition with history of significant weight loss. He was also diagnosed with major depression. Pelvic floor biofeedback was attempted along with inpatient psychiatric treatment of depression. He also spent 3 weeks in an intensive pain rehabilitation program aimed toward assisting the patient in managing his significant preoccupation with constipation and abdominal pain and to attempt refeeding. These interventions proved of little benefit and he subsequently underwent an ileostomy. Postsurgical evaluation at 6 months revealed no change in complaints of pain, constipation, ability to eat, or weight status. A diagnosis of anorexia nervosa was made with components of severe restriction in caloric intake reportedly due to pain and constipation, significant and sustained weight loss, inability to improve weight, and distorted body image. He was then referred to a formal eating disorders treatment program for aggressive refeeding and psychological treatment.

A 17-year-old female high school student presented with severe constipation and abdominal pain. Colon transit study was normal. Patient was diagnosed with constipation secondary to pelvic floor dysfunction. Current weight was 85 pounds. Psychological evaluation revealed a 2 1/2 year history of anorexia nervosa with no prior psychiatric treatment. Patient had severely restricted food intake, over-exercising, significant body image distortion, and much family turmoil surrounding her continued weight loss. In the past 6 months, family attempted to closely monitor food intake at which point constipation and abdominal pain became debilitating. Patient also appeared clinically depressed with suicidal ideation, no appetite, sleep disturbance, and significant preoccupation with food. In addition to the pelvic floor biofeedback program, the patient was referred to a formal adolescent eating disorders program, which could also address her significant depression.

INTERVENTIONS

Pharmacotherapy, behavioral therapy, and other types of psychosocial intervention as noted above can be extremely beneficial in the direct resolution of chronic constipation complaints. These interventions may also serve as an adjunct to other medical interventions enhancing treatment effectiveness.

Biofeedback is currently regarded as an effective approach, as well as the treatment of choice in well-selected patients with constipation resulting from pelvic floor dysfunction.[20,83–85] Rao recently reviewed outcome data resulting from 14 studies that examined the efficacy of biofeedback in the treatment of constipation resulting from obstructive defecation, and results revealed 44% to 100% improvement rates across studies.[86] Further, researchers have advocated the use of biofeedback in chronic constipation beyond the group of patients with normal transit and abnormal or paradoxical pelvic floor contraction during straining. Chiotakakou-Faliakou and colleagues reported long-term benefit in patients with biofeedback with slow transit constipation, as well as normal transit constipation and in patients with and without paradoxical contraction of the pelvic floor muscles upon straining.[87] Biofeedback is considered to be a safe and inexpensive intervention that is free of morbidity. A significant drawback is the lack of availability of this technique in treating the large numbers of patients that may respond to biofeedback.

A number of psychological interventions and pharmacologic agents have resulted in some improvement in IBS patients. Relaxation training, stress management, and a variety of psychotherapeutic approaches have been examined in the treatment of IBS.[88] The large number of interventions that seem to help these patients led a prominent researcher in the field to conclude, 'any treatment that is systematic and logical to the patient is likely to help at least 50% of IBS patients and possibly a higher percentage'.[89]

Given the high prevalence of psychological distress and co-morbid psychiatric diagnoses in this population, psychological screening is recommended for every patient presenting to a tertiary care center for complaints of chronic constipation. The evaluation and appropriate management of psychological distress or concurrent psychiatric diagnoses appears essential to the successful treatment of chronic constipation.

PELVIC PAIN AND SEXUAL DYSFUNCTION

In addition to disorders of elimination, pain and sexual dysfunction are common in pelvic floor disorders. Both of these problems are complex and involve physiological and psychological factors. The following sections will review recent epidemiologic, etiologic and treatment findings focusing on what is known about these problems and their relationship to the pelvic floor.

The psychological issues and approaches for pelvic pain and sexual dysfunctions vary slightly from those of constipation and IBS. As highlighted previously, patients with constipation and IBS have high rates of psychological distress that falls into categories of depression, anxiety, and eating disorders. They also exhibit changes in their behavior and habits that directly impact their medical condition. Patients with chronic pelvic pain may and do exhibit many of these problems. However, as we will discuss's their psychological distress and functional limitations closely mirror problems seen in other chronic pain populations. This section will also clarify research findings on the possible mechanisms of chronic pelvic pain and sexual dysfunctions using a psychophysiological and behavioral approach.

Chronic pelvic pain may have many origins including referred pain from the abdomen or reproductive organs, myofascial dysfunction, skeletal derangement, visceral/neurologic damage, and psychological distress. Because of these multiple etiological factors, the diagnosis and treatment of pelvic pain often involves multiple medical specialties. Historically, there has been a tendency to dichotomize the origin of pelvic pain syndromes as either organic or psychogenic. Fortunately, recent studies and treatment interventions have shown the limitations of this approach and the efficacy of considering both physical and psychological variables.[90]

There are many identified types of pain disorders related to the pelvic floor. The majority of these have been identified in women. There is increasing attention given to the identification and treatment of several pain disorders in men. The most widely identified pelvic pain disorders can be loosely called the 'dynias'. These include vulvodynia, prostatodynia, and orchialgia (testicular dynia).[91] In addition, two sexual dysfunctions, vaginismus and dyspareunia have functional and symptomatic components directly related to the pelvic floor.

Vulvodynia is perhaps the most widely reported of the pelvic pain disorders. Even so, the literature on its frequency, course, and treatment only dates back to the early 1980s. In 1984, The International Society for the Study of Vulvar Disease Task Force characterized vulvodynia as chronic vulvar discomfort with complaints of burning and stinging.[92] Vulvodynia has been reported in association with several conditions including vulvar dermatosis, cyclic vulvovaginitis, vulvar vestibulitis, and vulvar papillomatosis. Even though these conditions are associated with the complaint of vulvodynia, like other chronic pain problems the magnitude and interference of the symptoms is often greater than the identified pathology. Women with vulvodynia often have relatively benign medical histories other than their pain and possible mild gynecological problems. They do however, often exhibit psychological and functional complaints that are similar to patients with other chronic pain conditions.[93] As one might expect with the presence of pain in this region, there is also an increased risk for related pelvic floor and sexual dysfunctions including dyspareunia, and pelvic floor tension myalgia.

Two pain disorders are found in the male reproductive system, orchialgia, and prostatodynia. Orchialgia has an unknown incidence and prevalence, but has been reported across the age span with the greatest incidence in the mid to late thirties.[92] Although there are several secondary causes of orchialgia, in the majority of cases there is little in the way of identified organic pathology even after thorough medical evaluation. Many cases of orchialgia may be exacerbated by invasive tests and procedures. In a recent clinical review it was found that 74 different surgical procedures had been performed in a sample of 48 patients presenting with chronic orchialgia.[92] In 80% of these cases tissue samples revealed no identifiable pathology. Clearly this is a poorly understood condition that often leads the patient to seek invasive solutions. Such a pattern of care-seeking may indicate the level of emotional and physical distress that is experienced.

Prostatodynia is a subtype of 'prostatitis', a general descriptor of symptoms presumed to arise from the prostate gland. Pain presumed to generate from the prostate can lead to similar complaints and functional impact as other pelvic pain problems. Prostatitis is a presenting complaint in approximately 25% of visits by men for genitourinary tract disorders.[92] Typically, men with complaints of prostate pain have a normal prostate on physical exam and an unremarkable urological evaluation. However, there is often the finding of altered urodynamics and an implication that there is dyssynergy in the detrusor striated sphincter and abnormalities in urethral closing pressures. This observation may link prostatodynia to other pelvic floor disorders and lead to more focused treatment using biofeedback and behavioral interventions. None of the studies on these pain disorders reported rates of psychological distress or functional impairment. However, given the number of tests and interventions that are attempted, one can speculate that the impact is significant. Also with our understanding of psychological factors in other chronic pain syndromes, it would be surprising if these patients did not experience similar distress and dysfunction.

Normal sexual functioning is a variable and somewhat fragile phenomenon. By its very nature it involves both psychological and physiological mechanisms. Most healthy adults experience differing levels of sexual interest and ability during the course of their lifetimes. These changes can be due to normal effects of aging, psychological factors such as stress and relationship factors, and overall physical health. When an individual has chronic medical problems, sexual functioning can be greatly disrupted. This is particularly true when pain is a prevalent symptom and the pain is directly associated with sexual activity. Pelvic pain and sexual dysfunction are often inexorably linked in a clinical setting.

Patients with constipation, pelvic floor myalgias, endometriosis, and other conditions often report an alteration in their sexual functioning.

The diagnosis of specific sexual dysfunctions, according to DSM-IV,[66] is made on the basis of symptoms and complaints regarding sexual functioning. There is only one sexual dysfunction that is primarily based on a report of pain during sexual activity, that is dyspareunia. Vaginismus, the involuntary contraction of vaginal muscles during probing or penetration, may also be associated with pain. The other sexual disorders are dysfunctions in the psychophysiological aspects of sexual arousal and activity. Even if the diagnosis of dyspareunia or vaginismus cannot be made, attention should be given to other sexual problems that may relate to pain. When the body is chronically subjected to pain, emotional and physical resources are drawn away from other functions. Non-vital functions like sex are particularly affected. When questioned, patients will often admit to sexual difficulties, some of which may rise to a clinically significant level. In many cases the pain problem is adequately treated but sexual dysfunction remains because of anxiety and learned associations between sexual activity and pain. These too merit psychological attention and are often remedied with relatively straightforward behavioral interventions.

IMPACT

Throughout the medical literature, chronic pelvic pain is cited as a frequent presenting complaint. This is particularly true in reports focusing on gynecologic and urologic medicine. Recent, well-designed studies of the prevalence and impact of chronic pelvic pain suggest that approximately 15% of women surveyed reported pelvic pain of at least 6 months' duration.[94] This study was a telephone survey of randomly selected women, ages 18 to 50. In addition to estimates of prevalence, the authors also report that women with chronic pelvic pain report lower estimates of general health, and 61% had pelvic pain of unknown etiology. The impact of this problem was also demonstrated in economic terms. The estimated direct medical costs were $881.5 million per year, and reduced work productivity and capacity. High rates of pelvic pain are also found in primary care settings.[95] A sample of primary care patients was surveyed to determine the prevalence of dysmenorrhea, dyspareunia, pelvic pain, and IBS. A total of 581 women completed a medical history questionnaire. The reported prevalences were, dysmenorrhea, 90%, dyspareunia, 46%, pelvic pain, 39%, and IBS 12%. Pelvic pain was the most common complaint among women 26 to 30 years of age. These studies indicate the high prevalence of pelvic pain and related complaints and the impact of these symptoms on women in early to middle adulthood.

There are fewer reports on the prevalence and symptoms of pelvic pain in men. However, as mentioned, conditions such as prostatitis, rectal pain, scrotal pain, and testicular pain can be disruptive and often poorly controlled. A retrospective study of men with pelvic pain found pain was most common in the prostate and/or the perineal region (45.6%). Pain in the scrotum and testes was reported in 38.8% of the cases, penile pain and bladder pain each were reported in 5.8% of the cases, and lower abdomen and lower back 1.9% each.[96] A total of 88% of these patients demonstrated significant tenderness in the pelvic floor muscles and poor to absent pelvic floor function. Urodynamic functioning in these men was essentially normal. The results of this study highlight two important aspects of chronic pelvic pain, its presence in men and the specific role of the pelvic floor across a range of pain sites.

With regard to sexual functioning, estimates regarding the prevalence of dyspareunia have ranged widely. This is due in part to the relatively recent recognition of dyspareunia as a disorder that merits medical/psychological attention.[97] Early estimates of prevalence ranged from 4% to 55%. More recent data suggest that between 10% to 15% of sexually active women are affected.[98] Even with these more conservative estimates, it is clear that pain related to sexual functioning is common and should be addressed both medically and psychologically.

PSYCHOLOGICAL/PSYCHOPHYSIOLOGICAL FACTORS

Because causes of chronic pain in the pelvic floor often involve multiple medical disciplines, there has been a somewhat diverse and fragmented approach to assessment and management of psychological and functional factors. The most well established literature, from a psychological/psychosocial perspective has been in the area of sexual abuse and pelvic pain. The central theorem is that a history of sexual abuse predisposes one to developing chronic pelvic pain. This is based on a conceptualization of psychosomatic illness in which psychic trauma is expressed through somatic complaints.

The early literature on etiological factors of pelvic pain focused heavily on the high incidence of childhood sexual abuse and resultant adult psychopathology. Women with pelvic pain were viewed as neurotic and depressed with dysfunctional family histories. Methodological shortcomings and frequently biased assumptions limited these early reports. In an early attempt to support this hypothesis, Walker *et al.*[99] conducted a controlled study comparing women with chronic pelvic pain to women with other gynecological disorders. The subjects were given a psychiatric interview and laparoscopic exam. The pelvic pain group demonstrated higher levels of depression, substance abuse, sexual dysfunction, somatization, and a history of adult and childhood sexual abuse. The control group had a rate of childhood sexual abuse of 23% compared to 64% for the pelvic pain group. There was also a high correlation between childhood sexual abuse and adult sexual dysfunction. The authors found no differences in severity or type of organic pathology. From this they concluded that there was a distinct relationship between abuse history and the development of chronic pelvic pain. They further postulate that the pelvic pain develops as a defense against psychologically painful memories and conflicts.

More recent studies have refined the relationship between abuse history and pelvic pain, demonstrating a more complex psychophysiological relationship. In a survey of 36 patients with pelvic pain, 19 of 36 patients were found to have a history of abuse. There were no differences between the abused and non-abused groups in levels of pain, demographics, and functional impairment. There were significant differences in level of psychological distress. As expected, the abused group had higher levels of global distress, greater somatization, and less perceived life control.[100] The authors note that the rate of sexual abuse is similar to other chronic pain populations, and that both groups demonstrated a response to pain interference similar to other chronic pain populations. These findings begin to suggest that while there are high rates of sexual abuse in this population and there is a clear psychological consequence of sexual abuse, these patients appear to have similar functional difficulties as other chronic pain patients.

In order to control for bias and small sample sizes of previous studies, Jamieson and Steege[101] conducted a population-based study in a primary care setting. A total of 581 women were surveyed in a primary care practice. The survey included questions regarding pelvic pain, irritable bowel, dysmenorrhea, dyspareunia, and sexual abuse. In this population, the incidence of childhood sexual abuse was 26%, adult sexual abuse 28%, abuse as child or adult 40%, and abuse both as child and adult 13%. Both pelvic and non-pelvic pain complaints were more common in women with abuse histories. Data were analysed comparing those with a history of childhood sexual abuse versus a history of adult sexual abuse versus both childhood and adult sexual abuse. In the group with a childhood abuse history, only irritable bowel was more common than in the non-abused group. For women with a history of adult sexual abuse, dyspareunia, pelvic pain, irritable bowel, and multiple pelvic pain complaints were more common. These more recent studies seem to indicate that a history of sexual abuse is common among reproductive-aged women, but a history of abuse is by no means causal and other factors including the impact of chronic pain, functional limitations, and the person's current circumstances are also significant factors in this population. There have been no studies to date that examine these issues in men with pelvic pain.

Another series of investigations has looked at the relationship between pelvic pain and organic findings. In particular, patients with positive organic findings have been compared to patients with negative findings on a number of psychological and functional variables. Understanding the results of these investigations is crucial given the high number of diagnostic and therapeutic laparoscopies that are performed each year and the implication that negative findings indicate a psychogenic basis for the pain. As in other chronic pain populations, these assumptions can contribute to great frustration for physician and patient alike. It can also lead to further medical/surgical investigation and interventions that may worsen an already difficult problem.

Studies of laparoscopic findings in women with chronic pelvic pain have reported widely discrepant rates. The rates of organic abnormality have ranged from 8% to 88%, with pelvic adhesions and endometriosis the most commonly found pathology.[102] In a recent study, women with identified endometriosis were compared to those with negative laparoscopies on several psychosocial variables. There were no significant differences in level of distressed mood or personality characteristics. However, women with identified endometriosis did report greater levels of pain and social dysfunction.[103] In a similar study, women with positive surgical findings were compared to those without identifiable pathology. These women were assessed for psychological distress and ongoing physical symptoms following their operative laparoscopy. Both groups had ongoing complaints of psychological distress, including complaints of anxiety, depression, and somatic worries. They also both reported ongoing marital and sexual difficulty.[104] These studies indicate that like other chronic pain problems, the presence of correctable pathology does not preclude the patient from ongoing distress and interference from their pain.

Two other recent studies investigated the psychological impact of laparoscopy on women with pelvic pain. In the first, 71 women who underwent laparoscopy for pelvic pain were randomly assigned to two groups of different waiting times. There were no differences between the groups, and both exhibited improvement in pain after laparoscopy. Psychological variables of beliefs about the pain and seriousness of the medical condition predicted pain reduction. None of the medical variables including degree of pathology predicted pain relief.[105] The second study focused on changes in psychological symptoms and functioning in women undergoing laparoscopy for known medical conditions. Patients were given several measures of psychological and personality functioning before laparoscopic surgery and then at 3 months postoperatively. Following surgery, subjects reported a 53% reduction in pain severity and accompanying reductions in depression and pain-related psychological distress. They also reported a 24% increase in activity level. These results indicate that when pain can be effectively reduced, patients with chronic pelvic pain respond in a similar manner to other chronic pain populations with increased activity and improved psychological functioning. This would not be the case if the pain experience were solely a result of unresolved psychological issues or past sexual traumas.

In an effort to more thoroughly understand the mechanisms of chronic pelvic pain, several investigators have studied neurological and psychophysiological influences. In two studies of patients with IBS, researchers have found alterations in cerebral activity and regional pain signals that may account for some of the pain associated with this condition. In the first study, patients with IBS and healthy controls were compared on perception thresholds for discomfort and pain during stimulation in the rectum. A rectosigmoid colon balloon was placed, and subjects were asked to provide ratings of discomfort at different pressures. Subjects also completed psychological questionnaires. Subjects with IBS showed consistently lowered thresholds and hyperalgesia during the pressure stimulation indicating the presence of visceral sensitization. The results also indicate a possible mechanism in which stimuli such as stressful events may lead to sigmoid colon contractions that are exaggerated in IBS patients and result in pain and cramping.[106]

In an examination of central nervous system activity, Silverman *et al.*[107] measured cerebral activity during actual and anticipated painful rectal stimulation. Again, IBS patients were compared to a healthy control sample. Subjects underwent a protocol that included the placement of a rectal balloon and the real or anticipated expansion of the balloon with concurrent positron emission tomography (PET) scanning. Healthy controls exhibited activation of the anterior cingulate cortex with the administration of painful stimuli. IBS patients displayed activation of the left prefrontal cortex during both actual and anticipated stimulation conditions. Although preliminary, these data begin to suggest alterations in pain perception in cases of chronic pain and may further explain the influence of cerebral events in the experience of rectal and abdominal pain. Of further interest is the involvement of the prefrontal cortex, an area associated with vigilance. Involvement of this area may provide a link between neurological changes in response to chronic pain and psychological factors such as attention.

TREATMENT

As is evident from these lines of investigation our understanding of the interface between 'psychological' and 'physical' phenomena is improving. It does not seem prudent to simply divide patients into categories of organic versus psychogenic on the basis of lab or surgical findings. With the wider application of sophisticated brain studies and our broader understanding of psychological factors, better care for these patients can be achieved. Part of this change needs to occur in the communication between medical and surgical specialties as well as across disciplines. As this occurs a clearer understanding of the interrelated influences of the mind and body can be achieved.

The literature is clear that no one organic or psychological factor predicts the onset or course of pelvic pain. Patients without prominent organic findings do not consistently display one type of abuse history or set of psychological problems. Rather, like other chronic pain populations there is an amalgam of factors that may be highly individualized. Despite the set of unique factors that may have led to the individual patient's condition, we see the effects of chronic pain as a consistent pattern of emotional distress, functional impairment, and medical uncertainty. Untreated patients are often exposed to multiple medical evaluations and interventions that at best lead to frustration and distress, and at worst may permanently impair the patient. During this declining course, the patient's emotional, interpersonal and daily functioning deteriorates and their lives are often significantly altered. Because of this, judicious use of medical care with an early recognition of psychological factors can prevent further damage. The psychological factors that seem most important include depression, anxiety, coping and social/environmental support. In the patient with significant impairment a comprehensive pain rehabilitation approach is often necessary. This entails the use of physical and occupational therapy for physical reconditioning and improved tolerance of activities, as well as behavioral interventions targeting stressors, emotional distress, social disruption and adaptation to chronic pain.

CLINICAL CASE: ABDOMINAL PAIN

A 43-year-old, married female was referred for evaluation of chronic abdominal pain. Upon initial presentation to a tertiary medical center she reported a history of constipation, coccydynia, and osteoporosis. She was referred for a multi-specialty evaluation. She was ultimately diagnosed with pelvic floor tension myalgia with secondary constipation, dyspareunia, and coccydynia. She was placed in a combined program of pelvic floor biofeedback training and comprehensive pain rehabilitation. During the course of her treatment a number of psychosocial stressors were addressed as well as her significant anxiety. The patient reported significant, longstanding generalized anxiety as well as specific anxiety regarding possible audible flatulence and fecal incontinence in public. Following pain rehabilitation, she continued treatment for her anxiety and pelvic floor tension myalgia for 9 months. At the end of treatment her anxiety was significantly reduced despite ongoing (but reduced) abdominal and pelvic pain. The patient reported improved occupational and daily functioning. She also had improved marital and sexual functioning.

CLINICAL CASE: VAGINAL PAIN

A 28-year-old divorced female was referred for a pain rehabilitation evaluation. She initially presented to a tertiary medical center for treatment of vaginal and vulvar intraepithelial neoplasia and dysplasia. She had undergone as series of three laser surgeries to remove vaginal lesions. These procedures had resulted in poorly healing vaginal sores. The patient had a previous history of myxopapillary ependymoma. This was widely excised and had resulted in residual pain. Finally, the patient had been given the diagnosis of fibromyalgia for diffuse musculoskeletal pain. She was treated in a comprehensive pain rehabilitation program for 3 weeks. During this time a history of significant sexual abuse was reported. The abuse had occurred just prior to the onset of her medical problems and had resulted in post-traumatic stress disorder (PTSD). This was treated with behavior therapy during the pain rehabilitation program. Following dismissal from the program, the patient reported significant reduction in anxiety and an increase in social, occupational, and daily functioning.

CONCLUSION

We have chosen several disorders to highlight the behavioral and psychiatric complications that can be associated with pelvic floor dysfunction. We believe that the constipation disorders, pelvic pain and sexual dysfunction represent all the facets of psychological impact in this general area of medicine. Patients with any of these disorders are at risk for psychological morbidity and the development of psychiatric disorders such as anxiety, depression or eating disorders. The impact of pain or altered bowel function can greatly disrupt all areas of functioning and leave the patient quite impaired.

There is still much to be delineated about the etiology and treatment of these disorders. It is clear that behavioral and psychological factors are important. It is equally important to maintain a balance between identifying and understanding psychological factors while maintaining an appreciation of the complex mind–body relationships. When this is accomplished, patients, their physicians, and families will be best served.

REFERENCES

1. Drossman DA, Sandler RS, McKee DC *et al.* Bowel patterns among subjects not seeking health care. *Gastroenterology* 1982;**82**:529–34.
2. Milne JS, Williamson J. Bowel habits in older people. *Gerontol Clin* 1972;**14**:56–60.
3. Whitehead WE, Drinkwater D, Cheskin LJ, *et al.* Constipation in the elderly living at home. Definition, prevalence and relationship to lifestyle and health status. *J Am Geriatric Soc* 1989;**37**:429–9.
4. Surrenti E, Rath DM, Pemberton JH, *et al.* Audit of constipation in a tertiary referral gastroenterology practice. *Am J Gastroenterol* 1995;**90**(9):1471–5.
5. Thompson WG, Creed F, Drossman DA; *et al.* Functional bowel disease and functional abdominal pain. *Gastroenterol Int* 1992;**5**:75–91.
6. Shelton AA, Welton ML. The pelvic floor in health and disease. *West J Med* 1997;**167**(2):90–98.
7. Whitehead WE, Chaussade S, Corazziari E, *et al.* Report of an international workshop on management of constipation. *Gastroenterol Int* 1991;**4**:99–113.
8. Preston DM, Lennard-Jones JE. Anismus in chronic constipation. *Dig Dis Sci* 1985;**34**:1168–72.
9. Whitehead WE. Functional anorectal disorders. *Sem Gastrointest Dis* 1996;**7**(4):230–6.
10. Leroi AM, Berkelmans I, Denis P, *et al.* Anismus as a marker of sexual abuse. Consequences of abuse on anorectal motility. *Dig Dis Sci* 1995;**40**:1411–16.
11. Wald A, Chandra R, Gabel S. Evaluation of biofeedback in childhood encopresis. *J Pediatr Gastroentol Nutr* 1987; **6**:554–8.
12. Johanson JF, Sonnenberg A. The prevalence of hemorrhoids and chronic constipation: an epidemiological study. *Gastroenterology* 1990;**98**:380–86.
13. Sonneberg A, Koch TR. Epidemiology of constipation in the United States. *Dis Colon Rectum* 1989;**32**:1–8.
14. Hale WE, Perkins LL, May FE, *et al.* Symptom prevalence in the elderly. An evaluation of age, sex, disease, and medication use. *J Am Geriatric Soc* 1986;**34**:333–40.
15. Stewart RB, Moore MT, Marks RG, *et al.* Correlates of constipation in an ambulatory elderly population *Am J Gastroenterol* 1992;**87**:859–64.
16. Drossman DA, McKee DC, Sandler RS, *et al.* Psychosocial factors in the irritable bowel syndrome. A multivariate study of patients and nonpatients with irritable bowel syndrome. *Gastroenterology* 1988;**95**:701–708.
17. Whitehead WE, Bosmajian L, Zonderman AB, *et al.* Symptoms of psychological distress associated with irritable bowel syndrome. *Gastroenterology* 1988;**95**:709–14.
18. Kuijpers HC. Application of the colorectal laboratory in diagnosis and treatment of functional constipation. *Dis Colon Rectum* 1990;**33**:35–9.
19. Pemberton JH, Rath DM, Ilstrup DM. Evaluation and surgical treatment of severe chronic constipation. *Ann Surg* 1991;**214**:403–11.
20. Whitehead WE. Biofeedback treatment of gastrointestinal disorders. *Biofeedback Self Regul* 1992;**17**(1):59–76.
21. Everhart JE, Renault PF. Irritable bowel syndrome in office-based practice in the United States. *Gastroenterology* 1991;**100**:998–1005.

22. Switz DN. What the gastroenterologist does all day. *Gastroenterology* 1976;**70**:1048–50.
23. Ferguson A, Sircus W, Eastwood NA. Frequency of 'functional' gastrointestinal disorders. *Lancet* 1977;**2**:613–14.
24. Glia A, Lindberg G. Quality of life in patients with different types of functional constipation. *Scand J Gastroenterol* 1997;**32**(11):1083–9.
25. O'Keefe EA, Taley NJ, Zinsmeister AR, *et al.* Bowel disorders impair functional status and quality of life in the elderly: a population-based study. *J Gerontol, Ser A, Biol Sci Med Sci* 1995;**50A**(4):184–9.
26. Walker EA, Gelfand AN, Gelfand MD, *et al.* Psychiatric diagnoses, sexual and physical victimization, and disability in patients with irritable bowel syndrome or inflammatory bowel disease *Psychol Med* **25**(6):1995;1259–67.
27. Wald A. Colonic transit and anorectal manometry in chronic idiopathic constipation. *Arch Int Med* 1986;**146**:1713–16.
28. Wald A, Hinds J, Caruana B. Psychological and physiological characteristics of patients with severe idiopathic constipation. *Gastroenterology* 1989;**97**:932–7.
29. Derogatis LI. *The SCL-90-R Administration, Screening and Procedures Manual II*. Towson, MD: Clinical Psychometric Research, 1983.
30. Wald A, Burgio K, Holeva K, *et al.* Psychological evaluation of patients with severe idiopathic constipation. Which instrument to use? *Am J Gastroenterol* 1992;**87**:977–80.
31. Grotz RL, Pemberton JH, Talley NJ, *et al.* Discriminant value of psychological distress, symptom profiles, and segmental colonic dysfunction in outpatients with severe idiopathic constipation. *Gut* 1994;**35**:798–802.
32. Chattat R, Bazzocchi G, Balloni M, *et al.* Illness behavior, affective disturbances and intestinal transit time in idiopathic constipation. *J Psychosomatic Res* 1997;**42**(1):95–100.
33. Pilowsky I, Spence ND (eds). *Manual for the illness behavior questionnaire*, 2nd edn. Adelaide: University of Adelaide, 1982.
34. Folks DG, Cleveland Kinney F. The role of psychological factors in gastrointestinal conditions. A review pertinent to DSM-IV. *Psychosomatics* 1992;**33**:257–70.
35. Liss JL, Alpers D, Woodruff RA. The irritable colon syndrome and psychiatric illness. *Dis Nervous Syst* 1973;**34**:151–7.
36. Young SJ, Alpers DH, Norland CC, *et al.* Psychiatric illness and the irritable bowel syndrome. *Gastroenterology* 1976;**70**:162–6.
37. Blanchard EB, Scharff L, Schwarz SP, *et al.* The role of anxiety and depression in the irritable bowel syndrome. *Behav Res Ther* 1990;**28**:401–405.
38. Walker EA, Roy-Byrne PP, Katon WJ, *et al.* Psychiatric illness and irritable bowel syndrome: A comparison with inflammatory bowel disease *Am J Psychiat* 1990;**147**:1656–61.
39. Lydiard RB, Fossey MD, March W, *et al.* Prevalence of psychiatric disorders in irritable bowel syndrome. *Psychosomatics* 1993;**34**:229–34.
40. Blanchard EB. Irritable bowel syndrome. In: Gatchel RJ, Blanchard EB (eds). *Psychophysiological Disorders. Research and Clinical Applications.* American Psychological Association, 1993:23–62.
41. Schwarz SP, Blanchard EB, Berreman CF, *et al.* Psychological aspects of irritable bowel syndrome: Comparisons with inflamatory bowel disease and non-patient controls. *Behav Res Ther* 1993;**31**:297–304.
42. Gomborone J, Dewsnap P, Libby G, *et al.* Abnormal illness attitudes in patients with irritable bowel syndrome *J Psychosomat Res* 1995;**39**(2):227–30.
43. Bruce BK, Pemberton JH, Kvale SW, *et al.* Psychopathology among patients with chronic constipation. *Proceedings of the Society of Behavioral Medicine 12th Scientific Sessions*, 1991;**46**.
44. Nehra V, Camilleri, M, Pemberton JH, *et al. Psychological disorders in patients with evacuation disorders and constipation in a tertiary practice.* Paper presented at the 1999 annual meeting of the American Gastroenterological Association.
45. Preston DM, Pfeffer JM, Lennard-Jones, JE. Psychiatric assessment of patients with severe constipation. *Gut* 1984;**25**:A582.
46. Towers AL, Burgio KL, Locher JL, *et al.* Constipation in the elderly: Influence of dietary, psychological, and physiological factors. *J Am Geriat Soc* 1994;**42**:701–706.
47. Mehler P. Constipation: diagnosis and treatment in eating disorders. *Eating Disor* 1997;**5**(1):41–4.
48. Garvey M, Noyes R, Yates W. Frequency of constipation in major depression: Relationship to other clinical variables. *Psychosomatics* 1990;**31**(2):204–206.
49. Woodruff RA, Murphy CE, Herjouic M. The natural history of affective disorders: I. Symptoms of 72 patients at the time of index hospital admissions. *J Psychiat Res* 1967;**5**:255–63.
50. Baker M, Darzab J, Winokur G, *et al.* Depressive disease: Classification and clinical characteristics. *Comp Psychiat* 1972;**12**:354–65.
51. Nelson JD, Jatlow PI, Quinlan DM. Subjective complaints during desipramine treatment. *Arch Gen Psychiat* 1984;**41**:55–9.
52. Hatch ML. Conceptualization and treatment of bowel obsessions: Two case reports. *Behav Res Ther* 1997;**35**(3):253–7.
53. Lydiard RB, Laraia MT, Fossey M, *et al.* Possible relationship of bowel obsessions to panic disorder with agoraphobia. *Am J Psychiat* 1988;**145**:1324–5.
54. Barlow DH. The dimensions of anxiety disorders. In: Tuma AH, Maser JD (eds). *Anxiety and Anxiety Disorders.* Hillsdale, NJ: Lawrence Erlbaum Associates, 1985;479–500.
55. Pollard CA, Carmin CN. Agoraphobia without panic. *ADAA Rep* 1995; winter: 18–20.
56. Jenike MA, Baer L, Minichiello WE. *Obsessive–compulsive disorders: theory and management.* Chicago, IL: Year Book Medical, 1990.
57. Eisen AR, Silverman WK. Treatment of an adolescent with bowel movement phobia using self-control therapy. *Behav Ther Exp Psychiat* 1991;**22**:45–51.
58. North CS, Napier M, Alpers DH, *et al.* Complaints of constipation in obsessive–compulsive disorder. *Ann of Clin Psychiat* 1995;**7**(2):65–70.
59. Caballero R. Bowel obsession, response to clomipramine. *Am J Psychiat* 1988;**145**:650–51.

60. Jenike MA, Vitagliano HL, Rabinowitz J, *et al.* Bowel obsessions responsive to tricyclic antidepressant in four patients. *Am J Psychiat* 1987;**144**:1347–8.
61. Lyketsos CG. Successful treatment of bowel obsessions with nortriptyline. *Am J Psychiat* 1992;**149**:573.
62. Kahne GJ, Wray RW. Clomipramine for bowel obsessions. *Am J Psychia* 1989;**146**:120.
63. Ramchandani D. Trazodone for bowel obsession. *Am J Psychia* 1990;**147**:124.
64. Beidel DC, Bulik CM. Flooding and response prevention as a treatment for bowel obsessions. *J Anxiety Disord* 1990;**4**(3):247–56.
65. Maunder RG. Panic disorder associated with gastrointestinal disease: review and hypotheses. *J Psychosomat Res* 1998;**44**(1):91–105.
66. American Psychiatric Association. *Diagnostic and statistical manual of mental disorder (DSM-IV)*, 4th edn. Washington DC: APS, 1994:395.
67. Lydiard RB, Greenwald S, Weissman MM, *et al.* Panic disorder and gastrointestinal symptoms: findings from the NIMH Epidemiologic Catchment Area Project. *Am J Psychiat* 1994;**15**(1):64–70.
68. Noyes R Jr, Cook B, Garvey M, *et al.* Reduction of gastrointestinal symptoms with treatment of panic disorder. *Psychosomatics* 1990;**31**:75–9.
69. Greenbaum DS, Mayle JE, Vanegeren LE, *et al.* Effects of desipramine on irritable bowel syndrome compared with atropine and placebo. *Dig Dis Sci* 1987;**32**:257–66.
70. Marshall JR. Are some irritable bowel syndromes actually panic disorders? *Postgrad Med* 1988;**83**:206–209.
71. Lydiard RB, Laraia MT, Howell EF, *et al.* Can panic disorder present as irritable bowel syndrome? *J Clin Psychiat* 1986;**47**:470–73.
72. Eldridge GD, Walker JR, Holborn SW. Cognitive-behavioral treatment for panic disorder with gastrointestinal symptoms: a case study. *J Behav Ther Exp Psychiat* 1993;**24**:367–71.
73. American Psychiatric Association. *Diagnostic and statistical manual of mental disorder (DSM-IV)* 4th edn., Edition. Washington, DC: APS, 1994;435–6.
74. American Psychiatric Association. *Diagnostic and statistical manual of mental disorder (DSM-IV)* 4th edn. Washington, DC: APS, 1994;539–50.
75. Wardholtz BD, Anderson AE. Gastrointestinal symptoms in anorexia nervosa. *Gastroenterology* 1990;**98**:1415–19.
76. Chami TN, Andersen AE, Crowell MD, *et al.* Gastrointestinal symptoms in bulimia nervosa; effects of treatment. *Am J Gastroenterol* 1995;**90**(1):88–92.
77. Chun AB, Sokol MS, Kaye WH, *et al.* Colonic and anorectal function in constipated patients with anorexia nervosa. *Am J Gastroenterol* 1997;**92**(10):1879–83.
78. Pryor T, Wiederman MW, McGilley B. Laxative abuse among women with eating disorders: An indication of psychopathology? *Int J Eating Disord* 1996;**20**(1):13–18.
79. Mitchell JE. Bulimia: medical and physiological aspects. In: Brownell KD, Foreyt JP (eds). *Handbook of eating disorders. Physiology, psychology, and treatment of obesity, anorexia, and bulimia.* US: Basic Books, 1986:379–88.
80. Cummings JH. Progress report. Laxative abuse. *Gut* 1974;**15**:758–66.
81. Oster JR, Materson BJ, Rogers AI. Laxative abuse syndrome. *Am J Gastroenterol* 1980;**74**:451–8.
82. Baker EH, Sandle GI. Complications of laxative abuse. *Ann Rev Med* 1996;**47**:127–34.
83. Sagar PM, Pemberton JH. Anorectal and pelvic floor function. Relevance of continence, incontinence, and constipation. *Gastroenterol Clin North Am* 1996;**25**(1):163–82.
84. Ko CY, Tong J, Lehman RE, *et al.* Biofeedback is effective therapy for fecal incontinence and constipation. *Arch Surg* 1997;132(8):829–33.
85. Whitehead WE, Drossman DA. Biofeedback for disorders of elimination: fecal incontinence and pelvic floor dyssynergia. *Prof Psychol Res Prac* 1996;**27**(3):234–40.
86. Rao S. The technical aspects of biofeedback therapy for defecation disorders. *Gastroenterologist* 1998;**6**:96–103.
87. Chiotakakou-Faliakou E, Kamm MA, Storrie JB, *et al.* Biofeedback provides long-term benefit for patients with intractable, slow and normal transit constipation. *Gut* 1998;**42**(4):517–21.
88. Whitehead WE. Behavioral medicine approaches to gastrointestinal disorders. *J Consult Clin Psychol* 1992;**60**(4): 605–612.
89. Blanchard EB. Irritable bowel syndrome. In: Gatchel RJ, Blanchard EB (eds). *Psychophysiological disorders: research and clinical applications.* American Psychological Association, 1993:59.
90. Reiter R. Chronic pelvic pain. In: Block AR, Kremer EF, Fernandez E (eds). *Handbook of pain syndromes: biopsychosocial perspectives.* NY: Lawrence Erlbaum Associates, 1999:457–74.
91. Wesselmann U, Reich SG. The dynias. *Sem Neurol* 1996;**16**(1):63–74.
92. Wesselmann U, Burnett AL, Heinberg LJ. The urogenital and rectal pain syndromes. *Pain* 1997;**73**(3):269–94.
93. Bornstein J, Goldik Z, Alter Z, Zarfati D, Abramovici H. Persistent vulvar vestibulitis: the continuing challenge. *Obstet Gynecol Surv* 1998;**53**(1):39–44.
94. Mathias SD, Kuppermann M, Liberman RF, Lipschutz RC, Steege JF. Chronic pelvic pain: prevalence, health-related quality of life, and economic correlates. *Obstet Gynecol* 1996;**87**(3):321–7.
95. Jamieson DJ, Steege JF. The prevalence of dysmenorrhea, dyspareunia, pelvic pain, and irritable bowel syndrome in primary care practices. *Obstet Gynecol* 1996;**87**(1):55–8.
96. Zermann DH, Ishigooka M, Doggweiler R, Schmidt RA. Neurourological insights into the etiology of genitourinary pain in men. *J of Urol* 1999;**161**(3):903–908.
97. Meana M, Binik YM. Painful coitus: A review of female dyspareunia. *J Nerv Mental Dis* 1994;**182**(5):264–72.
98. Meana M, Binik YM, Khalife S, Cohen DR. Biopsychosocial profile of women with dyspareunia. *Obstet Gynecol* 1997;**90**(4pt1):583–9.
99. Walker E, Katon W, Harrop-Griffiths J, *et al.* Relationship of chronic pelvic pain to psychiatric diagnoses and childhood. *Am J Psychiat* 1988;**145**(1):75–80.
100. Toomey TC, Hermandez JT, Gittelman DF, *et al.* Relationship of sexual and physical abuse to pain and psychological assessment variables in chronic pelvic pain patients. *Pain* 1993;**53**(1):105–109.

101. Jamieson DJ, Steege JF. The association of sexual abuse with pelvic pain complaints in a primary care population. *Am J Obstet Gynecol* 1997;**177**(6):1408–1412.
102. Savidge, CJ, Slade P. Psychological aspects of chronic pelvic pain. *J Psychosoma Res* 1997;**42**(5):433–44.
103. Peveler R, Edwards J, Daddow J, Thomas E. Psychosocial factors and chronic pelvic pain: a comparison of women with endometriosis and with unexplained pain. *J Psychosomat Res* 1996;**40**(3):305–315.
104. Richter HE, Holley RL, Chandraiah S, *et al.* Laparoscopic and psychologic evaluation of women with chronic pelvic pain. *Internat J Psychiat Med* 1998;**28**(2):243–53.
105. Elcombe S, Gath D, Day A. The psychological effects of laparoscopy on women with chronic pelvic pain. *Psychol Med* 1997;**27**(5):1041–50.
106. Munakata J, Naliboff B, Harraf F, *et al.* Repetitive sigmoid stimulation induces rectal hyperalgesia in patients with irritable bowel syndrome. *Gastroenterology* 1997;**112**(1): 55–63.
107. Silverman DH, Munakata JA, Ennes H, *et al.* Regional cerebral activity in normal and pathological perception of visceral pain. *Gastroenterology* 1997;**112**(1):64–72.

Chapter 32

Sexually transmitted disease and the pelvic floor

Peter Sagar

INTRODUCTION

Since biblical times, the ano-rectum has been considered by some as an outlet for sexual satisfaction. The proportion of the population who regularly indulge in practices of genito-anal, oral–anal or other anal and pelvic floor based practices of an erotic nature appears to be on the increase. Most estimates suggest that about 5% of the adult male population in the UK and US are either homosexual or bisexual.[1] A promiscuous lifestyle is a major component of the homosexual population with perhaps 80–90% of this population practising outside of a monogamous relationship. The 'average', albeit stereotyped, homosexual has about 1000 sexual partners in a lifetime.[2] Even a homosexual who would consider himself only moderately active may have between 100 and 200 partners a year.[3] As many of these partners are casual pick-ups or anonymous, their sexual activity or background risk is not known. Clearly, such estimates of sexual activity are important and understandably the sexual transmission of disease involving the ano-rectum is a significant health problem within this population. It should be noted, however, that monogamous homosexuals carry no higher risk of sexually transmitted disease than monogamous heterosexuals. The conditions discussed in this chapter have become prevalent within the homosexual community. Collectively, they are referred to as the 'gay bowel syndrome' and the chapter will concentrate on the ano-rectal manifestations.

It is important to note that anal receptive intercourse is not confined to men. Surveys from gynecological clinics (which admittedly study select populations with inevitable bias) suggest that 25–30% of women have experienced genito-anal intercourse at least on one occasion and that 8–10% indulge on a regular basis.[4]

Ano-receptive intercourse is therefore the most common vector for transmission of ano-rectal sexually transmitted diseases. It permits direct inoculation of various pathogens into the rectal mucosa. The penis may serve as a passive conduit for infectious organisms. Initially, ano-receptive intercourse elicits a local reaction within the rectal mucosa that may then spread to affect the patient regionally and then systemically. The rectal mucosa is more fragile compared with the squamous mucosa of the vagina.[7] Ano-rectal innoculation depends on the interaction and method of invasion of the specific pathogen and the local anatomy. The intact skin of the perineum offers an effective barrier while the anal transitional zone and the rectal mucosa offer less resistance. This epithelium is more open to infectious agents and depends on the production of mucus, immunoglobulin A and specific populations of lymphocytes.[6] The already porous mucosa is made more so by the trauma of ano-receptive intercourse as this causes abrasions and compromises the integrity of the epithelial barriers. Infection is facilitated. Pathogens can be spread by the oral–anal route by the practice referred to as 'rimming' in homosexual circles. This practice tends to cause a more diffuse gastrointestinal pathology.

In addition to the infective conditions, anal receptive intercourse has direct effects on the anal sphincter complex that will cause clinical symptoms that may present to a colon and rectal specialist. The incidence of fecal seepage, fecal soilage and accidental bowel movements was found to be about 25% in a homosexual population that practised anal receptive intercourse compared with only 3% in an age and sex matched population.[5] Clinical physiological studies of the anal sphincter in this population have suggested that there is a reduction in the resting anal pressure and a shorter high-pressure zone. Anal sensation is diminished. Our own studies have indicated that there is also a reduction in the high pressure gradient of the anal sphincter complex (S. Stojkovic, personal communication). Such physiological changes may influence the type of surgical procedure offered to patients. For instance, a surgeon may be wary about carrying out a lateral subcutaneous sphincterotomy for a chronic anal fissure because of the concern about an increased risk of postoperative fecal incontinence.

DIAGNOSIS

Usually, it is the sexual activity and preferred practices of the patient that is the most significant factor for patients with sexually transmitted diseases. Sexual preference and degree of promiscuity provide a number of diagnostic clues. Although often a sensitive subject, careful and thorough questioning of the patient about sexual activity is very important as clinical symptoms and signs can be non-specific or subtle. Contrary to popular belief, homosexuals often do not show characteristics of dress or behavior that would automatically suggest their sexual leanings. Many are frightened or embarrassed to discuss their activities. Gentle sensitive coaxing is required. Discretion and assurances about confidentiality are needed when the sexual history is taken. The type of sexual practice (genito-anal, oro-anal, manual etc.) may direct the clinician to particular sites. The STDs most frequently found in homosexuals are gonorrhea/syphilis/herpes, chlamydia and condylomata acuminata (genital warts). Gastrointestinal manifestations of sexually transmitted diseases may occur anywhere from mouth to anus and the identification of one STD should prompt the clinician to look for others. If proctitis is identified, usually with pain and discharge, smears should be taken for microscopy, Gram stain and culture. In addition, serological tests for syphilis are required. Herpetic proctitis is associated with a burning rectal sensation, tenesmus and a low-grade fever. It is painful. Rectal ulcers may be seen at anoscopy and they may be confluent. In contrast, proctitis secondary to gonococcal and chlamydial infection is associated with erythema and friability of the anal canal with a purulent exudate. Certain strains of *Chlamydia trachomatis* may cause severe proctocolitis with bloody diarrhea. The rectal mucosa appears ulcerated, friable and mimics ulcerative colitis in the acute phase. Biopsies show a granulomatous reaction. Cultures need to be taken for *C. trachomatis* and serological testing for lymphogranuloma venereum (LGV) is required. Inflammation of the rectum may also be seen on proctoscopy in patients with syphilis. The severity varies and the mucosa may show discrete ulcers, friability or a mass. Serological testing for syphilis should be part of the routine investigation. A well-defined ulcer on the genital region, perianal skin or ano-rectum should suggest chancroid, herpes and LGV as the differential diagnosis. A mass in the ano-rectum should suggest an abscess, anal carcinoma, lymphoma or Kaposi's sarcoma.

The diagnosis of enteric sexually transmitted diseases requires a battery of diagnostic tests:

1. Spirochaetal pathogens (treponema pallidum) require dark field microscopy and VDRL serology.
2. Bacterial infection (*Neisseria gonorrhoea, C. trachomatis*) require microscopy, Gram stain, culture of discharge, stool culture and monoclonal antibody tests.
3. Viral infection (Condyloma acuminata, Herpes simplex, CMV, HIV) require biopsy, culture, monoclonal antibody testing and ELISA.
4. Yeast infection (*Candida*, Cryptosporidiosis) require culture, biopsy and acid-fast stain of stool specimens).
5. Protozoal infection (*Entamoeba histolytica, Giardia*) require stool culture.

The clinical responsibility should not end with the individual patient who is diagnosed with an STD. Rather the doctor has a duty to report the confirmed diagnosis to the local health authority and identify and counsel partners. Confidentiality must be assured and maintained throughout.

SPECIFIC SEXUALLY TRANSMITTED DISEASES

GONORRHEA

Incidence

As many as 55% of homosexual men who attend screening clinics may be infected with *Neisseria gonorrhoea.* The rectum is the sole site in almost half of these patients.[8] Rectal gonorrhea is present in 10–40% of homosexual men who attend genitourinary clinics[9] and 30–50% of women with positive cervical swabs for gonorrhea will have similarly infected rectal mucosa.[10] There was a significant downturn in the incidence of rectal gonorrhea in homosexual men from 1983 onwards almost certainly in response to health education programs and the consequent behavioral changes in response to the risk of HIV infection. Unfortunately, the incidence has been on the rise again over the past decade, perhaps because of complacency. There has also been an increase in the low-income heterosexual population.

Mode of transmission

Ano-receptive intercourse with a partner who has gonococcal urethritis may result in gonococcal proctitis. There is an incubation period of about a week. *N. gonorrhoea* infects columnar or transitional epithelium and therefore affects the mucosa of the anal canal and rectum. Within 36–48 hours of inoculation, the bacteria enter the submucosa by passing through epithelial cells. About 3% of infections develop into disseminated gonococcal infections with arthritis, dermatitis and tenosynovitis. Occasionally, systemic spread may cause pericarditis, perihepatitis and even meningitis.

Symptoms and signs

Many patients have no symptoms and are detected in partner screening clinics. Local symptoms include anal pain secondary to cryptitis, tenesmus, bloody discharge of mucus and pruritis ani. Intersphincteric abscesses may develop and cause more severe pain.

Diagnosis

Inflammation of the lower 10 cm of the rectal mucosa is seen on proctoscopy with a mucopurulent discharge. The mucosa is red and friable. Mucopus may be expressed with gentle pressure with the anoscope and sent for Gram stain and culture. If anoscopy is too uncomfortable, then a culture swab can be inserted into the anal canal and gently rotated. Gram-negative diplococci may be seen within either neurophils or colonic mucosal cells. Sensitivity increases when samples are taken under direct vision. Swabs are plated on Thayer–Martin culture medium. This is the best single method of diagnosis. The histology of rectal biopsies is usually non-specific. Edematous crypts and a mixed inflammatory cell infiltrate of polymorphs and lymphocytes within the lamina propria may be seen.

Treatment

Resistance has been developing and the usual recommendation of a penicillin based treatment has been replaced by a single dose of ceftriaxone 250 mg IM and then a 7-day course of doxycycline 100 mg twice daily. Ceftriaxone has the added advantage of also treating pharyngeal gonorrhea and doxycycline may treat any coexisting *C. trachomatis* infection. If symptoms persist, the rectum requires re-evaluation for other pathogens.

SYPHILIS

Incidence

Venereal syphilis is caused by the spirochaete treponema pallidum. The disease has systemic manifestations from the start and can affect almost the entire body. Syphilis was first described as long ago as 500 AD and has played an interesting role in our history. A significant rise in the incidence of syphilis was noted during World War II followed by a further rise in the 1950s. The prevalence rose again in the 1970s, mainly in the homosexual male population, but then awareness of the risk of HIV initially influenced homosexual behavior to such an extent that the incidence within this population declined in the 1980s. Conversely, there was a dramatic increase in the heterosexual population in the late 1980s, thought to be due to the use of crack cocaine at least in the US.

Mode of transmission

Direct penetration of the ano-rectum causes primary syphilitic infections. The first syphilitic lesion to appear is the primary chancre which emerges about 2–6 weeks after inoculation. It is usually painless.

Symptoms and signs

The primary chancre appears as a red macule. Quickly, it becomes papular and ulcerates. When fully developed, it is a hard, painless, indurated ulcer with regular well-demarcated margins. In contrast to other sites, an anal chancre may cause severe pain and be wrongly diagnosed as an anal fissure. Most chancres are single but they can be sited opposite each other in a 'kissing' arrangement. They can be multiple and oddly placed. A primary chancre can appear on the rectal wall and mimic a rectal carcinoma or a solitary rectal ulcer. Biopsies taken from a primary chancre will show ulceration, underlying granulation tissue and a heavy plasma cell and lymphocytic infiltration.

Local or inguinal lympadenopathy associated with the primary chancre is also often painless. Healing usually occurs over the next 3–6 weeks. Healing is by fibrosis. This leaves a small scar.

Six to eight weeks after the chancre has healed, the secondary manifestations of ano-rectal syphilis become apparent. The treponemal spriochaetes spread throughout the body. The patient may complain of tiredness, headaches, loss of weight, fever and muscular and joint pains. Skin lesions are variable and include a macular rash, and a papular rash with large fleshy masses in the warm and moist parts of the body – condyloma lata. These lesions appear as broad light brown or pink verrucous lesions usually around the anal and genital regions. They secrete mucus and have an unpleasant smell. Pruritus is then common. Condyloma lata contain many spirochaetes and are therefore highly infective. They occur in 10–20% of patients with secondary syphilis.[11] Rarely, there may be destructive pustular lesions. On mucous membranes a gray-white membrane can be seen with a dull-red margin seen particularly in the mouth, pharynx and larynx. 'Snail-track' ulcers may also be seen. Lymphadenitis, hepatitis, iritis, arthritis, bursitis and periostitis may develop. Patients then enter a latent phase in which they are asymptomatic for a year but are considered infectious in this period.

Progression on to tertiary syphilis leads to the gumma or inflammatory lesions in a number of tissues. The gumma is now rarely seen in the western world but, when seen, comprises a central core of structured necrosis with a surrounding zone of epithelioid cells and occasional giant cells. There is granulation tissue which is heavily infiltrated with plasma cells and lymphocytes, fibrosis and endarteritis obliterans. Lesions of tertiary syphilis found in bones provoke new bone formation, but later spread to cortical bone and have a destructive effect and lead to the worm eaten skull appearance. Gummas in the liver are followed by irregular fibrosis and this breaks the liver up into distorted lobes – 'hepar lobatum'.

Finally, quaternary or neurosyphilis produces changes within the spinal cord and involves the lower sensory neurons. Pathologically there is wasting of the posterior roots, thickening of the pia-arachnoid and gross demyelination of the dorsal columns. This tabes dorsalis can cause anal sphincter paralysis and severe perianal pain.

Diagnosis

Direct visualization with dark field illumination is the diagnosis of choice. Primary and secondary lesions are crowded with organisms. The treponemal spirochaetes are seen as cork-screw shaped and have a unique motility. They fluoresce yellowish-green. Serological tests are available. Four to six weeks after inoculation the fluorescent treponemal antibody (FTA) absorption test will be positive. The Venereal Disease Research Laboratory (VDRL) assay is positive about 4 to 7 days after the appearance of the primary lesion. As described above, biopsy of the lesions reveals an intense submucosal infiltrate with lymphocytes and destruction of the muscularis mucosa.

Treatment

A single intramuscular injection of 2.4 megaunits of penicillin G is effective, although patients with long-standing disease may need three injections at weekly intervals. All sexual partners from the previous 12 months will also require treatment. Infected individuals need to refrain from sexual activity until they demonstrate low VDRL titers. In the rare case of neurosyphilis, a 2-week course of intravenous penicillin G 2–4 million units every 4 hours is required.

Syphilis and HIV

Epidemiological studies have suggested that there is an interaction between HIV and syphilis. They relate positive HIV serology with positive syphilis serology. The majority of HIV positive patients have the appropriate serological response to syphilis. The early progression of both treated and non-treated HIV positive patients to neurosyphilis suggested that all syphilitic patients with neurological symptoms or signs should be treated for neurosyphilis. In all patients with HIV, VDRL tests should be carried out and repeated at 1, 2, and 3 months and 3-monthly thereafter until a satisfactory serological response is obtained. Cerebrospinal fluid samples should be obtained in non-responders.

CHLAMYDIA

Incidence

Chlamydia trachomatis is a common pathogen and is able to infect a number of organs. Chlamydial species are obligate intracellular parasites. Classic lymphogranulomatosis is endemic in tropical countries but chlamydial infections are regularly diagnosed wherever sexually transmitted diseases are evaluated. About 15% of asymptomatic homosexual men harbor chlamydial rectal infections. About 4 million chlamydial infections are reported each year in the US. The infection is on the increase and it is the most common STD.[12] There are 15 immunotypes of *Chlamydia trachomatis*. Types D and K are found most often in patients with genital and anal infections. The most serious, venereal lymphogranulomatosis (LGV), is associated with serotypes L1, L2 and L3. These subtypes are more invasive because they infect macrophages as opposed to the squamocolumnar cells favored by the non-LGV serotypes.

Mode of transmission

Primary inoculation of the ano-rectum occurs as a direct result of ano-receptive intercourse. Oro-anal sexual practices have also been incriminated. Chlamydial species cannot penetrate intact skin or mucous membranes. Entry is gained through abrasions and small lacerations. The incubation period is up to 6 weeks. Rectal infection may also result from lymphatic spread from penile or vaginal infection.

Symptoms and signs

In cases of lymphatic spread, the primary lesion of LGV may be a small papule that is asymptomatic. The papule may be found in the coronal sulcus within the urethra or on the scrotum. Small vesicles progress over several weeks and form an ulcer at the anal verge. Painful lymphadenopathy may develop in the inguinal regions either uni- or bilaterally. These may necrose into buboes and discharging sinuses. If the rectum is infected the draining sinuses affect nodes of the perirectal or iliac chain and cause lower abdominal and back pain. If both femoral and inguinal nodes are affected then a 'groove sign' appears in 20% of patients and is considered pathognomonic of LGV. Proctocolitis develops with enlargement of perirectal lymphatics, suppuration and the formation of fistulas. Strictures will eventually develop and the condition can therefore mimic Crohn's disease.

Diagnosis

A rectal biopsy will show crypt abscesses with giant cells and infectious granulomata. As well as histopathology, biopsies should be taken for culture. Special precautions need to be taken. The transport medium is sucrose based and the samples need to be maintained on ice for immediate tissue culture inoculation. Swabs of the rectal mucosa are unhelpful since chlamydia are obligate intracellular parasites. Complement fixation tests become positive 14 days after infection. A titer of more than 1:64 supports a diagnosis of LGV. It is usually worth aspirating affected lymph nodes but incisional biopsy should be avoided because of the risk of chronic sinus formation. A late manifestation of LGV infection is a rectal stricture.

Treatment

Chlamydial infections usually respond to tetracycline 500 mg four times a day for 7 to 14 days. Affected partners need to be screened and treated. Asymptomatic rectal strictures can be treated with longer courses of tetracycline but symptomatic strictures should be biopsied to exclude associated carcinoma.

HERPES SIMPLEX

Incidence and mode of transmission

The herpes simplex virus typically infects mucocutaneous sites and abrasions. It is a large enveloped DNA virus and is the most common pathogen isolated from the rectums of symptomatic homosexual men.[13] Over 95% of homosexual males have been infected with HSV type 2.[15] HSV 1 is spread by oro-anal contact while HSV 2 is spread by penile implantation. HSV 1 and HSV 2 cause an infection of similar severity although recurrence is more common after HSV 2. The viral particles are transported after replication to the neuronal nucleus where they lie dormant in a latent state. Recurrences may occur by active transport along the nerve to the mucocutaneous junction. Transmission risks for heterosexuals after sexual intercourse with an infected partner are about 10%.[14] The rate for homosexuals is unknown.

Symptoms and signs

The incubation period is between 5 and 20 days. Ano-rectal herpes causes pain and a burning sensation that is worse after defecation. Tenesmus is almost always present. Pruritis ani is common and patients may complain about a bloody or mucus discharge. A systemic viremia may occur especially during the prodrome. If the ganglia of the lumbosacral region become infected the patient may experience urinary dysfunction with impotence and parasthesia in the sacral distribution. Pain in the lower abdomen and lower limbs especially over the thighs and buttocks occur in half of homosexual men[16] and it may persist for many months.

Small vesicles are seen around the anus with surrounding erythema. They are painful and can prevent full examination unless anesthetic ointment is used. The vesicles may coalesce or rupture. Eventually they will crust over and heal. HSV proctitis is confined to the lower 8–9 cm of the rectum. Ulceration within the anal canal may become secondarily infected.

Diagnosis

Direct culture within viral culture media will give a positive result in one to four days. Cytological diagnosis is less sensitive. Scrapings taken from the base of the ulcers will show intranuclear inclusion bodies or multinucleate giant cells. Rectal biopsies will show crypt abscesses in about half of the infected individuals. HSV antigen detection with enzyme immunoassay is extremely accurate.[17]

Treatment

The primary drug treatment of choice is Acyclovir. This is an HSV DNA polymerase inhibitor. The recommended dose is 200 mg five times a day for 10 days. Symptomatic treatment includes warm baths, topical anesthetic preparations and analgesics. Attention to personal hygiene may reduce the risk of secondary infection. Patients who relapse are given a one year course of suppressive therapy – 400 mg twice daily.

HUMAN PAPILLOMA VIRUS (HPV)

Incidence

The perianal wart, condyloma acuminata, is caused by the human papilloma virus (HPV). Four types are sexually transmitted. While types 6 and 11 are benign types, types 16 and 18 are associated with the development of dysplasia and carcinoma. Such infected warts should therefore be considered to be premalignant.[18] There was a marked increase in the incidence of condyloma acuminata between the 1960s and 1980s. Homosexual and bisexual men are most commonly affected. As many as 70% may be affected.[19] Genital warts are seen more commonly in women with anal HPV with an incidence of about 80% compared with just 16% of men.[20]

Mode of transmission

Infection seems to begin with local trauma. This allows the HPV to gain access to the basal cells. The virus favors actively dividing cells such as those found in the anal transitional zone and cervix. As the basal cells mature, infectious viral particles are found in the more superficial epithelium. Close questioning of affected populations has suggested that 90% of patients with anal condyloma acuminata confess to anal receptive intercourse.[20] Direct spread from the genital area accounts for the others.

Symptoms and signs

The condylomas may appear as small cauliflower like lesions or flat papules. Small or subclinical lesions can be seen more easily if the skin is stained with 3% acetic acid and left on the skin surface for about 5 minutes. The infected zones appear white. Bleeding, itching, a damp feeling and discharge are common complaints. A macerated mass may form and produce a foul smell. Large lesions may form and keep growing into giant condylomata (Busche–Lowenstein's disease). These lesions may grow to almost obliterate the anal canal and are considered to be a low-grade verrucous carcinoma.

It is locally invasive and rarely metastasizes to regional lymph nodes.

Diagnosis

As well as an acetic acid tests, diagnosis may be helped by the use of magnification or colposcopy. Biopsies show marked acanthosis of the epidermis. Hyperplasia of the prickle cell layer is evident. There is an accompanying chronic cell infiltrate.

Treatment

Excise all lesions. Local or general anesthetic can be used with infiltration of the skin with a dilute adrenaline (1 in 100 000) solution to reduce blood loss and elevate the lesions. This facilitates scissor or diathermy excision. Although podophyllin is cytotoxic to the condyloma, it is also very irritant to the neighboring normal skin. It causes cell death by arresting mitosis. Application needs to be very careful as it causes an intense inflammatory reaction with subsequent crusting. Several applications are needed. It should be avoided for anal canal lesions because of the risk of stenosis or formation of fistulas. Podophyllin treatment can produce a dysplastic reaction within condyloma which mimics carcinoma *in situ*. Surgical excision has a lower recurrence rate compared with podophyllin treatment.[21] Alternative treatments include surgical destruction with cryotherapy or laser ablation and medical therapy with bichloroacetic acid which is less irritating than podophyllin. Immunotherapy with autologous injection of vaccine prepared from a sample of the patient's own condylomata and given IM over a 6-week period or interferon injected either intramuscularly or directly into the lesions have demonstrated benefit in a number of controlled trials.

HPV eradication in HIV patients

It is much more difficult to eliminate condyloma acuminata in patients who are HIV positive compared with HIV negative patients. Infection is more extensive. Individual therapy is required. Diathermy ablation controls about 50% of HIV positive patients as long as follow-up is close and thorough. Should any lesions progress to carcinoma *in situ* then excision with a 1 cm margin is recommended.

CHANCROID

Incidence

An infection with *Haemophilus ducreyi* causes a soft sore. The organism is an aerobic Gram-negative bacillus arranged in chains or clusters. The incidence had been on the decline until about 1985 but has recently begun to rise again. It is associated with poorer countries and developing economies. It is becoming a more common condition probably in association with the HIV epidemic. The condition is 10 times more prevalent in males compared with females. Females may however be asymptomatic and prostitutes are a major reservoir of infection. The condition rarely presents to a colon and rectal specialist as rectal infection is uncommon.

Symptoms and signs

The incubation period is between 3 and 7 days. Painful ulcers develop on the genitals and in the perineum. The ulcers are undermined, but can be difficult to differentiate from herpes ulcers. The perineal ulcers lead to abscess formation with associated regional lymphadenopathy which may require aspiration.

Diagnosis

Direct cultures of swab material are made on chocolate agar vancomycin media.

Treatment

Chancroid usually responds to a one week course of erythromycin 500 mg four times a day. Alternative drugs include amoxicillin and ciprofloxacin. Any sexual partner in contact with the patient over the previous 10 days also requires treatment.

ANO-RECTAL AND PELVIC FLOOR MANIFESTATIONS OF HIV INFECTION

Incidence

An outbreak of *Pneumocystis carinii* pneumonia and Kaposi's sarcoma was noted by the Center for Disease Control (CDC) in the US in 1981. A total of 26 cases of Kaposi's sarcoma and five cases of *Pneumocystis pneumonia* were reported. The outbreak involved young unmarried men and was associated with an acquired immunodeficiency state. By the end of that year, 316 patients had been reported.[22] From then on, the condition was referred to as AIDS. In 1982, cases were diagnosed in recipients of blood and blood products. The causative agent was originally labeled HTLV-III and then renamed human immunodeficiency virus (HIV) in 1986. Currently, it is estimated that one in 250 adults has been infected with HIV in the US. Homosexual and bisexual men account for about 70% of reported cases although the proportion has fallen with an increase in the incidence in intravenous drug abusers and heterosexual populations.[23] Male patients with HIV are nine times more common than women with HIV. In 1994, HIV infection was the leading cause of death in males aged between 25 and 44.

There has traditionally been an attitude of nihilism towards ano-rectal disease in patients with AIDS. This resulted from the publication of early data that showed a high morbidity and mortality in patients who underwent surgical intervention. The overall survival was short.[24] With the advent of newer treatment options and earlier diagnosis and intervention, it is essential that the many unpleasant and disabling conditions of the anorectum associated with HIV infection are recognized, diagnosed and treated.

Progression of the disease can be monitored by means of the CD4 count. Progressively lower CD4 counts lead to changes in the clinical state of the patient and associated pathological changes with a deterioration of the health of the patient. There is also now an HIV RNA assay which allows direct quantification of the viral load.[25]

Mode of transmission

HIV attacks mainly T-lymphocytes that carry the CD4 marker. This leads to their eventual destruction. These cells are helper T-cells and play a critical role in cell mediated immunity. They also facilitate humoral immunity. Their destruction therefore significantly compromises the defense of the host. The associated loss of antigen recognition interferes with the function of macrophages while B-cell production of immunoglobulins is compromised. The chance of the patient contracting infections or developing tumors is increased.

The spread of HIV is increased by direct contact with blood, semen and vaginal secretions that contain HIV virus. Direct inoculation with blood or blood products is the most effective mode of transmission which helps to explain the prevalence in the intravenous drug abuse community. Mother to child perinatal exposure also permits transmission.

Sexual activity carries a variable risk of transmission. There is a one in 100 risk of developing an infection with an act of penile–vaginal intercourse but ano-receptive intercourse carries a significantly higher, albeit poorly defined, risk. As the rectal mucosa is relatively fragile and has an excellent blood supply, small abrasions may occur in the course of anal receptive intercourse and permit the direct spread of HIV into the bloodstream.

After exposure there is a short viral-like illness which may last 3 to 15 days. Patients may then remain healthy for many years. The median time from HIV seroconversion to the development of AIDS is 8.3 years and the median time from AIDS to death is 17 months.[26] These data are from the 1980s and recent developments in antiretroviral treatment and prophylactic regimens have improved the outlook. Nevertheless, long-term prognosis remains poor.

Four stages of decline can be described:

Stage 1: Primary infection

There is rapid proliferation of the HIV in the blood and lymph nodes and the patient seroconverts.

Stage 2: Early immune deficiency

CD4 counts remain above 500 μl and there is some control of the virus by the lymphoid tissue. The patient exhibits no symptoms.

Stage 3: Intermediate immune deficiency (CD4 count 500 to 200 μl)

The immune mechanism begins to fail. Clinical signs of immunocompromise appear. The risk of opportunistic infection and malignancy is increased.

Stage 4: Advanced immune deficiency (CD4 level falls below 200 ml)

The virus overcomes the immune system. Major opportunistic infections and malignancies require significant intervention. Death is inevitable.

Symptoms and signs

Symptoms associated with the initial illness are non-specific and include sweats, fever, myalgia, arthralgia, headache and diarrhea. Sore throat may occur with lymphadenopathy and a maculopapular rash on the trunk. Occasionally, the central nervous system may be affected with peripheral neuropathy, meningoencephalitis or Guillain–Barré syndrome. The time from exposure to onset varies from 1 week to 3 months. Unfortunately, a large proportion of patients will remain symptom free and therefore not present for investigation. They may continue to infect others unknowingly. The history needs to include questions that relate to high risk behavior such as homosexual practices, intravenous drug abuse, travel to areas where AIDS is endemic and a past history of sexually transmitted disease.

About one third of patients with AIDS develop an ano-rectal condition in the course of their disease progression.[24] The intestinal mucosa has depressed numbers of CD4 cells in this group of patients and ano-rectal receptive intercourse may facilitate the development of the various colorectal manifestations of AIDS. Alloantigens present in sperm may be involved in immune suppression.[28]

Ano-rectal suppuration in HIV-positive patients may result from a number of bacterial pathogens which include *Mycobacterium tuberculosis* and *Mycobacterium avium*. The lack of inflammatory cells permit an insidious infection without the usual classic early signs. Anal or rectal pain with fever is the usual presenting symptom.

Anal fissures are difficult to evaluate in HIV-positive patients because of associated ulceration. The anal sphincter is characteristically hypotonic in such patients and the fissures are positioned more proximal than is usually the case. They can be aggressive and erode through the intersphincteric and trans-sphincteric planes. They resemble Crohn's ulcers. Collection of fecal matter in the ulcers leads to severe pain and pus collects in the eroded spaces.

Herpes simplex viral infection of the perianal skin in HIV-positive patients causes perianal pain, sacral radiculopathy and constipation with urinary tract disturbance. Since the usual vesicles are often absent a high index of suspicion is required.

Diagnosis

Seroconversion occurs when antibodies are produced against HIV. This usually occurs 2 to 6 weeks after exposure. Enzyme linked immunoabsorbent assay (ELISA) against HIV antibody is used as the initial screening test. If this is found to be positive then it is repeated and the positivity confirmed by means of Western blotting. This combination of tests has a sensitivity of 99%.[27] Originally, a definite diagnosis of AIDS was only made in patients infected with HIV who went on to develop one of the most common indicator conditions such as *Pneumocystis pneumonia*. The list of indicator conditions has expanded greatly over the last 10 years to include a variety of conditions. These include pulmonary or esophageal candidiasis, extrapulmonary cryptococcosis, cytomegalovirus disease, HIV related encephalopathy, disseminated histoplasmosis, toxoplasmosis of the brain, Kaposi's sarcoma and progressive multifocal leucoencephalopathy.

Treatment

Prompt treatment with drainage of ano-rectal suppuration is needed. Definitive treatment of a fistula tract can be carried out at initial operation or deferred to exam under anesthetic at a later date according to the state of the patient. Fistulotomy should be avoided for patients with troublesome diarrhea in case incontinence occurs.

Anal fissures and the associated ulceration require aggressive debridement under anesthetic. Pockets of pus or necrosis require deroofing. Direct injection of steroid preparation into the lesions is needed for patients with continuous symptoms. Internal sphincterotomy should be avoided. The results are disastrous with a high incidence of incontinence. Conversely, it is safe to perform sphincterotomy for patients with anal fissures proven to be associated with a high anal tone. Excision of anal ulcers with closure of the defect by means of an advancement flap will improve symptoms. HSV perianal disease can be treated with significant relief of symptoms with oral or topical acyclovir.

REFERENCES

1. Wilcox RR. The rectum as viewed by the venereologist. *Br J Venereal Dis* 1981;**57**:1–6.
2. Darrow WW, Barrett D, Jay K, Young A. The gay report on sexually transmitted diseases. *Am J Public Health* 1981;**71**:1004–1011.
3. William DC. The sexual transmission of parasitic infection in gay men. *J Homosexual* 1980;**5**:219–94.
4. Bolling DR. Prevalence, goals and complications of heterosexual anal intercourse in a gynecological population. *J Reprod Med* 1977;**19**:120–24.
5. Miles AJG. Pathophysiology of anoreceptive intercourse. In: Mersh A, Gottesman I (eds). *Anorectal disease in AIDS*. London: Edward Arnold, 1991:28–42.
6. Hodges JR, Wright R. Normal immune responses in the gut and liver. *Clin Sci* 1982;**63**:339–47.
7. Owen RJ. The role of biopsy in diagnosis of rectal infections. *Gastroenterology* 1986;**91**:770–74.
8. Janda WM, Bonhoff M, Morgello JA, Lerner SA. Prevalence and site-pathogen studies of *Neisseria meningitides* and *Neisseria gonorrhoea* in homosexual men. *JAMA* 1980;**244**:2060–64.
9. British Cooperative Clinical Group. Homosexuality and venereal disease in the United Kingdom. *Br J Venereal Dis* 1973;**49**:329–39.
10. Thin RN, Shaw EJ. Diagnosis of gonorrhoea in women. *Br J Venereal Dis* 1979;**55**:10–13.
11. Hutchinson CM, Hook EW. Syphilis in adults. *Med Clin North Am* 1990;**74**:1389–1416.
12. Centers for Disease Control and Prevention. Recommendations for the prevention and management of *Chlamydia trachomatis*. *MMWR* 1993;**42**:1.
13. Rompalo AM, Roberts PL, Honson K. Empiric therapy for the management of prostatis in homosexual men. *JAM* 1988;**260**:348–53.
14. Mertz GJ, Benedetti J, Ashley R. Risk factors for the sexual transmission of genital herpes. *Ann Intern Med* 1992;**116**:197–202.
15. Nerurkar L, Goedert J, Wallen W. Study of antiviral antibodies in sera of homosexual men. *Fed Proc* 1983;**42**:6109.
16. Samarasinghe PL, Oates JK, MacLennan IPB. Herpetic proctitis and sacral radiculopathy – a hazard for homosexual men. *Br Med J* 1979;**2**:365–6.
17. Baker DA, Gonik B, Milch PO. Clinical evaluation of a new herpes simplex virus ELISA: A rapid diagnostic test for herpes simplex virus. *Obstet Gynecol* 1989;**73**:322–5.
18. Palmer JG, Shepherd NA, Jass JR. Human papillomavirus type 16 DNA in anal squamous cell carcinoma. *Lancet* 1987;**2**:42–4.
19. Car G, William DC. Anal warts in a population of gay men in New York City. *Sex Transmit Dis* 1977;**4**:56–7.
20. Abcarian H, Sharon N. The effectiveness of immunotherapy in the treatment of anal condyloma acuminatum. *J Surg Res* 1977;**22**:231–6.
21. Jensen SL. Comparison of podophyllin application with simple surgical excision in clearance and recurrence of perianal condylom acuminatum. *Lancet* 1985;**2**:1146–8.
22. Centers for Disease Control and Prevention. Kaposi sarcoma and pneumocystis pneumonia among homosexual men, New York City and California. *MMWR* 1981;**30**:305–308.
23. Statistics from World Health Organization and Centers for Disease Control and Prevention 1993;**7**:1287–91.
24. Wexner SD, Smithy WB, Milsom JW. The surgical management of anorectal diseases in AIDS and pre-AIDS patients. *Dis Colon Rectum* 1986;**29**:719–23.

25. O'Brien WA, Hartigan PM, Martin D. Changes in plasma HIV-1 RNA and CD4 lymphocyte counts and risk of progression to AIDS. *N Engl J Med* 1996;**334**:426–31.
26. Veuglers PJ, Page KA, Tindall B. Determinates of HIV disease progression among homosexual men registered in the tricontinental seroconverter study. *Am J Epidemiol* 1994;**140**:747–58.
27. Bylund DJ, Siegner WHM, Hooper DG. Review of testing for human immunodeficiency virus. *Clin Lab Med* 1992;**12**:305–333.
28. Mavligit GM, Talpaz M, Hsia FT. Chronic immune stimulation by sperm alloantigens. *JAMA* 1984;**251**:237–41.

Chapter 33

Magnetic resonance imaging (MRI) of the pelvic floor

Lennox Hoyte, Eboo Versi

INTRODUCTION

Neurological, muscular and fascial components all play a role in the proper physiological functioning of the pelvic floor. The integrity of the pudendal nerve, levator ani, periurethral muscles, and the fascial attachments all contribute to pelvic floor function.[1] When there is damage to these tissues (e.g. due to childbirth injury), stress urinary incontinence and pelvic organ prolapse can result.[1] Additionally, estrogen may play a role in softening the urethral and vaginal epithelium[2,3] thus increasing urethral coaptation and possibly aiding urinary continence.[4]

Conservative therapy for genuine stress incontinence (GSI) is aimed at strengthening the levator muscles (Kegel exercises), increasing the urethral closure pressure (alpha agonist therapy), or thickening the urethral epithelium (estrogen therapy). When such therapy fails, surgical intervention is aimed at re-suspending the bladder neck and increasing its inferior support.[5] Commonly employed surgical procedures include the Burch colposuspension,[6] bladder neck sling,[7] needle urethropexy,[8] and the Kelly plication. These procedures have reported complication rates of 6–32%,[9] and failure rates of 3–40%.[9,10] These failures may result in part from failure to determine the specific anatomic defect causing the incontinence.

Procedures for correcting pelvic organ prolapse include the anterior colporrhaphy[11] and the paravaginal repair.[1] Despite surgery, prolapse can recur in up to 34% of cases.[12] It is possible that the recurrences may in part be due to failure to identify the causative lesion in the pelvic floor prior to surgery.

In either case, it would be helpful to be able to identify an anatomic basis for each clinical abnormality. Such anatomic bases could help guide therapy, possibly reducing the failure rates and may in themselves suggest novel surgical approaches. Magnetic resonance imaging (MRI) provides a technology for evaluating the soft tissues which may contribute to pelvic floor dysfunction. The steady improvements in MRI technology have increased our ability to discriminate between soft tissue structures at high resolution. MRI resolution (<1 mm pixels and 1.5–3 mm slice thickness) is superior to any ultrasound technique, and although computed tomography (CT) can have comparable resolution it cannot differentiate as finely between the different types of soft tissue which comprise the pelvic floor.

SUPINE MRI

MRI has been used to assess the normal anatomy of the female pelvic floor, as well as to study the anatomic determinants of pelvic organ dysfunction. Strohbehn *et al.* compared MRI findings with anatomy at dissection in two cadavers[13] (Fig. 33.1). They found that sagittal and axial MRI demonstrated the levator ani muscle from

Figure 33.2 Cadaveric and MR of levator path (c) showing midline sagittal view of the pelvis. (a) Cross-sectional anatomy. (b) Corresponding diagram. EAS: external anal sphincter muscle. (c) Fast spin-echo T2-weighted 1.5-tesla magnetic resonance imaging (MRI) of a 26-year-old living patient (repetition time 3600 milliseconds, echo delay time 85 milliseconds, field of view 24 cm, scan time 11:44 minutes). Incidental ovarian cyst (black arrow) is seen anterior to the uterus. BL: bladder; UT: uterus; R: rectum. (d) T2-weighted MRI of cadaver specimen at the same level. (*Note: The asterisk posterior to the symphysis on the cadaver MRI represents fixation artifact from a fluid collection in the space of Retzius in this and subsequent figures.) The fibers of the pubovisceralis muscle (puborectalis) that decussate behind the rectum are seen in relationship to the internal and external anal sphincter muscles. The image clarity is less in the patient MRI compared with the cadaver MRI because of motion artifact and shorter scan time, but the external anal sphincter muscle (*arrowhead*) and the pubovisceralis muscle (*open arrow*) are seen. From: Strohbehn, *Obstet Gynecol* 1996;**87**(2):279.

Coccygeus m.
Anococcygeus raphe
External anal sphincter

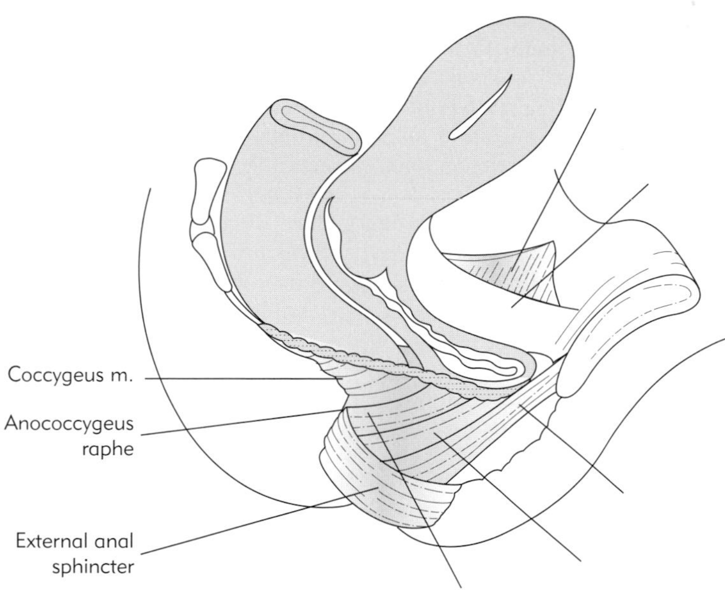

Figure 33.1 Cadaver based 3D pelvic reconstruction. From: Strohbehn, *Obstet Gynecol* 1996;**87**(2):278.

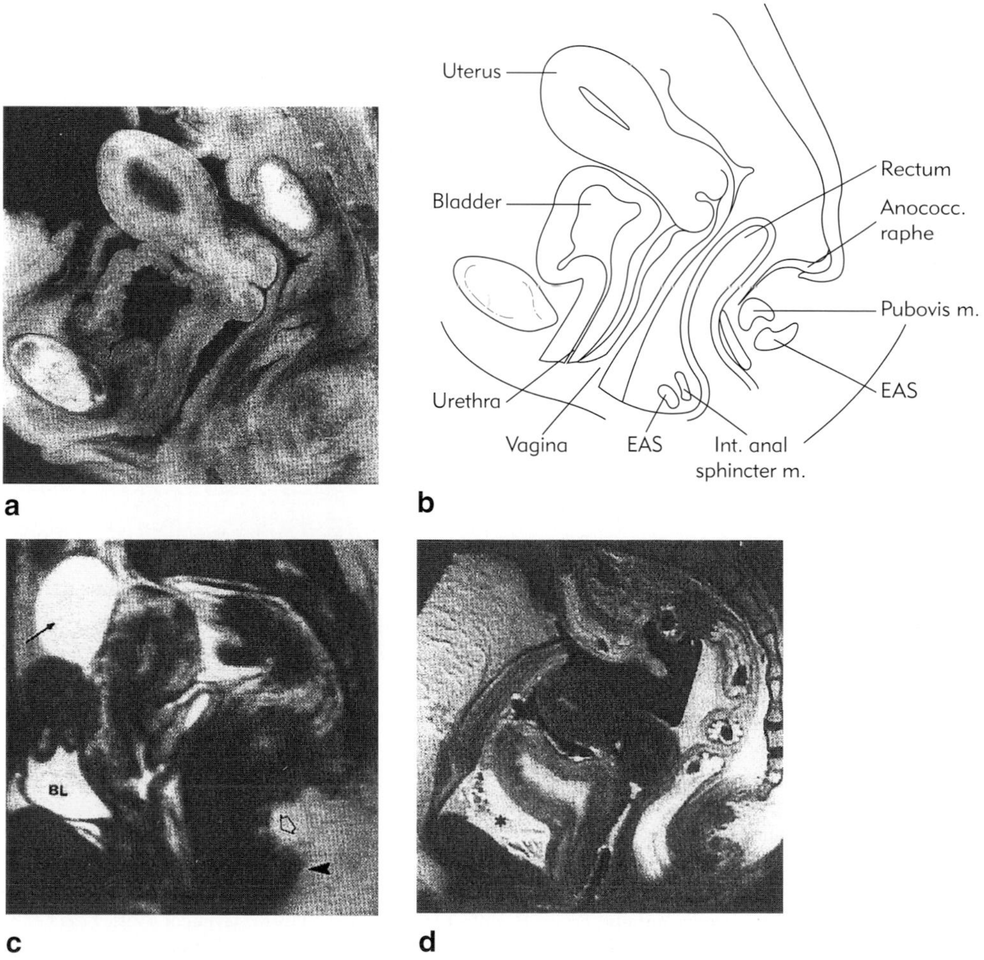

Uterus
Bladder
Urethra
Vagina
EAS
Int. anal sphincter m.
Rectum
Anococc. raphe
Pubovis m.
EAS
BL
a
b
c
d

its fascial origination at the pubic bone, along its course passing alongside the urethra, distal vagina, and posterior to the rectum, noting its insertion between the internal and external anal sphincters (Fig. 33.2). Further, MRI showed the iliococcygeus muscle attachment to the arcus tendineus laterally, as well as the relative thickness of the medial aspect of the levators, when compared to the thinner more lateral aspect. Their work demonstrated that MRI findings reflected actual anatomy. However they had the benefit of long MRI scan times which increased resolution without introducing the motion artifact which would limit scan times in living subjects.

Huddleston *et al.*[14] demonstrated MRI findings of three alterations in vaginal shape that were associated with clinical pelvic organ prolapse, demonstrating a relationship between pathological MR and clinical findings (Fig. 33.3). Kirschner-Hermanns *et al.* reported increased T1 signal intensity as evidence of muscle atrophy in 66% of their subjects with stress incontinence,[15] suggesting a relationship between levator weakness and stress urinary incontinence. Their conclusions were supported by Fielding *et al.*[16] who found a trend towards levator muscle laxity and thinning in women with stress urinary incontinence. However, it is possible that their results were a reflection of the wide normal range of levator muscle volume, and this bears further study.

Klutke *et al.* looked at bladder neck MRI findings taken in the supine position in normals compared to

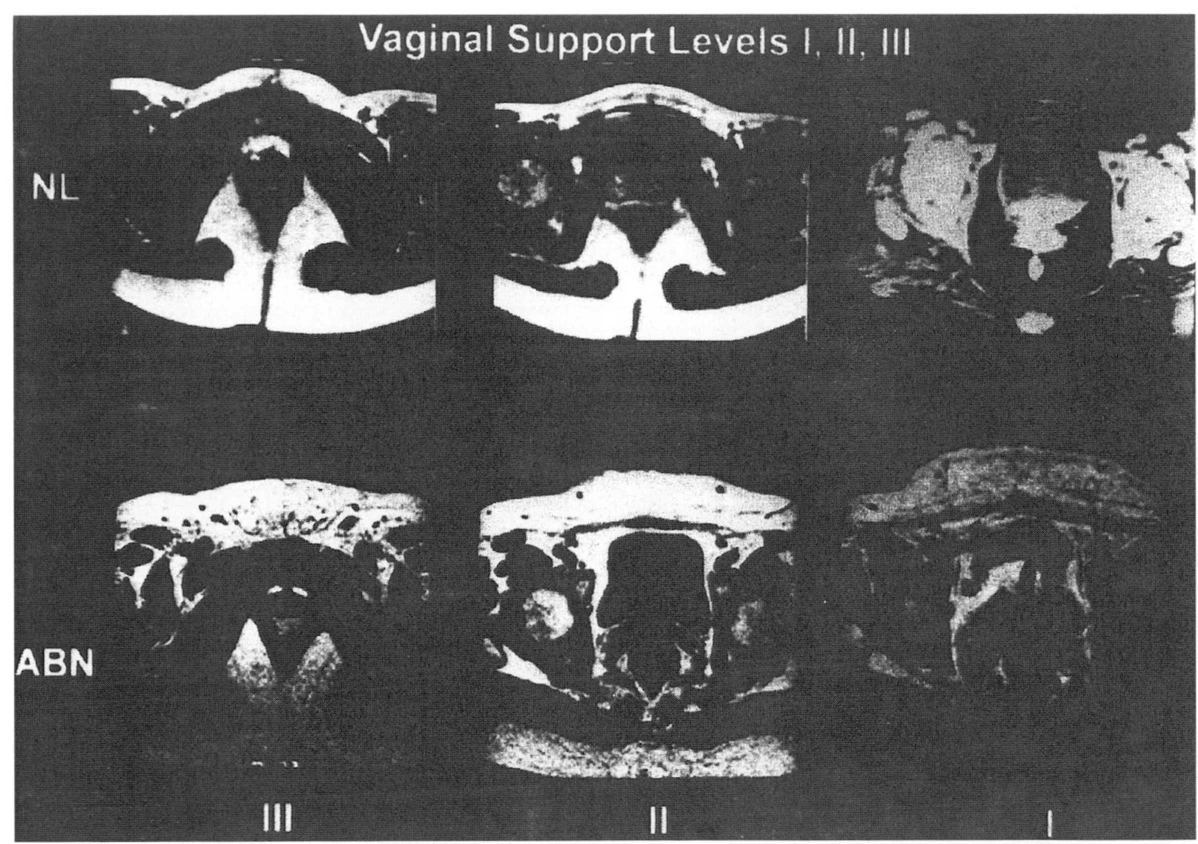

Figure 33.3 Composite of normal (NL) and abnormal (ABN) MRIs of levels I, II, and III. Upper panel, MRI of vaginal support levels I, II, and III in normal subjects. Note uplift of anterior vaginal wall in level III, where it is 'fused' to arcus tendineus fascia pelvis across the anterior pubococcygeus muscle fascia. Note horizontal anterior vagina in levels II and central position of cervix in level I. Uterosacral ligaments form faint white semicircular shadows down toward sacrospinus ligaments. Lower panel. Abnormal MRIs illustrating named defects from each of three levels are shown below corresponding normal view. Left to right. 'Mustache' sign formed by white fat in prevesical space against bilateral sag of detached vagina from arcus tendineus fascia pelvis (vagina is outlined by mineral oil): 'saddlebags' sign in level II is caused by displaced fluid-filled bladder wall into bilateral paravaginal defects; 'chevron' sign in level I is caused by bilateral paravaginal detachment at levels of ischial spines in posthysterectomy patient. From: Huddleston *et al. Am J Obstet Gynecol* 1995;**172**:1778–84.

those with a urodynamic diagnosis of genuine stress incontinence.[17] They found that, when compared to patients with GSI, normal subjects were characterized by MR findings of a bladder neck positioned close to the symphysis, a vaginal lumen with a widened 'H' shape, and nearly horizontal 'urethropelvic' ligaments. It should be noted that they considered the urethropelvic ligaments to attach the lateral aspect of the urethra to the medial aspect of the levator sling (Figs. 33.4 and 33.5).

Further pelvic MRI findings are given in Figs (33.6–33.8). A representative axial slice is given in Fig. 33.6. This is taken from a primiparous supine subject at the level of the mid-vagina, and demonstrates the periurethral striated muscle (p), vagina (v), rectum (r), and levator ani muscles (l). Figure 33.7 is taken from a multiparous subject with mild genuine stress urinary incontinence, similarly noted. In this case, a defect in the leftmost attachment of the pubo-urethral attachment is noted, leading to a droop in the vagina (d) on the ipsilateral side. An axial view from a 75-year-old subject is also presented in Fig. 33.8, demonstrating the bladder (b); bowed levators (l); and a uterine fibroid (f) which buttresses the bladder neck, probably kinking the urethra.

Taken together, these studies show that MRI can demonstrate findings associated with normal and abnormal pelvic floor anatomy, However, they fail to demonstrate specific anatomic markers which could serve as independent diagnostic determinants of pelvic floor dysfunction or which guide therapeutic choices.

UPRIGHT MRI

All the data discussed above were obtained from MRI machines where the subject lay in the imaging tube. This results in imaging in the supine position. However,

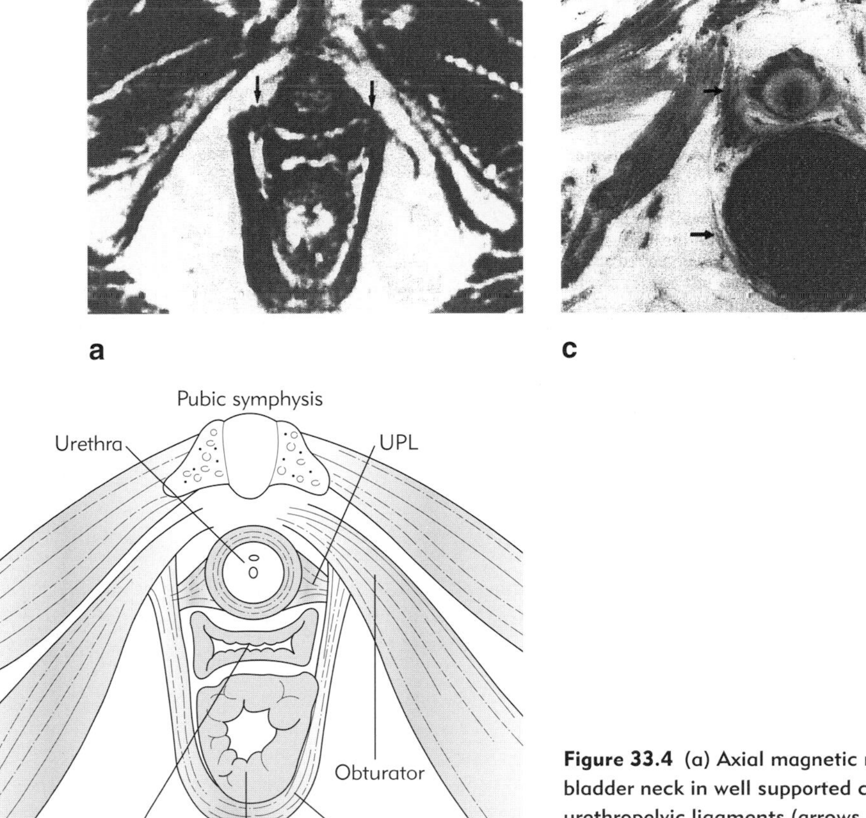

Figure 33.4 (a) Axial magnetic resonance image at level of bladder neck in well supported continent woman shows urethropelvic ligaments (arrows, UPL) supporting bladder neck. (b) and (c) Corresponding step-section at same level shows urethropelvic ligaments attaching to levator (arrows) at level of arcus tendineous. From: *J Urol* 1990;**143**:564.

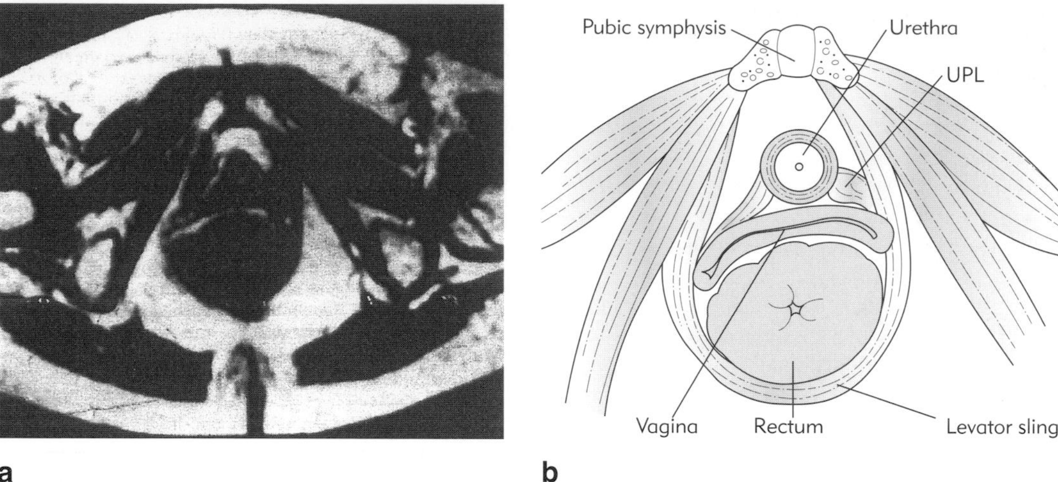

Figure 33.5 Abnormal MR findings in GSI. Axial magnetic resonance section at level of bladder neck in patient with genuine stress urinary incontinence. Bladder neck descent can be seen by increased distance between it and pubic symphysis. UPL: urethropelvic ligaments. From: *J Urol* 1990;**143**:564.

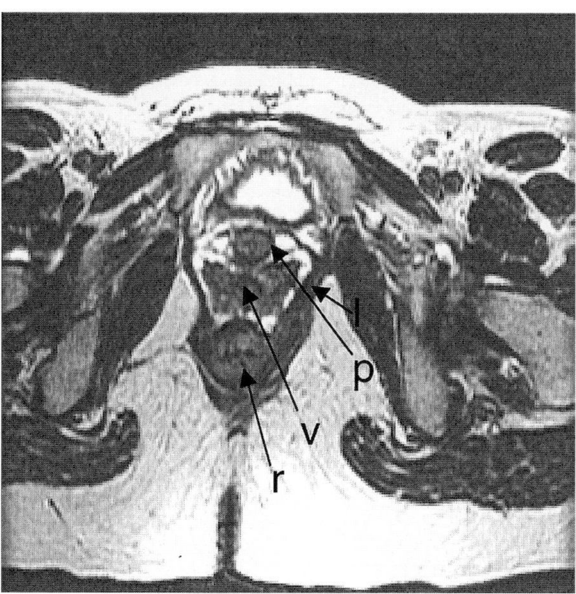

Figure 33.6 MR axial view; primiparous subject, asymptomatic. r: rectum, v: vagina, p: periurethral striated muscle, l: levator ani.

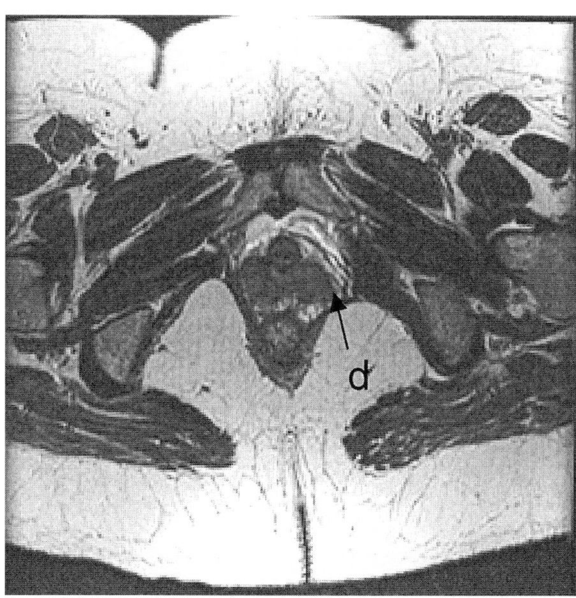

Figure 33.7 Axial MR, multiparous subject with GSI, and left pubo-urethral defect. d: descent of vagina due to pubo-urethral defect.

as pelvic floor dysfunction may, in part, result from humans adopting the upright posture, the value of such studies is limited. With the advent of interventional MRI, we[16] have been able to image in the sitting position. With the patient on a specialized commode, it is possible to image without artificial pelvic floor support and this technique allows the effects of gravity and physiologic activities to be included in the evaluation. Utilizing this technique we[18] have shown that images are completely different when imaged in the supine compared to the upright position especially when viewed in the sagittal plane (Fig. 33.9).

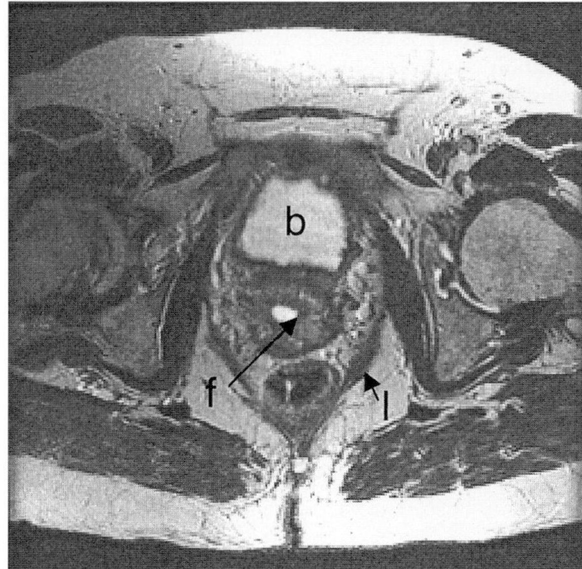

Figure 33.8 Axial MRI; 75 y/o subject, stage IV prolapse, with fibroid and bowing of levators. b: bladder, f: fibroid, l: levator.

MRI APPLICATIONS IN THE FEMALE PELVIS

In evaluating pelvic floor dysfunction, MRI could be used in several ways: (i) To determine the normal pelvic anatomy. (ii) To define the pathological variants of the anatomy and correlate them to known clinical findings. (iii) To evaluate changes in the pathological variants in order to track the effects of trophic medications (e.g. estrogens) and surgical or other therapies. The knowledge gained could be used to define clinically relevant pathologic markers which could be used to guide therapeutic choices. (iv) Finally, to aid visualization of the complex pelvic anatomy, with a view to surgical training.

Many of the published works to date have focused on the first two applications noted. However, quantification of the degree of pathology has not yet been documented. Furthermore, the role of the levator ani muscles in the pathogenesis of pelvic organ prolapse and stress incontinence remains to be elucidated. If bladder neck hypermobility and prolapse occur as a result of weakened or atrophic levator muscles, then muscle strengthening therapies should serve as effective treatment. If the condition stems from torn fascial attachments incurred during childbirth, then surgical reattachment would be ideal. On the other hand, if intact but stretched levator fascial attachments are the cause of the hypermobility and prolapse, then the results of Falconer *et al.* [19] would suggest that estrogen would have a tonic effect on the lax fascia, possibly alleviating the symptoms. Levator toning therapies might also be effective in this setting.

In evaluating the role of the levator ani, the relationship between muscle volume and normal versus pathologic cases must be determined. Muscle fascial attachments must be evaluated with respect to clinical findings to determine if torn or loose fascia may contribute to the pathology. MRI can facilitate both of these investigations. Muscle volume is computed by multiplying the levator ani muscle area on each MR slice by the slice thickness. The volumes for each slice are then

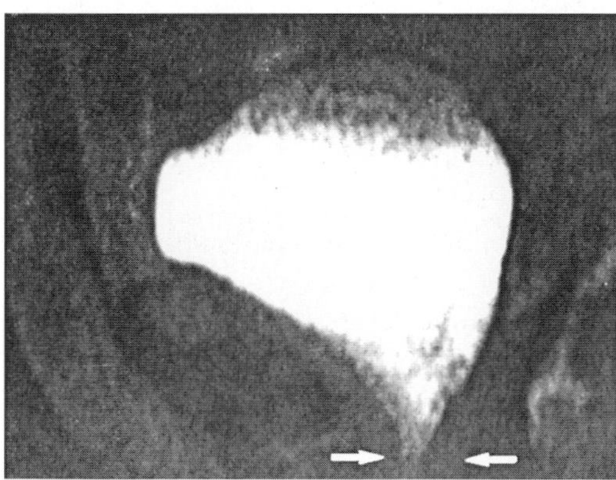

a

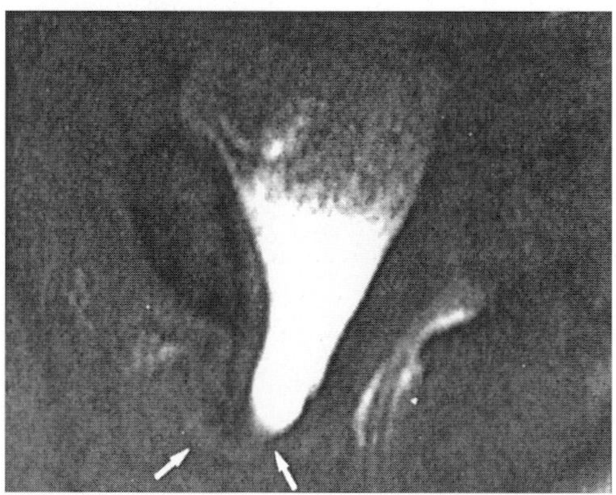

b

Figure 33.9 Comparison of supine and sitting MR images: 67-year-old woman with stress incontinence. (a) and (b) Sagittal T2-weighted MR images [TR/TE, 3000/105] were obtained at maximal strain in supine (a) and sitting (b) positions using inner volume-modified fast spin-echo pulse sequence. Cystocele and rotation of urethra (arrows) are of greater magnitude in sitting position. From: Fielding S. MR imaging of pelvic floor continence mechanisms in supine and sitting positions. *Am J Radiol* 1998;**171**:1607–1610.

added up to give the total volume. This technique is extremely time consuming when using conventional 2D MRI, but is made much easier when a 3-dimensional reconstruction technique is applied. The reconstructed 3D model also facilitates the evaluation of levator fascial attachment to the symphysis.

3D RECONSTRUCTION OF MRI

At our center, the 3D model is built up from a 2D MRI as follows: conventional 2D MRI studies are performed on each subject. T2-weighted source images are obtained in the axial and sagittal planes using a 1.5T magnet (General Electric Medical Systems, Milwaukee, WI) and a torso phased array coil wrapped around the pelvis. The following imaging parameters are employed: TR = 4200 ms, TE (eff) = 108 ms, 128 phase encodes, 24 cm field of view, 3 mm slice thickness, no gap, two acquisitions. The entire sequence is repeated adjusting the slice locations to obtain contiguous images 1.5 mm in thickness. Total scanning time is approximately 19 minutes.

After the MRI is completed, data are electronically transferred to a Sun UltraSparc-30 graphics computer workstation (Sun Microsystems, Mountain View, Ca). The data is first segmented into anatomically significant components, including bladder, urethra, uterus, vagina, rectum, muscles, and bones and then labeled using a combination of semi-automated and manual editing. From these images, 3D renderings of the pelvic viscera as well as supporting muscle, fascia and bones are reconstructed using the marching cubes algorithm and a surface rendering method.[20] Three dimensional surface models are generated using a pipeline consisting of dividing cubes, triangle reduction, and triangle smooth-

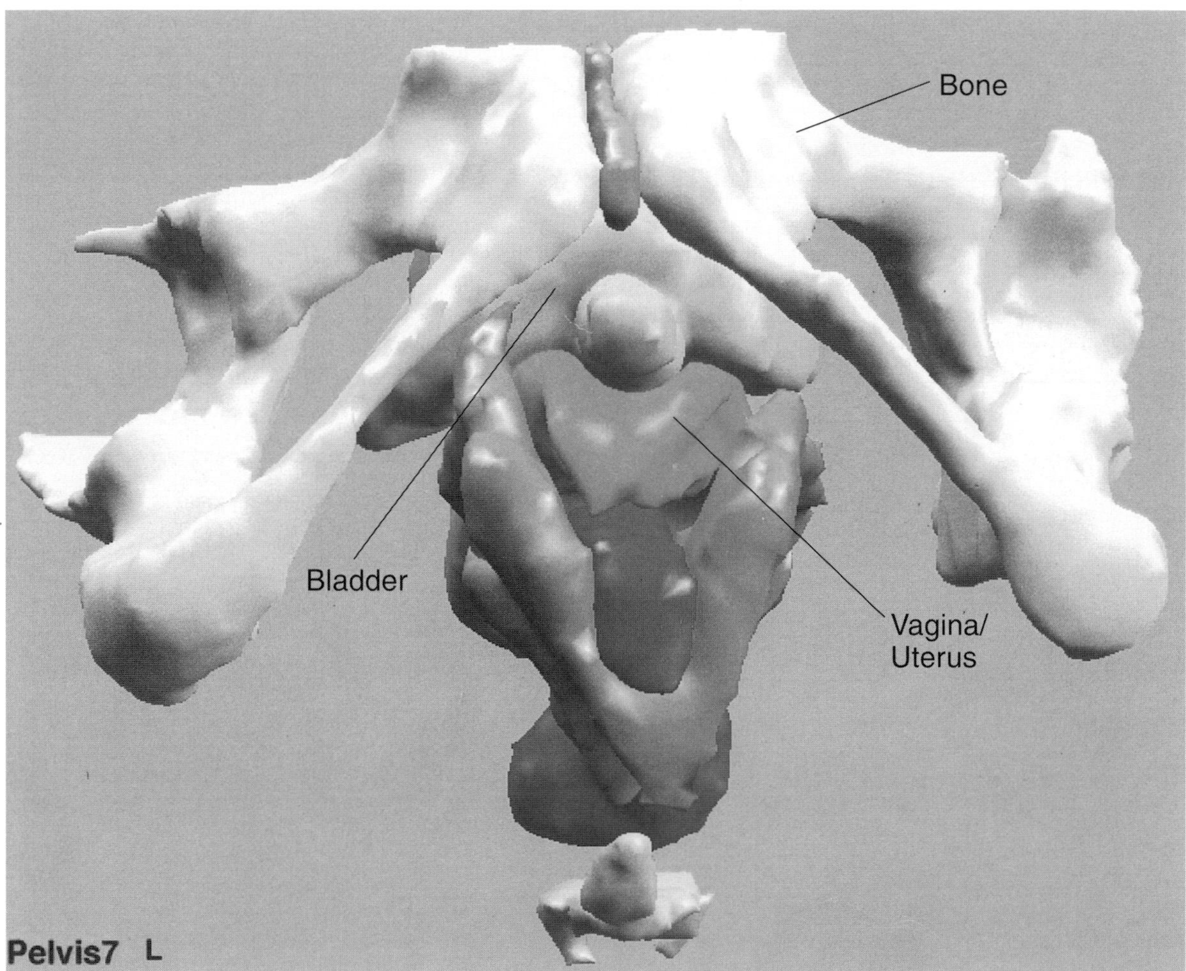

Figure 33.10 Reconstructed 3D view seen from the lithotomy position.

ing.[21,22] The final results are viewed on a workstation with graphics acceleration, and specialized measurement software is used to compute the linear and volume measurements of the on screen renderings.

Examples of the 3D renderings are shown in Figures 33.10–33.13. A representative 2D axial slice was given in Fig. 33.8. The patient is scanned in the supine position. A reconstructed 3D lithotomy view of this subject is shown in Fig. 33.10, and a sagittal view is given in Fig. 33.11 with the pelvic bones and obturator muscles removed.

The 3D model of the patient with massive prolapse and a fibroid is demonstrated in Figs 33.12–33.13. In Fig. 35.12, a lithotomy view is seen, with the prolapsed vaginal tissue noted. The sagittal view is given in Fig. 33.13, where the pelvic bones are removed. In Fig. 33.14, the levator and vagina are removed, demonstrating an elongated cervix and lower uterine segment, as well as an enlarged fibroid uterus which buttresses the bladder, and kinks the urethra, which is possibly the cause of this patient's urinary retention. Interestingly, this patient does not have a cystocele, probably because of the mass effect of the fibroid keeping it out of the pelvis.

From the 3D models, we can appreciate anatomic relationships which are not evident from the flat 2D images. This appreciation can possibly lead to a better understanding of the mechanisms of pelvic floor dysfunction, and perhaps lead to improved therapy for this disorder. For example, the shape of the levator muscle is primarily biconvex, in the nulliparous woman, and biconcave in the subject with massive prolapse. This suggests a laxity of the levator in the setting of prolapse. This preliminary but novel finding needs to be confirmed by other studies.

DISCUSSION

The value of MRI stems from its ability to accurately view critical pelvic floor structures in the living. Currently it is primarily a research tool, which has been successfully applied to demonstrate normal anatomy, and in limited ways, to look at anatomic findings in patients with GSI and prolapse. Independent, clinically relevant MRI markers remain to be elucidated, but the role of the levator ani in the pathogenesis of stress incontinence and prolapse is currently being studied with the help of MRI. MR based three-dimensional

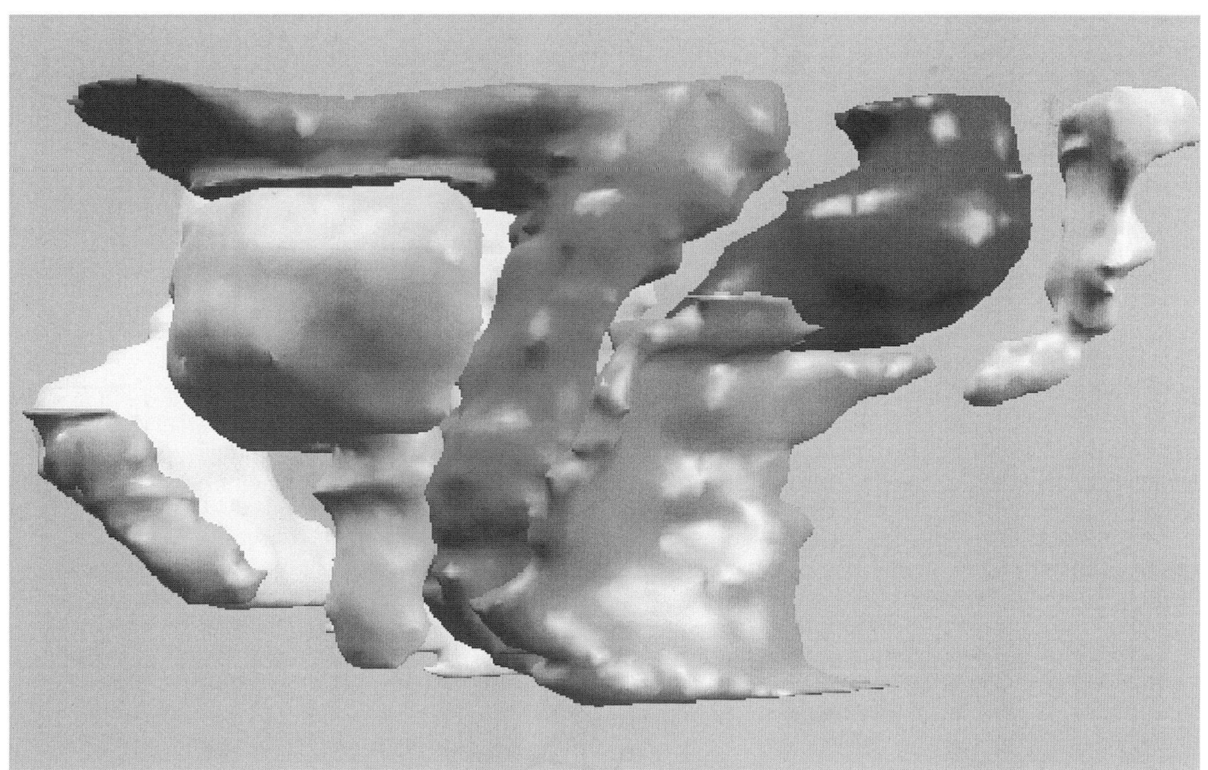

Figure 33.11 Sagittal 3D view with pelvic bones removed.

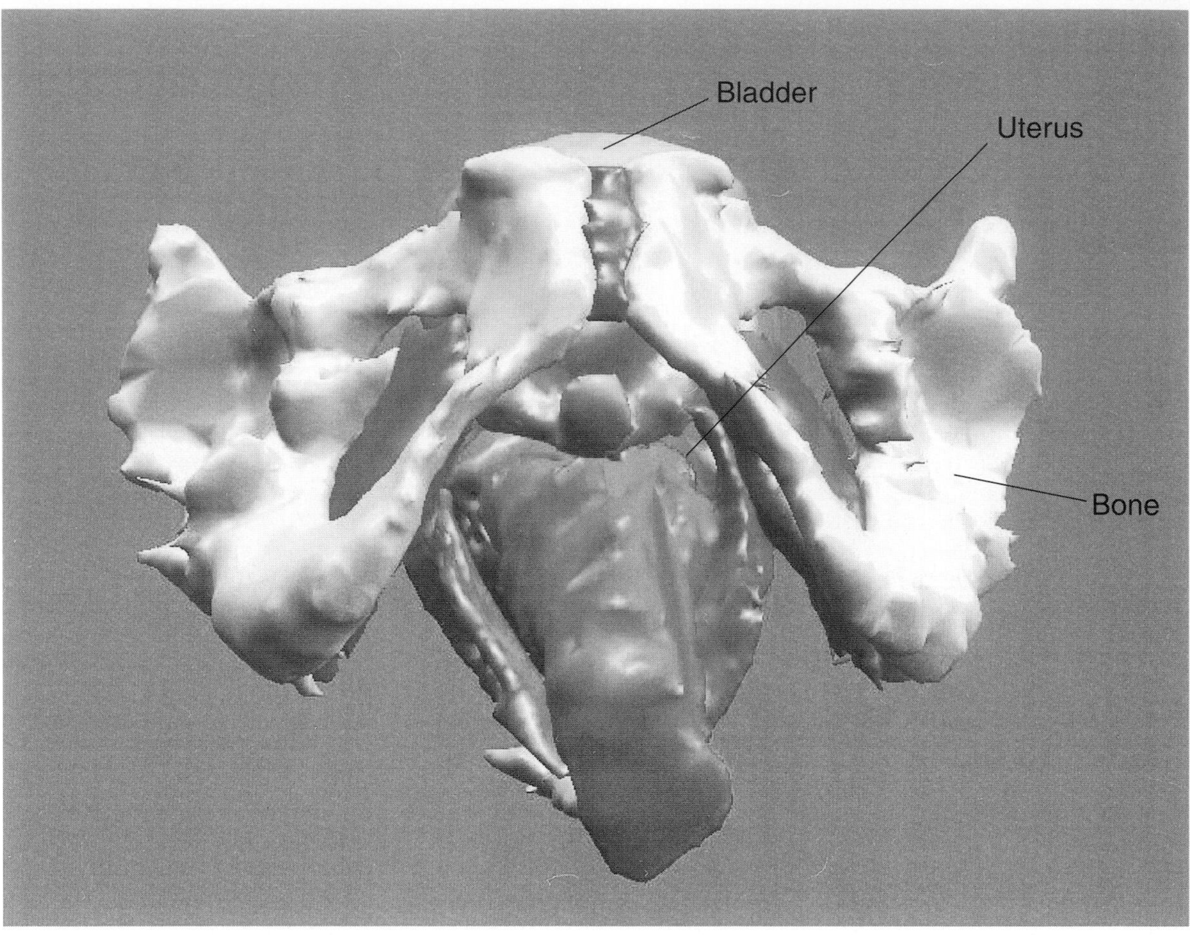

Figure 33.12 3D lithotomy view of subject with massive prolapse.

reconstruction techniques can aid visualization, possibly helping to better define the role of the levators, and to train students and pelvic surgeons. It is possible that 3D reconstruction can be used to correlate muscle volumes and attachments to the degree of pelvic dysfunction (e.g prolapse or genuine stress urinary incontinence). This may also help to determine why pelvic organ prolapse recurs after surgery in some patients and not in others. Perhaps further in the future, the 3D technique will permit pre-surgical evaluation of complex cases of pelvic organ dysfunction. It may also aid in designing appropriate surgical therapy, or even in stratifying patients for surgical versus non-surgical therapy.

There is a tradeoff between scan time and resolution. Relatively long scanning times (5–20 minutes) have previously limited the use of MRI in the evaluation of pelvic organs during Valsalva maneuvers, which can rarely be held consistently for more than a few seconds. Other techniques like spoiled gradient echo sequence, and fast spin echo can substantially reduce the scan times, which can facilitate rapid capture of the pelvic MRI under dynamic (e.g Valsalva) conditions. These techniques can facilitate further study of the mechanisms of stress incontinence and pelvic organ prolapse

Once the appropriate MR markers for pelvic dysfunction have been defined, MR changes could be used to document and monitor the effects of surgery, trophic medications and other therapies, giving further insight into guiding therapeutic choices based on MRI findings. In today's economic environment, MRI is too expensive to use for clinical management of pelvic floor dysfunction but who can predict what tomorrow will bring?

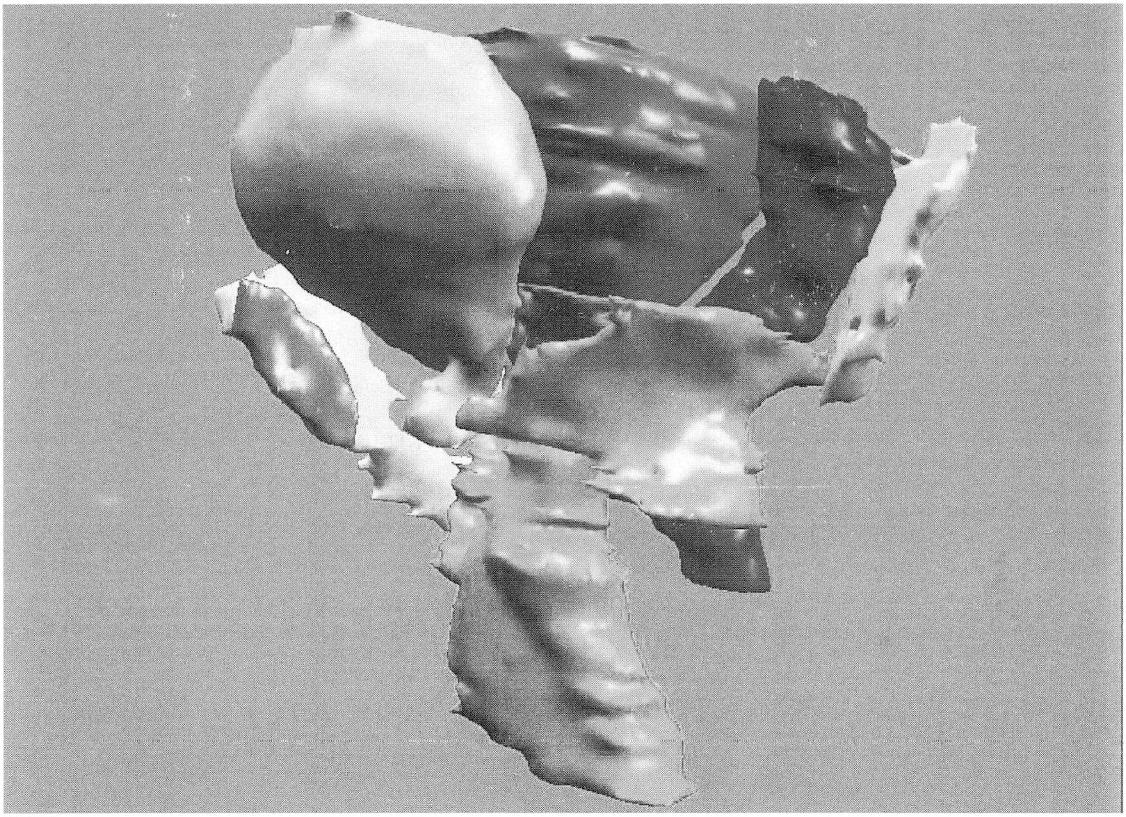

Figure 33.13 3D side view, shows elongated cervix and scant levator ani.

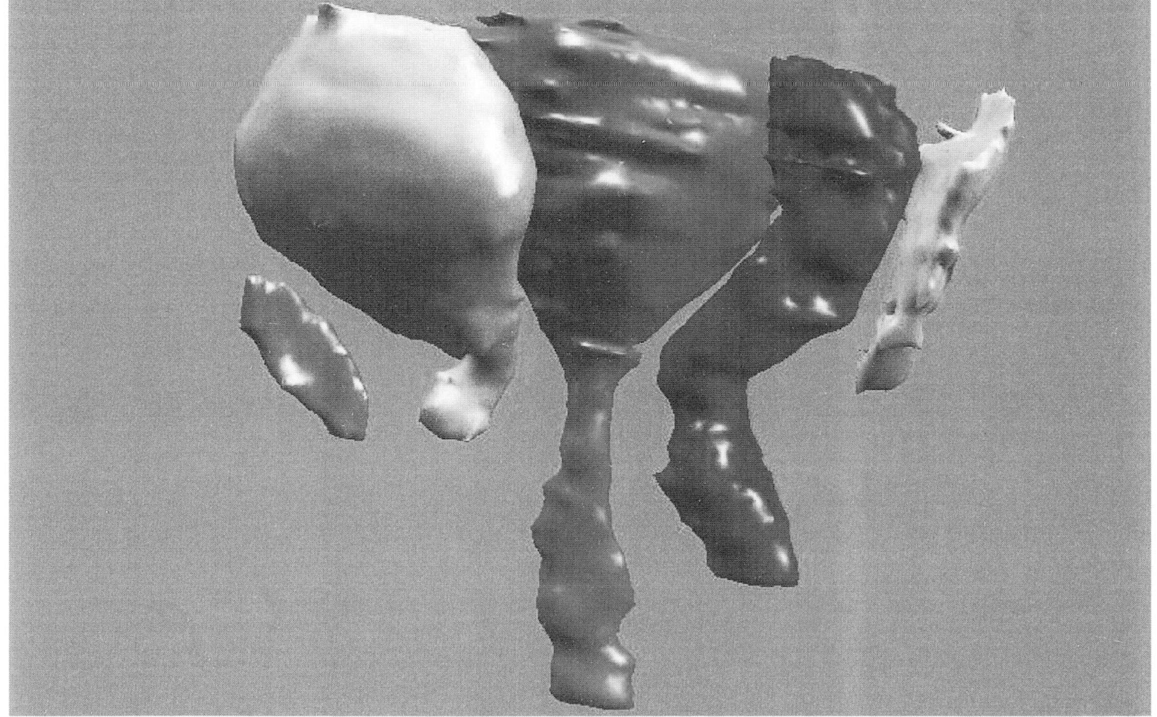

Figure 33.14 3D side view shows fibroid uterus which kinks bladder neck.

REFERENCES

1. Richardson AC, Lyon JB, Williams NL. A new look at pelvic relaxation. *Am J Obstet Gynecol*, 1976;**126**:568–73.
2. Zinner NN, Sterling AM, Ritter RC. The role of urethral softness in urinary incontinence. *Urology* 1980;**16**:115–7.
3. Zinner NN, Sterling AM, Ritter RC. Evaluation of inner urethral softness. *Urology* 1983;**22**:446–8.
4. Versi E. Incontinence in the climacteric. *Clin Obstet Gynecol* 1990;**33**:392–8.
5. Horbach N. Choosing the appropriate surgery for genuine stress incontinence. *Operat Tech Gynecol Surg* 1997;**2**(1):1–4.
6. Chen AH, Horbach NS. Abdominal retropubic urethropexy procedures. *Operat Tech Gynecol Surg* 1997;**2**(1):23–30.
7. Brubaker L. Suburethral sling procedures. *Operat Tech Gynecol Surg* 1997;**2**(1):44–50.
8. Griffiths DJ, Versi E. Needle urethropexies. *Operat Tech Gynecol Surg* 1997;**2**(1):35–43.
9. Nygaard IE, Kreder KJ. Complications of incontinence surgery. *Int Urogynecol J* 1994;**5**:353–60.
10. Shull BL, *et al.* A six year experience with paravaginal defect repair for stress urinary incontinence. *Am J Obstet Gynecol* 1989;**160**:1432–40.
11. Hurt WG Anterior colporraphy. *Operat Tech Gynecol Surg* 1997;**2**(1):17–22.
12. Shull BL, Benn SJ, Kuehl TJ. Surgical management of prolapse of the anterior vaginal segment: An analysis of support defects, operative morbidity, and anatomic outcome. *Am J Obstet Gynecol* 1994;**171**:1429–39.
13. Strohbehn K *et al.* Magnetic resonance imaging of the levator ani with anatomic correlation. *Obstet Gynecol* 1996;**87**:277–85.
14. Huddleston HT *et al.* Magnetic resonance imaging of defects in DeLancey's support levels I, II, and III. *Am J Obstet Gynecol* 1995;**172**:1778–84.
15. Kirshner-Hermanns R *et al.* The contribution of magnetic resonance imaging of the pelvic floor to the understanding of urinary incontinence. *Br J Urol* 1993;**72**:715–18.
16. Fielding JR, Versi E, Mulkern RV, Lerner MH, Griffiths DJ, Jolesz FA. MR imaging of the female pelvic floor in the supine and upright positions. *JMRI* 1996;**6**:961–3.
17. Klutke C *et al.* The anatomy of stress incontinence: magnetic resonance imaging of the female bladder neck and urethra. *J Urol* 1990;**143**:563–6.
18. Fielding JR, Griffiths DJ, Versi E, Mulkern RV, Lee MLT, Jolesz FA. MR imaging of pelvic floor continence mechanisms in the supine and sitting positions. *Am J Radiol* 1998;**171**:1607–10.
19. Falconer C *et al.* Paraurethral connective tissue in stress-incontinent women after menopause. *Acta Obstet Gynecol Scand* 1998;**77**(1):95–100.
20. Lorensen WCH. Marching cubes: a high resolution 3D surface construction algorithm. *Comput Graph* 1987;**21**: 163–89.
21. Schroeder WZJ, Lorenson W. Decimation of triangle meshes. *Comput Graph*, 1992;**26**:65–70.
22. Taubin G. Curve and surface smoothing without shrinkage. *IBM Res Rep* 1994;**RC-19536**.

Index

Page number in *italic* indicate figures and tables.

D

E

F

G